Type **2**
Diabetes

Type 2 Diabetes

Principles and Practice

Second Edition

Edited by

Barry J. Goldstein
Jefferson Medical College of Thomas Jefferson University
Philadelphia, Pennsylvania, USA

Dirk Müller-Wieland
Asklepios Clinic St. Georg
Hamburg, Germany

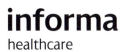

informa
healthcare

New York London

WK
810
T9917
2008

Informa Healthcare USA, Inc.
52 Vanderbilt Avenue
New York, NY 10017

International Standard Book Number-10: 0-8493-7957-1 (Hardcover)
International Standard Book Number-13: 978-0-8493-7957-4 (Hardcover)

Library of Congress Cataloging-in-Publication Data

Type 2 diabetes: principles and practice / edited by Barry J. Goldstein, Dirk Müller-Wieland. — 2nd ed.
   p. ; cm.
  Rev. ed. of: Textbook of type 2 diabetes. c2003.
  Includes bibliographical references and index.
  ISBN-13: 978-0-8493-7957-4 (hardcover : alk. paper)
  ISBN-10: 0-8493-7957-1 (hardcover : alk. paper) 1. Non-insulin-dependent diabetes.
I. Goldstein, Barry J. II. Müller-Wieland, Dirk. III. Textbook of type 2 diabetes.
  IV. Title: Type two diabetes.
  [DNLM: 1. Diabetes Mellitus, Type 2. WK 810 T9917 2007]
  RC662.18.T973 2007
  616.4'62—dc22   2007026823

Visit the Informa web site at
www.informa.com

and the Informa Healthcare Web site at
www.informahealthcare.com

To C. Ronald Kahn, an extraordinary mentor, who fostered our career interests in the molecular pathogenesis of diabetes and its complications.

To our families for their love and support.

To our patients, who suffer with the restrictions imposed by diabetes on their daily lives, with the hope that this book will help alleviate their burden.

Preface

The incidence and prevalence of type 2 diabetes mellitus have increased dramatically in modernized and developing nations over the past few decades—and this "epidemic" shows no signs of abating. Physicians and other healthcare professionals worldwide are well aware of this growing burden. The pathogenesis and management of the hyperglycemia of diabetes and its associated risk factors and morbidities, especially involving cardiovascular and microvascular complications, must be fully understood by all of the many providers that care for patients with diabetes worldwide.

Patients are always asking, "Isn't there anything new to help manage my diabetes?" This reflects the relative inadequacies of many of our attempts at lifestyle change, as well as some of the shortcomings of currently available medications for the long-term management of this disorder. Certainly, changes in lifestyle can be effective, but they are extremely difficult to implement over an extended period of time. Diabetes patient management is often implemented later in the course of the disease, since the disease can be asymptomatic and therefore can go unrecognized for many years. Recent studies have shown clearly that the onset of diabetes can be prevented or delayed and more aggressive, earlier treatment may also help to alter its course and, possibly, its chronic complications. Large clinical trials will help to answer these questions in the future.

In this second edition, we have thoroughly updated all existing chapters and developed new ones vital to the management of diabetes, while maintaining the international perspective and focus on clinical care found in the first edition. The entire clinical field is covered in succinct chapters written by recognized experts. The content spans from a current perspective on diabetes demographics and epidemiology, pathophysiology, disease monitoring, approaches to glucose control, and managing complications. New to this edition are chapters that expand on nonpharmacological management options; diabetes-related macrovascular conditions, including coronary heart disease and peripheral vascular disease; and discussions on rare forms of diabetes, polycystic ovarian syndrome, and non-alcoholic steatohepatitis. As before, this edition closes with a look at the future of new devices for glucose monitoring and diabetes management.

We hope this book will be used frequently and successfully in the management of this complex and widely prevalent disorder.

Barry J. Goldstein
Dirk Müller-Wieland

Contents

Contributors

Leon A. Adams School of Medicine, The University of Western Australia, Sir Charles Gairdner Hospital, Perth, Australia

Intekhab Ahmed Division of Endocrinology, Diabetes and Metabolic Diseases, Department of Medicine, Thomas Jefferson University, Philadelphia, Pennsylvania, U.S.A.

William E. Benson Retina Service, Wills Eye Hospital, Philadelphia, Pennsylvania, U.S.A.

David John Betteridge Department of Medicine, University College Hospital, London, U.K.

Christina Bratcher Department of Medicine, Section of Endocrinology, Tulane University Health Sciences Center, New Orleans, Louisiana, U.S.A.

Michael Camilleri Enteric Neuroscience Program, Mayo Foundation, Rochester, Minnesota, U.S.A.

Ramachandiran Cooppan Joslin Diabetes Center, Boston, Massachusetts, U.S.A.

Jill P. Crandall Diabetes Research and Training Center, Institute for Aging Research, Albert Einstein College of Medicine, Bronx, New York, U.S.A.

Philip E. Cryer Washington University School of Medicine, St. Louis, Missouri, U.S.A.

Samuel Dagogo-Jack Division of Endocrinology, Diabetes, and Metabolism, University of Tennessee Health Science Center, Memphis, Tennessee, U.S.A.

Tiina Dietz Department of Medicine, Division of Endocrinology, University Hospital of Essen Medical School, University of Duisburg-Essen, Essen, Germany

Steven V. Edelman Division of Endocrinology and Metabolism, San Diego Veterans Affairs Medical Center, San Diego, California, U.S.A.

Michael Edmonds Diabetic Foot Clinic, Kings College Hospital, Denmark Hill, London, U.K.

Erland Erdmann Clinic III of Internal Medicine, University of Cologne, Cologne, Germany

Vivian Fonseca Department of Medicine, Section of Endocrinology, Tulane University Health Sciences Center, New Orleans, Louisiana, U.S.A.

Juan P. Frias Amylin Pharmaceuticals, Inc., San Diego, California, U.S.A.

Baptist Gallwitz Department of Medicine, Eberhard-Karls University, Tübingen, Germany

Ruchira Glaser Department of Medicine, Cardiovascular Medicine Division, Hospital of the University of Pennsylvania, Philadelphia, Pennsylvania, U.S.A.

Barry J. Goldstein Division of Endocrinology, Diabetes and Metabolic Diseases, Department of Medicine, Jefferson Medical College of Thomas Jefferson University, Philadelphia, Pennsylvania, U.S.A.

Ioanna Gouni-Berthold Department of Internal Medicine, University of Cologne, Cologne, Germany

Susanne Hahn Endokrinologikum Ruhr, Center for Metabolic and Endocrine Diseases, Bochum-Wattenscheid, Germany

Markolf Hanefeld Center for Clinical Studies—Metabolism and Endocrinology, Technical University, Dresden, Germany

Hans-Ulrich Häring Department of Medicine, Division of Endocrinology, Metabolic and Vascular Medicine, University of Tübingen, Tübingen, Germany

Hans Hauner German Diabetes Research Institute, Heinrich-Heine Universität, Düsseldorf, Germany

Robert R. Henry Diabetes/Metabolism Section, VA San Diego Healthcare System and University of California at San Diego, San Diego, California, U.S.A.

Johannes Hensen Department of Medicine, Krankenhaus Nordstadt, Klinikum Region Hannover GmbH, Hannover, Germany

Alan M. Jacobson Behavioral and Mental Health Research, Joslin Diabetes Center, Boston, Massachusetts, U.S.A.

Onno E. Janssen Department of Medicine, Division of Endocrinology, University Hospital of Essen Medical School, University of Duisburg-Essen, Essen, Germany

Jeffrey I. Joseph Department of Anesthesiology, The Artificial Pancreas Center, Jefferson Medical College, Thomas Jefferson University, Philadelphia, Pennsylvania, U.S.A.

Birgit Knebel Institute of Clinical Biochemistry and Pathobiochemistry, German Diabetes Center, Heinrich Heine University Düsseldorf and Leibniz Center for Diabetes Research, Düsseldorf, Germany

Wilhelm Krone Department of Medicine, University College Hospital, London, U.K.

Markku Laakso Department of Medicine, Kuopio University Hospital, Kuopio, Finland

Axel Linke Department of Internal Medicine/Cardiology, University of Leipzig, Leipzig, Germany

Tilak Mallik Department of Medicine, Section of Endocrinology, Tulane University Health Sciences Center, New Orleans, Louisiana, U.S.A.

Jim I. Mann Department of Human Nutrition, University of Otago, Dunedin, New Zealand

Stephan Matthaei Diabetes Center, Quackenbrück, Germany

Anthony L. McCall Center for Diabetes and Hormone Excellence, University of Virginia, Charlottesville, Virginia, U.S.A.

Mary Kate McCullen Division of Endocrinology, Diabetes and Metabolic Diseases, Department of Medicine, Thomas Jefferson University, Philadelphia, Pennsylvania, U.S.A.

Carolé Mensing Diabetes Education Program, University of Connecticut Health Center, Farmington, Connecticut, U.S.A.

Carl Erik Mogensen Medical Department, Aarhus Sygehus, Aarhus University Hospital, Aarhus, Denmark

Pablo F. Mora Division of Endocrinology and Metabolism, Department of Internal Medicine, University of Texas, Southwestern Medical Center, Dallas, Texas, U.S.A.

Sunder Mudaliar Diabetes/Metabolism Section, VA San Diego Healthcare System and University of California at San Diego, San Diego, California, U.S.A.

Dirk Müller-Wieland Division of General Internal Medicine, Department of Endocrinology, Diabetes and Metabolism, Asklepios Clinic St. Georg and Teaching Hospital of the University of Hamburg, Hamburg, Germany

Michael Nauck Diabeteszentrum Bad Lauterberg, Bad Lauterberg, Germany

Ebenezer A. Nyenwe Division of Endocrinology, Diabetes, and Metabolism, University of Tennessee Health Science Center, Memphis, Tennessee, U.S.A.

Andreas F. H. Pfeiffer   Department of Endocrinology, Diabetes and Nutrition, University of Berlin, Berlin, Germany

Robert E. Ratner   MedStar Research Institute, Washington, D.C., U.S.A.

Carl D. Regillo   Department of Ophthalmology, Thomas Jefferson University Hospital and Wills Eye Hospital, Philadelphia, Pennsylvania, U.S.A.

Brett Rosenblatt   Long Island Vitreoretinal Consultants, Great Neck, New York, U.S.A.

Arlan L. Rosenbloom   Department of Pediatrics, Division of Endocrinology, University of Florida College of Medicine, Gainesville, Florida, U.S.A.

Gerit-Holger Schernthaner   Department of Medicine II, Medical University of Vienna, Vienna, Austria

Guntrum Schernthaner   Department of Medicine I, Rudolfstiftung Hospital, Vienna, Austria

Christian A. Schneider   Clinic III of Internal Medicine, University of Cologne, Cologne, Germany

Brock E. Schroeder   Amylin Pharmaceuticals, Inc., San Diego, California, U.S.A.

Gerhard Schuler   Department of Internal Medicine/Cardiology, University of Leipzig, Leipzig, Germany

Rhuna Shen   Department of Medicine, Cardiovascular Medicine Division, Hospital of the University of Pennsylvania, Philadelphia, Pennsylvania, U.S.A.

Michael Stumvoll   Department of Medicine, University of Leipzig, Leipzig, Germany

Susanne Tan   Department of Medicine, Division of Endocrinology, University Hospital of Essen Medical School, University of Duisburg-Essen, Essen, Germany

Tina K. Thethi   Department of Medicine, Section of Endocrinology, Tulane University Health Sciences Center, New Orleans, Louisiana, U.S.A.

Asha Thomas-Geevarghese   MedStar Research Institute, Washington, D.C., U.S.A.

Monika Toeller   German Diabetes Research Center, Heinrich-Heine University, Düsseldorf, Germany

Timon W. van Haeften   Department of Internal Medicine, University Medical Centre Utrecht, Utrecht, The Netherlands

Adrian Vella   Endocrine Research Unit, Division of Endocrinology, Mayo Clinic, Rochester, Minnesota, U.S.A.

Katie Weinger   Behavioral and Mental Health Research, Joslin Diabetes Center, Boston, Massachusetts, U.S.A.

Garry W. Welch   Behavioral and Mental Health Research, Joslin Diabetes Center, Boston, Massachusetts, U.S.A.

Susan E. Wiegers   Department of Medicine, Cardiovascular Medicine Division, Hospital of the University of Pennsylvania, Philadelphia, Pennsylvania, U.S.A.

Kathleen L. Wyne   Division of Endocrinology and Metabolism, Department of Internal Medicine, University of Texas Southwestern Medical Center, Dallas, Texas, U.S.A.

Dan Ziegler   Institute of Clinical Diabetes Research, German Diabetes Center, Leibniz Center for Diabetes Research, Heinrich Heine University, Düsseldorf, Germany

1 | Epidemiology of Type 2 Diabetes

Markku Laakso
Department of Medicine, Kuopio University Hospital, Kuopio, Finland

DIAGNOSTIC CRITERIA FOR DIABETES AND OTHER CATEGORIES OF ABNORMAL GLUCOSE TOLERANCE

Diabetes mellitus (DM) refers to a number of disorders that share the common feature of elevated blood glucose levels. The classification accepted by the World Health Organization (WHO) (1,2) and the American Diabetes Association (ADA) (3,4) combines both clinical stages of hyperglycemia and the etiological types. Two main subtypes of diabetes are type 1, either autoimmune or idiopathic, and type 2, attributable to insulin resistance, insulin secretion defects, or both. Although diabetes has been known for centuries our understanding of the etiology and pathogenesis of this disease is still incomplete. Type 1 is characterized by deficiency of insulin due to destructive lesions in pancreatic β-cells. It occurs typically in young subjects, but may affect people of any age. Type 2 diabetes comprises about 80% to 90% of all cases. Type 2 is a heterogenous, polygenic disorder resulting from interaction between susceptibility genes and lifestyle/environmental factors.

Diabetes affects currently about 5% of the world's population, and its prevalence is rapidly increasing, particularly in elderly subjects. There is a marked variation in the prevalence of diabetes among many national and ethnic populations. The spectrum ranges from very low prevalence of about 1% in tribes in Papua New Guinea, the Inuit, or the Chinese living in mainland China, to extremely high rates of 20% to 45% in Australian Aborigines, Nauruans of Micronesia, and Pima Indians of Arizona (5). Even within nations the variation in the prevalence is marked. For example, in the United States, African Americans have a twofold, Mexican Americans a 2.5-fold and Native Americans a fivefold increase in the risk of the development of type 2 diabetes compared with Caucasians (6). Large variation in the prevalence of type 2 diabetes in different populations probably results from environmental as well as genetic determinants.

Type 2 diabetes is usually preceded by a long period of asymptomatic hyperglycemia that may last for years. In this prediabetic state, postprandial or postglucose levels are mildly elevated whereas fasting blood glucose can usually be maintained within the near-normal range. The elevation of postglucose levels is used for the definition of impaired glucose tolerance (IGT), a nonspecific reversible stage. About 30% of these subjects progress to overt diabetes within 10 years (7). Elevation of fasting glucose is used for the definition of impaired fasting glucose (IFG). In some individuals beta-cells compensate for insulin resistance by increased insulin secretion, and type 2 diabetes does not develop. However, in a large number of prediabetic individuals multiple defects in insulin action and/or insulin secretion gradually lead to sustained hyperglycemia. As a consequence of insulin resistance, the beta-cell produces increased amounts of insulin, and compensatory hyperinsulinemia maintains normoglycemia. When beta-cell compensation to insulin resistance fails, decompensated hyperglycemic state develops. Thus, type 2 diabetic subjects have relative (rather than absolute) insulin deficiency. Usually these individuals do not need insulin treatment to survive.

Criteria for diagnosis of diabetes and other categories of glucose tolerance have changed considerably during the last 20 years (8,9). Table 1 shows the current criteria for normal glucose tolerance (NGT), IFG, IGT, and diabetes. Criteria proposed by the WHO (1,2) and the ADA (3,4) are different. The main difference between these new criteria is that the ADA does not recommend the use of an oral glucose tolerance test. The WHO defined a new subcategory of glucose tolerance, IGT, to describe subjects whose fasting glucose levels were normal but whose 2-hour postglucose challenge levels were elevated, although not diabetic. The 2 hour 75 g oral glucose tolerance test was recommended as the international standard for diabetes diagnosis. The cutoff point between IGT and diabetes was based on an increased risk of developing diabetic complications, primarily retinopathy, for these subjects with diabetes.

The ADA (but not the WHO) recommended that in epidemiological studies, estimates of diabetes prevalence and incidence should be based only on fasting glucose criteria. The fasting

TABLE 1 Criteria for Classification of Glucose Tolerance Status According to World Health Organization and the American Diabetes Association Criteria

Glucose tolerance status	Definition	Classification criteria (mmol/L)
Normal glucose tolerance (NGT)	WHO (1999)	FPG <6.1 and 2 h PG <7.8
	ADA (1997)	FPG <6.1
	ADA (2003)	FPG <5.6
Impaired fasting glucose (IFG)	WHO (1999)	FPG ≥6.1 and <7.0 and 2 h PG <7.8
	ADA (1997)	FPG ≥6.1 and <7.0
	ADA (2003)	FPG ≥5.6 and <7.0
Impaired glucose tolerance (IGT)	WHO (1999)	FPG <7.0 and 2 h PG ≥7.8 and <11.1
Diabetes mellitus (DM)	WHO (1999)	FPG ≥7.0 or 2 h PG ≥11.1
	ADA (1997)	FPG ≥7.0
	ADA (2003)	FPG ≥7.0

Abbreviations: DM, diabetes mellitus; IFG, impaired fasting glucose; IGT, impaired glucose tolerance; NGT, normal glucose tolerance. *Source*: From Refs. 1, 3, and 4.

glucose criteria for diagnosis were considered by the ADA to have good reproducibility, small variability, and easy application in clinical practice. IGT is defined by the WHO as a 2-hour plasma glucose concentration between 7.8 and 11.0 mmol/L. The ADA (3) also introduced a category of IFG, defined as fasting plasma glucose between 5.6 and 6.9 mmol/L, to replace IGT. IFG and IGT were considered to be metabolic stages intermediate between normal glucose homeostasis and diabetes. However, it is possible that IFG differs from IGT with respect to the relative contribution of insulin secretion defect and hepatic and peripheral insulin resistance. IFG and IGT are not clinical entities, but rather risk categories for future diabetes and/or cardiovascular disease. Normoglycemia is defined as plasma fasting glucose < 6.1 (WHO) (1) and 5.6 mmol/L (ADA) (3) and a 2-hour glucose < 7.8 mmol/L in an oral glucose tolerance test. The changes in diagnostic criteria for diabetes recognized results of epidemiological studies indicating that the risks of both retinopathy and cardiovascular disease start to increase at fasting plasma glucose values of about 6.0 mmol/L (10).

Both the ADA and WHO recommend a fasting plasma glucose concentration of 7.0 mmol/L for the diagnosis of diabetes, but according to the WHO criteria (1), diabetes can be also diagnosed if the 2-h glucose concentration is at least 11.1 mmol/L. For the asymptomatic person, at least one additional glucose test result with a value in the diabetic range is essential, from a random (casual) sample, or from the oral glucose tolerance test.

A number of studies summarized by Shawn et al. (11) have compared the WHO and ADA criteria for DM using fasting and 2-h definitions. These studies demonstrate both an increase and a decrease in people as having nearly diagnosed diabetes depending on the population studied. Compared to the WHO criteria, fasting glucose-based ADA criteria may underestimate glucose abnormalities more in older age than in younger age (12). Also the Cardiovascular Health Study demonstrated a 50% underestimation of diabetes prevalence in older adults (>65 years) comparing the ADA criteria with the WHO criteria (13). Furthermore, IGT may have higher sensitivity over IFG for predicting progression to type 2 diabetes (14).

In general the fasting criterion identifies different people as being diabetic compared to those identified by the 2-h criterion (15). In subjects without previously diagnosed diabetes, the DECODE study group from 16 different European populations (16) found that all subjects diagnosed by either the fasting or 2-h criteria, only 29% qualified as diabetic according to both criteria. This result was confirmed in the DECODA study group (17) including existing epidemiological data from 11 population-based studies collected from Asian people (*n*=17,666) between 30 and 89 years of age. The authors concluded that it would be inappropriate to use the ADA criteria alone for screening diabetes in Asian populations.

"EPIDEMIC" OF TYPE 2 DIABETES

Epidemiological studies had already identified "diabetes epidemic" in 1970s. The extraordinarily high prevalence of type 2 diabetes was reported in Pima Indians (18) and also in the Micronesian Nauruans in the Pacific (19), and subsequently in other Pacific and Asian island populations (20). These studies showed that transition from traditional lifestyle to Western way of life resulted in obesity, lack of exercise, profound changes in the diet, and finally to type 2 diabetes. Potential for a future global epidemic of diabetes were highlighted. Since the 1970s several other studies have shown that type 2 diabetes has reached epidemic proportions in several developing countries as well as in Australian Aboriginals (21), African-Americans, and Mexican Americans (22).

Table 2 shows the trends in the number of diabetic patients worldwide (23). Significant increase in the number of type 1 diabetic patients is expected, but the doubling of the number of diabetic subjects in the following 20 years is due to a huge increase in the number of type 2 diabetic patients. According to the estimation of the International Diabetes Federation (IDF) about 194 million people worldwide, or 5.1%, were estimated to have diabetes in the age group 20 to 79 years in 2003 (23). This estimate is expected to increase to some 333 million by 2025, or 6.3% of the adult population. Thus, the increase in the number of diabetic subjects will be almost twofold in the forthcoming 20 years. South East Asia has the most of the increase considering the size of the population (705 million in 2003 and 1081 million in 2025). People in Asia tend to develop diabetes with a lesser degree of obesity at younger ages. Similarly, childhood diabetes has increased substantially (24). The highest prevalence of diabetes was in 2003 in North America, and in 2025 about 10% of the people will have diabetes in this area of the world. Southeast Asia had the highest prevalence of IGT in 2003, and the percentage of people having IGT will be 13.5% in 2025. About 15% to 20% of people in different regions will have either DM or IGT in 2025.

The United States has the highest increase in the prevalence of DM on the basis of several follow-up studies. In the National Health and Nutrition Surveys (NHANES) II (1976–1980) the prevalence of diagnosed plus undiagnosed diabetes was 8.9%, but in the NHANES III (1988–1994) the prevalence was already 12.3% in the population 40 to 74 years of age (25). Prevalence of IFG increased from 6.5% to 9.7%. Figure 1 demonstrates a large difference between ethnic groups in diabetes prevalence in the U.S. population ≥20 years of age. The prevalence of diabetes (known plus undiagnosed) was particularly high in Mexican American men (13.1%) and women (14.5%). IFG or diabetes was present in about 20% of Mexican Americans. Diabetes has become one of the most common chronic diseases in the United States, where in subjects ≥60 years of age the prevalence is already 18.8%.

Until recently, type 2 diabetes was regarded as a disease of the middle-aged and elderly. However, evidence is accumulating that onset in subjects aged under 30 years is increasing. Even children and adolescent are diagnosed to have type 2 diabetes (26). For example, among children in Japan type 2 diabetes is already more common than type 1 and accounts for 80% of childhood diabetes (27). Between 8% and 45% of newly presenting children and adolescents in the United States have type 2 diabetes.

TABLE 2   Estimates of the Prevalence (%) of Diabetes Mellitus and Impaired Glucose Tolerance in the Age Group 20 to 79 Years in Different Regions of the World in 2003 and 2025

Region	2003		2025	
	DM	IGT	DM	IGT
Africa	2.4	7.3	2.8	7.3
Eastern Mediterranean and Middle East	7.0	6.8	8.0	7.4
Europe	7.8	10.2	9.1	10.9
North America	7.9	7.0	9.7	7.9
South and Central America	5.6	7.3	7.2	8.1
Southeast Asia	5.6	13.2	7.5	13.5
Western Pacific	3.1	5.7	4.3	6.9
Total	5.1	8.2	6.3	9.0

Abbreviations: DM, diabetes mellitus; IGT, impaired glucose tolerance.
Source: From Ref. 23.

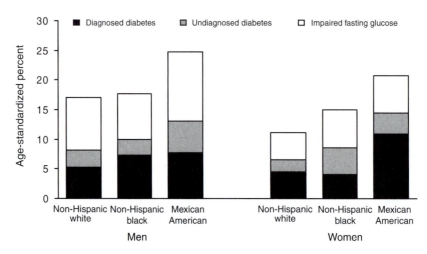

FIGURE 1   Age-standardized prevalence of diagnosed and underdiagnosed diabetes and impaired fasting glucose in the U.S. population >20 years of age, presented according to sex and racial or ethnic group, based on NHANES III. *Abbreviation*: NHANES, National Health and Nutrition Survey. *Source*: From Ref. 25.

Epidemic of type 2 diabetes is determined not only by an increase in the incidence but also by mortality rates. Although cardiovascular complications in nondiabetic subjects have significantly reduced in the United States during the last decades this is not the case in diabetic patients, particularly among women, as shown recently by Gu et al. (28). No reliable data on mortality rates are available from populations living in developing countries.

CRITERIA FOR TYPE 2 DIABETES AND CARDIOVASCULAR DISEASE

The chronic hyperglycemia of diabetes is associated with long-term complications, especially in the eyes, kidneys, nerves, heart, and blood vessels. Individuals with undiagnosed type 2 diabetes are at high risk of coronary heart disease, stroke, and peripheral vascular disease. More than half of type 2 diabetic patients die of cardiovascular causes (29).

From the perspective of cardiovascular complications of DM the diagnostic criteria have been too high. Already the Whitehall study showed an increased risk of cardiovascular disease when the 2-hour level exceeded 5.5 mmol/L, albeit after a 50 g glucose load (30). This study and several other population-based studies indicated that the risk for macrovascular complications starts at considerably lower levels of glycemia than has been included in the definition of diabetes.

Early diagnosis of diabetes aims to prevent long-term complications. Because cardiovascular disease is the main complication of type 2 diabetes recent studies have investigated the capability of new criteria to predict these complications. The association of hyperglycemia and cardiovascular disease is a crucial one on which to test the validity of the new criteria. The DECODE Study (31) showed that the 2-h criteria more accurately identifies people who are at increased risk of total and cardiovascular mortality compared to the ADA fasting criteria.

The DECODE study (31) analyzed 10 prospective European cohort studies including 15,388 men and 7,126 women, aged 30 to 89 years, who all had undergone a 2-h oral glucose tolerance test. The median follow-up was 8.8 years, and hazard ratios for deaths from all causes, cardiovascular disease, coronary heart disease, and stroke were estimated. Multivariate Cox regression analyses showed that the inclusion of fasting glucose did not add significant information on the prediction of 2-h glucose alone, whereas the addition of 2-h glucose to fasting glucose criteria significantly improved the prediction. Table 3 reports adjusted hazard ratios for deaths from cardiovascular disease, coronary heart disease, stroke,

TABLE 3 Adjusted Hazard Ratios from Cardiovascular Disease, Coronary Heart Disease, Stroke, and All Causes with Fasting and Two-Hour Glucose Categories in the Same Model: The DECODE Study[a]

	CVD	CHD	Stroke	All causes
Fasting glucose criteria				
IFG	1.01 (0.84–1.22)	1.01 (0.77–1.31)	1.00 (0.66–1.59)	1.03 (0.93–1.14)
Diabetes	1.20 (0.88–1.64)	1.09 (0.71–1.67)	1.64 (0.88–3.07)	1.21 (1.01–1.44)
2-h glucose criteria[b]				
IGT	1.32 (1.12–1.56)	1.27 (1.01–1.58)	1.21 (0.84–1.74)	1.37 (1.25–1.51)
Diabetes	1.40 (1.02–1.92)	1.56 (1.03–2.36)	1.29 (0.66–2.54)	1.73 (1.45–2.06)
Known diabetes[c]	1.96 (1.62–2.37)	1.94 (1.51–2.50)	1.73 (1.12–2.68)	1.82 (1.60–2.06)

[a] Adjusted for age, sex, center, total cholesterol, body mass index, systolic blood pressure, and smoking.
[b] Using fasting plasma glucose < 6.1 mmol/L as reference group.
[c] Using 2-h plasma glucose < 7.8 mmol/L as reference group.
Abbreviations: CHD, coronary heart disease; CVD, cardiovascular disease; IFG, impaired fasting glucose; IGT, impaired glucose tolerance.

and all causes with fasting and 2-h categories. IFG did not predict mortality. Diabetes based on fasting criteria predicted total mortality, but 2-h glucose criteria predicted mortality much better than fasting glucose criteria. IGT and diabetes predicted cardiovascular and coronary heart disease mortality as well as coronary heart disease mortality and total mortality. The highest hazard ratios for all categories of death were observed in known diabetic patients. The largest number of excess cardiovascular deaths was found in subjects with IGT who had a normal fasting glucose level, supporting the notion that IGT has prognostic importance. Also the Funaka Diabetes Study in Japan demonstrated that subjects with IGT had higher cardiovascular disease mortality than subjects with IFG (32). In contrast to these findings the Hoorn Study reported no clear differences in mortality risks for subjects classified as IGT, IFG, or newly diagnosed diabetes according to either set of criteria (33).

INSULIN RESISTANCE AND IMPAIRED INSULIN SECRETION AS PREDICTORS OF TYPE 2 DIABETES

Type 2 diabetes is caused by impaired insulin action (insulin resistance) and/or impaired insulin secretion. Insulin resistance is a characteristic metabolic defect in the great majority of patients, and it also precedes the development of frank hyperglycemia. Impaired insulin action is observed in several tissues, e.g., skeletal muscle, adipose tissue, and the liver. It leads to increased insulin secretion from the pancreas to overcome impaired insulin action. Compensatory hyperinsulinemia maintains glucose levels within the normal range but in individuals destined to develop diabetes, beta-cell function eventually declines and leads to hyperglycemic diabetic state. In a minority of subjects diabetes develops as a consequence of a primary defect in insulin secretion. Between 2% and 14% (on average about 5%) of people with IGT progress to type 2 diabetes each year (34). The progression rate is influenced by age, ethnicity, and the degree of glucose intolerance.

The degree of insulin resistance varies between different ethnic groups. For example, in the Insulin Resistance Atherosclerosis Study (35) including 1100 healthy subjects African-Americans and Mexican Americans had a lower insulin sensitivity than non-Hispanic whites. The first study to demonstrate that a combination of insulin resistance and impaired insulin secretion predicts type 2 diabetes was published on Pima Indians. Lillioja et al. (36) showed that low insulin secretory response and increased insulin resistance were both predictors of type 2 diabetes. Furthermore, both impaired insulin secretion and insulin resistance acted as an independent risk factor. Quite similar results were published on Mexican Americans. During the 7-year follow-up baseline high-fasting insulin level (indicator of insulin resistance) predicted the conversion to diabetes (37). Furthermore, low insulin secretion assessed by insulin response (30 min insulin minus fasting insulin divided by 30 min glucose minus fasting glucose) also predicted the development of diabetes. When these two parameters were combined they had an additive effect on the risk of developing diabetes. High degree of insulin resistance and normal insulin secretion increased the risk by 4.5-fold, and high insulin sensitivity but low insulin secretion increased the risk by 5.4-fold, whereas the combination of these two increased the risk by 13.9-fold (Fig. 2).

RISK FACTORS FOR TYPE 2 DIABETES

The identification of risk factors is essential for the successful implementation of primary prevention programs. Risk factors for type 2 diabetes can be classified as modifiable and nonmodifiable (Table 4). Subjects who subsequently develop diabetes have multiple adverse changes in risk factor levels. A good example is our study of 892 elderly Finnish subjects followed for 3.5 years (38). As shown in Figure 3 the highest risk of developing diabetes was associated with IGT and hyperinsulinemia. Furthermore, hypertriglyceridemia, central obesity, low high-density lipoprotein (HDL) cholesterol, high body mass index, hypertension, and a family history of diabetes were risk factors for diabetes.

Modifiable Risk Factors

Hu et al. (39) published results from the Nurses' Heath Study including 84,941 female nurses followed from 1980 to 1996, and who were free of diagnosed cardiovascular disease and diabetes at baseline. During the 16 years follow-up 3300 new cases of type 2 diabetes were diagnosed. As shown in Figure 4 obesity was the single most important predictor of diabetes. Women whose body mass index was at least $35.0 \, \text{km/m}^2$ had almost 40-fold risk of becoming diabetic compared to women whose body mass index was $< 23.0 \, \text{kg/m}^2$. Weekly exercised at least $7 \, \text{h/wk}$ reduced the risk of type 2 diabetes by 39% compared to women who exercise $< 0.5 \, \text{h/wk}$. Smoking of > 14 cigarettes/day increased the diabetes risk by 39%, but alcohol intake $> 10 \, \text{g/day}$ reduced the risk by 41%. The study also indicated that a diet high in cereal fiber and polysaturated fat and low in saturated and trans fats and glycemic load reduced the risk of developing diabetes. A combination of several lifestyle factors, including low body mass index ($< 25 \, \text{kg/m}^2$), a diet high in cereal fiber and polysaturated fat and low in saturated fat and trans fats and glycemic load, regular exercise, abstinence from smoking and moderate alcohol intake, was associated with a reduction of type 2 diabetes incidence by 90% compared to women without these factors.

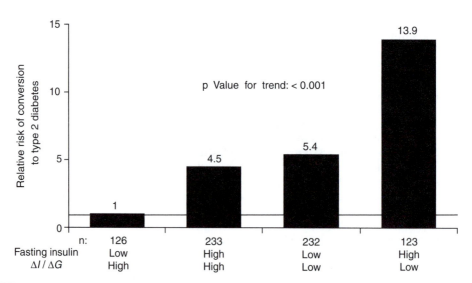

FIGURE 2   The risk of developing type 2 diabetes by fasting insulin concentration and insulin secretion (change in insulin divided by change in glucose concentrations over the first 30 minutes of an oral glucose tolerance test [$\Delta I_{30}/\Delta G_{30}$]). *Source*: From Ref. 35.

TABLE 4   Risk Factors for Type 2 Diabetes

Modifiable	Nonmodifiable
Obesity	Ethnicity
Central obesity	Age
Lack of physical activity	Sex
Smoking	Genetic factors
Alcohol abstinence	Family history of type 2 diabetes
Low fiber in the diet	Prior gestational diabetes
High saturated fat in the diet	Prior glucose intolerance
	History of cardiovascular disease
	History of hypertension
	History of dyslipidemia
	Low birth weight

Visceral adiposity precedes the development of type 2 diabetes. Boyko et al. (40) showed in their study of Japanese Americans that intra-abdominal fat area measured by computed tomography (CT) remained a significant predictor of diabetes incidence even after adjustment for body mass index, total body fat area, and subcutaneous fat area and other risk factors for diabetes. Interestingly, high insulin resistance and low insulin secretion predicted diabetes independently of directly measured visceral adiposity suggesting that visceral adiposity could contribute to the development of diabetes through actions independent of its effect on insulin sensitivity. Van Dam et al. (41) showed that in Dutch subjects the association between abdominal obesity (waist circumference) and hyperglycemia was stronger in the presence of a parental history of diabetes.

Physical inactivity is a major risk factor for the development of type 2 diabetes. For example, sedentary lifestyle, indicated by television viewing time, worsens glucose tolerance (42). Physical activity reduces insulin resistance and total and visceral fat mass (43). In contrast, the association of total dietary fat with type 2 diabetes or insulin sensitivity is less

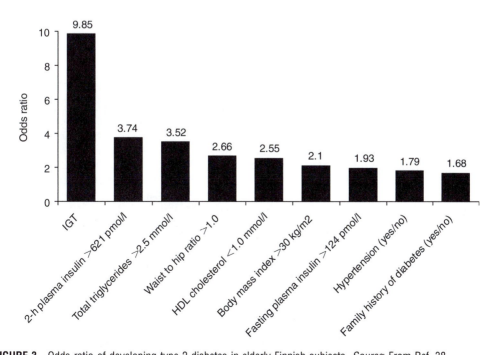

FIGURE 3   Odds ratio of developing type 2 diabetes in elderly Finnish subjects. *Source*: From Ref. 38.

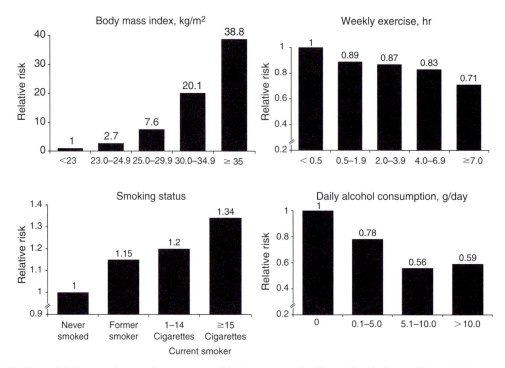

FIGURE 4   Relative risk of type 2 diabetes among 84,941 women in the Nurses' Health Study, 1980 to 1996. *Source:* From Ref. 39.

consistent. Meyer et al. (44) studied the relation between dietary fatty acids and diabetes in a prospective cohort study of 35,988 older women who initially did not have diabetes. Altogether 1890 new cases of diabetes occurred during 11 years of follow-up. Diabetes risk was negatively associated with dietary polysaturated fatty acids, vegetable fat, and trans fatty acids. Even after adjustment for confounding factors vegetable fat remained a significant predictor of new diabetes. Many studies show that high coffee consumption may protect from type 2 diabetes (45).

Nonmodifiable Risk Factors

The prevalence and incidence of type 2 diabetes are strongly related to age. In fact, about 50% of all type 2 diabetic patients are over 60 years old. Ethnicity is a strong determinant of diabetes occurrence. In Chinese the prevalence of type 2 diabetes is 1% whereas in Pima Indians it is >50% in adult population probably due to genetic influence or due to interaction between genes and environment. No systematic effect of gender on the prevalence and incidence of type 2 diabetes is observed but in some ethnic groups the occurrence of diabetes might depend on gender. Previous abnormality of glucose tolerance, a history of gestational diabetes and a family history of type 2 diabetes are all strong predictors of type 2 diabetes. Interestingly, also the presence of other disease states or conditions, for example hypertension and dyslipidemia increase the risk of type 2 diabetes. In recent years interest has been focused also on low birth weight as a risk factor for type 2 diabetes.

Associations between low birth weight and increased risk of type 2 diabetes in adult life have been reported in various populations (46). Several explanations for this relationship have been presented. Long-term effects of nutritional deprivation in utero could affect fetal growth and the development of the endocrine pancreas. Genetic factors could cause both low birth weight and later abnormalities of insulin secretion or insulin sensitivity. Whether the relationship between diabetes and low birth weight is mediated through impaired insulin sensitivity or impaired insulin secretion remains to be determined.

PREVENTION OF TYPE 2 DIABETES: IMPLICATIONS FOR SCREENING

Screening for diabetes may be appropriate under certain circumstances because early detection and prompt treatment may reduce the burden of type 2 diabetes and its complications. However, widespread screening for asymptomatic individuals for type 2 diabetes cannot be recommended. Screening may be appropriate if the subjects have one or more of the risk factors listed in Table 4.

The rationale for screening of type 2 diabetes must be based on the presence of factors having a significant effect on the risk of developing diabetes. Second, screening for diabetes is rational only if diabetes can be prevented by normalizing modifiable risk factors. Clinical trials have demonstrated the efficacy of lifestyle–intervention programs in the prevention of type 2 diabetes. Da Qing study from China (47) showed that exercise and diet resulted in a decrease of 42% to 46% an incidence of type 2 diabetes among 577 subjects with IGT. The Finnish Diabetes Prevention Program demonstrated that weight loss and regular exercise reduced the incidence of type 2 diabetes by 58% (48), and this preventive effect was observed even 3 years after the stopping the intervention (49). Similarly, the Diabetes Prevention Study in the United States showed that diet and regular exercise reduced the incidence of type 2 diabetes by 58% among 3234 subjects with IGT (50). Lifestyle intervention works as well in men and women and in all ethnic groups. Lifestyle was also effective in the Japanese (51) and Indian (52) trials. Accumulating evidence implies that lifestyle intervention is highly successful and screening should be targeted to subjects with high risk of developing diabetes.

The ADA has recommended the plasma fasting glucose measurements as a screening test because it is easier and faster to perform, more convenient and acceptable to patients, and less expensive (53). In contrast, the WHO criteria for diabetes still include a 2-h oral glucose tolerance test, which might be used in the screening of high-risk individuals. Recent studies indicating that 2-h glucose identifies better than fasting glucose values individuals with high risk of cardiovascular disease favors the use of a 2-h oral glucose tolerance test. However, the 2-h glucose tolerance test has the high within-test variability up to 25%. According to different studies when subjects were retested after an interval of up to 3 months 35% to 75% of the subjects who were IGT an the first test had reverted to normal when retested (54).

CONCLUDING REMARKS

In the next 20 years we will face a global epidemic of type 2 diabetes. Although the new cases of diabetes depend somewhat on the glucose criteria used to define diabetes, there has already been a true increase in the incidence and prevalence of type 2 diabetes. With increasing prevalence of obesity worldwide the epidemic of type 2 has emerged, and an "epidemic" of diabetes-related cardiovascular disease will follow (55). Incidence of diabetes in a population is tightly linked to the average weight of that population. Type 2 diabetes does not only cause micro- and macrovascular complications, excess mortality and morbidity, but it is also an expensive health problem. Therefore, socioeconomic, behavioral, nutritional, and public health issues relating to the epidemic of obesity and type 2 diabetes should be addressed. Furthermore, more funds are needed for continuing research aiming to reveal the unsolved issues in the pathophysiology and genetics of type 2 diabetes. Extremely important areas of research will be the identification of the genes responsible for the predisposition to type 2 diabetes, and the identification of environmental factors, which bring out this predisposition. Once these issues have been solved we will better understand the "epidemic" of type 2 diabetes, and target our nonpharmacological and pharmacological treatment modalities more effectively to prevent this continuously growing health problem and its devastating complications.

REFERENCES

1. WHO Consultation. Definition, diagnosis and classification of diabetes mellitus and its complications. Part 1: diagnosis and classification of diabetes mellitus. Report No. 99.2. Geneva: World Health Organization, 1999.

2. World Health Organization Study Group on Diabetes Mellitus. Technical Report Series 727. Geneva: World Health Organization, 1985.
3. Genuth S, Alberti KG, Bennett P, et al. Follow-up report on the diagnosis of diabetes mellitus. Diabetes Care 2003; 26:3160–7.
4. The Expert Committee on the Diagnosis and Classification of Diabetes Mellitus. Report of the Expert Committee on the Diagnosis and Classification of Diabetes Mellitus. Diabetes Care 1997; 20:1183–97.
5. King H, Rewers M. WHO Ad Hoc Diabetes Reporting Group: global estimates for prevalence of diabetes mellitus and impaired glucose tolerance. Diabetes Care 1993; 16:157–77.
6. Haffner SM. Epidemiology of type 2 diabetes: risk factors. Diabetes Care 1998; 21(Suppl. 3):C3–6.
7. Unwin N, Shaw J, Zimmet P, Alberti KG. Impaired glucose tolerance and impaired fasting glycaemia: the current status on definition and intervention. Diabet Med 2002; 19:708–23.
8. National Diabetes Data Group. Classification and diagnosis of diabetes mellitus and other categories of glucose intolerance. Diabetes 1979; 28:1039–57.
9. World Health Organization Expert Committee on Diabetes Mellitus. Second Report. Technical Report Series 646. Geneva: WHO, 1980.
10. Balkau B, Eschwege E, Tichet J, Marre M. Proposed criteria for the diagnosis of diabetes: evidence from a French epidemiological study. Diabet Metab 1997; 23:428–34.
11. Shaw JE, Zimmet PZ, McCarthy D, de Couten M. Type 2 diabetes worldwide according to the new classification and criteria. Diabetes Care 2000; 23 (Suppl. 2):B5–10.
12. Resnick HE, Harris MI, Brock DB, Harris TB. American Diabetes Association diabetes diagnostic criteria, advancing age, and cardiovascular disease risk profiles. Results from the Third Health and Nutrition Examination Survey. Diabetes Care 2000; 23:176–80.
13. Wahl PW, Savage PJ, Psaty BM, et al. Diabetes in older adults: comparison of 1997 American Diabetes Association classification of diabetes mellitus with 1985 WHO classification. Lancet 1998; 352:1012–5.
14. Shaw JE, Zimmet PZ, de Courten M, et al. Impaired fasting glucose or impaired glucose tolerance. What best predicts future diabetes in Mauritius? Diabetes Care 1999; 22:399–402.
15. Shaw JE, de Courten M, Boyko E, Zimmet PZ. Impact of new diagnostic criteria for diabetes on different populations. Diabetes Care 1999; 22:762–6.
16. DECODE Study Group. Is fasting glucose sufficient to define diabetes? Epidemiological data from 20 European studies. Diabetologia 1999; 42:647–54.
17. Qiao Q, Nakagami T, Tuomilehto J, et al. Comparison of the fasting and the 2-h glucose criteria for diabetes in different Asian cohorts. Diabetologia 2000; 43:1470–5.
18. Bennett PH, Burch TA, Miller M. Diabetes mellitus in American (Pima) Indians. Lancet 1971; ii:125–8.
19. Zimmet PZ, Taft P, Guinea A, et al. The high prevalence of diabetes mellitus on a Central Pacific island. Diabetologia 1977; 13:111–5.
20. Zimmet PZ. Kelly West Lecture: challenges in diabetes epidemiology: from West to the Rest. Diabetes Care 1992; 15:232–52.
21. O'Dea K. Westernisation, insulin resistance and diabetes in Australian Aborigines. Med J Aust 1991; 155:258–64.
22. Burke JP, Williams K, Haffner SM, et al. Elevated incidence of type 2 diabetes in San Antonio, Texas, compared with that of Mexico City, Mexico. Diabetes Care 2001; 24:1573–8.
23. International Diabetes Federation. Available at: http://www.idf.org.
24. Yoon K-H, Lee J-H, Kim J-W, et al. Epidemic obesity and type 2 diabetes in Asia. Lancet 2006; 368: 1681–8.
25. Harris MI, Flegal KM, Cowie CC, et al. Prevalence of diabetes, impaired fasting glucose, and impaired glucose tolerance in U.S. adults. Diabetes Care 1998; 21:518–24.
26. Alberti G, Zimmet P, Shaw J, Bloomgarden Z, Kaufman F, Silink M for the Consensus Workshop Group: Type 2 diabetes in the young: the evolving epidemic. Diabetes Care 2004; 27:1798–811.
27. Kitagawa T, Owada M, Urakami T, Yamanchi K. Increased incidence of non-insulin dependent diabetes mellitus among Japanese school children correlates with an increased intake of animal protein and fat. Clin Pediatr 1998; 37:111–6.
28. Gu K, Cowie CC, Harris MI. Diabetes and decline in heart disease mortality in US adults. J Am Med Assoc 1999; 281:1291–7.
29. Laakso M. Diabetes and cardiovascular disease in type 2 diabetes: challenge for treatment and prevention. J Intern Med 2001; 249:225–35.
30. Fuller J, Shipley MJ, Rose G, et al. Mortality from coronary heart disease and stroke in relation to degree of glycaemia: the Whitehall Study. BMJ 1983; 287:867–70.
31. The DECODE Study Group, on behalf of the European Diabetes Epidemiology Group. Glucose tolerance and cardiovascular mortality. Comparison of fasting and 2-hour glucose criteria. Arch Intern Med 2001; 161:397–404.
32. Tominaga M, Eguchi H, Manaka H, et al. Impaired glucose tolerance is a risk factor for cardiovascular disease, but not impaired fasting glucose: the Funagata Diabetes Study. Diabetes Care 1999; 22:920–4.

33. De Vegt F, Dekker JM, Stehouwer CDA, et al. Similar 9-year mortality risks and reproducibility for the World Health Organization and American Diabetes Association glucose tolerance categories. Diabetes Care 2000; 23:40–4.
34. Yudkin JS, Alberti KGMM, McLarty DS, Swai H. Impaired glucose tolerance. Is it a risk factor for diabetes or a diagnostic ragbag? BMJ 1990; 301:397–401.
35. Haffner SM, D'Agostino R, Saad MF, et al. Increased insulin resistance and insulin secretion in nondiabetic African-Americans and Hispanics compared with non-Hispanic whites: the Insulin Resistance Atherosclerosis Study. Diabetes 1996; 45:742–8.
36. Lillioja S, Mott DM, Spraul M, et al. Insulin resistance and insulin secretory dysfunction as precursors of non-insulin-dependent diabetes mellitus: prospective studies of Pima Indians. N Engl J Med 1993; 329:1988–92.
37. Haffner SM, Miettinen H, Gaskill SP, Stern MP. Decreased insulin secretion and increased insulin resistance are independently related to the 7-year risk of NIDDM in Mexican-Americans. Diabetes 1995; 44:1386–91.
38. Mykkänen L, Kuusisto J, Pyörälä K, Laakso M. Cardiovascular disease risk factors as predictors of type 2 (non-insulin-dependent) diabetes mellitus in elderly subjects. Diabetologia 1993; 36:553–9.
39. Hu FB, Manson JE, Stampfer MJ. Diet, lifestyle, and the risk of type 2 diabetes mellitus in women. N Engl J Med 2001; 345:790–7.
40. Boyko EJ, Fujimoto WY, Leonetti DL, Newell-Morris L. Visceral adiposity and risk of type 2 diabetes. A prospective study among Japanese Americans. Diabetes Care 2000; 23:465–71.
41. Van Dam RM, Boer JMA, Feskens EJM, Seidell JC. Parental history of diabetes modifies the association between abdominal adiposity and hyperglycemia. Diabetes Care 2001; 24:1454–9.
42. Dunstan DW, Salmon J, Healy GN, et al. for the AusDiab Steering Committee: Association of television viewing with fasting and 2-h postchallenge plasma glucose levels in adults without diagnosed diabetes. Diabetes Care 2007; 30:516–22.
43. Kay SJ, Fiatarone Singh MA. The influence of physical activity on abdominal fat: a systematic review of the literature. Obes Rev 2006; 7:183–200.
44. Meyer K, Kushi LH, Jacobs DR, Folsom AR. Dietary fat and incidence of type 2 diabetes in older Iowa women. Diabetes Care 2001; 24:1528–35.
45. Hu G, Jousilahti P, Meltonen M, Bidel S, Tuomilehto J. Joint association of coffee consumption and other factors to the risk of type 2 diabetes: a prospective study in Finland. Int J Obes 2006; 30:1742–9.
46. Barker DJ. The developmental origins of adult disease. J Am Coll Nutr 2004; 23 (6 Suppl):588S–95.
47. Pan X-R, Li G-W, Wang J-X, et al. Effects of diet and exercise in preventing NIDDM in people with impaired glucose tolerance: the Da Qing IGT and Diabetes Study. Diabetes Care 1997; 20:537–44.
48. Tuomilehto J, Lindström J, Eriksson JG, et al. Prevention of type 2 diabetes mellitus by changes in lifestyle among subjects with impaired glucose tolerance. N Engl J Med 2001; 344:1343–50.
49. Lindström J, Ilanne-Parikka P, Peltonen M, et al. Sustained reduction in the incidence of type 2 diabetes by lifestyle intervention: follow-up of the Finnish Diabetes Prevention Study. Lancet 2006; 368:1634–9.
50. The Diabetes Prevention Program Research Group. Reduction in the incidence of type 2 diabetes with lifestyle intervention or metformin. N Engl J Med 2002; 346:393–403.
51. Kosaka K, Noda M, Kuzuya T. Prevention of type 2 diabetes by lifestyle intervention: a Japanese trial in IGT males. Diab Res Clin Pract 2005; 67:152–62.
52. Ramachandran A, Snehalatha C, Mary S, et al. for the Indian Diabetes Prevention Programme (IDPP). The Indian Diabetes prevention Programme shows that lifestyle modification and metformin prevent type 2 diabetes in Asian Indian subjects with impaired glucose tolerance (IDPP-1). Diabetologia 2006; 49:289–97.
53. American Diabetes Association. Screening for type 2 diabetes. Diabetes Care 1998; 21 (Suppl. 1): S20–2.
54. Alberti KGMM. Impaired glucose tolerance—fact or fiction. Diabet Med 1996; 13:S6–8.
55. Ryden L, Standl E, Bartnik M, et al. Guidelines on diabetes, pre-diabetes, and cardiovascular disease: executive summary. The Task Force on Diabetes and Cardiovascular Diseases of the European Society of Cardiology (ESC) and of the European Association for the Study of Diabetes (EASD). Eur Heart J 2007; 28:88–136.

2 | Pathogenesis of Type 2 Diabetes

Michael Stumvoll
Department of Medicine, University of Leipzig, Leipzig, Germany

Barry J. Goldstein
Division of Endocrinology, Diabetes and Metabolic Diseases, Department of Medicine, Jefferson Medical College of Thomas Jefferson University, Philadelphia, Pennsylvania, U.S.A.

Timon W. van Haeften
Department of Internal Medicine, University Medical Centre Utrecht, Utrecht, The Netherlands

PATHOPHYSIOLOGY OF HYPERGLYCEMIA

An enormous amount of research has been dedicated to unraveling the pathophysiology of type 2 diabetes mellitus over the last 30 years. While a large number of reviews have been devoted to its description, this chapter follows the line of our recent seminar (1).

Insulin is the key hormone for regulating blood glucose. In general, normoglycemia is maintained by the balanced interplay between insulin secretion and the efficacy of insulin actions. In the fasting state, the major part of glucose is produced by the liver, and roughly half of it is used for brain glucose metabolism. The remainder is taken up by various tissues, mainly muscle and for a minor part adipose tissue. In this situation insulin levels are low, and have no appreciable effect on muscle glucose uptake. The normal liver is capable of increasing glucose production fourfold or more, and the main effect of the relatively low insulin levels is to restrain liver glucose production. After a meal, insulin is secreted in larger amounts, which diminishes liver glucose production even further and will lead to an enhancement of muscle (and adipose tissue) glucose uptake.

The normal pancreatic cell is capable of adapting to changes in insulin action, i.e., a decrease in insulin action is accompanied by upregulation of insulin secretion (and vice versa). Normal pancreas beta-cell adaptation precludes development of diabetes in a large number of insulin-resistant subjects. (Fig. 1) illustrates the curvilinear relationship between normal beta-cell function and insulin sensitivity (2). When the adaptation of the beta cell is insufficient ("deviation from the hyperbola"), the subjects will develop impaired glucose tolerance (IGT) or type 2 diabetes. Figure 1 shows how beta-cell function is inadequately low for a given degree of insulin sensitivity. Various studies (including follow-up studies in Pima Indians) have indeed shown that beta-cell dysfunction is critical in the pathogenesis of type 2 diabetes (3).

It is of note that even small increases in fasting (and postprandial) glucose occur in subjects with insulin resistance, which should stimulate insulin release (that is "traveling along" the hyperbola). Thus, when insulin action decreases (for example in increasing obesity) the system normally compensates by increasing beta-cell function, in the face of higher fasting and 2-hour glucose concentrations (4). Even if this increase is small, it now appears that this may be toxic to beta cells ("glucose toxicity").

INSULIN RESISTANCE

Insulin resistance is present when the biological effects of insulin are subnormal for both glucose disposal in skeletal muscle and suppression of endogenous glucose production primarily in liver (5). In the fasting state, however, muscle accounts for only a small proportion of glucose disposal (less than 20%) while endogenous glucose production is responsible for all of the glucose appearing in plasma. In patients with type 2 diabetes and in patients with impaired fasting glucose (IFG) endogenous glucose production is accelerated (6,7). Since many of these subjects may (still) have basal hyperinsulinemia, at least early in the disease, hepatic

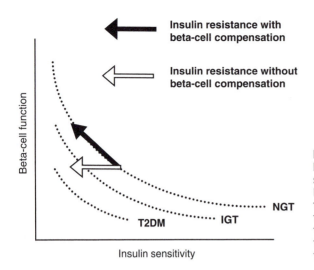

FIGURE 1 Hyperbolic relationship between beta-cell function and insulin sensitivity. In subjects with normal glucose tolerance a quasi-hyperbolic relationship exists between beta-cell function and insulin sensitivity. With deviation from this hyperbola, deterioration of glucose tolerance. *Abbreviations*: IGT, impaired glucose tolerance; NGT, normal glucose tolerance; T2DM, type 2 diabetes mellitus.

insulin resistance (with increased hepatic glucose production) is the driving force of hyperglycemia of type 2 diabetes.

Insulin resistance is strongly associated with obesity for which several mechanisms have been invoked. A number of circulating hormones, cytokines and metabolic fuels, such as nonesterified (free) fatty acids (NEFA) originate in the adipocyte and diminish insulin action (see below). In obese subjects, adipocytes are large, which renders them resistant to the ability of insulin to suppress lipolysis, especially in visceral or deep subcutaneous fat. This results in elevated release and circulating levels of NEFA and glycerol, both of which aggravate insulin resistance in skeletal muscle and liver (Fig. 2) (8).

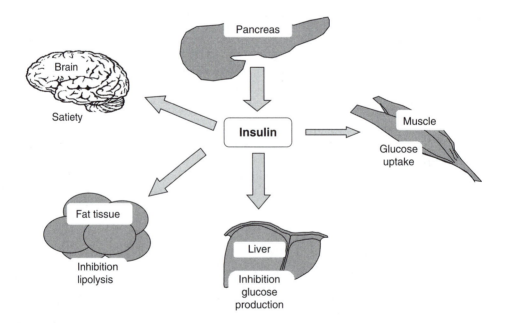

FIGURE 2 Schematic representation of normal effects of insulin. Insulin secretion from the pancreas normally reduces glucose output by the liver, enhances glucose uptake by skeletal muscle, and suppresses fatty acid release from fat tissue.

Tissue-Specific Insulin Receptor Knockout Models

In order to better understand whether severe insulin resistance can lead to frank diabetes, and to delineate the roles of the various insulin-sensitive tissues, the question has arisen whether it would be possible to induce diabetes in animal models harboring genetic defects leading to absence of insulin receptors in specific tissues (brain, muscle, liver, adipocytes, and pancreas islets). Therefore, animal models with "conditional knockouts of the insulin receptor" have been studied (Fig. 3). Although it had previously been widely thought that muscle insulin resistance would lead to diabetes, muscle-specific knockout models (9) did not develop diabetes, even if these animals did become obese. Similarly, neither adipocyte-specific (10) or brain-specific insulin receptor knockout animal models became diabetic (Fig. 2), although brain-specific animal models did become overweight, pointing to the physiological role of insulin as a (hypothalamic) satiety factor. However, liver-specific (11) and pancreas beta-cell-specific (12) knockout models did develop diabetes. The latter findings point to the great importance of insulin signaling within the beta cells for beta-cell growth and function.

However, the main positive conclusion of these studies is that even severe insulin resistance at the level of brain, muscle, or adipocyte does not lead to frank diabetes mellitus. The finding that severe insulin resistance in the liver or in the pancreas beta cells can lead to frank diabetes in itself cannot be taken as proof of the hypothesis that one or the other is an obligate part of the sequence of events of development of (human) type 2 diabetes.

Cellular Mechanisms

The insulin receptor is specific plasma membrane receptor with tyrosine kinase activity (13), to which insulin is bound. This kinase activates the insulin receptor substrate (IRS) proteins on multiple sites; these IRS proteins serve as binding scaffolds for a variety of adaptor proteins and lead to the downstream signaling cascade (Fig. 4) (14). Insulin activates a series of lipid and protein kinase enzymes linked to the translocation of glucose transporters to the cell surface, synthesis of glycogen, protein, mRNAs and to nuclear DNA that influences cell survival and proliferation. Insulin resistance presumably results from mechanisms blocking insulin signaling. It is of note that various normal biological processes can inhibit IRS protein activity via phosphorylation at specific serine and threonine residues within the IRS proteins. Other processes can interfere with insulin signaling by interfering with other proteins further

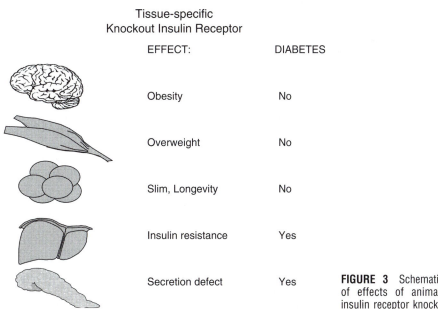

Tissue-specific
Knockout Insulin Receptor

	EFFECT:	DIABETES
	Obesity	No
	Overweight	No
	Slim, Longevity	No
	Insulin resistance	Yes
	Secretion defect	Yes

FIGURE 3 Schematic representation of effects of animal-tissue specific insulin receptor knockout models.

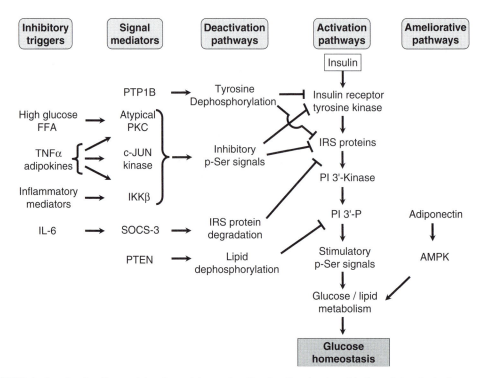

FIGURE 4 Insulin signaling and insulin resistance. Insulin signaling involves binding of insulin to its receptor followed by a cascade of intracellular events, depicted as activation pathways. Negative modulation of insulin action can be mediated via various pathways leading to insulin resistance: Various inhibitory triggers influence their respective signal modulators (partly via transcription factors), which lead via deactivating pathways (tyrosine phosphatases, serine kinases, lipid phosphatases, and degradation pathways) to inhibitory actions on insulin signaling (activation pathways). Adiponectin has an ameliorating function on glucose metabolism apart from insulin signaling.

downstream of the IRS proteins (for example, PKB/akt). Recent research indicates that several of these mechanisms underlie "insulin resistance."

The positive effects on downstream responses exerted by tyrosine phosphorylation of the receptor and the IRS proteins are opposed by dephosphorylation of these tyrosine side-chains by cellular protein-tyrosine phosphatases (PTPs) and by protein phosphorylation on serine and threonine residues (which often occur together) (15). PTP1B is a widely expressed PTP, which has been shown to play an important role in the negative regulation of insulin signaling (16).

Serine/threonine phosphorylation of IRS-1 reduces its ability to act as a substrate for the tyrosine kinase activity of the insulin receptor and inhibits its coupling to its major downstream effector systems. Multiple IRS serine kinases have been identified, including various mitogen-activated protein kinases (MAPK/ERK), c-Jun NH₃-terminal kinase (JNK), atypical protein kinase C, phosphatidylinositol 3′-kinase, among others (14). Signal down-regulation can also occur via internalization and loss of the insulin receptor from the cell surface and degradation of IRS proteins (17). Members of the "suppressor of cytokine signaling" (SOCS) family of proteins participate in IRS protein degradation through a ubiquitin proteosomal pathway (18).

Role of Adipocyte Products and Inflammation

Increased levels of NEFA and inflammatory cytokines (e.g., tumor necrosis factor α [TNFα] and interleukin 6 [IL-6]) released by expanded visceral adipose tissue adversely influence the insulin signaling cascade (19,20). NEFA inhibit insulin-stimulated glucose metabolism in skeletal muscle and suppress glycogenolysis in liver (21,22). NEFA activate cellular kinases, including atypical protein kinase C isoforms by increasing cellular diacylglycerol levels, which can activate the inflammatory kinases inhibitor κB kinase (IKK) and JNK, increasing serine/threonine phosphorylation of IRS-1 and reducing downstream IRS-1 signaling, as described above (23–25). TNFα enhances adipocyte lipolysis, which further increased NEFA levels, and also elicits its own direct negative effects on insulin signaling pathways (26). Neutralization of TNFα dramatically reverses insulin resistance in rodent models; however, the magnitude of its involvement in human insulin resistance is not entirely clear (27). The proinflammatory IL-6 inhibits the insulin signal by augmenting the expression of SOCS proteins (28,29).

While circulating NEFA and several adipokines are increased in visceral obesity, the levels of the adipose-specific protein adiponectin are decreased, reducing its insulin-sensitizing effects in liver and muscle (19,30). Adiponectin signals via AMP kinase, a stress-activated signaling enzyme implicated in a variety of metabolic responses, including suppression of hepatic gluconeogenesis, glucose uptake in exercising skeletal muscle, fatty acid oxidation, and inhibition of lipolysis, which may explain its beneficial metabolic effects (30–34).

A close connection between insulin resistance and classical inflammatory signaling pathways has also been recently identified. NF-κB is held in an inactive state in resting conditions by binding to an inhibitory partner, IκB (35). Phosphorylation of IκB by its kinase (IKK) leads to I B degradation, releasing NF-κB for translocation to the nucleus where it can influence the transcription of diverse genes involved in the inflammatory response. High doses of salicylates, which block IKK activity (36) can ameliorate hyperglycemia and insulin resistance in diabetes and obesity (37,38). More importantly, genetic disruption of IKKβ-normalized skeletal insulin resistance caused by NEFA via improvement in IRS-1 tyrosine phosphorylation and activation of its downstream signal cascade (39). Overall, this line of evidence suggests that IKK may be an important target for the development of new therapeutics in insulin resistance, especially in the setting of visceral adiposity.

In addition to their effects on insulin signaling, the circulating adipose tissue factors strongly influence vascular endothelial function, linking the increased vascular risk in the metabolic syndrome with mechanisms of cellular insulin resistance (30,40). Adipose secretory factors also recruit and activate inflammatory cells, which can further perpetuate a systemic inflammatory milieu that can strongly influence vascular function and atherogenesis (41).

Mitochondrial Metabolism

The accumulation of "ectopic" triglyceride in visceral depots has suggested a defect in mitochondrial lipid oxidation in patients with type 2 diabetes, who have impaired oxidative capacity and small mitochondria in skeletal muscle (42). Peroxisome proliferator-activated receptor-gamma (PPAR-γ) coactivator 1 (PGC-1), a transcription factor for genes involved in mitochondrial fatty acid oxidation and ATP synthesis, was decreased in young, lean, insulin-resistant offspring of parents with type 2 diabetes, suggesting that an inherited defect in mitochondrial oxidative phosphorylation could lead to cellular lipid accumulation (43). Gene expression profiling studies have also shown that decreased expression of PGC-1 and related gene products may affect mitochondrial function in subjects with insulin resistance and type 2 diabetes (44,45).

INSULIN EFFECTS IN THE CENTRAL NERVOUS SYSTEM

Insulin receptors are also expressed throughout the brain with particularly high concentrations in the hypothalamus, the hippocampus, and the cortex (46). In humans, however, positron emission tomography (PET) studies repeatedly failed to reveal effects of hyperinsulinemia on brain glucose uptake. Since glucose transport is probably not an important downstream effector of insulin in neurons because this is largely facilitated by GLUT3 and, to a minor extent, GLUT1 (an insulin-independent glucose transporter) the human brain has been traditionally regarded as an insulin-insensitive organ. Nevertheless, an insulin effect on neuronal glucose oxidation or glial glycogen metabolism can not be excluded. The most relevant neuronal insulin effect at the cellular level seems to be the inhibition of norepinephrine reuptake (47).

The resulting increase in synaptic cleft norepinephrine can have a variety of secondary effects, not only on the postsynaptic neuron but also on adjacent astrocytes (glial cells) via beta-adrenoceptor activation. Thus, insulin clearly has every potential to modulate central nervous system (CNS) activity.

Early work in animals suggested that insulin inhibits appetite at the CNS level (48). When given directly into the brain, insulin-induced suppression of food intake (49) and brain selective deletion of the insulin receptor resulted in hyperphagia, obesity, and metabolic insulin resistance in mice (50). Thus, the understanding of insulin regulation of appetite and its potential dysregulation in obesity should be of great relevance.

Given that insulin negatively regulates appetite in the CNS, the impact of CNS insulin on body weight regulation still remains widely unclear. In normal weight male subjects, insulin given intranasally over 8 weeks resulted in a weight loss of 1.3 kg and in a loss of 1.4 kg of body fat as determined by standard body impedance technique. Waist circumference decreased by 1.6 cm and plasma leptin levels dropped by an average of 27%. However, in normal weight female subjects, the same intervention yielded an increase of body weight by 1 kg mainly due to increased extracellular water (51).

A recent magnetoencephalography study demonstrated differential insulin effects in lean and overweight subjects (52). In this study, the stimulatory insulin effect (expressed as difference to the placebo experiment) on theta activity was significantly smaller in obese than in lean subjects. Moreover, the attenuation of insulin-induced changes in theta activity was inversely correlated with body mass index (BMI) in a multivariate analysis and positively with insulin-stimulated glucose disposal, i.e., metabolic insulin sensitivity in a univariate analysis. These early findings suggest that obesity is associated with reduced cerebrocortical insulin sensitivity.

BETA-CELL DYSFUNCTION

Although abnormalities of insulin secretion in the pathophysiology of diabetes have often been neglected, they occur already early during the disease and can often already be demonstrated in subjects with normal glucose tolerance (first-degree relatives of type 2 diabetes).

Normal Insulin Secretion

After uptake of glucose pancreatic beta-cell glucose is rapidly degraded in oxidative glucose metabolism, leading to ATP formation. ATP is involved in beta-cell membrane depolarization. The ADP/ATP ratio, the sulfonylurea receptor-1 (SUR 1) protein, which closes the adjacent potassium channel (potassium inward rectifier 6.2, KIR 6.2 channel). The closure of the potassium channels will decrease the membrane potential, which leads to opening of voltage-gated calcium channels; this induces the release of insulin-containing granules (Fig. 5). Upon stimulation with glucose, insulin is released with a short-lasting peak of a few minutes (so-called "first-phase") followed by a slowly evolving second phase; the second phase lasts as long as the plasma glucose level is elevated.

Insulin Secretion in Type 2 Diabetes

In patients with type 2 diabetes, plasma glucose levels are elevated; and consequently, fasting plasma insulin. Although the insulin levels sometimes increase slightly after a meal in patients with type 2 diabetes mellitus this is considerably less than normal. In studies in which glucose levels have been raised by glucose infusions (hyperglycemic clamps) to comparable levels in diabetic subjects and controls, it has become clear that second-phase insulin secretion is roughly 25% (IGT) to 50% decreased in type 2 diabetes (53). First-phase secretion is generally completely lost. In normoglycemic first-degree relatives insulin secretion is also diminished but to a lower extent, presumably on a genetic basis (54). It is suspected that upon acquaintance of insulin resistance (obesity, physical inactivity) the pancreas that has already lower secretory capabilities can adapt less than normal, which might lead to decreased glucose tolerance or diabetes. It has been widely suggested that various mechanisms might further

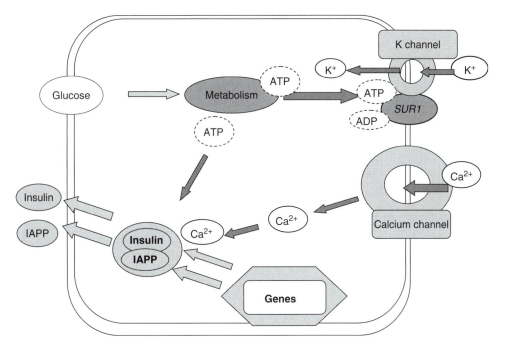

FIGURE 5   Insulin secretion. Schematic representation of normal glucose-induced insulin secretion. *Abbreviations*: ADP, adenosine dephosphate; ATP, adension triphosphate; IAAP, islet amyloid polypeptide.

aggravate beta-cell insulin secretory dysfunction, among which glucose toxicity, lipotoxicity, and amyloid deposition.

Glucose Toxicity

Since over time insulin secretion appears to decrease in most patients, it has been proposed that glucose itself is toxic to beta cells. This is in analogy with the situation in the "honeymoon period" in type 1 diabetes subjects: after the initial diagnosis of type 1 diabetes mellitus plasma glucose levels are lowered by injections with exogenous insulin. It has often been observed that dosages of exogenous insulin can be markedly decreased or even omitted during several months. It has been established that residual beta cells of these patients resume their insulin secretory function. Inevitably, in type 1 diabetes this is only a temporary improvement (due to the ongoing autoimmune destruction of remaining beta cells). It may well be that in type 2 diabetes glucose is toxic as well (55). In pancreas beta cells oxidative glucose metabolism will also lead to formation of reactive oxygen species (ROS), which would damage beta cells (Fig. 6). Indeed, beta cells have low amounts of catalase and superoxide dismutase, proteins which normally metabolize the ROS (56). ROS can activate NF-κB activity, which would be proapoptotic. Since it has been observed in an animal model of diabetes that pancreas duodenum homeobox-1 (PDX-1), a regulator of insulin gene transcription, is diminished by hyperglycemia, this could also be a mechanism of "glucose toxicity."

Yet another mechanism may involve upregulation of uncoupling protein 2 (UCP-2) by high glucose that would lead to uncoupling of oxidative glucose metabolism from ATP formation in the mitochondrion leading to lower ATP (57).

Lipotoxicity

Although free fatty acids (FFA), also termed NEFA, acutely increase insulin secretion, chronic FFA overload diminishes beta-cell function. Type 2 diabetes subjects have often increased FFA due to insulin resistance to (adipocyte) lipolysis. It is now clear that high glucose inhibits beta-cell fatty acid oxidation, which may lead to accumulation of long-chain

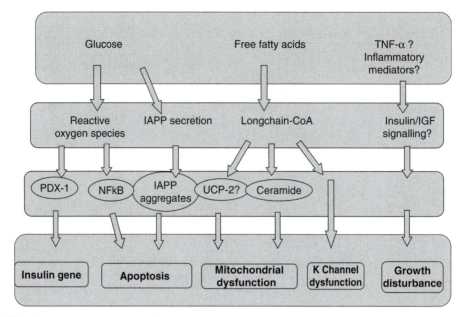

FIGURE 6 Schematic representation of possible negative influences of hyperglycemia and increased NEFA, and of various modulators involved in insulin resistance such as TNFα and inflammatory mediators on B-cell dysfunction. The pathways possibly involved are alteration in mitochondrial function and potassium channel function and IAPP aggregation and other pathways leading to B-cell apoptosis or altered gene transcription. *Abbreviations*: IAPP, islet amyloid polypeptide; NEFA, nonesterified fatty acids; TNFα, tumor necrosis factor alpha.

coenzyme A (LC-CoA) (58). This has been suggested to interfere with normal potassium channel activity, or to lead to activation of UCP-2, which would lead to uncoupling of oxidative glucose metabolism from ATP formation in the mitochondrion leading to lower ATP. FFA may diminish UCP-2 via augmentation of PPAR-gamma protein, which would lead to activation of UCP-2 (57). However, PPAR-gamma activation has numerous effects, and its overall importance in beta cells is therefore difficult to assess; for example, in animal models PPAR-gamma activation has been reported to enhance FFA oxidation in beta cells, which may in itself protect against lipotoxicity (59).

Yet another mechanism may involve synthesis of ceramide by FFA or generation of nitric oxide. In other tissues (muscle), degradation of ceramide has been shown to prevent FFA-induced insulin resistance almost completely (60); it is therefore conceivable that FFA act via ceramide formation in pancreas beta cells. Ceramide has been shown to inhibit insulin gene expression (61) and has been implied in apoptosis via various pathways. The importance of the insulin receptor signaling on insulin gene expression should not be underestimated, and may well harbor yet other mechanisms of lipotoxicity: via acyl-CoA FFA may inhibit insulin receptor signaling in beta cells via influences on IRS proteins, PI-3-kinase, or further downstream the insulin signaling cascade (62).

Islet Amyloid

It has been reported from postmortem studies in subjects with type 2 diabetes that most of the subjects' pancreas islets contain amyloid in considerable quantities.

Amyloid consists of islet amyloid polypeptide (IAPP), or amylin, deposits. IAPP is normally contained in the insulin granule, and therefore cosecreted together with insulin (in a 10-fold lower quantity). Although amyloid is also present in islets of monkeys and cats, which have developed diabetes, it is absent in diabetic rodents, although rodents do secrete IAPP (63). Small aggregates of IAPP are cytotoxic (in vitro), which has been suggested to be due to "channel formation" by aggregating IAPP molecules, which can lead to calcium influx into beta cells; another possibility is intracellular aggregation after interaction with liposomal membranes. While hyperglycemia itself may accelerate IAPP aggregation, FFA (or NEFA) may enhance cytotoxicity of the aggregates (64). Although it is tempting to speculate that increased insulin secretion automatically leading to more IAPP secretion in insulin-resistant subjects would lead to IAPP aggregation, the finding that first-degree relatives secrete less IAPP (and insulin) than controls contradicts this hypothesis (65). Since islet amyloid is absent in most insulin-resistant nondiabetic subjects, it seems more probable that amyloid formation is a relatively late occurrence during the pathophysiology of type 2 diabetes.

HEREDITY IN TYPE 2 DIABETES MELLITUS

The fact that more than half of obese insulin-resistant subjects will never develop diabetes points to susceptibility for the disease in some humans, while protective factors against the disease are present in others. Indeed, a positive family history confers a two- to threefold increased risk for the disease with a 15% to 30% risk to develop type 2 diabetes or IGT in first-degree relatives of type 2 diabetes subjects (66). The risk is even higher (around 60% by the age of 60 years) if both parents have diabetes (67). Similarly, if one twin has type 2 diabetes, the risk for type 2 diabetes mellitus in the other twin is higher in monozygotic (identical) twins (35% to 58%) as compared with dizygotic twins (around 20%) (68,69). A caveat is the presence of low birth weight in many twins, since low birth weight per se associates with increased risk of type 2 diabetes later in life (70,71).

GENETIC FACTORS

The polygenic nature of the disease has it made difficult to dissect individual genes conferring increased risk for diabetes. In general, two methods, the so-called candidate gene approach and the genome-wide scan approach have been used. The candidate gene approach examines specific genes with a plausible role in the disease process. The genome-wide scan locates genes through their chromosomal (genomic) position. In genetic studies the population-attributable risk is often given; this is the percentage of a disease that would be eliminated if the genetic factor were removed from the population.

CANDIDATE GENES

PPAR-Gamma

Currently, the most robust single candidate variant is the highly prevalent Pro12Ala polymorphism in PPAR-γ gene (72,73). PPARγ is a transcription factor (74,75); the isoform PPARγ_2 is specific for adipose tissue, where it plays a key role in regulating adipogenic differentiation (76). The proline allele of the P12A polymorphism in PPARγ_2 has a prevalence of 75% in Caucasian, and leads to a relative risk of 1.25 for diabetes (72,73,77), which leads to a population-attributable risk of 16%.

PGC1α

The Gly483Ser polymorphism in PPARγ coactivator (PGC1α), a transcriptional cofactor of PPARγ, is highly prevalent (around 38%). PGC1α is a regulator of oxidative phosphorylation in mitochondria, which has been shown to be diminished early in the disease and even in nondiabetic first-degree relatives of type 2 diabetes patients. A meta-analysis concludes to only a very modest relative risk of around 1.07 leading to a population-attributable risk of 2.5%.

HNF4Alpha

The discovery of MODY genes has rendered them candidate genes for type 2 diabetes. Genetic variation near or in the P2-promoter of the MODY-1 gene HNF4A (chromosome 20q) may relate to type 2 diabetes (see also Chapter 34) (78).

KCNJ11

Clearly, beta-cell potassium channels are candidates for genetic predisposition for type 2 diabetes. The E23K variant in the KCNJ11 gene (Potassium Inward Rectifier 6.2 (KIR6.2) channel) has been found in meta-analyses to confer a relative increased risk of 1.23 for heterozygotes and around 1.65 for homozygous carriers, presumably due to decreased insulin secretion (79). Since this variant is highly prevalent (15% to 20%), the population-attributable risk is around 7%.

GENOME-WIDE SCANS

A large number of genome-wide scans has been performed. Since initial positive findings have been replicated for over 20 genomic regions, the search for the genes responsible for the association with diabetes has proven to be difficult. However, three genes have now been found in this manner, calpain-10, ENPP1, and TCF7L2.

Calpain-10

The calpain-10 gene encodes for a cysteine protease reported to be responsible for the association of a region in chromosome 2 with diabetes (80,81). A recent meta-analysis indicates that several single-nucleotide polymorphisms (SNPs) are responsible for the association, each with only a modest effect with relative risks between 1.10 and 1.5 (82). Genetic variation in calpain-10 may affect sensitivity (83) or insulin secretion (84). It has also been shown to inhibit a protease involved in mitochondrial function, which might relate to mitochondrial dysfunction as is often observed in type 2 diabetes (85).

ENPP1

Genome-wide scans often lead to regions that are so wide that research is often directed also by candidate genes in that specific region. The 6q16-q24 region harbors the ectonucleotide pyrophosphate/phosphodiesterase 1 (ENPP1 or PC-1) gene, which is a candidate for insulin resistance since the gene product can interact with the insulin–insulin receptor complex, thereby diminishing receptor activation. One haplotype conferred a relative risk of roughly 1.50 for type 2 diabetes and for obesity (86). The highly prevalent K121Q polymorphism has been found in vitro to worsening inhibition of insulin–insulin receptor autophosphorylation by the ENPP protein. The prevalence of the ENPP1 K121Q polymorphism has been found to vary widely; for example in one study, it was found in 39% of type 2 diabetes versus 26% in nondiabetic Caucasian subjects, which would lead to a population-attributable risk of around 13% (87). Others have found a predominant effect of the polymorphism on (over-)weight with on average an increase in BMI of $1.3 \, kg/m^2$ (or 4 kg for an adult) for homozygotes (88).

The mechanism of its obesity and diabetes promoting action is uncertain; although it might be that it acts by virtue of diminished insulin-induced satiety in the brain and/or by inducing insulin resistance in muscle leading to "overflow" of nutrients to adipocytes thereby leading to obesity.

TCF7L2

The genome region 10q25 harbors the transcription factor 7-like 2 (TCF7L2) gene. In studies in three cohorts, it was shown that heterozygous (38%) and homozygous (7%) carriers of a prevalent intron microsatellite have relative risks of 1.4 and 2.4 for type 2 diabetes, respectively. Due to the high prevalence of this microsatellite the population-attributable risk for diabetes is around 18%. TCF7L2 is a transcription factor influencing the proglucagone gene; it is has been proposed to influence glucagon-like peptide 1 (GLP-1) levels. GLP-1 is one of the peptides encoded by this gene; it has stimulating effects both on insulin secretion per se, and on beta-cell growth (89). The importance of this gene can also be appreciated from studies showing that progression from IGT to diabetes was around 50% higher in homozygous carriers of each one of two polymorphisms in this gene (90).

ADIPOR2

The adiponectin receptor has also been considered a candidate gene for various reasons, including its presumed insulin sensitivity enhancing effect of adiponectin acting via IRS1. The adiponectin receptor 2 (ADIPOR2) presumably has major effects on the liver. In a meta-analysis of three case-control studies, the SNP rs767870 (*ADIPOR2*-SNP1) was estimated to confer a relative risk of 1.25 for type 2 diabetes. Its frequency of 19% would lead to a population-attributable risk of 5% (91).

REFERENCES

1. Stumvoll M, Goldstein BJ, Van Haeften TW. Type 2 diabetes: principles of pathogenesis and therapy. Lancet 2005; 365:1333–46.
2. Bergman RN. Lilly lecture 1989. Toward physiological understanding of glucose tolerance. Minimal-model approach. Diabetes 1989; 38:1512–27.
3. Weyer C, Bogardus C, Mott DM, Pratley RE. The natural history of insulin secretory dysfunction and insulin resistance in the pathogenesis of type 2 diabetes mellitus. J Clin Invest 1999; 104:787–94.
4. Stumvoll M, Tataranni PA, Stefan N, Vozarova B, Bogardus C. Glucose allostasis. Diabetes 2003; 52: 903–9.
5. Dinneen S, Gerich J, Rizza R. Carbohydrate metabolism in non-insulin-dependent diabetes mellitus. N Engl J Med 1992; 327:707–13.
6. Weyer C, Bogardus C, Pratley RE. Metabolic characteristics of individuals with impaired fasting glucose and/or impaired glucose tolerance. Diabetes 1999; 48:2197–203.
7. Meyer C, Stumvoll M, Nadkarni V, Dostou J, Mitrakou A, Gerich J. Abnormal renal and hepatic glucose metabolism in type 2 diabetes mellitus. J Clin Invest 1998; 102:619–24.
8. Boden G. Role of fatty acids in the pathogenesis of insulin resistance and NIDDM. Diabetes 1997; 46: 3–10.
9. Bruning JC, Michael MD, Winnay JN, et al. A muscle-specific insulin receptor knockout exhibits features of the metabolic syndrome of NIDDM without altering glucose tolerance. Mol Cell 1998; 2: 559–69.
10. Bluher M, Kahn BB, Kahn CR. Extended longevity in mice lacking the insulin receptor in adipose tissue. Science 2003; 299:572–4.
11. Michael MD, Kulkarni RN, Postic C, et al. Loss of insulin signaling in hepatocytes leads to severe insulin resistance and progressive hepatic dysfunction. Mol Cell 2000; 6:87–97.
12. Kulkarni RN, Bruning JC, Winnay JN, Postic C, Magnuson MA, Kahn CR. Tissue-specific knockout of the insulin receptor in pancreatic beta cells creates an insulin secretory defect similar to that in type 2 diabetes. Cell 1999; 96:329–39.
13. Kido Y, Nakae J, Accili D. Clinical review 125: the insulin receptor and its cellular targets. J Clin Endocrinol Metab 2001; 86:972–9.
14. White MF. IRS proteins and the common path to diabetes. Am J Physiol Endocrinol Metab 2002; 283: E413–22.
15. Zick Y. Insulin resistance: a phosphorylation-based uncoupling of insulin signaling. Trends Cell Biol 2001; 11:437–41.
16. Goldstein BJ. Protein-tyrosine phosphatases and the regulation of insulin action. In: LeRoith D, Taylor SI, Olefsky JM, eds. Diabetes mellitus: A Fundamental and Clinical Text. Philadelphia: Lippincott, 2003:255–68.
17. Zhande R, Mitchell JJ, Wu J, Sun XJ. Molecular mechanism of insulin-induced degradation of insulin receptor substrate 1. Mol Cell Biol 2002; 22:1016–26.
18. Rui L, Yuan M, Frantz D, Shoelson S, White MF. SOCS-1 and SOCS-3 block insulin signaling by ubiquitin-mediated degradation of IRS1 and IRS2. J Biol Chem 2002; 277:42394–8.
19. Rajala MW, Scherer PE. Mini review: the adipocyte—at the crossroads of energy homeostasis, inflammation, and atherosclerosis. Endocrinology 2003; 144:3765–73.
20. Ravussin E, Smith SR. Increased fat intake, impaired fat oxidation, and failure of fat cell proliferation result in ectopic fat storage, insulin resistance, and type 2 diabetes mellitus. Ann NY Acad Sci 2002; 967:363–78.
21. Boden G, Shulman GI. Free fatty acids in obesity and type 2 diabetes: defining their role in the development of insulin resistance and b-cell dysfunction. Eur J Clin Invest 2002; 32(Suppl. 3):14–23.
22. Shulman GI. Cellular mechanisms of insulin resistance. J Clin Invest 2002; 106:171–6.
23. Griffin ME, Marcucci MJ, Cline GW, et al. Free fatty acid-induced insulin resistance is associated with activation of protein kinase C theta and alterations in the insulin signaling cascade. Diabetes 1999; 48:1270–4.
24. Itani SI, Ruderman NB, Schmieder F, Boden G. Lipid-induced insulin resistance in human muscle is associated with changes in diacylglycerol, protein kinase C, and I kappa B-alpha. Diabetes 2002; 51:2005–11.

25. Gao Z, Zhang X, Zuberi A, et al. Inhibition of insulin sensitivity by free fatty acids requires activation of multiple serine kinases in 3T3-L1 adipocytes. Mol Endocrinol 2004; 18:2024–34.

26. Hotamisligil GS. Molecular mechanisms of insulin resistance and the role of the adipocyte. Int J Obes Relat Metab Disord 2000; 24(Suppl. 4):S23–7.

27. Moller DE. Potential role of TNF-alpha in the pathogenesis of insulin resistance and type 2 diabetes. Trends Endocrinol Metab 2000; 11:212–7.

28. Senn JJ, Klover PJ, Nowak IA, et al. Suppressor of cytokine signaling-3 (SOCS-3), a potential mediator of interleukin-6-dependent insulin resistance in hepatocytes. J Biol Chem 2003; 278: 13740–6.

29. Krebs DL, Hilton DJ. A new role for SOCS in insulin action. Suppressor of cytokine signaling. Sci STKE 2003:E6.

30. Goldstein BJ, Scalia R. Adiponectin: a novel adipokine linking adipocytes and vascular function. J Clin Endocrinol Metab 2004; 89:2563–8.

31. Yamauchi T, Kamon J, Minokoshi Y, et al. Adiponectin stimulates glucose utilization and fatty-acid oxidation by activating AMP-activated protein kinase. Nat Med 2002; 8:1288–95.

32. Tomas E, Tsao TS, Saha AK, et al. Enhanced muscle fat oxidation and glucose transport by ACRP30 globular domain: acetyl-CoA carboxylase inhibition and AMP-activated protein kinase activation. Proc Natl Acad Sci USA 2002; 99:16309–13.

33. Wu X, Motoshima H, Mahadev K, Stalker TJ, Scalia R, Goldstein BJ. Involvement of AMP-activated protein kinase in glucose uptake stimulated by the globular domain of adiponectin in primary rat adipocytes. Diabetes 2003; 52:1355–63.

34. Ruderman NB, Cacicedo JM, Itani S, et al. Malonyl-CoA and AMP-activated protein kinase (AMPK): possible links between insulin resistance in muscle and early endothelial cell damage in diabetes. Biochem Soc Trans 2003; 31:202–6.

35. Karin M, Delhase M. The I kappa B kinase (IKK) and NF-kappa B: Key elements of proinflammatory signalling. Semin Immunol 2000; 12:85–98.

36. Yin MJ, Yamamoto Y, Gaynor RB. The anti-inflammatory agents aspirin and salicylate inhibit the activity of I (kappa) B kinase-beta. Nature 1998; 396:77–80.

37. Kim JK, Kim YJ, Fillmore JJ, et al. Prevention of fat-induced insulin resistance by salicylate. J Clin Invest 2001; 108:437–46.

38. Yuan M, Konstantopoulos N, Lee J, et al. Reversal of obesity- and diet-induced insulin resistance with salicylates or targeted disruption of Ikkbeta. Science 2001; 293:1673–7.

39. Shoelson SE, Lee J, Yuan M. Inflammation and the IKK beta/I kappa B/NF-kappa B axis in obesity- and diet-induced insulin resistance. Int J Obes Relat Metab Disord 2003; 27(Suppl. 3):S49–52.

40. Havel PJ. Control of energy homeostasis and insulin action by adipocyte hormones: leptin, acylation stimulating protein, and adiponectin. Curr Opin Lipidol 2002; 13:51–9.

41. Wellen KE, Hotamisligil GS. Obesity-induced inflammatory changes in adipose tissue. J Clin Invest 2003; 112:1785–8.

42. Kelley DE, He J, Menshikova EV, Ritov VB. Dysfunction of mitochondria in human skeletal muscle in type 2 diabetes. Diabetes 2002; 51:2944–50.

43. Petersen KF, Dufour S, Befroy D, Garcia R, Shulman GI. Impaired mitochondrial activity in the insulin-resistant offspring of patients with type 2 diabetes. N Engl J Med 2004; 350:664–71.

44. Patti ME, Butte AJ, Crunkhorn S, et al. Coordinated reduction of genes of oxidative metabolism in humans with insulin resistance and diabetes: potential role of PGC1 and NRF1. Proc Natl Acad Sci USA 2003; 100:8466–71.

45. Mootha VK, Lindgren CM, Eriksson KF, et al. PGC-1alpha-responsive genes involved in oxidative phosphorylation are coordinately down regulated in human diabetes. Nat Genet 2003; 34:267–73.

46. Hopkins DF, Williams G. Insulin receptors are widely distributed in human brain and bind human and porcine insulin with equal affinity. Diab Med 1997; 14:1044–50.

47. Boyd FT, Clarke DW, Muther TF, Raizada MK. Insulin receptors and insulin modulation of norepinephrine uptake in neuronal cultures from rat brain. J Biol Chem 1985; 15:15880–4.

48. Woods S, Lotter E, McKay L, Porte DJ. Chronic intracerebroventricular infusion of insulin reduces food intake and body weight of baboons. Nature 1979; 282:503–5.

49. Porte D Jr, Seeley RJ, Woods SC, Baskin DG, Figlewicz DP, Schwartz MW. Obesity, diabetes and the central nervous system. Diabetologia 1998; 41:863–81.

50. Bruning JC, Gautam D, Burks DJ, et al. Role of brain insulin receptor in control of body weight and reproduction. Science 2000; 289:2122–5.

51. Hallschmid M, Benedict C, Schultes B, Fehm HL, Born J, Kern W. Intranasal insulin reduces body fat in men but not in women. Diabetes 2004; 53:3024–9.

52. Tschritter O, Preissl H, Hennige AM, et al. The cerebrocortical response to hyperinsulinemia is reduced in overweight humans: a magneto encephalographic study. Proc Natl Acad Sci USA 2006.

53. Gerich JE. The genetic basis of type 2 diabetes mellitus: impaired insulin secretion versus impaired insulin sensitivity. Endocr Rev 1998; 19:491–503.

54. Pimenta W, Korytkowski M, Mitrakou A, et al. Pancreatic beta-cell dysfunction as the primary genetic lesion in NIDDM. JAMA 1995; 273:1855–61.
55. Yki-Järvinen H. Glucose toxicity. Endocr Rev 1992; 13:415–31.
56. Robertson RP, Harmon J, Tran PO, Tanaka Y, Takahashi H. Glucose toxicity in beta-cells: type 2 diabetes, good radicals gone bad, and the glutathione connection. Diabetes 2003; 52:581–7.
57. Patane G, Anello M, Piro S, Vigneri R, Purrello F, Rabuazzo AM. Role of ATP production and uncoupling protein-2 in the insulin secretory defect induced by chronic exposure to high glucose or free fatty acids and effects of peroxisome proliferator-activated receptor-gamma inhibition. Diabetes 2002; 51:2749–56.
58. Robertson RP, Harmon J, Tran PO, Poitout V. Beta-cell glucose toxicity, lipotoxicity, and chronic oxidative stress in type 2 diabetes. Diabetes 2004; 53(Suppl. 1):S119–24.
59. Shimabukuro M, Zhou YT, Lee Y, Unger RH. Troglitazone lowers islet fat and restores beta cell function of diabetic fatty rats. J Biol Chem 1998; 273:3547–50.
60. Chavez JA, Holland WL, Bar J, Sandhoff K, Summers SA. Acid ceramidase over expression prevents the inhibitory effects of saturated fatty acids on insulin signaling. J Biol Chem 2005; 280:20148–53.
61. Kelpe CL, Moore PC, Parazzoli SD, Wicksteed B, Rhodes CJ, Poitout V. Palmitate inhibition of insulin gene expression is mediated at the transcriptional level via ceramide synthesis. J Biol Chem 2003; 278:30015–21.
62. Haber EP, Ximenes HM, Procopio J, Carvalho CR, Curi R, Carpinelli AR. Pleiotropic effects of fatty acids on pancreatic beta-cells. J Cell Physiol 2003; 194:1–12.
63. Hoppener JW, Ahren B, Lips CJ. Islet amyloid and type 2 diabetes mellitus. N Engl J Med 2000; 343: 411–9.
64. Hull RL, Westermark GT, Westermark P, Kahn SE. Islet amyloid: a critical entity in the pathogenesis of type 2 diabetes. J Clin Endocrinol Metab 2004; 89:3629–43.
65. Knowles NG, Landchild MA, Fujimoto WY, Kahn SE. Insulin and amylin release are both diminished in first-degree relatives of subjects with type 2 diabetes. Diabetes Care 2002; 25:292–7.
66. Pierce M, Keen H, Bradley C. Risk of diabetes in offspring of parents with non-insulin-dependent diabetes. Diabet Med 1995; 12:6–13.
67. Tattersal RB, Fajans SS. Prevalence of diabetes and glucose intolerance in 199 offspring of thirty-seven conjugal diabetic parents. Diabetes 1975; 24:452–62.
68. Kaprio J, Tuomilehto J, Koskenvuo M, et al. Concordance for type 1 (insulin-dependent) and type 2 (non-insulin-dependent) diabetes mellitus in a population-based cohort of twins in Finland. Diabetologia 1992; 35:1060–7.
69. Newman B, Selby JV, King MC, Slemenda C, Fabsitz R, Friedman GD. Concordance for type 2 (non-insulin-dependent) diabetes mellitus in male twins. Diabetologia 1987; 30:763–8.
70. Hales CN, Barker DJ. Type 2 (non-insulin-dependent) diabetes mellitus: the thrifty phenotype hypothesis. Diabetologia 1992; 35:595–601.
71. Hattersley AT, Tooke JE. The fetal insulin hypothesis: an alternative explanation of the association of low birth weight with diabetes and vascular disease. Lancet 1999; 353:1789–92.
72. Parikh H, Groop L. Candidate genes for type 2 diabetes. Rev Endocrinol Metab Disord 2004; 5: 151–76.
73. Lohmueller KE, Pearce CL, Pike M, Lander ES, Hirschhorn JN. Meta-analysis of genetic association studies supports a contribution of common variants to susceptibility to common disease. Nat Genet 2003; 33:177–82.
74. Olefsky JM. Treatment of insulin resistance with peroxisome proliferator-activated receptor gamma agonists. J Clin Invest 2000; 106:467–72.
75. Schoonjans K, Auwerx J. Thiazolidinediones: an update. Lancet 2000; 355:1008–10.
76. Auwerx J. PPARgamma, the ultimate thrifty gene. Diabetologia 1999; 42:1033–49.
77. Memisoglu A, Hu FB, Hankinson SE, et al. Prospective study of the association between the proline to alanine codon 12 polymorphism in the PPARgamma gene and type 2 diabetes. Diabetes Care 2003; 26:2915–7.
78. Silander K, Mohlke KL, Scott LJ, et al. Genetic variation near the hepatocyte nuclear factor-4 alpha gene predicts susceptibility to type 2 diabetes. Diabetes 2004; 53:1141–9.
79. Gloyn AL, Weedon MN, Owen KR, et al. Large-scale association studies of variants in genes encoding the pancreatic beta-cell KATP channel subunits Kir6.2 (KCNJ11) and SUR1 (ABCC8) confirm that the KCNJ11 E23K variant is associated with type 2 diabetes. Diabetes 2003; 52:568–72.
80. Cox NJ. Challenges in identifying genetic variation affecting susceptibility to type 2 diabetes: examples from studies of the calpain-10 gene. Hum Mol Genet 2001; 10:2301–5.
81. Horikawa Y, Oda N, Cox NJ, et al. Genetic variation in the gene encoding calpain-10 is associated with type 2 diabetes mellitus. Nat Genet 2000; 26:163–75.
82. Tsuchiya T, Schwarz PE, Bosque-Plata LD, et al. Association of the calpain-10 gene with type 2 diabetes in Europeans: results of pooled and meta-analyses. Mol Genet Metab 2006.
83. Baier LJ, Permana PA, Yang X, et al. A calpain-10 gene polymorphism is associated with reduced muscle mRNA levels and insulin resistance. J Clin Invest 2000; 106:R69–73.

84. Sreenan SK, Zhou YP, Otani K, et al. Calpains play a role in insulin secretion and action. Diabetes 2001; 50:2013–20.
85. Arrington D, Van Vleet T, Schnellmann R. Calpain 10: a mitochondrial calpain and its role in calcium-induced mitochondrial dysfunction. Am J Physiol Cell Physiol 2006.
86. Meyre D, Bouatia-Naji N, Tounian A, et al. Variants of ENPP1 are associated with childhood and adult obesity and increase the risk of glucose intolerance and type 2 diabetes. Nat Genet 2005; 37: 863–7.
87. Abate N, Chandalia M, Satija P, et al. ENPP1/PC-1 K121Q polymorphism and genetic susceptibility to type 2 diabetes. Diabetes 2005; 54:1207–13.
88. Matsuoka N, Patki A, Tiwari HK, et al. Association of K121Q polymorphism in ENPP1 (PC-1) with BMI in Caucasian and African-American adults. Int J Obes (Lond) 2006; 30:233–7.
89. Grant SF, Thorleifsson G, Reynisdottir I, et al. Variant of transcription factor 7-like 2 (TCF7L2) gene confers risk of type 2 diabetes. Nat Genet 2006; 38:320–3.
90. Florez JC, Jablonski KA, Bayley N, et al. TCF7L2 polymorphisms and progression to diabetes in the Diabetes Prevention Program. N Engl J Med 2006; 355:241–50.
91. Vaxillaire M, Dechaume A, Vasseur-Delannoy V, et al. Genetic analysis of ADIPOR1 and ADIPOR2 candidate polymorphisms for type 2 diabetes in the Caucasian population. Diabetes 2006; 55:856–61.

3 | Rationale and Goals for Glucose Control in Diabetes Mellitus and Glucose Monitoring

Ramachandiran Cooppan
Joslin Diabetes Center, Boston, Massachusetts, U.S.A.

Diabetes mellitus is a chronic disease that results in major morbidity and mortality. As with any chronic illness the goals of therapy are to alleviate the acute symptoms and complications and then focus on preventing the long-term consequences. While the initial goals can be reasonably achieved in most instances, the long-term complications can prove to be more of a challenge. This is in part due to the fact that the disease is not a single entity but a complex metabolic syndrome that results in hyperglycemia. This can be due to an absolute deficiency of insulin or either defects in insulin secretion and insulin action or a combination of both. Clinically, it is convenient to classify the patient as having either type 1 or type 2 diabetes mellitus. This approach is based more on the underlying pathophysiology than on treatment, since many patients with type 2 diabetes will eventually require insulin for treatment.

Several different pathogenic processes may cause the development of diabetes and range from an autoimmune destruction of the beta cells in type 1 diabetes mellitus to alterations in insulin secretory capacity and peripheral insulin resistance in type 2 diabetes. In general type 1 diabetes develops in younger individuals while type 2 disease occurs in adults. However, there is a recent increase in the prevalence of type 2 diabetes mellitus in children. In the Pima Indians the prevalence has increased from 1% in subjects aged 15 to 24 1979 to 5%, and has also emerged in the 10- to 15-year-olds (1). In addition there has been an increase in African American and Mexican American youth. This increase is also seen in other parts of the world such as Japan, Bangladesh, Libya, and New Zealand (2). The issue of an increase in type 2 diabetes in the young makes it even more important to diagnose and treat the disease earlier as the long-term microvascular complications are related to both the degree of hyperglycemia as well as the duration of the disease. Dating the onset of clinical type 1 diabetes may be easier because of the acute onset of symptoms in general. However it is more difficult to do this in type 2 diabetes because the onset of symptoms is preceded by many years of asymptomatic hyperglycemia. Many patients with adult type 2 diabetes already have evidence of complications at diagnosis (3). It is estimated that these patients have had their disease for at least 10 years before it is diagnosed.

Another major issue that challenges our strategies and overall approach to therapy has to do with the long-term complications of diabetes. While microvascular disease affecting the eye, kidney, and nerves can occur in both type 1 and type 2 diabetes, patients with type 2 disease have a greater risk of developing macrovascular disease, especially coronary artery disease. Cardiovascular disease is the most important cause of death in patients with type 2 diabetes and the risk starts very early during the stage of impaired glucose tolerance well before the clinical diagnosis of diabetes mellitus (4).

These clinical issues therefore have important implications as we address the issue of glycemic control and the goals we set for our patients. If controlling the blood glucose to normal levels resulted in preventing the development and progression of both microvascular and macrovascular disease then the situation would be clear. We could approach our patients with confidence and encourage them to control the disease, while reassuring them that the time and effort they put in would be rewarded with no complications. However, the data is not as clear-cut as this, especially in regard to macrovascular disease, though recent data indicates that early glycemic control can affect the later development of heart disease in type 1 patients. The situation for the microvascular disease is far more compelling, especially with data from studies completed in the last decade.

MICROVASCULAR DISEASE

To better understand the rationale for glucose control it is useful to review the role of hyperglycemia in the development of the long-term microvascular complications. After the discovery of insulin it was noted that patients with insulin-dependent diabetes who lived longer tended to develop retinopathy. It was not clear at the time as to whether these were usual changes of the disease or whether they were related to the level of hyperglycemia. Early pathological studies in animals indicated a relationship between elevated blood glucose levels and retinopathy. Currently a number of different mechanisms have been implicated in the pathogenesis of the microvascular disease and this has been studied extensively in diabetic retinopathy and nephropathy. Chronic duration of the disease, a number of metabolic abnormalities including hyperglycemia, and genetic factors all play a role in causing the microangiopathy. Diabetic retinopathy has been most thoroughly studied because it is one of the first complications that can be detected clinically. The early changes of diabetic retinopathy include the formation of capillary microaneurysms with increased permeability and thickening of the capillary basement membrane. However, even before these changes are evident, there are changes in endothelial cell function that can affect capillary blood flow. With poor glycemic control there is progression of the retinopathy from background changes to preproliferative and then proliferative retinopathy. Eventually this can lead to bleeding from rupture of the neovascularization with the end stage of blindness.

PATHOGENESIS OF MICROVASCULAR DISEASE

From a pathogenic viewpoint a number of different molecular mechanisms have been proposed for the development of the various manifestations of diabetic retinopathy. The underlying abnormalities may also play a role in the microvascular disease that results in nephropathy and possibly neuropathy. Many of these theories have been studied extensively in animals and humans using both in vitro and in vivo methods. The primary goal of these studies was to try and identify the underlying mechanisms through which hyperglycemia and other metabolic factors cause damage to vascular cells, that in turn lead to specific organ damage and ultimately the long-term complications.

This type of evidence is very important and will provide the clinician with a scientific basis for advocating tight glycemic control. This in turn will also be a major factor in shaping the healthcare policies for patients with diabetes. However, it is also apparent that our current therapies do not allow us to optimally control the blood sugars into the normal range for prolonged periods. Therefore an understanding of the basis for the microvascular disease can have far-reaching implications. If we can identify other areas where hyperglycemia induces further metabolic changes that lead to vascular damage, inhibiting or blocking the enzymes or products that cause this damage can become additional therapies. This approach can be additive to the initial goal of trying to achieve normoglycemia by the traditional treatments. It is of interest that there have been reports in the literature of patients who develop all the microvascular complications but who do not have overt clinical diabetes at the time (5). Abdella et al. reported on a 47-year-old man who presented with the nephrotic syndrome and renal failure with proliferative retinopathy on fundoscopy. The patient did not have overt hyperglycemia but did have impaired glucose tolerance on testing. These case reports serve to remind us that while hyperglycemia is critical to the development of diabetic complications, milder degrees of glucose intolerance can also play a role through other mechanisms.

PATHOGENIC MECHANISMS FOR MICROVASCULAR DISEASE
The Formation of Advanced Glycosylated End Products (AGEs)

The effects of glucose in causing damage to the vascular cells can occur through the metabolism of glucose or through chemical changes that do not involve any enzyme activation. A high glucose concentration can lead to glycosylation of amino groups in proteins. The ultimate effect is the formation of advanced glycosylation end products (AGE). These AGEs can also form in other diseases like renal failure and normal aging. In diabetes mellitus the production and deposition of these products are thought to contribute to the development of the long-term microvascular complications. The AGE formation occurs especially with long half-life proteins like basement membrane. The AGEs bind to receptors and cause changes in signal transduction in macrophages or vascular endothelial cells. This in turn can lead to the release of various cytokines such as tumor necrosis factor, as well as oxidants. Recently AGEs and oxidants have been implicated in the increased expression of vascular endothelial growth factor (VEGF), which can increase vascular permeability and cause retinal angiogenesis (6,7).

Increased Aldose Reductase Activity

The aldose reductase pathway has been extensively studied because of the presence of the enzyme in the retina, kidney, and nerves. These are all targets for the long-term complications and would present a unified model for the damage caused by chronic hyperglycemia. The enzyme increases its activity in the presence of high blood glucose levels and causes increased levels of sorbitol. Sorbitol dehydrogenase metabolizes the sorbitol that is then postulated to lead to other metabolic changes that can cause neuropathy and retinopathy. This pathway has been best studied in relation to diabetic neuropathy (8). Despite this understanding of the possible underlying role for this mechanism, trials of aldose reductase inhibitors in slowing down the development or progression of retinopathy and neuropathy have not been very effective.

Formation of Excessive Oxidants

Currently there is a great deal of interest in the role of oxidative stress in diabetes. Increases in oxidant formation are derived from many different sources such as glucose autooxidation, protein glycation, and free radical formation. These oxidants can affect many cellular processes including increases in oxidized low-density lipoprotein (LDL), cross-linked proteins, and DNA. In addition this increase in oxidants can lead to reduction of nitric oxide (NO), which can result in vasoconstriction and hypoxia. These mechanisms may play a very significant role in the increased macrovascular disease that is found in patients with diabetes. In one recent study of diabetic retinopathy, vitamin E was used in a dose-dependent manner (1000–2000 IU/day) and resulted in the normalization of the retinal blood flow changes in type 1 diabetic patients (9). Further long-term studies will be needed to fully assess the significance of these findings.

Alteration in the Signal Transduction Pathway

This last theory may once again provide a conceptual framework to link the various clinical manifestations of the complications. While AGEs and oxidants can play a role, the diacylglycerol, protein kinase C (DAG-PKC) activation pathway has been best studied. The presence of hyperglycemia increases DAG and PKC actions that through multiple intermediary substances can result in many cellular abnormalities. These include such changes as basement membrane thickening, increased permeability, coagulation and contractibility abnormalities as well as increased angiogenesis and cardiomyopathy. These changes are all found clinically in diabetic patients so it is reasonable to try to block the PKC by inhibitors to see if this would reduce or reverse the abnormalities. The use of a specific PKC beta isoform inhibitor, LY333531, has been studied and a delay in the hemodynamic changes seen in diabetic retinopathy, nephropathy, and cardiovascular disease has been observed. The drug is now being studied clinically in patients with macular edema and neovascularization to see if visual loss can be prevented (10).

A recent study noted that the oral administration of ruboxistaurin (RBX) mesylate, a selective PKC beta inhibitor, in a dose of 16 mg twice daily, the diabetes induced increase in retinal circulation time was ameliorated. No serious safety problems were identified in the 28-day trial. This is the first direct human evidence of the effects of an oral PKC beta inhibitor and more long-term data is awaited (44).

In another study RBX was used to treat patients with diabetes and diabetic peripheral neuropathy. This was a randomized, PHASE 11, double-blind placebo-controlled parallel-group trial of 205 patients and used 32 or 64 mg of RBX for 1 year. Overall there were no significant changes in vibration detection threshold or neuropathy total symptom score between the groups. However a subgroup with less severe neuropathy did benefit with relief of sensory symptoms and improved nerve function (45).

From the many theories that have been advanced to play a role in the pathogenesis of the microvascular complications of diabetes, it is evident that the one common abnormality in all theories is the presence of an elevated blood glucose level. Therefore it is very important to try and correct this abnormality optimally using all currently available therapies and then to add other therapies that will be of additional benefit as they become available.

MACROVASCULAR DISEASE

Cardiovascular disease, that includes coronary heart disease (CHD) rebrovascular disease, and peripheral vascular disease, is the leading cause of mortality in people with diabetes. The majority of deaths are due to CHD, where the risk is two- to fourfold greater in patients, especially women with diabetes, when compared with age-matched subjects without diabetes (11). The relative importance of the problem has been highlighted by recent studies. Gu et al. compared adults with diabetes with those without diabetes for time trends in mortality from all causes, heart disease, and ischemic heart disease. They based the data on the First National Health and Nutrition Examination Survey (NHANES) conducted between 1971 and 1975 and the NHANES follow-up conducted between 1982 and 1984. The nondiabetic men had a 36.4% decline in age-adjusted heart disease mortality compared with a 13.1% decline in diabetic men. In the nondiabetic women it declined 27% but in the diabetic women the rate increased 23%. The suggestions for this trend were that risk factors for cardiovascular disease in patients with diabetes may have declined less or the patients with diabetes may have benefited less from improved medical care for heart disease. Another suggestion was that the overall rates of cardiovascular disease could have declined less in those with diabetes (12). Haffner and colleagues compared the mortality from CHD in Finland in a recent paper. They studied 1059 subjects with type 2 diabetes and 1373 nondiabetic subjects with and without previous myocardial infarction (MI) (13). The 7-year incidence rates of MI in the nondiabetic group at baseline were 18.8% and 3.5%, respectively. The 7-year rates of MI in the diabetic subjects at baseline were 45% and 20.2% respectively. Even after adjusting for age, sex, total cholesterol, hypertension, and smoking the risk was similar in both groups. This suggests that patients with type 2 diabetes without a prior MI have the same risk as someone without diabetes and a prior myocardial infarct. This study clearly reveals the enormous risk of heart disease in patients with type 2 diabetes and emphasizes the need for aggressive risk factor treatment. In fact after the first cardiac event, 50% of patients with diabetes die within one year, and half die before they can reach a hospital (14). This very high mortality suggests that a primary prevention strategy is needed to reduce the risk. Multiple studies have now been done that show the benefit of lowering cholesterol and blood pressure in patients with diabetes. The Scandanvian Simvastatin Survival Study (4S) and the Cholesterol and Recurrent Events (CARE) (15,16) both showed a reduction in cardiovascular mortality in small numbers of patients with diabetes that were included in these studies. The 4S was a secondary prevention randomized control trial that reduced CHD death or nonfatal MI. There were 22.9% events in the intervention group compared with 43.8% in the control group. The CARE trial included similar endpoints as well as revascularization, and there were 28.7% events in the intervention group compared to 36.8% in the control group. The Hypertension Optimal Treatment Trial (HOT) and the United Kingdom Prospective Diabetes Study (UKPDS) (17,18) also demonstrated a significant reduction in cardiovascular events as well as a reduction in microvascular events in the UKPDS, with blood pressure control. In the HOT trial there was a 4.4% event rate in the treatment group compared to 9% in the control group. This was a more than 50% reduction with a target diastolic pressure of 80 mmHg. In the UKPDS tight blood pressure control resulted in 14.1% acute myocardial infarction (AMI) events compared to 21.3% in the less-tight control group.

More recent data comes from the Heart Protection Study (HPS) and the Collaborative Atorvastatin Diabetes Study (CARDS). The HPS was a secondary prevention trial with 5,963 patients with diabetes and 14,573 with arterial occlusive disease and no known diabetes. The use of 40 mg of simvastatin resulted in a 22% reduction in first occurrence of any major vascular event in patients on simvastatin treatment and a 27% reduction in participants whose pretreatment LDL cholesterol was below 3.0 mmol (116 mg/dL). Furthermore there was a 25% reduction in other subgroups studied including duration of diabetes, age over 65 years, control of diabetes or presence of hypertension (46).

The CARDS trial is significant because it is a primary prevention trial in 2838 patients with type 2 diabetes with out high-LDL cholesterol levels. At study entry the subjects had not documented previous cardiovascular disease, LDL cholesterol of 4.14 mmol or less, a fasting triglyceride of 6.78 mmol or less and at least one of the following: retinopathy, albuminuria, current smoking, or hypertension. The trial was terminated 2 years earlier as the use of 10 mg of atorvastatin resulted in a 37% reduction in at least one major cardiovascular event over the 3.9 years of the trial. In addition stroke was reduced by 48%.This trial in patients with type 2 diabetes without elevated LDL cholesterol raises the question of whether all patients with type 2 diabetes and one other risk factor should be on statin therapy (47).

In both type 1 and type 2 diabetes accelerated macrovascular disease is a problem and the etiology is multifactorial, with hyperglycemia playing a significant role. In the type 2 patient there are multiple cardiovascular risk factors that form part of the insulin resistance syndrome. There are abnormalities in lipid metabolism, derangements in the coagulation system, the effects of hyperglycemia, and the potential role of hyperinsulinemia. To this list can be added increasing age, the development of obesity, and hypertension. It is beyond the scope of this chapter to review in detail the various abnormalities, but one issue deserves attention and that is the role of hyperglycemia. There is considerable debate in the medical literature on the role of hyperglycemia as an independent risk factor for CHD. Balkau et al. reviewed the question by examining the mortality data from the Paris Prospective Study. This was a study of 7018 men, aged 44 to 55 years who were not known to have diabetes at baseline. They found no clear thresholds for fasting or 2 h glucose concentrations above which, all cause and CHD mortality increased sharply. They did find, that in the upper levels of glucose distributions, the risk for death progressively increased with increasing fasting and 2 h glucose levels (19). A subject with a fasting glucose level of 7.8 mmol/L had a risk of death 40% greater than one with fasting glucose of 6.0 mmol/L. The lowest risk was found in the 4.5 to 5.5 mmol/L range. For the 2 h glucose, a level of 11.1 mmol/L carried a 55% greater risk than for a level of 7.7 mmol/L. The lowest risk was in the 5.5 to 6.5 mmol/L range for the 2 h glucose. After adjustments for other risk factors the 2 h glucose was still significantly associated with both all causes and CHD mortality, whereas the fasting correlated with all causes of death. One limitation of the study is that it is done on men and the relationship of these results to women is unclear at present.

In a metaregression analysis of 20 recent studies involving 95,783, nondiabetic subjects, Coutinho et al. (20) revisit this question. While acknowledging the limitations of the different types of study design, varying methods of glucose measurements, and different glucose loads for the tolerance tests, they did find that a high fasting, 1 and 2 h glucose increased risk for cardiovascular events. A fasting level of 6.1 mmol/L increased the relative risk 1.33 compared with a fasting level of 4.2 mmol/L. Similarly the 2 h glucose of 7.8 mmol/L was associated with a relative risk of 1.58. The DECODE Study included over 25,000 patients with a mean follow-up time was 7.3 years (20a). This study showed that a high blood glucose concentration 2 h after a glucose load was associated with increased risk of death, independently of fasting blood glucose. These studies do not imply a cause and effect relationship, but do suggest that with increasing glucose levels there may be worsening of the underlying risk factors for cardiovascular disease. In patients with impaired glucose tolerance there is an increased risk for cardiovascular disease.

RESULTS OF STUDIES OF GLYCEMIC CONTROL AND MICROVASCULAR DISEASE

The ultimate proof that glycemic control is worthwhile has to come from long-term randomized-controlled trials (RCT). We are fortunate that after many decades of observational or retrospective studies, we now have one systematic review and three long-term RCTs showing the benefits of glucose control in both type 1 and type 2 diabetes. There is one major type 1 study and two type 2 studies that will be briefly reviewed. The systematic review by Groeneveld et al. (21) looked at 16 small RCTs in type 1 diabetes, that had a follow-up of 8 to 60 months. The overall conclusion of these studies was that glycemic control was important in reducing the microvascular complications.

The Diabetes Control and Complications Trial (DCCT) was a landmark trial that was designed to finally answer the glycemic control and complications question (22). This was a large multicenter trial with enough statistical power to answer the issue conclusively. The study involved 1441 patients with type 1 diabetes who were randomized to either intensive glucose control or conventional treatment. The intensive therapy regimen was designed to achieve blood glucose levels close to the normal range as possible with three or more daily injections of insulin or an insulin pump. The conventional therapy consisted of one or two insulin injections. The cohorts were studied to answer two different questions that were related to the control and complications debate. One of the study questions was, whether intensive therapy would prevent the development of diabetic retinopathy (primary prevention) and the other whether intensive therapy would affect the progression of early diabetic retinopathy (secondary prevention). While retinopathy was the main outcome, renal, neurologic, cardiovascular, and neuropsychological outcomes and adverse effects of the two treatments were also studied (Table 1). There were 726 patients in the primary arm and 715 in the secondary prevention arm and the mean follow-up was 6.5 years. In the primary prevention cohort the intensive treatment reduced the adjusted mean risk for developing retinopathy by 76% as compared to the conventional therapy group. In the secondary prevention cohort, intensive therapy slowed retinopathy progression by 54% and also reduced the development of proliferative or severe nonproliferative retinopathy by 47%. Furthermore there was a reduction in microalbuminuria (>40 mg/24h) by 39% and of albuminuria (>300 mg/24h) by 54%. Clinical neuropathy was also reduced 60%. However, it was noted that patients on the intensive treatment did have a three times greater increase in the number of severe hypoglycemic episodes. The hypoglycemia did not result in death or stroke and the mortality did not differ in the two treatment cohorts. Despite the hypoglycemia difference there was no clinically important changes in neuropsychological function between the groups. The patients appeared to adjust well to the demands of the intensive therapy program. Weight gain was a problem in the intensively treated group with a mean gain of 4.6 kg at 5 years. There was no increase in the ketoacidosis rates in either group. This benefit was achieved in the intensive treatment group with a mean blood glucose of 155 mg/dL and HbA$_{1c}$ of ~7.2% with a normal average glucose being ~110 mg/dL and the HbA$_{1c}$ <6.05%.

Another important outcome of the DCCT was the finding that there is no glycemic threshold for the development of long-term complications. In a retrospective Joslin clinic study (23), it has been suggested that a threshold exists for microalbuminuria and that it increases substantially around an HbA$_{1c}$ of ~8%. The prospective Stockholm Study (24), also showed that the risk for microalbuminuria increased substantially once the HbA$_{1c}$ was more than 8.9% to 9%. However, the data from the DCCT refute this idea and indicate that for every 10% reduction in HbA$_{1c}$ there is a 39% reduction in the risk of retinopathy progression throughout the HbA$_{1c}$ range. The relationship also holds for developing microalbuminuria as well as neuropathy, and is continuous but nonlinear. However, the magnitude of the risk reduction (RR) is greater at higher HbA$_{1c}$ levels and at the same time as control improves the risk of hypoglycemia increases with the lower HbA$_{1c}$ levels (25).

In a follow-up study of the DCCT, the Epidemiology of Diabetes Interventions and Complications (EDIC) study found that the benefits of intensive treatment, persists over the

TABLE 1 Risk Reduction (RR) in Microvascular Complications in the Diabetes Control and Complications Trial

	Retinopathy	Severe diabetic retinopathy	Laser surgery	Microalb	Severe microalb	Albuminuria	Neuropathy
RR	76%	61%	56%	43%	51%	56%	64%

Abbreviations: DDCT, Diabetes Control and Complications Trial; RR, risk reduction.

4 years of follow-up (26). After the initial study was completed the patients in the control group were offered intensive therapy and all patients now received care from their own physicians. Retinopathy and nephropathy were assessed based on fundus photographs and urine specimens, respectively. The median HbA_{1c}, which was on average 9.1% and 7.2% in the control and intensive therapy groups in the DCCT narrowed during this follow-up. The median during the 4 years was 8.2% in the control group and 7.9% in the intensive therapy group. Despite this worsening in the glycemic control in the intensive treatment group the proportion of patients having worsening of retinopathy, including proliferative changes as well as macula edema, and the need for laser treatment was less. There was also a significantly lower increase in urinary albumin excretion in the intensive treatment group. Therefore, in contrast to the DCCT, where the benefits of intensive therapy were not evident until 3 or 4 years of treatment, in the EDIC the benefits persisted despite an increase in the HbA_{1c}. Another interesting finding of the DCCT was that for primary prevention of the complications intensive therapy should be started within the first 5 years of the onset of the disease.

In another study Ohkubo and colleagues from Kumamoto, Japan also demonstrated the benefits of intensive insulin therapy in a group of thin type 2 patients (27). A total of 110 patients with type 2 diabetes were randomized to intensive treatment with multiple insulin injections (MIT) or conventional insulin therapy (CIT). The MIT consisted of premeal rapid acting insulin and intermediate insulin at bedtime and goals of fasting glucose of less than 140 mg/dL and postprandial levels of 200 mg/dL or less. In addition the HbA_{1c} goal was 7% or less. The CIT group was treated with one or two injections of intermediate insulin and was to try and keep the fasting glucose close to less than 140 mg/dL. There was a primary prevention and secondary prevention group based on the presence of diabetic retinopathy and urinary albumin excretion. After 6 years the mean HbA_{1c} was 7.1% in the intensive group and 9.4% in the control group. In the primary prevention cohort there was a 7.7% development of retinopathy in MIT group after 6 years compared with 32% in the CIT group. In addition in the secondary prevention cohort, in the MIT group, 19.2% had progression of retinopathy compared to 44% in the CIT group. Similar reductions in both the primary as well as secondary cohorts were found for nephropathy and neuropathy. Overall the investigators stated that from this study the glycemic threshold to prevent the onset and progression of diabetic microangiopathy was an $HbA_{1c} < 6.5\%$, fasting blood glucose < 110 mg/dL and a 2 h postprandial blood glucose of < 180 mg/dL. Over the entire study period 6 patients in the MIT group and 4 patients in the CIT group had one or more, mild hypoglycemic reactions with no coma or seizures or need for assistance from another person.

After the publication of these two studies there was still an ongoing discussion on the applicability of the results to the larger group of patients with type 2 diabetes mellitus. In part the issue has to do with the complications as they develop in type 2 diabetes mellitus. As noted earlier most patients with this form of diabetes die from cardiovascular disease and to date we have no data like the DCCT to support the role of glucose control alone in reducing the risk. On the other hand the long-term microvascular complications are identical in both type 1 and type 2 diabetes. Overall the prevalence of these complications is similar and the major difference is that at the time of diagnosis more patients with type2 diabetes have evidence of complications. This is due to the fact that they tend to have the disease for at least 5 to 7 years before clinical diagnosis. The higher prevalence of macrovascular disease is probably due in part to the older age of the patients as well the associated risk factors like hypertension, dyslipidemia, obesity, and the changes in fibrinolysis and coagulation, that are part of the insulin resistance syndrome.

However, we are now able to answer this issue of microvascular complications with another landmark study led by Robert Turner from Oxford, which studied patients with type 2 diabetes. The UKPDS is the largest type 2 diabetes study ever done (28). This clinical study was designed to assess the effects of intensive treatment with four pharmacological monotherapies versus a diet only control group, on cardiovascular and microvascular complications of type 2 diabetes (Table 2). In the study 3867 patients with newly diagnosed type 2 diabetes were randomly assigned to two treatment groups: one group, the intensive treatment policy took one of three oral sulfonylurea drugs (cholorpropamide, glibenclamide, or glipizide) or insulin; and a second group, whose only initial treatment was dietary

TABLE 2 U.K. Prospective Diabetes Study. Risk Reduction for Diabetes-Related Endpoints During Intensive Therapy with Sulfonylureas and Insulin

	Risk reduction[a]	*P* value
Any diabetes-related endpoint	12%	0.029
Myocardial infarction	16%	0.052
Microvascular disease	25%	0.0099
Retinopathy progression (at 12 years)	21%	0.015
Cataract extraction	24%	0.046
Microalbuminuria (at 12 years)	33%	< 0.001

[a] Compared with conventional therapy.

restriction. The goal of the intensive treatment was a fasting plasma glucose of less than 108 mg/dL while in the diet treated group the aim was the best achievable fasting glucose and oral drugs were added if there were hyperglycemic symptoms or the fasting plasma glucose was over 270 mg/dL. Three end points were used in the study to assess effect of treatment: any diabetes-related clinical endpoint, diabetes-related death and all cause mortality. The analysis was by intention to treat. Over 10 years the HbA_{1c} was 7.0% in the intensive group compared with HbA_{1c} 7.9% in the control group, a 11% reduction. There was no difference in between the different agents in the intensive therapy. Compared to the control group, any diabetes-related end point was 12% lower, diabetes-related death was 10% lower and all cause mortality 8% lower. Most of the reduction in diabetes-related endpoints was in a 25% reduction in microvascular endpoints, including the need for laser photocoagulation. For every percentage point reduction in HbA_{1c} there was a 35% reduction in the risk of complications. No glycemic threshold was found for any microvascular complication. Patients on intensive treatment had more major hypoglycemic episodes per year (1.0% with cholorpropamide, 1.4% with glibenclamide, and 1.8% with insulin) compared to the control group (0.7%).

Weight gain was also significantly greater with the intensive treatment (mean 2.9 kg) than the conventional group and patients on insulin had the greatest increase of 4.0 kg compared to 2.6 kg for cholorpropamide and 1.7 kg with glibenclamide. There was no statistically significant decrease in macrovascular events (16%) but events were not increased with the intensive treatment therapies. However, the epidemiological analysis of the study also clearly demonstrated that there was a continuous association between the risk of cardiovascular complications and glycemia. For every percentage point decrease in HbA_{1c} there was a 25% decrease in diabetes-related deaths, 7% reduction in all cause mortality and 18% reduction in combined fatal and nonfatal MI. While there have been discussions about the design and treatment assignments and therapy cross-over in the trial, the primary conclusion that glycemic control in type 2 diabetes is beneficial is accepted. In a second publication (29), the results of subgroup of obese patients treated with metformin showed a 32% reduction in any diabetes-related endpoint, 42% reduction for diabetes-related death, and 36% reduction for all cause mortality. The HbA_{1c} was 7.4% compared to the conventional group of 8.0%. Among the patients allocated to intensive therapy, metformin showed greater effect on any diabetes-related endpoint and all cause mortality, than any of the other oral sulfonylureas or insulin. The authors of the study concluded that metformin was the treatment of choice in the overweight type 2 patient. However, later in the study 537 patients, obese and normal weight on sulfonylurea, unable to maintain their glucose control, were assigned to combination therapy. In this group there was an increased risk of diabetes-related death of 96% when compared to sulfonylurea alone. A combined analysis of the main and supplementary studies actually showed fewer metformin-treated patients having diabetes-related clinical endpoints, a 19% RR. In addition, the epidemiological assessment of the possible association of combination therapy in 4415 patients showed no increased risk of diabetes-related death in patients treated with metformin and a sulfonylurea. This observation also generated considerable discussion but in its position statement on the implications of the UKPDS, the American Diabetes Association (ADA) has reviewed the study and its results. The statement accepted the important role of glucose control in reducing the incidence of microvascular complications as it has endorsed in type 1 diabetes (30). However, the statement while accepting the relationship of cardiovascular disease to hyperglycemia felt that the UKPDS did not conclusively prove the benefits on intensive glycemic control and cardiovascular complications. In regard to the conflicting results on metformin use as monotherapy and as combination therapy with sulfonylureas, the ADA did not recommend any change in the use of this specific combination. It did raise the issue of the lack of a placebo control in this substudy and the use of meta-analysis to reconcile the different outcomes. An important observation of the study was also the fact that after 3 years there was a slow increase in the HbA_{1c} in all the oral medication treatment groups indicating a steady deterioration in beta cell function over the follow-up period. This finding has important implications for making an earlier diagnosis of type 2 diabetes and for more aggressive therapy. The reduction of the effects of glucose toxicity on beta cell function and insulin action with either combination oral treatment or early insulin use may help preserve the beta cell.

The results of these three randomized and controlled studies now give us the outcome data we need to accept the role of glycemic control in not only primary prevention of microvascular complications but also for the reduction in progression of existing early complications. One further study is worth mentioning in this regard. Our goal for control is to strive for euglycemia and to replace insulin in type 1 patients in a physiological manner. While there is a growing body of literature on beta cell replacement we still are not within sight of a solution that will benefit the many thousands of patients with type1 diabetes. Nonetheless this is a high-priority goal for patients with type 1 disease. In this regard the pancreatic transplantation literature is quite enlightening and shows us the kind of results we can expect once beta cell replacement becomes a reality for our patients. The study by Fioretto et al., from the University of Minnesota looked at the effects of pancreas transplantation on diabetic nephropathy (31). They studied renal function and performed renal biopsies before pancreas transplantation and then 5 and 10 years after in 8 patients with type1 diabetes mellitus who had no uremia and mild to advanced diabetic nephropathy. All the patients had normal glycosylated hemoglobin values after transplantation and the albumin excretion dropped from 103 mg per day to 30 mg per day after 5 years. By 10 years the albumin excretion was down to 20 mg per day and the glomerular and tubular basement thickening while not changed at 5 years was also decreased significantly. Similar changes were noted in mesangial fractional volume and it was the conclusion of the study that pancreas transplantation can reverse lesions of diabetic nephropathy but that reversal requires more than 5 years of normoglycemia. This study clearly demonstrates the primary role of hyperglycemia in causing the microvascular complications and the need to obtain glucose control early in diabetes and to maintain this for prolonged periods.

Finally another area where glucose control is stressed is during pregnancy in patients with diabetes mellitus. In fact because of the adverse effects of poorly controlled diabetes in increasing congenital abnormalities and perinatal mortality there are now recommended guidelines for screening and treatment from national diabetes organizations. The ADA and others have stressed not only meticulous glucose control during pregnancy but also in the preconception period. Gestational diabetes mellitus (GDM) complicates approximately 7% of all pregnancies and results on more than 200,000 cases annually (32). Gestational diabetes is associated with increased risk of fetal macrosomia, neonatal hypoglycemia, hyperbilirubinemia, hypocalcemia, and polycythemia. Furthermore the children of mothers with GDM are at greater risk for childhood obesity and diabetes as young adults (33). Because of the importance of this problem all women should be evaluated for possible GDM and those at high risk should be screened as soon as possible and for all others testing should be done between 24 weeks to 28 weeks. If GDM is diagnosed, the goal of treatment is fasting plasma glucose goal is 105 mg/dL or less, 1 h postmeal 155 mg/dL or less and the 2 h value 130 mg/dL or less. This can be accomplished with nutritional counseling and self-blood glucose monitoring (SBGM). If these goals cannot be met then the patient is started on insulin therapy.

In patients with known diabetes mellitus perinatal mortality is two to seven times more common than in nondiabetic women. Apart from strict blood glucose control these women need close follow-up because the pregnancy can be associated with worsening of diabetic retinopathy and renal disease. All women with diabetes should attempt to maintain blood glucose levels in the nondiabetic range and HbA_{1c} levels more than 140% of the upper limit of normal nonpregnant women must be avoided. While treatment into the nondiabetic range is recommended, this must be done without significant increase in severe hypoglycemia. With these approaches there has been a reduction in the fetal loss and congenital abnormality rates (34).

MACROVASCULAR DISEASE AND GLUCOSE CONTROL

As noted earlier in the discussion on macrovascular disease, there are many studies showing the benefit of lipid and blood pressure control in patients with diabetes. The issue of the direct benefit of glucose control has not been settled to date in a study where other risk factors are controlled and glucose control is the major outcome. The study by Balkau (19) and a metaanalysis by Couthinho (20) demonstrates that increasing fasting as well as postprandial glucose levels is associated with cardiovascular disease. The Veterans Affairs Cooperative Study on Glycemic Control and Complications in type 2 Diabetes (VACSDM) was a feasibility trial in 153 adult men with type 2 diabetes (35). The patients had a mean HbA_{1c} of 9.8%, and were either on insulin or failing oral therapy and judged to need insulin. In addition, 38% of them had prior cardiovascular events. The goal of the standard treatment arm was to keep the HbA_{1c} within two standard deviations on the mean of the outpatient diabetic clinics of the participating hospitals. The intensive therapy aimed for normal fasting glucose (80–120 mg/dL) and preprandial glucose (<130 mg/dL) and HbA_{1c} of <6.1%. The glucose control was achieved via a four stepped phases treatment plan. Therapy started with evening insulin and then had an oral sulfonylurea, glipizide added and progressed to twice daily insulin and no oral medication and ended with multiple daily insulin injections. Efforts were made to control blood pressure, lipids, obesity, and smoking in both groups. The intensively treated patients had more hypoglycemia, required larger insulin doses and had more statistically nonsignificant cardiovascular events. Interestingly these events occurred in the group with HbA_{1c} levels between 5.5% and 8%. The total mortality rate and cardiovascular mortality was identical in both treatment groups. This study does not answer the question of glycemic control and cardiovascular disease because of the high number of patients who already had cardiovascular events before entry.

The results of glucose control and macrovascular outcome are summarized in the table below (Table 3). These studies are not comparable and they vary in design and main outcomes studied. Apart from the VACSDM, all the other studies showed no increase in cardiovascular risk as blood glucose control was improved. The UKPDS and Kumamoto were studies primarily of glycemic control and microvascular disease, while the Diabetes Insulin Glucose Acute Myocardial Infarction (DIGAMI) study looked at the effects of intensive insulin therapy in the situation of an acute MI.

The data from the table indicate that there is a cardiovascular benefit in lowering the blood glucose that ranges from a relative risk reduction (RRR) of 16% to 46%. But the problem with this observation is that the data comes from multiple sources and what is now needed, is study that is specifically designed to address the question. The new Action to Control Cardiovascular Risk in Diabetes (ACCORD) Trial has been designed to address the issue in

TABLE 3 Glucose Lowering in Type 2 Diabetes Mellitus and Cardiovascular Disease Risk

	Treatment	HbA$_{1c}$ change	Outcome	Relative risk reduction
UKPDS	Insulin/Su[a]	0.9%	MI	16%
UKPDS	Metformin	0.6%	MI	39%
Kumamoto	Insulin	2.3%	CV	46%
VACSDM	Insulin/Su[a]	2.2%	CV	−40%
DIGAMI	Insulin	.8%	CV	29%

[a] Su, sulfonylurea.

Abbreviations: DIGAMI, Diabetes Insulin Glucose Acute Myocardial Infarction; UKPDS, U.K. Prospective Diabetes study; VACSDM, Veterans Affairs Cooperative Study on Glycemic Control and Complications in Type 2 Diabetes.

patients with type 2 diabetes with high risk for cardiovascular disease. Ten thousand patients will be studied comparing an HbA_{1c} of <6.0 % versus <7.5% as well as studies on controlling blood pressure and lipids. The results of this important study should answer this important question. In the meanwhile it is essential to continue to control the blood glucose as close to normal as possible and to be aggressive about risk factor reduction.

The recent EDIC trial data is a landmark trial in type 1 diabetes on the effects of tight glycemic control and cardiovascular disease. The 11th year follow-up data showed a 42% reduction in nonfatal MI, stroke and a 57% reduction in cardiovascular death in the intensively treated DCCT group compared to conventional treatment. This result strongly suggests that the tight glycemic control during the DCCT trial with a mean AIC of 6.5% had sustained benefits even though the glycemic control was not maintained during the EDIC trial (48).

A recent meta-analysis of randomized trials of glycemic control and macrovascular disease in type 1 and type 2 diabetes showed a reduction in cardiac and peripheral vascular events with type 1 diabetes and a reduction in stroke and peripheral vascular events in type 2 diabetes with better control. Thus it appears effects of glucose control on specific manifestations of macrovascular disease may be different between type 1 and type 2 diabetes (49).

GLUCOSE MONITORING

Self Blood Glucose Monitoring

In order to obtain blood glucose control and to maintain this on a daily basis, it is essential for patients with diabetes to do SBGM. The DCCT and other studies clearly demonstrated the importance of this approach and it is now considered as one of the cornerstones of therapy. However one of the findings of the DCCT was that with intensive therapy the number of severe hypoglycemic episodes increase. The data obtained from monitoring are used to assess the efficacy of the treatment program and the frequency of hypoglycemia, to make adjustments to the program that will involve medication change as well as reviewing medical nutrition therapy and the effects of exercise. A great deal of progress has been made in the accuracy and ease of use of the glucose monitoring equipment. Monitors are now available that need very small amounts of blood and can record and store many blood glucose results with date, time of test and even provide 14-day averages of selected tests. Some of the monitors can be downloaded into personal computers and can provide a number of presentations of the data, including pie charts, line diagrams, and bar graphs. It is not clear if presenting data in this way is superior to patient records done manually. For the visually impaired, specific monitors are also available so that almost every patient or care giver has access to this type of information to aid in obtaining the best control possible safely. In its position statement the ADA made a number of recommendations (36). It states that most patients with type 1 diabetes can only obtain blood glucose close to normal with SBGM because of the increased risk of hypoglycemia with intensive therapies. Therefore not only should all insulin treated patients monitor but patients on sulfonylureas also need monitoring to avoid asymptomatic hypoglycemia. The optimal frequency for testing is actually dictated by the needs and goals of the individual patient (Table 4). For type 1 patients tests should be done

TABLE 4   Recommended Targets for Blood Glucose

	Goal
Preprandial capillary plasma glucose (mg/dL)	90–130
Peak postprandial capillary plasma glucose (mg/dL)	<180
HbA_{1c} (%)	<7.0
	<6.5

Source: From Refs. 50 and 51.

four times daily, a fasting test and then before each meal and bedtime. Some patients on more intensive treatment programs may need to do block tests one day a week consisting of the above frequency with additional testing after meals and possibly at 3 a.m. to check for nocturnal hypoglycemia. The exact frequency of testing in type 2 patients on oral medication is not known but testing must be individualized to meet the needs of the patient and the goals set for the degree of control. The role of SBGM in stable diet controlled type 2 patients is unknown at present. A recent report by Harris using data from the NHANES 111 noted that the frequency of SBGM was more common as the HbA_{1c} increased (37). The report also noted that most patients treated with oral medications or diet rarely monitored their blood glucose. The data obtained from 1480 subjects found that 29% patients treated with insulin, 65% treated with oral agents and 80% of those treated with diet alone had never monitored their blood glucose or did it less than once a month. It was also noted that 39% of insulin treated and 5% to 6% of oral agent or diet controlled patients monitored at least once daily. Part of this low-monitoring rate may be a reflection of the policy of Medicare reimbursing monitoring strips and monitors only in insulin treated patients during the years 1988 to 1994. However, data obtained in 1998, after Medicare started to reimburse the costs of monitoring regardless of insulin treatment, a survey from 1997 to 1999, showed that the number of patients monitoring at least once daily increased by 44% over the earlier period. It is obvious that the costs of monitoring plays an important role in the level of patient acceptance and utilization. Not only are these cost issues pertinent but also the health care beliefs of the patients and providers in using this approach. In addition the issues of pain, discomfort, and inconvenience of testing all need to be addressed and will determine the degree of success. The role of government and third party payers in improving this situation is readily apparent given the enormous burden of diabetes in all countries.

In order to use SBGM properly, each patient should be taught by a diabetes nurse educator, who can evaluate the correct testing technique and use of the monitor selected. Most of the new blood glucose monitors are calibrated to reflect plasma glucose levels that have become the standard measurement in most laboratories. Since the plasma glucose is 10% to 15% higher than whole blood, patients need to know what they are measuring in the event their meter still reads whole blood. To use SBGM optimally requires proper interpretation of the data and this has to be taught to the patient. They need to use the data to assess the effects of nutrition, exercise, and their pharmacological therapy. The use of newer oral drugs, rapid acting insulin analogues, and basal insulin also make it important to test more often. These treatments have specific actions and effects on blood glucose. Rapid acting insulin is used to control postmeal glucose levels and basal insulin to provide up to 24 h coverage. Therefore to obtain the best control it is necessary for the patient to test at specific times to maximize the benefits of the treatment and to avoid hypoglycemia. As noted above a major concern with the use of more intensive therapy is the risk for severe hypoglycemia and its consequences. A report by Cox in 1994 determined whether severe hypoglycemia could be predicted by the results of SBGM, blood glucose variability and the HbA_{1c} (38). They found that patients who recorded variable and frequent low blood glucose readings during routine SBGM were at higher risk for subsequent severe hypoglycemia.

The ADA also has recommendations for glucose testing by health-care providers for routine outpatient management of diabetes. It states that laboratory glucose testing should be available for use as needed as in diet controlled or certain patients taking oral medication. Management of the patient is done with the SBGM data in conjunction with the HbA_{1c} results. The laboratory glucose can also be useful if it is done simultaneously with the patients monitor test to check the accuracy of the patient results. If this is done using portable capillary testing devices rather than the laboratory, then rigorous quality control measures must be used to ensure the validity of the results.

GLYCOSYLATED HEMOGLOBIN (HBA$_{1c}$)

The development of the glycosylated hemoglobin assay has become one of the major advances in taking care of patients with diabetes mellitus. The glycohemoglobin measurement correlates with fasting blood glucose, postprandial glucose, the glucose peak during an oral glucose tolerance test and the mean glucose levels over many weeks. Currently most laboratories use the HbA$_{1c}$ measurement but this is not universal. After the results of the DCCT were published the use of the HbA$_{1c}$ level in setting a goal for optimal glucose control was firmly established. However in a consensus statement by Marshall, it was apparent that standardization of the assay was an issue (39). In this consensus statement it was recommended that a DCCT-aligned HbA$_{1c}$ assay should be used since this as well as the UKPDS and Kumamoto study were the best data available on the relationship between control and complications. Furthermore, the availability of a standardized assay will be important for educating patients on the goals of treatment as well for the standards for glycemic control set by national diabetes associations. It will also be important for designing future studies in diabetes where the question of control and complications are studied.

The glycated hemoglobin is a series of stable minor hemoglobin components formed slowly and nonenzymatically from glucose and hemoglobin. The rate of formation of this product is directly related to the level prevailing glucose concentration and is irreversible. Because the red blood cells where the reaction takes place have an average life span of 120 days the test reflects the prior 2 to 3 months of glycemic control. However, most of the reaction takes place over the last 2 to 3 weeks before the measurement. Many types of assay methods are available to the routine laboratory. These methods vary in the glycated components measured, interferences, and the nondiabetic range. It is important for the clinician to know what the laboratory being used measures and what the normal ranges are. In the United States there is the National Glycohemoglobin Standardization Program that is in part sponsored by the ADA. This is an attempt to standardize HbA$_{1c}$ determinations to the DCCT values. Manufacturers of HbA$_{1c}$ assays are given an annual "certificate of traceability to the DCCT reference method" if they pass the criteria for accuracy and precision.

In the United States more than 98% of laboratories use the NGSP certified methods and report results as either HbA$_{1c}$ or HbA$_{1c}$ equivalents. However, changes are on the way. More recently the International Federation of Clinical Chemistry (IFCC) Working Group on HbA$_{1c}$ Standardization has recommended a new reference method that results in a lower normal range (2.8%–3.8%) which is 1.3% to 1.9% lower across the range compared to the NGSP results. An international working group of the ADA/EASD/IDF has recommended that the IFCC reference be adopted as the new global standard for calibration of HbA$_{1c}$ by manufacturers. However the current DCCT/EDIC results will be in place until data linking HbA$_{1c}$ to mean blood glucose can be obtained and public and professional education is done on the new reporting system (52).

According to the ADA position statement testing of the HbA$_{1c}$ should be performed routinely in all patients with diabetes to document the level of their glycemic control. In general the test should be repeated three to four times a year, but the actual frequency will vary based on the individual patient and the goals set. In a study to test the usefulness of HbA$_{1c}$ measurements in type 1 patients, Lytken Larsen and colleagues randomly assigned 240 matched patients with type 1 diabetes mellitus to either a 3 monthly measurement of HbA$_{1c}$ or blood glucose and urine testing to monitor treatment (40). Treatment was modified based on the results of the tests and after one year in the group having the HbA$_{1c}$ measured, the mean HbA$_{1c}$ dropped from 10.1% to 9.5%. In the control group the values were 10.0% and 10.1%, respectively. As a result the proportion of patients in poor control, defined as an HbA$_{1c}$ value above 10% decreased from 46% to 30%. Another interesting study by Chase and colleagues, looked at the issue of severe hypoglycemic episodes in type 1 patients after the introduction of rapid acting lispro insulin in 1996 (41). The DCCT study resulted in an increase in severe hypoglycemia with intensive therapy. They used the DCCT definition of hypoglycemia and studied patients <5 years of age to >18 years. They found additional reduction in the HbA$_{1c}$ levels with no increase in the number of severe hypoglycemic episodes. While it is reasonable to measure the HbA$_{1c}$ three to four times a year in type 1 patients the optimal frequency in type 2 diabetes is not clear, especially in stable patients who are diet treated. In the absence of definitive studies, stable patients should have the HbA$_{1c}$ measured twice a year and probably quarterly in those who are not in control or are having therapy changes.

It is extremely important that patients and caregivers understand the basis for the test and how to use the information. Rather than have fixed goals for all patients based on the studies discussed so far, it is better to individualize the approach. The ability of the patient to participate in the treatment program is crucial for optimal control. Focusing only on the HbA_{1c} levels without addressing such issues as, the stresses of adolescence, puberty, the home environment, ageing, depression, and economic issues, will create a counterproductive situation. This is especially important when setting goals in the elderly where comorbidities and many psychosocial and economic issues will determine the goals (42). Caregivers also need to be aware that the glycohemoglobin values we use today to set the goals of treatment come from the DCCT and only assays that are referenced to this method are valid. Other assays cannot be used in the same way since they lack the data showing a relationship of the complications of diabetes to the glycohemoglobin. The ADA suggests an HbA_{1c} goal of <7% and that the treatment regimen be revaluated if the level is >8%. It may be argued that based on the data from the UKPDS, where a 0.9% difference is the glycohemoglobin resulted in a 25% reduction in microvascular complications that anything above 7% requires revaluation.

There has also been increased use of point of service AIC assays where a result is obtained during the visit from a finger stick blood sample and changes in treatment made as needed. The advantages to this are obvious as the patient is available to interact with the provider. One issue is the accuracy of these methods compared to the DCCT/EDIC reference assay. In a recent study the DCA 2000 assay was compared to the DCCT/EDIC assay in 200 youth with type 1 diabetes. The DCA 2000 results strongly correlated with the reference test ($r = 0.94$, $p < .001$), was slightly higher with a mean difference of $+0.2\%$. This test therefore can be used in clinical care and results are available in about 6 min (53).

Apart from the glycohemoglobin, a glycated serum protein (GSP) and glycated serum albumin (GSA) assay are also available. Because of the much shorter half-life of serum albumin (14–20 days) this assay can reflect an index of glycemia for shorter periods of time. In general the assays correlate well with the HbA_{1c} measurements. These assays can be useful in situations where the HbA_{1c} cannot be measured, as with hemolytic anemia. The fructosamine assay is one such test that is widely used. However, the results can be affected in situations where synthesis or clearance of these proteins is altered such as, systemic illness and liver disease. In general these assays reflect the glycemic control over a 1 to 2 week period whereas the HbA_{1c} provides an index over 2 to 3 months. One area where these shorter tests may be useful is in pregnancy or after major treatment changes. However these tests are not equivalent to the HbA_{1c} in setting the goals of treatment as they have not been shown to be related to the development or progression diabetic complications.

After many decades of questioning the role of glucose control in preventing the long-term complications of diabetes mellitus we now have some data that indicate the benefits of good control. The long-term trials that have been done to date are not many, but the question has been satisfactorily answered and what is needed is to implement the results into clinical practice. We cannot control all our patients equally well but we need to improve all of them. Any decrease in the HbA_{1c} that can be obtained safely is important. The ideal is to keep the patients in the nondiabetic range. Until beta cell transplantation or regeneration becomes widely available for type 1 diabetes the best approach is to use all our current resources optimally. For the global epidemic of type 2 diabetes, it is now apparent that the early treatment of patients with impaired glucose tolerance with lifestyle measures can have a major impact on progression to clinical disease. The situation with regard to macrovascular disease in type 2 diabetes is being addressed by a long-term trial. To improve diabetes care and spread the message of glycemic control will involve a major effort to educate both physicians and patients. All will need to know about the evidence and the importance of good blood glucose control, and to be aware of the standards of care and goals set out by their national diabetes organizations. It will also require close collaboration between the government and health care providers. There are major human and financial costs from the complications of diabetes and to have evidence that control matters should inspire all involved in diabetes care to improve our efforts. We need to balance our need to control glucose to set goals with the realities of the daily life of our patients and the psychological stresses of living with a chronic disease. While the evidence is very persuasive for controlling diabetes mellitus to glycohemoglobin and fasting and postprandial goals, it is extremely important that the goals be set and adjusted to the individual patient. This situation should serve to foster greater understanding of patients and their problems and the need to continue to build long-term relationships with effective communications and support systems.

REFERENCES

1. Rosenbloom AL. The cause of the epidemic of type 2 diabetes in children. Curr Opin Endocrinol Diab 2000; 7:191–6.
2. Rosenbloom Al, Joe JR, Young RS, Winter WE. The emerging epidemic of type 2 diabetes mellitus in youth. Diabetes Care 1999; 22:345–54.
3. UK Prospective Diabetes Study group. Intensive blood-glucose control with sulfonylureas or insulin compared with conventional treatment and risk of complications in patients with type 2 diabetes. Lancet 1998; 352:837–53.
4. Haffner SM, Stern MP, Hazuda P, et al. Cardiovascular risk factors in confirmed prediabetic individuals. N Engl J Med 1990; 263:2893–8.
5. Abdella N, Salman A, Moro M. Classical microangiopathic diabetic complications in the absence of overt diabetes mellitus. Diab Res Clin Pract 1990; 8:283–6.
6. Aiello LP, Avery RL, Arrigg PG, et al. Vascular endothelial growth factor in ocular fluid of patients with diabetic retinopathy and other retinal disorders. N Engl J Med 1994; 331:1480–7.
7. Brownlee M, Cerami A, Vlassara H. Advanced glycosylation end products in tissue and the biochemical basis of diabetic complications. N Eng J Med 1988; 318:1315–21.
8. Greene DA, Lattimer SA, Sima AAF. Pathogenesis and prevention of diabetic neuropathy. Diabetes/Metab Rev 1988; 4:201–21.
9. Bursell SE, Clermont AC, Aiello LP, et al. High dose vitamin E supplementation normalizes retinal blood flow and creatinine clearance in patients with type 1 diabetes. Diabetes Care 1999; 22:1245–51.
10. Bursell SE, King GL. Can protein kinase C inhibition and vitamin E prevent the development of diabetic vascular complications. Diab Res Clin Pract 1999; 45:169–82.
11. American Diabetes Association. Consensus development conference on the diagnosis of coronary heart disease in people with diabetes. Diabetes Care 1998; 21:1551–9.
12. Gu K, Cowie CC, Harris MI. Diabetes and decline in heart disease mortality in US adults. JAMA 1999; 281:1291–7.
13. Haffner SM, Lehto S, Ronnemaa T, Pyorala K, Laakso M. Mortality from coronary heart disease in subjects with type 2 diabetes and in nondiabetic subjects with and without prior myocardial infarction. N Engl J Med 1998; 339:229–34.
14. Miettinen H, Lehto S, Salomaa V, et al. Impact of diabetes on mortality after the first myocardial infarction. Diabetes Care 1998; 21:69–75.
15. Pyorala K, Pedersen TR, Kjekshus J, et al. Cholesterol lowering with simvastatin improves prognosis of diabetic patients with coronary heart disease: a subgroup analysis of the Scandanavian simvastatin survival study (4S). Diabetes Care 1997; 20:614–20.
16. Sacks FM, Pfeffer MA, Moye LA, et al. The effects of pravastatin on coronary events after myocardial infarction in patients with average cholesterol levels. N Engl J Med 1996; 335:1001–9.
17. Hansson L, Zanchetti A, Carruthers SG, et al. The effects of intensive blood-pressure lowering and low-dose aspirin in patients with hypertension: principal results of the hypertension optimal treatment (HOT) randomized trial. Lancet 1998; 351:1755–62.
18. Turner RC, Millins H, Neil HA, et al. for the United Kingdom prospective diabetes study group. Risk factors for coronary disease in non-insulin dependent diabetes mellitus: United Kingdom prospective diabetes study. BMJ 1998; 316:823–8.
19. Balkau B, Bertrais S, Ducimetiere P, Eschwege E. Is there a glycemic threshold for mortality risk? Diabetes Care 1999; 22:696–9.
20. Coutinho M, Gerstein HC, Wang Y, Yusuf S. The relationship between glucose and incident cardiovascular events: a metaregression analysis of published data from 20 studies of 95,783 individuals followed for 12.4 years. Diabetes Care 1999; 22:233–40.
21. The DECODE study group on behalf of the European diabetes epidemiology group. Glucose tolerance and mortality: comparison of WHO and American Diabetes Association diagnostic criteria. Lancet 1999; 354:617–25.
22. Groeneveld Y, Petri H, Hermans J, Springer MP. Relationship between blood glucose level and mortality in type 2 diabetes mellitus: a systematic review. Diabet Med 1999; 16:2–13.
23. The Diabetes control and complications trial research group. The effect of intensive treatment of diabetes on the development and progression of long-term complications in insulin-dependent diabetes mellitus. N Engl J Med 1993; 329:977–86.

24. Krolweski AS, Laffel LMB, Krolweski M, et al. Glycosylated hemoglobin and the risk of microalbuminuria in patients with insulin dependent diabetes mellitus. N Eng J Med 1995; 332: 1251–5.

25. Reichard P. Are there any glycemic thresholds for the serious microvascular diabetic complications? J Diabet Complications 1995; 9:25–30.

26. The diabetes control and complications trial research group. The absence of a glycemic threshold for the development of long-term complications: THE perspective of the diabetes control and complications trial. Diabetes 1996; 45:1289–98.

27. The Diabetes control and complications trial/epidemiology of diabetes interventions and Complications research group. Retinopathy and nephropathy in patients with type1 diabetes four years after a trial of intensive therapy. N Engl J Med 2000; 342:381–9.

28. Ohkubo Y, Kishikawa H, Araki E, et al. Intensive insulin therapy prevents the progression of diabetic microvascular complications in Japanese patients with non-insulin-dependent diabetes mellitus: a randomized prospective 6-year study. Diab Res Clin Pract 1995; 28:103–17.

29. UK Prospective Diabetes Study (UKPDS) Group. Intensive blood-glucose control with sulfonylureas or insulin compared with conventional treatment and risk of complications in patients with type 2 diabetes (UKPDS 33). Lancet 1998; 352:837–53.

30. UK Prospective Diabetes Study (UKPDS) Group. Effect of intensive blood glucose control with metformin on complications in overweight patients with type 2 diabetes (UKPDS 34). Lancet 1998; 352:854–65.

31. American Diabetes Association. Implications of the United Kingdom prospective diabetes study. Diabetes Care 1998; 21:2180–4.

32. Fioretto P, Steffes MW, Sutherland DER, et al. Reversal of lesions of diabetic nephropathy after pancreatic transplantation. N Eng J Med 1998; 339:69–75.

33. American Diabetes Association. Gestational diabetes mellitus. Diabetes Care 2001; (Suppl. 1):S77–9.

34. Pettit DJ, Baird HR, Aleck KA, et al. Excessive obesity in offspring of Pima Indian women with diabetes during pregnancy. N Eng J Med 1983; 308:242–5.

35. Canadian Diabetes Association. 1998 clinical practice guidelines for the management of diabetes in Canada. CMAJ 1998; 159 (Suppl. 8):SS18–9.

36. Abraira C, Colwell JA, Nuttall F, et al, for the VA CSDM Group. Cardiovascular events and correlates in the Veterans affairs diabetes feasibility trial. Arch Intern Med 1997; 157:181–8.

37. Tests of Glycemia in Diabetes. The American Diabetes Association. Diabetes Care 2001; 24:S80–2.

38. Harris MI. Frequency of blood glucose monitoring in relation to glycemic control in patients with type 2 diabetes. Diabetes Care 2001; 24:979–82.

39. Cox DJ, Kovatchev BP, Julian DM, et al. Frequency of severe hypoglycemia in insulin dependent diabetes mellitus can be predicted from self -blood monitoring blood glucose data. J Clin Endo Metab 1994; 79:1659–62.

40. Marshall SM, Barth JH. Standardization of HbAic measurements—a consensus statement. Diabetic Med 2000; 17:5–6.

41. Lytken Larsen M, Horder M, Mogensen EF. Effect of long-term monitoring of glycosylated hemoglobin levels in insulin-dependent diabetes mellitus. N Engl J Med 1990; 323:1021–5.

42. Chase P, Lockspeiser T, Peery B, et al. The impact of the diabetes control and complications trial and Humalog insulin on glycohemoglobin levels and severe hypoglycemia in type 1 diabetes. Diabetes Care 2001; 24:430–4.

43. Cooppan R. Diabetes in the elderly: implications of the diabetes control and complications trial. Comprehen Ther 1996; 22:286–90.

44. Aiello LP, Clermont A, Arora V, Davis MD, Sheetz MJ, Bursell SE. Inhibition of PKC beta by oral administration of RBX is well tolerated and ameliorates diabetes-induced retinal hemodynamic abnormalities in patients. Invest Ophthamol Vis Sci 2006; 47:86–92.

45. Vinik AI, Bril V, Kempler P, et al. Treatment of symptomatic diabetic peripheral neuropathy with the protein kinase C beta-inhibitor ruboxistaurin mesylate during a 1 year, randomized, placebo-controlled, double blind clinical trial. Clin Ther 2005; 27:1164–80.

46. Collins R, Armitage J, Parish S, Sleigh P, Peto R. Heart Protection Study Collaborative Group. MRC/BHF Heart Protection Study of cholesterol-lowering with simvastatin in 5963 people with diabetes: a randomized placebo controlled trial. Lancet 2003; 361:2005–16.

47. Colhoun HM, Betteridge DJ, Durrington PN, et al. Primary prevention of cardiovascular disease with atovarstatin in type 2 diabetes in the Collaborative Atovarstatin Diabetes Study (CARDS): multicenter randomized placebo-controlled trial. Lancet 2004; 364:685–96.

48. The Diabetes Control and Complications Trial/Epidemiology of Diabetes Interventions and Complications(DCCT/EDIC). Study Research Group. Intensive diabetes treatment and cardiovascular disease in patients with type 1 diabetes. N Engl J Med 2005; 353:2643–53.

49. Stettler C, Allemann S, Juni P, et al. Glycemic control and macrovascular disease in types 1 and 2 diabetes mellitus:metaanalysis of randomized trials. Am Heart J 2006; 152:27–38.

50. American Diabetes Association. Diabetes Care. 2006; 29:(Suppl.):S10.

51. European Diabetes Policy Group. Diabetic Med. 1999; 16:716–73.
52. Sacks DB for the ADA/EASD/IDF Working Group of the HbA$_{1c}$ Assay. Global Harmonization of Hemoglobin A$_{1c}$. Clin. Chem 2005; 51:681–3.
53. The Diabetes Research in Children Network (DirecNet) Study Group. Comparison of finger stick hemoglobin A1c levels assayed by DCA 2000 with the DCCT/EDIC central laboratory assay: results of a DirecNet Study. Pediatric Diabetes 2005; 6:13–6.

4 | The Role of the Diabetes Educator in the Education and Management of Diabetes Mellitus

Carolé Mensing
Diabetes Education Program, University of Connecticut Health Center, Farmington, Connecticut, U.S.A.

INTRODUCTION

Diabetes self-management education (DSME) has long been revered as the cornerstone of care for all persons affected by diabetes. The diabetes educator provides this valuable service as an integral part of the healthcare delivery team. A large body of evidence supports the effectiveness of diabetes education (1) and, although there are variances in delivery methods, the educational process is universal. Since 1983, educators have focused on delivery of a formalized educational content. This content, as well as the process of DSME, is defined by the National Standards of DSME (2) and more recently supported by the Diabetes Self-Management Outcomes Continuum (3).

Other factors have also influenced the enhancement and effectiveness of diabetes self-management. These contributions include the shift from an acute medical management care model to a more public health view, reflective of diabetes as a chronic, progressive disease. Two models depict this shift. They are Wagner's chronic disease management model (4) and the ecological model, providing a framework for the multiple influences on health behavior by the community (5).

The overall combined goals of diabetes care and education continue to be to optimize health and metabolic control, prevent or delay complications, and improve or optimize the patient's quality of life (6). *Healthy People 2010* supports these goals and plans to increase the proportion of individuals with diabetes who receive formal diabetes education from 40% to 60% (7). However, at present there continues to be significant knowledge and skill deficits in 50% to 80% of individuals with diabetes (5), and there are still under-served populations, i.e., only a small percentage of the people affected by diabetes attend educational events (8).

THE BROAD ROLE OF THE DIABETES EDUCATOR

The diabetes educator serves a pivotal role in the management of people with diabetes. The role is multidimensional, with boundaries for accountability that interface with both other members of the healthcare team, and internal and external customers (10). The general scope of practice of a diabetes educator (Table 1) has changing dimensions because of the multidisciplinary nature of the healthcare professionals who provide this service and the changing healthcare delivery system. Each professional who practices as a diabetes educator brings a unique focus to the educational process. This phenomenon can have significant impact on the scope of practice for an individual educator, and is appropriate within the boundaries of each professional discipline. Diabetes educators are of diverse nature and bring varied skill-sets to the healthcare system. They frequently assume extended and complementary roles, such as in program, case or clinical management; as healthcare consultants; in public and professional education, or public health and wellness promotion; as well as researching diabetes management and education. The educator has a vital supportive role in the multidisciplinary team.

THE MULTIDISCIPLINARY TEAM HISTORY

Over a decade or more ago, the multidisciplinary team began to be recognized as an effective and efficient method of care delivery and provider of the educational support demanded by

TABLE 1   Guidelines for Scope of Practice for Diabetes Educators

American Nurses Association, Scope and Standards of Diabetes Nursing, 1998
American Association of Diabetes Educators, Scope of Practice for Diabetes Educators and the Standards of Practice for Diabetes Educators, 2005
American Dietetic Association, Standards of Professional Practice for Dietetics Professionals, 2005
American Diabetes Association, Clinical Practice Recommendations, 2006
Task Force on the Delivery of Diabetes Self-Management Education and Medical Nutrition Therapy, 1998 report

diabetes. This team approach does not eliminate the primary practitioner or sole practitioner (8), but instead supports the variety of skills, timing, assistance and prerequisites brought by each of its members. The team brings a variety of services, interventions and assistance to fully integrate into a person's lifestyle as needed. Effective teams serve the population whether they are rural, inner city, small or large practice, inpatient or clinic-based, special population needs, etc. They may have a patient-centered or population-based focus. Few other diseases demand such a level of attention. In general, the less the person is educated, the less adherent they are to treatment, and the more (team) effort is required (12). The team is formed by a stepwise process:

- Ensure commitment of leadership
- Gain support from care-providers
- Identify team members
- Identify the patient population
- Stratify the patient population
- Assess resources
- Develop a system for coordinated, continuous, quality care

This process focuses on common goals, each member airing opinions and contributing to decisions about patient care and education. Efficient care delivery to all patients focuses on care delivery itself, mechanisms of identifying high-risk patients, cost-effective methods of education, and treatment in the outpatient setting (12).

Team Definition

The 'gold standard' is a clearly defined team assisting diabetes self-management. Most teams work under the auspices of a physician or nurse practitioner to meet standards of care and for reimbursement. Diabetes care is often symptom-focused, and managed according to the acute presenting symptoms—this is the medical model. However, education is now viewed as an ongoing strategy, helping people to manage their diabetes with continuous, proactive, planned care (13). Patient-centered care is now more appropriate than provider-centered care (14). Numerous publications now support a chronic disease model for diabetes and there is evidence to support team care as an effective method of chronic disease management for diabetes (13). The benefits of a team approach have been well-documented (15). "The role of the health care provider is to deliver appropriate treatment, including comprehensive medical care (prevention, detection, treatment of acute and chronic conditions related to diabetes) AND self-management educations, including medical nutrition therapy, directed toward helping the person with diabetes make informed choices regarding self care (16)."

Team Management

Team management is a coordinated multidisciplinary approach. It is crucial to share information to develop and implement a patient's care plan, and to evaluate success. The composition of the team will vary depending on the setting. Typically, a physician, or advanced practice provider, initiates direction and supervises medical care. A nurse or nutritionist participates in assessments, and other disciplines are utilized as available. A more comprehensive team (health psychologist or behavioralist, social worker, podiatrist, pharmacist, etc.) may also be involved. The team usually consists of three or four healthcare providers with complementary skills who are committed to one common goal or approach (13) and includes a physician or other primary-care provider, a nurse and a dietitian, and it is recommended that at least one member is a Certified Diabetes Educator [(CDE) requiring the passing of an exam administered by the National Certification Board for Diabetes Education] (2). The team is multidimensional, with accountability as defined by their individual discipline's scope of practice. A multidisciplinary team offers a variety of skills, experience that contributes to a common purpose (13).

Primary care physicians often provide the majority of diabetes care, augmented and enhanced by other healthcare professionals and community partners and services. In the USA, a primary care practitioner, advanced nurse practitioner, or physician assistant often take on the coordinating care role. Nurse practitioners have been shown to produce similar clinical outcomes to physicians in a primary care setting (17). A primary care team consists of medical and educational managers. It is essential that a key individual coordinates the care effort between primary care providers, CDE, and other healthcare providers.

The diabetes control and complications trial (DCCT) was a large clinical trial of people with type 1 diabetes mellitus, and included medicine, nursing, nutrition, education, and counselling (18,19). The UK Prospective Diabetes Study (UKPDS), a clinical trial of people with type 2 diabetes, included teams of physicians, nurses, and dietitians (20). O'Connor summarizes primary care setting progress towards the goal of better diabetes care (21). Successful interventions need to utilize the strategy of:

- Identify
- Monitor
- Prioritize
- Intensify

Not every team member needs to be involved with every patient, but will be guided by the assessed needs, selected by age grouping of the person (from pediatric to geriatric); special needs (language, literacy, learning abilities, family interactions, etc.); level of information required (basic survival skills to advanced level); the intensity of management (meal planning to infusion pump); and availability. All these factors will influence the frequency of contact and amount of time allotted. Literature/publications can support both short and long-term health outcomes: increasing patient and provider satisfaction, improving the quality-of-life, decreasing risk of complications, and costs.

In each case, the team is needed to provide the ongoing care and education, glycemic management, health promotion, reduction of risks, telephone interventions, etc., which are guided by principles (13), clinical guidelines (3) and standards (2), as well as the 'process' of team education.

PROCESS OF TEAM EDUCATION

The gold standard, based on insurance reimbursement, is a coordinated team, often physician-led and nurse/dietitian supported. The role of the diabetes educator is recognized as an integral part of the instructional team. A 'diabetes educator' is defined as any qualified health professional, CDE, or clinical diabetes specialist involved in the education process. Some patients with complications require a more intense application of resources, increasing the cost per visit, amount of physician and allied health professional's time, and variety of initiatives needed to improve healthcare (12). This involves a move from recording simple vitals and giving a pamphlet, to complex patient education and counseling. Norris et al. suggest that behavior-change strategies were 'more effective' than a didactic approach when combined with healthcare provider adjustments and reinforcement of educational messages (1). In summary, the goal of diabetes team management is to individualize care and treatment, maximizing adherence. The diabetes educator clinician role emerges from this. The educator role convenes and coordinates the following team services: clinical, educational coordinating, consulting, and advocacy roles.

THE DIABETES EDUCATOR

Role Description

All clinicians and educators need good clinical and educational backgrounds, and experiential expertise to fill certain requirements. Experience is needed in current clinical practice of diabetes care and management, and the principles of teaching–learning. These roles demand much flexibility, as the populations served and the settings (inpatient, outpatient, clinical, research) vary. Diabetes educators offer support and a valuable service to the team, often fulfilling a role that it is difficult for a single physician or clinical care professional to provide because of time and availability constraints. Mensing and Norris advise that educators be familiar with and utilize a number of educational skill sets as outlined in Table 2.

After initial instruction, educators provide continued personal and telephone or electronic contact for follow through and assessment of progress. Many people require repeated instruction and teaching. Educators have the expertise, experience and, often, more scheduled time to assess, instruct and assist patients with the learning process, and working through the personal barriers to learning, such as language, reading levels, disabilities, etc. Scheduling of education, length and timing are often left to the educator, although new legislation promotes use of more group experience. Instruction in the basics for survival and more advanced learning are common approaches. The standards currently identify 10 basic content areas to be delivered; educators are prepared to develop these as needed:

- Diabetes disease process
- Nutritional management
- Physical activity
- Medications
- Monitoring
- Complications
- Risk reduction
- Goal setting/problem solving
- Psychosocial adjustment
- Preconception care, pregnancy, gestational diabetes management

More recently, the AADE 7 Self-Care Behaviors (3) have been introduced and offer a similar content structure incorporating the 10 basic content areas described in the revised standards. The AADE 7 content areas are:

- Being Active
- Healthy Eating
- Taking medications
- Monitoring
- Problem Solving
- Reducing Risks
- Healthy Coping

All members of the team are key players. Newer members of the clinical team are the CDE, the clinical nurse specialist (CNS), advanced practice nurse (APN), and those with the advanced clinical role with the newest credentials: the Board Certified Advanced Diabetes Management (BC-ADM) certification. Each of these members has a strong basis in diabetes

TABLE 2 Educator Skill Set

Preparation: topics, materials, audio-visuals
Delivery: demonstratons, visits, discussion, empowerment, Powerpoint, homework
Assessment: individualized, readiness, confidence, conviction
Documentation: handwritten, automated medical record, phone and e-mail forms

disease-specific practice, together with an expanded role. These are performed and guided by written procedures and policies, clinical practice guidelines, and evidence-based research (24). In conclusion, the CDE role is an important part of the integration of clinical care into a more formal educational approach to diabetes. Patients must learn to be skilled and knowledgeable in diabetes self-care, able to access care, and facilitate ongoing decision-making related to their ongoing medical and self-care practices. They are at the center of their own team. As the clinical role solidifies, educational programming and service development needs arise. The educator then assumes the role of coordinating these services, utilizing both business skills and quality management.

Clinician Role

The clinical role of the diabetes educator is a critical first encounter. Clinical background, including knowledge of the Clinical Practice Standards (3), facilitates recommendations for patient education and implementation of the treatment plan; it also fosters independence and access to the healthcare team. Clinical services (Table 3) provided often include objective analysis of current healthcare practices, preferences, and knowledge base, and assisting the person with diabetes to achieve metabolic control, following the DCCT goal *Metabolic Control Matters* (18). The person's understanding of personal clinical status, acquisition of technical skills, communication with clinicians, and observation of physical and emotional challenges, etc. are crucial to the development of a plan for care, guidance in achievement, and educational planning. This clinician educator role may occur in the inpatient or outpatient setting, through referral from the same or a different clinical setting, and the service can be delivered in a variety of creative ways (person to person, electronically, via the mail service, etc.). The clinical delivery alternatives also imply a modified team, which may include a variety of providers and specialists. Addressing risk reduction is a primary focus and the average patient will need hugely complex medical regimes involving multiple antidiabetic, antihypertensive, dlp's and lipid-lowering agents to achieve target. Management strategies consider (19):

- Minimizing cost
- Minimizing weight gain
- Minimal injections (using a combination of pills, plus)
- Minimal circulating insulin (order of introduction of agents)
- Minimal patient effort (improves adherence, increases motivation, minimizes effort)
- Hypoglycemia avoidance
- Postprandial targeting (better control achievement)

Family practice physicians appear to recognize and incorporate clinical and educational care into their diabetes-related visits. Chronic illness provides multiple opportunities for patient education over time and chronic illness visits can be used as 'teachable moments' to facilitate collaborative care (21). Diabetes care requires distinctly different visits than an acute care illness (probably also life style versus other chronic diseases). A direct observational study found that 2.5 patient visits redo content and readdress physical needs, versus 2.1 visits for other chronic diseases, and 1.8 visits for acute care. More problems result in more visits. The amount of time spent on chronic topics, such as diet (meal planning), advice, negotiation, assessment of compliance, (achievement) exercise (activity planning), etc., is more for advanced patients and less for patients undergoing procedures (21).

TABLE 3   Organizing Diabetes Care: Strategies

1. Accurately *identifying* patients with diabetes
2. *Monitoring* one or more important clinical parameters, such as A1C or cholesterol levels
3. *Prioritizing* patients based on their clinical status and readiness to change
4. *Intensifying* care through active outreach or visit planning

DSME Coordinator Role

Diabetes educators often find themselves faced with the challenge of starting a diabetes education program/service or they are hired to manage one. For many educators with varying levels of clinical competence, starting, coordinating or managing a diabetes self-management program poses many challenges, and the development of additional skills for diabetes educators has become as important as clinical skills. These skills include:

- Program development
- Strategic and business planning
- Marketing
- Financial management
- Human resource management
- Continuous quality improvement (CQI)
- Outcomes management

The development of a strategic marketing analysis plan, when starting a DSME program, will increase the potential for long-term success. Along with a thorough market analysis, the educator needs to conduct a financial analysis of the proposed service, and be prepared to present this to the sponsoring organization or community supporter. Budgeting is an important aspect of program development and will continue to be an important component of ongoing program management.

Familiarity with the National Standards for Diabetes Self-Management Education or other applicable standards (Table 4) is essential for coordinators in the early stage of starting a program. The National Standards define quality DSME that can be implemented in diverse settings and which will facilitate improvement in healthcare outcomes for people with diabetes. They comprise ten evidence-based standards, which address structure, process and outcomes. The first national standard states that DSME must have documentation which describes its organizational structure, mission statement, and overall goals. It also states that quality must be an integral component of the program. There is strong scientific evidence in the business and healthcare literature which suggests that establishing a commitment to a strong organizational infrastructure which supports all of the above elements results in efficient and effective provision of services (25–28).

After the standards have been reviewed and 'homework' done, which includes community assessment, competitive analysis, target population and resource identification, a simple business plan is developed. It does not need to be complex, but serves as a guide for the leader and the team. According to the Joint Commission on Accreditation of Health Care Organizations (JCAHO), this type of documentation is important to both small and large organizations (29). Once the target population, their needs, and the resources needed have been identified, a team will need to be formed. This 'core' clinical team usually consists of three or four healthcare professionals with complementary skills who are committed to a common goal and approach (30). The diabetes educator may be the person who champions the case for diabetes education, but the organization's decision makers must demonstrate their commitment to a multidisciplinary team, along with the resources and infrastructure that enables the team to function (13).

The diabetes education team will be the most important resource of the DSME. Without knowledgeable and competent diabetes educators, there will not be a program. The studies on diabetes education and diabetes care have rarely studied the characteristics of who actually

TABLE 4 Clinician Educator Role

Self-care and family-care assessment, patient education skills
Communication, contact (acute/ongoing)
Review of clinical progress, problem-solving
Care trends, research, equipment, insurance team coordination
Care/case management

provides the diabetes education, and what the outcome measures are of provider efficacy (31). The studies have been clear that the provision of diabetes care and education always require a team. The national standards state that DSME must be provided by a multifaceted educational instructional team, which may include a behaviorist, exercise physiologist, ophthalmologist, optometrist, pharmacist, physician, podiatrist, registered dietician, registered nurse, other professional, and paraprofessionals in the community.

They must be collectively qualified to teach all content areas, and must include, at a minimum, a registered dietitian and registered nurse (16,32). All instructors must be either a CDE or have recent didactic and experiential preparation in education and diabetes management. The research to date has shown that DSME is most effective when delivered by a multidisciplinary team with a comprehension plan of care (30–34). If the program aims to become an ADA Education Recognized Program (ERP), the minimum team, as described in the national standards and adopted by the ADA ERP, must be in place (39).

Following the market survey, a mission statement and goals should be developed before beginning to develop the team and program's services. There are several ways of approaching this. One common approach is to go back to the national standards and develop a curriculum based on Standard 7, which states that a written curriculum with criteria for successful learning outcomes is required, and the assessed needs of the individual will determine which content areas are delivered (Table 5). There are also a number of curricula already developed that meet the national standards criteria (Table 6).

For predicting success, program services must be based on the selected curriculum, as well as on the needs of the target population (Table 7). Demographics are analyzed for age, type of diabetes, payer mix (Medicare and some other insurers will mandate the delivery modality), and ethnic background. Clear descriptions of program services are important in order to market your program. There is still a widespread belief that 1:1 DSME is the best delivery modality, and that group teaching is a compromise made in response to economic pressure. However, there is data to support that group DSME is just as effective as individual education when utilized appropriately. The dilemma becomes not whether to provide quality DSME programs in a group format, but whether diabetes educators have acquired the skills and strategies to provide effective educational, behavioral, and clinical interventions in a group format. The diabetes educator who has assumed a role as program coordinator will need to be comfortable with applying change strategy not only for the patients but also for the staff. Quality management is also necessary to support the service.

Quality is a management philosophy that supports a continuous striving for service excellence and an unrelenting commitment to customer satisfaction. As individuals and organizations in healthcare began to attempt to define quality, hundreds of definitions came into existence. The definitions include terms such as quality assurance, quality assessment, total quality management and continuous quality improvement. The two models of quality activities most frequently cited have been the traditional structure, process, and outcome model of quality assurance, as described by Donebedian, and the industrial model of quality described by Deming, and Juran (40–42). Quality is fundamentally a philosophy, and there is no one prescription for application. It is the concepts that need to be applied to the goal of striving for service excellence. There are a number of quality methodologies, with continuous quality improvement (CQI) being one of the most utilized. Two other frequently used methodologies are quality planning and quality measurement (43). Understanding CQI is an important aspect for all diabetes educators, but especially for those who have assumed the coordinator role for program services. The steps in the CQI process are:

TABLE 5 National Education Standards Resources

Canadian Diabetes Association, Diabetes Educator Section, Standards for Diabetes Education in Canada
U.S. Department of Health and Human Services, Medicare Program; Expanded Coverage of Outpatient Diabetes Self-management Training Services
International Diabetes Federation Consultive Section on Education, International Consensus Standards of Practice for Diabetes Education
U.S. National Standards for Diabetes Self-Management Education

TABLE 6   Curriculum References

American Association of Diabetes Educators (AADE). The Art and Science of Diabetes Education-A Desk Reference for Health
   Professionals
American Diabetes Association (ADA): Life With Diabetes: A Series of Teaching Outlines by the Michigan Diabetes Research
   and Training Center.
International Diabetes Center, Type 2 Diabetes Curriculum Guide.

- Identify problem/opportunity
- Data collection
- Data analysis
- Identify alternative solutions
- Generate recommendations
- Implement recommendations
- Evaluate actions improvement

Implementing a CQI program for DSME has now become one of the national standards for DSME, and has been adopted by the ADA ERP (2,20). Outcome measures form part of CQI; these are reviewed below.

Coordinator of professional, community education/consultant/advocate. Educators are often sought to provide professional and community intervention, together with prevention education, for a variety of groups ranging from other diabetes specialists to staff nurses, case managers, office nurses, pharmacists, primary care providers, and the general public. Educators develops their skill sets based on their current practice environment and their personal areas of interest (Table 2). Topics that they may be called on to present are diverse, and range from the core content areas in the National Standards to clinical management, and less traditional areas, such as program development, quality management, and behavior change strategies. They may include support group and screening activities, school and camp programs, or work-site or faith-based presentations. The topic areas are as diverse and multidimensional as the role of the diabetes educator itself. Use of talking circles, promoters, parish nurses and other community based programs offer a number of resources and opportunities for educators to help their patients access comfortable information and support resources.

Coordinator of disease/case management is a new term. In recent years there has been an effort to identify new models of care for chronic diseases such as diabetes. The traditional model of acute care has been shown to inadequately address the needs of people with diabetes. A recent survey of patients who received their diabetes care from primary care providers showed that they were receiving 64 to 74% of the ADA Provider Recognition Program recommended services (47). The new models apply some recurring themes, such as systems approach, population based; preventive services, evidenced-based medicine; and outcomes management through IS solutions. These new models of care are often called disease and case management (51). The diabetes educator has often been identified as a health professional with the requisite skill-set to coordinate such a model of care.

OUTCOME MEASUREMENT

Outcome measures have been defined as data that describe a patient's health status. Patient health outcomes have been measured for years, and their use has been increasing as researchers are beginning to see these outcomes as the best way to improve the performance of

TABLE 7   Predictors of Successful Management

Duration of the intervention
Regular reinforcement. Proven more effective than one-time or short-term education (not limited to diabetes)
Not just unusual or novel, but personalized, repeated contact using every feasible delivery system

providing healthcare. Donebedian defines outcomes as "A measurable product and is the changed state or condition of an individual as a consequence of health care over time" (41). An outcome is a change that occurs as a result of some intervention—it is not a single point in time. The chronic care model (3) also supports the need for identification of essential elements to show improvement in outcomes of service delivery. The need to examine these outcomes in healthcare and diabetes care has been reinforced by mandates from Healthcare Financing Administration (HCFA—now renamed CMS, Centers for Medicaid and Medicare Services), Agency for Health Care Policy and Research (AHCPR), and accrediting bodies, such as the JCAHO, National Council on Quality Assurance (NCQA), and the American Diabetes Association Education and Provider Recognition programs.

Healthcare outcomes cross the healthcare continuum. They include educational, behavioral, clinical and long-term health status outcomes. Several outcome measurement instruments exist for assessing patient behavior, functional status, and QOL, for example: SF–36, PAID, and the Diabetes-Self-Management Assessment Report tool (D-SMART) (42–45) Other outcomes that are important to different customers are cost outcomes, such as cost effectiveness (ratio of costs of a program or process to the effects).

Evaluation is critical to the future of DSME programs. The effectiveness of interventions must be documented in order to have a better understanding of which interventions are the most appropriate for a specific population. Diabetes education has long been held by many to be the cornerstone of effective diabetes care. Yet in 1997, when diabetes educators were asked by HCFA to provide specific evidence of what the attributes of effective education were, diabetes educators could give little specificity. In 1999, at the AADE Research Summit, the question was asked: "Is diabetes education effective and what methods are the best?" The answer is: it depends on the following factors, what treatment, for what population, delivered by whom, under what set of conditions, for what outcome, and how did it come about (46)? Outcome measures associated with diabetes education programs include clinical (medical), educational (learning and behavioral), and psychosocial (QOL, coping, efficacy, etc.) (52). Through an extensive review of the literature and a process of expert consensus, the AADE Outcomes Task Force determined that health related behaviors are the unique and measurable outcomes of effective diabetes education (51,56). As the profession of diabetes education has evolved, it has begun to shift focus from 'Did we deliver the right content' to 'Did we achieve the desired patient outcomes?' Research in diabetes education has not yet provided specificity in characteristics of 'best practice' in diabetes education. More detail is required about what steps in the process of diabetes education are important, including variables such as characteristics about the providers, population, delivery methodologies, and healthcare environment. The process of assessing patient characteristics and determining what interventions are associated with the best outcomes is called clinical practice improvement (CPI) (57). CPI is in many ways complementary to the CQI process as well as RCT, as it creates a permanent feedback loop aimed at all clinicians involved in the process of care delivery. It provides them with data about their daily practice, and the information necessary to understand and modify their interventions. The CPI framework is the basis for the AADE National Diabetes Education Outcomes System (NDEOS), which resulted from the work of the AADE Outcomes Task Force. Based on expert consensus, a comprehensive review of the literature, and a customer analysis of the AADE membership, the Outcomes Team determined that health-related behavior changes are the unique and measurable outcomes of diabetes education (44). These behavior changes (which are compatible with the 10 DSME categories listed above) can be categorized in the following outcome areas:

- Physical activity (exercise)
- Food choices (eating)
- Medication administration
- Monitoring of blood glucose
- Problem solving for blood glucose: highs, lows, and sick days
- Risk-reduction activities
- Psychosocial adaptation

Finding a definition of DSME that conveys your message in a clear and articulate way is important to the marketing of your program. One definition that has been used widely is the following; "Diabetes self-management education (including medical nutrition therapy) is an interactive, collaborative, ongoing process involving the person with diabetes and the educator. It is a four-step process:

- Assess individual's education needs
- Identify individual's specific diabetes self-management goals
- Educate individual to achieve identified self-management goals
- Evaluate attainment of goals (51).

Utilizing this information assists the diabetes education coordinator in developing and implementing a quality educational product. As the product expands, other educator roles may be identified and become appropriate.

SUMMARY

Many physicians or health provider practices do not have access to a full comprehensive, multidisciplinary team, a diabetes educator in this expanded role, or this type of case and care management model. Contacting ADA or AADE can help identify educators in your local area. Regardless of practice setting, providers need to incorporate basic diabetes SM skills into routine office practice. A variety of materials and support supplies may be used to reinforce education. These may be obtained from ADA, AADE, CDC, etc. Reading level targeted material, larger print, graphics, models, sample products, audio, visual, and computer aids can all assist the learning process. A more balanced approach, especially for type 2 diabetes, emphasizes risk reduction as well as glycemic control (58).

The appropriate allocation of the team educator role, as well as adequate teaching time, is necessary to facilitate the learning process. Skills demonstration, information repetition and situational problem solving are excellent tools for advancing the learning process. Content concepts should be limited, and specific behavioral instructions are better retained. General office staff reinforcement and encouragement help provide success. Standards that include guidelines for curriculum, minimum professional expertise and training, advisory bodies, and systematic review of outcomes, are readily available to promote acceptable quality education nationwide for all people with diabetes. The voluntary recognition of ADA has created a template process. CMS has implemented accreditation for third party reimbursement, guided by these standards and the role of the educator.

As a result of the rapidly changing environment of healthcare financing and reimbursement, as well as the results of the DCCT and UKPDS, providers are faced with challenges of medical and educational care. Diabetes care and education has evolved into a highly specialized field with a focus on advanced practice, education and training requirements, and continuing to deliver care and education. The diabetes educator is the 'gold standard' for maintaining the educational process and the future holds the promise of easier implementation of therapies, together with the possibility that people with diabetes mellitus can live longer and better with education (59–64).

APPENDIX
Definitions

CDE-Certified Diabetes Educator passing an exam administered by the National Certification Board for Diabetes Education. (AADE Scope of Practice)

Clinical teaching is communication, facilitates learning, provides structure, clients assume responsibility to improve health through changes in attitudes and behaviors (57,58). The teaching role is generally accepted of all professionals. Process is: assessment, analysis, planning, implementation, evaluation.

Diabetes education a "planned series of events or experiences which include counseling, teaching of information, experiential skill-building, discussions, problem solving, and assistance in reviewing one's life and determining if lifestyle changes necessary to support different, better health practices." The primary role of the educator is to educate the person with diabetes and their family and support about diabetes self-management and related issues (10 Curriculum).

Diabetes Clinical Specialist or advanced practitioner professional with a master's degree and/or certification in a specialty practice. They have training, expertise, autonomy and in many areas licensing with prescriptive ability. (ACCN/AADE)

Education the interactive, collaborative, ongoing process involving the person with diabetes and the educator. (AADE Scope of Practice.)

Educator healthcare professional who has mastered the core knowledge and skills (biological and social sciences, communication, counseling, education) and has current experience in the care of people with diabetes.

Goal meet the academic, professional, experiential requirements to become a CDE. (AADE)

Patient education expanding and evolving, now central to achieving adequate outcomes of care. Integrated throughout the care to individuals and groups, in all settings. Diagnostic–intervention– evaluation process model is used to practice patient education (59).

REFERENCES

1. Norris SL, Engelgau MM, Narayan KMV. Effectiveness of self-management teaching in type 2 diabetes: a systematic review of randomized trials. Diabetes Care 2001; 24:561–87.
2. Mensing CR, Boucher J, Cypress M, et al. National standards for diabetes self-management education. Diabetes Care 2006; 29 Suppl 1:578–85.
3. Mulcahyk, Marynuik M, Peeples M, et al. Diabetes self-mangement education core outcomes measures. Diabetes Educ 2003: 29:768–88. J Am Diet Assoc. 2003; 103 (8):1061–72; AADE.
4. Wagner, EH, Austin, BT, Von Korff, M. Improving outcomes in chronic illness. Managed care Quarterly 1196; 4:12–25.
5. ADA. DC. 2002; 25:599–606.
6. American Diabetes Association. Clinical practice recommendations 2001. Diabetes Care 2001; 24 (Suppl 1).
7. United States Department of Health and Human Services PHS. Healthy people 2010. Washington DC: United States Department of Health and Human Services, 2000.
8. Clement S. Diabetes self-management education. Diabetes Care 1995; 18:1204–14.
9. American Association of Diabetes Educators. Executive summary of the diabetes educational and behavioral research summit 2001. Chicago, IL: American Association of Diabetes Educators, 2001, 6.
10. American Association of Diabetes Educators. The 2006 scope of practice for diabetes educators and the standards of practice for diabetes educators. Diabetes Ed, 2006; 32:25 Chicago, IL: American Association of Diabetes Educators, 2000.
11. American Association of Diabetes Educators. Intensive diabetes management. The team approach. Chicago, IL: American Association of Diabetes Educators, 1995.
12. Leichter SB, Cost and reimbursement as determinants of the quality of diabetes care: I. direct cost determinants. Cl Diab 2001; 19:142–4.
13. Centers for Disease Control and Prevention. Team care: comprehensive lifetime management for diabetes. National Diabetes Education Program (NDEP–36). Atlanta, Georgia: US Department of Health and Human Services, 2001.
14. Etzwiler DD. Chronic care: a need in search of a system. Diabetes Ed 1997; 23:569–73.
15. Lebovitz H. Therapy for diabetes mellitus and related disorders. In: Farkas-Hirsch R, editor. The role of diabetes education in patient management. 3rd edn. American Diabetes Association, 1998.
16. Franz MJ, Monk A, Barry B, et al. Effectiveness of medical nutrition therapy provided by dieticians in the management of non-insulin-dependent diabetes mellitus: a randomized, controlled trial. J Am Diet Assoc 1995; 95:1009–17.
17. Mundinger MO, Kane RL, Lenz ER, et al. Primary care outcomes in patients treated by nurse practitioners or physicians: a randomized trial. J Am Med Assoc 2000; 283:59–68.
18. Diabetes Control and Complications Trial Research Group. The effect of intensive treatment of diabetes on the development and progression of long-term complications in insulin dependent diabetes mellitus. N Engl J Med 1993; 329:986–97.

19. National Institute of Diabetes and Digestive and Kidney diseases. Metabolic control matters. Nationwide translation of the diabetes control and complications trial: analysis and recommendations. NIH publication no. 94–3773. Bethesda, MD: US Department of Health and Human Services, 1994.

20. United Kingdom Prospective Diabetes Study Group. Intensive blood-glucose control with sulfonylureas or insulin compared with conventional treatment and risk of complications in patients with type 2 diabetes (UKPDS 33). Lancet 1998; 352:837–53.

21. O'Connor PJ. Organizing diabetes care: identify, monitor, prioritize, intensify [editorial]. Diabetes Care 2001; 24:1515–6.

22. Buse JB. Progressive use of medical therapies in type 2 diabetes. Diabetes Spectrum 2000; 13:2000.

23. Yawn B, Zyzanski SJ, Goodwin MA, et al. Is diabetes treated as an acute or chronic illness in a community family practice? Diabetes Care 2001; 24:1390–6.

24. American Nurses Credentialing Center, www.Nursingworld.org/ancc/. Visited 13th March 2002.

25. American Association of Diabetes Educators, www.aadenet.org. Visited 13th March 2002.

26. Fox CH, Mahoney MC. Improving diabetes preventive care in a family practice residency program: a case study in continuous quality improvement. Family Med 1998; 30:441–5.

27. Gilroth BE. Management of patient education in US hospitals: evolution of a concept. Patient Ed Couns 1990; 15:101–11.

28. Heins JM, Nord WR, Cameron M. Establishing and sustaining state-of the art diabetes education programs: research and recommendations. Diabetes Ed 1992; 18:501–8.

29. Mangan M. Diabetes self-management education programs in the Veterans Health Administration. Diabetes Ed 1997; 23:87–695.

30. Joint Commission on Accreditation of Healthcare Organizations. Framework for improving performance. Oakbrook Terrace, IL: Joint Commission on Accreditation of Healthcare Organizations, 1994.

31. National Institute of Diabetes and Digestive and Kidney Diseases. Metabolic control matters. Nationwide translation of diabetes control and complications trial: analysis and recommenda-tions. NIH publication no. 94–3773. Bethesda MD: US Department of Health and Human Services, 1994.

32. Young-Hyman D. Provider impact in diabetes education: what we know, what we would like to know, paradigms for asking. Diabetes Ed 1999; 25(Suppl):34–42.

33. Aubert RE, Herman WH, Waters J, et al. Nurse case management to improve glycemic control in diabetic patients in a health maintenance organization. Ann Intern Med 1998; 129:605–12.

34. Abourizk NN, O'Conner PJ, Crabtree BF, Schnatz JD. An outpatient model of integrated diabetes treatment and education: functional, metabolic, and knowledge outcomes. Diabetes Ed 1994; 20:416–21.

35. Etzweiler D. Chronic care: a need in search of a system. Diabetes Ed 1997; 23:569–73.

36. Shamoon H, Vaccaro-Olko MJ. Diabetes education teams. Professional education in diabetes. In: Proceedings of the DRTC Conference. National Diabetes Information Clearinghouse and National Institute of Diabetes and Digestive and Kidney Diseases, NIH, 1980.

37. Koproski J, Pretto Z, Poretsky L. Effects of an intervention by a diabetes team in hospitalized patients with diabetes. Diabetes Care 1997; 20:1553–5.

38. Levetan CS, Salas JR, Wilets IF. Impact of endocrine and diabetes team consultation on hospital length of stay for patients with diabetes. Am J Med 1995; 99:22–8.

39. American Diabetes Association, Education Recognition Program. Available at: http://www.diabetes.org. Visited June, 2006.

40. Rickheim PL, Weaver TW, Flader J. Group versus individual education: a randomized study. Submitted for publication.

41. Donabedian A. The definition of quality: a conceptual exploration. Ann Arbor: Health Admini-stration Press, 1980.

42. Deming WE. Out of crisis. Cambridge, MA: MITCAES; 1986.

43. Juran JM. Juran's quality control handbook. 4th edn. New York: McGraw-Hill, 1988.

44. Juran JM. Reengineering processes for competitive advantage: business process quality management Wilton, CT: Juran Institute, 1994.

45. US Department of Health and Human Services, Agency for Health Care Policy and Research. Washington, DC: 1995. DHHS publication 95–0045.

46. Anderson RM, Fitzgerald JT, Wisdom K, et al. A comparison of global versus disease-specific quality of life measures in patients with diabetes. Diabetes Care 1997; 20:299–305.

47. Ware JEJ, Sherbourne CD. The MOS 36–item short-form health survey (SF–36): Conceptual framework and item changes. Med Care 1992; 30:473–83.

48. Polonsky WH, Welch GM. Listening to our patient's concerns: understanding and addressing diabetes-specific emotional distress. Diabetes Spectrum 1997; 9:8–11.

49. Peeples M, Mulcahy K, Tomky D, Weaver T. The conceptual framework on the National Diabetes Outcomes System (NDEOS). Diabetes Ed 2001; 27:547–62.

50. Mulcahy KA, Peeples M, Tomky D, et al. National diabetes education outcomes system: application to practice. Diabetes Ed 2000.
51. American Association of Diabetes Educators. Diabetes educational and behavioral research summit. Diabetes Ed 1999; 25(Suppl).
52. American Diabetes Association. Task force. Diabetes Spectrum 1999; 12:45.
53. Glasgow RE, Strycker LA. Preventive care practices for diabetes management in two primary care samples. Am J Prev Med 2000; 19:9–14.
54. Peyrot M. Evaluation of patient education programs: how to do it and how to use it. Diabetes Spectrum 1996; 9:86–93.
55. Brown SA. Predicting metabolic control in diabetes: a pilot study using meta-analysis to estimate a linear model. Nursing Res 1994; 43:362–8.
56. Glasgow R. Evaluating diabetes education. Diabetes Care 1992; 15:1423–32.
57. McGlynn E. Choosing and evaluating clinical performance measures: The Joint Commission. 1998; 24:470–9.
58. Peyrot M, Rubin R. Modeling the effect of diabetes education on glycemic control. Diabetes Ed 1994; 20:143–8.
59. Horn SD, Hopkins DSP. Clinical practice improvement a new technology for developing cost-effective quality care. New York: Faulkner and Gray; 1994.
60. Pronk N, Goodman M, O'Connor PJ, Martinson B: Relationship between modifiable risks and short-term health care charges. J Am Med Assoc 1999; 282:2235–39.
61. American Diabetes Association. Annual review of diabetes. American Diabetes Association, 2001.
62. Babcock D, Miller M. Client education, theory and practice. Mosby, 1994.
63. Pender NJ. Health promotion in nursing practice. Norwalk, CN; Appleton-Century Crofts, 1987.
64. Redman BK. The practice of patient education. 8th edn. Mosby, 1997.

5 | Nutrition in the Etiology and Management of Type 2 Diabetes

Monika Toeller
German Diabetes Research Center, Heinrich-Heine University, Düsseldorf, Germany

Jim I. Mann
Department of Human Nutrition, University of Otago, Dunedin, New Zealand

INTRODUCTION

The prevalence of type 2 diabetes is increasing rapidly in many countries (1–3). As there is currently no cure for diabetes, all measures that could contribute to prevention or treatment of the metabolic disturbances that precede or characterize the disease should be exploited. The important role of nutritional modifications in the prevention and treatment of type 2 diabetes is now well recognized (4–7).

Most persons with type 2 diabetes are overweight and/or insulin-resistant. Many of them also have dyslipidemia and hypertension, both of which are frequently present before type 2 diabetes is diagnosed. Nutritional intervention should therefore be started early enough to achieve the benefits that can be expected from medical nutritional treatment. This chapter describes the potential of nutritional measures to prevent or treat type 2 diabetes mellitus and its complications. These measures are based on the best available evidence derived from scientific literature and clinical experience from expert groups (8–11).

THE ROLE OF NUTRITION IN THE ETIOLOGY OF TYPE 2 DIABETES

Energy Intake

There is now a considerable amount of evidence to suggest that rapid acculturation is associated with increased rates of type 2 diabetes (11). Several characteristics of the Western lifestyle predispose to overnutrition and obesity, which in turn increases the risk of developing insulin resistance and type 2 diabetes—particularly in individuals or populations with a genetic predisposition for diabetes. Physical inactivity and high intakes of energy-dense foods lead to an energy intake in excess of requirements (2,12).

An impressive decline in diabetes death rates in several places was reported during World Wars I and II in locations affected by food shortages. The contribution of overnutrition to risk of diabetes has also been demonstrated. When food consumption per capita rose sharply in Japan, Taiwan, and some Pacific islands, there was also a sharp rise in the prevalence of type 2 diabetes (11).

A number of studies have demonstrated improvements in metabolic parameters among people with impaired glucose tolerance (IGT) after interventions aimed at reducing energy intake and increasing physical activity, suggesting that it may be possible to reduce the incidence of type 2 diabetes (13–15). Indeed, some recent intervention studies have demonstrated the potential for weight loss to reduce the risk of progression from IGT to type 2 diabetes. The Finnish Diabetes Prevention study included 522 overweight persons with IGT, randomized to a control group or to intensive lifestyle intervention. The cumulative incidence of type 2 diabetes after 4 years was 11% in the intervention group and 23% in the control group. The risk of type 2 diabetes was reduced by 58%, and this outcome was directly related to changes in lifestyle (17,18).

The Diabetes Prevention Program in the United States included 3234 persons of diverse ethnic background with IGT (19). Participants in the intensive lifestyle program reduced their risk of developing type 2 diabetes by 58% over 3 years of follow-up, and the risk reduction was 71% among persons over the age of 60 years. Of interest is the finding that metformin, the pharmacological agent tested in this study, resulted in a risk reduction of 31%, which was less than the risk reduction observed for lifestyle intervention (20).

Excess body fat is perhaps the most important modifiable risk factor for the development of type 2 diabetes (11,15). It is estimated that the risk of type 2 diabetes attributable to obesity is as great as 75%. However, it is important to emphasize that in most intervention studies aimed at weight reduction there are major difficulties in disentangling the potential benefits of weight loss from the effects of altering intakes of individual foods and nutrients and increasing physical activity, all of which have the potential to reduce diabetes risk. Energy intake is difficult to assess adequately in large-scale epidemiological studies, even when the best available instruments are employed, and it has been demonstrated that overweight or obese persons underestimate their energy intake. Nevertheless, the consistency of beneficial effects shown in intervention studies in which body weight was reduced strengthens the recommendation: energy intake in excess of requirement and overweight should be avoided, particularly among those with a familial predisposition. In addition, the Finnish Diabetes Prevention study recently could show beneficial effects of high fiber, low-fat diets in the prediction of long-term weight loss as well as in the risk reduction of type 2 diabetes (18). Such advice probably offers the best hope of reducing the risk of developing resistance to the action of insulin and progression to type 2 diabetes (8,14,21).

Carbohydrate and Fiber

Many studies have examined the role of sucrose and sugars in the etiology of type 2 diabetes. A few have suggested a positive association, but the majority of studies have shown no association. Some have even suggested an inverse association between diabetes incidence and sucrose intake (11,14). Poor assessment of dietary intake, inability to disentangle dietary and other confounding factors, as well as overinterpretation of data derived from observational studies characterize many of these studies. Despite the lack of direct evidence for the role of sugars in the etiology of type 2 diabetes, it is conceivable that excessive sucrose intake might predispose to obesity, and thus sucrose indirectly may be a predisposing factor for type 2 diabetes. This has been suggested particularly in those who prefer to consume large amounts of sugar-sweetened beverages (22,23).

There is support for the suggestion that foods rich in slowly digested starch or high in fiber might be protective. Countries with high intakes of these foods have low rates of type 2 diabetes. In a cross-sectional study of normoglycemic men, intake of pectin was inversely associated with postprandial blood glucose levels, independent of total energy intake and body mass index (BMI) (5). In the Health Professionals' Follow-up study and the Nurses' Health study, diets low in cereal fiber and with high-glycemic loads were associated with an increased risk of type 2 diabetes after adjustment for other risk factors (13). In the Iowa Women's Health study the risk of self-reported diabetes was highest in the group with the lowest whole-grain intake. In contrast, a higher consumption of refined grains was associated with an increased risk of type 2 diabetes after adjustment for age and total energy intake. The ratio of whole grain to refined grain was related to a significantly lower risk of diabetes, suggesting a potential benefit for replacing refined grains with whole grains (24).

It is of interest that, in the studies quoted, cereal fiber appeared to contribute most to the protective effect; however, experimental studies have repeatedly demonstrated a more marked beneficial effect of soluble fibers than insoluble fibers on several measures of carbohydrate and lipid metabolism. Thus, fiber from fruit and vegetables might have been expected to have exerted a more marked protective effect than cereal fiber. Although further research is needed to investigate the effects of different types and sources of fiber, it seems to be prudent to encourage an increased consumption of total dietary fiber from different sources: whole grains, fruits, vegetables, and legumes.

Types of Fat

In the San Luis Valley Diabetes Study a high intake of fat was associated with an increased risk of IGT and type 2 diabetes. In the 1 to 3 year follow-up of this study, fat consumption predicted the progression to type 2 diabetes in persons with IGT (25). A positive association has also been found between saturated fat and hyperglycemia or glucose intolerance in cross-sectional studies (5,25). However, large cohort studies with diagnosed type 2 diabetes as an end point did not show an appreciable association with saturated fat intake (26). Conversely, a high intake of vegetable fat was inversely associated with the risk of type 2 diabetes during 6 years of follow-up among participants in the Nurses' Health Study who were not obese (26). With the exception of the San Luis Valley Diabetes Study, other epidemiological studies did not find a significant association between intakes of monounsaturated fat and risk of type 2 diabetes (25). However, fats of a different nature are often highly correlated in the diets, and therefore confounding by one type of fat may have hindered the analysis for another type of fat. The relationship between nature of dietary fat and type 2 diabetes has been studied in persons with IGT and undiagnosed type 2 diabetes patients who were reported to have higher proportions of saturated fatty acids in serum cholesterol esters than persons with normal glucose tolerance (27).

Perhaps the best evidence for the potentially deleterious effect of saturated fatty acids comes from the KANWU Study. In this study, replacing an appreciable proportion of dietary saturated fatty acids with monounsaturated fatty acids was associated with an increase in insulin sensitivity (28). It is also of interest to note that both in the Finnish Diabetes Prevention Study and in the US Diabetes Prevention Project, which showed a reduced risk of progression from IGT to type 2 diabetes, the dietary recommendations included advice to appreciably reduce saturated fatty acids. No studies are yet available to suggest conclusive associations between trans-fatty acids and the risk of type 2 diabetes.

The suggestion that $n - 3$ polyunsaturated fatty acids may also play a role in the development of type 2 diabetes came from a prospective study of 175 elderly men and women who were habitual fish eaters. They were shown to have a 50% lower risk of developing glucose intolerance over a follow-up period of 4 years compared with persons who were not regular fish eaters (29).

It now appears that the effects of various fatty acids on the risk of type 2 diabetes are similar to their effects on lipoprotein-mediated risk of coronary heart disease (30–32). According to the available data, modifying intake of dietary fats towards consuming less saturated fat and more unsaturated fats may reduce the risk of developing type 2 diabetes—in addition to reducing cardiovascular risk.

Other Nutritional Factors

There are no firm epidemiological data with regard to the role of dietary protein in the etiology of type 2 diabetes. Although vegetarians present with lower rates of type 2 diabetes compared with persons who eat meat, it is impossible to disentangle the association of animal protein with the risk of type 2 diabetes from other dietary factors, such as saturated fat and fiber intake (11). The relationship between alcohol and other dietary variables similarly complicates attempts to evaluate a potential role for alcohol in the etiology of type 2 diabetes. In the Rancho Bernardo Study, increasing intakes of alcohol in obese men were associated with an increased risk of type 2 diabetes (33). On the other hand, moderate alcohol intake has been shown to be associated with enhanced insulin sensitivity (34,35).

So far, no epidemiological studies have provided convincing support for the role of micronutrients in the etiology of type 2 diabetes. The suggestion that low-birth weight infants, especially those who show rapid catch-up growth, are at increased risk of developing IGT and type 2 diabetes later in life is fairly consistent, but the possible relation of this phenomenon to maternal malnutrition needs further research.

Recent knowledge regarding the potential of nutritional factors in the prevention of type 2 diabetes can be summarized as follows:

- Structured programs on lifestyle modification that emphasize a reduction in total energy and saturated fat intake, and encourage an increase in fiber consumption, together with increased physical activity and regular contact with the healthcare team, are the most promising approaches to reducing the risk of developing type 2 diabetes.

- Avoiding being overweight, treating overweight and obesity as well as prevention of weight regain once weight loss has been achieved are particularly important for those with a familial predisposition for type 2 diabetes.

MEDICAL NUTRITION TREATMENT IN THE MANAGEMENT OF TYPE 2 DIABETES

Goals of Nutrition Therapy for Type 2 Diabetes

Nutritional management aims to help optimize metabolic control and reduce risk factors for chronic complications of diabetes. This includes the achievement of blood glucose and glycosylated hemoglobin (HbA_{1c}) levels as close to normal as is safely possible, and lipid and lipoprotein profiles, as well as blood pressure values, that may be expected to reduce the risk of macrovascular disease. Individual nutritional needs and the quality of life of the person with diabetes also have to be considered when defining nutritional objectives (7–10,14,16,36). The nutritional recommendation for an individual patient should include practical advice regarding appropriate food choices and quantities. However, it should be stressed that nutritional recommendations for people with type 2 diabetes are similar to those aimed at the population as a whole for the promotion of good health and the prevention of metabolic disorders and vascular complications. Thus, the food for persons with diabetes should not differ appreciably from that recommended for other family members (37–39).

Energy Restriction and Body Weight

Many individuals with type 2 diabetes are overweight. Insulin resistance increases with increasing body weight, and obesity may also aggravate hyperlipidemia and hypertension (Fig. 1). Many short-term studies have demonstrated that weight loss, especially of intra-abdominal fat, in persons with type 2 diabetes is associated with decreased insulin resistance, improved glycemic control, reduced blood pressure and improvement of dyslipidemia (Table 1) (35,40). Thus, energy restriction and weight loss are important therapeutic objectives for obese individuals with type 2 diabetes (7,8,10). However, long-term data are still scarce to assess the extent to which metabolic improvements by means of weight loss can be maintained in people with type 2 diabetes. Long-term weight loss is often difficult to achieve, and it has to be considered that genetic factors may play an important role in determining body weight.

Environmental factors also often make losing weight difficult for those genetically predisposed to obesity. Nevertheless, the potential of structured weight loss programs should be exploited in obese persons with type 2 diabetes to achieve the possible beneficial effects.

The U.K. Prospective Diabetes Study (UKPDS) reported that the initial glucose response in persons with type 2 diabetes was particularly related to the decreased energy intake. Once energy intake was increased, fasting glucose levels increased even when weight loss was maintained (41). Prevention of weight regain seems to be an important target in those who lose weight, but evidently a long-term restricted energy intake is necessary to sustain the metabolic improvements. Nevertheless, even modest weight loss of under 10% body weight improves

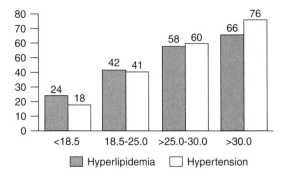

FIGURE 1 Prevalence of hyperlipidemia and hypertension ($n\%$) by categories of BMI (kg m^{-2}) in a sample of 1988 persons with diabetes [930 male, 1058 female; mean age 57 ± 13 years; mean diabetes duration 8 (1–56) years].

TABLE 1 Nutritional Factors and their Possible Impact on Insulin Resistance

Total energy reduction	$\downarrow\downarrow\downarrow$
Increased fiber intake	$\downarrow$
Low-glycemic index food	$\downarrow$
Small amounts of alcohol	$\downarrow$
Saturated fat intake	$\uparrow\uparrow$
Total fat	$\uparrow$
Salt	$\uparrow$

$\downarrow$decrease, $\uparrow$increase

insulin sensitivity and glucose tolerance and reduces lipid levels and blood pressure. Weight loss may lead to greater improvements in cardiac risk factors in persons with a high waist circumference (42).

Those who are overweight should be encouraged to reduce caloric intake so that their BMI moves towards the recommended range of 18.5 to 24.9 kg m^{-2}. Advice concerning the reduction of high fat and energy-dense foods, in particular those high in saturated fat and free sugars will usually help to achieve a weight loss. Fiber intake should be encouraged. If such measures do not result in a desired weight reduction, it may be necessary to offer specific weight reduction programs, which also include increased physical activity and behavior modification approaches (6,40). The use of very low-energy diets should be restricted to persons with a BMI > 35 kg m^{-2} (6).

Carbohydrate and Type 2 Diabetes

The recommended intake of carbohydrate for people with diabetes is 45% to 60% of total energy intake (Table 2). Provided that foods rich in fiber and with low-glycemic index predominate, there are no known deleterious effects with this range of carbohydrate intake. When carbohydrate intakes are at the upper end of the proposed range, restriction of carbohydrate to around 45% of total energy and a partly replacement of carbohydrate by monounsaturated fat may be tried for some patients with unsatisfactory glycemic control. However, there is concern that increased fat intake might promote weight gain and potentially contribute to insulin resistance. The advice for carbohydrate intake should therefore be individualized, based on nutrition assessment, metabolic results and treatment goals, however, there is no justification for the recommendation of very low-carbohydrate diets in persons with diabetes (8,43).

Vegetables, legumes, fresh fruit, and whole-grain cereal-derived foods are the preferred sources of carbohydrate. They are rich in fiber, micronutrients, and vitamins, and help to ensure the recommended intakes of other nutrients. However, many individuals with diabetes do not consume such foods on a regular basis (Fig. 2).

A number of factors influence glycemic response to carbohydrate-containing foods, including the nature of the starch (amylose, amylopectin, resistant starch), the amount of dietary fiber and the type of sugar. Different carbohydrates have different glycemic responses and, clearly, the amount of carbohydrate is one important factor in postprandial glucose levels. However, foods with a low-glycemic index may confer benefits not only for postprandial glycemia in persons with type 2 diabetes, but also for their lipid profile (44–48). Foods with a low-glycemic index (e.g., legumes, pasta, parboiled rice, whole-grain breads, oats, certain raw fruits) should therefore be substituted when possible for those with a high-glycemic index (e.g., mashed potatoes, white rice, white bread and rolls, sugary drinks).

People with diabetes should be encouraged to choose a variety of fiber-containing foods. It has been shown that increased fiber intake results in benefits for glycemic control, hyperinsulinemia and serum lipids (49–51). Dietary fiber intake should ideally be more than 40 g/day, about half of which should be soluble, however, beneficial effects are also obtained with lower, and for some, more acceptable amounts (8). The available evidence from controlled clinical studies demonstrates that moderate intake of dietary sucrose in diets with

TABLE 2   Recommended Nutrient Intakes for Persons with Diabetes

Carbohydrate 45% to 60% total energy/day	Metabolic characteristics (HbA$_{1c}$, blood glucose levels, serum lipids) suggest the most appropriate intakes within this range: 225 to 300 g in a 2000 kcal diet; 170 to 225 g in a 1500 kcal diet
	Foods rich in fiber and with low-glycemic index should be preferred (e.g., legumes, vegetables, fresh fruit, whole-grain cereals, parboiled rice, pasta)
Dietary fiber ideally 40 g/day (20 g/1000 kcal)	Naturally occurring foods rich in dietary fiber are encouraged (e.g., 5 servings of fiber-rich vegetables or fruits/day, 4 servings of legumes/week; whenever possible whole-grain cereal-based foods)
Glycemic index	Carbohydrate-rich, low-glycemic index foods are a suitable choice provided also other attributes of the foods are appropriate
Sucrose and other free sugars < 10% total energy	Monosaccharides and disaccharides added to foods or sugars naturally present in honey, syrup or fruit juice ≤ 50 g in a 2000 kcal diet; ≤ 37 g in a 1500 kcal diet
Total dietary fat ≤ 35% energy/day	≤ 75 g in a 2000 kcal diet; ≤ 55 g in a 1500 kcal diet
Saturated fatty acids plus trans-unsaturated fatty acids < 10% total energy	If LDL-cholesterol is elevated < 7% total energy (trans-fats are present in several manufactured foods that contain partly hydrogenated fats → see labeling)
Polyunsaturated fatty acids ($n-6$) up to 10% total energy	Corn, sunflower, soya bean oils, and seeds
Consider $n-3$ unsaturated fatty acids	Oily fish (2–3 servings/week) and rapeseed oil, soya bean oil, nuts
(Cis-) Monounsaturated fatty acids 10% to 20% total energy	Olive oil, rapeseed oil
Cholesterol < 300 mg/day	If LDL-cholesterol is elevated < 200 mg/day
Protein 10% to 20% total energy/day	≤ 100 g in a 2000 kcal diet; ≤ 75 g in a 1500 kcal diet (beneficial effects of restricted intakes to 0.8 g/kg desirable body weight have been shown in persons with type 1 diabetes with macroalbuminuria)
Alcohol < 20 g/day for men < 10 g/day for women	1 to 2 small drinks/day (e.g., wine or beer)
Antioxidant nutrients, vitamins, minerals, and trace elements	Foods naturally rich in dietary antioxidants (tocopherols, carotenoids, vitamin C, flavonoids, polyphenols, phytic acid) should be encouraged
Supplements and functional foods	No recommendations are offered. Further research is needed.

an appreciable amount of fiber—with the sucrose displacing other fiber-depleted carbohydrate-containing food—does not worsen glycemic control in persons with diabetes (52–54). Thus, sucrose and other added sugars may be included in moderation in the diets of people with type 2 diabetes, however, the bulk of dietary carbohydrate should be derived from foods with a low-glycemic index and/or rich in fiber. It is of interest that low-glycemic index foods and fiber-rich foods appear to have an effect independent of other attributes; but many high-fiber foods do indeed have a low-glycemic index, and vice versa.

Fructose produces a reduction in postprandial glycemia when it replaces sucrose, however, this potential benefit is tempered by the fact that higher amounts of fructose may

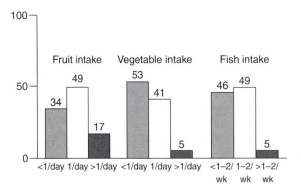

FIGURE 2   Frequency of fresh fruit, vegetable, and fish intake (n%) in a sample of 1988 persons with diabetes [930 male, 1058 female; mean age 57 ± 13 years; mean diabetes duration 8 (1–56) years] in Germany in 2000.

adversely effect plasma lipids by increasing triglycerides. But there is no reason to recommend that persons with diabetes avoid naturally occurring fructose, e.g., in fruits, vegetables and other foods. A moderate intake of fructose (up to 30 g/day) appears to have no deleterious effects on plasma insulin and lipids in persons with type 2 diabetes (8). Adding fructose, sugar alcohols, and other nutritive sweeteners, all of which are energy sources, does not have substantial advantage over added sucrose as a sweetener for people with diabetes and therefore should not to be encouraged (6,7,10). Intake of food containing sugar alcohols has been reported to cause diarrhea. Furthermore, it is unlikely that sugar alcohols in the amounts likely to be ingested in foods or meals will contribute to a significant reduction in total energy or carbohydrate intake, although they are only partially absorbed from the small intestine.

Approved nonnutritive sweeteners may be used by people with diabetes to sweeten beverages, desserts, fruits, etc. (6,14,55). The recommended acceptable daily intake (ADI), defined as the amount of a food additive that can be safely consumed on a daily basis over a person's lifetime without risk, should be considered when nonnutritive sweeteners are chosen. However, it is unknown whether the use of nonnutritive sweeteners improves glycemic control or assists in weight loss in persons with diabetes.

For individuals with type 2 diabetes treated with insulin, to avoid hypoglycemia and excessive postprandial hyperglycemia it is important that the timing and dose of insulin match the amount, type, and time of carbohydrate-containing food intake (8,9). Individuals receiving intensive insulin therapy should adjust their premeal insulin dose based on the content and glycemic load of carbohydrate-containing snacks and meals. In persons with type 2 diabetes postprandial glucose responses to a variety of carbohydrates are similar if the amount of carbohydrate is constant (14). Patients should therefore try to be consistent in day-to-day carbohydrate intake when they are treated with fixed daily insulin doses or with high doses of sulfonylurea or glitinides to avoid hypoglycemic episodes. Self-monitoring of blood glucose is helpful in determining the most appropriate timing of food intake and optimal food choices for the individual patient. There are no general principles regarding the optimum frequency of snacks and meals. Individual preferences, the needs of different treatment regimes and total energy requirements are the main determinants of meal frequency and portion sizes (6).

Fat Modification

The primary goal regarding dietary fat intake in individuals with type 2 diabetes is to decrease intake of saturated fatty acids. Compared with the nondiabetic population, persons with diabetes have an increased risk of cardiovascular disease and the intake of saturated fat is already undesirably high in most countries with a western way of life. To assist in achieving optimal low-density lipoprotein (LDL)-cholesterol levels (<100 mg dL^{-1}) it is recommended that the intake of saturated fatty acids plus trans-unsaturated fatty acids be limited to no more than 10% of total energy intake, and the amount of dietary cholesterol to <300 mg/day (6–10,56). In patients with elevated LDL-cholesterol, a further reduction of saturated fat to $<7\%$, and of dietary cholesterol to <200 mg/day, have been recommended for nondiabetics with dyslipidemia. Although specific studies in persons with diabetes are not available to conclusively demonstrate the effects of these limits, the goals for patients with diabetes remain the same as for other high-risk groups (Table 3).

For those on weight-maintaining diets, the debate has focused on what is the best energy source alternative to saturated fat. Several studies suggest that saturated fat could be replaced by carbohydrate food rich in fiber and/or by *cis*-monounsaturated fatty acids (6,7,57). Diets high in *cis*-mono-unsaturated fatty acids, or low in fat and high in fiber-rich carbohydrate result in improvements in glycemia and lipid levels compared with diets high in saturated fat.

Controversial results have been reported from the few studies that evaluated the effects of polyunsaturated fat and glycemic control and serum lipid levels in persons with type 2 diabetes. It is currently recommended that intake should be $<10\%$ of total energy, based upon the potential adverse consequences of increased lipid oxidation and reduced levels of high-density lipoprotein associated with high intakes (8,9).

$N - 3$ polyunsaturated fat (omega-3 fatty acids) has the potential to reduce serum triglyceride levels, particularly in persons with hypertriglyceridemia, and to have beneficial

TABLE 3   Dietary Modifications to Reduce Cardiovascular Risk Factors in Type 2 Diabetes

When body weight is high (overweight: BMI ≥ 25 to $29.9\,kg\;m^{-2}$; obesity: BMI $\geq 30\,kg\;m^{-2}$) and/or waist circumference suggests an increased or markedly increased risk for cardiovascular disease (males >94 or $>102\,cm$, females >80 or $>88\,cm$):
Reduce caloric intake (e.g., minus $500\,kcal/day$)- Increase physical activity (e.g., at least 30 min at 3–4 days/week)
Reduce energy-dense foods, particularly those high in saturated fat and free sugars
Increase foods rich in fiber
Reduce consumption of alcoholic drinks
When blood pressure is elevated ($\geq 130/80\,mmHg$):
Reduce salt intake to target of $<6\,g/day$ (particularly if salt sensitive)
Avoid added salt
Avoid obviously salted foods (particularly processed foods)
Prefer meals cooked directly from natural ingredients
When serum cholesterol is elevated (total cholesterol $>170\,mg/dL$ or LDL-cholesterol $>100\,mg/dL$)
Restrict intakes of saturated fat and trans-fatty acids ($<7\%$ total energy) and dietary cholesterol intake ($<200\,mg/day$)
Substitute mono-unsaturated fat for saturated fat
Increase intake of fiber
Choose meat, cold meat and sausage with a lower fat content
Consume skimmed milk and fat-reduced milk products
Restrict the consumption of high-fat snacks (e.g., potato chips, chocolate, cakes, and cookies)
Prefer use of vegetable oils, particularly oils rich in mono-unsaturated fat
Use fat and oils only in small quantities
Consume five portions of vegetables or fruits per day
Give preference to whole-meal or whole-grain cereals and cereal products

effects on platelet aggregation and thrombogenicity (58). Although studies of the effects of $n\,-3$ fatty acids in patients with diabetes have primarily used fish-oil supplements, there is evidence from the general population that foods containing $n\,-\,3$ fatty acids have cardioprotective effects. Food sources of $n\,-\,3$ polyunsaturated fat include fatty fish and plant sources, such as rapeseed oil, soya bean oil, and nuts. The consumption of at least 2–3 helpings of oily fish each week will contribute to ensuring an adequate intake of $n\,-\,3$ fatty acids (6,8,11).

Trans-unsaturated fatty acids are produced during the hydrogenation of unsaturated fats and are found in many manufactured products, such as biscuits, cakes, confectionery, soups, and some margarines. When studied independently of other fatty acids the effect of trans-fatty acids is similar to that of saturated fats in raising LDL-cholesterol. The intake of trans-fatty acids therefore should be minimized (7,8).

Dietary Protein

A few studies suggest that persons with type 2 diabetes have an increased need for protein during moderate hyperglycemia, and an altered adaptive mechanism for protein-sparing during weight-loss, resulting in an increased protein requirement. However, in many countries the protein intake for persons with diabetes is relatively high and exceeds by far the recommended dietary allowance (RDA) of $0.8\,g\;kg^{-1}$ desirable body weight for adults. On average, protein intake was 21% of daily energy in the UKPDS. In general, there seems to be little concern that persons with diabetes may develop a deficiency in protein intake (59). The current recommendation for people with diabetes is that protein may provide 10% to 20% of total energy intake. In individuals with controlled type 2 diabetes, ingested protein does not increase glucose concentrations (14).

An association between dietary protein intake and renal disease has been shown in a large-scale cross-sectional study of people with type 1 diabetes. Those with a protein intake above 20% of total energy intake had abnormal albumin excretion rates (AER $>20\,\mu g\;min^{-1}$), particularly when hypertension was present (59). This suggests that a very high-protein intake may have undesirable effects on renal function, and it may be prudent to avoid a very high protein intake.

Several studies have focused on reversing or retarding the progression of proteinuria, and preventing nephropathy. Only a few studies have evaluated nutritional modifications, particularly a reduction of protein intake in patients with type 2 diabetes. With reductions in protein intake, to $0.8\,g\,kg^{-1}$ body weight, AER were reduced in patients with microalbuminuria (60,61), however, the studies were of short duration and do not allow a general recommendation for this kind of protein restriction in microalbuminuric persons with type 2 diabetes. Whether substituting vegetable protein for protein from animal sources might result in beneficial effects has also been explored; however, there is still insufficient evidence to make firm recommendations regarding the nature of dietary protein in individuals with diabetes.

Alcohol

Precautions regarding alcohol intake that apply to the general population also apply to people with type 2 diabetes. If persons with diabetes choose to drink alcohol, intake should be no more than 10 g/day for adult women and 20 g/day for adult men. This corresponds to approximately one or two small drinks of wine or beer per day (8,9). The cardioprotective effect of alcohol appears not to be determined by the type of the alcoholic beverages consumed. However, alcohol is an important energy source in overweight persons with type 2 diabetes, and alcohol consumption can be associated with raised blood pressure and hypertriglyceridemia. In individuals with diabetes, chronic intake of moderate amounts (5–15 g/day) of alcohol was associated with a decreased risk of coronary heart disease. However, conversely, a strong association between excessive habitual intake (> 30–60 g/day) of alcohol and raised blood pressure was found in both men and women (62).

Alcohol can have both hypoglycemic and hyperglycemic effects in people with diabetes, depending on the amount of alcohol acutely ingested. In studies where alcoholic beverages were consumed with carbohydrate-containing food by people with diabetes, no acute effects were seen on blood glucose or insulin levels. Alcohol should therefore be consumed with food to reduce the risk of hypoglycemia and persons with diabetes are advised not to omit food when choosing to drink a moderate amount of alcoholic beverages (8,9).

Vitamins and Minerals

Individuals with diabetes should be advised about the importance of acquiring daily vitamin and mineral requirements from natural food sources. Regular consumption of a variety of vegetables, fresh fruit (five or more servings of vegetables or fruits per day), legumes, low-fat milk, vegetable oils, nuts, whole-grain breads, and oily fish should be encouraged to ensure that recommended intakes are met (8,14). On the other hand, people with diabetes should be advised to restrict salt intake to under 6 g/day, particularly when elevated blood pressure is a problem.

Persons with diabetes may have increased oxidative stress, there has therefore been interest in recommending intake of antioxidant vitamins. However, placebo-controlled trials have failed to show a clear benefit from antioxidant supplementation and, in some cases, adverse effects have been suggested e.g., for beta-carotene supplements (14).

The role of folate supplementation in reducing cardiovascular events is still under further investigation. Vitamin and mineral supplementation in pharmacological dosages should be viewed as a therapeutic intervention, and recommended only in case of proven deficiencies (6,8). There is no clear evidence of benefit from vitamin or mineral supplementation in people who do not have underlying deficiencies. Evaluation of the micronutrient status of a person with type 2 diabetes begins with a careful dietary history, as laboratory evaluation is often confounded by methodological problems. However, measurements of serum folate, vitamin B12, vitamin D, calcium, potassium, magnesium, and iron concentrations may be clinically useful to define micronutrient deficiencies (14).

TABLE 4 Nutritional Management as Part of the Continuing Treatment and Education Process in Persons with Type 2 Diabetes

Nutritional review and individual recommendations
At diagnosis
At each consultation if the patient is overweight or vascular risk factors are not well controlled
Every year as a routine
At the beginning of insulin therapy
On special request

Check
Is healthy eating a part of lifestyle? Is energy intake appropriate for attaining or maintaining a desirable body
  weight (BMI <25 kg m^{-2})?
Is alcohol intake moderate, or could it be exacerbating hypertension, hypertriglyceridemia, or contributing to hypoglycemia?
Is money being spent unnecessarily on special diabetic food products?
Does the distribution of meals or snacks reflect the glucose-lowering medication?
Does raised blood pressure suggest a benefit from salt (<6 g/day) restriction?

Advise
Carbohydrate intake should be higher and fat intake lower than presently consumed in most countries—reducing saturated
  fats and/or trans-fats (e.g., in cream, chocolates, fast foods, high-fat cheese, sausages, meat, spreads, and fatty bakery)
The use of fresh fruit and vegetables (5 servings a day)
Consuming preferably whole-grain breads and cereals, parboiled rice, pasta, legumes
The use of vegetable oils (e.g., olive oil, rapeseed oil, soya bean oil), nuts, seeds and oily fish
Sugar does not need to be excluded but should be limited
Alcoholic beverages, if desired, should be consumed as part of the total caloric intake (no more than 1–2 small drinks/day)
Meals, snacks, and food choices should match individual therapeutic needs, preferences and culture

NUTRITIONAL ADVICE AND STRUCTURED TRAINING

Each patient with type 2 diabetes needs individual advice and structured training by his or her physician and other members of the healthcare team, to enable them to translate the principles of nutrition in type 2 diabetes into specific actions in daily life (Table 4). A balance must be achieved among the demands of metabolic control, risk factor management, and the patient's well-being and safety. The therapeutic needs of an individual person will change with time and, therefore, continuing nutritional education must be provided (38,39). To improve compliance, the main aspects of dietary advice given to a person with diabetes should also have a potential benefit for family members and should be acceptable to them.

A nutritional history should be taken at diagnosis, as well as at visits whenever the patient is not well controlled and it is thought that nutritional factors might have contributed to the unsatisfactory metabolic results. A nutritional review and individual nutritional recommendations should be provided at least once a year, or more often on special request (38).

Individual advice can be combined with structured group training. Since the clinical picture and the personal situation of the individual with diabetes may change during the course of the disease, different priorities are required in the training programs.

All steps in the nutritional management of a person with type 2 diabetes should be documented and the outcome evaluated by means of important markers, such as body weight, waist circumference, blood pressure, HbA$_{1c}$, fasting, and/or postprandial blood glucose (self-) monitoring, serum-lipids, AER and well-being or quality of life.

REFERENCES

1. American Diabetes Association. Type 2 diabetes in children and adolescents. Consensus statement. Diabetes Care 2000; 23:381–9.
2. Seidell JC. Obesity, insulin resistance and diabetes—a world wide epidemic. Br J Nutr 2000; 83 (Suppl. 1):5S–8S.
3. Dunstan DN, Zimmet PZ, Welborn TA, et al. The rising prevalence of diabetes and impaired glucose tolerance: the Australian Diabetes, Obesity, and Lifestyle Study. Diabetes Care 2002; 25:829–34.

4. Hadden DR, Blair ALT, Wilson EZ, et al. Natural history of diabetes presenting at age 40–69 years: a prospective study of the influence of intensive dietary therapy. QJM 1986; 59:579–98.

5. Feskens EJ, Virtanen SM, Räsänen L, et al. Dietary factors determining diabetes and impaired glucose tolerance: a 20-year follow-up of the Finnish and Dutch cohorts of the Seven Countries Study. Diabetes Care 1995; 18:1104–12.

6. Mann J, Lean M, Toeller M, et al. on behalf of the Diabetes and Nutrition Study Group (DNSG) of the European Association for the Study of Diabetes (EASD). Recommendations for the nutritional management of patients with diabetes mellitus. Eur J Clin Nutr 2000; 54:353–5.

7. American Diabetes Association. Evidence-based nutrition principles and recommendations for the treatment and prevention of diabetes related complications. Position statement. Diabetes Care 2002; 25:202–12.

8. Mann J, De Leeuw I, Hermansen K, et al. on behalf of the Diabetes and Nutrition Study Group (DNSG) of the European Association for the Study of Diabetes (EASD). Evidence-based nutritional approaches to the treatment and prevention of diabetes mellitus. Nutr Metab Cardiovasc Dis 2004; 14:373–94.

9. American Diabetes Association. Nutritional principles and recommendations in diabetes. Diabetes Care 2004; 27(Suppl. 1):S36–46.

10. Nutrition Subcommittee of the Diabetes Care Advisory Committee of Diabetes UK. The implementation of nutritional advice for people with diabetes. Diabetic Medicine 2003; 20:786–807.

11. Mann J, Toeller M. Type 2 diabetes: aetiology and environmental factors. In: Ekoe J-M, Zimmet P, Williams R, eds. The Epidemiology of Diabetes Mellitus. Chichester, John Wiley & Sons, 2001:133–40.

12. Turner RC, Millns H, Neil HA, et al. Risk factors for coronary artery disease in non-insulin dependent diabetes mellitus: United Kingdom Prospective Diabetes Study (UKPDS: 23). BMJ 1998; 316:823–8.

13. Liu S, Manson JE, Stampfer MJ, et al. A prospective study of whole grain intake and risk of type 2 diabetes mellitus in US women. Am J Public Health 2000; 90:1409–15.

14. Franz MJ, Bantle JP, Beebe CA, et al. Evidence-based nutrition principles and recommendations for the treatment and prevention of diabetes and related complications. Technical review. Diabetes Care 2002; 25:148–98.

15. Hu FB, van Dam RM, Liu S. Diet and risk of type 2 diabetes: the role of types of fat and carbohydrate. Diabetologia 2002; 44:805–17.

16. McAuley KA, Williams SM, Mann JI, et al. Intensive lifestyle changes are necessary to improve insulin sensitivity: a randomized controlled trial. Diabetes Care 2002; 25:445–52.

17. Tuomilehto J, Lindstrom J, Eriksson JG, et al. Prevention of type 2 diabetes mellitus by changes in lifestyle among subjects with impaired glucose tolerance. N Engl J Med 2001; 344:1343–50.

18. Lindström J, Peltonen M, Eriksson JE, et al. High fibre, low fat diets predict long-term weight loss and decreased type 2 diabetes risk. The Finnish Diabetes Prevention Study. Diabetologia 2006; 49: 912–20.

19. The Diabetes Prevention Program Research Group. The Diabetes Prevention Program: design and methods for a clinical trial in the prevention of type 2 diabetes. Diabetes Care 1999; 22:623–31.

20. Knowler WC, Barrett-Connor E, Fowler SE, et al. for the Diabetes Prevention Program Research Group. Reduction in the incidence of type 2 diabetes with lifestyle intervention or metformin. N Engl J Med 2002; 346:393–403.

21. Ha TKK, Lean MEJ on behalf of the Diabetes and Nutrition Study Group (DNSG) of the European Association for the Study of Diabetes (EASD). Technical review: recommendations for the nutritional management of patients with diabetes mellitus. Eur J Clin Nutr 1998; 52:467–81.

22. Bray GA, Nielsen SJ, Popkin BM. Consumption of high-fructose corn syrup in beverages may play a role in the epidemic of obesity. Am J Clin Nutr 2004; 79:537–43.

23. Schulze MB, Manson JE, Ludwig DS, et al. Sugar sweetened beverages, weight gain and incidence of type 2 diabetes in young and middle-aged women. JAMA 2004; 292:927–34.

24. Jacobs DR, Meyer KA, Kushi LH, Folsom AR. Whole grain intake may reduce the risk of ischemic heart disease death in postmenopausal women: the Iowa Women's Health Study. Am J Clin Nutr 1998; 68:248–57.

25. Marshall JA, Hoag S, Shetterly S, Hamman RF. Dietary fat predicts conversion from impaired glucose tolerance to NIDDM. The San Luis Valley Diabetes Study. Diabetes Care 1994; 17:50–6.

26. Colditz GA, Manson JE, Stampfer MJ, et al. Diet and risk of clinical diabetes in women. Am J Clin Nutr 1992; 55:1018–23.

27. Vessby B, Aro A, Skarfors E, et al. The risk to develop NIDDM is related to the fatty acid composition of the serum cholesterol esters. Diabetes 1994; 43:1353–7.

28. Vessby B, Uusitupa M, Hermansen K, et al. Substituting dietary saturated fat with monounsaturated fat impairs insulin sensitivity in healthy men and women: the KANWU Study. Diabetologia 2001; 44: 312–9.

29. Feskens EJ, Bowles CH, Kromhout D. Inverse association between fish intake and risk of glucose tolerance in normoglycemic elderly men and women. Diabetes Care 1991; 14:935–41.

30. Haffner SM. Management of dyslipidemia in adults with diabetes. Technical review. Diabetes Care 1998; 21:160–78.
31. Svethey LP, Simons-Morton D, Vollmer WM, et al. for the DASH Collaborative Research Group. Effects of dietary patterns of blood pressure: subgroup analysis of the Dietary Approaches to Stop Hypertension (DASH). Randomized clinical trial. Arch Intern Med 1999; 159:285–93.
32. Adler A, Stevens RJ, Neil A, et al. UKPDS 59: hyperglycaemia and other potentially modifiable risk factors for peripheral vascular disease in type 2 diabetes. Diabetes Care 2002; 25:894–9.
33. Holbrook TL, Barrett-Connor E, Wingard DL. A prospective population-based study of alcohol use and non-insulin-dependent diabetes mellitus. Am J Epidemiol 1990; 132:902–9.
34. Facchini F, Chen J, Reaven GM. Light to moderate alcohol intake is associated with enhanced insulin sensitivity. Diabetes Care 1994; 17:115–9.
35. Riccardi G, Rivellese AA. Dietary treatment of the metabolic syndrome: the optimal diet. Br J Nutr 2000; 83 (Suppl. 1):S143–8.
36. Toeller M. Well-being in non-insulin-dependent diabetic patients–a long term follow-up. In: Lefèbvre PJ, Standl E, eds. New Aspects in Diabetes. Berlin, New York: Walter de Gruyter, 1992; 127–43.
37. Coulston AM, Mandelbaum D, Reaven GM. Dietary management of nursing home residents with non-insulin-dependent diabetes mellitus. Am J Clin Nutr 1990; 51:62–71.
38. European Diabetes Policy Group. A desktop guide to type 2 diabetes mellitus. Diabetic Medicine 1999; 16:716–30.
39. American Diabetes Association. Position Statement. Standards of medical care in diabetes. Diabetes Care 2005; 28 (Suppl. 1):S4–6.
40. Astrup A, Grunwald GK, Melanson EL, et al. The role of low-fat diets in body weight control: a meta-analysis of ad libitum dietary intervention studies. Int J Obes Relat Metab Disord 2000; 24: 1545–52.
41. UKPDS Group. UK Prospective Complications Study: response of fasting plasma glucose to diet therapy in newly presenting type 2 patients with diabetes. Metabolism 1990; 39:905–12.
42. WHO. Technical Report Series 916. Diet, nutrition and the prevention of chronic diseases. Report of a Joint FAO/WHO Expert Consultation. Geneva, Switzerland: World Health Organization, 2003.
43. American Diabetes Association. Statement. Dietary carbohydrate (amount and type) in the prevention and management of diabetes. Diabetes Care 2004; 27:2266–71.
44. Frost G, Wilding J, Beecham J. Dietary advice based on the glycaemic index improves dietary profile and metabolic control in type 2 diabetic patients. Diabet Med 1994; 11:397–401.
45. Järvi AE, Karlström BK, Granfeldt YE, et al. Improved glycemic control and lipid profile and normalized fibrinolytic activity on a low glycemic index diet in type 2 diabetes mellitus patients. Diabetes Care 1999; 22:10–8.
46. Bouché C, Rizkalla SW, Luo J, et al. Five-week, low-glycemic index diet decreases total fat mass and improves plasma lipid profile in moderately overweight nondiabetic men. Diabetes Care 2002; 25: 822–8.
47. Mann J, Hermansen K, Vessby B, Toeller M. Evidence-based nutritional recommendations for the treatment and prevention of diabetes and related complications. A European perspective (letter). Diabetes Care 2002 2s:1256–58.
48. Brand-Miller J, Hayne S, Petocz P, Colagiuri S. Low-glycemic index diets in the management of diabetes. A meta-analysis of randomized controlled trials. Diabetes Care 2003; 26:2261–7.
49. Brown L, Rosner B, Willett WW, Sacks FM. Cholesterol lowering effects of dietary fiber: a meta-analysis. Am J Clin Nutr 1999; 69:30–42.
50. Chandalia M, Garg A, Lutjohann D, et al. Beneficial effects of high dietary fiber intake in patients with type 2 diabetes. N Engl J Med 2000; 342:1392–8.
51. Jenkins DJA, Kendall CWC, Vuksan V, et al. Soluble fiber intake at a dose approved by the US Food and Drug Administration for a claim of health benefits: serum lipid risk factors for cardiovascular disease assessed in a randomized controlled crossover trial. Am J Clin Nutr 2002; 75:834–9.
52. Peterson DB, Lambert J, Gerring S, et al. Sucrose in the diet of diabetic patients–just another carbohydrate? Diabetologia 1986; 29:216–20.
53. Toeller M. Dietary programmes and the use of sweeteners in diabetes. In: Mogensen CE, Standl E, eds. Concepts for the ideal diabetes clinic. Berlin, New York: Walter de Gruyter, 1992; 153–70.
54. Nadeau J, Koski KG, Strychar I, Yale JF. Teaching subjects with type 2 diabetes how to incorporate sugar choices into their daily meal plan promotes dietary compliance and does not deteriorate metabolic profile. Diabetes Care 2001; 24:222–7.
55. Toeller M. Diet and diabetes. Diabetes/Metabolism Reviews 1993; 9:93–108.
56. Laitinen JH, Ahola IE, Sarkkinen ES, et al. Impact of intensified dietary therapy on energy and nutrient intakes and fatty acid composition of serum lipids with recently diagnosed non-insulin dependent diabetes mellitus. Am J Diet Assoc 1993; 93:276–83.
57. Garg A. High-monounsaturated fat diets for patients with diabetes mellitus: a meta-analysis. Am J Clin Nutr 1998; 67:577S–82S.

58. Friedberg CE, Janssen MJEM, Heine RJ, Grobbee DE. Fish oil and glycemic control in diabetes: a meta-analysis. Diabetes Care 1999; 21:494–500.
59. Toeller M, Buyken AE. Dietary modifications in patients with diabetic nephropathy. In: Hasslacher C, ed. Diabetic Nephropathy. Chichester, New York: John Wiley & Sons, 2001; 265–76.
60. Kasiske BL, Lakatua JDA, Ma JL, Louis TA. A meta-analysis of the effects of dietary protein restriction on the rate of decline in renal function. Am J Kidney Dis 1998; 31:954–61.
61. Pijls LTJ, de Vries H, Donker AJM, van Eijk JTM. The effect of protein restriction on albuminuria in patients with type 2 diabetes mellitus: a randomized trial. Nephrol Dial Transpl 1999; 14:1445–53.
62. Bell RA, Mayer-Davis EJ, Martin MA, et al. Associations between alcohol consumption and insulin sensitivity and cardiovascular disease risk factors: the Insulin Resistance and Atherosclerosis Study. Diabetes Care 2000; 53:1630–6.

6 | Diabetes and Exercise

Gerhard Schuler and Axel Linke
Department of Internal Medicine/Cardiology, University of Leipzig, Leipzig, Germany

EXERCISE AND PRIMARY PREVENTION

The first systematic investigation on the effect of regular physical exercise as a protective factor against coronary artery disease was published more than 60 years ago (1). It showed a negative correlation between the amount of physical work performed and the incidence of myocardial infarction in London bus drivers. Since then this finding has been confirmed by a great number of studies conducted on thousands of patients. More than 3000 healthy, nondiabetic volunteers participated in the U.S. railroad study, which established a linear, inverse relation between the amount of energy spent during leisure time physical activity and the risk to develop coronary artery disease (2). The lowest risk was calculated for the most active persons who consumed more than 3000 kcal/week, which requires roughly 6 hours of training at medium intensity. The optimal level of intensity has been a matter of considerable controversy and contradictory recommendations. In the U.S. railroad study 100 kcal/week spent in the form of intensive exercise weighed as much as 1000 kcal/week of moderate exercise with regard to its protective effect, i.e., intensive physical exercise was 10 times more effective than moderate exercise, whereas walking was associated with beneficial effects in other trials (3, 4).

An interesting trial has been published under the name Harvard Alumni study (5); in 16,936 college alumni the amount of leisure time physical activity was estimated from questionnaires and structured interviews. After an observation time between 12 and 16 years participants in the most active group reduced their cardiovascular risk by 50% as compared to inactive persons. All of the above studies determined physical activity by questionnaire with an inherent degree of error. A recently published trial used the maximal work capacity on a treadmill to determine "physical fitness" as a hard parameter in more than 6000 patients referred for evaluation of various angina-like symptoms. Cardiovascular risk in the fittest quintile was only one-quarter of the risk in the quintile with the lowest fitness (6). In total there are more than 30 publications with nearly 250,000 enrolled patients, followed for an average of 10 years, documenting the efficacy of regular physical exercise to reduce cardiovascular risk in primary prevention. Accordingly the ACC/AHA task force on primary prevention determined that there is sufficient evidence to make exercise a class I recommendation for primary prevention of coronary artery disease without the need for further studies in this field.

EFFECTS OF EXERCISE IN DIABETICS

Metabolic Effects

During exercise at maximal levels energy demands may be 20-fold increased as compared to resting conditions. In order to maintain homeostasis and prevent hypoglycemia several regulatory mechanisms are activated. Initially skeletal muscles break down their own stores of glycogen, triglycerides, and free fatty acids derived from adipose tissue. In order to mobilize extramuscular stores adjustments on a hormonal basis are necessary. In the early phase of exercise hepatic glucose production is increased by a reduction of insulin levels in the presence of unchanged glucagon levels. In subsequent stages glucagon and catecholamine levels are elevated. As a result, glucose levels in healthy individuals remain fairly constant during exercise. In patients with diabetes type 2 exercise of moderate or high intensity regularly decreases blood glucose levels as a result of insulin-independent activation of glucose transport (7) as well as increased insulin sensitivity (8). Due to an exaggerated counter-regulatory response in the postexercise period hyperglycemia and hyperinsulinemia is frequently encountered in patients with type 2 diabetes.

Following a meal most of the glucose contained in it is rapidly taken up by skeletal muscle and deposited as glycogen. In addition, exercise per se is a powerful stimulator of glucose uptake; part of this action is explained by the increase of skeletal muscle glucose transporter protein (GLUT4) in healthy individuals as well as in patients with type 2 diabetes; it is responsible for insulin-independent glucose transport into skeletal muscle. Following a session of exercise with total depletion of muscular glycogen stores sufficient amounts of glucose need to be absorbed in order to replenish the stores resulting in an increase of insulin sensitivity for more than 72 hours. Conversely, after 6 months of training insulin sensitivity returned to baseline after only 72 hours of sedentary lifestyle, underlining the importance of persistent and regular exercise (9).

Regular physical activity is associated with changes in body composition with a reduction in body fat, increase in muscle mass, and maximal oxygen uptake in healthy individuals; insulin sensitivity is closely correlated to these factors. Corresponding results are obtained in patients with diabetes type 2 who engage in a structured exercise program. Improvements of insulin sensitivity are independently correlated to a reduction in abdominal obesity and an increase in muscle cross-sectional area (10). The benefits of exercise, however, are only maintained for short periods of time; they attenuate 3 to 6 days after the last exercise session stressing the importance of persistent lifestyle changes (11–13). By adding resistance training to aerobic exercise muscle mass may be increased, particularly in elderly patients who tend to loose muscle mass as a result of aging (10, 14).

Correction of Endothelial Dysfunction

Coronary macroangiopathy is preceded by endothelial dysfunction by many years; a reduction in endothelium-dependent vasodilation is a hallmark of nearly all patients with diabetes type 2 and predicts cardiovascular events (Fig. 1) (10, 15). Endothelial-dependent responses become abnormal very early in the course of the disease and therefore they can be substituted as surrogate markers in interventional trials (16). The quality of vascular reactivity is determined by the balance between NO-production and NO inactivation. NO is elaborated from L-arginin by the endothelial NO-synthase (eNOS) and degraded mainly by free oxygen radicals (ROS); it reaches vascular smooth muscle cell by rapid diffusion and causes a fall of intracellular Ca^{++} concentration resulting in vasodilation. Endothelial dysfunction in diabetes and coronary atherosclerosis can be detected on the basis of paradox vasoconstriction following application of acetylcholine. It is the result of multifactorial process, which eventually leads to reduced concentrations of NO (17). Endothelial NO production is hampered by reduced bioavailability of the precursor L-arginin, by an increased concentration of asymmetric dimethylarginin (ADMA), which inhibits eNOS activity, as well as by alterations of the eNOS protein structure found in patients with polymorphisms (18–23).

Free oxygen radicals that are produced by a number of enzymes particularly in patients with diabetes are capable of destroying NO. Superoxide anions, elaborated by the

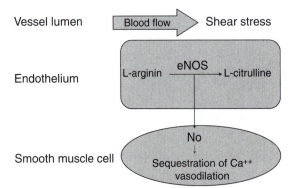

FIGURE 1 Blood flow in the coronary vessel causes deformation of the endothelial cell. In response to shear stress, endothelial NO synthase elaborates NO from L-arginin, which diffuses rapidly into smooth muscles in the vessel wall and results in sequestration of intracellular Ca^{++} and consecutive vasodilation.

NADPH-oxidase and xanthin-oxidase, are responsible for NO-degradation in the first line (24, 25). In addition ROS oxidate tetrahydrobiopterin, an essential cofactor of eNOS. This leads to an uncoupling of eNOS, which now starts to produce oxygen radicals instead of NO, further aggravating endothelial dysfunction (17, 26).

To counterbalance premature NO degradation a number of enzymatic and nonenzymatic protective mechanisms are available within the endothelium; the most important are superoxide dismutase (SOD), extracellular SOD, glutathionperoxidase, catalase, and thioredoxin/thioredoxin-reductase.

A previously published study showed that endothelial dysfunction may be corrected by regular physical exercise in patients with congestive heart failure or atherosclerotic heart disease (Fig. 2) (27). Patients with stable angina pectoris were randomized between an active intervention group, which exercised on stationary bicycles, and an inactive control group. At baseline endothelial function was assessed by intracoronary infusion of acetylcholine, which was highly abnormal in both groups. Following 4 weeks of submaximal exercise paradox vasoconstriction in response to acetylcholine was reduced by 54%. Peak blood flow velocity in response to intracoronary adenosine, representing coronary vasodilatory reserve, improved by 64%. This finding may in part explain the reduction of anginal symptoms frequently observed in patients exercising on a regular basis.

Mobilization of Endothelial Precursor Cells

Apoptosis of endothelial cells in diabetes type 2 and atherosclerosis eventually results in loss of integrity of the endothelial lining with the consequences described above (Fig. 3). Until recently it was accepted that repair of these defects could only be accomplished by local endothelial cells. Recently published observations, however, indicate that certain subpopulations of bone marrow stem cells, circulatory endothelial progenitor cells (CPCs), can be mobilized in response to various stimuli, such as exercise and growth factors (28). After leaving the bone marrow they home in to vessels with defective endothelial lining; they attach to these defective areas and become competent and functional endothelial cells. Their concentration in the peripheral circulation can be increased by regular physical exercise; moreover, their functional capabilities as reflected by their migratory capacity are improved, and their concentration has been associated with future cardiovascular events. However, their survival and functional integrity in the peripheral circulation is greatly diminished by hyperglycemic states (28, 29).

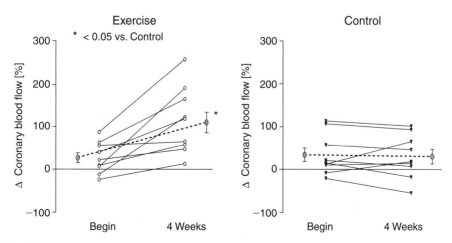

FIGURE 2 Changes in coronary blood flow following 4 weeks of regular physical exercise in patients with coronary artery disease as determined by Doppler sonography in response to acetylcholine. An increase of 68% is noted, significantly different from sedentary control patients. *Source*: From Ref. 27.

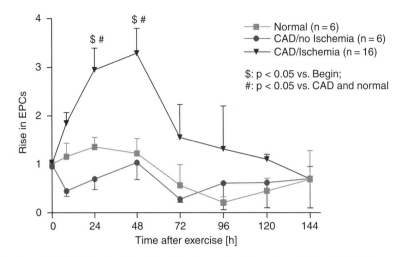

FIGURE 3   Release of EPCs following a bout of physical exercise. There is a significant rise in the number of EPCs detected in the peripheral circulation in patients with ischemia during exercise; no change is detected in normals or in patients with coronary artery disease but without stress-induced ischemia, indicating that ischemia may represent an adequate stimulus for release of EPCs from the bone marrow. *Abbreviation*: EPC, endothelial progenitor cells. *Source*: From Ref. 28.

Does Exercise Correct Overweight/Obesity?

In the metabolic syndrome/diabetes type 2 overweight and physical inactivity are the most conspicuous problems (Fig. 4). Theoretically, overweight could be corrected by an increase of physical activity; in order to burn 0.1 kg of fat 700 kcal need to be expended, i.e., 90 min of bicycle exercise at an intensity of 100 Watts. Requirements to loose significant amounts of weight (>10 kg) and maintain it by exercise only are impressive: 2500 to 2800 kcal need to be expended per week requiring a minimum of 5 to 6 h of exercise at moderate levels (500 kcal/h) (30–35). It is quite obvious that only exceptionally motivated patients are willing to invest the time and the effort to achieve this goal. Moreover, as a result of excessive overweight many patients have lost the capability to undergo such demanding exercise programs. After having been inactive for the better part of their life it would be quite unrealistic to expect radical changes from patients after the age of 50. Thus, most studies relying on exercise only to reduce weight have yielded disappointing results (35,36). Long-term reduction and maintenance of weight can only be achieved by the combination of exercise and reduction of caloric intake. Even after a highly successful and promising start it is difficult for most patients to maintain it for longer periods of time, the daily routines of life slowly erode the initial success and lead to a relentless increase in body weight (37,38). Despite widespread public awareness this epidemic has spread to the younger generation; it can be safely assumed that more than 25% of the school children are overweight at the present time (39,40).

HOW TO PREPARE THE PATIENT WITH DIABETES FOR EXERCISE

Cardiovascular System

The incidence of vascular problems such as coronary artery disease is greatly elevated in patients with type 2 diabetes as compared to a healthy population. Moreover, due to impaired sensation of anginal pain in many individuals uncontrolled exercise may precipitate grave consequences. Cardiac autonomic neuropathy may be suspected in patients with resting tachycardia (>100/min), orthostasis (fall in blood pressure >20 mmHg during upright standing), or signs of autonomous nervous system dysfunction (skin, pupils, gastrointestinal, genitourinary systems). In order to minimize harmful side effects of physical exercise in patients with type 2 diabetes they should undergo a careful evaluation prior to increasing their level of physical activity on a regular basis.

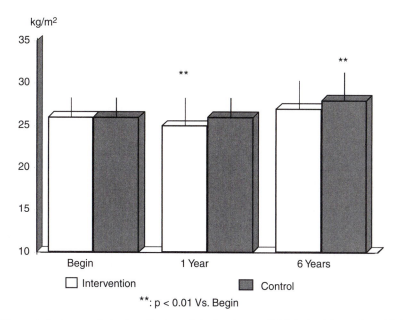

kg/m²

FIGURE 4 Change in body mass index in patients participating in a multirisk factor intervention trial. Initial weight loss of nearly 10% at one year in the intervention group is slowly eroded over time; at 6 years the body mass index tends to be higher as compared to beginning with a gain of 4% (p:n.s.). In the control group there is a significant increase in body mass index by 8% (*p* < 05). *Source*: From Ref. 55.

The following recommendations have been modified from the *Health Professional's Guide to Diabetes and Exercise*. A graded treadmill exercise test should be performed in all patients in order to detect myocardial ischemia, and to determine the individual cardiopulmonary fitness and exercise tolerance. The optimal training heart rate is determined as 80% of the maximal symptom free heart rate. In patients with questionable results alternative stress tests (stress echocardiography, radionuclide stress test) can be employed to increase the diagnostic precision. In patients with typical anginal symptoms or significant ST-segment changes invasive diagnostic coronary angiography is indicated. Patients with hemodynamically significant coronary lesions should undergo either interventional or surgical treatment as indicated prior to embarking on an exercise program.

Long-standing diabetes may result in significant impairment of myocardial function and cause symptoms and signs of congestive heart failure (diabetic cardiomyopathy) (35, 41). Myocardial hypertrophy combined with an increase in interstitial fibrosis may cause diastolic heart failure, indistinguishable from systolic heart failure on clinical grounds. Echocardiography is used to assess left ventricular performance, rule out valvular heart disease and determine left ventricular compliance in patients with myocardial hypertrophy. The magnitude of left ventricular hypertrophy is correlated to the degree and duration of hyperinsulinemia, whereas the degree of left ventricular dysfunction seems to be mainly the result of hyperglycemia.

Peripheral Arterial Disease

Intermittent claudication and trophic changes of the feet are indicators of peripheral arterial disease and should prompt evaluation by duplex sonography and treadmill testing. The presence of palpable pulses does not rule out microangiopathy.

Retinopathy

Patients with proliferative diabetic retinopathy are at risk to develop vitreous hemorrhage or traction retinal detachment during strenuous physical exercise. Their activity should be tailored to their individual need and avoid anaerobic, strenuous exercises. Swimming, walking, or bicycle ergometry are alternative activities recommended for these patients.

Peripheral Neuropathy

Loss of peripheral sensation particularly in the feet may ultimately result in skin ulcerations and fractures. Peripheral neuropathy can be detected by evaluating the tendon reflexes, the vibratory sense, and touch sensation. Weight bearing and repetitive exercises should be limited in these patients.

EFFECTS OF EXERCISE IN DIABETES TYPE 2: CLINICAL STUDIES

Previous studies in nondiabetic patients have shown that exercise reduces hypertension, dyslipidemia, insulin resistance, and hyperglycemia (38, 42–45). In diabetics a number of small studies have been published, however, apart from lacking statistical power, their results were not uniform, and no large-scale studies have been performed so far. A meta-analysis of 14 trials, extracted from a total of 2700 potential articles, included 504 participants. Selection of the studies was based on a predetermined program of physical exercise lasting for a minimum of 8 weeks, supervision of exercise, and presence of type 2 diabetic control group (46). Of the 14 trials, 11 were randomized controlled trials, and 3 were case-control trials. The mean age of the participants was 55.0 ± 7 years, duration of diabetes was 4.3 ± 4.6 years; 50% of the participants were women. The exercise interventions consisted of three workouts per week lasting for a mean of 53 ± 17 min. Exercise consisted of walking or cycling of light to moderate intensity.

Postintervention HbA_{1C} was reduced by 0.66% in the intervention groups as compared to the nonexercise groups; in contrast body mass index remained unchanged. The magnitude of this reduction is comparable to the results of the U.K. Prospective Diabetes study (47), where patients received intensive treatment with insulin or sulfonylureas. In this study HbA_{1C} decreased from 7.9% to 7.0% ($p < .001$), and was associated with a reduction in clinical endpoints from 46 events to 40.9 events per 1000 patient years ($p < .03$).

A more recent meta-analysis of interventional studies using exercise was published in the Cochrane Database (48); 14 studies were included in the analysis comprising 377 patients. There is considerable overlap with the analysis published by Boulé in 2001, and not surprisingly the results and the conclusions are not dissimilar. It is common to all studies that although the benefit of any form of exercise has been proven beyond doubt, adherence to these programs is short and haphazard. The therapeutic benefit offered by this form of treatment is utilized only to a very small degree rendering its efficiency in daily practice insignificant.

EFFECTS OF EXERCISE IN PREDIABETIC SYNDROMES (INSULIN RESISTANCE SYNDROME)

The insulin resistance syndrome has been recognized as an important new risk factor associated with premature coronary artery disease. There seems to be a genetic trait because the underlying abnormality can also be demonstrated in offsprings of parents affected by this syndrome (49, 50). Cardiovascular risk factors, such as hypertension, glucose intolerance, elevated levels of triglycerides combined with low levels of high-density lipoproteins (HDL), and impaired fibrinolytic activity, are detected with a higher frequency in these individuals than expected. There is also considerable evidence that impaired aerobic exercise capacity is an important component of this syndrome. Muscle biopsies obtained from these individuals exhibit a reduction of mitochondrial and capillary density, not totally dissimilar from patients with congestive heart failure (51). It has been speculated that the limited aerobic capacity of skeletal muscles may induce these patients to select a more sedentary lifestyle. Aerobic exercise in sufficient quantity has consistently been shown to ameliorate the effects of this syndrome and prevent progression to overt clinical disease.

PREVENTION OF DIABETES

Several large studies were published on prevention of diabetes type 2 by exercise combined with other interventions such as weight loss and intensified medical treatment. In one study 3234 nondiabetic patients with impaired glucose tolerance were randomly assigned to either placebo, metformin (850 mg twice daily), and lifestyle-modification program with the goals of a minimum of 7% weight loss and 150 min physical activity per week (52). Physical activity was only recommended, not supervised; adherence to the intervention was assessed by a log book kept by the patient. The mean age of the participants was 51 years and average follow-up was 2.8 years. By the end of the curriculum (24 weeks) 50% of the participants in the lifestyle-intervention group had reached the goal of 7% weight loss, which decreased to 38% at the most recent visit, however. The proportion of participants who met the goal of 150 min physical activity per week was 74% at 24 weeks, and 58% at the most recent visit.

Patients assigned to the lifestyle intervention had a much greater weight loss and greater increase in leisure time physical activity than did participants assigned to placebo or metformin. The average weight loss was 0.1, 2.1, and 5.6 kg in the placebo, metformin, and lifestyle-intervention groups, respectively ($p < .001$).

The incidence of diabetes was reduced by 58% in the lifestyle-intervention group, and by 31% in the metformin group, as compared to placebo. Rates of adverse events, hospitalizations, and mortality were similar in both groups. The number needed-to-treat was 6.9 for the lifestyle-intervention, and 13.9 for the metformin group.

Combined effects of lifestyle factors were examined in a large study for which 84,941 nurses were recruited between 1980 and 1996 (53). During 16 years of follow-up 3300 new cases of diabetes type 2 were documented. Overweight or obesity were the single most important predictor of diabetes, but lack of exercise, poor diet, and current smoking were also associated significantly with an increased risk of diabetes. The risk of developing diabetes type 2 could be lowered by 90% by adhering consistently to lifestyle characteristics such as maintaining a body mass index below 25, exercising regularly, eating a prudent diet, abstaining from smoking, and consuming alcohol moderately.

In a large study from China 577 individuals with impaired glucose tolerance were randomized to four different groups: diet only, exercise only, diet plus exercise, and control (54). At 6 years the cumulative incidence of diabetes was 67.7% in the control group as compared to 43.8% in the diet group, 41.1% in the exercise group, and 46.0% in the diet plus exercise group ($p < .05$).

CONCLUSIONS

Physical inactivity has been identified as one of the most important risk factors for developing diabetes type 2. Ninety percent of type 2 cases can be accounted for by a combination of physical inactivity, overweight, and dietary problems. A number of mechanisms have been clarified by which regular exercise is capable of repairing or at least ameliorating the effects of the western lifestyle: expression of eNOS in endothelial cells, mobilization of endothelial precursor cells from the bone marrow, increasing insulin sensitivity in skeletal muscles, and normalizing and maintaining body weight. However, the therapeutic value of physical exercise, although proven beyond any doubt, is severely limited by the inability of the vast majority of patients to implement and maintain lifestyle changes without constant supervision. Adherence to any interventional program advocating regular physical exercise and weight reduction is short-lived and haphazard. Moreover, it can be safely assumed that patients recruited for such a trial represent a positive selection from the large pool of patients not even considering to participate.

In the face of a relentless and accelerating increase of the incidence of type 2 diabetes new strategies are urgently needed to deal with this problem. We have to face the fact that the majority of trials conducted in adults have yielded disappointing long-term results, demonstrating that patient motivation is the limiting factor in these interventions.

Impressive results are usually limited to a brief period of close supervision only to be eroded slowly as soon as the patient returns to normal life. Now it is time to shift the focus of attention to the young generation. The epidemic of overweight and physical inactivity has already arrived in this age bracket, but there is still hope that changes in lifestyle achieved in school children or even in kindergarten may be longer lasting and perhaps permanent.

REFERENCES

1. Morris JN, Heady JA, Raffle PA, Roberts CG, Parks JW. Coronary heart-disease and physical activity of work. Lancet 1953; 265(6796):1111–20.
2. Slattery ML, Jacobs DR Jr, Nichaman MZ. Leisure time physical activity and coronary heart disease death. The US Railroad Study. Circulation 1989; 79(2):304–11.
3. Bijnen FC, Caspersen CJ, Feskens EJ, Saris WH, Mosterd WL, Kromhout D. Physical activity and 10-year mortality from cardiovascular diseases and all causes: the Zutphen Elderly Study. Arch Intern Med 1998; 158(14):1499–505.
4. Hakim AA, Curb JD, Petrovitch H, et al. Effects of walking on coronary heart disease in elderly men: the Honolulu Heart Program. Circulation 1999; 100(1):9–13.
5. Paffenbarger RS Jr, Hyde RT, Wing AL, Hsieh CC. Physical activity, all-cause mortality, and longevity of college alumni. N Engl J Med 1986; 314(10):605–13.
6. Myers J, Prakash M, Froelicher V, Do D, Partington S, Atwood JE. Exercise capacity and mortality among men referred for exercise testing. N Engl J Med 2002; 346(11):793–801.
7. Wallberg-Henriksson H, Holloszy JO. Contractile activity increases glucose uptake by muscle in severely diabetic rats. J Appl Physiol 1984 ; 57(4):1045–9.
8. Burstein R, Epstein Y, Shapiro Y, Charuzi I, Karnieli E. Effect of an acute bout of exercise on glucose disposal in human obesity. J Appl Physiol 1990; 69(1):299–304.
9. Schneider SH, Amorosa LF, Khachadurian AK, Ruderman NB. Studies on the mechanism of improved glucose control during regular exercise in type 2 (non-insulin-dependent) diabetes. Diabetologia 1984; 26(5):355–60.
10. Cuff DJ, Meneilly GS, Martin A, Ignaszewski A, Tildesley HD, Frohlich JJ. Effective exercise modality to reduce insulin resistance in women with type 2 diabetes. Diabetes Care 2003; 26(11): 2977–82.
11. Dela F, Larsen JJ, Mikines KJ, Ploug T, Petersen LN, Galbo H. Insulin-stimulated muscle glucose clearance in patients with NIDDM. Effects of one-legged physical training. Diabetes 1995; 44(9): 1010–20.
12. King DS, Baldus PJ, Sharp RL, Kesl LD, Feltmeyer TL, Riddle MS. Time course for exercise-induced alterations in insulin action and glucose tolerance in middle-aged people. J Appl Physiol 1995; 78(1): 17–22.
13. Segal KR, Edano A, Abalos A, et al. Effect of exercise training on insulin sensitivity and glucose metabolism in lean, obese, and diabetic men. J Appl Physiol 1991; 71(6):2402–11.
14. Dunstan DW, Daly RM, Owen N, et al. High-intensity resistance training improves glycemic control in older patients with type 2 diabetes. Diabetes Care 2002; 25(10):1729–36.
15. Lerman A, Zeiher AM. Endothelial function: cardiac events. Circulation 2005; 111(3):363–8.
16. Luscher TF, Noll G. Endothelial function as an end-point in interventional trials: concepts, methods and current data. J Hypertens 1996; 14(2 Suppl):S111–9.
17. Mehta JL, Rasouli N, Sinha AK, Molavi B. Oxidative stress in diabetes: a mechanistic overview of its effects on atherogenesis and myocardial dysfunction. Int J Biochem Cell Biol 2006; 38(5–6):794–803.
18. Adams V, Linke A, Krankel N, et al. Impact of regular physical activity on the NAD(P)H oxidase and angiotensin receptor system in patients with coronary artery disease. Circulation 2005; 111(5):555–62.
19. Erbs S, Baither Y, Linke A, et al. Promoter but not exon 7 polymorphism of endothelial nitric oxide synthase affects training-induced correction of endothelial dysfunction. Arterioscler Thromb Vasc Biol 2003; 23(10):1814–9.
20. Hambrecht R, Adams V, Erbs S, et al. Regular physical activity improves endothelial function in patients with coronary artery disease by increasing phosphorylation of endothelial nitric oxide synthase. Circulation 2003; 107(25):3152–8.
21. Harrison D, Griendling KK, Landmesser U, Hornig B, Drexler H. Role of oxidative stress in atherosclerosis. Am J Cardiol 2003; 91(3A):7A–11.
22. Ito A, Tsao PS, Adimoolam S, Kimoto M, Ogawa T, Cooke JP. Novel mechanism for endothelial dysfunction: dysregulation of dimethylarginine dimethylaminohydrolase. Circulation 1999; 99(24): 3092–5.

23. Lu TM, Ding YA, Charng MJ, Lin SJ. Asymmetrical dimethylarginine: a novel risk factor for coronary artery disease. Clin Cardiol 2003; 26(10):458–64.
24. Griendling KK, FitzGerald GA. Oxidative stress and cardiovascular injury. Part I: basic mechanisms and in vivo monitoring of ROS. Circulation 2003; 108(16):1912–6.
25. Spiekermann S, Landmesser U, Dikalov S, et al. Electron spin resonance characterization of vascular xanthine and NAD(P)H oxidase activity in patients with coronary artery disease: relation to endothelium-dependent vasodilation. Circulation 2003; 107(10):1383–9.
26. Landmesser U, Dikalov S, Price SR, et al. Oxidation of tetrahydrobiopterin leads to uncoupling of endothelial cell nitric oxide synthase in hypertension. J Clin Invest 2003; 111(8):1201–9.
27. Hambrecht R, Wolf A, Gielen S, et al. Effect of exercise on coronary endothelial function in patients with coronary artery disease. N Engl J Med 2000; 342(7):454–60.
28. Adams V, Lenk K, Linke A et al. Increase of circulating endothelial progenitor cells in patients with coronary artery disease after exercise-induced ischemia. Arterioscler Thromb Vasc Biol 2004; 24(4): 684–90.
29. Krankel N, Adams V, Linke A, et al. Hyperglycemia reduces survival and impairs function of circulating blood-derived progenitor cells. Arterioscler Thromb Vasc Biol 2005; 25(4):698–703.
30. Jakicic JM, Marcus BH, Gallagher KI, Napolitano M, Lang W. Effect of exercise duration and intensity on weight loss in overweight, sedentary women: a randomized trial. JAMA 2003; 290(10): 1323–30.
31. Jolliffe JA, Rees K, Taylor RS, Thompson D, Oldridge N, Ebrahim S. Exercise-based rehabilitation for coronary heart disease. Cochrane Database Syst Rev 2001; (1):CD001800.
32. Schoeller DA, Shay K, Kushner RF. How much physical activity is needed to minimize weight gain in previously obese women? Am J Clin Nutr 1997; 66(3):551–6.
33. Weinsier RL, Hunter GR, Desmond RA, Byrne NM, Zuckerman PA, Darnell BE. Free-living activity energy expenditure in women successful and unsuccessful at maintaining a normal body weight. Am J Clin Nutr 2002; 75(3):499–504.
34. Wing RR. Physical activity in the treatment of the adulthood overweight and obesity: current evidence and research issues. Med Sci Sports Exerc 1999; 31(11 Suppl.):S547–52.
35. Wing RR, Hill JO. Successful weight loss maintenance. Ann Rev Nutr 2001; 21:323–41.
36. Zachwieja JJ. Exercise as treatment for obesity. Endocrinol Metab Clin North Am 1996; 25(4): 965–88.
37. Niebauer J, Hambrecht R, Velich T, et al. Attenuated progression of coronary artery disease after 6 years of multifactorial risk intervention: role of physical exercise. Circulation 1997; 96(8):2534–41.
38. Schuler G, Hambrecht R, Schlierf G, et al. Regular physical exercise and low-fat diet. Effects on progression of coronary artery disease. Circulation 1992; 86(1):1–11.
39. Pontiroli AE. Type 2 diabetes mellitus is becoming the most common type of diabetes in school children. Acta Diabetol 2004; 41(3):85–90.
40. James PT, Rigby N, Leach R. The obesity epidemic, metabolic syndrome and future prevention strategies. Eur J Cardiovasc Prev Rehabil 2004; 11(1):3–8.
41. Poornima IG, Parikh P, Shannon RP. Diabetic cardiomyopathy: the search for a unifying hypothesis. Circ Res 2006; 98(5):596–605.
42. Hambrecht R, Walther C, Mobius-Winkler S, et al. Percutaneous coronary angioplasty compared with exercise training in patients with stable coronary artery disease: a randomized trial. Circulation 2004; 109(11):1371–8.
43. Despres JP. Visceral obesity, insulin resistance, and dyslipidemia: contribution of endurance exercise training to the treatment of the plurimetabolic syndrome. Exerc Sport Sci Rev 1997; 25:271–300.
44. Kelley DE. The regulation of glucose uptake and oxidation during exercise. Int J Obes Relat Metab Disord 1995; 19(4 Suppl.):S14–7.
45. Physical Activity/Exercise and Diabetes Mellitus. Diabetes Care 2003; 26(90001):73S–7.
46. Boule NG, Haddad E, Kenny GP, Wells GA, Sigal RJ. Effects of exercise on glycemic control and body mass in type 2 diabetes mellitus: a meta-analysis of controlled clinical trials. JAMA 2001; 286(10): 1218–27.
47. Implications of the United Kingdom Prospective Diabetes Study. Diabetes Care 2000; 23(1 Suppl.): S27–31.
48. Thomas DE, Elliott EJ, Naughton GA. Exercise for type 2 diabetes mellitus. Cochrane Database Syst Rev 2006; 3:CD002968.
49. Perseghin G, Ghosh S, Gerow K, Shulman GI. Metabolic defects in lean nondiabetic offspring of NIDDM parents: a cross-sectional study. Diabetes 1997; 46(6):1001–9.
50. Haffner SM, Stern MP, Hazuda HP, Mitchell BD, Patterson JK. Increased insulin concentrations in nondiabetic offspring of diabetic parents. N Engl J Med 1988; 319(20):1297–301.
51. Marin P, Andersson B, Krotkiewski M, Bjorntorp P. Muscle fiber composition and capillary density in women and men with NIDDM. Diabetes Care 1994; 17(5):382–6.
52. Diabetes Prevention Program Research Group. Reduction in the incidence of type 2 diabetes with lifestyle intervention or metformin. N Engl J Med 2002; 346(6):393–403.

53. Hu FB, Manson JE, Stampfer MJ, et al. Diet, lifestyle, and the risk of type 2 diabetes mellitus in women. N Engl J Med 2001; 345(11):790–7.
54. Pan XR, Li GW, Hu YH, et al. Effects of diet and exercise in preventing NIDDM in people with impaired glucose tolerance. The Da Qing IGT and Diabetes Study. Diabetes Care 1997; 20(4):537–44.
55. Schuler G, Schlierf G, Wirth A, et al. Low-fat diet and regular, supervised physical exercise in patients with symptomatic coronary artery disease: reduction of stress-induced myocardial ischemia. Circulation 1988; 77(1):172–81.

7 | Psychosocial Issues and Type 2 Diabetes

Garry W. Welch, Alan M. Jacobson, and Katie Weinger
Behavioral and Mental Health Research, Joslin Diabetes Center, Boston, Massachusetts, U.S.A.

INTRODUCTION

This chapter briefly discusses the social and cultural forces that are driving up both obesity and type 2 diabetes rates to epidemic levels in the United States. It also provides a review of the considerable psychological and social impacts on the individual living with type 2 diabetes and includes a discussion of current intervention approaches.

CULTURAL CHANGES AND THE RISE OF TYPE 2 DIABETES

Type 2 diabetes accounts for 90% to 95% of the nearly 21 million diabetes cases in the United States (1,2). The disease is nearing epidemic proportions due, in part, to our aging population, but mostly as a result of a sharp increase in the prevalence of obesity and its associated insulin resistance (3). Results from the 2003 to 2004 National Health and Nutrition Examination Survey (NHANES), reported that an estimated 66% of U.S. adults are either overweight or obese, up from 45% in 1991 (4–6). Approximately 80% of those with type 2 diabetes are overweight or obese (7).

The three most important risk factors in the pathogenesis of this disease—sedentary lifestyle, poor dietary habits, and changes in body composition—are essentially modifiable risks, related to a set of profound social and cultural changes that have taken place recently in our society. Nestle and Jacobson (8) and others, including the Federation of American Societies for Experimental Biology (9), Schumann (10,11), Battle and Brownell (12), Burros (13), Bar-Or et al. (14), USDA (15), WHO (16), and Tufts University Health & Nutrition Newsletter (17), have highlighted some of these social and cultural changes:

- The greater use of labor-saving devices and the automobile for transportation have reduced habitual activity levels. More than 60% of American adults are not regularly physically active. In fact, 25% of all adults are not active at all.
- Greater access to mass-produced high-calorie foods that are relatively inexpensive and heavily advertised, with recent emphasis on larger portion sizes. There has been a rapid growth of the food industry and its use of sophisticated marketing and merchandizing campaigns to stimulate food consumption, including fast foods, snacks, and drinks. For example, the McDonalds fast-food chain spends over a billion dollars a year on promotion of its products. The Centers for Disease Control analyzed data from four NHANES, which took place between the years of 1971 and 2000. Their analyses indicated that during this time, the average daily energy intake for men increased from 2450 to 2618 kcal ($p < .01$), and from 1542 to 1877 kcal ($p < .01$) for women (18). Put simply, Americans are eating more.
- The more hectic pace of modern life, longer working hours, and changes in family roles that reward convenience in terms of eating patterns, and limited time available for recreation and outside activities.

Reversing these recent cultural trends that impact eating and exercise habits will require a multifaceted public health policy approach focusing on the prevention of weight gain as early in life as possible as a key strategy (8,14). In recent years, three highly powered clinical trials have shown that moderate dietary adjustments and exercise can help reduce the risk of developing type 2 diabetes in adults who are most at risk (19,20). By exercising moderately 30 minutes a day and losing 5% to 7% of body weight, high-risk study participants in both the Diabetes Prevention Program (DPP) and Finnish Diabetes Prevention Study, were able to reduce their odds of developing type 2 diabetes by 58% (21,22). Participants in these studies had glucose intolerance at entry and were at high risk for developing type 2 diabetes. Enhancing physical activity through a moderate exercise program, even without weight loss, has been found to decrease incidence of type 2 diabetes in at-risk populations by 44% (23). The social and cultural causes of obesity and type 2 diabetes suggest that a dramatic shift is needed from our current medical and behavioral models to a public health model involving prevention and public policy initiatives supported by medical and behavioral strategies. Indeed, current strivings for a medical cure of the multisystem defects inherent in type 2 diabetes involving the pancreas, liver, and peripheral tissues ignore the underlying social problems that are at the heart of the recent growth in obesity and type 2 diabetes rates.

THE PSYCHOLOGICAL AND SOCIAL IMPACT OF TYPE 2 DIABETES

The patient with type 2 diabetes must adjust to a demanding treatment regimen and the eventual onset of diabetes-related complications (24–28). In this section we discuss some of these psychosocial issues and provide an update on treatment approaches in these areas. Most of the research on psychosocial issues in diabetes in the United States has been carried out on Caucasians, principally in academic clinics and hospital diabetes centers, rather than in primary care settings, where most type 2 diabetes care is delivered. Despite these limitations, there is a sizeable body of research available that can help us understand the psychosocial impact of type 2 diabetes, and identify clinically useful interventions to manage patient problem areas.

Type 2 diabetes is consistently described in clinical reports as demanding and complex from the patient's perspective (29–32). Reflecting clinician time constraints, their training focus, institutional support, and reimbursement practices, most clinical interviews in diabetes practice focus largely on medical or educational aspects of type 2 diabetes, and concentrate little on psychosocial features that, for a subgroup of patients, should be at the forefront of priorities (33). Psychosocial issues in type 2 diabetes have a significant influence on both patient outcomes and quality-of-life. High blood sugar levels, associated with poor blood sugar control, cause a range of medical complications (e.g., cardiovascular disease, retinopathy, neuropathy, nephropathy) that can impact many areas of the patients life, including ability to work, family functioning, quality-of-life, and sexual functioning (24,25,34).

As with other chronic medical conditions, the patient needs to carry out many daily treatment-related tasks if adequate blood glucose control is to be achieved. While a sound medical plan is important (e.g., a patient on oral agents who is undermedicated will find food and exercise regimens relatively ineffective), a good medical plan is a necessary but not sufficient condition to ensure good blood glucose control. Diet and exercise, blood glucose monitoring, timing and dosage of prescribed diabetes medications (insulin and/or oral agents), hypoglycemia management and prevention, foot care, sick day management, clinic visits, and various necessary medical screenings and education activities must all be successfully incorporated into life roles and any unexpected crises (33,35). Changes to food habits can be particularly difficult to achieve and sustain. Also, diabetes regimen changes must be maintained by the individual patient within the context of helpful or unhelpful peer and social pressures, domestic and economic responsibilities, and distracting life events (36). Self-care behavior change must be sustained over time to translate into improved blood glucose control and a reduction or slowing down of diabetes complications progression (37). Type 2 diabetes typically emerges in middle adulthood, a period of life where lifestyle patterns and behaviors have become firmly established and may require greater effort to change. Also, during the precomplications phase of type 2 diabetes, and even in the early phase of complications, the patient is often asymptomatic. Driving forces that might motivate a patient to seek medical care—unpleasant symptoms and awareness and fear of a serious illness—are therefore not present to provide a sufficient level of threat and motivation to make changes.

DIABETES-RELATED EMOTIONAL DISTRESS

It is common for patients to experience emotional distress from living with diabetes and the impact of its complications. The terms "diabetes burnout" (32) and "diabetes overwhel-mus"

(30) have been coined to capture this distress. The types of specific emotional problem faced by type 2 diabetes patients have been reported in several studies (38–40). Approximately one third reported "worry about the future and the possibility of diabetes complications" as a serious issue. Other areas endorsed as "serious" by approximately 15% to 20% of patients included:

- Guilt and anxiety at being off-track with treatment
- Scared about living with diabetes
- Not knowing if mood or feelings were related to diabetes
- Being constantly concerned about food and eating
- Feeling deprived around food
- Feeling depressed living with diabetes

The questionnaire used in these surveys is the problem areas in diabetes (PAID) scale (see Fig. 1) (40,41). This is a brief, one-page screening tool that can be used by busy diabetes clinicians to gather information about patient concerns that may affect their self-care behaviors. It can be given to patients routinely, to screen for overall high emotional distress related to living with type 1 or type 2 diabetes. A total score (overall emotional distress) is generated by simply adding the 0 to 4 values endorsed by the patient for each of the 20 questions in the PAID. This sum is then multiplied by 1.25 to provide a total score of 0 to 100. A cutoff score of 50 denotes a high level emotional distress that warrants further professional attention. Individual questions scored as "serious" (i.e., scored 4 on a scale of 0–4) identify individual areas that a patient finds difficult. These are specific "hot spots" with which the patient is currently struggling emotionally. For patients scoring high on the total score or individual questions, the clinician might consider investing additional time exploring feelings and practical barriers to good diabetes self-care. It is rare in medical settings for patients to be asked even briefly about their illness-related feelings—despite the great value of this exercise to clinician for patients troubled with the emotional burden of diabetes (30,31).

A key task for the clinician is to give the patient a brief opportunity (i.e., a few minutes) to talk about how he or she feels about living with diabetes. The aim is to talk with the patient about feelings openly and in a safe way (supportive, nonjudgmental). Good listening skills start with open questions, to stimulate the patient to talk about his or her feelings. For example, if a patient scores high on the PAID (above 50), the clinician may say:

> It sounds as if you have been feeling overwhelmed with your diabetes care. Could you tell me a little more about how you have felt lately?

Close-ended questions that simply require a "yes" or "no" response tend to close down conversation rather than opening it up. Avoid interrupting at this point, providing information, or showing personal reactions to what the patient has said. Some other suggestions: be aware of your own "mental chatter" and try to simply listen to what the patient is saying when he or she talks. Be aware also of the patient's body language (tone of voice, facial expressions, use of hands and body posture, pauses and hesitations during difficult moments, etc.). Maintain good eye contact and use small encouraging body signals (nod your head, say "yes, go on" or "hmm" to show you are staying with the patient's story). Then briefly summarize what you have heard from the patient both in terms of the specific emotions (e.g., guilt, anxiety, feeling alone, etc.) and the reasons the patient gives for feeling that way. Check with the patient that what you have said is accurate:

> If I've heard you correctly, you've felt … because … Does that sound accurate?

Look for a response from the patient that might "fine tune" your summary if needed. A patient who feels he or she has been heard by an empathic healthcare professional about the emotional distress of living with diabetes, even for a brief period, will feel less distressed and be more motivated to make any behavior changes that may be needed. Good listening enhances the therapeutic bond between patient and healthcare team member and can be used

Instructions: *Which of the following diabetes issues are currently a problem for you?*
Circle the number that gives the best answer for you. Please provide an answer for each question.

	Not a problem ▼	Minor problem ▼	Moderate problem ▼	Somewhat serious problem ▼	Serious problem ▼
1 Not having clear and concrete goals for your diabetes care?	0	1	2	3	4
2 Feeling discouraged with your diabetes treatment plan?	0	1	2	3	4
3 Feeling scared when you think about living with diabetes?	0	1	2	3	4
4 Uncomfortable social situations related to your diabetes care (e.g. people telling you what to eat)?	0	1	2	3	4
5 Feelings of deprivation regarding food and meals?	0	1	2	3	4
6 Feeling depressed when you think about living with diabetes?	0	1	2	3	4
7 Not knowing if your mood or feelings are related to your diabetes?	0	1	2	3	4
8 Feeling overwhelmed by your diabetes?	0	1	2	3	4
9 Worrying about low blood sugar reactions?	0	1	2	3	4
10 Feeling angry when you think about living with diabetes?	0	1	2	3	4
11 Feeling constantly concerned about food and eating?	0	1	2	3	4
12 Worrying about the future and the possibility of serious complications?	0	1	2	3	4
13 Feelings of guilt or anxiety when you get off track with your diabetes management?	0	1	2	3	4
14 Not 'accepting' your diabetes?	0	1	2	3	4
15 Feeling unsatisfied with your diabetes physician?	0	1	2	3	4
16 Feeling that diabetes is taking up too much of your mental and physical energy every day?	0	1	2	3	4
17 Feeling alone with your diabetes?	0	1	2	3	4
18 Feeling that your friends and family are not supportive of your diabetes management efforts?	0	1	2	3	4
19 Coping with complications of diabetes?	0	1	2	3	4
20 Feeling 'burned out' by the constant effort needed to manage diabetes?	0	1	2	3	4

FIGURE 1 Problem areas in diabetes scale. *Source*: From Ref. 41.

regularly to good effect in all areas of diabetes management. Referral can be made if appropriate to a diabetes nurse educator or other available member of the diabetes clinical team to tackle specific practical issues arising from the emotional concerns identified by the patient (e.g., fear of complications, difficulties with the diet plan). The U.K. Prospective Diabetes Study (UKPDS) (37) has demonstrated the benefit of improved blood glucose control on progression of complications in type 2 diabetes. Screening for diabetes emotional distress and intervening where a high level of distress is present will support patient self-care efforts that, in turn, will contribute to improved blood glucose control (30). Recently, the diabetes attitudes, desires, and needs (DAWN) study was launched across 13 countries with the goal to enhance communication between people with diabetes and their healthcare providers using a brief empathic listening intervention (understanding what the patient is saying, thinking, and feeling through open questions, reflective listening, and brief summaries of what was heard) (42). A focus on understanding the patient's perspective is an important first step in providing support to the patient experiencing high emotional distress living with diabetes as this strengthens rapport and trust and can help identify the most important issues to focus on from the patient's perspective.

STRESS AND BLOOD GLUCOSE CONTROL

Psychological stress has significant effects on the metabolism on individuals without diabetes by increasing counterregulatory hormones, which could result in elevated blood sugars, among other impacts. In type 2 diabetes it is thought that stress can exert an effect on blood glucose control, either directly through these hormones or indirectly by disruption of the diabetes self-care regimen. Although the laboratory and clinical research to date does not appear to support a consistent stress-blood glucose response across all patients, there is evidence that some individuals with diabetes are "stress responders" (43). Individuals with type 1 diabetes may have idiosyncratic responses to stress, with some showing increases in blood glucose levels and others decreases. However, for type 2 diabetes the effects of stress are more likely to result in increases in blood glucose, secondary to sympathetic activity (43,44).

Evidence from animal models also suggests a role for stress in the onset of type 2 diabetes (45). Ineffective coping (e.g., avoidance, denial, detachment, anger) has been shown to be associated with poorer metabolic control in diabetes and adaptive coping (e.g., active problem solving and ability to obtain social support) with a stress-buffering role (46), highlighting the role of patient perceptions of stressful events. It is unclear whether relaxation training (e.g., biofeedback) produces glycemic benefits in type 2 diabetes (47). Generally, there is a paucity of studies on stress in type 2 diabetes.

PSYCHIATRIC ILLNESSES

Patients with diabetes have elevated levels of psychiatric illnesses compared with the general population and similar to those found in other chronic illnesses. The most common psychiatric disorder in type 2 diabetes is major depression, while other significant disorders include anxiety disorders, alcohol and substance use disorders, and eating disorders, principally binge-eating syndrome (28,48–51). Lifetime prevalence of recent (i.e., within 6 months) psychiatric disorders among individuals with chronic illnesses, such as cancer, arthritis, and heart disease, has been found to be 40%, which is higher than for those without such illnesses (52). A number of studies have been conducted recently to estimate psychiatric illnesses in type 2 diabetes. This chapter concentrates on major depression, but also discusses briefly anxiety disorders, alcohol abuse and dependence, and binge-eating disorder (BED), which are commonly associated with obesity.

MAJOR DEPRESSION

Major depression is the most severe form of depression. The essential feature of major depression is depressed mood, or loss of interest in usual activities, which is experienced most of the day and nearly every day, for a period of at least 2 weeks. Accompanying these symptoms are appetite disturbance and weight change, sleep problems, either physical agitation or slowing down, decreased energy, feelings of worthlessness or excessive guilt, difficulty concentrating or thinking, and recurrent suicidal thoughts. Major depression is present in 15% to 20% of patients with diabetes, regardless of diabetes type (53). Several studies have found glycemic control significantly worse among depressed versus nondepressed diabetes patients (54–56). The course of the illness is generally chronic; even after successful treatment it will reoccur in as many as 80% of diabetic patients and reoccur on an average of four episodes during a subsequent 5-year period (57). Depression is recognized and treated in only one third of cases. Depression also doubles the risk of type 2 diabetes onset, independent of its association with other risk factors (58–61). Randomized controlled trials have shown both psychotherapy (i.e., cognitive behavioral therapy that targets negative thought patterns) and psychopharmacy [i.e., tricyclics and selective serotonin-reuptake inhibitors (SSRIs)] to have significant beneficial effects on both mood and glycemic control (53,62). A meta-analysis of relevant studies demonstrated a significant and consistent association of diabetes complications and depressive symptoms (63). Both diabetes complications and hyperglycemia are associated with diminished response to depression treatment and with an increased risk of recurrence. This suggests that optimal relief of depression in diabetes may require vigorous, simultaneous treatment of both the blood sugar control and psychiatric conditions.

Dysthymia, defined as persistent presence with fewer symptoms of depression, can occur in the absence of major depression. Moreover, it is commonly found in patients with chronic medical conditions, and is responsive to depression treatments. Patients with dysthymia may seem like chronic complainers and so their depressions may be misread as "personality problems."

There are a number of barriers that make detection of depression particularly challenging for the physician in the medical setting (64). These include:

- Lack of time (i.e., brief visits)
- Somatization (patient presents the physical symptoms of depression such as fatigue, appetite change, or sleep disruption, but not the affective or cognitive symptoms)
- Stigmatization (which inhibits explicit questioning)
- Comorbid medical conditions (camouflage depression by sharing somatic symptoms)

In the latter case, special attention should be paid to the affective components of depression such as mood, loss of interest in usual activities, guilt, or suicidal thoughts the patient may also be experiencing. If time constraints are a particular problem, a single question "Have you felt depressed or sad much of the time in the past year?" has been found to have a sensitivity of 85% and specificity of 66% (65).

ANXIETY

Although not as well studied in diabetes, some research suggests anxiety disorders are more common in adults with type 2 diabetes than the general population (66–68) and anxiety symptoms are linked with worse glycemic control (67). Demographic comparisons parallel depression, in that women, African-Americans, and those with less education are more likely to report anxiety symptoms (28).

Formal anxiety disorders include panic disorder, which involves repeated episodes of intense fear that strikes often and without warning. Physical symptoms include chest pain, heart palpitations, shortness of breath, dizziness, abdominal distress, feelings of unreality, and fear of dying. Obsessive-compulsive disorder is characterized by repeated, unwanted thoughts or compulsive behaviors that seem impossible to stop or control. Phobias include two major types of phobias: social phobia and specific phobia. Social phobia involves the experience of an overwhelming and disabling fear of scrutiny, embarrassment, or humiliation in social situations, which leads to avoidance of many potentially pleasurable and meaningful activities. Specific phobias can produce extreme, disabling and irrational fear of something that poses little or no actual danger, the fear effectively leads to avoidance of these objects or situations and can cause people to limit their lives unnecessarily. Finally, generalized anxiety disorder (GAD) involves exaggerated, worrisome thoughts and tension about everyday routine life events and activities, lasting at least 6 months. Individuals with GAD always anticipate the worst, even though there is little reason to expect it and the fear is accompanied by physical symptoms, such as fatigue, trembling, muscle tension, headache, or nausea.

Two clinically proven forms of psychotherapy used to treat anxiety disorders are behavioral therapy and cognitive-behavioral therapy. Cognitive-behavioral therapy teaches patients to understand and change negative thinking patterns, so the individual can react differently to the situations that cause them anxiety. In diabetes, behavioral interventions have reduced anxiety and improved glycemic control (69,70). Psychopharmacological agents can be effective in the treatment of anxiety disorders and treatment with SSRIs is becoming increasingly popular. Okada et al. (71) found reduced anxiety levels with fludiazepam, a benzodiazepine, in a study involving a small patient group, and glycemic control was improved in another study that focused on anxiety symptoms (72). There is relatively little information on benzodiazepine use in type 2 diabetes, although one study found that antidepressant treatment reduced blood glucose levels in a sample of obese type 2 diabetics

(28,73). Anxiety symptoms may be confused with the symptoms of low blood sugars among patients treated with sulfonylureas and insulin. Self-monitoring of blood glucose concentrations can help the anxious patient discriminate between hypoglycemia and anxiety (74). When emotional and behavioral symptoms (e.g., persistent fears, worries, obsessions, compulsions) are predominant, as opposed to physical symptoms (e.g., palpitations and sweating), the diagnosis of anxiety disorder is more readily made (29).

ALCOHOL DEPENDENCY AND ABUSE

Alcohol use disorders involve four problem areas:

- A strong need, or urge, to drink (craving)
- Not being able to stop drinking once drinking has begun (loss of control)
- Withdrawal symptoms, such as nausea, sweating, shakiness, and anxiety after stopping drinking (physical dependence)
- The need to drink greater amounts of alcohol to get "high" (tolerance).

Alcohol dependence (alcoholism) refers to a repetitive pattern of excessive alcohol use with serious adverse consequences, often including lack of control, tolerance, and withdrawal. Alcohol abuse is a milder category that refers to continued drinking despite adverse consequences, in the absence of dependence (75). Data from the 2001 to 2002 National Epidemiologic Survey on Alcohol and Related Conditions (NESARC) showed that alcohol use disorders have an annual prevalence rate of 7.35% in the United States (76). As many as 5 out of 6 patients who meet diagnostic criteria for abuse or dependence go unrecognized in primary care settings (77). When diabetes and alcohol use disorders coexist, they represent a considerable clinical challenge. Alcohol-induced fasting hypoglycemia can occur 6 to 36 h after alcohol intake in the context of low food intake. Fasting depletes liver glycogen stores and alcohol impairs gluconeogenesis. Neuroglycopenic symptoms are predominate and can include stupor and coma (78).

Chronic alcohol use can create medical and behavioral problems, including: blackouts, chronic abdominal pain, depression, liver dysfunction, hypertension, sexual dysfunction, sleep disorders, and work or interpersonal problems (79). It can also affect nutritional status in type 2 diabetes, through direct changes to carbohydrate, lipid, and protein metabolism, but also indirectly by changing eating habits (e.g., meals become irregular or skipped). Chronic use can also promote hyperglycemia by the extra calories consumed and by enhancing insulin resistance and glucose intolerance (80). Early detection is important and can be supported by use of the widely used CAGE assessment (81). After asking the patient whether or not they drink alcohol and if the answer is 'yes' then establishing the types, amounts, and frequency of drinking, the following four questions are presented to the patient:

- C: Have you ever felt you should CUT down on your drinking?
- A: Have people ANNOYED you by criticizing your drinking?
- G: Have you ever felt bad or GUILTY about your drinking?
- E: Have you ever had a drink first thing in the morning as an EYE OPENER?

CAGE can reveal problem areas that should be further explored. Individuals at risk include those with one or more positive CAGE responses. Alcohol dependence requiring referral is likely if the patient gives 3 to 4 positive responses for the past year (79).

EATING DISORDERS

Although community prevalence rates of 1% for anorexia nervosa and 3% for bulimia nervosa can occur among young women, these disorders are not common in the older age group (over 40 years) when type 2 diabetes typically emerges. However, BED is an eating disorder found among 70% of obese individuals, and 80% of type 2 diabetes patients are obese. The diabetes clinician will likely uncover BED if he or she is actively looking for it and asks questions about uncontrolled eating binges. BED is different from binge-purge syndrome (bulimia nervosa), as individuals with BED usually do not purge afterward by use of vomiting, laxative abuse, diuretic abuse, or insulin omission. In contrast to other eating disorders, where 90% or more of cases are female, one third of all patients with BED are men (82). In the general population the prevalence of BED is around 1% to 2%. Among mildly obese people in self-help or commercial weight-loss programs, 10% to 15% have BED. A recent study found that among a sample of type 2 diabetics, 20% displayed eating disorders and BED was the prevailing diagnosis (10%) (83). A BED prevalence of 25.6% in a group of type 2 diabetes patients attending a diabetes clinic at an academic medical center has also been found, but BED remains a neglected area of clinical research in type 2 diabetes. BED does not appear to be associated with worse blood glucose control (49,84). However, people with BED are typically extremely distressed by their binge eating. Most feel ashamed and try to hide their problem. Often they are so successful at this that close family members and friends do not know they binge eat. Several methods are being used to treat BED (85). At this early stage of research we do not know which method or combination of methods is the most effective in caring for BED patients:

- Cognitive-behavioral therapy teaches patients techniques to monitor and change their eating habits, as well as to change the way they respond to difficult situations.
- Interpersonal psychotherapy helps people examine their relationships with friends and family and to make changes in problem areas.
- Treatment with antidepressants may be helpful for some individuals.
- Self-help groups also may be a source of support.

SOCIAL SUPPORT

Social support can be defined as the availability of close family, friends, and other significant people in the individual's life that is provided through the individual's social network (86). There is general agreement that there are several distinct types of social support (87,88):

- Instrumental support (practical help).
- Informational (provision of information).
- Emotional (lending a good listening ear, showing understanding, helping talk over problems, or make difficult decisions).
- Approval (giving verbal support).

Low perceived level of diabetes-related support has been related to a number of factors, including: lack of diabetes knowledge among individuals in the support network, resistance to making changes that would support improved patient self-care, the presence of serious interpersonal conflicts, and lack of specific requests for help from the individual with diabetes (32). There is strong empirical support for the value of good social support to health and longevity. For example, a large study of men tracked for 4 years (89) showed higher cardiovascular disease, accident, and suicide-related deaths among those classified as socially isolated (i.e., not married, fewer than six friends or relatives, no membership in community groups). In diabetes, reviews have shown moderate positive correlations between social support and markers of self-care such as glycosylated hemoglobin (HbA_{1c}) (35). One study showed health-related quality-of-life is affected by the marital status of both type 1 and type 2 diabetic patients, with separated and divorced individuals generally experiencing lower levels of quality-of-life (34). Weissberg-Benchell and Pichert (90) have provided some simple questions for the diabetes clinician interested in exploring social support:

- Who helps you care for your diabetes and how do they help?
- Are there things they do or say that make it harder for you to care for your diabetes?
- Who do you talk to for emotional support for having diabetes? Are they good listeners?

Social support is generally conceived of as a positive influence on health, although some support can be negative in type 2 diabetes if the patient fears being nagged or harassed about their self-care behaviors (91). The "diabetes police" is a term that has been coined to describe a pattern of behavior by family, friends, and others in the diabetes patient's social network where they monitor the patient's self-care behavior intrusively, and try to pressure the patient to improve self-care through persuasion, advice, criticism, and threats (32).

SEXUAL FUNCTIONING

Impaired sexual functioning is a well-recognized complication of type 2 diabetes in men and women. The prevalence of erectile dysfunction (ED) in the overall population between the ages of 40 and 70 years is 52%, while the prevalence in men with diabetes is as high as 75% (92–95). Moreover, diabetic men develop ED at an earlier age than men without diabetes (2). In women, type 2 diabetes has been shown to impact sexual desire, orgasmic capacity, lubrication, sexual satisfaction, sexual activity, and relationship with sexual partner (96). Relationship problems may be a primary or aggravating factor in sexual functioning (97). Performance anxieties and relationship problems have been identified as potential problem areas that may need sensitive investigation (98). Sildenafil citrate and related medications are well-tolerated and effective in improving ED in men with type 2 diabetes, even in patients with poor glycemic control and chronic complications (99). The rates of adverse events, such as headache, flushing, dyspepsia, and dizziness, is similar to that for nondiabetic individuals (100).

COGNITIVE FUNCTIONING

Early research in cognitive functioning focused on type 2 diabetes as a theoretical model of accelerated aging [e.g., Kent (101)] but, more recently, there has been interest in potential changes in cognition that might make patient adherence to treatment more difficult (102). Both chronically elevated high blood sugars and recurrent low blood sugar levels have the potential to independently contribute to cognitive dysfunction, for example through changes to the blood–brain barrier transport of glucose. Verbal learning and memory skills may be especially disrupted in type 2 diabetes, but mainly for patients older than 60 years of age (103–105). Other cognitive skills, such as attention, executive function, and psychomotor efficiency, were less affected. Although most research on cognition in diabetes has been conducted with type 1 patients, studies show that middle-aged type 2 individuals are apparently protected, insofar as researchers have only infrequently reported learning and memory impairments in that age group. It is likely that older adults have an increased risk of diabetes-associated memory dysfunction as a consequence of a synergistic interaction between diabetes-related blood glucose changes and the structural and functional changes occurring in the central nervous system that are part of the normal aging process (106,107).

Multiple diabetes-related comorbid conditions (i.e., hyperinsulinaemia, hypertension, hypercholesterolaemia) may individually and synergistically impact learning and memory skills [see review by Ryan and Geckle (104)]. For example, hyperinsulinaemia may independently affect the central nervous system. Insulin levels usually rise with age, and are strong predictors of cognitive impairment in adults without diabetes. Data from the Framingham study showed that both hypertension and diabetes independently affect cognition generally, and memory skills in particular. Given their high rates in type 2 diabetes, it is notable that hypertension and hypercholesterolaemia interacts with hyperinsulinemia to disrupt memory. Generally, there is evidence to support the view that verbal learning and memory skills are particularly vulnerable to disruption in type 2 diabetes compared with other cognitive skills as a result of diabetes and its comorbidities. Recent data has indicated a link between insulin resistance and Alzheimer's disease (AD). Although the mechanism linking these conditions is unclear, the predominate hypothesis is that insulin resistance, accompanied by hyperinsulinemia and subsequent glucose metabolism disturbances, leads to neurodegeneration, and ultimately, AD (108–110). This association suggests that future AD treatments should focus on reversing or preventing insulin abnormalities (111,112).

While mild and severe hypoglycemia rates are lower in type 2 diabetes compared with type 1, due to residual insulin production in type 2, patients who use sulfonylureas or progress to insulin therapy can experience acute low blood sugars (113). Such episodes cause both autonomic and neuroglycopenic changes. Neuroglycopenia appears to impact the cerebral cortex more than the deeper brain structures, in terms of cognitive functioning. Complex, attention-demanding and speed-dependent responses are most impaired, with accuracy often preserved at the expense of speed. Cognitive function does not recover fully until 40 to 90 min after blood glucose is returned to normal. Hypoglycemia also provokes changes in mood, including anxiety and depression, and increases fear of further hypoglycemia, which in turn can modify self-care behavior (e.g., over-treating with food) and thus blood sugar control (114).

In summary, there are a wide range of psychosocial issues important to address in the clinical management of type 2 diabetes. For some patients, these issues are serious enough to warrant active treatment by the clinician, or referral to other healthcare professionals. This chapter briefly discussed some of these psychosocial issues and suggested practical, patient-centered strategies to aid the busy clinician. We should not lose sight of the fact that both obesity and type 2 diabetes are preventable diseases that have major public health implications. As a society, we need to focus on the profound social and cultural changes that have occurred in our daily lives. These involve reduced habitual activity and increased food intake. Practical preventive strategies at the societal and cultural level must be generated to reverse these trends. This may be the greatest challenge we face in tackling the current epidemic of type 2 diabetes.

REFERENCES

1. American Diabetes Association. Diabetes Statistics. Alexandria, VA: American Diabetes Association, 2006.
2. American Diabetes Association. Medical Management of Type 2 Diabetes. Alexandria, VA: American Diabetes Association, 1998.
3. Diabetes Research Working Group. Congressional report on National Institutes of Health implementation of the recommendations of the Congressionally-directed Diabetes Research Working Group, 1998.
4. Mokdad AH, Ford ES. Diabetes trends in the U.S.: 1990–1998. Diabetes Care 2000; 23:1278–83.
5. Ogden CL, Carroll MD. Prevalence of overweight and obesity in the United States, 1999–2004. JAMA 2006; 295:1549–55.
6. Flegal KM, Carroll MD, Ogden CL, Johnson CL. Prevalence and trends in obesity among US adults, 1999–2000. JAMA 2002; 288:1723–7.
7. Tan AS, Brietzke SA, Gardner OW, Sowers JR. In: Mantzoros CS, ed. Obesity, Diabetes, and Hypertension. Totowa, NJ: Humana Press Inc., 2006:169–92.
8. Nestle M, Jacobson MF. Halting the obesity epidemic: a public health policy approach. Public Health Rep 2000; 115:12–24.
9. Federation of American Societies for Experimental Biology, LSRO. Executive summary from the third report on nutrition monitoring in the United States. J Nutr 1996; 126:1907S–36.
10. Schumann M. Megabrands: top brands hold the line in 2001. Advertising Age 2002; S1–9:200–12.
11. USDA. 1994–96 Continuing survey of food intakes by individuals. USDA 2002:10–7.
12. Battle EK, Brownell KD. Confronting a rising tide of eating disorders and obesity: treatment vs. prevention and policy. Addict Behav 1996; 21:755–65.
13. Burros M. Losing count of calories as plates fill up. New York Times 2 April 1997; Section C:4.
14. Bar-Or O, Foreyt J. Physical activity, genetic, and nutritional considerations in childhood weight management. Med Sci Sports Exerc 1998; 30:2–10.
15. USDA. Data tables: Results from USDAs 1994–96. Continuing Survey of Food Intakes by Individuals and 1994–96 Diet and Health Knowledge Survey. USDA 1997.
16. World Health Organization. Obesity: preventing and managing a global epidemic. Report of a WHO Consultation. 2000. Geneva, WHO: WHO Technical Report Series 894. 1999.
17. Tufts University. Special Report: Portion Distortion. Tufts University Health & Nutrition Newsletter 2002; 18:4–5.
18. Center for Disease Control. Trends in intake of energy and macronutrients—United States, 1971–2000. CDC 2004; 11–8–2006.
19. Wylie-Rosett J, Herman WH, Goldberg RB. Lifestyle intervention to prevent diabetes: intensive and cost effective. Curr Opin Lipidol 2006; 17:37–44.

20. Pan XR, et al. Effects of diet and exercise in preventing NIDDM in people with impaired glucose tolerance. The Da Qing IGT and Diabetes Study. Diabetes Care 1997; 20:537–44.
21. Tuomilehto J, Lindstrom J. Prevention of type 2 diabetes mellitus by changes in lifestyle among subjects with impaired glucose tolerance. N Engl J Med 2001; 344:1343–50.
22. Diabetes Prevention Program Research Group. Reduction in the incidence of type 2 diabetes with lifestyle intervention or metformin. N Engl J Med 2002; 346:403.
23. Hamman RF, Wing RR. Effect of weight loss with lifestyle intervention on risk of diabetes. Diabetes Care 2006; 29:2102–7.
24. Bradley C. Handbook of Psychology and Diabetes: A Guide to Psychological Measurement in Diabetes Research and Practice. London: Harwood Academic Publishers, 1994.
25. Rubin RR, Peyrot M. Quality of life and diabetes. Diabetes Metab Res Rev 1999; 15:205–18.
26. Snoek FJ, Skinner TC. Psychology in Diabetes Care. New York: John Wiley & Sons, 2000.
27. Glasgow RE, Hiss RG. Report of the health care delivery work group: behavioral research related to the establishment of a chronic disease model for diabetes care. Diabetes Care 2001; 24:124–30.
28. Rubin RR, Peyrot M. Psychological issues and treatments for people with diabetes. J Clin Psychol 2001; 57:457–78.
29. Jacobson AM. The psychological care of patients with insulin-dependent diabetes mellitus. N Engl J Med 1996; 334:1249–53.
30. Rubin RR. Counselling and Psychotherapy in Diabetes Mellitus. In: Snoek FJ, Skinner TJ, eds. Psychology in Diabetes Care. New York, NY: Wiley, 2000:235–63.
31. Funnell MF, Anderson RM. Patient Empowerment. In: Snoek FJ, ST eds. Psychology in Diabetes Care. New York: Wiley, 2000.
32. Polonsky WH. Diabetes burnout. What to do when you can't take it anymore. Alexandria, VA: American Diabetes Association, 2000.
33. Day JL. Diabetic patient education: determinants of success. Diabetes Metab Res Rev 2000; 16 (Suppl. 1):S70–4.
34. Jacobson AM, de Groot M, Samson JA. The evaluation of two measures of quality of life in patients with type I and type II diabetes. Diabetes Care 1994; 17:267–74.
35. Glasgow RE. Medical Office-Based Interventions. In: Snoek FJ, Skinner TC, eds. Psychology in Diabetes Care. New York, NY: Wiley, 2000:141–68.
36. Clark M, Asimakopoulou K. Diabetes in Older Adults. In: Snoek FJ, Skinner TC, eds. Psychology in Diabetes Care. New York, NY: Wiley, 2000.
37. UK Prospective Diabetes Study Group. Intensive blood glucose control with sulfonylureas or insulin compared with conventional treatment and risk of complications with type 2 diabetes (UKPDS). Lancet 1998; 352:837–53.
38. Welch GW, Jacobson AM, Polonsky WH. The problem areas in diabetes scale. An evaluation of its clinical utility. Diabetes Care 1998; 20:760–6.
39. Snoek FJ, Pouwer F, Welch GW, Polonsky WH. Diabetes-related emotional distress in Dutch and U.S. diabetic patients: cross-cultural validity of the problem areas in diabetes scale. Diabetes Care 2000; 23:1305–9.
40. Welch GW, de Groot M, Buckland GT, Chipkin S. Risk stratification of diabetes patients using diet barriers and self care motivation in an inner city hospital setting. Diabetes 1999; 48(Suppl).
41. Polonsky WH, Anderson BJ. Assessment of diabetes-related emotional distress. Diabetes Care 1995; 18:754–60.
42. Peyrot M, Rubin RR. Psychosocial problems and barriers to improved diabetes management: results of the cross-national diabetes attitudes, wishes and needs (DAWN) Study. Diabet Med 2005; 22:1379–85.
43. Delamater AM, Cox DJ. Psychological stress, coping, and diabetes. Diabetes Spect 1994; 7:46–9.
44. Surwit RS, Schneider MS. Role of stress in the etiology and treatment of diabetes mellitus. Psychosom Med 1993; 55:380–93.
45. Surwit RS, Schneider MS, Feinglos MN. Stress and diabetes mellitus. Diabetes Care 1992; 15:1413–22.
46. Peyrot MF, McMurry JF Jr. Stress buffering and glycemic control. The role of coping styles. Diabetes Care 1992; 15:842–6.
47. Aikens JE, Kiolbasa TA, Sobel R. Psychological predictors of glycemic change with relaxation training in non-insulin-dependent diabetes mellitus. Psychother. Psychosom 1997; 66:302–6.
48. Cohen ST, Welch G, Jacobson AM, de Groot M, Samson J. The association of lifetime psychiatric illness and increased retinopathy in patients with type I diabetes mellitus. Psychosomatics 1997; 38: 98–108.
49. Crow S, Kendall D, Praus B, Thuras P. Binge eating and other psychopathology in patients with type 2 diabetes mellitus. Int J Eat Dis 2001; 30:222–6.
50. Pouwer F, Beekman AT. Rates and risks for co-morbid depression in patients with type 2 diabetes mellitus: results from a community-based study. Diabetologia 2003; 46:892–98.
51. Anderson RJ, Freedland KE, Clouse RE, Lustman PJ. The prevalence of comorbid depression in adults with diabetes: a meta-analysis. Diabetes Care 2001; 24:1069–78.

52. Wells KB, Golding JM, Burnam MA. Psychiatric disorder in a sample of the general population with and without chronic medical conditions. Am J Psychiatry 1988; 145:976–81.
53. Lustman PJ, Griffith LS. Effects of nortriptyline on depression and glycemic control in diabetes: results of a double-blind, placebo-controlled trial. Psychosom Med 1997; 59:241–50.
54. Mazze RS, Lucido D, Shamoon H. Psychological and social correlates of glycemic control. Diabetes Care 1984; 7:360–6.
55. de Groot M, Jacobson AM, Samson JA, Welch G. Glycemic control and major depression in patients with type 1 and type 2 diabetes mellitus. J Psychosom Res 1984; 46:425–35.
56. Lustman PJ, Griffith LS, Freedland KE, Clouse RE. The course of major depression in diabetes. Gen Hosp Psychiatry 1997; 19:138–43.
57. Lustman PJ, Griffith LS, Freedland KE, Kissel SS, Clouse RE. Cognitive behavior therapy for depression in type 2 diabetes mellitus: a randomized, controlled trial. Ann Intern Med 1998; 129:613–21.
58. Kawakami N, Takatsuka N, Shimizu H, Ishibashi H. Depression symptoms and occurrence of type 2 diabetes among Japanese men. Diabetes Care 1999; 22:1071–6.
59. Eaton WW, Armenian H, Gallo J, Pratt L, Ford DE. Depression and risk for onset of type II diabetes. A prospective population-based study. Diabetes Care 1996; 19:1097–102.
60. Arroyo C, Hu FB. Depressive symptoms and risk of type 2 diabetes in women. Diabetes Care 2004; 27:129–33.
61. Golden SH, Williams JE. Depressive symptoms and the risk of type 2 diabetes: the atherosclerosis risk in communities study. Diabetes Care 2004; 27:429–35.
62. Lustman PJ, Freedland KE, Griffith LS, Clouse RE. Fluoxetine for depression in diabetes: a randomized double-blind placebo-controlled trial. Diabetes Care 2000; 23:618–23.
63. de Groot M, Anderson R, Freedland KE, Clouse RE, Lustman PJ. Association of depression and diabetes complications: a meta-analysis. Psychosom Med 2001; 63:619–30.
64. Kroenke K. Discovering depression in medical patients: reasonable expectations. Ann Intern Med 1997; 126:463–5.
65. Williams JW Jr, Mulrow CD. Case-finding for depression in primary care: a randomized trial. Am J Med 1999; 106:36–43.
66. De Groot M, Jacobson AM, Samson JA. Psychiatric illness in patients with type 1 and type 2 diabetes mellitus. Psychosom Med 1994; 56:176A.
67. Peyrot M, Rubin RR. Levels and risks of depression and anxiety symptomatology among diabetic adults. Diabetes Care 1997; 20:585–90.
68. Green L, Feher M, Catalan J. Fears and phobias in people with diabetes. Diabetes Metab Res Rev 2000; 16:287–93.
69. Surwit RS, van Tilburg MA. Stress management improves long-term glycemic control in type 2 diabetes. Diabetes Care 2002; 25:30–4.
70. Yoo JS, Kim EJ, Lee SJ. The effects of a comprehensive life style modification program on glycemic control and stress response in type 2 diabetes. Taehan Kanho Hakhoe Chi 2006; 36:751–60.
71. Okada S, Ichiki K. Effect of an anxiolytic on lipid profile in non-insulin-dependent diabetes mellitus. J Int Med Res 1994; 22:338–42.
72. Lustman PJ, Griffith LS. Effects of alprazolam on glucose regulation in diabetes. Results of double-blind, placebo-controlled trial. Diabetes Care 1995; 18:1133–9.
73. Svacina S. Our experience with antidepressant treatment in the obese and type 2 diabetics. Prague Med Rep 2005; 106:291–6.
74. Cox D, Gonder-Frederick L. A multicenter evaluation of blood glucose awareness training-II. Diabetes Care 1995; 18:523–8.
75. American Psychiatric Association. Diagnostic and Statistical Manual of Mental Disorders. Washington, DC: American Psychiatric Association, 1994.
76. Stinson FS, Grant BF. Comorbidity between DSM-IV alcohol and specific drug use disorders in the United States: results from the National Epidemiologic Survey on Alcohol and Related Conditions. Drug Alcohol Depend 2005; 80:105–16.
77. McQuade WH, Levy SM, Yanek LR, Davis SW, Liepman MR. Detecting symptoms of alcohol abuse in primary care settings. Arch Fam Med 2000; 9:814–21.
78. Avogaro A, Tiengo A. Alcohol, glucose metabolism and diabetes. Diabetes Metab Rev 1993; 9: 129–46.
79. National Institute on Alcohol Abuse and Alcoholism. Eighth Special Report to the U.S. Congress on Alcohol and Health. Washington, DC: Secretary of Health and Human Services, 1993.
80. Emanuele NV, Swade TF, Emanuele MA. Consequences of alcohol use in diabetics. Alcohol Health Res World 1998; 22:211–9.
81. Ewing JA. Detecting alcoholism. The CAGE questionnaire. JAMA 1984; 252:1905–7.
82. National Institute of Mental Health. Eating disorders: facts about eating disorders and the search for solutions. NIH Publication No. P01 4901 2001.
83. Papelbaum M, Appolinario JC. Prevalence of eating disorders and psychiatric comorbidity in a clinical sample of type 2 diabetes mellitus patients. Rev Bras Psiquiatr 2005; 27:135–8.

84. Wing RR, Nowalk MP, Marcus MD, Koeske R, Finegold D. Subclinical eating disorders and glycemic control in adolescents with type I diabetes. Diabetes Care 1986; 9:162–7.
85. Wolff GE, Clark MM. Changes in eating self-efficacy and body image following cognitive-behavioral group therapy for binge eating disorder: a clinical study. Eat Behav 2001; 2:97–104.
86. Kaplan RM, Sallis JF, Patterson TL. Health and Human Behavior. New York: McGraw-Hill, 1993.
87. House JS, ed. Work Stress and Social Support. Reading, MA: Addison-Wesley, 1981:13–40.
88. Lazarus RS, Folkman S. Stress, Appraisal, and Coping. New York: Springer, 1984.
89. Kawachi I, Colditz G. A prospective study of social networks in relation to total mortality and cardiovascular disease in men in the USA. J Epidemiol Community Health 1996; 50:245–51.
90. Weissberg-Benchell J, Pichert JW. Counseling techniques for clinicians and educators. Diabetes Spect 1999; 12(2):103–7.
91. Boehm S, Schlenk EA, Funnell MM, Powers H, Ronis DL. Predictors of adherence to nutrition recommendations in people with non-insulin-dependent diabetes mellitus. Diabetes Educ 1997; 23: 157–65.
92. Hakim LS, Goldstein I. Diabetic sexual dysfunction. Endocrinol Metab Clin North Am 1996; 25: 379–400.
93. Chu NV, Edelman SV. Erectile dysfunction and diabetes. Curr Diab Rep 2002; 2:60–6.
94. Israilov S, Shmuely J. Evaluation of a progressive treatment program for erectile dysfunction in patients with diabetes mellitus. Int J Impot Res 2005; 17:431–6.
95. Doggrell SA. Comparison of clinical trials with sildenafil, vardenafil and tadalafil in erectile dysfunction. Expert Opin Pharmacother 2005; 6:75–84.
96. Schreiner-Engel P, Schiavi RC, Vietorisz D, Smith H. The differential impact of diabetes type on female sexuality. J Psychosom Res 1987; 31:23–33.
97. Veves A, Webster L, Chen TF, Payne S, Boulton AJ. Aetiopathogenesis and management of impotence in diabetic males: four years experience from a combined clinic. Diabet Med 1995; 12:77–82.
98. Guay AT. Safety and tolerability of sildenafil citrate for the treatment of erectile function in men with type 1 and type 2 diabetes [abstract]. Diabetes 2000; 49(Suppl. l):363.
99. Boulton AJ, Selam JL, Sweeney M, Ziegler D. Sildenafil citrate for the treatment of erectile dysfunction in men with type II diabetes mellitus. Diabetologia 2001; 44:1296–301.
100. Blonde L. Sildenafil citrate for erectile dysfunction in men with diabetes and cardiovascular risk factors: a retrospective analysis of pooled data from placebo-controlled trials. Curr Med Res Opin 2006; 22:2111–20.
101. Kent S. Is diabetes a form of accelerated aging? Geriatrics 1976; 31:140–54.
102. Perlmuter LC, Hakami MK. Decreased cognitive function in aging non-insulin-dependent diabetic patients. Am J Med 1984; 77:1043–8.
103. Strachan MWJ, Deary IJ, Ewing FME, Frier BM. Is type 2 (non-insulin dependent) diabetes mellitus associated with an increased risk of cognitive dysfunction? Diabetes Care 1997; 20:438–45.
104. Ryan CM, Greckle M. Why is learning and memory dysfunction in type 2 diabetes limited to older adults. Diabetes Metab Res Rev 2000; 16:308–15.
105. Debling D, Amelang M, Hasselbach P, Sturmer T. Diabetes and cognitive function in a population-based study of elderly women and men. J Diabetes Complications 2006; 20:238–45.
106. Manschot SM, Brands AM. Brain magnetic resonance imaging correlates of impaired cognition in patients with type 2 diabetes. Diabetes 2006; 55:1106–13.
107. Akisaki T, Sakurai T. Cognitive dysfunction associates with white matter hyperintensities and subcortical atrophy on magnetic resonance imaging of the elderly diabetes mellitus Japanese elderly diabetes intervention trial (J-EDIT). Diabetes Metab Res Rev 2006; 22:376–84.
108. Steen E, Terry BM. Impaired insulin and insulin-like growth factor expression and signaling mechanisms in Alzheimer's disease—is this type 3 diabetes? J Alzheimers Dis 2005; 7:63–80.
109. Biessels GJ, Kappelle LJ. Increased risk of Alzheimer's disease in type II diabetes: insulin resistance of the brain or insulin-induced amyloid pathology? Biochem Soc Trans 2005; 33:1041–4.
110. Rasgon N, Jarvik L. Insulin resistance, affective disorders, and Alzheimer's disease: review and hypothesis. J Gerontol A Biol Sci Med Sci 2004; 59:178–83.
111. Craft S. Insulin resistance syndrome and Alzheimer's disease: age- and obesity-related effects on memory, amyloid, and inflammation. Neurobiol Aging 2005; 26(Suppl 1):65–9.
112. Sun MK, Alkon DL. Links between Alzheimer's disease and diabetes. Timely. top. Med Cardiovasc Dis 2006; 10:E24.
113. Marcus AO. Safety of drugs commonly used to treat hypertension, dyslipidemia, and type 2 diabetes (the metabolic syndrome): Part 1. Diabetes Technol Ther 2000; 2:101–10.
114. Frier BM. Hypoglycaemia and cognitive function in diabetes. Int J Clin Pract 2001; (Suppl):30–7.

8 | Oral Hypoglycemic Agents: Sulfonylureas and Meglitinides

Andreas F. H. Pfeiffer
Department of Endocrinology, Diabetes and Nutrition, University of Berlin, Berlin, Germany

INTRODUCTION

For many years sulfonylureas have been the mainstay of oral antidiabetic therapy based on their insulinotropic action on beta cells in the pancreatic islets of Langerhans. Several alternative oral agents have now become available, broadening the spectrum of therapeutic alternatives. However, insulinotropic agents target one of the deficits that characterize diabetes mellitus type 2, namely a relative insufficiency of insulin secretion. Their therapeutic efficacy has been proven in several smaller trials, and in a large randomized prospective trial in type 2 diabetes—the U.K. Prospective Diabetes Study (UKPDS)—and was shown to be similar to the administration of insulin (1). A recent study in the United States compared the glucose-lowering potential of insulin with sulfonylureas in a setting of treatment by family practitioners, and found similar potency for either treatment (2). Insulin lowered the glycosylated hemoglobin (HbA$_{1c}$) by 0.8% and the sulfonylurea by 1.1%, which is comparable to the outcome observed in the UKPDS.

A number of different insulinotropic agents have been developed, which differ in their insulinotropic potency, duration of action, routes of elimination, and noninsulinotropic additional and side effects (3). Very recently, an additional group of insulinotropic agents acting on the sulfonylurea receptor has become available. These compounds are termed meglitinides, and presently consist of the benzoic acid derivative repaglinide and the tryptophane derivative nateglinide.

MECHANISM OF ACTION

Sulfonylureas and meglitinides (repaglinide and nateglinide) bind to a subunit of a potassium channel (K$_{ATP}$-channel) on beta cells named SUR1 (for sulfonylurea). SUR1 is a subunit of a potassium channel of the inward rectifier (IR) type, together with the channel-forming subunit named Kir6.2 (4). This channel is physiologically regulated by adenosine triphosphate (ATP). ATP is generated by oxidative phosphorylation in the mitochondria and is derived from glucose metabolism. ATP closes the K$_{ATP}$-channel, which normally allows efflux of K$^+$ from the beta cell, thereby generating the normal hyperpolarized membrane potential. Closure of the K$_{ATP}$-channel depolarizes the cell and activates voltage-driven Ca^{2+} channels. The ensuing influx of Ca^{2+} into the cell promotes fusion of insulin granules with the cell membrane, causing insulin release (5). Sulfonylureas and the "glinides," i.e., the meglitinides repaglinide and nateglinide, promote closure of the K$_{ATP}$-channel complex by binding to the SUR1 subunit. They can thereby enhance the effect of ATP, but also cause closure of the channels on their own. Sulfonylureas, therefore, cause an increase in basal insulin secretion and enhance glucose- or nutrient-induced insulin secretion. The degree to which basal and meal-stimulated insulin release is enhanced may differ between compounds.

Recently glimepiride and glybenclamide were shown to activate the nuclear transcription factor PPARγ in vitro, which is thought to mediate the insulin-sensitizing action of thiazolidinediones (6). Their maximal potency was about 60% of that of pioglitazone. This provides a novel explanation for insulin-sensitizing actions of SUs, which may thus be caused by a partial agonism at these nuclear receptors. Two clinical studies reported that glimepiride increases adiponectin and reduced inflammatory cytokines such as TNFα, which is increased by activation of PPARγ (7).

THE INDICATION FOR SULFONYLUREA TREATMENT

Treatment goals for diabetes demand near-normal glucose levels if possible in view of patient compliance and ability to follow therapeutic recommendations. This should be achieved with diet and exercise whenever possible. In the early phase of type 2 diabetes, insulin secretion typically is elevated (8), compared with healthy subjects, in an attempt to compensate for insulin resistance. Nevertheless, the chronically elevated levels of glucose, as occurs in manifest type 2 diabetes, indicate relative deficiency of insulin.

Insulinotropic agents are considered first-choice treatment in insulin-deficient patients who are not overweight, i.e., have a body mass index (BMI) $<25 \, kg/m^2$ (9). In overweight patients, metformin and alpha glucosidase inhibitors are recommended first-choice treatment and insulinotropic agents can be added where blood glucose control is insufficient. In obese patients with type 2 diabetes, sulfonylureas are considered second-choice treatments since an increase in body weight of 2 to 4 kg was observed in most studies with either sulfonylureas or with insulin, but not with metformin. In obese patients, the use of sulfonylureas is indicated if hyperglycemia is not controlled by other agents, and many diabetologists will add a sulfonylurea to metformin.

EFFICACY

Sulfonylureas will decrease blood glucose on average by 30 to 60 mg/dL (1.5–3 mmol/L) and lower HbA_{1c} by about 1.0% to 2.5%. The glucose-lowering potency of sulfonylureas is directly related to the initial glucose concentration at the onset of treatment, and is greater the higher the initial glucose concentration (2,6). In the UKPDS, the starting HbAlc concentration was around 9% and was lowered to about 7% by diet during the run-in period. The HbA_{1c} was lowered on average by 0.9% using chlorpropamide or glibenclamide (identical to glyburide in the United States) compared with the diet group, and this difference persisted during the 10 years of the study in patients controlled by sulfonylureas (1). Over this time, the mean HbA_{1c} of all treatment groups increased by about 2%, reflecting the overall loss of beta-cell function. However, this increase in HbA_{1c} was seen in all treatment groups and was not a consequence of sulfonylurea treatment, but rather was a consequence of the disease itself. Clearly, increased efforts are required to achieve good glucose control over time in patients with type 2 diabetes.

About 25% of the patients treated with sulfonylureas after diagnosis of type 2 diabetes will achieve a fasting plasma glucose $< 140 \, mg/dL$, which is still above the recommended ideal range of 80 to 120 mg/dL of fasting glucose (2,6). A good response is predicted by a moderately elevated fasting blood glucose of 140 to 220 mg/dL before onset of treatment, and a high-fasting plasma C-peptide and absence of markers of type 1 diabetes (GAD65 and/or IA2 antibodies). About 50% to 75% of newly diagnosed patients will require a second agent apart from lifestyle changes to achieve a blood glucose control of $< 140 \, mg/dL$ or 7.8 mmol/L, and thus are regarded as partial responders.

Patients with no or a poor response often have antibodies to GAD65 and belong to the group with latent autoimmune diabetes of adults' (LADA), which is a type 1 diabetes and represents about 10% of patients. Their age at onset of LADA is above 50 years and the BMI was around 23 to 25 kg/m^2 in several studies, thus was lower than in type 2 diabetes where BMI of 27 to 30 kg/m^2 are frequently reported. C-peptide in these patients is usually $<1 \, ng/mL^1$, while this is elevated in type 2 diabetes.

Patients with a good initial response to sulfonylureas usually show a declining response over time, resulting in a failure rate of about 5% per year. Within 10 years of treatment the majority of patients with type 2 diabetes appear to develop an insufficient response to sulfonylureas, termed "secondary failure." Clinical causes may be an increased need of insulin due to weight gain, chronic inflammation, immobilization or dietary factors. However, a decline in beta cell function has been observed in long-term studies, independent of the agents used for treatment, and represents a presently unmodifiable aspect of type 2 diabetes. The pathophysiology of this process is unknown. Early studies suggested that sulfonylureas may stress beta cells by increased demand, possibly causing secondary beta cell failure.

The UKPDS followed patients over about 9 years and documented that beta cell failure occurs independently of the type of treatment and was observed with metformin and with insulin to a similar degree as with sulfonylureas (10). Beta cell failure must apparently be regarded as an inherent aspect of the pathogenic process of type 2 diabetes. A recent trial compared monotherapy with glibenclamide, metformin, and rosiglitazone in 4360 newly diagnosed type 2 diabetes patients. Monotherapy treatment failure at 5 years, defined as a fasting plasma glucose above 180 mg/dcl, occurred at a rate of 34% with glibenclamide, 21% with metformin, and 15% with rosiglitazone. This is the first study suggesting different rates of beta cell failure related to the type of antidiabetic agent used (11).

A possible cofactor causing a decline of beta cell function may be seen in the chronic challenge of beta cells by supranormal levels of glucose, termed glucose toxicity, which permanently activates the secretory signaling pathways, thereby leading to their desensitization. This includes the signaling pathway activated by K_{ATP}-channel inhibitors. The disturbances in lipid metabolism typical of type 2 diabetes with elevated free fatty acids provide another putatively toxic component, termed by analogy "lipotoxicity," which should be improved with thiazolidinediones.

DRUG TYPES

Sulfonylureas were developed over 50 years ago and the first-generation agents, such as tolbutamide, chlorpropamide, and tolazamide, have a lower potency than the second-generation agents (glipizide, glibenclamide/gliburide, gliclazide, glisoxepide) (4). Potency correlates quite well with the affinity for the sulfonylurea receptor, and second-generation agents have a higher affinity for the sulfonylurea receptor. Glimepiride was proposed to possess some extrapancreatic effects and has therefore been termed a third-generation agent. However, with the development of a wide range of different sulfonylureas and meglitinides, the classification into different generations is more a marketing aspect than a meaningful characterization. The pharmacokinetic properties are summarized in Table 1.

The meglitinides differ structurally from the sulfonylureas and do not contain the sulfonylurea chemical motif. Repaglinide is a benzoic acid derivative, and nateglinide is derived from the amino acid tryptophane. Both compounds have substantially shorter duration of action than glibenclamide or glimepiride and have no active metabolites.

All these compounds bind to the sulfonylurea receptor and share the mechanism of action, i.e., all close the ATP-dependent potassium channel. The exact binding sites may differ somewhat, leading to complex displacement curves of radiolabeled glibenclamide (12), but the clinical significance of such rather subtle differences is unclear. Nateglinide has low affinity for the ATP-dependent potassium channel and, therefore, has rapid kinetics of association and dissociation, while repaglinide is intermediate between the high-affinity ligands glibenclamide or glimepiride and nateglinide.

DOSING SCHEDULE

With all compounds one should start treatment with the lowest effective dose and titrate upward until sufficient control or a maximal dose is achieved. The drug dose can be increased every 1 to 2 weeks. The first-generation compounds tolbutamide (500–2500 mg), tolazamide (100–1000 mg), and chlorpropamide (100–500 mg) required larger doses to be effective. Glipizide requires 5 to 20 mg, with 20 mg being the maximally effective dose, although doses of up to 40 mg have been approved. Glibenclamide (gliburide in the United States) can be given once daily, or in a divided dose of 1.75 to 10.5 mg for the micronized preparation, or up to 15 mg/day for the conventional, larger particle preparation. Glimepiride is given once daily in doses of 1 to 4 mg. Higher doses (8 mg) have been approved, but do not afford additional effects.

Gliquidon is administered once daily until a dose of 30 mg, higher doses, up to 120 mg, are given in a divided dose twice daily. The dose is also divided for patients with advanced renal impairment. Gliclazide was recently offered in a new once-daily formulation (MR)

TABLE 1 Pharmacokinetic Properties of Sulfonylureas

Sulfonylurea	Enteral resorption	Bioavailability (%)	C_{max} [a] (h)	$T_{1/2}$ [b] (h)	Plasma-protein binding (%)	Placental passage	Dose per day	Onset of effect (min)	Max. effect (h)	Duration of effect (h)	Hepatic metabolism	Excretion by the kidney (%)	Other ways of excretion
Tolbutamide	Fast	85–100	2–5	6–8	93–99	Yes	0.5–2.0 g	60	2–5	12–18	80%, active metabolite	>75%, <1% unchanged	9% via feces
Chlorpropamide	Fast	>90	2–4	35	>87	Yes	0.125–05 g			>24	80%	>90%, 20% unchanged	Little via feces
Tolazamide	Slow	85–90	4–6	7	87–94	Yes	0.125–05 g	100	6	6–12 (–116)	93%, five metabolites, three active	85	6% via feces
Glibenclamide (Gliburide)	Fast	>95	1–3	8–10	99	Yes	1.75–10.5	30	2–5	15–24	Complete to inactive metabolites	50, almost 0% unchanged	50% via feces
Glibomurid	Fast	91–98	3–4	5–11	95–97	Yes	12.5–75 mg				100%, six inactive metabolites	60–72, 0% unchanged	
Glisoxepide	Fast	>95	1	1.7	~93	Yes	2–16 mg	30–35	1	5–10	50% inactive metabolites	70–80, 50% unchanged	15–25% via feces
Gliquidon	Fast	>95	2–3	4–6	99	Yes	15–120 mg	60–90	2–3		100% inactive metabolites	0–5	>95% via feces
Glipizide	Fast	>95	1–2	2.7–4	97–99	Yes	2.5–30 mg	30	1	8–10	>9% inactive metabolites	64–87, 3–10% unchanged	15% via feces
Gliclazide	Slow	95	4–8	♂♀11	85–97	Yes	40–320 mg		2	6	99%, seven inactive metabolites	60–70	10–20 via feces
Gliclazide MR	Fast	>95	6	12–20	97	Yes	30–120 mg	60–120	4–6	24	99% inactive metabolites	60–70	10–20% via feces
Glimepiride	Fast	>95	2.5	5–8	99	Yes	1–8 mg	30–60	2–6	24 h	100%, two metabolites	84	10% via feces
Meglitinides													
Nateglinide	Fast	>75%	1	1.5	97–99		180–360 mg	15–30	30 min	3–4 h	Inactive metabolites	90	10% via feces
Repaglinide	Fast	>90%	1	1.5	>90		1.5–8 mg	30 min	30 min	3–4 h	Inactive metabolites	<10%	90% via feces

[a] C_{max}, maximum serum concentration.
[b] $T_{1/2}$, half-life.

requiring lower doses of 30 to 120 mg, instead of 80 to 320 mg with the old twice daily formulation (13).

Repaglinide and nateglinide are administered immediately before meals 2 to 4 times daily. Repaglinide is available in doses of 0.5 to 2 mg/meal and patients should be started with the lowest dose. Nateglinide is usually given in the dose of 120 mg/meal, although a 60 mg tablet is available (14–19).

EXTRAPANCREATIC EFFECTS OF SULFONYLUREAS AND MEGLITINIDES

Sulfonylureas cause a moderate improvement in the lipid profile due to improvement of lipid metabolism by increased levels of insulin and lowered level of glucose, which is considered an indirect effect.

Large randomized trials, such as the UKPDS, usually showed a weight gain of 2 to 4 kg with longer acting sulfonylureas, e.g., glibenclamide and chlorpropamide. This weight gain can be avoided by dietary advice if patients are compliant. Indeed, no weight gain was observed in smaller studies with glipizide, glimepride, and the shorter acting substances (20). Weight gain is apparently related to the increase in insulin and its antilipolytic and trophic action on fat cells, and is probably enhanced by the addition of further agents inhibiting lipolysis, such as beta-blockers or the thiazolidinediones, which promote fat cell differentiation and proliferation.

Glimepiride was shown to translocate glucose transporters to the cell membrane by a direct action in several experimental systems. In human, a modest effect on insulin sensitivity was shown in euglycemic clamps and insulin levels were slightly lower in glimepiride compared with glibenclamide-treated patients (21). A recent report compared glimepiride, glibenclamide, and gliclazide in hyperinsulinemic euglycemic clamps and described an enhanced insulin action for glimepiride and somewhat less for glibenclamide compared with gliclazide (22).

Chlorpropamide has two unique effects: it can cause a flushing reaction after ingestion of alcohol, by inhibiting the metabolism of acetaldehyde, and it sometimes causes a syndrome of inappropriate antidiuretic hormone (ADH) action (SI ADH), by enhancing its effects. Chlorpropamide is not now used in Europe and the United States.

Gliclazide was shown to have potent antioxidative actions in vitro and in vivo. Theoretically, this might be advantageous in patients with type 2 diabetes, but there are no studies with hard endpoints that demonstrate this.

Some studies, such as the University Group Diabetes Program (UGDP) (23) in 1976, suggested that sulfonylureas are associated with a poor outcome after a myocardial infarction, but these studies have been heavily criticized (24), and do not correspond with current standards. Theoretically, sulfonylureas might close ATP-dependent potassium channels possessing a SUR2a/b subunit, which are present on cardiomyocytes and coronary and arterial vessel smooth muscle cells, thereby preventing adaptive changes and relaxation of cardiomyocytes and vascular smooth muscle cells in response to hypoxia. This would occur by preventing smooth muscle cell hyperpolarization caused by potassium efflux, due to the closure of K_{ATP}-channels by the sulfonylurea, which might enlarge the infarct area. Although sulfonylureas bind the SUR1 on beta cells with much higher affinity than SUR2a/b, some activation appears possible. Glimepiride and nateglinide show much lower affinity for the cardiac SUR2b sulfonylurea receptor than for beta cell SUR1 and are a safer choice in this respect. Most of the increased deaths after myocardial infarction in diabetes appear to be due to poor left ventricular function. There is no convincing evidence for negative effects of sulfonylureas from clinical trials. Moreover, the UKPDS has not provided evidence for an increased mortality of patients treated with glibenclamide or chlorpropamide, which would be expected to become apparent in such a large study. However, in conditions of hypoxia, such as after a myocardial infarction or during coronary interventions, negative effects have not been sufficiently studied. It therefore appears prudent to withdraw high-affinity ligands of SUR2a/b in this condition (25).

SAFETY

Hypoglycemia is the major safety concern with sulfonylureas. Large studies have provided numbers for hypoglycemic episodes associated with some of the sulfonylureas used. The longer the duration of action and the more potent a compound, the higher the risk of hypoglycemia. Typically, elderly nonobese patients with type 2 diabetes who are given long-acting sulfonylureas and may miss a meal after having received the treatment are at highest risk. The presence of renal and/or hepatic insufficiency enhances the risk, due to impaired gluconeogenesis. In renal insufficiency, accumulation of compounds may occur due to decreased elimination.

There are few detailed studies about the use of sulfonylureas in renal impairment. Moderate reductions in creatinine clearance (up to 60 mL/min) require dose reductions, but allow the use of most sulfonylureas, whereas more severely compromised kidney function represents a contraindication. Gliquidone is almost completely eliminated in the feces after hepatic metabolism to inactive metabolites, and <5% are eliminated via the kidney. This is therefore the safest agent to use for type 2 diabetes treatment in renal insufficiency (26,27).

The shorter acting meglitinides may possess a lower risk of hypoglycemia simply because of the short duration of action and intake with meals, although not all studies have confirmed this assumption (16,28). Observational studies have suggested that glimepiride is less frequently associated with severe hypoglycemia than glibenclamide, but this was not shown in prospective controlled trials.

A COMPARISON OF DIFFERENT SULFONYLUREAS AND MEGLITINIDES

Among sulfonylureas, no definitive advantages have been demonstrated for one compound compared with others in trials with hard endpoints. The potent long-acting sulfonylureas bear a higher risk of protracted hypoglycemias in elderly people who may miss meals, and in poorly controlled conditions. Shorter acting and less potent insulin releasers may be advantageous under these circumstances (16,28). Specific advantages have been proposed for gliclazide, due to its antioxidant actions, and glimepiride, due to its insulin sensitizing effects, both of which are of unknown significance (29,30).

Meglitinides have been compared with glibenclamide and glipizide with regard to effects on average glucose- and meal-related insulin secretion. Indeed, repaglinide and nateglinide caused a more rapid increase in meal-related insulin secretion compared with glibenclamide, and achieved a more potent lowering of postprandial increases in glucose. Studies with nateglinide performed in patients with a fasting glucose slightly above 200 mg/ dL also showed that nateglinide was less potent in lowering fasting plasma glucose. Used as a single agent, the therapeutic effect is relatively small and HbA_{1c} was lowered by 0.6%. Thus, the drug appears most suitable for use in early diabetes. With more pronounced elevations of fasting glucose, combination with metformin was effective. This is, however, true for all combinations of sulfonylureas with metformin (see below). The faster acting meglitinides may achieve better postprandial control of blood glucose in combination with metformin or insulin sensitizers. It is unproven whether this difference of postprandial glucose results in advantages for the patient with regard to the risk of macrovascular disease.

Increases in postprandial glucose were shown to be associated with elevated risk of cardiovascular disease in impaired glucose tolerance (Lancet Decode 1999). This was not shown as well among patients with manifest type 2 diabetes. The extrapolation of studies in impaired glucose tolerance suggest that near-normal control of glucose, both fasting and postprandial, should decrease the cardiovascular risk associated with type 2 diabetes back to the normal range. Although this is plausible, and is expressed in the current treatment guidelines, it has not yet been proven in prospective trials. Such trials would have to overcome the difficulty that it is presently much harder to lower blood glucose into the normal range than to lower blood pressure or elevated cholesterol levels. However, the impact of clinical studies demonstrating a substantial advantage of normalizing—and not just lowering—blood glucose would be enormous and would change current treatment practices.

A reduction of postprandial glucose levels, however, is most likely to be successful in a setting of normalized fasting glucose levels i.e., 80 to 120 mg/dL. Advantages of better control of postprandial glucose are of unknown relevance with permanently elevated fasting glucose levels.

ORAL COMBINATION THERAPY

The combination of sulfonylureas with other noninsulinotropic agents results in additive effects and potently lowers blood glucose. The combination of metformin with sulfonylureas or meglitinides is frequently used, and additionally lowers HbA_{1c} by 1% to 2%, depending on the dose of metformin added. A dose-related increase has been shown to occur to a ceiling of 2 g metformin added to the insulin releaser per day in two doses (31). However, the mortality in the combination therapy group was increased compared with sulfonylurea monotherapy in the UKPDS (32). This has been attributed to an exceptionally low mortality in the sulfonylurea monotherapy group. However, similar trends were observed in a population-based observational study, indicating an urgent need for further studies of this combination (33). Similar improvements of blood glucose were reported for the combination of meglitinides with metformin (18) and for combinations of thiazolidinediones or α-glucosidase inhibitors and sulfonylureas. In all combinations, HbA_{1c} was lowered by 1% to 2%, in addition to the effect of the insulinotropic agent.

Most patients will, in fact, require more than one agent to achieve treatment goals of HbA_{1c} <7%. The choice may be individualized, depending on body weight, compliance, kidney function, and individual response to the treatment. The combination of insulinotropic agents with thiazolidinediones is highly effective in lowering blood glucose, but also additively increases body weight by 2 to 6 kg. The combination with α-glucosidase inhibitors was also shown to lower HbAlc by about 1%, but the lowering of fasting plasma glucose takes several weeks—for unknown reasons. This combination causes no additive weight gain. A combination with rimonabant, an inverse agonist of the cannabinoid receptor type 1 (CB1), was shown to lower HbA_{1c} and body weight by about 5 kg.

Since all diabetes trials observed a positive relation between blood glucose and the occurrence of late complications, this approach is rational and well-justified, based on current evidence.

COMBINATION THERAPY WITH INSULIN

An effective approach for narrow control of blood glucose once other combinations fail or are unwanted for other reasons is the use of evening administration of a long-acting insulin and an insulinotropic agent during the day. The evening dose of insulin should be titrated to achieve near normoglycemic blood glucose levels, while the insulinotropic agent improves postprandial blood glucose control during the daytime (34). Remarkably, a fair control may be achieved in some patients with type 2 diabetes, even when evening doses of 40 or more units of insulin are required. This scheme exploits the endogenous capacity for regulation of blood glucose still present with advanced type 2 diabetes, and may be tried before starting a multiple injection plan. However, this combination also is prone to cause substantial increases in body weight.

REFERENCES

1. UK Prospective Diabetes Study (UKPDS) Group. Intensive blood-glucose control with sulphonylur-eas or insulin compared with conventional treatment and risk of complications in patients with type 2 diabetes (UKPDS 33). Lancet 1998; 352:837–53.
2. Hayward RA, Manning WG, Kaplan SH, et al. Starting insulin therapy in patients with type 2 diabetes: effectiveness, complications, and resource utilization. Am Med Assoc 1997; 278:1663–9.
3. Schatz H, Mark M, Ammon H. Antidiabetika: Diabetes mellitus und Pharmakotherapie. Stuttgart: Wissenschaftliche Verlagsgesellschaft mbH Stuttgart, 1986.

4. Hu S, Wang S, Fanelli B, et al. Pancreatic beta-cell K(ATP) channel activity and membrane-binding studies with nateglinide: a comparison with sulfonylureas and repaglinide. Pharmacol Exp Ther 2000; 293:444–52.
5. Panten U, Schwanstecher M, Schwanstecher C. Sulfonylurea receptors and mechanism of sulfonylurea action. Exp Clin Endocrinol Metab 1996; 104:1–9.
6. Fukuen S, Iwaki M, Yasui A, Makishima M, Matsuda M, Shimomura I. Sulfonylurea agents exhibit peroxisome proliferator-activated receptor gamma agonistic activity. J Biol Chem 2005; 280:23653–9.
7. Tsunekawa T, Hayashi T, Suzuki Y, et al. Plasma adiponectin plays an important role in improving insulin resistance with glimepiride in elderly type 2 diabetic subjects. Diabetes Care 2003; 26:285–9.
8. DeFronzo RA. Pharmacologic therapy for type 2 diabetes mellitus. Ann Intern Med 1999; 131: 281–303.
9. European Diabetes Policy Group 1999. A desktop guide to type 2 diabetes mellitus. Diabet Med 1999; 16:716–30.
10. United Kingdom Prospective Diabetes Study Group. United Kingdom Prospective Diabetes Study 24: A 6-year, randomized, controlled trial comparing sulfonylurea, insulin, and metformin therapy in patients with newly diagnosed type 2 diabetes that could not be controlled with diet therapy. Ann Intern Med 1998; 128:165–75.
11. Kahn SE, Haffner SM, Heise MA, et al. Glycemic durability of rosiglitazone, metformin, or glyburide monotherapy. N Engl J Med 2006; 355:2427–43.
12. Fuhlendorff J, Rorsman P, Kofod H, et al. Stimulation of insulin release by repaglinide and glibenclamide involves both common and distinct processes. Diabetes 1998; 47:345–51.
13. Drouin P. Diamicron MR once daily is effective and well tolerated in type 2 diabetes: a randomized, double-blind, multi-national study. Diabet Comp 2000; 14:185–91.
14. Moses RG, Gomis R, Frandsen KB, et al. Flexible meal-related dosing with repaglinide facilitates glycemic control in therapy-naive type 2 diabetes. Diabetes Care 2001; 24:11–15.
15. Owens DR, Luzio SD, Ismail I, Bayer T. Increased prandial insulin secretion after administration of a single preprandial oral dose of repaglinide in patients with type 2 diabetes. Diabetes Care 2000; 23:518–23.
16. Landgraf R, Frank M, Bauer C, Dieken ML. Prandial glucose regulation with repaglinide: its clinical and lifestyle impact in a large cohort of patients with type 2 diabetes. Int J Obes Relat Metab Disord 2000; 24(Suppl. 3):S38–44.
17. Keilson L, Mather S, Walter YH, et al. Synergistic effects of nateglinide and meal administration on insulin secretion in patients with type 2 diabetes mellitus. Clin Endocrinol Metab 2000; 85:1081–6.
18. Horton ES, Clinkingbeard C, Gatlin M, et al. Nateglinide alone and in combination with metformin improves glycemic control by reducing mealtime glucose levels in type 2 diabetes. Diabetes Care 2000; 23:1660–5.
19. Hollander PA, Schwartz SL, Gatlin MR, et al. Importance of early insulin secretion: comparison of nateglinide and glyburide in previously diet-treated patients with type 2 diabetes. Diabetes Care 2001; 24:983–8.
20. Simonson DC, Kourides IA, Feinglos M, et al. Efficacy, safety, and dose-response characteristics of glipizide gastrointestinal therapeutic system on glycemic control and insulin secretion in NIDDM. Results of two multicenter, randomized, placebo-controlled clinical trials. The Glipizide Gastrointestinal Therapeutic System Study Group. Diabetes Care 1997; 20:597–606.
21. Clark HE, Matthews DR. The effect of glimepiride on pancreatic beta-cell function under hyperglycaemic clamp and hyperinsulinaemic, euglycaemic clamp conditions in non-insulin-dependent diabetes mellitus. Horm Metab Res 1996; 28:445–50.
22. Sato J, Ohsawa I, Oshida Y, et al. Comparison of the effects of three sulfonylureas on in vivo insulin action. Arzneimittelforschung 2001; 51:459–64.
23. Kilo C, Miller JP, Williamson JR. The crux of the UGDP. Spurious results and biologically inappropriate data analysis. Diabetologia 1980; 18:179–85.
24. Genuth S. Exogenous insulin administration and cardiovascular risk in non-insulin-dependent and insulin-dependent diabetes mellitus. Ann Intern Med 1996; 124(1 Pt 2):104–9.
25. Garrat K, Brady P, Hassinger N, et al. Sulfonylurea drugs increase early mortality in patients with diabetes mellitus after direct angioplasty for acute myocardial infarction. Am Coll Cardiol 1999; 33:119–24.
26. Harrower AD. Pharmacokinetics of oral antihyperglycaemic agents in patients with renal insufficiency. Clin Pharmacokinet 1996; 31:111–9.
27. Dedov II, Demidova I, Pisklakov SV, Antokhin EA. Use of glurenorm in patients with non-insulin-dependent diabetes mellitus and liver diseases. Probl Endokrinol (Mosk) 1993; 39:6–8.
28. Landgraf R. Meglitinide analogues in the treatment of type 2 diabetes mellitus. Drugs Aging 2000; 17:411–25.
29. Vallejo S, Angulo J, Peiro C, et al. Prevention of endothelial dysfunction in streptozotocin-induced diabetic rats by gliclazide treatment. Diabetes Compl 2000; 14:224–33.

30. Elhadd TA, Newton RW, Jennings PE, Belch JJ. Antioxidant effects of gliclazide and soluble adhesion molecules in type 2 diabetes. Diabetes Care 1999; 22:528–30.
31. Riddle M. Combining sulfonylureas and other oral agents. Am J Med 2000; 108:15S–22S.
32. Effect of intensive blood-glucose control with metformin on complications in overweight patients with type 2 diabetes (UKPDS 34). UK Prospective Diabetes Study (UKPDS) Group. Lancet 1998; 352: 854–65.
33. Olsson J, Lindberg G, Gottsater M, et al. Increased mortality in type 2 diabetic patients using sulfonylurea and metformin combination. Diabetologia 2000; 43:558–60.
34. Riddle M. Combined therapy with a sulfonylurea plus evening insulin: safe, reliable and becoming routine. Horm Metabol Res 1996; 28:430–3.

9 | Metformin

Michael Stumvoll
Department of Medicine, University of Leipzig, Leipzig, Germany

Hans-Ulrich Häring
Department of Medicine, Division of Endocrinology, Metabolic and Vascular Medicine, University of Tübingen, Tübingen, Germany

Stephan Matthaei
Diabetes Center, Quakenbrück, Germany

HISTORICAL ASPECTS AND INTRODUCTION

The glucose-lowering potential of guanides was first described in medieval times when extracts of Galega officinalis (goat's rue or French lilac) were used as treatment of diabetes in Europe (1). In 1957, metformin, a dimethylated biguanide, and phenformin, a phenetylated biguanide were introduced for the therapy of type 2 diabetes mellitus (Fig. 1). Because of the strong association with lactic acidosis, phenformin was withdrawn in the 1970s in most countries including the United States (2). In contrast, metformin continued to be used in Europe, Canada, and many other countries but was not approved by the U.S. Food and Drug Administration until 1995 (3). There is now a large body of data documenting the clinical efficacy of metformin in the treatment of type 2 diabetes (4) and most of its clinical, pharmacological, and basic cellular aspects have been addressed in several excellent reviews published during the past 20 years (5–12). Recently, the U.K. Prospective Diabetes Study (UKPDS) showed that metformin is particularly effective in type 2 diabetic subjects with obesity, a condition commonly associated with insulin resistance (13). Moreover, in essentially all clinical studies the improvement of hyperglycemia with metformin occurred in the presence of unaltered or reduced plasma insulin concentrations, e.g. (14,15). Taken collectively, these findings indicate the potential of metformin as an insulin-sensitizing drug and form the basis for metformin's current role in the treatment of type 2 diabetes (Fig. 2) (16).

CELLULAR MECHANISM OF ACTION

For almost 40 years of research, the precise cellular mechanism of metformin action has been a mystery. While depending on the researcher's background, the experimental system used or the available assay, a great many cellular mechanisms have been described but a single unifying site of action such as a receptor, an enzyme, or a transcription factor, had stubbornly escaped detection. Throughout this quest it was generally undisputed that metformin had no effect on the pancreatic beta cell in stimulating insulin secretion (8) and its main site of action had to be on the insulin action end.

The enzyme AMP-activated protein kinase (AMPK) is considered a cellular masters-witch in the control of whole-body energy and substrate metabolism. It plays a major role in the control of hepatic metabolism by integrating nutritional and hormonal signals. AMPK maintains energy balance by switching on catabolic pathways and switching off ATP-consuming pathways, both by short-term effects on phosphorylation of regulatory proteins and by long-term effects on gene expression. Activation of AMPK in the liver leads to the stimulation of fatty acid oxidation and inhibition of lipogenesis, glucose production, and protein synthesis. Metformin, like adiponectin and exercise is a potent stimulator of AMPK activity (17). Activation of AMPK results in many of the well-known cellular effects of metformin: inhibition of key enzymes of gluconeogenesis and glycogen synthesis in hepatocytes, and stimulation of insulin signaling and glucose transport in muscle cells (18).

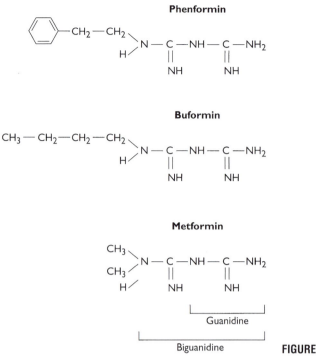

FIGURE 1 Chemical structure of biguanides.

One important upstream kinase of the AMPK cascade is the tumor suppressor LKB1, which was originally identified for its role in Peutz-Jegher's syndrome (19). Interestingly, deletion of the gene-encoding LKB1 in the liver leads to marked hyperglycemia as a consequence of increased gluconeogenic gene expression and hepatic glucose output. More importantly, the absence of LKB1 in the liver abolishes the effect of lowering glucose level caused by metformin (20). These findings establish LKB1 as the molecular target of metformin by which it increases AMPK activity which in turn regulates the key metabolic pathways of metformin action (Fig. 3).

MECHANISMS OF ACTION IN HUMANS

Glucose Production

Accelerated endogenous glucose production is thought to be a key factor in the development of fasting hyperglycemia in type 2 diabetes (21,22). In patients with type 2 diabetes metformin has been shown to inhibit endogenous glucose production in most (23–29), but not all studies (summarized in Ref. 30) to various degrees (from a nonsignificant ~10% up to a significant ~30% (Fig. 4) (30). This could largely be accounted for by inhibition of gluconeogenesis (24,31) although an additional inhibitory effect of metformin on glycogen breakdown is likely (24,25). The observation in many studies that in the basal postabsorptive state overall glucose disposal (metabolic plasma clearance rate of glucose) did not change while endogenous glucose production decreased (23–25,28,29,32) suggests that the improvement in glycemic control is largely attributable to the effect of metformin on glucose production.

Peripheral Glucose Metabolism

Most (23,26,28,29,33–35), but not all studies (25,27,32,36) using the hyperinsulinemic–eugly-cemic clamp technique have shown a metformin-induced increase in insulin-stimulated glucose disposal in patients with type 2 diabetes varying from ~15% up to ~40% (Fig. 5) (30). Since muscle represents a major site of insulin-mediated glucose uptake (21,37), metformin must, either directly or via indirect mechanisms, have an insulin-like or insulin-sensitizing

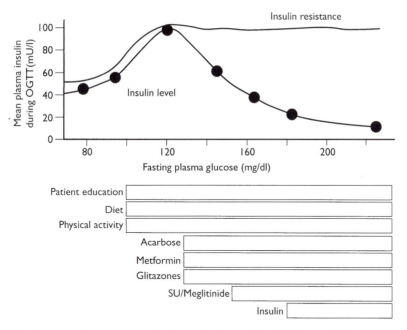

FIGURE 2 Starling's curve of the pancreas and rational treatment of type 2 diabetes mellitus. Starling's curve of the pancreas as originally described by DeFronzo et al. (22), indicating the relationship of mean plasma insulin levels during an oral glucose tolerance test (OGTT) and fasting plasma glucose levels of subjects with normal glucose tolerance, impaired glucose tolerance (IGT), and type 2 diabetes. The depicted therapeutic options should be selected according to the pathophysiological stage of the individual patient. *Abbreviations*: IGT, impaired glucose tolerance; OGTT, oral glucose tolerance test; SU, sulfonylureas. *Source*: From Refs.16 and 22.

effect on this tissue. In humans, the increase in insulin-stimulated glucose disposal is mostly accounted for by nonoxidative pathways (29,34,38). Nonoxidative glucose metabolism includes storage as glycogen, conversion to lactate, and incorporation into triglycerides. While no effect on lactate production is observed (24,25) implications on net triglyceride synthesis cannot be drawn. Nevertheless, it appears reasonable to propose that in human muscle glucose transport and possibly as a consequence, glycogen syntheses are the major targets of metformin action in the insulin-stimulated state. However, in the basal state, metformin had no effect on glucose clearance or whole-body glucose oxidation although the proportion of glucose turnover undergoing oxidation was increased (24). Moreover, forearm glucose uptake in the postabsorptive state was not significantly altered (24).

Metabolic Effects Independent of Improved Glycemia

The interpretation of the above experiments is limited by the fact that treatment with metformin was always accompanied by improvement in glycemic control and sometimes also by reduction of body weight. It can not be excluded; therefore, that the effects on endogenous glucose production and glucose disposal at least in part were secondary to reduced glucose toxicity (39) and/or weight loss (40) rather than metformin per se. Only four studies have examined the metabolic actions of metformin in the absence of any changes in glycemic control or body weight.

In one study 1 g of metformin was administered acutely to patients with type 2 diabetes and after 12 hours no effect on insulin-stimulated glucose disposal was seen while the excessive endogenous glucose production in the basal state was significantly reduced (32). This suggests that in patients with type 2 diabetes improvement in insulin-stimulated glucose disposal is predominantly due to alleviation of glucose toxicity while endogenous glucose production is immediately affected by metformin. In another study lean, normal glucose-tolerant, insulin-resistant first-degree relatives of patients with type 2 diabetes acutely received 1 g of metformin and the exact opposite was observed (38). In subjects with impaired glucose tolerance (IGT) 6-week metformin treatment improved basal homeostasis model

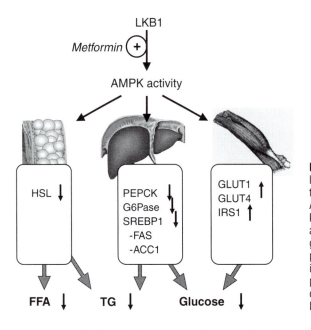

FIGURE 3 Mechanisms of metformin action on lipid and carbohydrate metabolism in adipose tissue, liver, and skeletal muscle. *Abbreviations*: ACC1, acetyl-CoA carboxylase 1; AMPK, AMP-kinase; FAS, fatty acid synthase; FFA, free fatty acids; GLUT1, glucose transporter 1; GLUT4, glucose transporter 4; G6Pase, glucose-6-phosphatase; IRS 1, HSL, hormone-sensitive lipase; insulin receptor substrate 1; LKB1, tumor suppressor gene; PEPCK, phosphoenolpyruvate carboxylase; SREBP1, sterol regulatory element-binding protein 1; TG, triglycerides.

assessment (HOMA), but not insulin-stimulated glucose disposal or glucose oxidation (41). In this study both fasting glucose and insulin decreased significantly. In android obese subjects with IGT increased insulin sensitivity (using an intravenous glucose tolerance) was observed after only 2 days of metformin treatment (1700 mg/day) (42). In obese women with the polycystic ovarian syndrome (PCOS) 6 months treatment with metformin also significantly improved insulin-stimulated glucose disposal (43,44). In another study in obese women with PCOS the decrease in serum insulin levels was associated with an increased ovulatory response to clomiphene (45). Glucose production was not assessed in the latter study. These apparent discrepancies could be explained by differences in the type of insulin resistance. In the highly selected group of lean, first-degree relatives and women with PCOS mechanisms may contribute to insulin resistance, which are different than those in garden-variety type 2 diabetes where insulin resistance is predominantly the result of obesity and longstanding hyperglycemia. Moreover, the reduction in endogenous glucose production after metformin treatment may only be seen in subjects in whom it was increased to begin with, such as patients with type 2 diabetes. The latter is supported by observations showing that metformin alone does not cause hypoglycemia or lowers blood glucose in nondiabetic subjects (46,47). The effect of metformin on endogenous glucose production in nondiabetic humans has not been studied yet.

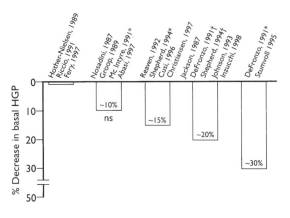

FIGURE 4 Summary of the effect of metformin on basal hepatic glucose production in type 2 diabetic patients. *Abbreviations*: HGP, hepatic glucose production. *Source*: From Ref. 30.

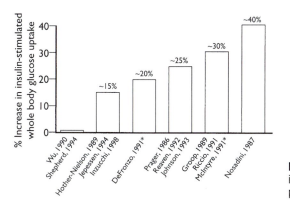

FIGURE 5 Summary of the effect of metformin on insulin-stimulated glucose disposal in type 2 diabetic patients. *Source*: From Ref. 30.

Additional evidence for improved insulin action comes from studies combining insulin therapy and metformin. It was shown that requirements of exogenous insulin are reduced (by ~30%) by addition of metformin in obese patients with type 2 diabetes (48–50) and in some patients with type 1 diabetes in whom glycemic control was unaltered (51–53).

Other Mechanisms of Action

It has been suggested that part of the antihyperglycemic effect of metformin is due to decreased release of free fatty acids (FFA) from adipose tissue and/or decreased lipid oxidation (32,54). However, reduced FFA levels after metformin treatment have only been shown in some (28,36,54) but not all studies (24,25,38). Moreover, in vitro studies have shown that metformin does not enhance the antilipolytic action of insulin on adipose tissue (55). Only two studies have examined FFA turnover using isotope techniques and found either no difference (24) or a 17% reduction (34) after metformin treatment. In the latter study the effect was only seen in the basal state but not in the insulin-stimulated state where FFA flux was largely suppressed. Thus, the metformin effect on peripheral glucose uptake may, at least in part, be mediated by suppression of FFA and lipid oxidation. In contrast, a causal relationship with endogenous glucose production is unlikely, since distinctly greater reductions in circulating FFA levels with acipimox failed to lower glucose production (56,57).

Evidence for other proposed mechanisms of metformin action is less convincing. Increased intestinal utilization of glucose has been suggested by animal studies (58–60). More

TABLE 1 In Vitro Studies—Effect of Metformin on Insulin-Mediated Glucose Metabolism

Effect cell/tissue type	Administration	Comment	Author (Ref)
Glucose transport			
↑ I Adipocytes humans	In vitro		Cigolini (26)
↑ I Adipocytes, rat	In vivo	Hyperglycemia after injury	Frayn (47)
↑ I Muscle strips, DM,N	In vitro	Effect only in insulin resistant subjects	Galuska (48,49)
↑ I Adipocytes, rat	In vitro/in vivo	Stimulation of GLUT1 and GLUT4 translocation	Matthaei (31,32)
↑ I L6 myotubes	In vitro	Stimulation of GLUT1 but not GLUT4 translocation	Hundal (50)
↑ I Muscle, mouse	In vivo	Streptozotocin, no effect in non-diabetic animals	Bailey (51)
↑ I Muscle, rat	In vitro	Alloxan diabetes, no effect in non-diabetic animals	Frayn (52)
↑ BI Adipocytes, rat	In vitro	Prevention of GLUT4 down -regulation	Kozka (53)
↑ BI Myotubes, humans	In vitro	Stronger effect with 25 mM versus 5 mM glucose	Sarabia (54)
NC Adipocytes, DM	In vitro		Pedersen (23)
Glycogen synthesis			
↑ I Muscle, mouse	In vivo	Streptozotocin diabetes	Bailey (51)
↑ I Muscle, rat	In vivo	Streptozotocin diabetes	Rossetti (30)
Glucose oxidation			
↑ I Muscle, mouse	In vivo	Streptozotocin diabetes	Bailey (51)
NC Muscle, mouse	In vitro	Streptozotocin diabetes	Wilcock (85)

Abbreviations: B, basal; 1, insulin-stimulated; DM, patients with type 2 diabetes, N, normal subjects.

TABLE 2 Metabolic Studies in Humans with Type 2 Diabetes—Effects of Metformin

Author	N	Dose, duration (mg daily, wks)	FG (mg/dL)	FI (μ/U/ml)	Basal MCR	Insulin-stimulated MCR	Basal glucose production
Prager (42)	12, obese	1.7/4	244 → 160	–	–	↑	↓
Nosadini (25)	7, obese	2.55/4	156 → 113*	15 → 9*	NC	↑	↓
Jackson (43)	10, lean	2.0–2.5/12	172 → 103*	23 → 23	–	NC	↓
Hother-Nielsen (56)	9, obese	2.0–2.5/12	205 → 184*	50 → 43	↑	↑	–
Wu (57)	12, obese	2.5/> 12	~220 → ~180*	~13 → ~11	–	NC	–
DeFronzo (44)	14, lean/obese	2.5/12	207 → 158*	19 → 13*	NC	↑	↓
Riccio (59)	6, non-obese	1.7/4	~163 → ~143*	NC	–	↑	–
McIntyre (65)	12, obese	3/6	175 → 103*	14.9 → 15.7	↑	↑	NC
Johnson (45)	8, obese	2.55/12	149 → 122*	15.8 → 11.3	NC	↑	↓
Perriello (46)	21, lean/obese	1.0/acute	–	–	NC	NC	↓
Stumvoll (40)	10, obese	2.55/15	220 → 155*	12 → 10*	NC	–	↓
Cusi (41)	20, obese	2.55/16	196 → 152*	17 → 14	NC	NC	↓
Fery (134)	9, obese	1.7/3	148 → 119*	19 → 15	↑	–	NC
Abbasi (78)	11, lean/obese	2.5/12	224 → 175*	13 → 12	↑	–	NC

Abbreviations: * indicates significant change; DM2, type 2 diabetes; FDR, first degree relatives of patients with type 2 diabetes; FG, fasting glucose; FI, fasting insulin; MCR, metabolic clearance rate of glucose; NC, no change; PCO, women with polycystic ovary syndrome; ~ indicates values taken from a figure.

recently, in vivo treatment with metformin increased gene expression of the energy-dependent sodium-glucose cotransporter (SGLT1) in rat intestine (61). However, such a mechanism has not been confirmed in humans (27).

Weight Loss

Unlike other pharmacological therapies for type 2 diabetes (sulfonylureas, insulin) metformin treatment is not associated with weight gain. Consistently, clinical studies have shown either a small but significant decrease in body weight (28,62) or a significantly smaller increase in body weight compared to other forms of treatment (48). One study has shown that weight loss during metformin treatment was largely accounted for by loss of adipose tissue (24). This was explained by differential effects of metformin on adipose tissue and muscle. While metformin improves insulin sensitivity in muscle, it does not affect the antilipolytic action of insulin on adipose tissue (63). The overall effect of metformin on body weight is attributed to a reduction in caloric intake (48,64) rather than an increase in energy expenditure (24,32,65). Since

TABLE 3 Metabolic Studies in Humans without Type 2 Diabetes—Effects of Metformin

Author	N	Dose, duration (g daily, weeks)	FG (mg/dL)	FI (μU/mL)	Basal MCR	Insulin-stimulated MCR	Basal glucose production
Morel (68)	19, obese, IGT	1.7/6	112 → 104	15.9 → 11.9	–	NC	–
Nestler (72)	35, obese, PCO	0.5/5	78 → 81	19 → 14	–	–	–
Moghetti (71)	23, obese PCO	1.5/26	85 → 79	15 → 10*	–	↑	–
Widen (66)	9, lean (FDR)	1.0/acute	–	–	NC	↑	NC
Diamanti (70)	16, PCO	1.7/26	86 → 88	21 → 19	–	↑	–

Abbreviations: * indicates significant change; FDR, first degree relatives of patients with type 2 diabetes; FG, fasting glucose; FI, fasting insulin; MCR, metabolic clearance rate of glucose; NC, no change; PCO, women with polycystic ovary syndrome; ~ indicates values taken from a figure.

reduction in body weight per se reduces insulin resistance this may also represent a mechanism by which metformin improves insulin resistance.

To summarize, the partly divergent observations from the numerous metabolic studies regarding metformin's effect on muscle and liver (Fig. 4 and 5) may reflect different mechanisms of metformin action in the basal versus the insulin-stimulated state. In the basal, postabsorptive state the improvement of fasting hyperglycemia is mostly due to a decrease of the accelerated endogenous glucose production. This results from inhibition of both gluconeogenesis and glycogen breakdown. Direct or indirect effects on regulatory enzymes are likely to be involved. No data are available for suppression of glucose production during experimental hyperinsulinemia. However, the fact that reduction in basal glucose production occurs in the presence of lower or unaltered insulin levels suggests that glucose production in liver and kidney (66,67) is more sensitive to the restrictive action of insulin after treatment with metformin.

In the insulin-stimulated state during the clamp peripheral glucose disposal is increased even in the absence of improved fasting glycemia indicating a reduction in insulin resistance. This is thought to be mainly a result of enhanced glucose transport and storage in muscle. The effect on glucose transport is most likely due to a potentiation of insulin-stimulated translocation of glucose transporters and an increase in their intrinsic activity (68,69). Glycogen synthesis is increased as a result of stimulatory effects of metformin on the signaling chain to activation of glycogen synthase. Moreover, the in vivo effect on muscle may in part be due to a reduction in FFA oxidation. Finally, in insulin-resistant subjects the effect on muscle appears to be more pronounced suggesting a reversal of insulin resistance rather than a mere improvement in insulin sensitivity.

CLINICAL EFFICACY OF METFORMIN IN PATIENTS WITH TYPE 2 DIABETES MELLITUS

Glycemic Control

The glucose-lowering effect of metformin, monotherapy or in combination, has been extensively reviewed (70–72). In a meta-analysis (73) all randomized, controlled clinical trials comparing metformin with placebo (29,62,74–80) and sulfonylurea (62,74,81–87) were evaluated. The weighted mean difference between metformin and placebo after treatment (median treatment duration 4.5 months) for fasting blood glucose was –2.0 mM and for HbA_{1c} –0.9%. Body weight was not significantly changed after treatment. Sulfonylureas and metformin lowered blood glucose (–2.0 and –1.8 mM, respectively) and HbA_{1c} (–1.1% and –1.3%, respectively) equally (median treatment duration 6 months). However, while after sulfonylurea treatment body weight increased by 2.9 kg there was a decrease of 1.2 kg after metformin. In a retrospective study of 9875 patients with type 2 diabetes mellitus who attended a large health maintenance organization metformin treatment improved the mean HbA_{1c} by 1.41% over a 20 months period (88).

Among obese patients allocated intensive blood glucose control within in the UKPDS, metformin showed a significantly greater effect than chlorpropamide, glibenclamide, or insulin for any diabetes-related endpoint, all-cause mortality, and stroke (74). In summary, metformin is as effective as sulfonylureas in improving glycemic control but, especially in overweight/obese patients, advantageous with respect to body weight, diabetes-related endpoints, and frequency of hypoglycemia.

Lipid Profile and Cardiovascular System

In addition to improving glycemic control metformin has been shown to reduce serum lipid levels. Metformin treatment results in a moderate (10–20%) reduction in circulating triglyceride levels, particularly in patients with marked hypertriglyceridemia and hyperglycemia (24,36,89), and also in nondiabetic subjects (90,91). This has been attributed to a reduction in hepatic very low-density lipoprotein (VLDL)-synthesis (36,78,92). Small (5–10%)

decreases in total circulating cholesterol have also been reported (67,75–77), which were essentially attributed to reductions in LDL levels (93–95) since high-density lipoprotein (HDL)-cholesterol were either increased (90) or unchanged (95).

In addition to the improvement of the lipid profile, metformin appears to have potentially beneficial hemostaseological effects. Fibrinolysis is increased (91,93,94) and the fibrinolysis inhibitor plasminogen-activator inhibitor 1 (PAI-1) is decreased (78,91,96).

Moreover, a decrease in platelet aggregability and density has been demonstrated (82,97). These additional effects of metformin that have been extensively reviewed elsewhere (70,71) may explain the advantage of metformin over sulfonylurea or insulin treatment with respect to macrovascular endpoints shown in the UKPDS (74), and in other randomized clinical trials that have been recently reviewed in a Cochrane meta-analysis (98).

Combination Therapies: Metformin Plus Sulfonylureas, Metformin Plus Glitazones, and Metformin Plus Insulin

Metformin is also used in combination with other antihyperglycemic agents. Because of its unique mechanisms of action a synergistic effect on glycemic control has been observed in combination with sulfonylureas (62,99,100), glitazones (101,102), and insulin where a dose-sparing effect was consistently demonstrated (48–50,103–105). Interestingly, in patients in whom sulfonylurea therapy has failed to satisfactory control glycemic, the combination of bedtime NPH-insulin. with metformin was advantageous compared to other combinations (105). In contrast to insulin alone, insulin plus sulfonylurea, and sulfonylurea alone, combining bedtime NPH-insulin with metformin achieved a decrease in HbA$_{1c}$ without significant weight gain (104,105).

Adverse Effects

While mild gastrointestinal disturbances are the most common side effects, lactic acidosis, though rare, is the most serious side effect of metformin treatment (106). In 9875 patients one case of probable lactic acidosis was observed in 20 treatment months (88). The incidence of lactic acidosis is 10 to 20 times lower than with phenformin. This is explained by the necessity to hydroxylate phenformin prior to renal excretion, a step which is genetically defective in 10% of whites (107,108). Metformin, in contrast, is excreted unmetabolized. In addition, in contrast to phenformin (109), metformin does neither increase peripheral lactate production nor decrease lactate oxidation (24,25) making lactate accumulation unlikely.

One study investigating individual cases of metformin-associated lactic acidosis showed that in these patients metformin should either have never been started or discontinued with the onset of acute illness (110). Thus, strict adherence to the exclusion criteria of metformin treatment [renal (creatinine clearance <60 mL/min) and hepatic disease, cardiac (NYHA III-IV) or respiratory insufficiency, severe infection, alcohol abuse, history of lactic acidosis, pregnancy, use of intravenous radiographic contrast) should minimize the risk of metformin-induced lactic acidosis.

Guidelines for the Clinical Use of Metformin

As recently recommended in a consensus statement of the American Dental Association (ADA) and the European Association for the Study of Diabetes (EASD) metformin should be initiated together with diet and exercise when patients have been diagnosed with type 2 diabetes (111). Metformin appears to be the drug of choice to start pharmacological treatment in insulin resistant and overweight/obese diabetic subjects (70,74,112). However, since the antihyperglycemic effects of metformin are similar in lean and obese subjects it can also be recommended as first-line treatment in the absence of obesity. It has been shown that the maximal antihyperglycemic effect of metformin is obtained using 2 g/day (Fig. 6) (113). Addition of metformin to sulfonylureas in patients with secondary sulfonylurea failure appears reasonable in view of their synergistic mechanisms of action and has been shown to improve glycemic control. Furthermore, especially in overweight/obese patients the addition

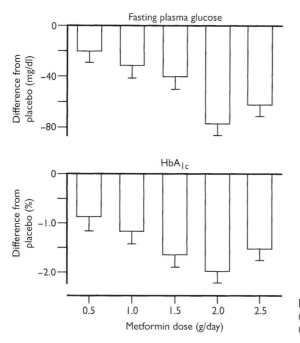

Fasting plasma glucose

HbA$_{1c}$

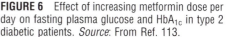

Metformin dose (g/day)

FIGURE 6 Effect of increasing metformin dose per day on fasting plasma glucose and HbA$_{1c}$ in type 2 diabetic patients. *Source*: From Ref. 113.

of metformin to insulin is advantageous compared to insulin alone (114). Moreover, in the Diabetes Prevention Program metformin has been shown to reduce the risk to develop type 2 diabetes in subjects with IGT by 31% (112), but it is not yet approved for use in subjects with IGT.

The above-described favorable effects of metformin in patients with type 2 diabetes have lead to the widespread recommendation in evidence-based guidelines in many countries to use metformin as first-line drug.

REFERENCES

1. Bailey CJ, Day C. Traditional plant medicines as treatments for diabetes. Diabetes Care 1989; 12: 553–64.
2. Luft D, Schmülling R, Eggstein M. Lactic acidosis in biguanide-treated diabetics: a review of 330 cases. Diabetologia 1978; 14:75–8.
3. Colwell J. Is it time to introduce metformin in the U.S.? Diabetes Care 1993; 16:653–5.
4. Johansen K. Efficacy of metformin in the treatment of NIDDM. Diabetes Care 1999; 22:33–7.
5. Bailey CJ, Turner RC. Metformin. N Engl J Med 1996; 334:574–9.
6. Dunn CJ, Peters DH. Metformin. A review of its pharmacological properties and therapeutic use in non-insulin-dependent diabetes mellitus. Drugs 1995; 49:721–49.
7. Davidson MB, Peters AL. An overview of metformin in the treatment of type 2 diabetes mellitus. Am J Med 1997; 102:99–110.
8. Bailey CJ. Biguanides and NIDDM. Diabetes Care 1992; 15:755–72.
9. Klip A, Leiter L. Cellular mechanism of action of metformin. Diabetes Care 1990; 13:696–704.
10. Bailey C. Metformin revisited: its actions and indications for use. Diabet Med 1988; 5:315–20.
11. Hermann L. Biguanides and sulfonylureas as combination therapy in NIDDM. Diabetes Care 1990; 13:37–41.
12. Bailey C, Nattrass M. Treatment—metformin. Baillieres Clin Endocrinol Metab 1988; 2:455–76.
13. U.K. Prospective Diabetes Study Group. Effect of intensive blood-glucose control with metformin on complications in overweight patients with type 2 diabetes (UKPDS 34). Lancet 1998; 352:854–65.
14. DeFronzo RA, Goodman AM, The Multicenter Metformin Study Group. Efficacy of metformin in patients with non-insulin-dependent diabetes mellitus. N Engl J Med 1995; 333:541–9.
15. Hermann LS, Kjellström T, Nilsson-Ehle P. Effects of metformin and glibenclamide alone and in combination on serum lipids and lipoproteins in patients with non-insulin-dependent diabetes mellitus. Diabet Metab 1991; 17:174–9.

16. Matthaei S, Stumvoll M, Kellerer M, Häring HU. Pathophysiology and pharmacological treatment of insulin resistance. Endocr Rev 2000; 21:585–618.

17. Zhou G, Myers R, Li Y, et al. Role of AMP-activated protein kinase in mechanism of metformin action. J Clin Invest 2001; 108:1167–74.

18. Viollet B, Foretz M, Guigas B, et al. Activation of AMP-activated protein kinase in the liver: a new strategy for the management of metabolic hepatic disorders. J Physiol 2006; 574(Pt 1):41–53.

19. Carling D. LKB1: a sweet side to Peutz-Jeghers syndrome? Trends Mol Med 2006; 12:144–7.

20. Shaw RJ, Lamia KA, Vasquez D, et al. The kinase LKB1 mediates glucose homeostasis in liver and therapeutic effects of metformin. Science 2005; 310:1642–6.

21. Dinneen S, Gerich J, Rizza R. Carbohydrate metabolism in non-insulin-dependent diabetes mellitus. N Engl J Med 1992; 327:707–13.

22. DeFronzo RA, Bonadonna RC, Ferrannini E. Pathogenesis of NIDDM. Diabetes Care 1992; 15: 318–68.

23. Nosadini R, Avogaro A, Trevisian R, et al. Effect of metformin on insulin-stimulated glucose turnover and insulin binding to receptors in type II diabetes. Diabetes Care 1987; 10:62–7.

24. Stumvoll M, Nurjhan N, Perriello G, Dailey G, Gerich JE. Metabolic effects of metformin in non-insulin-dependent diabetes mellitus. N Engl J Med 1995; 333:550–4.

25. Cusi K, Consoli A, DeFronzo RA. Metabolic effects of metformin on glucose and lactate metabolism in noninsulin-dependent diabetes mellitus. J Clin Endocrinol Metab 1996; 81:4059–67.

26. Prager R, Schernthaner G, Graf H. Effect of metformin on peripheral insulin sensitivity in non-insulin-dependent diabetes mellitus. Diabet Metab 1986; 12:346–50.

27. Jackson R, Hawa M, Jaspan J, et al. Mechanism of metformin action in noninsulin-dependent diabetes. Diabetes 1987; 36:632–40.

28. DeFronzo RA, Barzilai N, Simonson DC. Mechanism of metformin action in obese and lean noninsulin-dependent diabetic subjects. J Clin Endocrinol Metab 1991; 73:1294–301.

29. Johnson AB, Webster JM, Sum CF, et al. The impact of metformin therapy on hepatic glucose production and skeletal muscle glycogen synthase activity in overweight type II diabetic patients. Metabolism 1993; 42:1217–22.

30. Cusi K, DeFronzo RA. Metformin: a review of its metabolic effects. Diabet Rev 1998; 6:89–131.

31. Hundal RS, Krssak M, Dufour S, et al. Mechanism by which metformin reduces glucose production in type 2 diabetes. Diabetes 2000; 49:2063–9.

32. Perriello G, Misericordia P, Volpi E, et al. Acute antihyperglycemic mechanisms of metformin in NIDDM. Evidence for suppression of lipid oxidation and hepatic glucose production. Diabetes 1994; 43:920–8.

33. Hother-Nielsen O, Schmitz O, Andersen PH, Beck-Nielsen H, Pedersen O. Metformin improves peripheral but not hepatic insulin action in obese patients with type II diabetes. Acta Endocrinol (Copenh) 1989; 120:257–65.

34. Riccio A, Del Prato S, Vigili de Kreutzenberg S, Tiengo A. Glucose and lipid metabolism in non-insulin-dependent diabetes. Effect of metformin. Diabet Metab 1991; 17:180–4.

35. McIntyre HD, Ma A, Bird DM, Paterson CA, Ravenscroft PJ, Cameron DP. Metformin increases insulin sensitivity and basal glucose clearance in type 2 diabetes mellitus. Aust N Z J Med 1991; 21: 714–9.

36. Wu M, Johnston P, Sheu W, et al. Effect of metformin on carbohydrate and lipoprotein metabolism in NIDDM patients. Diabetes Care 1990; 13:1–8.

37. DeFronzo RA. The triumvirate: B-cell, muscle, and liver: a collusion responsible for NIDDM. Diabetes 1988; 37:667–87.

38. Widen E, Eriksson J, Groop L. Metformin normalizes nonoxidative glucose metabolism in insulin-resistant normoglycemic first-degree relatives of patients with NIDDM. Diabetes 1992; 41:354–8.

39. Yki-Järvinen H. Glucose toxicity. Endocr Rev 1992; 13:415–31.

40. Wing RR, Koeske R, Epstein LH, Norwalk MP, Gooding W, Becker D. Long-term effects of modest weight loss in type II diabetic patients. Arch Intern Med 1987; 147:1749–53.

41. Morel Y, Golay A, Pernegert T, et al. Metformin treatment leads to an increase in basal, but not insulin-stimulated, glucose disposal in obese patients with impaired glucose tolerance. Diabet Med 1999; 16:650–5.

42. Scheen AJ, Letiexhe MR, Lefebvre PJ. Short administration of metformin improves insulin sensitivity in android obese subjects with impaired glucose tolerance. Diabet Med 1995; 12: 985–9.

43. Diamanti Kandarakis E, Kouli C, Tsianateli T, Bergiele A. Therapeutic effects of metformin on insulin resistance and hyperandrogenism in polycystic ovary syndrome. Eur J Endocrinol 1998; 138: 269–74.

44. Moghetti P, Castello R, Negri C, et al. Metformin effects on clinical features, endocrine and metabolic profiles, and insulin sensitivity in polycystic ovary syndrome: a randomized, double-blind, placebo-controlled 6-month trial, followed by open, long-term clinical evaluation. J Clin Endocrinol Metab 2000; 85:139–46.

45. Nestler JE, Jakubowicz DJ, Evans WS, Pasquali R. Effects of metformin on spontaneous and clomiphen-induced ovulation in the polycystic ovary syndrome. N Engl J Med 1998; 338:1876–80.
46. Hermann L. Metformin: a review of its pharmacologic properties and therapeutic use. Diabet Metab 1975; 5:233–45.
47. McLelland J. Recovery from metformin overdose. Diabet Med 1985; 2:410–1.
48. Mäkimattila S, Nikkilä K, Yki-Järvinen H. Causes of weight gain during insulin therapy with and without metformin in patients with type II diabetes. Diabetologia 1999; 42:406–12.
49. Giugliano D, Quatraro A, Consoli G, et al. Metformin for obese, insulin-treated diabetic patients: improvement in glycaemic control and reduction of metabolic risk factors. Eur J Clin Pharmacol 1993; 44:107–12.
50. Robinson AC, Johnston DG, Burke J, Elkeles RS, Robinson S. The effect of metformin on glycemic control and serum lipids in insulin-treated NIDDM patients with suboptimal metabolic control. Diabet Care 1998; 21:701–5.
51. Gin H, Messerchmitt C, Brottier E, Aubertin J. Metformin improved insulin resistance in type I, insulin-dependent, diabetic patients. Metabolism 1985; 34:923–5.
52. Pagano G, Tagliaferro V, Carta Q, et al. Metformin reduces insulin requirements in type 1 (insulin-dependent) diabetes. Diabetologia 1983; 24:351–4.
53. Gin H, Slama G, Weissbrodt P, et al. Metformin reduces post-prandial insulin needs in type I (insulin-dependent) diabetic patients: assessment by the artificial pancreas. Diabetologia 1982; 23: 34–6.
54. Abbasi F, Carantoni M, Chen YD, Reaven GM. Further evidence for a central role of adipose tissue in the antihyperglycemic effect of metformin. Diabet Care 1998; 21:1301–5.
55. Cigolini M, Bosello O, Zancanaro C, Orlandi PG, Fezzi O, Smith U. Influence of metformin on metabolic effects of insulin in human adipose tissue in vitro. Diabet Metab 1984; 10:311–5.
56. Puhakainen I, Yki-Järvinen H. Inhibition of lipolysis decreases lipid oxidation and gluconeogenesis from lactate but not fasting hyperglycemia or total hepatic glucose production. Diabetes 1993; 42: 1694–9.
57. Saloranta C, Taskinen M, Widen E, Harkonen M, Melander A, Groop L. Metabolic consequences of sustained suppression of free fatty acids by acipimox in patients with NIDDM. Diabetes 1993; 42: 1559–66.
58. Wilcock C, Bailey CJ. Sites of metformin-stimulated glucose metabolism. Biochem Pharmacol 1990; 39:1831–4.
59. Penicaud L, Hitier Y, Ferre P, Girard J. Hypoglycaemic effect of metformin in genetically obese (fa/fa) rats results from an increased utilization of blood glucose by intestine. Biochem J 1989; 262: 881–5.
60. Bailey CJ, Mynett KJ, Page T. Importance of the intestine as a site of metformin-stimulated glucose utilization. Br J Pharmacol 1994; 112:671–5.
61. Wilcock C, Bailey CJ. Accumulation of metformin by tissues of the normal and diabetic mouse. Xenobiotica 1994; 24:49–57.
62. DeFronzo RA, Goodman AM, The Multicenter Metformin Study Group. Efficacy of metformin in patients with non-insulin-dependent diabetes mellitus. N Engl J Med 1995; 333:541–9.
63. Bellomo R, McGrath B, Boyce N. In vivo catecholamine extraction during continuous hemofiltration in inotrope-dependent patients. ASAIO Trans 1991; 37:M324–5.
64. Lee A, Morley JE. Metformin decreases food consumption and induces weight loss in subjects with obesity with type II non-insulin-dependent diabetes. Obes Res 1998; 6:47–53.
65. Leslie P, Jung RT, Isles TE, Baty J. Energy expenditure in non-insulin dependent diabetic subjects on metformin or sulfonylurea therapy. Clin Sci 1987; 73:41–5.
66. Stumvoll M, Meyer C, Mitrakou A, Nadkarni V, Gerich J. Renal glucose production and utilization. New aspects in humans. Diabetologia 1997; 40:749–57.
67. Meyer C, Stumvoll M, Nadkarni V, Dostou J, Mitrakou A, Gerich J. Abnormal renal and hepatic glucose metabolism in type 2 diabetes mellitus. J Clin Invest 1998; 102:619–24.
68. Matthaei S, Hamann A, Klein HH, et al. Association of metformin's effect to increase insulin-stimulated glucose transport with potentiation of insulin-induced translocation of glucose transporters from intracellular pool to plasma membrane in rat adipocytes. Diabetes 1991; 40: 850–7.
69. Matthaei S, Reibold JP, Hamann A, et al. In vivo metformin treatment ameliorates insulin resistance: evidence for potentiation of insulin-induced translocation and increased functional activity of glucose transporters in obese (fa/fa) Zucker rat adipocytes. Endocrinology 1993; 133: 304–11.
70. Bailey CJ, Turner RC. Metformin. N Engl J Med 1996; 334:574–9.
71. Dunn CJ, Peters DH. Metformin. A review of its pharmacological properties and therapeutic use in non-insulin-dependent diabetes mellitus. Drugs 1995; 49:721–49.
72. Davidson MB, Peters AL. An overview of metformin in the treatment of type 2 diabetes mellitus. Am J Med 1997; 102:99–110.

73. Johansen K. Efficacy of metformin in the treatment of NIDDM. Diabetes Care 1999; 22:33–7.
74. UK Prospective Diabetes Study Group. Effect of intensive blood-glucose control with metformin on complications in overweight patients with type 2 diabetes (UKPDS 34). Lancet 1998; 352:854–65.
75. Lalor BC, Bhatnagar D, Winocour PH, et al. Placebo-controlled trial of the effects of guar gum and metformin on fasting blood glucose and serum lipids in obese, type 2 diabetic patients. Diabet Med 1990; 7:242–5.
76. Teupe B, Bergis K. Prospective randomized two-years clinical study comparing additional metformin treatment with reducing diet in type 2 diabetes. Diabet Metab 1991; 17:213–7.
77. Dornan T, Heller S, Peck G, Tattersall R. Double-blind evaluation of efficacy and tolerability of metformin in NIDDM. Diabetes Care 1991; 14:342–4.
78. Nagi D, Yudkin J. Effects of metformin on insulin resistance, risk factors for cardiovascular disease, and plasminogen activator inhibitor in NIDDM subjects. Diabetes Care 1993; 16:621–9.
79. Tessari P, Biolo G, Bruttomesso D, et al. Effects of metformin treatment on whole-body and splanchnic amino acid turnover in mild type 2 diabetes. J Clin Endocrinol Metab 1994; 79:1553–60.
80. Grant PJ. The effects of high- and medium-dose metformin therapy on cardiovascular risk factors in patients with type II diabetes. Diabetes Care 1996; 19:64–6.
81. Rains S, Wilson G, Richmond W, Elkeles R. The effect of glibenclamide and metformin on serum lipoproteins in type 2 diabetes. Diabet Med 1988; 5:653–8.
82. Collier A, Watson HH, Patrick AW, Ludlam CA, Clarke BF. Effect of glycaemic control, metformin and gliclazide on platelet density and aggregability in recently diagnosed type 2 (non-insulin-dependent) diabetic patients. Diabet Metab 1989; 15:420–5.
83. Josephkutty S, Potter JM. Comparison of tolbutamide and metformin in elderly diabetic patients. Diabet Med 1990; 7:510–4.
84. Noury J, Nandeuil A. Comparative three-month study of the efficacies of metformin and gliclazide in the treatment of NIDD. Diabet Metab 1991; 17:209–12.
85. Boyd K, Rogers C, Boreham C, Andrews WJ, Hadden DR. Insulin, glibenclamide or metformin treatment for non insulin dependent diabetes: heterogenous responses of standard measures of insulin action and insulin secretion before and after differing hypoglycaemic therapy. Diabetes Res 1992; 19:69–76.
86. Hermann LS, Kjellström T, Schersten B, Lindgärde F, Bitzen P, Melander A. Therapeutic comparison of metformin and sulfonylurea, alone and in various combinations. Diabetes Care 1994; 17:1100–9.
87. Campbell IW, Menzies DG, Chalmers J, McBain AM, Brown IR. One year comparative trial of metformin and glipizide in type 2 diabetes mellitus. Diabet Metab 1994; 20:394–400.
88. Selby JV, Ettinger B, Swain BE, Brown JB. First 20 months' experience with use of metformin for type 2 diabetes in a large health maintenance organization. Diabetes Care 1999; 22:38–44.
89. Reaven G, Johnston P, Hollenbeck C, et al. Combined metformin-sulfonylurea treatment of patients with noninsulin-dependent diabetes in fair to poor glycemic control. J Clin Endocrinol Metab 1992; 74:1020–6.
90. Giugliano D, De Rosa N, Di Maro G, et al. Metformin improves glucose, lipid metabolism, and reduces blood pressure in hypertensive, obese women. Diabetes Care 1993; 16:1387–90.
91. Landin K, Tengborn L, Smith U. Treating insulin resistance in hypertension with metformin reduces both blood pressure and metabolic risk factors. J Intern Med 1991; 229:181–7.
92. Schneider J, Erren T, Zöfel P, Kaffarnik H. Metformin-induced changes in serum lipids, lipoproteins, and apoproteins in non-insulin-dependent diabetes mellitus. Atherosclerosis 1990; 82:97–103.
93. Landin K, Tengborn L, Smith U. Metformin and metoprolol CR treatment in non-obese men. J Intern Med 1994; 235:335–41.
94. Landin K, Tengborn L, Smith U. Effects of metformin and metoprolol CR on hormones and fibrinolytic variables during a hyperinsulinemic, euglycemic clamp in man. Thromb Haemost 1994; 71:783–7.
95. Pentikainen PJ, Voutilainen E, Aro A, Uusitupa M, Penttila I, Vapaatalo H. Cholesterol lowering effect of metformin in combined hyperlipidemia: placebo controlled double blind trial. Ann Med 1990; 22:307–12.
96. Grant PJ, Stickland MH, Booth NA, Prentice CR. Metformin causes a reduction in basal and post-venous occlusion plasminogen activator inhibitor-1 in type 2 diabetic patients. Diabet Med 1991; 8: 361–5.
97. Gin H, Freyburger G, Boisseau M, Aubertin J. Study of the effect of metformin on platelet aggregation in insulin-dependent diabetics. Diabetes Res Clin Pract 1989; 6:61–7.
98. Saenz A, Fernandez-Esteban J, Mataix A, et al. Metformin monotherapy for type 2 diabetes mellitus. Cochrane Database Syst Rev 2005; 20:CD002966.
99. Marena S, Tagliaferro V, Montegrosso G, Pagano A, Scaglione L, Pagano G. Metabolic effects of metformin addition to chronic glibenclamide treatment in type 2 diabetes. Diabet Metab 1994; 20: 15–9.

100. Groop L, Widen E. Treatment strategies for secondary sulfonylurea failure. Should we start insulin or add metformin? Is there a place for intermittent insulin therapy? Diabet Metab 1991; 17:218–23.
101. Weissman P, Goldstein BJ, Rosenstock J, et al. Effects of rosiglitazone added to submaximal doses of metformin compared with dose escalation of metformin in type 2 diabetes: the EMPIRE Study. Curr Med Res Opin 2005; 21:2029–35.
102. Waugh J, Keating GM, Plosker GL, et al. Pioglitazone: a review of its use in type 2 diabetes mellitus. Drugs 2006; 66:85–109.
103. Hanuschak LN. Metformin useful in combination with exogenous insulin [letter]. Diabetes Care 1996; 19:671–2.
104. Aviles-Santa A, Sinding J, Raskin P. Effects of metformin in patients with poorly controlled, insulin treated type 2 diabetes. Ann Int Med 1999; 131:182–8.
105. Yki-Järvinen H, Ryysy L, Nikkilä K, Tulokas T, Vanamo R, Heikkilä M. Comparison of bedtime insulin regimens in patients with type 2 diabetes mellitus. Ann Int Med 1999; 130:389–96.
106. Misbin RI, Green L, Stadel BV, Gueriguian JL, Gubbi A, Fleming GA. Lactic acidosis in patients with diabetes treated with metformin. N Engl J Med 1998; 338:265–6.
107. Oates NS, Shah RR, Idle JR, Smith RL. Influence of oxidation polymorphism on phenformin kinetics and dynamics. Clin Pharmacol Ther 1983; 34:827–34.
108. Kreisberg R, Pennington L, Boshell B. Lactate turnover and gluconeogenesis in obesity: effect of phenformin. Diabetes 1970; 19:64–9.
109. Lalau JD, Lacroix C, Compagnon P, et al. Role of metformin accumulation in metformin-associated lactic acidosis. Diabetes Care 1995; 18:779–84.
110. Nathan DM. Some answers, more questions, from UKPDS. Lancet 1999; 352:832–3.
111. Nathan DM, Buse JB, Davidson MB, et al. Management of hyperglycemia in type 2 diabetes: a consensus algorithm for the initiation and adjustment of therapy: a consensus statement from the American Diabetes Association and the European Association for the Study of Diabetes. Diabetes Care 2006; 29:1963–72.
112. Knowler WC, Barrett-Connor E, Fowler SE, et al. Reduction in the incidence of type 2 diabetes with lifestyle intervention or metformin. N Engl J Med 2002; 346:393–403.
113. Garber A, Duncan T, Goodman A, Mills D, Rohlf J. Efficacy of metformin in type-II diabetes: results of a double-blind, placebo-controlled, dose–response trial. Am J Med 1997; 102:491–7.
114. Buse J Combining insulin and oral agents. Am J Med 2000; 108 (Suppl. 1):23–32.

10 | Alpha-Glucosidase Inhibitors

Markolf Hanefeld
Center for Clinical Studies—Metabolism and Endocrinology, Technical University, Dresden, Germany

INTRODUCTION

There is a strong role for impaired insulin secretion in the development and progression of type 2 diabetes, in particular due to a deficit in the early phase response to glucose load, as well as increasing insulin resistance (1,2). It is believed that most subjects developing type 2 diabetes pass through a phase of impaired glucose tolerance (IGT). In this process—following the glucose toxicity theory—excessive postprandial hyperglycemia may act in a vicious circle (7), with harmful effects on both the insulin-producing beta-cells (3) and insulin sensitivity (4), leading to chronic hyperglycemia and progressive deterioration of diabetes, as shown in the U.K. Prospective Diabetes Study (UKPDS) (5).

There is increasing evidence that postprandial or 2 h postchallenge hyperglycemia is an independent risk factor for cardiovascular disease (6,7) and all-cause mortality (8–10). Excessive postprandial glucose excursion initiates a cascade of proatherogenic events: increased insulin resistance, activation of low-grade inflammation and blood coagulation as well as oxidative stress. Among other factors (Table 1), postprandial hyperglycemia strongly depends on the amount and of absorbed monosaccharides and velocity of absorption in the small intestine. Carbohydrates should account for ~50% of the daily supply of calories in type 2 diabetes. Monosaccharides play only a minor role as dietary carbohydrates since they consist mainly of complex carbohydrates, such as starch (~60%), and disaccharides, such as sucrose (~30%). Complex carbohydrates and disaccharides must be hydrolyzed by intestinal and pancreatic enzymes before they can be transported through the mucosa of the bowel. Thus, any medication that delays breakdown of complex carbohydrates should decrease postprandial hyperglycemia and improve insulin sensitivity, as well as protecting the beta-cells of the pancreas.

The digestion of complex carbohydrates in the lower parts of the small intestine and upper part of colon, as is the case with natural eating habits, has a stronger stimulating effect on gastrointestinal hormones, such as glucagon-like peptide 1 (GLP1) (12) than consumption of refined carbohydrates as typical for modern fast food. Alpha-glucosidase inhibitors (AGIs—acarbose, miglitol, voglibose) are oral antidiabetics that specifically inhibit α-glucosidases in the brush border of the small intestine. These enzymes are essential for the release of glucose from more complex carbohydrates (14,15).

STRUCTURE AND MODE OF ACTION OF AGIs

The concept of AGI was developed by Puls et al. (14), as a method of controlling the release of glucose from starch and sucrose—the major carbohydrate components in western diet. Inhibition affects both degradation of complex carbohydrates and digestion of disaccharides. An appropriate agent (acarbose) of microbial origin (culture filtrates of actinoplanes) was first described in 1977 by Schmidt et al. (13), and this inhibitor was introduced onto the market in 1990. Three AGIs are now in therapeutic use worldwide (Fig. 1), and are frequently prescribed in Central and south Europe and Asia.

Acarbose is a pseudotetrasaccharide with a nitrogen bound between the first and second glucose unit. This modification of a natural tetrasaccharide is important for its high affinity for active centers of alpha-glucosidases of the brush border of the small intestine, and for its stability. 1-Desoxynojirimycin is the parent compound of other AGIs such as miglitol which, in contrast with acarbose, is a small molecule, similar to glucose. Voglibose is produced by reductive alkylation of valiolamine (16,17).

TABLE 1 Determinants of Postprandial Glucose Excursion

Fasting plasma glucose
Insulin secretion (early phase)
Hepatic gluconeogenesis
Insulin sensitivity of target tissues
Meal composition and quantity
Additives to meal (alcohol, spices, fibers)
Gastric emptying, intestinal digestion and absorption
Duration of the meal
Gut hormones (enteroinsular axis)
Medication affecting insulin sensitivity (beta-blockers, angiotensin converting-enzyme inhibitors, etc.)
Physical activity

AGIs act as competitive inhibitors because of their high affinity for alpha-glucosidases, they block the enzymatic reaction particularly because of their nitrogen component. Thus, AGIs must be present at the site of enzymatic action at the same time as the carbohydrates. The effect on postload glucose excursion and insulin after a starch-containing mixed meal is shown in Figure 2. In principle, all three AGIs act in the same way, by inhibiting alpha-glucosidase enzymes in the brush border of the upper part of the small intestine. There are, however, some differences with respect to the inhibitory efficiency on various alpha-glucosidases, which may be responsible for differences in the frequency of side effects. Acarbose is most effective on glucoamylase, followed by sucrase, maltase, and dextranase (15). It also has a degree of inhibition of alpha-amylase, but has no effect on beta-glucosidases, such as lactase. Miglitol is a more potent inhibitor of disaccharide digesting enzymes, such as sucrase and maltase, than acarbose, and is also active on isomaltase but has no effect on alpha-amylase (18). It also weakly interacts as a pseudomonosaccharide with the intestinal sodium-dependent glucose transporter, without having a clinically relevant effect on glucose absorption (19). Voglibose is isolated from *Streptomyces* culture broths. It is a strong AGI with little effect on alpha-amylase.

PHARMACOLOGY OF AGIs

Acarbose is poorly absorbed (0.5–1.7%), and is degraded in the large intestine by bacterial enzymes into glucose, maltose, and acarviosine. A nonabsorbed fraction of 60% to 80% is excreted via feces (Table 2). About 35% of an oral dose appears as degradation products in the urine (16); this may be clinically relevant in cases of impaired kidney function. Miglitol is rapidly absorbed and transported in the intestine in the same way as glucose. It is

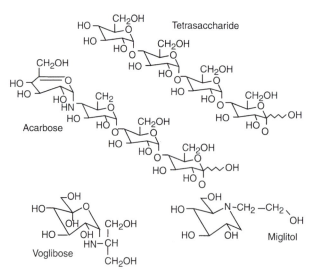

FIGURE 1 Structures of AGIs in clinical use.

TABLE 2 Summary of Pharmacological Characteristics of AGIs in Clinical Use

	Acarbose	Miglitol	Voglibose
Extent of absorption	Low	High, dose dependent	Low, dose dependent
Unchanged drug	<2%	>96%	<6%
Metabolites	<35%		
Bioavailability	<2%	>96%	<6%
Clearance	Mainly renal by glomerular filtration	Mainly renal by glomerular filtration	Mainly renal
Protein binding	Low to high species-dependent saturable	Low	Low to high species-dependent saturable
Distribution	Extracellular low tissue affinity	Extracellular Low tissue affinity	Low tissue affinity
Metabolism	Extrasystemic in the intestine	None	None
Excretion			
Fecal	>65%	Low	Almost complete
Renal	<35%	>96%	<5%
Biliary	<5%	<0.2%	–

Source: From Ref. 16.

concentrated in the brush border of the small intestine. Miglitol is unchanged, absorbed and excreted dose-dependently by the kidneys. Only 3% to 5% of voglibose is absorbed, and it is almost completely excreted via the feces. After oral administration, about 90% unchanged drug remains. By extrapolation, the most striking differences between AGIs in clinical use are with respect to absorption. Neither acarbose nor voglibose are absorbed in their active form, whereas miglitol is almost completely absorbed in the upper part of the small intestine, it has a long-lasting presence in the mucosa. It is not known whether this is relevant for comparative safety.

EFFECT ON CARBOHYDRATE METABOLISM

When AGIs are given orally, they reduce the digestion of carbohydrates in the upper half of the small intestine, so that a larger proportion is digested in the lower part and in the colon (Fig. 2). The rise in postprandial hyperglycemia is immediately diminished when AGIs are taken with the first bites of a meal (20). The amount of carbohydrate reaching the colon, and the alpha-glucosidase activity in the lower small intestine, determines the frequency and severity of gastrointestinal side effects, such as meteorism, flatulence, and diarrhea, due to fermentation gases and short-chain fatty acids (21). The quantity of undigested carbohydrates reaching the colon can be determined by measurement of breath hydrogen. The therapeutic effects, as well as side effects, therefore strongly depend on the amount and type of carbohydrates in the diet. It has been shown that acarbose is more effective in a diet rich in starch, because it has its strongest effect on glucoamylase (22).

There is a great variety of individual and racial intestinal enzyme patterns, which may explain the striking differences in efficacy and acceptance in different areas, and among different population groups. In Asia with a nutrition rich in complex carbohydrates (rice) AGIs are frequently used as first-line oral antidiabetics with few gastrointestinal side effects. With western nutrition habits low in starch and crude fibers—only small amounts of undigested carbohydrates reach the lower part of the small intestine. Unadapted exposure of the ileum and colon to greater amounts of these undigested carbohydrates after administration of AGIs leads to the side effects listed in Figure 3. Controlled studies (23) have shown that side effects can be minimized by dose titration, starting with doses of 25 mg of acarbose or miglitol twice a day. Over 1 to 3 months, the alpha-glucosidase content of the lower part of the small intestine increases, and the frequency of gastrointestinal side effects reduces (24).

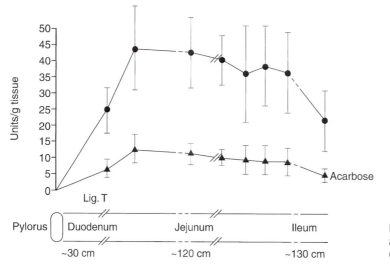

FIGURE 2 Mode of action of acarbose on postprandial glucose excursion.

Effect on Insulin and Enterohormones

There is no evidence of any direct effect of AGIs on insulin secretion and action. However, an improvement in insulin sensitivity may be achieved by control of postprandial hyperglycemia, which protects the beta-cells of the pancreas. This is supported by the results of the STOP-NIDDM trial (25) and 5-year follow-up data on clinical type 2 diabetes, which reveals an increasing efficacy in reduction of glycosylated hemoglobin (HbA_{1c}) over time (26). Three studies (two with acarbose (27,28) and one with voglibose (29)) in subjects with IGT directly measured insulin resistance and found an increase in insulin sensitivity. However, in type 2 diabetes this effect was only marginal, and was without statistical significance in investigations with CLAMP (30,31).

A recently published paper on elderly type 2 diabetes presents data by HOMA that indicates an improvement in insulin sensitivity (32). Consistent data from all three AGIs have shown a reduction in postprandial insulin excursion lasting $\geq 3\,h$ (33,34). So far, no data are available with respect to impact on the early insulin secretion phase. Two studies in IGT (27,28)

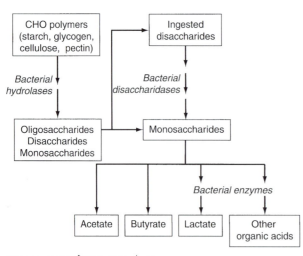

Consequences: ↑ Osmolarity, ↓ pH

FIGURE 3 Pathogenesis of gastrointestinal side effects after intake of AGIs; relationship of dosage and time after start of therapy. *Source*: From Ref. 44.

and one with 24 h profiles in type 2 diabetes (35), show a reduction in proinsulin levels postprandium, which may be indicative of an improved beta-cell function, following protection of the beta-cells from postprandial glucose spikes.

Inhibition of carbohydrate digestion by AGIs in the upper part of the small intestine affects release of two gut hormones: gastric inhibitory polypeptide (GIP) and GLP1. GIP is produced in the duodenum and upper jejunum, dependent on transmembranal glucose transport (36); it stimulates gastric emptying. The decrease in postprandial glucose absorption by AGI intake causes a decrease in GIP release after a carbohydrate-rich meal, which leads to a slower gastric emptying supporting the action of AGIs on postprandial glucose rise (37). The impact on GLP1 release seems to be even more important (36,37). GLP1 is mainly produced in the cells of the ileum and colon. AGIs trigger a long-lasting increase in GLP1 secretion in the late postprandial phase (60 to >240 min) when glucose excursion is already back at baseline. It is postulated that long-lasting increase in GLPa via the enteroinsular axis may support the therapeutic effects of AGIs (38,39).

Effect on Energy Balance and Components of the Metabolic Syndrome

AGIs delay the release of glucose but cause no malabsorption. In long-term studies (40,41) an average reduction in body weight of 0.7 to 0.9 kg was observed. However, no significant changes in eating pattern and energy intake were seen (22,41). In healthy volunteers, treatment with miglitol caused no significant loss of carbohydrates, proteins, and fat measured in the feces (15). The small weight loss registered in most long-term observations may therefore be a secondary phenomenon resulting from improved insulin sensitivity. AGIs have little or no effect on low-density lipoprotein (LDL)- and high-density lipoprotein (HDL)-cholesterol levels (42). However, recently published investigations in people with IGT treated with acarbose revealed a decrease in small dense LDL together with a lower lag time what is indicative of an ameliorated atherogenecity of LDLs (43).

The major effect is on fasting and postprandial triglycerides (44), with a reduction of about 15%. Furthermore, elevated LDL-cholesterol was lowered with acarbose (42) and with miglitol as adjuvant to sulfonylurea treatment (45). These weak effects on dyslipidemia may also be secondary results of improved insulin sensitivity.

In a placebo-controlled study on insulin resistance in obese hypertensive subjects with normal glucose tolerance the HOMA index in the acarbose group declined from 5.36 to 4.10 (p=.001) without a significant change in body mass index (BMI). This strong effect on insulin resistance may also be explained by reduction in postprandial glucose excursion (46).

In the STOP-NIDDM study in people with IGT the incidence of newly diagnosed hypertension was reduced by 34% versus placebo. In the MERIA meta-analysis systolic blood pressure decreased by 2.7 mmHg (p=.024). The effect of acarbose was compared to long-acting insulin secretagogue glibenclamide in type 2 diabetes patients with mild hypertension using automatic 24 h blood pressure measurements. After 6 months systolic blood pressure was lowered by 5.2 mmHg with acarbose versus 1.6 mmHg with glibenclamide ($p < .01$) whereas glibenclamide was more effective in lowering diastolic blood pressure. These results indicate that acarbose has beneficial effects on elevated systolic blood pressure. There are some new results that show that acarbose may have anti-inflammatory potentials. Significant reductions of hsCRP in people with IGT treated with acarbose have recently been published. Furthermore a decrease in fibrinogen after treatment with acarbose has been reported.

Thus by extrapolation AGIs, with best evidence for acarbose exhibit beneficial effects on all components of the metabolic syndrome and low-grade inflammation in patients with prediabetes and type 2 diabetes.

CLINICAL EFFICACY AND USE OF AGIs IN PATIENTS WITH TYPE 2 DIABETES

AGIs have been in clinical use for 10 years and are now registered worldwide. They are among the best-studied oral antidiabetics, with data from controlled studies and long-term clinical investigations for all three clinically used compounds. AGIs are used as first-line drugs in early type 2 diabetes, as well as in combination with nearly all established oral antidiabetics and insulin. In some cases of type 1 diabetes, with rapid postprandial glucose rise, and in cases of premeal hypoglycemia, AGIs may be introduced as adjunct therapy (36).

AGIs in Type 2 Diabetes Insufficiently Treated with Lifestyle Improvement

Acarbose (47,48) and miglitol (49) have been studied in drug naive patients in multinational European- and US-trials in dosages of 25 to 600 mg three times a day (Table 3). These studies have shown a dose–response relationship for acarbose and miglitol between 25 and 200 mg three times a day, with a plateau at 50 and 100 mg, with respect to both postprandial hyperglycemia and HbA_{1c}. However, side effects strongly increase at dosages of > 100 mg three times a day. Acarbose at a dosage of 100 mg seems to have more gastrointestinal side effects than miglitol at the same dosage (49).

Efficacy studies show that AGIs mainly act on postprandial hyperglycemia, with an effect on fasting plasma glucose occurring after 8 to 12 weeks. In clinical practice, glucose monitoring should therefore include measurements 2 h after major meals. In a meta-analysis of 13 controlled clinical trials with acarbose, the mean reduction in fasting glucose was 24 ± 7.2 mg/dL, in postprandial glucose it was 54 ± 15.8 mg/dL and in HbA_{1c} 0.90% $\pm 0.25\%$. The efficacy of therapeutic doses of miglitol is in the same range, with a somewhat higher effect on HbA_{1c} at a dosage of 50 mg three times per day, versus the same dose of acarbose (50). Fewer data are available for voglibose. Comparative studies with other oral antidiabetics show a weaker effect on HbA_{1c} than for metformin (34), except for one study that showed a similar efficacy (46). Except in one publication (51), a stronger effect of tolbutamide (52) and glibenclamide at 24 to 56 weeks follow-up has been consistently shown (36). It is a consistent finding that metformin and the sulfonylureas were more effective on fasting blood glucose control, whereas the AGIs were superior in the control of postprandial hyperglycemia. No reliable data have been published comparing the "prandial" insulin-secretagogues repaglinide and nateglinide with AGIs in face-to-face investigations.

A Cochrane review of 22 placebo-controlled studies with 1895 type 2 patients found a 0.78 (95% CI—0.93 – 0.63) overall reduction in HbA_{1c}. Compared to glibenclamide the efficacy was equal. Only one study reported a face-to-face comparison with metformin (53).

Combination Therapy of AGIs With Oral Antidiabetics and Insulin in Type 2 Diabetes

AGIs are frequently used as add-on therapy in patients insufficiently treated with sulfonylurea or metformin monotherapy. Less data exist on add-on therapy with AGIs as the first-line

TABLE 3 Dose–Response of Efficacy of Acarbose and Miglitol on Plasma Glucose (PG) and HbA_{1c} after 24 Weeks Treatment

Change (%)	Fasting PG	1 h postprandial PG	2 h postprandial PG	HbA_{1c}
Placebo	−0.4	−1.5	−2.7	7.83
Acarbose				
(three times per day)				
25 mg	−4.3	−11.6	−11.3	7.37
50 mg	−11.8	−15	−15.5	7.08
100 mg	−7.5	−13	−12.5	6.98
200 mg	−15	−19.4	−22.5	6.79
Placebo	NA	NA	+ 3.6	+ 0.29
Miglitol				
25	NA	NA	−8.4	−0.08
50	NA	NA	−17.7	−0.18
100	NA	NA	−28.9	−0.60
				HbA_{1c} initial
				(6.1–10.4%)

Abbreviation: NA, not available.
Source: From Refs. 48 and 73.

treatment. Recently, early combinations of oral antidiabetics with AGIs, to achieve perfect control of the glucotriad with lower dosage of the single drug and fewer side effects, have been discussed. Coadministration of AGIs to patients treated with metformin has an effect complementary to the major action of metformin, reducing hepatic gluconeogenesis and improving peripheral glucose disposal. There is now evidence from long-term studies that the add-on therapy with acarbose (54) or miglitol (55) to metformin results in an average decrease of HbA_{1c} of 0.8% to 0.9% in placebo-controlled long-term trials. The addition of metformin to patients on acarbose was particularly useful in fasting hyperglycemia (56).

Titration of metformin therapy should be started with a bedtime tablet, to optimize the effect on gluconeogenesis after midnight. Long-acting sulfonylureas, such as glibenclamide and glimepiride, are still in widespread use as first-line drugs. Addition of AGIs in subjects insufficiently treated with these insulin secretagogues has a synergistic effect to better control postprandial hyperglycemia. As consistently shown in controlled trials (52,56), an average reduction in HbA_{1c} of 0.8% to 0.9% can be achieved with this combination. Long-term data so far available suggest that add-on therapy with AGIs may delay the chronic progression of beta-cell failure, by protecting them from postprandial glucose spikes (25,26). Information comparing combination treatment of sulfonylurea plus metformin with the combination of either drugs with AGIs is scarce. An additive effect of acarbose on postprandial glucose excursions in type 2 patients treated by prandial insulin secretagogue repaglinide has been shown (57). Less favorable results are available on the combination of AGIs with insulin treatment in type 2 diabetes (58). The only moderately successful option in this trial was the combination of daytime AGI with bedtime injection of a long-acting insulin.

AGIs AS ADJUNCT IN TYPE 1 DIABETES

AGIs have been used as adjunct in type 1 diabetic patients whose postprandial glucose excursions cannot be adequately controlled with an insulin regimen (59). They reduce rapid rise in the early postprandial phase, and prevent spikes and troughs in the premeal phase (60). This smoothing effect is beneficial to avoid hypoglycemic episodes and acute hunger attacks before meals, due to delayed gastric emptying. A reduction of 0.5% in HbA_{1c}, by addition of acarbose, was shown in a 24-week placebo-controlled study, but no significant impact on frequency of hypoglycemic episodes was shown. In another study (59), nocturnal hypoglycemia was shown to be prevented when acarbose was given before dinner (60). Insulin dosage remained unchanged in the majority of cases. AGIs may therefore be helpful in brittle diabetes if best efforts to control postprandial glucose spikes by insulin regimen adjustment do not give an adequate control of postprandial glucose excursions. The same applies for excessive premeal hunger and nocturnal hypoglycemia.

Cardiovascular Effects

As already described AGIs have beneficial effects on a broad spectrum of cardiovascular risk factors inclusive low-grade inflammation and blood coagulation (61). In animal experiments increased platelet activation in Zucker rats with IGT was corrected by acarbose (62). Cardiac ischemia injury could be prevented by reducing postprandial hyperglycemia with AGI acarbose (63). In patients with IGT control of postprandial hyperglycemia with acarbose was associated with a significant improvement in flow-mediated vasodilation (64). Impressive cardiovascular preventive effects have been reported from the STOP-NIDDM trial where cardiovascular events were a secondary objective. In this study with IGT patients an overall reduction of cardiovascular events by 49% was observed inclusive 12:1 newly registered myocardial infarctions (65). In a substudy of STOP-NIDDM, which measured intima media thickness (IMT) as surrogate parameter of atherosclerosis progression IMT was reduced by ~50% comparable to people with normal glucose tolerance.

In a meta-analysis with seven controlled studies comprising 2180 patients with type 2 diabetes with a follow-up time of ≥1 year treatment with acarbose was associated with a 65% lower incidence of myocardial infarction and 35% less overall cardiovascular events. Thus these data suggest that AGIs, with preliminary evidence so far only for acarbose, have vasoprotective potentials. Two prospective studies with cardiovascular events as primary objective are under way to confirm these beneficial results.

SAFETY AND SIDE EFFECTS

AGIs are the safest oral antidiabetics, but are associated with a rather high frequency of gastrointestinal side effects because they inhibit digestion of carbohydrates. With >1 million patients having taken acarbose for >1 year, no serious adverse event has been reported. As antihyperglycemic agents they carry no risk of causing hypoglycemia. When given in combination with oral insulin secretagogues, the frequency of hypoglycemic episodes was reduced (52) and there was no increase in hypoglycemias observed in insulin-treated patients (54). A minor weight loss is observed in monotherapy with AGIs, and the weight gain caused by sulfonylureas is reduced if AGIs are added to this treatment regimen (52).

Gastrointestinal side effects frequently noted by patients are meteorism, flatulence, diarrhea (Table 4) or simple "abdominal discomfort (7)." Gastrointestinal complaints exhibit strong interindividual and regional differences, depending on nutrition habits, diet compliance, and advice from medical staff. During the first weeks of treatment, and within the first 3 months, the enzyme content of the lower part of the small intestine increases and most of the carbohydrates reaching this part of the bowel can be digested here. This is indicated by a decrease in gastrointestinal side effects to <10% in long-term follow-up studies (26). No malabsorption of carbohydrates is observed, together with fermentative digestion of carbohydrates in the colon. Thus, weight remains nearly unchanged, with a maximal weight loss of 0.7 to 0.9 kg in long-term follow-up studies (26,40). Gastrointestinal side effects diminish after 4 to 6 weeks (Fig. 4) (48), as has been consistently shown in controlled studies. In the UKPDS follow-up of a dosage of 100 mg of acarbose three times a day, 49% (diet alone), 43% (with sulfonylureas), and 39% (with metformin combinations) still took the drug at 3 years, compared with 70%, 60%, and 58%, respectively taking the placebo (40). On the other hand, in a large 2-year follow-up clinical trial with 1907 patients, 7.5% reported gastrointestinal side effects and the dropout rate resulting from gastrointestinal adverse events was only 2.5% (66). In a follow-up after 5 years, the incidence of acarbose-associated side effects was 4.7% (26).

The good compliance rate in motivated subjects and physicians was confirmed in the STOP-NIDDM study, a primary prevention trial in 1429 subjects with IGT. In the placebo arm, 2.5% of patients stopped taking the "drug" during 3.4 years follow-up because of adverse gastrointestinal events, versus 13.0% in the acarbose arm (25). In combination treatment, no increase in gastrointestinal side effects and drug interaction was observed if combined with sulfonylurea or insulin (52,54). The incidence of gastrointestinal side effects with metformin plus acarbose (54) and metformin plus miglitol (55) was not significantly different from that observed for monotherapy with either AGIs or metformin, although the rate of discontinuations was higher for the combination with metformin—as observed in the UKPDS. Flatulence (30% vs. 12%) and diarrhea (16% vs. 8%) were the major reasons for noncompliance with acarbose treatment in the UKPDS (40). In a face-to-face comparison, miglitol intake was

TABLE 4 Gastrointestinal and Other Side Effects, Extrapolation from Controlled and Surveillance Studies

Effect	Percentage
Meteorism	15–60
Flatulence	20–70
Diarrhea	5–16
Spasm and abdominal discomfort	3–4
Constipation	<1
Headache	<1
Nausea and vomiting	≈5

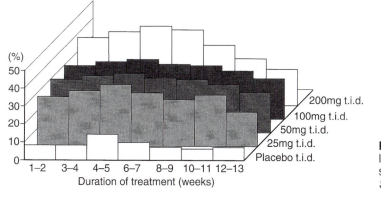

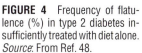

(%)

Duration of treatment (weeks)

FIGURE 4 Frequency of flatulence (%) in type 2 diabetes insufficiently treated with diet alone. *Source*: From Ref. 48.

associated with a lower frequency of gastrointestinal symptoms (49). On the other hand, elderly patients, particularly women with constipation, may benefit from the soft stools and report fewer problems with constipation.

AGIs in general have no liver toxic effects. In all controlled studies the incidence of transaminase elevations was at the level of the placebo group (47–49). In a safety review from the United States and Japan, 6/100,000 transient transaminase elevations were reported with AGIs (67). Two cases of severe hepatotoxic reactions during treatment with acarbose have been described recently. Both patients fully recovered and the reaction was interpreted as idiosyncratic (68). Acarbose degradation products may accumulate in cases of renal insufficiency, but no clinical complications have so far been reported. The upper limit for the use of acarbose where there is renal dysfunction was set for a creatinine level of >3.5 mg/ dL. Hematological studies with AGIs have not shown any changes in blood cells and bleedings. No effect on urine excretion of minerals or blood concentration levels of sodium and potassium has been observed (15).

Drug Interactions

A slight, clinically nonrelevant, reduction was seen in beta-acetyldigoxin and propranolol after coadministration of miglitol in healthy volunteers (15). Comedication with acarbose resulted in subtherapeutic plasma level of digitoxin in two cases of cardiac failure (69). AGIs do not interfere with the absorption of sulfonylureas, ACE inhibitors, beta-blockers or warfarin. The clinical bioavailability of metformin was marginally reduced by comedication with acarbose (70). In clinical practice this was not relevant for any AGIs.

INDICATIONS FOR AGIs AND CLINICAL PRACTICE

AGIs can be used as first-line drugs in newly diagnosed type 2 diabetes insufficiently treated with diet and exercise alone (34,73), as well as in combination with all oral antidiabetics and insulin if monotherapy with these drugs fails to achieve the targets for HbA_{1c} and postprandial blood glucose. As first-line drugs, AGIs are particularly useful in newly diagnosed type 2 diabetes with an excessive postprandial hyperglycemia, because of their unique mode of action in controlling the release of glucose from complex carbohydrates and disaccharides. In these cases, they lower postprandial blood glucose level peaks by >50 mg/ dL, resulting in an average reduction of HbA_{1c} by 0.7% to 1.2%. Table 5 summarizes subgroups of type 2 diabetes that may preferentially benefit from the use of AGIs as first-line treatment. Among them are elderly obese women. High percentages of who exhibit postchallenge hyperglycemia as the dominant abnormality of glucose homeostasis. Since AGIs are very safe and have very few contraindications and drug interactions, they also may be considered in polymorbid patients with beginning renal and hepatic dysfunction. Their weak weight-reducing effect could be an advantage over oral insulin secretagogues for some patients. As antihyperglycemic agents, AGIs have no risk of causing hypoglycemia, they are therefore a rational alternative for patients who experience hypoglycemic episodes with insulin secretagogues. In newly diagnosed type 2 diabetes with high-fasting plasma-glucose and high postprandial glucose, an early combination of either metformin or long-acting insulin secretagogues, such as glibenclamide and glimepiride, should be considered. This approach has the advantage of increasing efficacy and reducing side effects if low doses of either drug is used for the combination.

Many patients on monotherapy with either metformin or sulfonylureas do not reach HbA_{1c} levels <6.5% to 7%. A further reduction of HbA_{1c} of 0.5% to 1% can be achieved by add-on therapy with AGIs (26,36). There is increasing evidence (71,72) that postprandial hyperglycemic excursions add to the risk of progression of type 2 diabetes and its cardiovascular complications. In this context, AGIs are also useful adjuncts if postprandial glucose levels cannot be controlled sufficiently with metformin, sulfonylureas, or insulin. A meta-analysis (36) revealed an additional effect of 0.7% of acarbose given after metformin pretreatment, and 0.85% when added to sulfonylurea treatment. Extrapolation of controlled clinical trials with AGIs as add-on therapy showed an additional reduction in postprandial glucose of >40 mg/dL. The additional reduction in fasting blood glucose is >20 mg/dL. Little is known so far about combination therapy with thiazolidinediones and "prandial oral insulin secretagogues," such as nateglinide and repaglinide. Scarce information exists on the clinical use of AGIs in combination with bedtime administered long-acting insulin injections in type 2 diabetes. With AGIs as add-on therapy, a further reduction of HbA_{1c} of 0.4% to 0.54% was obtained. This combination may be useful in avoiding weight gain and to achieve better control of postprandial hyperglycemia.

PRACTICALITIES

Efficacy, side effects, and compliance strongly depend on rational indications, education of patients on how to use the drug, and good dietary advice. Even with good clinical practice, a considerable variation in response and side effects is seen. Side effects depend, among other things, on the dose and time intervals for titration of optimal therapeutic dosage. It is essential to start with low doses of 25 mg of acarbose or miglitol twice a day, with a stepwise increase in 2 to 3 week intervals. A study in type 2 diabetes patients treated with sulfonylurea compared the tolerability of stepwise increase with an initial dose of 100 mg three times per day of acarbose (23). The stepwise increase in dosage reduced specific side effects from 70% to 31%. The maximum dosage for acarbose and miglitol is usually 100 mg three times per day. There are, however, controlled studies that show that 200 mg three times per day is more effective, but has a higher adverse event rate (48).

After 3 to 4 weeks gastrointestinal side effects diminish to <20% in almost all studies. In long-term studies, the great majority of discontinuations because of side effects happen during the first 3 months. It is important to reinforce dietary advice before treatment and if side effects occur. A high content of raffined carbohydrates, and a diet rich in fat and protein are causes of gastrointestinal discomfort. Patients should be made aware that side effects are due to the mode of action, are mostly transient, and can be prevented by prudent diet. Table 6 summarizes some guidelines for patients to help overcome difficulties.

Patients should also take blood glucose levels twice a week at 1 to 2 h postprandial to see the benefit of treatment. With AGI treatment, fasting blood glucose levels in the first month of treatment is not indicative of therapy success.

TABLE 5   Indications for AGIs as First-Line Drug Treatment in Type 2 Diabetes

Newly diagnosed patients insufficiently treated with diet and dominating postprandial hyperglycemia
Elderly multimorbid patients
Elderly patients with weight gain or hypoglycemia under treatment with insulin secretagogues
Hepatic and renal dysfunction

Abbreviation: AGIs, alpha-glucosidase inhibitors.

TABLE 6   Advice to Patients to Overcome Difficulties with AGIs

Start low, go slow
Prefer nutrients with complex carbohydrates (rice, pasta, full bread, vegetables, fruits)
Avoid refined carbohydrates (sugar, sweets). Take only three meals per day
Avoid laxatives, such as sugar alcohols (sorbitol)
Control your postprandial blood glucose to experience the efficacy of treatment
In most cases gastrointestinal side effects are transient

Abbreviation: AGIs, alpha-glucosidase inhibitors.

USE OF AGIs IN PRIMARY PREVENTION OF TYPE 2 DIABETES

IGT is an accepted risk factor for both conversion to diabetes and cardiovascular disease. Prevalence of IGT in all nations with westernized lifestyles is > 15% in subjects aged > 40 years. Primary prevention efforts with lifestyle modification are therefore of high priority. In terms of medical intervention in subjects with IGT, AGIs have been shown to improve insulin sensitivity and reduce proinsulin secretion (27,28). In the STOP-NIDDM trial, a large placebo-controlled multinational study of 1429 subjects with IGT, acarbose reduced the annual incidence of diabetes by 36% in the intention to treat analysis (25). Acarbose is now registered in 26 countries as a drug for treatment of IGT. This was associated with a significantly lower event-rate of cardiovascular comorbidities. No serious adverse event associated with acarbose was observed during the 3 to 4 year follow-up.

CONTRAINDICATIONS

AGIs have very few contraindications. They should not be given to patients with diverticulosis, large hernia, acute gastrointestinal diseases, colitis, inclusive and obstructive diseases of the bowel because of their adverse effects on gas production in the bowel, particularly in the colon. Pregnancy and lactation period are contraindications. For acarbose, but not for miglitol, severe renal insufficiency (serum creatinine >3.5 mg/dL) is a contraindication. Bile acid adsorbents, such as cholestyramine, antacid agents, and digestive enzymes, may decrease the efficacy of these drugs. Clinical experience has shown that combination with the lipase inhibitor orlistat can exaggerate the gastrointestinal side effects of both drugs, but no controlled data are available. Laxatives and sugar alcohols, such as sorbitol with its high osmotic activity, increase gastrointestinal adverse reactions and should not be taken with AGI treatment.

REFERENCES

1. Haffner SM, Miettinen H, Gaskill SP, Stern MP. Decreased insulin action and insulin secretion predict the development of impaired tolerance. Diabetologia 1996; 39:1201–7.
2. Tripathy D, Carlsson M, Almgren P, et al. Insulin secretion and insulin sensitivity in relation to glucose tolerance. Lessons from the Bothnia study. Diabetes 2000; 49:975–80.
3. Pratley RE, Weyer C. The role of impaired early insulin secretion in the pathogenesis of type II diabetes mellitus. Diabetologia 2001; 44:929–45.
4. Gerich JE. Is insulin resistance the principal cause of type II diabetes? Diabet Obes Metab 1999; 1:257–63.
5. UK Prospective Diabetes Study (UKPDS) Group. Intensive blood-glucose control with sulphonylureas or insulin compared with conventional treatment and risk of complications in patients with type II diabetes (UKPDS 33). Lancet 1998; 352:837–53.
6. Smidt N, Barzilay J, Shaffer D, et al. Fasting and 2-hour postchallenge serum glucose measures and risk of incident cardiovascular events in the elderly. The Cardiovascular Health Study. Arch Intern Med 2002; 162:209–16.
7. de Vegt F, Dekker JM, Ruhe HG, et al. Hyperglycaemia is associated with all cause and cardiovascular mortality in the Hoorn population: the Hoorn Study. Diabetologia 1999; 42:926–31.
8. Hanefeld M, Schmechel H, Schwanebeck U, Lindner J. [The DIS-Group]. Predictors of coronary heart disease and death in NIDDM: the Diabetes Intervention Study experience. Diabetologia 1997; 40:123–4.

9. DECODE Study group on behalf of the European Diabetes Epidemiology Study Group. Glucose tolerance and mortality: comparison of WHO and American Diabetic Association diagnostic criteria. Lancet 1999; 354:617–21.

10. Leiter LA, Ceriello A, Davidson JA, et al. International Prandial Glucose Regulation (PGR) Study Group. Postprandial glucose regulation: new data and new implications. Clin Ther 2005; 27(Suppl. 2): S42–56.

11. Temelkova-Kurktschiev T, Koehler C, Henkel E, Hanefeld M. Leukocyte count and fibrinogen are associated with carotid and femoral intima-media thickness in a risk population for diabetes. Cardiovasc Res 2002; 56:277–83.

12. Goke B, Herrmann C, Goke R, et al. Intestinal effects of alpha-glucosidase inhibitors: absorption of nutrients and enterohormonal changes. Eur J Clin Invest 1994; 24(Suppl. 3):25–30.

13. Schmidt DD, Frommer W, Junge B, et al. Alpha-glucosidase inhibitors. New complex oligosaccharides of microbial origin. Naturwissenschaften 1977; 64:535–6.

14. Puls W, Keup U, Krause HP, et al. Glucosidase inhibition. A new approach to the treatment of diabetes, obesity and hyperlipoproteinemia. Naturwissenschaften 1977; 64:536–7.

15. Puls W. Pharmacology of glucosidase inhibitors Oral Antidiabet 1996; 119:497–525.

16. Krause HP, Ahr HJ. Pharmacokinetics and metabolism of glucosidase inhibitors. In: Kuhlmann J, Puls W, eds. Handbook of Experimental Pharmacology: Oral Antidiabetics, vol. 119. Berlin: Springer, 1996:541–5.

17. Taylor R, Bardolph E. Clinical evaluation of glucosidase inhibitors. Oral Antidiabet 1996; 119: 633–46.

18. Junge B, Matzke M, Stoltefuss J. Chemistry and structure-activity relationships of glucosidase inhibitors. In: Kuhlmann J, Puls W, eds. Handbook of Experimental Pharmacology: Oral Antidiabetics, vol. 119. Berlin: Springer, 1996:541–5.

19. Joubert PH, Venter HL, Foukaridis GN. The effect of miglitol and acarbose after an oral glucose load: a novel hypoglycaemic mechanism. Br J Clin Pharmacol 1990; 30:391–6.

20. Caspary WF. Sucrose malabsorption in men after ingestion of alpha-glucosidase hydrolase inhibitor. Lancet 1978; i:1231–3.

21. Holt RR, Atillasoy E, Lindenbaum J, et al. Effects of acarbose on fecal nutrients, colonic pH, and short chain fatty acids and rectal proliferative indices. Metabolism 1996; 45:1179–87.

22. Toeller M. Modulation of intestinal glucose absorption: postponement of glucose absorption by alpha-glucosidase inhibitors. In: Mogensen CE, Standl E, eds. Pharmacology of Diabetes. Berlin: De Gruyter, 1991:93–112.

23. May C. Efficacy and tolerability of step wise increasing dosage of acarbose in patients with non-insulin-dependent diabetes (NIDDM) treated with sulfonylureas. Diabetes Stoffwechsel 1995; 4:3–7.

24. Caspary WF, Lembke B, Creutzfeldt W. Inhibition of human intestinal alpha-glucoside hydrolase activity by acarbose and clinical consequences. In: Creutzfeldt W, ed. Proceedings First International Symposium on Acarbose, Montreux, October 1981. Amsterdam: Excerpta Medica, 1981:27–37.

25. Chiasson JL, Josse RG, Gomis R, et al. For the STOP-NIDDM trial research group. Acarbose can prevent the progression of impaired glucose tolerance to type 2 diabetes mellitus: the STOP-NIDDM trial. Lancet 2002; 359:2072–7.

26. Mertes G. Safety and efficacy of acarbose in the treatment of type 2 diabetes: data from 5-year surveillance study. Diabetes Res Clin Pract 2001; 2:193–204.

27. Chiasson JL, Josse RG, Leiter LA, et al. The effect of acarbose on insulin sensitivity in subjects with impaired glucose tolerance. Diabetes Care 1996; 19:1190–3.

28. Laube H, Linn T, Heyen P. The effects of acarbose on insulin sensitivity and proinsulin in overweight subjects with impaired glucose tolerance. Exp Clin Endocrinol Diabetes 1998; 106:231–3.

29. Shinozaki K, Suzuki M, Ikebuchi M, et al. Improvement of insulin sensitivity and dyslipidemia with a new alpha-glucosidase inhibitor, voglibose, in non-diabetic hyperinsulinemic subjects. Metabolism 1996; 45:731–7.

30. Schnack C, Prager RJF, Winkler J, et al. Effect of 8 week a-glucosidase inhibition on metabolic control, C-peptide secretion, hepatic glucose output and peripheral insulin sensitivity in poorly controlled type 2 diabetic patients. Diabetes Care 1989; 12:537–43.

31. Calle-Pascal A, Garcia-Honduvilla J, Martin Alvarez PJ, et al. Influence of 16-week monotherapy with acarbose on cardiovascular risk factors in obese subjects with non-insulin-dependent diabetes mellitus: a controlled, double-blind comparison study with placebo. Diabetes Metab 1996; 22:201–2.

32. Meneilly G, Ryan EA, Radziuk J, et al. Effect of acarbose on insulin sensitivity in elderly patients with diabetes. Diabetes Care 2000; 23:1162–7.

33. Hillebrand I, Boehme K, Frank G, et al. Effects of the glycoside hydrolase inhibitor (BAY g 5421) on post-prandial blood glucose, serum insulin and triglycerides levels in man. In: Creutzfeldt, ed. Frontiers of Hormone Research: The Entero-Insular Axis. Basel: Karger, 1979; 7:290–1.

34. Hanefeld M, Fischer S, Schulze, et al. Therapeutic potentials of acarbose as first-line drug in NIDDM insufficiently treated with diet alone. Diabetes Care 1991; 14:732–7.

35. Hanefeld M, Haffner SM, Menschikowski M, et al. Different effects of acarbose and glibenclamide on proinsulin and insulin profiles in people with type 2 diabetes. Diabetes Res Clin Pract 2002; 55:221–7.
36. Leboritz HE. A-glucosidase inhibitors as agents in the treatment of diabetes. Diabetes Rev 1998; 6: 132–45.
37. Qualmann C, Nauck MA, Hoist JJ, et al. Glucagon-like peptide 1 (GLP-1) [17-36 amide] secretion in response to luminal sucrose from the upper and lower gut: a study using a-glucosidase inhibition (acarbose). Scand J Gastroenterol 1995; 30:892–6.
38. Goke B, Fuder H, Wieckhorst G, et al. Voglibose is an efficient alpha-glucosidase inhibitor and mobilize the endogenous GLP-1 reserve. Digestion 1995; 56:493–501.
39. Goke B, Herrmann C, Goke R, et al. Intestinal effects of alpha-glucosidase inhibitors: absorption of nutrients and enterohormonal changes. Fur Clin Invest 1994; 24(Suppl. 3):25–30.
40. Holman RR, Turner RC, Cull CA, et al. A randomised double-blind trial of acarbose in type 2 diabetes shows improved glycemic control over 3 years (UK Prospective Diabetes Study 44). Diabetes Care 1999; 22:960–4.
41. Wolever TMS, Chiasson JL, Josse RG, et al. Small weight loss on long-term acarbose therapy with no change in dietary pattern or nutrient intake of individuals with non-insulin-dependent diabetes. Int J Obes Relat Metab Disord 1997; 21:756–63.
42. Leonardt W, Hanefeld M, Fischer S, et al. Beneficial effects on serum lipids in noninsulin-dependent diabetics by acarbose treatment. Arzt Forschung 1991; 41:735–8.
43. Shinoda Y, Inoue I, Nakano T, et al. Acarbose improves fibrinolytic activity in patients with impaired glucose tolerance. Metabolism 2006; 55:935–9.
44. Hanefeld M, Cagatay M, Petrowitsch T, Neuser D, Petzinna D, Rupp M. Acarbose reduces the risk for myocardial infarction in type 2 diabetic patients: meta-analysis of seven long-term studies. Eur Heart J 2004; 25:10–6.
45. Johnston PS, Feig PU, Coniff RF, et al. Chronic treatment of African-American type 2 diabetes patients with type 2 diabetic patients with alpha-glucosidase inhibition. Diabetes Care 1998; 21:416–21.
46. Rachmani R, Bar-Dayan Y, Ronen Z, Levi Z, Slavachevsky I, Ravid M. The effect of acarbose on insulin resistance in obese hypertensive subjects with normal glucose tolerance: a randomized controlled study. Diabetes Obes Metab 2004; 6:63–8.
47. Coniff RF, Shapiro JA, Robbins D, et al. Reduction in glycosylated hemoglobin and postprandial hyperglycemia by acarbose in patients with NIDDM: a placebo-controlled dose comparison study. Diabetes Care 1995; 18:817–24.
48. Fischer S, Hanefeld M, Spengler M, et al. European study on dose-response relationship of acarbose as a first-line drug in non-insulin-dependent diabetes mellitus: efficacy and safety of low and high doses. Acta Diabetol 1998; 35:34–40.
49. Rybka J, Goke B, Sissmann. European comparative study of 2 a-glucosidase inhibitors, miglitol and acarbose [abstract]. Diabetes 1999; 44(Suppl. 1):101.
50. Hoffmann J, Spengler M. Efficacy of 24-week monotherapy with acarbose, metformin or placebo in dietary-treated NIDDM patients: the Essen II Study. Am J Med 1997; 103:483–90.
51. Hoffmann J, Spengler M. Efficacy of 24-week monotherapy with acarbose, glibenclamide, or placebo in NIDDM patients. The Essen study. Diabetes Care 1994; 17:561–6.
52. Coniff RF, Shapiro JA, Seaton TB, Bray GA. Multicenter, placebo-controlled trial comparing acarbose with placebo, tolbutamide and tolbutamide-plus-acarbose in non-insulin-dependent diabetes mellitus. Am J Med 1998; 98:443–51.
53. Hofmann J, Spengler M. Efficacy of 24-week monotherapy with acarbose, metformin, or placebo in dietary-treated NIDDM patients: the Essen-II-Study. Am J Med; 103:483–90.
54. Chiasson JL, Josse RG, Hunt JA, et al. The efficacy of acarbose in the treatment of patients with non-insulin-dependent diabetes mellitus: a multicenter controlled clinical trial. Ann Intern Med 1994; 121:928–35.
55. Chiasson JL, Naditch L and The Miglitol Canadian University Investigator Group. The synergistic effect of miglitol plus metformin combination therapy in the treatment of type 2 diabetes. Diabetes Care 2001; 24:989–94.
56. Hanefeld M, Bar K. Effizienz und Sicherheit der Kombinationsbehandlung von IT type 2-Diabetikern mit Acarbose und Metformin. Diabetes Stoff 1998; 7:186–90.
57. Rosak C, Hofmann U, Paulwitz O. Modification of beta-cell response to different postprandial blood glucose concentrations by prandial repaglinide and combined acarbose/repaglinide application. Diabetes Nutr Metab 2004; 17:137–42.
58. Kelley DE, Schimel D, Bidot P, et al. Efficacy and safety of acarbose in insulin-treated patients with type 2 diabetes. Diabetes Care 1998; 21:2056–61.
59. Dimitriadis G, Hatziagellki E, Alexopoulos E, et al. Effects of a-glucosidase inhibition on meal glucose-tolerance and timing of insulin administration in patients with type I diabetes mellitus. Diabetes Care 1991; 14:393–8.
60. Hollander P, Pi-Sunyer X, Coniff RF. Acarbose in the treatment of type 1 diabetes. Diabetes Care 1997; 20:248–53.

61. Ceriello A, Taboga C, Tonutti L, et al. Post-meal coagulation activation in diabetes mellitus: the effect of acarbose. Diabetologia 1996; 39:469–73.
62. Schafer A, Widder J, Eigenthaler M, Bischoff H, Ertl G, Bauersachs J. Increased platelet activation in young Zucker rats with impaired glucose tolerance is improved by acarbose. Thromb Haemost 2004; 92:97–103.
63. Frantz S, Calvillo L, Tillmanns J, et al. Repetitive postprandial hyperglycemia increases cardiac ischemia/reperfusion injury: prevention by the alpha-glucosidase inhibitor acarbose. FASEB J 2005; 19:591–3.
64. Wascher TC, Schmoelzer I, Wiegratz A, et al. Reduction of postchallenge hyperglycaemia prevents acute endothelial dysfunction in subjects with impaired glucose tolerance. Eur J Clin Invest 2005; 35: 551–7.
65. Chiasson JL, Josse RG, Gomis R, Hanefeld M, Karasik A, Laakso M, STOP-NIDDM Trial Research Group. Acarbose treatment and the risk of cardiovascular disease and hypertension in patients with impaired glucose tolerance: the STOP-NIDDM trial. JAMA 2003; 290:486–94.
66. Mertes G. Efficacy and safety of acarbose in the treatment of type 2 diabetes: data from a 2-year surveillance study. Diab Res Clin Pract 1998; 40:63–70.
67. Hollander PA. Safety profile of acarbose and alpha glucosidase inhibitor. Drugs 1992; 44(Suppl. 3): 47–53.
68. Gentile S, Turco S, Guarino G, et al. Aminotransferase activity and acarbose treatment in patients with type 2 diabetes. Diabetes Care 1999; 22:12–7.
69. Ben-Am H, Krivo N, Nagachandran P, et al. Interaction between digoxin and acarbose. Diabetes Care 1999; 22:860–1.
70. Scheen AJ, Ferreira Alves de Megalheas AC, Salvatore T, et al. Reduction of the acute bioavailability of metformin by the a-glucosidase inhibitor acarbose in normal man. Eur J Clin Invest 1994; 24 (Suppl. 3):50–4.
71. Hanefeld M, Fischer S, Julius U, et al. and the DIS Group. Risk factors for myocardial infarction and death in newly detected NIDDM: the Diabetes Intervention Study, 11-year follow-up. Diabetologia 1996; 39:1577–83.
72. Temelkova-Kurktschiev T, Kohler C, Henkel E, et al. Post-challenge plasma glucose and glycemic spikes are more strongly associated with atherosclerosis than fasting glucose or HbA$_{1c}$ level. Diabetes Care 2000; 23:1830–4.
73. Drent ML. Miglitol as single oral hypoglycemic agent in type 2 diabetes [abstract]. Diabetologia 1994; 37(Suppl. 1):211.

11 | Thiazolidinediones

Sunder Mudaliar and Robert R. Henry

Diabetes/Metabolism Section, VA San Diego Healthcare System and University of California at San Diego, San Diego, California, U.SA.

INTRODUCTION

Type 2 diabetes is a burgeoning epidemic associated with substantial morbidity and mortality and afflicting more than 150 million people worldwide (1,2). Intensive control of blood glucose significantly reduces and ameliorates the microvascular complications of retinopathy, nephropathy, and neuropathy. However, up to 80% of patients with type 2 diabetes die from the macrovascular complications of cardiovascular disease. This increased incidence of accelerated atherosclerosis disease is closely associated with insulin resistance, which is a major pathophysiologic abnormality in type 2 diabetes and is known to be intricately involved in the development of not only hyperglycemia, but also dyslipidemia, hypertension, hypercoagulation, vasculopathy, and accelerated atherosclerotic cardiovascular disease. This cluster of metabolic abnormalities has been variously termed the insulin resistance or metabolic syndrome (3,4). The effects of thiazolidinediones, through their peroxisome proliferator-activated receptor γ (PPAR-γ) agonist, not only improve insulin sensitivity and glycemic control with reduced insulin requirements, but also have other potentially favorable effects on components of the insulin resistance or metabolic syndrome. These effects on lipid and adipose tissue metabolism and vascular endothelial function have the potential to modify pro-atherogenic metabolic processes and improve cardiovascular risk. A thiazolidine 2-4 dione structure is common to all thiazolidinediones, and they differ in their side chain, which alters their pharmacologic and side-effect profiles. Two compounds in this class are presently approved for use in the United States and around the world—rosiglitazone and pioglitazone. The first agent in this class, troglitazone, was withdrawn in March 2000, after reports of fulminant hepatotoxicity associated with its use. In clinical use so far, rosiglitazone and pioglitazone appear to be devoid of idiosyncratic, fulminant hepatotoxicity.

MECHANISM OF ACTION

The thiazolidinediones are highly selective and potent agonists for the PPAR-γ (Fig. 1) (5,6). These receptors are important regulators of adipocyte differentiation, lipid homeostasis, insulin action, and vascular endothelial function and are found not only in key target tissues for insulin action, such as adipose tissue, skeletal muscle, and liver, but also in the vascular endothelium, macrophages and other cell types (5,6). The thiazolidinediones act, at least in part, by binding with PPAR-γ in various tissues to influence/alter the expression of a number of genes encoding proteins involved in glucose and lipid metabolism, endothelial function and atherogenesis (5–7). The glucose-lowering effects of the thiazolidinediones involve the alteration of the expression of several genes involved in glucose and lipid metabolism, including glucose transporter (GLUT)1, GLUT4, leptin, tumor necrosis factor-α, hepatic glucokinase, Phosphoenolpyruvate carboxykinase (PEPCK), fatty acid (FA) binding protein, FA transport protein, and acyl CoA oxidase. These changes lead to improved metabolic effects, such as improved adipose tissue insulin sensitivity resulting in decreased free fatty acid (FFA) release and increased adiponectin release; improved hepatic insulin sensitivity, decreased gluconeogenesis and decreased hepatic glucose production; and improved muscle insulin sensitivity with increased tissue glucose uptake. Perhaps the most exciting development in the field of adipocyte biology and thiazolidinedione action has been the identification and characterization of the adipocyte-derived hormone

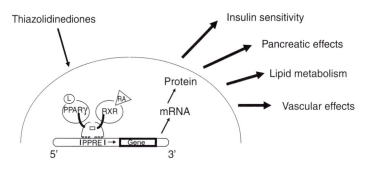

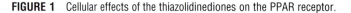

L = Ligand, RA = Retinoic acid, RXR = Retinoid-X receptor

PPRE = PPARγ responsive element, mRNA = messenger RNA

FIGURE 1   Cellular effects of the thiazolidinediones on the PPAR receptor.

adiponectin (8). Adipose tissue expression of adiponectin is lower in insulin-resistant states and lower plasma levels of adiponectin have been documented in human subjects with obesity, type 2 diabetes, or coronary artery disease (CAD). Studies in humans demonstrate a close correlation between changes in plasma levels of adiponectin after thiazolidinedione treatment and measures of insulin-mediated glucose metabolism and adipose tissue distribution (8).

Currently, it is still not clear if the thiazolidinediones produce in vivo insulin-sensitizing effects by altering expression of adipocyte genes, which, in turn, convey some signal (metabolic or non-metabolic) to other insulin-sensitive tissues, and/or they exert direct effects on these tissues. Since the thiazolidinediones potently induce adipocyte differentiation, it is possible that the primary action of thiazolidinediones is in fat cells, with secondary effects on skeletal muscle and other insulin-sensitive tissue to improve insulin action, possibly through a thiazolidinedione-mediated changes in circulating FFA levels, adiponectin secretion, or some other signal (Fig. 2).

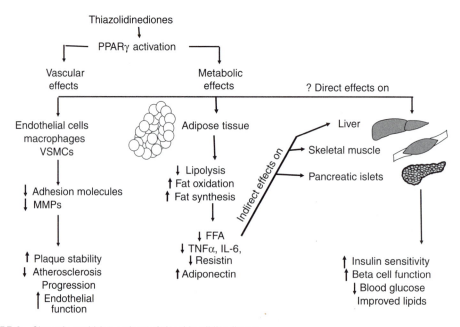

FIGURE 2   Sites of sensitizing actions of the thiazolidinediones.

CLINICAL INDICATIONS

In the United States, rosiglitazone and pioglitazone are approved by the FDA for use as monotherapy and in combination with the sulfonylureas, metformin and with insulin. In Europe however, the thiazolidinediones are not approved for use in combination with insulin. The usual starting dose of rosiglitazone is 4 mg orally as a single dose once daily or in divided doses twice daily (9). For pioglitazone, initial therapy may be initiated at 15 or 30 mg p.o. once daily and the dose increased to 45 mg p.o. once daily (10). In combination therapy, the maximum approved dose of pioglitazone is 30 mg daily and for rosiglitazone, the maximum approved dose is 8 mg daily, except in combination with insulin, where the dose is 4 mg daily. The thiazolidinediones should not be used in adolescents and children, since their safety in these age groups has not yet been established. Thiazolidinedione use is contraindicated in pregnancy and lactating women.

GLYCEMIC EFFECTS

As potent insulin sensitizers, the thiazolidinediones have significant effects on glucose metabolism that result in lower blood glucose levels in insulin-resistant patients with type 2 diabetes (Table 1). Several studies have documented the glucose-lowering effects of rosiglitazone and pioglitazone when used as monotherapy agents and in combination with sulfonylureas, metformin, and insulin.

Thaizolidinedione Monotherapy

In large, multicenter studies, rosiglitazone and pioglitazone significantly improve glycemic control. In a 26-week study with 408 type 2 diabetic patients (11), treatment with 15, 30, or 45 mg pioglitazone significantly decreased the HbA_{1c} by 1.00% to 1.60%

TABLE 1 Relative Efficacy of Rosiglitazone and Pioglitazone

	Reduction in fasting plasma glucose, mean change from the control group	Reduction in HbA_{1c} (%)
Monotherapy		
Rosiglitazone 4 mg	43–58	0.9–1.2
Rosiglitazone 8 mg	62–76	1.5
Pioglitazone 15 mg	39	1.0
Pioglitazone 30 mg	41–58	1.0–1.5
Pioglitazone 45 mg	65–68	1.5–1.6
Combination with sulfonylureas		
Rosiglitazone 4 mg	39–47	0.9–1.13
Pioglitazone 15 mg	39	0.9
Pioglitazone 30 mg	58	1.3
Combination with metformin		
Rosiglitazone 4 mg	40	1.0
Rosiglitazone 8 mg	53	1.5
Pioglitazone 30 mg	38	0.8
Combination with insulin		
Rosiglitazone 4 mg	41	0.7
Rosiglitazone 8 mg	45	1.3
Pioglitazone 15 mg	35	1.0
Pioglitazone 30 mg	40	1.3

Note: Since the above data was not obtained from simultaneous trials, the comparative data is only a rough approximation of the relative effectiveness as stage, severity of hyperglycemia and type of patients studied varied in the above studies.
Source: From Refs. 11,12,15,16,19,20–25.

and fasting plasma glucose (FPG) 39 to 65 mg/dL as compared to placebo. Decreases in FPG occurred as early as the second week of therapy with maximal decreases seen after 10 to 14 weeks and maintained until the end of therapy. In addition, in all pioglitazone groups, there were significant beneficial effects on lipids. Of interest, the subset of patients naive to oral antidiabetic therapy had greater improvements in HbA_{1c} and FPG compared with previously treated patients. In a similar 26-week study with 493 patients (12), rosiglitazone 2 and 4 mg twice daily reduced FPG concentrations relative to placebo by 58 and 76 mg/dL and mean HbA_{1c} levels by 1.2% and 1.5%, respectively. In this study, there were also beneficial changes in measures of insulin sensitivity, β-cell function, and microalbuminuria. The overall adverse event profile of pioglitazone and rosiglitazone in these large studies was similar to that of placebo.

In the context of monotherapy, it is noteworthy that in the UKPDS, there was a progressive failure of all glucose-lowering therapies (metformin, sulfonylureas, and insulin) to maintain glycemic control (13). Since the thiazolidinediones increase insulin sensitivity and improve β-cell function, it is expected that glycemic control with these agents would be enduring. In the ADOPT study (A Diabetes Outcome Progression Trial), 4360 type 2 diabetic subjects were randomized to either rosiglitazone, metformin or glyburide as initial monotherapy and evaluated for monotherapy failure (defined as a confirmed FPG level of >180 mg/dL) (14). After 5 years, the cumulative incidence of monotherapy failure in the rosiglitazone group was 15%, compared to 21% with metformin and 34% with glyburide. The annual rate of decline in β-cell function (after the first 6 months) was 6.1% in the glyburide group, 3.1% in the metformin group, and 2% in the rosiglitazone group. As expected, rosiglitazone was associated with more weight gain and edema than metformin or glyburide. Surprisingly, glyburide was associated with a lower risk of cardiovascular events [including congestive heart failure (CHF)] than was rosiglitazone ($P < 0.05$), and the risk associated with metformin was similar to that with rosiglitazone.

Thiazolidinedione and Sulfonylurea Combination Therapy

The thiazolidinediones are useful glucose lowering agents when used in combination therapy in patients with type 2 diabetes failing existing sulfonylurea therapy (15,16). In a large international, 26-week, open-label study, 348 patients with type 2 diabetes were randomized to receive 2 mg b.i.d. rosiglitazone or placebo daily, in addition to existing sulfonylurea therapy (15). After 26 weeks, the addition of rosiglitazone to existing sulfonylurea therapy significantly reduced the mean HbA_{1c} from 9.1% to 7.9% as compared to no change in the control group. Although adverse events were similar in both groups, more patients in the rosiglitazone + sulfonylurea group reported mild hypoglycemia. Similar glycemic benefits have been reported when pioglitazone is used in combination with sulfonylureas (17). Results from these studies highlight the fact that combination thiazolidinedione + sulfonylurea treatment improves glycemic control and is well-tolerated in patients with type 2 diabetes from across the world.

In studies so far, there does not appear to be any differences between rosiglitazone and pioglitazone in terms of their glucose-lowering and insulin-sensitizing properties. This was confirmed in a double-blind study in which 87 type 2 diabetic patients with the metabolic syndrome were randomized to the addition of pioglitazone 15 mg/day or rosiglitazone 4 mg/day along with glimepiride, 4 mg/day (18). After 12 months, there were similar decreases in HbA_{1c} in both the thiazolidinedione groups (from 7.8% to 6.7% in the rosiglitazone + glimepiride group and from 7.9% to 6.8% in the pioglitazone + glimepiride group). In both treatment groups there was an improvement in insulin sensitivity as measured by the homeostasis model assessment index (HOMA). Of note, triglycerides decreased significantly in the pioglitazone + glimepiride group as compared to a significant increase in triglycerides in the rosiglitazone + glimepiride group. These possible lipid differences between the thiazolidinediones are discussed later in the lipids section.

Thiazolidinedione and Metformin Combination Therapy

In obese type 2 diabetic patients inadequately controlled on metformin alone, the addition of a thiazolidinedione further improves insulin sensitivity, glucose control and β-cell function. In a large, U.S. multicenter, double-blind study, 348 patients [mean body mass index (BMI) 30.1 kg/m^2, FPG 216 mg/dL and HbA$_{1c}$ level 8.8%], were randomized to receive 2.5 g/day of metformin plus either placebo, 4 or 8 mg of rosiglitazone (19). After 26 weeks, metformin–rosiglitazone therapy significantly improved glucose control, insulin sensitivity, and β-cell function significantly in a dose-dependent manner. The mean levels of HbA$_{1c}$ significantly decreased by 1.0% and 1.2% in the 4 and 8 mg metformin–rosiglitazone groups, respectively, as compared with the metformin–placebo group. Interestingly, in this study, while those in the control group experienced a mean decrease in weight of 1.2 kg from baseline, those in the rosiglitazone groups experienced a significant mean increase of 0.7 kg in the 4-mg and 1.9 kg in the 8-mg rosiglitazone groups. There were no significant differences in waist-to-hip ratios among groups.

Like rosiglitazone, pioglitazone also improves insulin sensitivity and glucose control when added to metformin. In a 16-week study (followed by a 1.5-year open-label extension), 328 patients with type 2 diabetes who had suboptimal control on maximum doses of metformin (20) were randomized to either pioglitazone + metformin or placebo + metformin and 249 subjects completed the study. After 16 weeks, patients receiving pioglitazone 30 mg + metformin had significant decreases in FPG levels by 38 mg/dL and HbA$_{1c}$ by 0.83% compared with the placebo + metformin group. In the 72-week open-label extension of this study, 154 patients received open-label pioglitazone 30 mg + metformin and this resulted in a sustained mean decrease from baseline of 1.36% in HbA$_{1c}$ and 63 mg/dL in FPG.

Of note, in an analysis of 550 patients of varying BMI, the improvement in glycemia, insulin sensitivity (HOMA) and β-cell function resulting from the addition of rosiglitazone to maximum dose metformin was most pronounced in the more obese patients (21).

Triple Oral Agent Combination Therapy

Thiazolidinedione treatment is also effective when used late in the course of type 2 diabetes and a thiazolidinedione is added to a failing regimen of a sulfonylurea and metformin—triple oral agent combination therapy. In a prospective observational study, 35 patients with type 2 diabetes were followed after the addition of pioglitazone or rosiglitazone to a failing regimen of a sulfonylurea and metformin (22). At a mean follow-up of 72 months, 51% of patients remained well controlled on triple oral therapy (mean HbA$_{1c}$ 6.9%). In the remaining patients, triple oral therapy failed (mean HbA$_{1c}$ 8%) and the use of insulin was necessary after a mean duration of 38 months. Of note, stimulated C-peptide levels increased significantly in the triple therapy group and did not increase or decrease non-significantly at the time of insulin initiation in the insulin-requiring group. Thus even when used late in the course of type 2 diabetes, thiazolidinediones result in improved and enduring glycemic control which persists for up to 6 years and is dependent on preserved or improved β-cell function.

Thiazolidinedione and Insulin Combination Therapy

In the United States, both pioglitazone and rosiglitazone are approved for use in combination with insulin. However, since thiazolidinedione and insulin combination therapy is associated with an increased incidence of edema and a potentially greater propensity for patients to develop CHF, the thiazolidinediones should be used prudently in patients with pre-existing edema, especially in those who have evidence of milder degrees of heart failure (NYHA Class 1 and 2). In patients with NYHA Class 3 and 4 cardiac status, treatment with rosiglitazone or pioglitazone is currently not recommended.

Two large, multicenter studies have evaluated the efficacy and safety of the thiazolidinediones in insulin-treated patients with type 2 diabetes (23,24). In one 26-week study, 319 type 2 diabetic patients (mean $HbA_{1c} > 7.5\%$) on twice-daily insulin therapy (total daily dose $> 30\,U$) (23) were randomized to rosiglitazone 4 or 8 mg daily or placebo. In an intent-to-treat analysis, rosiglitazone plus insulin treatment resulted in a significant mean reduction in HbA_{1c} from baseline of 0.6% and 1.2% in the 4 and 8 mg groups, respectively, despite a 6% and 12% mean reduction of insulin dosage in the two groups. The most common adverse event was symptoms consistent with hypoglycemia and edema. However, no case of edema was considered to be a serious and no patients were withdrawn from the study due to edema.

In the other large, double-blind, placebo-controlled, randomized, multicenter study, 566 patients with type 2 diabetes on stable insulin regimens for > 30 days and HbA_{1c} $> 8.0\%$ (24) received either 15 or 30 mg pioglitazone, or placebo. After 16 weeks, pioglitazone 15 and 30 mg significantly decreased the mean HbA_{1c} from baseline by 1.0% and 1.3%, respectively. As in the study with rosiglitazone and insulin, the incidence of weight increase, hypoglycemia and edema were higher among patients receiving insulin plus pioglitazone.

Since thiazolidinedione treatment is associated with variable amounts of weight gain, it would be expected that when these agents are used in morbidly obese patients with type 2 diabetes, there would be excessive weight gain, especially since these patients require large quantities of insulin to maintain glucose control. In one study (25), eight morbidly obese patients (median BMI $42\,kg/m^2$) with type 2 diabetes on large doses of insulin (median daily dose 204 U) and poor glycemic control (median HbA_{1c} 8.1%) were treated with combination insulin and maximum doses of rosiglitazone. At 24 weeks, there was a median weight gain of 3 kg, a fall in median HbA_{1c} from 8.1% to 6.7% and a reduction in median insulin dose from 204 to 159 U/day (23% reduction from baseline). Peripheral edema was the only significant side-effect seen in five of the eight patients. Thus, the combination of insulin and rosiglitazone is effective in morbidly obese patients with type 2 diabetes without excessive weight gain but with a high incidence of peripheral edema.

Thiazolidinediones and Type 1 Diabetes

At the outset, it should be noted that insulin is the mainstay of treatment in type 1 diabetes and thiazolidinediones are not approved for use in these patients. However, it is being increasingly recognized that although insulin resistance is common in type 2 diabetes, overweight and normal-weight adults with type 1 diabetes can have peripheral and hepatic insulin resistance. Type 1 diabetic subjects with a family history of type 2 diabetes who undergone intensive insulin therapy have a greater tendency toward expressing the markers of insulin resistance, such as weight gain, increased insulin requirements, and dyslipidemia (26).

In a recent randomized, double-blind study in 50 adult type 1 diabetic subjects with BMI $> 27\,kg/m^2$, rosiglitazone 4 mg b.i.d. in combination with insulin improved glycemic control and blood pressure (BP) without an increase in insulin requirements, compared with the insulin- and placebo-treated subjects, whose improved glycemic control required an 11% increase in insulin dose. Weight gain and hypoglycemia were similar in both groups. The greatest effect of rosiglitazone occurred in subjects with more pronounced markers of insulin resistance. Clearly, there is need for more investigation into the long-term effects of the thiazolidinediones on glycemic control and cardiovascular risk factors in type 1 diabetic individuals with features of insulin resistance (27).

EFFECTS ON INSULIN SENSITIVITY

The thiazolidinediones improve peripheral insulin action not only in patients with type 2 diabetes, but also in other insulin resistant states like impaired glucose tolerance (IGT), polycystic ovary disease, previous gestational diabetes and Werner's syndrome (28–31).

In studies using either the hyperinsulinemic–euglycemic clamp study which is currently considered the "gold standard" to evaluate peripheral insulin sensitivity, or other less direct methods like the frequently sampled intravenous glucose tolerance test, the insulin tolerance test, the oral glucose tolerance test and the HOMA (S), the thiazolidinediones consistently improve insulin-mediated peripheral glucose utilization in obese and lean insulin-resistant, type 2 diabetes patients by approximately 30% to 100% (32). In all these studies, the improvements in insulin sensitivity with the thiazolidinediones has consistently resulted in improved glycemia, lower HbA$_{1c}$ levels and in the case of insulin-resistant IGT/impaired fasting glucose (IFG) subjects, regression from IGT/IFG to normoglycemia, besides improvement in the lipid profile and other cardiovascular risk markers (33).

In one study, 29 diet-treated diabetic patients were randomly assigned to either rosiglitazone, 8 mg/day or placebo (34). After 12 weeks, rosiglitazone improved the FPG (195–150 mg/dL) and HbA$_{1c}$ (8.7–7.4%), significantly suppressed endogenous glucose production by 13% and increased whole-body glucose uptake (measured by the insulin clamp technique) by 37%. Other beneficial changes included a decrease in FFA levels which occurred despite an increase in both body weight and total fat mass of 4 kg. There were significant correlations between measures of insulin sensitivity and plasma FFA levels and the authors concluded that rosiglitazone increases hepatic and peripheral (muscle) tissue insulin sensitivity and reduces FFA turnover despite increased total body fat mass and suggest that the beneficial effects of rosiglitazone on glycemic control are mediated, in part, by the drug's effect on FFA metabolism (34).

Pioglitazone has also been shown to improve peripheral insulin sensitivity. In a large, international study in 205 patients with recently diagnosed, treatment-naïve type 2 diabetes, after 24 weeks, pioglitazone was comparable to metformin in improving glycemic control and FPG (decreases in HbA$_{1c}$ of ~1.3% and FPG of ~54 mg/dL, respectively) (35). However, insulin sensitivity (assessed by HOMA-S) increased significantly by 17.4% in the pioglitazone group as compared with an increase of only 8.9% in the metformin group.

EFFECTS ON β-CELL FUNCTION

Along with insulin resistance, β-cell dysfunction is also a cardinal feature of type 2 diabetes. Data from the UKPDS and other studies suggest that β-cell function decreases with duration of type 2 diabetes in all treatment groups (13,36). Since PPAR-γ is expressed in human islet endocrine cells, it is possible that thiazolidinediones may have direct effects on human pancreatic endocrine cells (37). Improvements in β-cell function after thiazolidinedione treatment may also be secondary to increased insulin sensitivity and concomitant decrease in hyperglycemia. There is growing evidence from several studies that thiazolidinedione therapy improves β-cell function (38–42). These studies have evaluated β-cell function using both surrogate measures and also direct measurements of β-cell function like intravenous glucose tolerance tests, hyperglycemic clamps with arginine stimulation, assessment of baseline high-frequency insulin pulsatility, and glucose-entrained insulin pulsatility. A surrogate measure of β-cell function is the ratio of proinsulin (PI) to immunoreactive insulin (IRI). An elevated ratio of PI to IRI is often present in type 2 diabetes and may reflect dysfunctional β-cell processing of the prohormone and associated reduced β-cell secretory capacity (38). Treatment with the thiazolidinediones is associated with a decrease in PI/IRI ratio suggestive of direct effects on the β cell (38,39). In a study using direct measures of β-cell function, although rosiglitazone treatment for 3 months in type 2 diabetic patients exerted no action on insulin secretion per se, it did improve glucose-entrained high-frequency insulin pulsatility, thereby suggesting an increased ability of the β cell to sense and respond to glucose changes within the physiological range (40). Improvements in β-cell function have also been demonstrated in the TRIPOD (Troglitazone In Prevention Of Diabetes) and the PIPOD (Pioglitazone In Prevention Of Diabetes) studies in Hispanic women with prior gestational diabetes and extremely high risk for progression to diabetes (41,42).

In the ADOPT study, β-cell function (by the HOMA-S method) was determined in 4360 type 2 diabetic subjects who were randomized to either rosiglitazone, metformin or glyburide as initial monotherapy and evaluated for monotherapy failure (defined as a confirmed FPG level of >180 mg/dL) (14). After 5 years, the cumulative incidence of monotherapy failure in the rosiglitazone group was 15%, compared to 21% with metformin and 34% with glyburide. In this study, although there was a durable and robust improvement in insulin sensitivity with rosiglitazone, effects on β-cell function were less robust with the annual rate of decline in β-cell function after 6 months being 2% in the rosiglitazone group compared to 6.1% in the glyburide group and 3.1% in the metformin group.

EFFECTS ON DIABETES PREVENTION

Given the substantial morbidity and excess mortality associated with diabetes, the prevention of type 2 diabetes is a major public-health issue (43). It is well known that subjects with IGT (those with a plasma glucose between 140 and 199 mg/dL 2 hours after a 75 g oral glucose load) are insulin resistant and at high risk to progress on to type 2 diabetes (44). As potent insulin sensitizers, the thiazolidinediones have the potential to prevent type 2 diabetes in high-risk individuals. In the first study to demonstrate this effect (TRIPOD study) (41), Buchanan et al. observed that treatment with troglitazone 400 mg daily for up to 5 years delayed or prevented the onset of type 2 diabetes in high-risk Hispanic women with a history of gestational diabetes by about 50%. This protective effect was associated with the preservation of pancreatic β-cell function and persisted for 8 months after study medications were stopped (41). Women who completed the TRIPOD study were offered participation in the PIPOD study and in these women, 3 years of pioglitazone treatment was associated with stable pancreatic β-cell function and the same diabetes prevention effect seen in the TRIPOD study (42).

The diabetes-prevention effect of the thiazolidinediones was confirmed in the landmark Diabetes Prevention Program, in which more than 4000 subjects with IGT and high FPG were randomized to either intensive lifestyle intervention, metformin 850 mg b.i.d., troglitazone 400 mg daily or placebo (44). In this study, troglitazone was discontinued early due to reports of idiosyncratic hepatotoxicity associated with its use. However, in the subjects who received troglitazone for a mean of 0.9 years, there was a robust 75% reduction in the incidence of diabetes compared to the placebo group. In the same period, there was a 57% reduction in the intensive lifestyle group and a 44% reduction in the metformin group (45). An interesting aspect of this study was that after troglitazone withdrawal, the diabetes incidence rate increased to that of the placebo group, thereby indicating that the protective effect did not persist after the drug was stopped. This is in contrast to the findings from the study conducted by Buchanan et al. in Hispanic women with GDM, in whom the effects of troglitazone persisted for up to 8 months after discontinuation (41).

The DREAM trial (Diabetes REduction Assessment with ramipril and rosiglitazone Medication) is the largest completed diabetes prevention trial and was designed to assess whether rosiglitazone reduces the frequency of diabetes in individuals with IGT or IFG, or both (33). A total of 5269 adults aged 30 years or more with IGT/IFG, or both, and no previous cardiovascular disease were randomly assigned to receive rosiglitazone 8 mg daily or placebo (in this study, ramipril was also studied in a 2×2 factorial design). After a median of 3 years, rosiglitazone substantially reduced incident type 2 diabetes by 62% and increased the likelihood of regression to normoglycemia. Cardiovascular event rates were much the same in both groups, although 0.5% of participants in the rosiglitazone group and 0.1% in the placebo group developed heart failure ($P = 0.01$). Of note, in this study, ramipril failed to reduce the progression to type 2 diabetes. The DREAM trial confirms the results of the earlier studies and strongly suggests that diabetes progression can be altered with thiazolidinedione therapy in high-risk individuals with IGT/IFG. Early treatment with a thiazolidinedione may represent a useful treatment option to effectively prevent or delay the progression of diabetes and its complications. However, the greater benefits in high-risk individuals will have to be balanced against the increased risk of heart failure. Nevertheless, treatment with a thiazolidinedione may be an option in people at high risk of diabetes in whom lifestyle intervention (diet and exercise) and metformin therapy has failed or is not indicated.

EFFECTS ON LIPIDS

Patients with type 2 diabetes manifest a characteristic dyslipidemic profile with an elevation in triglyceride-rich lipoproteins, a decrease in high-density lipoprotein (HDL) cholesterol concentrations and moderately elevated low-density lipoprotein (LDL) cholesterol levels (mostly of the pro-atherogenic type B or small dense LDL type) which is prone to glycation and oxidation (46). This diabetic dyslipidemic profile is closely related to underlying insulin resistance and may, in part, be responsible for the increased incidence of cardiovascular disease in type 2 diabetic patients (47). Since the thiazolidinediones are insulin sensitizers, it is expected that these drugs favorably influence diabetic dyslipidemia.

The effects of the thiazolidinediones on LDL cholesterol are complex. Both pioglitazone and rosiglitazone increase LDL cholesterol levels by ~10% to 15% (9,10,32,48,49). Although this may appear to be detrimental, LDL sub-particle analysis reveal that despite an increase in LDL cholesterol levels, there is a marked shift in the LDL particle size resulting in more of the less atherogenic, buoyant type A LDL particle and a decrease in the pro-atherogenic, small dense type B LDL particle levels (48,49). Following thiazolidinedione treatment, the LDL particles are also less prone to oxidative modification (48–50). As regards HDL cholesterol, both pioglitazone and rosiglitazone increase HDL cholesterol levels by about 10% to 15% (9,10,48,49,51).

There appears to be a difference between the thiazolidinediones in their effects on triglycerides. In a double-blind, head-to-head study, 802 subjects with type 2 diabetes (treated with diet alone or monotherapy) and dyslipidemia (not treated with lipid-lowering agents) were randomized to either pioglitazone 45 mg or rosiglitazone 8 mg (52). At the end of the study (24 weeks), glycemic control was similar between groups (decline in HbA_{1c} of ~0.7%). Triglyceride levels were reduced by 51.9 mg/dL with pioglitazone, but increased by 13.1 mg/dL with rosiglitazone ($P < 0.001$ between treatments). Additionally, the increase in HDL cholesterol was greater (5.2 vs. 2.4 mg/dL; $P < 0.001$) and the increase in LDL cholesterol was less (12.3 vs. 21.3 mg/dL; $P < 0.001$) for pioglitazone compared with rosiglitazone, respectively. LDL particle concentration was also reduced with pioglitazone and increased with rosiglitazone ($P < 0.001$), while LDL particle size increased more with pioglitazone ($P < 0.005$). Thus in this study, pioglitazone and rosiglitazone had significantly different effects on plasma lipids independent of glycemic control or concomitant lipid-lowering or other anti-hyperglycemic therapy. At this time, the clinical significance of these changes is not known.

Another aspect of thiazolidinedione effect on lipids that needs clarification is their effect on the atherogenic lipoprotein, Lp(a). There have been reports in the past that Lp(a) levels increased significantly after troglitazone treatment (53). However, in a recent report, pioglitazone treatment was not associated with an increase in Lp(a) levels (54). Since Lp(a) may be associated with the development of CAD, further studies are needed to confirm and evaluate the significance of changes in Lp(a) levels in thiazolidinedione-treated diabetic patients.

EFFECTS ON ADIPOSE TISSUE

In all clinical studies to date, type 2 diabetic patients treated with thiazolidinediones tend to gain weight and accumulate adipose tissue (55). It would appear paradoxical that a drug which improves insulin sensitivity and glucose and lipid profiles would at the same time increase adiposity and body weight. Considerable research has focused on the reasons for this paradox, especially the sites and nature of thiazolidinedione-induced weight gain. The thiazolidinediones, through PPAR-γ activation cause preadipocytes to differentiate into mature fat cells and also induce key enzymes involved in lipogenesis (56). However, in vitro studies demonstrate that the thiazolidinediones specifically promote the differentiation of pre-adipocytes into adipocytes only in subcutaneous fat and not in omental fat (57). Thiazolidinedione-associated increase in fat mass occurs predominantly in the more insulin responsive subcutaneous fat depots and not in the insulin-resistant visceral body compartments which secrete increased quantities of cytokines. Early clinical studies with CT scans confirmed that thiazolidinedione treatment produces a shift in adipose tissue distribution from the more deleterious omental depot to the more insulin sensitive subcutaneous compartment (58,59). Recent studies with determinations of fat distribution using abdominal magnetic resonance imaging (MRI) and dual energy x-ray absorptiometry (DEXA) after rosiglitazone and pioglitazone therapy confirm that there is greater accumulation in the subcutaneous adipose tissue compartment as compared to a decrease or no change in visceral fat (60). In these and other studies, thiazolidinedione treatment is also associated with a decrease in hepatic lipid content (measured by CT or MRI) and this is consistent with a shift in fat storage not only away from omental/visceral fat, but also away from ectopic storage sites such as the liver to subcutaneous fat tissue.

This putative mechanism is elegantly demonstrated in a study which examined the effects of rosiglitazone treatment in nine subjects with type 2 diabetes (61). After 3 months of rosiglitazone treatment, there were significant improvements in insulin-stimulated glucose metabolism by 68% and 20% during low- and high-dose insulin clamps, respectively. This was associated with significant reductions in plasma FA concentration and hepatic triglyceride content, a 39% increase in extramyocellular lipid content and a 52% increase in the sensitivity of peripheral adipocytes to the inhibitory effects of insulin on lipolysis (as assessed by glycerol release in microdialysis from SQ fat). These results support the hypothesis that thiazolidinediones enhance insulin sensitivity in patients with type 2 diabetes by promoting increased insulin sensitivity in peripheral adipocytes, which results in lower plasma FA concentrations and a redistribution of intracellular lipid from insulin responsive organs into peripheral adipocytes.

CARDIOVASCULAR EFFECTS

The thiazolidinediones have multiple beneficial effects on the cardiovascular system and these are detailed below and in Table 2.

Effects on Cardiac Structure and Function

Left ventricular hypertrophy (LVH) and LV diastolic dysfunction are both common cardiac consequences of hypertension and independently predict cardiovascular morbidity and mortality. In early rodent studies, troglitazone caused reversible increases in heart weight at high doses (62). However, in later animal studies, thiazolidinedione treatment inhibited LVH and improved LV function (63,64). In humans, treatment with troglitazone 800 mg for 48 weeks produced no significant changes in left ventricular mass index. Indeed, compared to the control glyburide group, troglitazone-treated patients demonstrated significant increases in cardiac stroke volume and cardiac index and decreases in diastolic pressure and peripheral vascular resistance (62). Another study

TABLE 2   Cardiovascular Risk Factor Reduction with Thiazolidinedione Treatment

Improve dyslipidemia (↑HDL-C,↓TG, ↓LDL density)
Decrease microalbuminuria, blood pressure
Decrease vascular inflammation, C-reactive protein, endothelin-1, MMP-9, MCP-1 levels
Improve vascular reactivity, endothelial function
Increase thrombolysis, decrease PAI-1 activity
Reduce neointimal/vascular smooth muscle cell proliferation, macrophage migration
Reduce carotid intimal medial thickness

assessed the effects of long-term treatment with rosiglitazone versus glyburide on cardiac structure/function and glycemic control in patients with type 2 diabetes. After 52 weeks of treatment, although small significant increases from baseline in left ventricular mass index (LVMI) were observed in the rosiglitazone group, these changes occurred primarily by week 28 and did not progress further at week 52 (65). In addition, the change in LVMI in the rosiglitazone group was not statistically significantly different to that in the glyburide group.

In a recent study in non-diabetic, insulin-resistant hypertensive patients, pioglitazone treatment significantly improved LV diastolic function without LV mass regression, in proportion to the amelioration of insulin resistance in these patients (66).

Effects on Myocardial Metabolism

Glucose is an important substrate for the myocardial cells, especially during ischemia and an improvement in myocardial metabolic function may play a role in improved cardiac function in diabetic patients treated with thiazolidinediones. A study using positron emission tomography scanning demonstrated that 26 weeks of rosiglitazone treatment significantly increased insulin-stimulated myocardial glucose uptake by 38% and whole-body glucose uptake by 36%, while metformin treatment had no significant effect on these parameters. In this study, myocardial glucose uptake correlated inversely with FFA concentrations and interleukin (IL)-6 concentrations (67). Similar findings were reported in another study in which rosiglitazone therapy significantly increased insulin sensitivity and improved myocardial glucose uptake in type 2 diabetic patients with CAD (68). However, in a study in subjects with insulin-requiring type 2 diabetes and no CAD, pioglitazone treatment for 12 weeks had no demonstrable effect on myocardial blood flow despite metabolic improvements. The lack of any effect in this study may be due to differences in study subject selection and study duration (12 weeks vs. 16–26 weeks) (69).

Effects of Blood Pressure

The prevalence of hypertension in patients with diabetes is up to twofold higher than in non-diabetic individuals (70). In type 2 diabetes and other insulin-resistant states there is blunted insulin-mediated vasodilation caused by several factors including endothelial dysfunction, increased activation of sympathetic nervous system and enhancement of renal sodium reabsorption (71). It is possible that by improving insulin sensitivity, the thiazolidinediones enhance the tonic vasodilator response to insulin pressure, leading to reduced peripheral vascular resistance and BP. Further, by reducing hyperinsulinemia and plasma insulin levels, it is possible that the thiazolidinediones attenuate the potential BP-raising actions of insulin, such as renal sodium retention (72) and increased sympathetic activity. In a study using ^{123}I-meta-iodobenzylguanidine cardiac imaging to evaluate cardiac sympathetic nervous function, troglitazone had a beneficial effect on cardiac sympathetic nervous function through a decrease in insulin resistance in patients with essential hypertension (73).

In most clinical studies so far, the thiazolidinedione have consistently been shown to lower both systolic and diastolic BP. In a meta-analysis of 37 clinical trials, when compared with baseline, the thiazolidinediones lowered systolic BP by 4.70 mmHg [95% confidence interval (CI), –6.13 to –3.27] and diastolic BP by 3.79 mmHg (95% CI, –5.82 to –1.77). When compared with placebo, thiazolidinediones lowered systolic BP by 3.47 mmHg (95% CI, –4.91 to –2.02) and diastolic BP by 1.84 mmHg (95% CI, –3.43 to –0.25) (74).

Effects on Glomerular Function and Albuminuria

Microalbuminuria (urinary albumin excretion rate between 30 and 300 mg/24 hr) is widely regarded as a marker of impaired vascular integrity in type 2 diabetic patients and is not only considered to be an early indicator of renal and cardiovascular disease risk, but also confers an increased risk for all-cause mortality (75). The presence of microalbuminuria is an indication for aggressive intervention to improve glycemic and BP control and reduce cardiovascular risk factors.

In a study from Japan (76), 45 type 2 diabetes patients with microalbuminuria were randomized to either pioglitazone 30 mg, glibenclamide 5 mg or voglibose 0.6 mg (an alpha-glucosidase inhibitor). After 3 months, only pioglitazone was effective in reducing urinary albumin excretion and urinary endothelial-1 (ET-1) concentrations. An increase in circulating ET-1 is known to precede microalbuminuria in diabetic patients. In another 52-week, open-label study, patients with type 2 diabetes were randomized to treatment with rosiglitazone 4 mg b.i.d. or glyburide. At week 28, significant reductions from baseline in albumin/creatinine ratio (ACR) were observed in both treatment groups. However, at week 52, only the rosiglitazone group showed a significant reduction from baseline. For patients with microalbuminuria at baseline, reductions in ACR did not correlate strongly with glycemic control, but showed strong correlation with changes in mean 24-h systolic and diastolic BP in rosiglitazone-treated patients (77). Of note, PPAR-γ receptors are present in the renal mesangial cells and in cultured mesangial cells, PPAR-γ activation by thiazolidinediones attenuates TGF-β (1)-induced fibronectin accumulation observed in the glomerular mesangium in cases of glomerulosclerosis (78).

Anti-Atherogenic Effects

The vascular endothelial cells, the monocyte/macrophage cells and the vascular smooth muscle cells all play a crucial role in the development of accelerated atherosclerosis (79). There is growing evidence from both in vitro and animal studies that the thiazolidinediones as PPAR-γ agonists modify the risk of atherosclerosis progression through beneficial effects on all these components. Several studies have documented that the thiazolidinediones inhibit the expression of the endothelial cellular adhesion molecules (MCP-1, ICAM-1 and VCAM-1) (80), negatively regulate macrophage activation (81,82); regulate macrophage lipid homeostasis through activation of the ABCA-1-mediated reverse cholesterol pathway (83); and reduce the expression and release of tissue factors (84). Through these effects, the thiazolidinediones modify the vascular pathology and thrombogenicity associated with atherosclerosis and improve the stability of the atherosclerotic plaque. The effects of these changes on biochemical markers and surrogate markers of atherosclerosis progression like carotid intimal medial thickening have been favorable (84,85). Cardiac intravascular ultrasound studies have also shown a significant reduction in neointimal tissue proliferation after coronary stent implantation in diabetic patients treated with thiazolidinediones (86).

However, the "gold standard" to determine the cardiovascular benefits of a drug is a randomized, double-blind, placebo-controlled study. In the Prospective Pioglitazone Clinical Trial in Macrovascular Events Study (PROactive Study), 5238 patients with type 2 diabetes and evidence of pre-existing cardiovascular disease were randomized to pioglitazone 45 mg daily, or placebo in addition to their usual glucose-lowering medications (87). In order to assess the effect of pioglitazone on CAD, independent of its glucose lowering effects, all patients were treated to optimal glucose, lipid and BP goals. After an average follow up of ~3 years, pioglitazone treatment was associated with a modest 10% (not statistically significant, $P = 0.09$), reduction in the risk of the primary composite endpoint, which consisted of all-cause mortality, nonfatal myocardial infarction, stroke, acute coronary syndrome, and revascularization or amputation. However, the "main secondary endpoint" (defined before the unblinding of the data) and consisting of certain of the primary outcome measures, namely all-cause mortality, myocardial infarction, and stroke, was significantly reduced by 16%. Of note, pioglitazone treatment was associated with an increase in CHF and hospitalization for CHF. However, the criteria for heart failure were not clearly defined and it is unclear whether the frequency of this diagnosis was confounded by an increased presence of peripheral edema in the pioglitazone group. On the other hand, it is reassuring that mortality from heart failure was not increased.

Although the PROActive study results demonstrated a reduction in all-cause mortality, myocardial infarction, and stroke with pioglitazone, the study was not designed to determine the mechanism(s) for this benefit. This could have resulted from the lower HbA$_{1c}$ of 0.5% in the pioglitazone group, a small but significant reduction in BP, or changes in the lipid profile. Given the multiple beneficial effects of the thiazolidinediones on improving insulin sensitivity and on traditional and non-traditional risk factors, it is tempting to speculate that these anti-atherogeneic effects contributed to the results. Also, it is not known if thiazolidinediones reduce vascular events in the setting of optimal BP, lipid and glucose control. This is being studied in the National Institutes of Health funded ACCORD study, a 7-year, 10,000-patient study designed to evaluate the effects of tight BP, lipid and glucose control (using insulin sensitizers, insulin secretagogues and insulin), on cardiovascular events in patients with type 2 diabetes (88); and the RECORD study, a 6-year study designed to evaluate whether rosiglitazone, in combination with metformin or sulfonylurea, affects CAD outcomes and progression of diabetes in the long term (89).

EFFECTS IN NON-DIABETES CONDITIONS

In addition to being present in the classic insulin responsive tissues and the vascular endothelium, PPAR-γ is also found in other cell types. Several studies (in vitro and in vivo) have shown that the thiazolidinediones have beneficial effects in polycystic ovary syndrome (PCOS), HIV disease, various cancers and inflammatory diseases.

Polycystic ovary syndrome is characterized by hyperandrogenism, chronic anovulation, and insulin resistance. Consistent with their role as insulin sensitizers, the thiazolidinediones have been shown to have both insulin-sensitizing and ovulation-inducing effects in women with PCOS (90–92). Highly active antiretroviral therapy (HAART) is associated with several metabolic complications including fat redistribution (lipodystrophy), insulin resistance, and increased incidence of diabetes mellitus, hyperlipidemia, and hypertension (93). In several studies, the thiazolidinediones have been shown to improve insulin sensitivity and body fat distribution in HAART-treated AIDS patients (94–96).

PPAR-γ is expressed in several human cancer cell lines and the thiazolidinediones have been shown to have antitumor effects in several types of human malignant neoplasms, including colon, breast, pancreatic, prostate and leukemia cell lines (98) through PPAR-γ receptor-dependent and -independent effects (99) and also direct and indirect anti-angiogenic effects (100). However, the promising data from in vitro studies have not been replicated in clinical studies. In studies in patients with metastatic colorectal cancer and recurrent prostate carcinoma (101,102), the thiazolidinediones did not retard disease progression. Also, it should be noted that there is some evidence of tumor-inducing effects of the thiazolidinediones in a murine model for familial adenomatous polyposis and sporadic colon cancer (103). Hence it is prudent that these drugs not be prescribed in people with a family history of adenomatous polyposis coli. Long-term studies are needed to monitor effects on the development of sporadic colon tumors.

The thiazolidinediones exert anti-inflammatory effects through several mechanisms including inhibition of proliferation of activated T cells, inhibition of the NF-kappaB pathway, inhibition of IL-2 secretion and/or the induction of apoptosis (81,104,105). In a study in patients with active ulcerative colitis (106) rosiglitazone treatment was associated with clinical and endoscopic disease remission in several patients.

Activation of PPAR-γ by thiazolidinediones may result in lower bone mass. In a recent 4-year observational study, it was noted that each year of thiazolidinedione use was associated with additional bone loss of 0.61% per year at the whole body level, 1.23% at the lumbar spine, and 0.65% at the trochanter in women, but not men, with diabetes (97). These results were confirmed in the recently published ADOPT study, where examination of data on adverse events during the 5 years of the study, identified a higher rate of fractures in women (but not men) in the group receiving rosiglitazone as compared to those on metformin or glyburide. Lower limb fractures were primarily increased in the foot. However, the number of women with hip fractures did not differ between the groups (14). Although these observational results suggest that thiazolidinediones may cause bone loss in older women, this needs to be tested in a randomized trial.

DRUG INTERACTIONS

There are significant differences in drug interactions among the thiazolidinediones. Pioglitazone is metabolized by the cytochrome P450 isoform CYP3A4 (10). Thus, safety and efficacy could possibly be affected when pioglitazone is co-administered with other drugs metabolized by this enzyme and hence, blood-glucose should be monitored more carefully in such patients (10,107). in vitro data demonstrate that rosiglitazone is predominantly metabolized by CYP2C8, and to a lesser extent, 2C9.

SIDE EFFECTS

Both rosiglitazone and pioglitazone have now been in clinical use worldwide with several million patients treated with these drugs. The vast majority of these patients have tolerated these agents well and have shown clinical improvement in their glycemic status (9,10). Overall in these studies, the types of adverse experiences reported with rosiglitazone and pioglitazone were similar to placebo, except for hypoglycemia and edema. Importantly, the incidence of withdrawals from clinical trials due to an adverse event other than hyperglycemia was similar for patients receiving placebo or a thiazolidinedione.

Edema

In clinical trials and post-marketing surveillance, both pioglitazone and rosiglitazone have been associated with an increased incidence of edema which varied from about 3.0% to 7.5% with the thiazolidinediones compared with 1.0% to 2.5% with placebo or other oral antidiabetic therapy (9,10). The highest incidence of edema has been reported when thiazolidinediones are used in combination with insulin. In clinical studies, patients treated with insulin plus pioglitazone or insulin plus rosiglitazone have an incidence of edema of 15.3% and 14.7%, respectively (compared with 7.0% and 5.4% in the insulin-only groups). Of clinical concern, in a very small minority of patients, the thiazolidinediones lead to significant peripheral edema and in some patients possibly precipitation/worsening of CHF (87,108).

It is still not clear by what precise mechanism(s) the thiazolidinediones cause edema or whether the edema is related to decompensation of cardiac function (108). In studies in non-diabetic volunteers, the thiazolidinediones increase plasma volume by about 6% to 7% (10). As PPAR-γ is predominantly expressed in the renal medullary collecting ducts, a critical site for fluid reabsorption, activation of PPAR-γ in the distal nephron may serve as the primary mechanism responsible for thiazolidinedione-induced fluid retention. In rodent models, thiazolidinedione-induced weight gain and edema was blocked by the collecting duct-specific diuretic amiloride. In addition, thiazolidinedione-induced fluid retention was prevented by deletion of PPAR-γ from the collecting duct, using a specific mouse model (109,110).

Whether it is an increase in plasma volume that leads to edema or other causes such as increased renal tubular sodium reabsorption, or even reflex sympathetic activation, alteration of intestinal ion transport, or increased production of VEGF (a potent tissue permeability factor) is not clear at present (Fig. 3). Studies into the pathophysiology of edema associated with thiazolidinediones are ongoing, since it is important to elucidate the mechanism(s) responsible for the causation of edema in patients with type 2 diabetes treated with thiazolidinediones, and even more important to determine if it is possible to identify those patients susceptible to development of edema and CHF. Knowledge of the mechanisms of edema formation could lead to effective preventative or therapeutic modalities. There are anecdotal reports of improvement in thiazolidinedione-associated edema with diuretics.

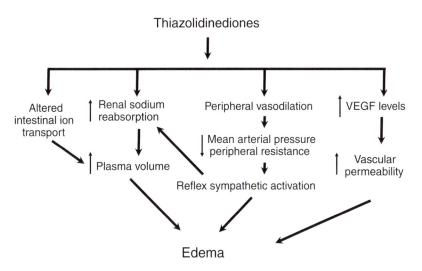

FIGURE 3 Multi-factorial mechanisms of edema formation with thiazolidinediones.

Weight Gain

In clinical use, treatment with thiazolidinediones is associated with weight gain (9,10). In the 26-week rosiglitazone approval clinical trials, the mean weight gain in patients treated with rosiglitazone monotherapy was 1.2 kg (on 4 mg daily) and 3.5 kg (on 8 mg daily). When rosiglitazone was combined with metformin, weight gain was blunted at 0.7 kg (on 4 mg daily) and 2.3 kg (on 8 mg daily). In these studies, there was a mean weight loss of about 1 kg in the placebo and metformin groups. In a longer 52-week glyburide-controlled study, the mean weight gain with 4 and 8 mg of rosiglitazone daily was 1.75 and 2.95 kg, respectively, versus 1.9 kg in glyburide-treated patients (62). Pioglitazone treatment also is accompanied by weight gain in a dose-related manner (10). The mean weight gain in placebo-controlled monotherapy trials ranged from 0.5 to 2.8 kg for pioglitazone-treated patients compared to a weight loss 1.3 to 1.9 kg in placebo-treated patients (these patients remained glycosuric and hence lost weight). In combination with a sulfonylurea, pioglitazone treatment was associated with an increase in weight of 1.9 kg (15 mg) and 2.9 kg (30 mg), versus –0.8 kg for placebo. When pioglitazone was combined with insulin, the mean weight gain was 2.3 and 3.7 kg for 15 and 30 mg of pioglitazone, respectively, and no weight change for placebo. In these studies, combination pioglitazone and metformin therapy resulted in mean weight gain of 1.0 kg versus –1.4 kg for placebo. Thus, both thiazolidinediones are associated with weight gain that occurs in a dose-dependent manner and is highest in combination with insulin and minimal in combination with metformin, which appears to blunt thiazolidinedione-associated weight gain. As already discussed in the section on adipose tissue, the thiazolidinediones preferentially increase fat accumulation in the metabolically beneficial subcutaneous fat depot and reduce fat accumulation in the metabolically harmful intra-abdominal region.

At the present time, it is not clear how much of the thiazolidinedione-induced weight gain is due to adipose tissue accumulation versus fluid retention. In a recent study, when pioglitazone and glipizide were given in doses sufficient to achieve equivalent glycemic control in patients with type 2 diabetes, pioglitazone 45 mg significantly increased total body water by 2.4 L, thus accounting for 75% of the total weight gain 3.1 kg. In addition, pioglitazone therapy tended to decrease visceral and abdominal fat content, BP and systemic vascular resistance (111).

Hypoglycemia

The thiazolidinediones do not stimulate insulin secretion and hence when used as monotherapy, are not expected to cause hypoglycemia. However, mild to moderate hypoglycemia can occur and has been reported during combination therapy with sulfonylureas or insulin (9,10). Hypoglycemia was reported in 1% of placebo-treated patients and 2% of patients receiving pioglitazone in combination with a sulfonylurea. In combination with insulin, hypoglycemia was reported for 5% of placebo-treated patients, 8% for patients treated with pioglitazone 15 mg, and 15% for patients treated with pioglitazone 30 mg.

Anemia

In studies conducted in non-diabetic volunteers, thiazolidinedione treatment is associated with an increase in plasma volume of ~6% to 8% (9) and it is to be expected that due to a dilutional effect, there will be decreases in hemoglobin and hematocrit. In U.S. double-blind studies, anemia was reported in 0.3% to 1.6% of pioglitazone-treated patients and 0% to 1.6% of placebo-treated patients (10). In clinical use so far, there have not been any reports of significant hematologic effects with thiazolidinedione treatment. Of note, there are also reports of thiazolidinedione-treated patients experiencing slight decreases in white blood cell counts possibly related to the increased plasma volume (9,10).

MONITORING REQUIREMENTS/PRECAUTIONS/CONTRAINDICATIONS

Liver Function

Troglitazone, the first glitazone marketed in the United States was associated with idiosyncratic hepatotoxicity and rare cases of liver failure, liver transplants, and death which lead to its recall from clinical use in March 2000. Hence, until recently, periodic monitoring of liver function tests was mandatory with the use of both pioglitazone and rosiglitazone. However, in all clinical trials with rosiglitazone and pioglitazone, the incidence of hepatotoxicity and ALT elevations is similar to placebo (9,10) and there have only been very rare reports of hepatotoxicity associated with rosiglitazone and pioglitazone (112,113) in sick patients with other confounding factors. In a recent large analysis of data from several large studies of rosiglitazone use, no evidence of hepatotoxic effects was observed in studies that involved 5006 patients taking rosiglitazone as monotherapy or combination therapy for 5508 person-years (114). These findings suggest that the idiosyncratic liver toxicity observed with troglitazone is unlikely to be a thiazolidinedione or a PPAR-γ agonist class effect. In fact, poorly controlled patients with type 2 diabetes may even have moderate elevations of serum ALT that decrease with improved glycemic control during treatment with rosiglitazone or other antihypergly-cemic agents (114). There are also reports that the thiazolidinediones improve biochemical and histological features in patients with nonalcoholic steatohepatitis (NASH). In a recent proof-of-concept study, the administration of pioglitazone for 6 months, led to significant metabolic and histologic improvement in subjects with NASH (115).

It is currently recommended that liver enzymes be checked prior to the initiation of therapy with rosiglitazone or pioglitazone in all patients and periodically thereafter at the discretion of the clinician (9,10).

Congestive Heart Failure

As already discussed in the section on edema, in a small minority of patients, thiazolidinedione therapy is associated with significant peripheral edema and in some patients possibly precipitation/worsening of CHF due to several putative causes including an increase in plasma volume, increased renal tubular sodium reabsorption, reflex sympathetic activation, alteration of intestinal ion transport, and increased production of VEGF (a potent tissue permeability factor). In two large 26-week clinical trials in the United States with 611 patients with longstanding type 2 diabetes and a high prevalence of pre-existing medical conditions, an increased incidence of heart failure and other cardiovascular events was seen with rosiglitazone in combination with insulin as compared to patients treated with insulin and placebo (9). Patients who experienced heart failure in these studies were on average older, had a longer duration of diabetes and were mostly on the higher 8 mg daily dose of rosiglitazone. In this population however, it was not possible to determine specific risk factors that could be used to identify all patients at risk of heart failure on combination therapy with rosiglitazone and insulin. Of note, heart failure developed in some patients not known to have prior CHF or pre-existing cardiac conditions.

A recent retrospective cohort study compared new users of thiazolidinedione with all other diabetic patients being treated with oral hypoglycemic agents and reported that thiazolidinedione use was associated with an increased risk of incident CHF [hazard ratio (HR) 1.7; $P < 0.001$] (116). However, this study did not measure or adjust for levels of glycemia, a known risk factor for CHF in diabetes, and also in this study there was the potential for residual confounding by indication/severity of disease. When these factors are adjusted for, thiazolidinedione use does not appear to be associated with increased CHF risk, as demonstrated in the study by Karter et al. who conducted a cohort study of all patients in the Kaiser Permanente Northern California Diabetes Registry with type 2 diabetes who initiated any diabetes pharmacotherapy ($n = 23,440$) between October 1999 and November 2001. After adjusting for demographic, behavioral and clinical factors, relative to patients initiating sulfonylureas, there were no significant increases in the incidence of hospitalization for CHF in those initiating pioglitazone (HR $= 1.28$; 95% CI: 0.85–1.92). There was a significantly higher incidence among those initiating insulin (HR $= 1.56$; 95% CI: 1.00–2.45) and lower incidence among those initiating metformin (HR $= 0.70$; 95% CI: 0.49–0.99). Thus, this study of patients with type 2 diabetes failed to find evidence that short-term pioglitazone use was associated with an elevated risk of hospitalization for CHF relative to the standard, first-line diabetes therapy (117).

Despite the above, it is prudent that rosiglitazone and pioglitazone be used with caution in patients with pre-existing edema, especially in those who have milder degrees of heart failure (NYHA Class 1 and 2) (9,10,118). In patients with NYHA Class 3 and 4 cardiac status, treatment with rosiglitazone or pioglitazone is not recommended. In all other patients, rosiglitazone or pioglitazone therapy should be initiated with a low dose and patients should be evaluated early for edema (within several weeks) (Fig. 4). If edema does occur, dose reduction may be attempted. In those who develop symptoms of CHF, it may be prudent to discontinue the drug altogether, since in the published case reports of

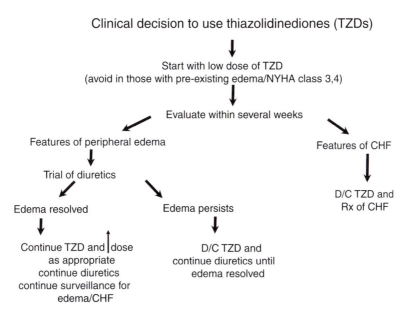

FIGURE 4 Proposed algorithm to treat edema associated with the use of thiazolidinediones.

pulmonary edema, clinical improvement did not occur with diuretics and inotropes, while the thiazolidinedione agent was still continued (32). In those with peripheral edema who do not respond to conventional doses of diuretics, it may be wise to discontinue the thiazolidinedione agent permanently and use other oral agents or insulin. As yet, treatment of thiazolidinedione-associated edema has not been systematically evaluated and treatment must be guided by clinical judgment.

OTHER PRECAUTIONS

Caution should also be exercised when using pioglitazone or rosiglitazone in pre-menopausal anovulatory females with insulin resistance who may resume ovulation as a result of thiazolidinedione therapy. These patients may be at risk of becoming pregnant if adequate contraception is not used. In the case of pioglitazone, those who use oral contraceptive therapy may also be at risk due to CYP3A4 enzyme induction.

CONCLUSION

The thiazolidinediones agents belong to a unique class of oral antidiabetic agents that exert direct effects on the mechanisms of insulin resistance, which is a major pathophysiologic abnormality in type 2 diabetes. Through effects on PPAR-γ, the thiazolidinediones regulate the expression of numerous genes affecting carbohydrate and lipid metabolism and vascular function. These effects result in improved glycemia and lower insulin requirements in type 2 diabetics. Preliminary evidence also suggests that the thiazolidinediones improve other components of the insulin-resistance syndrome and thereby may be able to prevent or delay premature atherosclerotic cardiovascular disease, morbidity, and death. However, in a small minority of patients, weight gain and edema remain undesirable side effects of these agents and the thiazolidinediones should not be used in patients with advanced degrees of CHF. In the future, it is possible to envisage the availability of tailored thiazolidinedione or even non-thiazolidinedione compounds which through their selective agonist effects will have enhanced beneficial effects on glucose, lipid and vascular endothelial metabolism and through their partial agonist, or even selective antagonist effects, do not possess the unwanted side effects of weight gain and fluid retention. The ultimate goal in the treatment of diabetes is the prevention of the disease. Preliminary evidence suggests that the thiazolidinediones have the potential to delay or even prevent the development of type 2 diabetes in high-risk individuals.

ACKNOWLEDGMENTS

This work was supported by the Department of Veterans Affairs and the VA San Diego Healthcare System, San Diego, CA, Grant DK-58291 from the NIDDK and Grant MO1 RR-00827 from the General Clinical Research Branch, Division of Research Resources, National Institutes of Health.

REFERENCES

1. Zimmet P, Alberti KG, Shaw J. Global and societal implications of the diabetes epidemic. Nature 2001; 414:782–7.
2. King H, Aubert RE, Herman, W. Global burden of diabetes, 1995–2025: prevalence, numerical estimates, and projections. Diabetes Care 1998; 21:1414–31.
3. Reaven G. The metabolic syndrome or the insulin resistance syndrome? Different names, different concepts, and different goals. Endocrinol Metab Clin North Am 2004; 33(2):283–303.
4. Expert Panel on Detection, Evaluation and Treatment of High Blood Cholesterol in Adults. Executive summary of the Third Report of the National Cholesterol Education Program (NCEP) of High Blood Cholesterol in Adults (Adult Treatment Panel III). JAMA 2001; 285:2486–97.
5. Desvergne B, Michalik L, Wahli W. Be fit or be sick: peroxisome proliferator-activated receptors are down the road. Mol Endocrinol 2004; 18(6):1321–32.

6. Kersten S, Desvergne B, Wahli W. Role of PPARs in health and disease. Nature 2000; 405:421–4.
7. Bogacka I, Xie H, Bray GA, Smith SR. The effect of pioglitazone on peroxisome proliferator-activated receptor-γ target genes related to lipid storage in vivo. Diabetes Care 2004; 27(7):1660–7.
8. Kadowaki T, Yamauchi T, Kubota N, et al. Adiponectin and adiponectin receptors in insulin resistance, diabetes, and the metabolic syndrome. J Clin Invest 2006; 116(7):1784–92.
9. Avandia [package insert]. Research Triangle Park, NC: GlaxoSmithKline, 2005.
10. Actos (Prescribing information). Lincolnshire, IL: Takeda; Indianapolis, IN: Elli Lilly Company, 2002.
11. Aronoff S, Rosenblatt S, Braithwaite S, et al. Pioglitazone hydrochloride monotherapy improves glycemic control in the treatment of patients with type 2 diabetes: a 6-month randomized placebo-controlled dose–response study. The Pioglitazone 001 Study Group. Diabetes Care 2000; 23(11): 1605–11.
12. Lebovitz HE, Dole JF, Patwardhan R, et al. The Rosiglitazone Clinical Trials Study Group. Rosiglitazone monotherapy is effective in patients with type 2 diabetes [erratum appears in J Clin Endocrinol Metab 2001; 86(4):1659]. J Clin Endocrinol Metab 2001; 86(1):280–8.
13. UK Prospective Diabetes Study Group. 1995 UK Prospective Diabetes Study 16. Overview of 6 years' therapy of type II diabetes: a progressive disease. Diabetes 1995; 44:1249–58.
14. Kahn SE, Haffner SM, Heise MA, et al. for the ADOPT Study Group. Glycemic durability of rosiglitazone. N Engl J Med 2006; 355:2427–43.
15. Vongthavaravat V, Wajchenberg BL, Waitman JN, et al. 125 Study Group. An international study of the effects of rosiglitazone plus sulphonylurea in patients with type 2 diabetes. Curr Med Res Opin 2002; 18(8):456–61.
16. Barnett AH, Grant PJ, Hitman GA, et al. Indo-Asian Trial Investigators. Rosiglitazone in Type 2 diabetes mellitus: an evaluation in British Indo-Asian patients. Diabet Med 2003; 20(5):387–93.
17. Hanefeld M, Brunetti P, Schernthaner GH, et al. QUARTET Study Group. One-year glycemic control with a sulfonylurea plus pioglitazone versus a sulfonylurea plus metformin in patients with type 2 diabetes. Diabetes Care 2004; 27(1):141–7.
18. Derosa G, Cicero AF, Gaddi A, et al. A comparison of the effects of pioglitazone and rosiglitazone combined with glimepiride on prothrombotic state in type 2 diabetic patients with the metabolic syndrome. Diabetes Res Clin Pract 2005; 69(1):5–13.
19. Fonseca V, Rosenstock J, Patwardhan R, et al. Effect of metformin and rosiglitazone combination therapy in patients with type 2 diabetes mellitus: a randomized controlled trial. JAMA 2000; 283 (13):1695–702.
20. Einhorn D, Rendell M, Rosenzweig J, et al. Pioglitazone hydrochloride in combination with metformin in the treatment of type 2 diabetes mellitus: a randomized, placebo-controlled study. The Pioglitazone 027 Study Group. Clin Ther 2000; 22(12):395–409.
21. Jones TA, Sautter M, Van Gaal LF, et al. Addition of rosiglitazone to metformin is most effective in obese, insulin-resistant patients with type 2 diabetes. Diabetes Obes Metab 2003; 5(3):163–70.
22. Bell DS, Ovalle F. Long-term glycaemic efficacy and weight changes associated with thiazolidinediones when added at an advanced stage of type 2 diabetes. Diabetes Obes Metab 2006; 8(1): 110–5.
23. Raskin P, Rendell M, Riddle MC, et al. The Rosiglitazone Clinical Trials Study Group. A randomized trial of rosiglitazone therapy in patients with inadequately controlled insulin-treated type 2 diabetes. Diabetes Care 2001; 24(7):1226–32.
24. Rosenstock J, Einhorn D, Hershon K, et al. Pioglitazone 014 Study Group. Efficacy and safety of pioglitazone in type 2 diabetes: a randomized, placebo-controlled study in patients receiving stable insulin therapy. Int J Clin Pract 2002; 56(4):251–7.
25. Buch HN, Baskar V, Barton DM, et al. Combination of insulin and thiazolidinedione therapy in massively obese patients with Type 2 diabetes. Diabet Med 2002; 19(7):572–4.
26. Purnell JQ, Dev RK, Steffes MW, et al. Relationship of family history of type 2 diabetes, hypoglycemia, and autoantibodies to weight gain and lipids with intensive and conventional therapy in the Diabetes Control and Complications Trial. Diabetes 2003; 52:2623–9.
27. Strowig SM, Raskin P. The effect of rosiglitazone on overweight subjects with type 1 diabetes. Diabetes Care 2005; 28(7):1562–7.
28. Suter SL, Nolan JJ, Wallace P, et al. Metabolic effects of new oral hypoglycemic agent CS-045 in NIDDM subjects. Diabetes Care 1992; 15:193–203.
29. Nolan JJ, Ludvik B, Beerdsen P, et al. Improvement in glucose tolerance and insulin resistance in obese subjects treated with troglitazone. N Eng J Med 1994; 331:1188–98.
30. Dunaif A, Scott D, Finegood D, et al. The insulin-sensitizing agent troglitazone improves metabolic and reproductive abnormalities in the polycystic ovary syndrome. J Clin Endocrinol Metab 1996; 81:3299–306.
31. Takino H, Okuno S, Uotani S, Yano M, Matsumoto K, Kawasaki E, Takao Y, Yamasaki H, Yamaguchi Y, Akazawa S. Increased insulin responsiveness after CS-045 treatment in diabetes associated with Werner's syndrome. Diabetes Res Clin Pract 1994; 24:167–72.

32. Mudaliar S, Henry RR. New oral therapies for type 2 diabetes—the thiazolidinediones or insulin sensitizers. Annu Rev Med 2001; 52:239–57.
33. The DREAM Trial Investigators. Effect of rosiglitazone on the frequency of diabetes in patients with impaired glucose tolerance or impaired fasting glucose: a randomized controlled trial. Lancet 2006; 368:1096–105.
34. Miyazaki Y, Glass L, Triplitt C, et al. Effect of rosiglitazone on glucose and non-esterified fatty acid metabolism in Type II diabetic patients. Diabetologia 2001; 44(12):2210–9.
35. Pavo I, Jermendy G, Varkonyi TT, et al. Effect of pioglitazone compared with metformin on glycemic control and indicators of insulin sensitivity in recently diagnosed patients with type 2 diabetes. J Clin Endocrinol Metab 2003; 88(4):1637–45.
36. Levy J, Atkinson AB, Bell PM, et al. β-cell deterioration determines the onset and rate of progression of secondary dietary failure in Type 2 diabetes mellitus: the 10-year follow-up of the Belfast diet study. Diabet Med 1998; 15:290–6.
37. Dubois M, Pattou F, Kerr-Conte J, et al. Expression of peroxisome proliferator-activated receptorγ (PPARγ) in normal human pancreatic islet cells. Diabetologia 2000; 43(9):1165–9.
38. Prigeon RL, Kahn SE, Porte D. Effect of troglitazone on B cell function, insulin sensitivity and glycemic control in subjects with type 2 diabetes mellitus. J Clin Endo Metab 1998; 83(3):819–923.
39. Kubo K. Effect of pioglitazone on blood proinsulin levels in patients with type 2 diabetes mellitus. Endocr J 2002; 49(3):323–8.
40. Juhl CB, Hollingdal M, Porksen N, et al. Influence of rosiglitazone treatment on β-cell function in type 2 diabetes: evidence of an increased ability of glucose to entrain high-frequency insulin pulsatility. J Clin Endocrinol Metab 2003; 88(8):3794–800.
41. Buchanan TA, Xiang AH, Peters RK, et al. Preservation of pancreatic β-cell function and prevention of type 2 diabetes by pharmacological treatment of insulin resistance in high-risk Hispanic women. Diabetes 2002; 51:2796–803.
42. Xiang AH, Peters RK, Kjos SL, et al. Effect of pioglitazone on pancreatic β-cell function and diabetes risk in Hispanic women with prior gestational diabetes. Diabetes 2006; 55(2):517–22.
43. Venkat Narayan KM. The diabetes pandemic: looking for the silver lining. Clin Diabetes 2005; 23: 51–2.
44. The Diabetes Prevention Program Research Group. The Diabetes Prevention Program. Reduction in the incidence of type 2 diabetes with lifestyle intervention or metformin. N Engl J Med 2002; 346(6): 393–403.
45. Knowler WC, Hamman RF, Edelstein SL, et al. Diabetes Prevention Program Research Group. Prevention of type 2 diabetes with troglitazone in the Diabetes Prevention Program. Diabetes 2005; 54(4):1150–6.
46. Garg A. Dyslipoproteinemia and diabetes. Endocr Metab Clin North Am 1998; 27(3):613–26.
47. Ginsberg HN. Insulin resistance and cardiovascular disease. J Clin Invest 2000; 106:453–8.
48. Freed MI, Ratner R, Marcovina SM, et al. Rosiglitazone Study 108 investigators. Effects of rosiglitazone alone and in combination with atorvastatin on the metabolic abnormalities in type 2 diabetes mellitus. Am J Cardiol 2002; 90(9):947–52.
49. Aronoff S, Rosenblatt S, Braithwaite S, et al. Pioglitazone hydrochloride monotherapy improves glycemic control in the treatment of patients with type 2 diabetes: a 6-month randomized placebo-controlled dose-response study. The Pioglitazone 001 Study Group. Diabetes Care 2000; 23(11): 1605–11.
50. Crawford RS, Mudaliar SR, Henry RR, Chait A. Inhibition of LDL oxidation in vitro but not ex vivo by troglitazone. Diabetes 1999; 48(4):783–90.
51. Rosenblatt S, Miskin B, Glazer NB. Pioglitazone 026 Study Group. The impact of pioglitazone on glycemic control and atherogenic dyslipidemia in patients with type 2 diabetes mellitus. Coron Artery Dis 2001; 12(5):413–23.
52. Goldberg RB, Kendall DM, Deeg MA, et al. GLAI Study Investigators. A comparison of lipid and glycemic effects of pioglitazone and rosiglitazone in patients with type 2 diabetes and dyslipidemia. Diabetes Care 2005; 28(7):1547–54.
53. Matsumoto K, Miyake S, Yano M, et al. Increase of lipoprotein (a) with troglitazone. Lancet 1997; 350:1748–9.
54. Nagai Y, Abe T, Nomura G. Does pioglitazone, like troglitazone, increase serum levels of lipoprotein(a) in diabetic patients? Diabetes Care 2001; 24:408–9.
55. Yki-Jarvinen H. Thiazolidinediones. N Engl J Med 2004; 351(11):1106–18.
56. Spiegelman BM. PPAR : adipogenic regulator and thiazolidinedione receptor. Diabetes 1998; 47: 507–14.
57. Adams M, Montague CT, Prins JB, et al. Activators of peroxisome proliferator-activated receptor-γ have depot-specific effects on human preadipocyte differentiation. J Clin Invest 1997; 100:3149–53.
58. Mori Y, Murakawa Y, Okada K, et al. Effect of troglitazone on body fat distribution in type 2 diabetic patients. Diabetes Care 1999; 22(6):908–12.

59. Kelly IE, Han TS, Walsh K, et al. Effects of a thiazolidinedione compound on body fat and fat distribution of patients with type 2 diabetes. Diabetes Care 1999; 22(2):288–93.

60. Carey DG, Cowin GJ, Galloway GJ, et al. Effect of rosiglitazone on insulin sensitivity and body composition in type 2 diabetic patients. Obes Res 2002; 10(10):1008–15.

61. Mayerson AB, Hundal RS, Dufour S, et al. The effects of rosiglitazone on insulin sensitivity, lipolysis, and hepatic and skeletal muscle triglyceride content in patients with type 2 diabetes. Diabetes 2002; 51(3):797–802.

62. Ghazzi MN, Perez JE, Antonucci TK, et al. The Troglitazone Study Group: cardiac and glycemic benefits of troglitazone treatment in NIDDM. Diabetes 1997; 46:433–9.

63. Asakawa M, Takano H, Nagai T, et al. Peroxisome proliferator-activated receptor γ plays a critical role in inhibition of cardiac hypertrophy in vitro and in vivo. Circulation 2002; 105(10): 1240–6.

64. Shiomi T, Tsutsui H, Hayashidani S, et al. Pioglitazone, a peroxisome proliferator-activated receptor-γ agonist, attenuates left ventricular remodeling and failure after experimental myocardial infarction. Circulation 2002; 106(24):3126–32.

65. St John Sutton M, Rendell M, Dandona P, et al. A comparison of the effects of rosiglitazone and glyburide on cardiovascular function and glycemic control in patients with type 2 diabetes. Diabetes Care 2002; 25(11):2058–64.

66. Horio T, Suzuki M, Suzuki K, et al. Pioglitazone improves left ventricular diastolic function in patients with essential hypertension. Am J Hypertens 2005; 18(7):949–57.

67. Hallsten K, Virtanen KA, Lonnqvist F, et al. Enhancement of insulin-stimulated myocardial glucose uptake in patients with Type 2 diabetes treated with rosiglitazone. Diabet Med 2004; 21 (12):1280–7.

68. Lautamaki R, Airaksinen KE, Seppanen M, et al. Rosiglitazone improves myocardial glucose uptake in patients with type 2 diabetes and coronary artery disease: a 16 week randomized, double-blind, placebo-controlled study. Diabetes Care 2005; 54(9):2787–94.

69. McMahon GT, Plutzky J, Daher E, et al. Effect of a peroxisome proliferator-activated receptor-γ agonist on myocardial blood flow in type 2 diabetes. Diabetes Care 2005; 28(5):1145–50.

70. Simonson DC. Etiology and prevalence of hypertension in diabetic patients. Am J Hypertens 1995; 8:316–20.

71. Sarafidis PA, Lasaridis AN. Actions of peroxisome proliferator-activated receptors-γ agonists explaining a possible blood pressure-lowering effect. Am J Hypertens 2006; 19(6):646–53.

72. Baron AD. Hemodynamic actions of insulin. Am J Physiol 1994; 267:E187–202.

73. Watanabe K, Komatsu J, Kurata M, et al. Improvement of insulin resistance by troglitazone ameliorates cardiac sympathetic nervous dysfunction in patients with essential hypertension. J Hypertens 2004; 22(9):1761–8.

74. Qayyum R, Adomaityte J. A meta-analysis of the effect of thiazolidinediones on blood pressure. J Clin Hypertens (Greenwich) 2006; 8(1):19–28.

75. American Diabetes Association. Position statement: diabetic nephropathy. Diabetes Care 2000; 23 (Suppl. 1):S69–72.

76. Nakamura T, Ushiyama C, Shimada N, et al. Comparative effects of pioglitazone, glibenclamide, and voglibose on urinary endothelin-1 and albumin excretion in diabetes patients. J Diabetes Complications 2000; 14(5):250–4.

77. Bakris G, Viberti G, Weston WM, et al. Rosiglitazone reduces urinary albumin excretion in type II diabetes. J Hum Hypertens 2003; 17(1):7–12.

78. Maeda A, Horikoshi S, Gohda T, et al. Pioglitazone attenuates TGF-β (1)-induction of fibronectin synthesis and its splicing variant in human mesangial cells via activation of peroxisome proliferator-activated receptor (PPAR)γ. Cell Biol Int 2005; 29(6):422–8.

79. Duez H, Fruchart JC, Staels B. PPARs in inflammation, atherosclerosis and thrombosis. J Cardiovasc Risk 2001; 8(4):187–94.

80. Hsueh WA, Javkson S, Law RE. Control of vascular cell proliferation and migration by PPARg. Diabetes Care 2001; 24(2):392–7.

81. Ricote M, Li AC, Willson TM, et al. The peroxisome proliferator-activated receptor-g is a negative regulator of macrophage activation. Nature 1998; 391:79–82.

82. Jiang C, Ting AT, Seed B. PPAR-g agonists inhibit production of monocyte inflammatory cytokines. Nature 2001; 391:82–6.

83. Chawla A, Boisvert WA, Lee CH, et al. A PPAR g-LXR-ABCA1 pathway in macrophages is involved in cholesterol efflux and atherogenesis. Mol Cell 2001; 7(1):161–71.

84. Haffner SM, Greenberg AS, Weston WM, et al. Effect of rosiglitazone treatment on nontraditional markers of cardiovascular disease in patients with type 2 diabetes mellitus. Circulation 2002; 106(6): 679–84.

85. Koshiyama H, Shimono D, Kuwamura N, et al. Inhibitory effect of pioglitazone on carotid arterial wall thickness in type 2 diabetes. J Clin Endocrinol Metab 2001; 86:3452–6.

86. Choi D, Kim SK, Choi SH, et al. Preventative effects of rosiglitazone on restenosis after coronary stent implantation in patients with type 2 diabetes. Diabetes Care 2004; 27(11):2654–60.
87. Dormandy JA, Charbonnel B, Eckland DJ, et al. The PROactive investigators. Secondary prevention of macrovascular events in patients with type 2 diabetes in the PROactive Study (PROspective pioglitAzone Clinical Trial In macroVascular Events): a randomized controlled trial. Lancet 2005; 366:1279–89.
88. http://www.nih.gov/news/pr/feb2003/nhlbi-20.htm.
89. Home PD, Pocock SJ, Beck-Nielsen H, et al. Rosiglitazone Evaluated for Cardiac Outcomes and Regulation of Glycaemia in Diabetes (RECORD): study design and protocol. Diabetologia 2005; 48 (9):1726–35.
90. Dunaif A, Scott D, Finegood D, et al. The insulin-sensitizing agent troglitazone improves metabolic and reproductive abnormalities in the polycystic ovary syndrome. J Clin Endocrinol Metab 1996; 81 (9):3299–306.
91. Brettenthaler N, De Geyter C, Huber PR, et al. Effect of the insulin sensitizer pioglitazone on insulin resistance, hyperandrogenism, and ovulatory dysfunction in women with polycystic ovary syndrome. J Clin Endocrinol Metab 2004; 89(8):3835–40.
92. Rautio K, Tapanainen JS, Ruokonen A. Endocrine and metabolic effects of rosiglitazone in overweight women with PCOS: a randomized placebo-controlled study. Hum Reprod 2006; 21(6): 1400–7.
93. Hadigan C, Miller K, Corcoran C. Fasting hyperinsulinemia and changes in regional body composition in human immunodeficiency virus-infected women. J Clin Endocrinol Metab 1999; 84: 1932–7.
94. Gelato MC, Mynarcik DC, Quick JL, et al. Improved insulin sensitivity and body fat distribution in HIV-infected patients treated with rosiglitazone: a pilot study. J Acquir Immune Defic Syndr 2002; 31(2):163–70.
95. Walli R, Michl GM, Muhlbayer D, et al. Effects of troglitazone on insulin sensitivity in HIV-infected patients with protease inhibitor-associated diabetes mellitus. Res Exp Med 2000; 199(5):253–62.
96. van Wijk JP, de Koning EJ, Cabezas MC, et al. Related comparison of rosiglitazone and metformin for treating HIV lipodystrophy: a randomized trial. Ann Intern Med 2005; 143(5):337–46.
97. Schwartz AV, Sellmeyer DE, Vittinghoff E, et al. Thiazolidinedione use and bone loss in older diabetic adults. J Clin Endocrinol Metab 2006; 91(9):3349–54.
98. Giannini S, Serio M, Galli A. Pleiotropic effects of thiazolidinediones: taking a look beyond antidiabetic activity. J Endocrinol Invest 2004; 27(10):982–91.
99. Chaffer CL, Thomas DM, Thompson EW, et al. PPARγ independent induction of growth arrest and apoptosis in prostate and bladder carcinoma. BMC Cancer 2006; 6:53.
100. Panigrahy D, Singer S, Shen LQ, et al. PPARγ ligands inhibit primary tumor growth and metastasis by inhibiting angiogenesis. J Clin Invest 2002; 110(7):923–32.
101. Kulke MH, Demetri GD, Sharpless NE, et al. A phase II study of troglitazone, an activator of the PPARγ receptor, in patients with chemotherapy-resistant metastatic colorectal cancer. Cancer J 2002; 8(5):395–9.
102. Smith MR, Manola J, Kaufman DS, et al. Rosiglitazone versus placebo for men with prostate carcinoma and a rising serum prostate-specific antigen level after radical prostatectomy and/or radiation therapy. Cancer 2004; 101:1569–74.
103. Seed B. PPAR- and colorectal carcinoma: conflicts in a nuclear family. Nat Med 1998; 4:1004–5.
104. Clark RB. The role of PPARs in inflammation and immunity. J Leukoc Biology 2002; 71(3):388–400.
105. Chinetti G, Fruchart JC, Staels B. Peroxisome proliferator-activated receptors (PPARs): nuclear receptors at the crossroads between lipid metabolism and inflammation. Inflamm Res 2000; 49(10): 497–505.
106. Lewis JD, Lichtenstein GR, Stein RB, et al. An open-label trial of the PPAR-γ ligand rosiglitazone for active ulcerative colitis. Am J Gastroenterol 2001; 96(12):3323–8.
107. Deng L, Wang F, Li H. Effect of gemfibrozil on the pharmacokinetics of pioglitazone. Eur J Clin Pharmacol 2005; 61(11):831–6.
108. Mudaliar S, Henry RR. Thiazolidinediones, peripheral edema and type 2 diabetes: incidence, pathophysiology and clinical implications. Endocr Pract 2003; 9(5):406–16.
109. Zhang H, Zhang A, Kohan DE, et al. Related Collecting duct-specific deletion of peroxisome proliferator-activated receptor γ blocks thiazolidinedione-induced fluid retention. Proc Natl Acad Sci U S A 2005; 102(26):9406–11.
110. Guan Y, Hao C, Cha DR, et al. Thiazolidinediones expand body fluid volume through PPARγ stimulation of ENaC-mediated renal salt absorption. Nat Med 2005; 11(8):861–6.
111. Basu A, Jensen MD, McCann F, Mukhopadhyay D, Joyner MJ, Rizza RA. Effects of pioglitazone versus glipizide on body fat distribution, body water content, and hemodynamics in type 2 diabetes. Diabetes Care 2006; 29(3):510–4.
112. Al-Salman J, Arjomand H, Kemp DG. Hepatocellular injury in a patient receiving rosiglitazone. A case report. Ann Int Med 2000; 132(2):121–4.

113. Pinto AG, Cummings OW, Chalasani N. Severe but reversible cholestatic liver injury after pioglitazone therapy. Ann Intern Med 2002; 137(10):857.
114. Lebovitz HE, Kreider M, Freed MI. Evaluation of liver function in type 2 diabetic patients during clinical trials: evidence that rosiglitazone does not cause hepatic dysfunction. Diabetes Care 2002; 25(5):815–21.
115. Belfort R, Harrison SA, Brown K, et al. A placebo-controlled trial of pioglitazone in subjects with nonalcoholic steatohepatitis. N Engl J Med 2006; 355:2297–307.
116. Delea TE, Edelsberg JS, Hagiwara M, et al. Use of thiazolidinediones and risk of heart failure in people with Type 2 diabetes: a retrospective cohort study. Diabetes Care 2003; 26:2983–9.
117. Karter AJ, Ahmed AT, Liu J, et al. Pioglitazone initiation and subsequent hospitalization for congestive heart failure. Diabet Med 2005; 22(8):986–93.
118. ADA/AHA CONSENSUS, Nesto RW, Bell D, Bonow RO, et al. Thiazolidinedione use, fluid retention, and congestive heart failure. A consensus statement from the American Heart Association and American Diabetes Association. Circulation 2003; 108:2941–8.

12 | Treatment Strategies for Type 2 Diabetes Based on Incretin Action

Baptist Gallwitz
Department of Medicine, Eberhard-Karls University, Tübingen, Germany

Michael Nauck
Diabeteszentrum Bad Lauterberg, Bad Lauterberg, Germany

THE DISCOVERY OF THE INCRETIN HORMONES GASTRIC INHIBITORY POLYPEPTIDE AND GLUCAGON-LIKE PEPTIDE-1

Early in the first half of the 20th century it was already hypothesized that gastrointestinal hormones are important for glucose homeostasis and stimulation of insulin secretion after a meal (1,2). In the late 1960s it was finally shown that orally administered glucose leads to a greater insulin response than intravenously administered glucose dosed to lead to identical serum glucose excursions (3). This difference in insulin secretion is termed the "incretin effect." The gastrointestinal hormones promoting the pronounced insulin response after an oral glucose load are called "incretins." The incretin effect is responsible for approximately 30% to 60% of the postprandial C-peptide response depending on the amount of glucose consumed. In patients with type 2 diabetes the incretin effect is markedly reduced (4,5).

Gastric inhibitory polypeptide (GIP) was discovered as an incretin in 1970 and accounts for approximately 60% of the total incretin effect (6). It is synthesized by the K cells in the upper small intestine (6,7) and released in response to a carbohydrate- or fat-rich meal. Mice lacking the GIP receptor show an impairment in glucose tolerance and interestingly also a resistance to nutrient-induced weight gain by hypercaloric feeding (8,9).

Glucagon-like peptide-1 (GLP-1) was discovered in 1985 after the cloning of the glucagon gene and is generated by tissue-specific post-translational processing of proglucagon in neuroendocrine L cells of the lower small intestine and the hypothalamus (10), while glucagon is the major product of the proglucagon processing in alpha cells of the pancreatic islet (11). GLP-1 is a physiological incretin (6,11,12). It is a 29 amino acids containing peptide and has a high sequence similarity with GIP, glucagon and other peptides of the glucagon family of hormones (13).

PHYSIOLOGICAL EFFECTS OF GLP-1 AND GIP

GLP-1 enhances glucose-induced insulin secretion and contributes to the incretin effect. Plasma concentrations of GLP-1 increase after a carbohydrate-rich meal three- to eightfold (12). The contribution of GIP to the incretin effect exceeds that of GLP-1 at typical postprandial plasma concentrations in healthy subjects (14).

Since GLP-1 lowers postprandial glycemia not only by its effect on endocrine pancreatic secretion, but also by a significant deceleration of gastric emptying (15–18), the physiological contribution of both hormones to the maintenance of normoglycemia after meal ingestion may be considered to be similar (19). GLP-1, but not GIP action is essential for the control of fasting glycemia, as acute antagonism (studies with the GLP-1-antagonist exendin(9-39)) or genetic disruption of GLP-1 action (studies in GLP-1 receptor knockout mice) leads to increased levels of fasting glucose in rodents (20). Additionally, GLP-1 is essential for glucose homeostasis also in humans, as studies with GLP-7 antagonist exendin (9-39) demonstrate impaired glucose-stimulated insulin secretion, reduced glucose clearance, increased levels of glucagon and more rapid gastric emptying (21). The actions of GLP-1 and GIP on the control of blood glucose have lead to considerable interest in the use of these agents for the treatment of type 2 diabetes.

However, GIP has lost most of its insulinotropic potency in type 2 diabetes (22,23). The majority of pharmaceutical efforts directed at potentiation of incretin action for the treatment of type 2 diabetes have focused on GLP-1 for this reason.

The GLP-1 receptor is expressed in the islet alpha and beta cells and in peripheral tissues including the central and peripheral nervous system, heart, lung and gastrointestinal tract (24). Activation of GLP-1 and GIP receptors leads to increases of cyclic AMP and intracellular calcium, followed by insulin exocytosis, in a glucose-dependent manner (25). More sustained incretin receptor signaling is associated with protein kinase A activation, induction of gene transcription, enhanced levels of insulin biosynthesis, and stimulation of β-cell proliferation (26).

DEFECTS IN THE INCRETIN EFFECT IN TYPE 2 DIABETES

The incretin effect is absent or diminished in type 2 diabetes. GLP-1 still stimulates insulin secretion in type 2 diabetic patients at higher plasma concentrations, whereas GIP has lost most of its insulinotropic activity (27–29). The reason for the loss of the insulinotropic action of GIP has not completely been elucidated yet. Specific defects in GIP signaling and general secretory defects of the beta cell are most likely responsible. GLP-1 secretion as well as GLP-1 action is diminished in type 2 diabetes, but supraphysiological concentrations of GLP-1 by exogenous administration of GLP-1 can restore the defects in the incretin effect. The therapeutic potential of GLP-1 as a pharmacological tool for treating type 2 diabetes has been suggested in the 1990s (29,30). The insulinotropic effect of GLP-1 is only present under hyperglycemic conditions providing the possibility of glucose normalization without the risk of hypoglycemias (29,31). GLP-1 has further physiological actions that may be advantageous in type 2 diabetes therapy.

FAVORABLE GLP-1 ACTIONS IN TYPE 2 DIABETES BEYOND THE INSULINOTROPIC EFFECT

GLP-1 inhibits glucagon secretion (32,33). In type 2 diabetes, excessive glucagon secretion in relation to the plasma glucose aggravates fasting hyperglycemia by stimulating hepatic glucose output (34). Exogenous administration of GLP-1 in type 2 diabetic patients leads to a significant suppression of glucagon secretion together with a normalization in fasting plasma glucose (29). The counterregulatory response of glucagon secretion in hypoglycemia is unaffected by GLP-1 administration (35). GLP-1-based therapies will therefore not bear an intrinsic risk for hypoglycemia (36).

Concerning gastrointestinal functions, GLP-1 slows gastric emptying and inhibits gastric acid secretion (18). In the central nervous system, GLP-1 acts as a neurotransmitter in the hypothalamus and stimulates satiety directly (37). Continuous GLP-1 application over 6 weeks in type 2 diabetic patients produced significant weight loss due to reduced food intake and increased satiety (37,38). Whether the effects of GLP-1 on satiety in humans are mainly mediated by the retardation of gastric emptying through a feedback loop or are centrally mediated is not completely clear yet (39,40).

In animal studies as well as in vitro studies including studies with human islets GLP-1 causes an increase of beta cell mass. This increase is explained by a stimulation of islet cell neogenesis (41–43) from precursor cells as well as an inhibition of apoptosis of beta cells (42,44). In man, the effect of GLP-1 on the beta cell mass cannot easily be quantified, but indirect measures of beta cell function have shown an improvement after GLP-1 application (45). in vitro, in isolated human islets, GLP-1 improves insulin secretion and islet cell morphology (46).

THE ANTIDIABETIC PROPERTIES OF GLP-1 IN TYPE 2 DIABETES AND LIMITATIONS TO ITS THERAPEUTIC USE

In patients with type 2 diabetes, the incretin effect is reduced or absent (47). GLP-1 secretion is diminished in type 2 diabetic subjects, possibly contributing to the reduced incretin effect (48). A continuous intravenous GLP-1 infusion stimulates insulin secretion and normalizes both fasting and postprandial blood glucose in patients with type 2 diabetes (29,49). A continuous subcutaneous administration for 6 weeks reduced diurnal glucose concentrations and HbA_{1c} by 1.3% and suppressed glucagon secretion (38). Furthermore, the patients treated with GLP-1 lost approximately 2 kg of weight (Fig. 1) (38,50).

The multiple actions of GLP-1 constitute a novel and attractive therapeutic principle for the treatment of type 2 diabetes by improving the postprandial metabolic situation and eliminating hypoglycemic events (Table 1) (38). The risk of hypoglycemia observed in patients treated with GLP-1 is minimal because GLP-1 only stimulates insulin secretion under hyperglycemic conditions (33,51). Intravenous infusions of GLP-1 can normalize plasma glucose in patients with type 2 diabetes. Hepatic glucose production is lowered due to the inhibition of glucagon secretion (29) and the effects on body weight are also desirable.

Effects of a single subcutaneous injection of GLP-1, however, were disappointing due to the very rapid degradation of GLP-1 in vivo (52). GLP-1 (and the other incretin, GIP) is degraded within a few minutes by the enzyme dipeptidyl peptidase-4 (DPP-4) (53,54). Due to the enzymatic degradation, only approximately 20% of the GLP-1 administered by an intravenous infusion reaches circulation intact and in a biologically active form (38,54).

Generally, either DPP-4-resistant GLP-1 receptor agonists or substances inhibiting DPP-4 could be used to utilize the therapeutic potential of GLP-1 (55).

Peptidergic GLP-1 receptor agonists (GLP-1 analogs, also termed "incretin mimetics") are currently being introduced into type 2 diabetes therapy as injectable compounds (26,55–58). On the other hand, various orally active DPP-4 inhibitors are also evaluated in clinical trials or approved in single countries (26).

GLP-1 ANALOGUES—INCRETIN MIMETICS

The first "incretin mimetic" available in the United States for the therapy of type 2 diabetic patients not optimally controlled with an oral antidiabetic therapy (sulfonylureas and/or metformin) is exenatide [Byetta®; Eli Lilly (Indianapolis, IN, U.S.A.) & Amylin Pharmaceuticals (San Diego, CA, U.S.A.)]. Exenatide is the synthetic recombinant form of the naturally occurring peptide exendin-4. Exendin-4 was discovered in the salivary gland of the Gila monster (Heloderma suspectum). It has a high amino acid sequence similarity to GLP-1 and is not cleaved by DPP-4. Exendin-4 has physiological effects comparable to GLP-1 and a biological half-life of several hours making a therapy with twice daily injections feasible (59). In clinical studies exenatide showed a significant

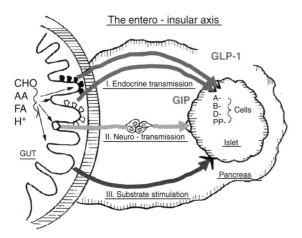

FIGURE 1 The entero-insular axis. Postprandially, insulin secretion is directly stimulated by substrates and by the strong endocrine stimulation through incretin hormones. *Abbreviations*: AA, amino acids; CHO, carbohydrates; FA, fatty acids; H^+, protons from gastric acid. *Source*: From Ref. 1.

TABLE 1   Organ-Specific Effects of GLP-1

Organ/cell system	GLP-1 effect
Endocrine pancreas	Beta cells ■ Stimulation of insulin secretion ■ Stimulation of insulin gene expression ■ Stimulation of growth, regeneration, and neogenesis of beta cells ■ Inhibition of apoptosis of beta cells Alpha cells ■ Inhibition of glucagon secretion Delta cells ■ Stimulation of somatostatin secretion
Stomach	Deceleration of gastric emptying Inhibition of gastric acid secretion
Ileum	GLP-1 synthesis; secretion is stimulated by carbohydrate- or fat-rich meals
Central nervous system (CNS)	Nucleus tractus solitarii ■ GLP-1 production Hypothalamus (GLP-1 receptors) ■ Inhibition of appetite; inhibition of food and water intake ■ Stimulation of satiety Note: Circumventricular organs that have access to circulating GLP-1 and GLP-1 from the gastrointestinal tract can reach the CNS via afferent fibers of the vagus nerve
Liver, muscle, adipose tissue	Indirect effects ■ Stimulation of glucose uptake ■ Stimulation of glycogen synthesis (predominantly liver)

improvement of glycemic control without weight gain and an improvement in beta-cell function without causing hypoglycemia in monotherapy or in combination with metformin (Fig. 2) (45,60–64,66). Hypoglycemia occurred only in patients receiving a combination of exenatide and sulfonylureas (45,62,65,66). Patients in an open extension of the studies comparing the efficacy and safety of exenatide to placebo receiving 10 μg exenatide b.i.d. subcutaneously had a sustained reduction of their HbA_{1c}-concentrations over a period of 2 years and also a reduction of their fasting glucose concentrations (63). The patients (mean BMI >30 kg/m^2) also continuously lost weight (63). In a head to head comparison of a combination therapy of oral antidiabetic drugs plus insulin glargine with a combination therapy of oral antidiabetic drugs plus exenatide, the exenatide-treated patients had less hypoglycemic events, less variations in their diurnal glucose concentrations and a significant weight loss compared to the patients receiving insulin glargine. Both treatment arms were equally effective in lowering HbA_{1c} (64). Exenatide also restores the diminished first phase of insulin secretion during an intravenous glucose load in patients with type 2 diabetes (67). Currently, a long acting release form of exenatide (exenatide LAR) designed for a once weekly injection is tested in clinical trials. Exenatide LAR reduces HbA_{1c} and body weight very effectively, with approximately 85% of patients reaching an HbA_{1c} of <7% (68).

A synthetic GLP-1 analog, liraglutide (NN2211) (Novo Nordisk Pharmaceuticals, Copenhagen, Denmark) is DPP-4-resistant and possesses a biologically longer half-life than native GLP-1 due to the addition of a fatty acid side chain to the peptide molecule. The mechanism of protraction is a combination of albumin binding and self-association in vivo, resulting in slow absorption after injection, stability against dipeptidyl-peptidase-4, and a long plasma half-life. It is suitable for once-daily injection. Liraglutide also improves plasma glucose and HbA_{1c} without an intrinsic risk for hypoglycemia and promotes weight loss (50,69). Animal studies using primary neonatal rat islets showed that native GLP-1 and liraglutide similarly inhibited both cytokine- and free fatty acid-induced apoptosis in a dose-dependent manner, suggesting that liraglutide may be useful for retaining beta-cell mass in both type 1 and type 2 diabetic patients (70). An increase of beta-cell mass and an improvement of beta-cell function in experimental animal models have been shown for exenatide and liraglutide likewise (70–73).

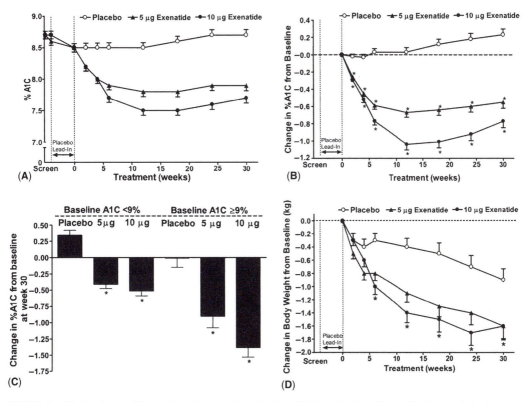

FIGURE 2 Effects of exenatide on glycemic control and body weight in subjects with type 2 diabetes. Patients were treated with metformin and sulfonylurea plus exenatide or placebo. (**A**) HbA$_{1c}$ values over the course of the study. (**B**) Change in HbA$_{1c}$ over 30 weeks. (**C**) Week 30 change in HbA$_{1c}$ stratified by baseline HbA$_{1c}$. (**D**) Effects of exenatide on body weight. Subjects in all treatment arms were maintained on metformin–sulfonylurea therapy. *< 0.001 compared with placebo treatment. Data are mean $\pm$ SE. *Source*: From Ref. 66.

Unlike insulin therapy that requires frequent dose adjustment, standard doses of GLP-1 receptor agonists facilitate diabetes treatment, additionally the probability of hypoglycemia is low.

Treatment with GLP-1 analogs is safe and adverse reactions are rare. There were no clinically relevant changes in hematology, clinical chemistry, or urinalysis analyte values in any of the studies. Side effects are mostly gastrointestinal in nature, nausea and fullness being the most frequent side effects occurring in approximately 40% of the patients (55,56,62). Nausea occurs most likely during the beginning of treatment, but usually ceases within a few days to weeks. Nausea is less prominent, when GLP-1 analogs are dose-titrated starting with a lower dose in the beginning. The majority (>90%) of the reported nausea and all hypoglycemic cases were mild or moderate in intensity, with no reports of hypoglycemia requiring the assistance of another individual. Hypoglycemia only occurred in patients who were taking a sulfonylurea (45). In patients treated with exenatide, formation of antibodies to the drug that are not cross-reacting with GLP-1 and that are not neutralizing antibodies was observed in approximately 45% of patients (63). In clinical studies with liraglutide no antibody formation has been observed so far (74).

DPP-4 INHIBITORS

Endogenous GLP-1 concentrations can be raised two- to threefold by inhibiting GLP-1 degradation via DPP-4. Support for this approach to therapy also comes from the observations that glucose tolerance is improved in animals in which the enzyme has been genetically deleted (75) and in animals treated with DPP-4 inhibitors (76). Various substances with DPP-4 inhibition properties are currently being tested in preclinical and clinical trials. The two compounds have reached approval in several countries are sitagliptin (MK0431, Januvia®; Merck Pharmaceuticals, Whitehouse Station, NJ, U.S.A.) and vildagliptin (LAF 237, Galvus®; Novartis Pharmaceticals, Basel, Switzerland) (77). Saxagliptin and further substances are presently also in clinical studies (78). In clinical studies, vildagliptin lowered HbA_{1c}, fasting and postprandial glucose in type 2 diabetic patients not sufficiently treated with metformin and other oral antidiabetic drugs (79). In monotherapy, vildaglitpin lead to a sustained HbA1 reduction almost similar to metformin. Sitagliptin also effectively lowers the HbA_{1c} and reduces diurnal fluctuations in glucose concentrations (58,80). In clinical studies, DPP-4 inhibitors improve beta-cell secretory capacity and suppress glucagon secretion from the alpha cells. In contrast to incretin mimetics, DPP-4 inhibitors have been weight neutral in clinical studies so far (58,79) (Fig. 3).

The application of DPP-4 inhibitors retards endogenous GLP-1 degradation, but there is still some uncertainty, whether all effects of DPP-4 inhibitors are exclusively mediated by the prolongation of the biological half-life of the peptide (81–83). One puzzling finding might support this: in patients with type 2 diabetes, concentrations of active GLP-1 after meal ingestion are doubled by DPP-4 inhibition (compared with placebo), and glucose control improves (79). In contrast, when similar increases in GLP-1

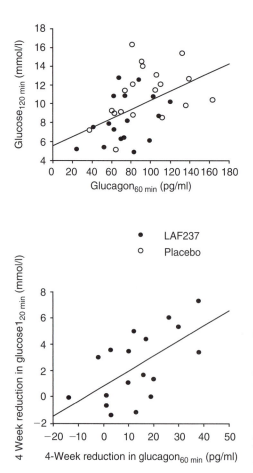

FIGURE 3 Inhibition of glucagon secretion after a test meal in patients with type 2 diabetes treated with Vildagliptin (LAF237). (*Upper panel*) Correlation between the 60-min glucagon levels and the 120-min glucose levels after ingestion of breakfast after 4 weeks of treatment with placebo (n=19) or LAF237 (vildagliptin) at 100 mg daily (n=18) in subjects with type 2 diabetes. (*Lower panel*) Correlation between the 4-week reduction in 60-min glucagon and the 4-week reduction in 120-min glucose after treatment with LAF237 at 100 mg daily (n=18) in subjects with type 2 diabetes. Linear correlations are shown. *Source*: From Ref. 91.

TABLE 2   Favorable Effects of GLP-1-Based Therapies in Type 2 Diabetes

Potential for normalizing glucose/HbA$_{1c}$
Glucose-dependent effect, no intrinsic hypoglycemias
Various principles of action (e.g., glucagonostatic effect)
No dose titration—"one size fits all"
Moderate weight loss possible or weight neutral
No severe side effects/broad therapeutic range
Results from animal and in vitro studies: positive effect on islet mass (neogenesis, proliferation, apotosis)

levels are produced by exogenous infusion, these have little or no effect on insulin secretion or glucose levels (22). This suggests that mediators other than GLP-1 may contribute to the therapeutic effect of DPP-4 inhibition. For instance, DPP-4 inhibition also blocks the inactivation of the other major incretin hormone GIP (81). Furthermore, various neuropeptides may contribute to the actions of DPP-4 inhibitors in diabetes like pituitary adenylate cyclase-activating peptide (PACAP), which is localized to islet nerves and has several actions relevant to glucose homeostasis (84). For example, PACAP is a powerful stimulator of insulin secretion and may, like GLP-1, be of importance for islet mass. PACAP may play a leading role in contributing to the prandial, neurally dependent cephalic phase of insulin secretion. Furthermore, it enhances glucose uptake in adipocytes and augments the antilipolytic action of insulin (81,85). Since PACAP is also a substrate for DPP-4, it is reasonable to speculate that this neuropeptide may contribute to the therapeutic benefits of DPP-4 inhibition. However, it is not yet known whether neuropeptides such as PACAP are substrates of DPP-4 in humans under physiological conditions, and this remains a weakness in this line of argument (81).

Because DPP-4 is involved in the degradation of many peptide hormones, the action of DPP-4 inhibitors is less specific than that of GLP-1 receptor agonists. Along with this, long-term immunological effects of DPP-4 inhibitors in humans are not known yet, since DPP-4 is also expressed on lymphocytes as CD26 (86,87). So far, however, DPP-4 inhibitor treatment did not show serious side effects and in human and animal studies no immunological changes have been observed.

In summary, the therapeutic principle of GLP-1 using incretin mimetics is a novel and attractive treatment option with multiple favorable actions for type 2 diabetes (Table 2) (55,56). Table 3 highlights the major differences between GLP-1 receptor agonists and DPP-4 inhibitors.

OUTLOOK AND PERSPECTIVES

The therapeutic principle of GLP-1 with the multiple mode of action besides its glucose-normalizing effect adds a new and attractive perspective to diabetes therapy. Since incretin mimetics and GLP-1 analogs are peptides, they have to be injected. This fact and their potential costs will probably give them a place in clinical practice for patients who have failed on oral therapy and in whom insulin therapy is not an alternative due to weight problems or possible hypoglycemia. Theoretically, GLP-1-like agents may be also

TABLE 3   Major Differences between GLP-1 Receptor Agonists and DPP-4 Inhibitors

Important pharmacological action of drug class	GLP-1 receptor agonists	DPP-4 inhibitors
Mechanism of stimulation of insulin secretion exclusively by GLP-1	Yes	Probably not only GLP-1 (GIP?, PACAP?, others?)
Restoration of lack of biphasic insulin secretion	Yes (Exanatide)	Not tested
Counterregulation by glucagon preserved in hypoglycemia	Yes	Not tested
Inhibition of gastric emptying	Yes	Marginal
Effect on body weight	Weight loss	Weight neutral
Predominant adverse effects	Nausea	None
Mode of administration	Subcutaneous	Oral

useful in slowing the progression of type 2 diabetes or to be used as anti-obesity agents due to their effects on body weight and beta-cell mass and function (88), but here lifestyle intervention and metformin are also effective (89). Incretin mimetics have the advantage of exclusively activating the GLP-1 receptor and therefore exerting exclusively the desired GLP-1-like effects (Table 1) in comparison to DPP-4 inhibitors. DPP-4 inhibitors have the benefit of being oral (and maybe less costly) agents, but their multiple effects besides raising endogenous GLP-1 concentrations are currently not completely elucidated (81). So far, only data from clinical trials covering a timeframe of 1 to 2 years are available. Long-term effects of GLP-1 analogs, incretin mimetics and DPP-4 inhibitors, e.g., on beta-cell proliferation and on the brain have to be followed in clinical practice (90).

REFERENCES

1. Creutzfeldt W. The incretin concept today. Diabetologia 1979; 16:75–85.
2. Zunz E, LaBarre J. Contibutions à l'étude des variations physiologiques de la sécrétion externe et interne du pancréas. Arch Int Physiol Biochim. 1929; 31:20–44.
3. Unger RH, Eisentraut AM. Entero-insular axis. Arch Intern Med 1969; 123:261–66.
4. Nauck MA, Homberger E, Siegel EG, et al. Incretin effects of increasing glucose loads in man calculated from venous insulin and C-peptide responses. J Clin Endocrinol Metab 1986; 63:492–98.
5. Creutzfeldt W. Entero-insular axis and diabetes mellitus. Horm Metab Res 1992; Suppl 26:13–8.
6. Meier JJ, Nauck MA, Schmidt WE, Gallwitz B. Gastric inhibitory polypeptide: the neglected incretin revisited. Regul Pept 2002; 107:1–13.
7. Pederson RA, Schubert HE, Brown JC. The insulinotropic action of gastric inhibitory polypeptide. Can J Physiol Pharmacol 1975; 53:217–23.
8. Miyawaki K, Yamada Y, Yano H, et al. Glucose intolerance caused by a defect in the entero-insular axis: a study in gastric inhibitory polypeptide receptor knockout mice. Proc Natl Acad Sci U S A 1999; 96:14843–47.
9. Miyawaki K, Yamada Y, Ban N, et al. Inhibition of gastric inhibitory polypeptide signaling prevents obesity. Nat Med 2002; 8:738–42.
10. Bell GI, Sanchez-Pescador R, Laybourn PJ, Najarian RC. Exon duplication and divergence in the human preproglucagon gene. Nature 1983; 304:368–71.
11. Holst JJ, Bersani M, Johnsen AH, Kofod H, Hartmann B, Orskov C. Proglucagon processing in porcine and human pancreas. J Biol Chem 1994; 269:18827-33.
12. Kreymann B, Williams G, Ghatei MA, Bloom SR. Glucagon-like peptide-1 7-36: a physiological incretin in man. Lancet 1987; 2:1300–04.
13. Schmidt WE, Siegel EG, Creutzfeldt W. Glucagon-like peptide-1 but not glucagon-like peptide-2 stimulates insulin release from isolated rat pancreatic islets. Diabetologia 1985; 28:704–7.
14. Nauck MA, Bartels E, Orskov C, Ebert R, Creutzfeldt W. Additive insulinotropic effects of exogenous synthetic human gastric inhibitory polypeptide and glucagon-like peptide-1-(7-36) amide infused at near-physiological insulinotropic hormone and glucose concentrations. J Clin Endocrinol Metab 1993; 76:912–17.
15. Wettergren A, Schjoldager B, Mortensen PE, Myhre J, Christiansen J, Holst JJ. Truncated GLP-1 (proglucagon 78-107-amide) inhibits gastric and pancreatic functions in man. Dig Dis Sci 1993; 38: 665–73.
16. Nauck MA, Niedereichholz U, Ettler R, et al. Glucagon-like peptide 1 inhibition of gastric emptying outweighs its insulinotropic effects in healthy humans. Am J Physiol 1997; 273:E981–88.
17. Schirra J, Kuwert P, Wank U, et al. Differential effects of subcutaneous GLP-1 on gastric emptying, antroduodenal motility, and pancreatic function in men. Proc Assoc Am Physicians 1997; 109:84–97.
18. Meier JJ, Gallwitz B, Salmen S, et al. Normalization of glucose concentrations and deceleration of gastric emptying after solid meals during intravenous glucagon-like peptide 1 in patients with type 2 diabetes. J Clin Endocrinol Metab 2003; 88:2719–25.
19. Vilsboll T, Krarup T, Madsbad S, Holst JJ. Both GLP-1 and GIP are insulinotropic at basal and postprandial glucose levels and contribute nearly equally to the incretin effect of a meal in healthy subjects. Regul Pept 2003; 114:115–21.
20. Scrocchi LA, Brown TJ, MaClusky N, et al. Glucose intolerance but normal satiety in mice with a null mutation in the glucagon-like peptide 1 receptor gene. Nat Med 1996; 2:1254–58.
21. Schirra J, Sturm K, Leicht P, Arnold R, Goke B, Katschinski M. Exendin(9-39)amide is an antagonist of glucagon-like peptide-1(7-36)amide in humans. J Clin Invest 1998; 101:1421–30.
22. Nauck MA, Heimesaat MM, Orskov C, Holst JJ, Ebert R, Creutzfeldt W. Preserved incretin activity of glucagon-like peptide 1 [7-36 amide] but not of synthetic human gastric inhibitory polypeptide in patients with type-2 diabetes mellitus. J Clin Invest 1993; 91:301–7.

23. Meier JJ, Hucking K, Holst JJ, Deacon CF, Schmiegel WH, Nauck MA. Reduced insulinotropic effect of gastric inhibitory polypeptide in first-degree relatives of patients with type 2 diabetes. Diabetes 2001; 50:2497–2504.
24. Lam NT, Kieffer TJ. The multifaceted potential of glucagon-like peptide-1 as a therapeutic agent. Minerva Endocrinol 2002; 27:79–93.
25. Drucker DJ, Philippe J, Mojsov S, Chick WL, Habener JF. Glucagon-like peptide I stimulates insulin gene expression and increases cyclic AMP levels in a rat islet cell line. Proc Natl Acad Sci U S A 1987; 84:3434–38.
26. Drucker DJ. The biology of incretin hormones. Cell Metab 2006; 3:153–165.
27. Gutniak M, Orskov C, Holst JJ, Ahren B, Efendic S. Antidiabetogenic effect of glucagon-like peptide-1 (7-36)amide in normal subjects and patients with diabetes mellitus. N Engl J Med 1992; 326: 1316–22.
28. Nathan DM, Schreiber E, Fogel H, Mojsov S, Habener JF. Insulinotropic action of glucagon-like peptide-I-(7-37) in diabetic and nondiabetic subjects. Diabetes Care 1992; 15:270–76.
29. Nauck MA, Kleine N, Orskov C, Holst JJ, Willms B, Creutzfeldt W. Normalization of fasting hyperglycaemia by exogenous glucagon-like peptide 1 (7-36 amide) in type 2 (non-insulin-dependent) diabetic patients. Diabetologia 1993; 36:741–44.
30. Holst JJ. Glucagon-like peptide-1, a gastrointestinal hormone with a pharmaceutical potential. Curr Med Chem 1999; 6:1005–17.
31. Vilsboll T, Krarup T, Madsbad S, Holst JJ. No reactive hypoglycaemia in Type 2 diabetic patients after subcutaneous administration of GLP-1 and intravenous glucose. Diabet Med 2001; 18:144–49.
32. Matsuyama T, Komatsu R, Namba M, Watanabe N, Itoh H, Tarui S. Glucagon-like peptide-1 (7-36 amide): a potent glucagonostatic and insulinotropic hormone. Diabetes Res Clin Pract 1988; 5: 281–84.
33. Meier JJ, Nauck MA. The potential role of glucagon-like peptide 1 in diabetes. Curr Opin Investig Drugs 2004; 5:402–10.
34. DeFronzo RA. Lilly lecture 1987. The triumvirate: beta-cell, muscle, liver. A collusion responsible for NIDDM. Diabetes 1988; 37:667–87.
35. Nauck MA, Heimesaat MM, Behle K, et al. Effects of glucagon-like peptide 1 on counterregulatory hormone responses, cognitive functions, and insulin secretion during hyperinsulinemic, stepped hypoglycemic clamp experiments in healthy volunteers. J Clin Endocrinol Metab 2002; 87:1239–46.
36. Gallwitz B. Glucagon-like peptide-1-based therapies for the treatment of type 2 diabetes mellitus. Treat Endocrinol 2005; 4:361–70.
37. Turton MD, O'Shea D, Gunn I, et al. A role for glucagon-like peptide-1 in the central regulation of feeding. Nature 1996; 379:69–72.
38. Zander M, Madsbad S, Madsen JL, Holst JJ. Effect of 6-week course of glucagon-like peptide 1 on glycaemic control, insulin sensitivity, and beta-cell function in type 2 diabetes: a parallel-group study. Lancet 2002; 359:824–30.
39. Gutzwiller JP, Degen L, Matzinger D, Prestin S, Beglinger C. Interaction between GLP-1 and CCK-33 in inhibiting food intake and appetite in men. Am J Physiol Regul Integr Comp Physiol 2004; 287: R562–67.
40. Gutzwiller JP, Degen L, Heuss L, Beglinger C. Glucagon-like peptide 1 (GLP-1) and eating. Physiol Behav 2004; 82:17–19.
41. Perfetti R, Hui H. The role of GLP-1 in the life and death of pancreatic beta cells. Horm Metab Res 2004; 36:804–10.
42. Brubaker PL, Drucker DJ. Minireview: Glucagon-like peptides regulate cell proliferation and apoptosis in the pancreas, gut, and central nervous system. Endocrinology 2004; 145:2653–59.
43. Drucker DJ. Glucagon-like peptides: regulators of cell proliferation, differentiation, and apoptosis. Mol Endocrinol 2003; 17:161–71.
44. Wang Q, Li L, Xu E, Wong V, Rhodes C, Brubaker PL. Glucagon-like peptide-1 regulates proliferation and apoptosis via activation of protein kinase B in pancreatic INS-1 beta cells. Diabetologia 2004; 47: 478–87.
45. Fineman MS, Bicsak TA, Shen LZ, et al. Effect on glycemic control of exenatide (synthetic exendin-4) additive to existing metformin and/or sulfonylurea treatment in patients with type 2 diabetes. Diabetes Care 2003; 26:2370–77.
46. Farilla L, Bulotta A, Hirshberg B. et al. Glucagon-like peptide 1 inhibits cell apoptosis and improves glucose responsiveness of freshly isolated human islets. Endocrinology 2003; 144:5149–58.
47. Nauck M, Stockmann F, Ebert R, Creutzfeldt W. Reduced incretin effect in type 2 (non-insulin-dependent) diabetes. Diabetologia 1986; 29:46–52.
48. Vilsboll T, Krarup T, Deacon CF, Madsbad S, Holst JJ. Reduced postprandial concentrations of intact biologically active glucagon-like peptide 1 in type 2 diabetic patients. Diabetes 2001; 50:609–13.
49. Nauck MA, Sauerwald A, Ritzel R, Holst JJ, Schmiegel W. Influence of glucagon-like peptide 1 on fasting glycemia in type 2 diabetic patients treated with insulin after sulfonylurea secondary failure. Diabetes Care 1998; 21:1925–31.

50. Madsbad S, Schmitz O, Ranstam J, Jakobsen G, Matthews DR. Improved glycemic control with no weight increase in patients with type 2 diabetes after once-daily treatment with the long-acting glucagon-like peptide 1 analog liraglutide (NN2211): a 12-week, double-blind, randomized, controlled trial. Diabetes Care 2004; 27:1335–42.

51. Holz GGt, Kuhtreiber WM, Habener JF. Pancreatic beta-cells are rendered glucose-competent by the insulinotropic hormone glucagon-like peptide-1(7-37). Nature 1993; 361:362–65.

52. Nauck MA, Wollschlager D, Werner J, Holst JJ, Orskov C, Creutzfeldt W, et al. Effects of subcutaneous glucagon-like peptide 1 (GLP-1 [7-36 amide]) in patients with NIDDM. Diabetologia 1996; 39:1546–53.

53. Mentlein R, Gallwitz B, Schmidt WE. Dipeptidyl-peptidase IV hydrolyses gastric inhibitory polypeptide, glucagon-like peptide-1(7-36)amide, peptide histidine methionine and is responsible for their degradation in human serum. Eur J Biochem 1993; 214:829–35.

54. Deacon CF, Johnsen AH, Holst JJ. Degradation of glucagon-like peptide-1 by human plasma in vitro yields an N-terminally truncated peptide that is a major endogenous metabolite in vivo. J Clin Endocrinol Metab 1995; 80:952–57.

55. Meier JJ, Gallwitz B, Nauck MA. Glucagon-like peptide 1 and gastric inhibitory polypeptide: potential applications in type 2 diabetes mellitus. BioDrugs 2003; 17:93–102.

56. Joy SV, Rodgers PT, Scates AC. Incretin Mimetics as Emerging Treatments for Type 2 Diabetes (January). Ann Pharmacother 2005; 39(1):110–18.

57. Baggio LL, Huang Q, Brown TJ, Drucker DJ. A recombinant human glucagon-like peptide (GLP)-1-albumin protein (albugon) mimics peptidergic activation of GLP-1 receptor-dependent pathways coupled with satiety, gastrointestinal motility, and glucose homeostasis. Diabetes 2004; 53:2492–2500.

58. Bergman AJ, Stevens C, Zhou Y, et al. Pharmacokinetic and pharmacodynamic properties of multiple oral doses of sitagliptin, a dipeptidyl peptidase-IV inhibitor: a double-blind, randomized, placebo-controlled study in healthy male volunteers. Clin Ther 2006; 28:55–72.

59. Goke R, Fehmann HC, Linn T, et al. Exendin-4 is a high potency agonist and truncated exendin-(9-39)-amide an antagonist at the glucagon-like peptide 1-(7-36)-amide receptor of insulin-secreting beta-cells. J Biol Chem 1993; 268:19650-55.

60. Kolterman OG, Buse JB, Fineman MS, et al. Synthetic exendin-4 (exenatide) significantly reduces postprandial and fasting plasma glucose in subjects with type 2 diabetes. J Clin Endocrinol Metab 2003; 88:3082–89.

61. DeFronzo RA, Ratner RE, Han J, Kim DD, Fineman MS, Baron AD. Effects of exenatide (exendin-4) on glycemic control and weight over 30 weeks in metformin-treated patients with type 2 diabetes. Diabetes Care 2005; 28:1092–1100.

62. Buse JB, Henry RR, Han J, Kim DD, Fineman MS, Baron AD. Effects of exenatide (exendin-4) on glycemic control over 30 weeks in sulfonylurea-treated patients with type 2 diabetes. Diabetes Care 2004; 27:2628–35.

63. Barnett AH. Exenatide. Drugs Today (Barc) 2005; 41:563–578.

64. Heine RJ, Van Gaal LF, Johns D, Mihm MJ, Widel MH, Brodows RG. Exenatide versus insulin glargine in patients with suboptimally controlled type 2 diabetes: a randomized trial. Ann Intern Med 2005; 143:559–69.

65. Kolterman OG, Kim DD, Shen L, et al. Pharmacokinetics, pharmacodynamics, and safety of exenatide in patients with type 2 diabetes mellitus. Am J Health Syst Pharm 2005; 62:173–81.

66. Kendall DM, Riddle MC, Rosenstock J. et al. Effects of exenatide (exendin-4) on glycemic control over 30 weeks in patients with type 2 diabetes treated with metformin and a sulfonylurea. Diabetes Care 2005; 28:1083-91.

67. Fehse F, Trautmann M, Holst JJ. et al. Exenatide augments first- and second-phase insulin secretion in response to intravenous glucose in subjects with type 2 diabetes. J Clin Endocrinol Metab 2005; 90:5991–97.

68. Kim D, Macconell L, Zhuang D. et al. Safety and Effects of a Once-Weekly, Long-Acting Release Formulation of Exenatide over 15 Weeks in Patients with Type 2 Diabetes. Diabetes 2006; 55 (Suppl. 1):A116.

69. Mark M. NN-2211 Novo Nordisk. IDrugs 2003; 6:251–58.

70. Bregenholt S, Moldrup A, Blume N, et al. The long-acting glucagon-like peptide-1 analogue, liraglutide, inhibits beta-cell apoptosis in vitro. Biochem Biophys Res Commun 2005; 330:577–84.

71. Sturis J, Gotfredsen CF, Romer J, et al. GLP-1 derivative liraglutide in rats with beta-cell deficiencies: influence of metabolic state on beta-cell mass dynamics. Br J Pharmacol 2003; 140:123–32.

72. Gedulin BR, Nikoulina SE, Smith PA, et al. Exenatide (exendin-4) improves insulin sensitivity and {beta}-cell mass in insulin-resistant obese fa/fa Zucker rats independent of glycemia and body weight. Endocrinology 2005; 146:2069–76.

73. Kim JG, Baggio LL, Bridon DP, et al. Development and characterization of a glucagon-like peptide 1-albumin conjugate: the ability to activate the glucagon-like peptide 1 receptor in vivo. Diabetes 2003; 52:751–9.

74. Feinglos MN, Saad MF, Pi-Sunyer FX, An B, Santiago O. Effects of liraglutide (NN2211), a long-acting GLP-1 analogue, on glycaemic control and bodyweight in subjects with Type 2 diabetes. Diabet Med 2005; 22:1016–23.

75. Marguet D, Baggio L, Kobayashi T, et al. Enhanced insulin secretion and improved glucose tolerance in mice lacking CD26. Proc Natl Acad Sci U S A 2000; 97:6874–79.

76. Reimer MK, Holst JJ, Ahren B. Long-term inhibition of dipeptidyl peptidase IV improves glucose tolerance and preserves islet function in mice. Eur J Endocrinol 2002; 146:717–27.

77. Mest HJ. Dipeptidyl peptidase-IV inhibitors can restore glucose homeostasis in type 2 diabetics via incretin enhancement. Curr Opin Investig Drugs 2006; 7:338–43.

78. Augeri DJ, Robl JA, Betebenner DA, et al. Discovery and preclinical profile of Saxagliptin (BMS-477118): a highly potent, long-acting, orally active dipeptidyl peptidase IV inhibitor for the treatment of type 2 diabetes. J Med Chem 2005; 48:5025–37.

79. Ahren B, Gomis R, Standl E, Mills D, Schweizer A. Twelve- and 52-week efficacy of the dipeptidyl peptidase IV inhibitor LAF237 in metformin-treated patients with type 2 diabetes. Diabetes Care 2004; 27:2874–80.

80. Kim D, Wang L, Beconi M, et al. (2R)-4-oxo-4-[3-(trifluoromethyl)-5,6-dihydro[1,2,4]triazolo[4,3-a] pyrazin -7(8H)-yl]-1-(2,4,5-trifluorophenyl)butan-2-amine: a potent, orally active dipeptidyl peptidase IV inhibitor for the treatment of type 2 diabetes. J Med Chem 2005; 48:141–51.

81. Ahren B. What mediates the benefits associated with dipeptidyl peptidase-IV inhibition? Diabetologia 2005; 48:605–7.

82. Nauck MA, El-Ouaghlidi A. The therapeutic actions of DPP-IV inhibition are not mediated by glucagon-like peptide-1. Diabetologia 2005; 48:608–11.

83. Holst JJ, Deacon CF. Glucagon-like peptide-1 mediates the therapeutic actions of DPP-IV inhibitors. Diabetologia 2005; 48:612–15.

84. Filipsson K, Kvist-Reimer M, Ahren B. The neuropeptide pituitary adenylate cyclase-activating polypeptide and islet function. Diabetes 2001; 50:1959–69.

85. Akesson L, Ahren B, Manganiello VC, Holst LS, Edgren G, Degerman E. Dual effects of pituitary adenylate cyclase-activating polypeptide and isoproterenol on lipid metabolism and signaling in primary rat adipocytes. Endocrinology 2003; 144:5293–99.

86. Villhauer EB, Brinkman JA, Naderi GB, et al. 1-[[(3-hydroxy-1-adamantyl)amino]acetyl]-2-cyano-(S)-pyrrolidine: a potent, selective, and orally bioavailable dipeptidyl peptidase IV inhibitor with antihyperglycemic properties. J Med Chem 2003; 46:2774–89.

87. Deacon CF, Holst JJ. Dipeptidyl peptidase IV inhibition as an approach to the treatment and prevention of type 2 diabetes: a historical perspective. Biochem Biophys Res Commun 2002; 294:1–4.

88. Meier JJ, Gallwitz B, Schmidt WE, Nauck MA. Glucagon-like peptide 1 as a regulator of food intake and body weight: therapeutic perspectives. Eur J Pharmacol 2002; 440:269–79.

89. Knowler WC, Barrett-Connor E, Fowler SE, et al. Reduction in the incidence of type 2 diabetes with lifestyle intervention or metformin. N Engl J Med 2002; 346:393–403.

90. Nielsen LL. Incretin mimetics and DPP-IV inhibitors for the treatment of type 2 diabetes. Drug Discov Today 2005; 10:703–10.

91. Ahren B, Landin-Olsson M, Jansson PA, Svensson M, Holmes D, Schweizer A. Inhibition of dipeptidyl peptidase-4 reduces glycemia, sustains insulin levels, and reduces glucagon levels in type 2 diabetes. J Clin Endocrinol Metab 2004; 89:2078–84.

13 | Pramlintide Acetate in the Treatment of Type 2 Diabetes

Steven V. Edelman
Division of Endocrinology and Metabolism, San Diego Veterans Affairs Medical Center, San Diego, California, U.S.A.

Brock E. Schroeder and Juan P. Frias
Amylin Pharmaceuticals, Inc., San Diego, California, U.S.A.

INTRODUCTION

The pivotal role that multiple pancreatic and gut hormones play in the maintenance of glucose homeostasis has become increasingly apparent over the past several years (1,2). We know today that in patients with diabetes, hyperglycemia results not only from factors beyond absolute or relative insulin deficiency and insulin resistance, but also from abnormalities in secretion and action of a number of hormones including the α-cell hormone glucagon, the incretin glucagon-like-peptide-1, and the β-cell hormone amylin (1,2). This chapter focuses on the hormone amylin and the therapeutic use of the amylin analog pramlintide in the management of insulin-using patients with type 2 diabetes.

AMYLIN THE HORMONE

Amylin is a 37-amino acid β-cell hormone, which is co-located and co-secreted with insulin in response to nutrient intake. In persons without diabetes, the pattern of amylin and insulin secretion throughout the day is similar: low fasting concentrations that rapidly increase following meals (Fig. 1) (3–6). Preclinical experiments in rodents have demonstrated that amylin exerts its effects as a neuroendocrine hormone, activating specific amylin receptors in the brain (7,8). Via this central binding, amylin stimulates three key actions that together help control the rate of glucose appearance into the circulation during the postprandial period. Amylin suppresses postprandial glucagon secretion (9–12), modulates the rate of gastric emptying (13,14), and attenuates feeding behavior (15,16). Since one of the primary actions of insulin in the postprandial period is promotion of glucose disappearance (into peripheral tissues), amylin, with its effects on glucose appearance, can be considered a partner or complementary hormone to insulin, with both hormones contributing to the maintenance of normal postprandial glucose concentrations (Fig. 2). Given the characteristics of β-cell dysfunction in diabetes, there is an absolute deficiency of insulin and amylin in patients with type 1 diabetes and a progressive decline of insulin and amylin secretory capacity in patients with type 2 diabetes (Fig. 3) (3,5,17).

PRAMLINTIDE

Because of amylin's insolubility and tendency to aggregate, pramlintide, a synthetic, soluble, non-aggregating analog of amylin with similar mechanisms of action, was developed as a pharmaceutical agent (18,19). Pramlintide acetate injection is indicated in the United States as an adjunct to mealtime insulin in patients with type 2 and type 1 diabetes who have failed to achieve desired glucose control despite optimal insulin therapy, with or without a concurrent sulfonylurea agent and/or metformin in patients with type 2 diabetes (20). In patients with diabetes, pramlintide induces many of the same actions as amylin, including suppression of inappropriately elevated postprandial glucagon secretion, slowing of gastric emptying, and enhancement of satiety. Collectively, these mechanisms of action result in lowering of postprandial glucose concentrations.

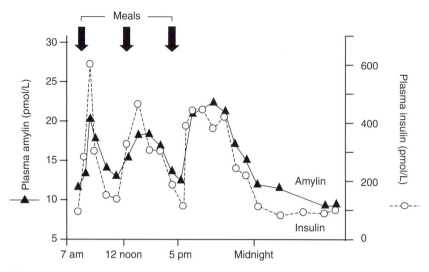

FIGURE 1 Twenty-four hour plasma profile of amylin and insulin in healthy subjects. Insulin and amylin have similar diurnal secretory patterns, with low basal levels and robust increases after nutrient intake. *Source*: From Ref. 17.

Glucagon serves as the primary signal for hepatic glucose production and release. While glucagon is normally secreted in times of fasting and suppressed after meals, in patients with diabetes there is often inadequate suppression or even a paradoxical increase of glucagon secretion following meals, contributing to postprandial hyperglycemia (21). Pramlintide suppresses this abnormal rise in postprandial glucagon (21). Given that insulin-induced hypoglycemia is a major concern for patients with diabetes, and that pramlintide is

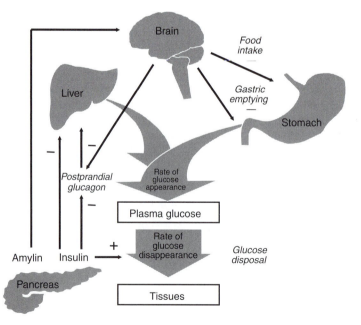

FIGURE 2 Proposed model of amylin and insulin action. Insulin is the major hormone involved in regulation of postprandial glucose disappearance. Amylin complements the effects of insulin by regulating the rate of glucose appearance into the bloodstream. *Source*: Model derived from animal studies.

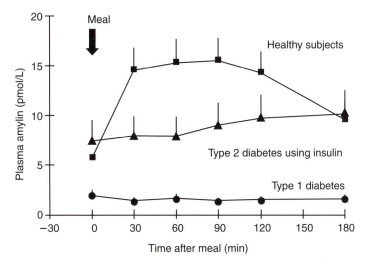

FIGURE 3 Mean amylin (±SE) plasma concentration versus time after a liquid Sustacal® meal. Amylin secretion is absent in patients with type 1 diabetes and impaired in patients with type 2 diabetes. *Source*: From Ref. 17.

administered as an adjunct to insulin, it is important to note that pramlintide's glucagon-suppressing effect is overridden in the presence of hypoglycemia (22).

An additional mechanism of action of pramlintide is control of the rate of gastric emptying. Gastric emptying may be accelerated in patients with diabetes (23–25); furthermore, early postprandial plasma glucose increases in direct proportion to the rate of gastric emptying (26). In studies utilizing both solid and liquid meals, pramlintide prolonged the half-gastric emptying time by 60 to 90 minutes, without any carry-over effect to the subsequent meal (27,28).

A third mechanism of action involves a satiogenic effect, resulting in reduced food intake. In a placebo-controlled, crossover study of patients with type 2 diabetes, pramlintide administration (120 µg) 1 hour before an ad libitum buffet meal resulted in a reduction in caloric intake of approximately 23% compared with placebo (29). Reduction in food intake was independent of nausea, which can accompany pramlintide treatment. This satiogenic effect may help explain the weight loss observed in the long-term clinical trials (30,31).

Short-Term Clinical Studies Assessing Postprandial Glucose Control

Given pramlintide's mechanisms of action which collectively reduce the appearance of glucose into the circulation during the postprandial period, one of its most important effects is a reduction of postprandial glucose concentrations and daily glucose fluctuations. These effects have been examined in several clinical trials in patients with type 2 diabetes treated with mealtime insulin (32,33). In patients using insulin lispro, pramlintide administered immediately prior to a standardized meal significantly reduced postprandial glucose excursions compared with mealtime insulin therapy alone (Fig. 4) (33). Pramlintide achieved this effect with an average reduction in mealtime insulin of approximately 17% (33).

Long-Term, Placebo-Controlled Clinical Studies

Long-term (26–52 weeks), placebo-controlled clinical studies designed to assess the safety and efficacy of pramlintide as an adjunct to mealtime insulin in patients with type 2 diabetes consistently demonstrated improvements in glycemic control with reduction in body weight. Adjunctive pramlintide therapy (120 µg) significantly reduced A_{1c} by −0.6% (vs. −0.2% for placebo, $P < 0.05$), and did so despite a reduction in daily insulin (Fig. 5) (30,31).

Weight gain is associated with most traditional antihyperglycemic therapies (34). In contrast, the improvement in glycemic control in pramlintide-treated patients was associated with a significant ($P < 0.0001$) and sustained ($P < 0.0001$) reduction in body weight. Following

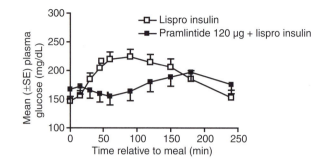

FIGURE 4 Pramlintide-reduced postprandial glucose concentrations. Patients with type 2 diabetes ($n = 19$) were administered placebo or 120 μg pramlintide and rapid-acting insulin lispro immediately prior to a meal. Pramlintide significantly reduced glucose concentrations in the postprandial period compared to placebo ($P < 0.05$). *Source*: From Ref. 33.

6 months of pramlintide treatment, patients with type 2 diabetes lost an average of -1.5 kg compared with an average gain of $+0.2$ kg in placebo-treated patients (Fig. 5) (30,31). Weight reductions were sustained for up to 1 year. Stratification of patients based on baseline body mass index demonstrated that body weight reductions were greatest in those who were overweight or obese (35). Furthermore, weight reduction in pramlintide-treated patients occurred without prescribed modification of diet or exercise routines (30,31) and was independent of nausea, a common side effect of pramlintide treatment (30).

In these initial long-term, placebo-controlled clinical trials investigators and patients were encouraged to maintain stable insulin dosages when pramlintide was introduced in order to isolate the effects of pramlintide. Additionally, the dose of pramlintide was not slowly up-titrated to the maintenance dose, in contrast to what is recommended today (20). As a result, an increased rate of severe hypoglycemia during the initial 3 months of pramlintide therapy was observed when compared to placebo (30,31). It is important to note that although pramlintide itself does not cause hypoglycemia, the addition of pramlintide to an insulin-based regimen can increase the risk of insulin-induced severe hypoglycemia. Therefore, proper mealtime insulin dose adjustments upon initiation of pramlintide therapy are very important to reduce the risk of hypoglycemia.

A subsequent 29-week, placebo-controlled, non-inferiority study was conducted in patients with type 1 diabetes using intensive insulin therapy (multiple daily injections or insulin pump) in order to determine a method of pramlintide initiation that would mitigate the increased risk of severe hypoglycemia (36). During initiation of therapy, pramlintide was escalated from 15 to 60 μg per meal in 15-μg increments over 4 weeks and mealtime insulin was reduced by 30% to 50% on pramlintide initiation. The insulin dose was subsequently adjusted to optimize glycemic control in both the pramlintide- and placebo-treated groups. As expected, since both study arms were targeting similar glycemic parameters, A_{1c} decreased comparably in the pramlintide + insulin group and the placebo + insulin group (-0.4% and -0.5%, respectively), despite reductions in insulin doses in the pramlintide-treated group (mealtime insulin: 28%; total daily insulin: 12%). Pramlintide-treated patients also experienced significant reductions in postprandial glucose excursions and had significant weight loss (-1.3 kg vs. $+1.2$ kg) compared to subjects in the placebo group. These changes were all observed in the context of an improved safety profile compared with the previous long-term clinical studies. Patients with type 2 diabetes were not examined in this study; however, the study supports the pramlintide dose escalation and initial mealtime insulin dose reduction recommended upon pramlintide initiation in patients with type 2 diabetes (20).

Open-Label Clinical Study

This method of pramlintide initiation was assessed in a 6-month open-label clinical practice study. Patients with type 2 diabetes were instructed to reduce mealtime insulin by 30% to 50% upon pramlintide (120 μg) initiation. In this study, despite significant reductions in mealtime and total insulin doses of -10.3% and -6.4%, respectively ($P < 0.05$), significant A_{1c} reductions

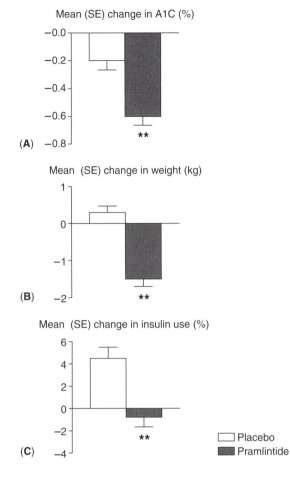

Mean (SE) change in A1C (%)

(A)

Mean (SE) change in weight (kg)

(B)

Mean (SE) change in insulin use (%)

(C)

☐ Placebo
■ Pramlintide

FIGURE 5 Mean changes (±SE) in A_{1c} (**A**), body weight (**B**), and insulin use (**C**) at 26 weeks in ITT populations in the combined long-term, placebo-controlled clinical studies of pramlintide in insulin-using patients with type 2 diabetes after 26 weeks of treatment. Patients were treated with 120 µg pramlintide b.i.d. ($n = 292$) versus placebo ($n = 284$). **$P < 0.01$. *Source*: From Refs. 30 and 31.

from baseline of −0.56 % were observed ($P < 0.05$). Self-monitored blood-glucose profiles at baseline and after 6 months of adjunctive pramlintide therapy revealed significantly ($P < 0.05$) reduced postprandial glucose concentrations, resulting in smoother daily glucose profiles (Fig. 6) (37). As in the earlier long-term clinical trials, glycemic improvements also were accompanied by significant weight loss (-2.76 kg, $P < 0.05$) (37).

Pramlintide in Type 2 Patients Using Basal Insulin (Without Mealtime Insulin)

The potential benefits of pramlintide in patients with type 2 diabetes using basal insulin alone (without mealtime insulin) were assessed via two post-hoc analyses. Patients with type 2 diabetes ($n = 18$) from a placebo-controlled, 52-week study, using pramlintide (120 µg b.i.d.) as an adjunct to basal insulin (Lente, Ultralente, or NPH) experienced greater reductions in A_{1c} (−1.16% vs. −0.48%) and greater weight loss (-2.3 kg vs. −0.9 kg) compared to placebo-treated patients (38). In patients ($n = 10$) treated with insulin glargine (± oral antidiabetic agents) and enrolled in an open-label study, similar changes were observed (39). At 52 weeks, A_{1c} was reduced by 1.0%, despite an 18% reduction in insulin glargine dose, and patients had an average weight loss of −3 kg. Importantly, no pramlintide-treated patient in either analysis experienced an episode of severe hypoglycemia.

Oxidative Stress

Oxidative stress, the imbalance between free radical production and antioxidant consumption, is increasingly regarded as a significant factor in the pathogenesis of diabetes complications (40,41). Moreover, it is well documented that hyperglycemia generates oxidative stress (42,43).

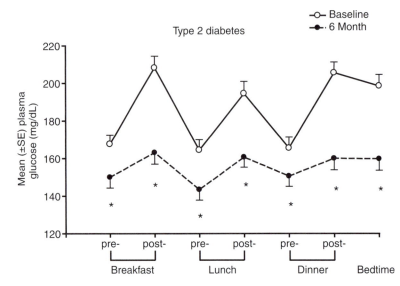

FIGURE 6 Postprandial glucose fluctuations were reduced by pramlintide. Patients with type 2 diabetes self-monitored blood glucose before and after the three major meals of the day and at bedtime at baseline and after 6 months of pramlintide treatment. Pramlintide significantly reduced blood glucose following all three major meals in patients with type 2 diabetes ($n = 166$). *$P < 0.05$. *Source*: From Ref. 37.

Given that pramlintide decreases postprandial glucose excursions, oxidative stress markers were studied in a post-hoc analysis of a short-term, crossover study. In 19 patients with type 2 diabetes, pramlintide treatment (120 μg) led to a reduction in oxidized LDL cholesterol and a significant ($P < 0.05$) reduction in postprandial nitrotyrosine. In addition, total radical-trapping antioxidant parameter was protected from consumption ($P < 0.05$) (44). Significant correlations were also present between postprandial glucose concentrations and markers of oxidative stress. These findings support further investigation into the potential effects of pramlintide treatment on the development of cardiovascular disease in patients with diabetes.

Safety and Tolerability

Pramlintide was generally well-tolerated in the clinical trials (30,31). No pramlintide-associated alterations were observed in cardiac function, laboratory tests, vital signs; and there was no evidence of renal or hepatic toxicity. Nausea and hypoglycemia were the most frequently cited adverse effects.

Gastrointestinal Side Effects

Aside from hypoglycemia, the most common side effects that were reported more frequently with pramlintide treatment than with placebo in the clinical trials (30,31) were gastrointestinal in nature (30,31). Nausea was reported by approximately 30% of patients treated with pramlintide. It generally occurred early in the course of therapy, was mild to moderate in intensity, and decreased over time.

Hypoglycemia

As mentioned above, while pramlintide alone does not cause hypoglycemia, when added to insulin therapy, pramlintide increases the risk of insulin-induced severe hypoglycemia, particularly in patients with type 1 diabetes (2). The event rate of severe hypoglycemia requiring medical assistance that was observed in studies where pramlintide was initiated at a fixed dose without proactive reduction in mealtime insulin was mitigated in subsequent studies in which mealtime insulin dose was initially reduced (Fig. 7) (36,37).

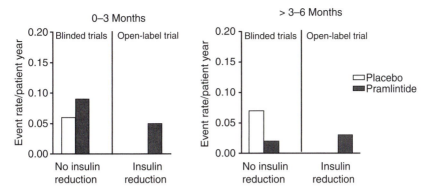

FIGURE 7   Annual event rate of medically assisted severe hypoglycemia in patients with type 2 diabetes from long-term, placebo-controlled, blinded clinical trials and an open-label clinical practice study. *Source*: From Refs. 30, 31, and 37.

INDICATION AND TREATMENT GUIDELINES

Pramlintide acetate injection is approved in the United States for use as an adjunct to mealtime insulin in patients with type 2 and type 1 diabetes who are unable to achieve glycemic goals despite optimized insulin therapy. In insulin-using patients with type 2 diabetes, pramlintide can be used concurrently with metformin and/or sulfonylureas. Pramlintide is supplied as a clear solution in a vial (5 mL, 0.6 mg/mL) and is administered just before mealtimes by subcutaneous injection using a standard insulin syringe. Because pramlintide is formulated with a pH of 4.0 and most insulin formulations have a neutral pH, mixing the two in the same syringe may lead to alterations in the pharmacokinetic and/or pharmacodynamic character-istics of either pramlintide or insulin (20,45). Thus, pramlintide and insulin should not be mixed. In addition, pramlintide should be administered via a separate syringe, and at a site separate from the concurrent insulin injection.

In patients with type 2 diabetes, pramlintide should be initiated at a dose of 60 μg with major meals and titrated to 120 μg based on tolerability of nausea. If the 120-μg dose is not well-tolerated, a maintenance dose of 60 μg can be used. During initiation of pramlintide treatment, mealtime insulin doses should be proactively reduced by 50%, and patients should carefully self-monitor blood glucose concentrations. Once pramlintide treatment is estab-lished, it is important that insulin dose be adjusted, based on self-monitoring of blood glucose, to achieve individual glycemic targets.

The choice of mealtime insulin used with pramlintide (e.g., regular insulin vs. a rapid-acting analog) and the timing of mealtime insulin administration should also be taken into consideration. Pramlintide reduces postprandial glucose concentrations, in part by slowing gastric emptying, and thus also affects the rate of nutrient absorption. When pramlintide is administered concurrently with a rapid-acting insulin analog, this may result in an initial reduction of postprandial glucose, followed by a late, gradual increase during the period of time following peak mealtime insulin action. Administering the rapid-acting analog after the meal, using regular human insulin, or using an extended wave bolus feature (in insulin pump-treated patients) may prevent this late postprandial rise in glucose and further improve overall glycemia in patients treated with pramlintide.

CONCLUSIONS

Pramlintide, an analog of the naturally occurring β-cell hormone amylin, is the first agent in the new amylinomimetic class. As an adjunct to mealtime insulin in patients with type 2 or type 1 diabetes, pramlintide improves postprandial and overall glycemic control (A_{1c}). These glycemic improvements are generally achieved with lower insulin doses and, importantly, with weight loss, as opposed to the weight gain observed with most other antidiabetic agents.

Though pramlintide can increase the risk of insulin-induced hypoglycemia, this risk can be mitigated by appropriate insulin dose adjustments. Given these characteristics, pramlintide represents an effective and physiologically relevant therapeutic option for patients with type 2 diabetes who are unable to achieve glycemic control with insulin therapy alone.

REFERENCES

1. Drucker DJ. Biologic actions and therapeutic potential of the proglucagon-derived peptides. Nat Clin Pract Endocrinol Metab 2005; 1(1):22–31.
2. Edelman SV, Weyer C. Unresolved challenges with insulin therapy in type 1 and type 2 diabetes: potential benefit of replacing amylin, a second β-cell hormone. Diabetes Technol Ther 2002; 4:175–89.
3. Koda JE, Fineman M, Rink TJ, et al. Amylin concentrations and glucose control. Lancet 1992; 339: 1179–80.
4. Koda JE, Fineman MS, Kolterman OG, et al. 24 hour plasma amylin profiles are elevated in IGT subjects vs. normal controls [abstract 876]. Diabetes 1995; 44(Suppl. 1):238A.
5. Fineman MS, Giotta MP, Thompson RG, et al. Amylin response following Sustacal® ingestion is diminished in type II diabetic patients treated with insulin [abstract 556]. Diabetologia 1996; 39 (Suppl. 1):A149.
6. Weyer C, Maggs DG, Young AA, et al. Amylin replacement with pramlintide as an adjunct to insulin therapy in type 1 and type 2 diabetes mellitus: a physiological approach toward improved metabolic control. Curr Pharm Des 2001; 7(14):1353–73.
7. Young A, Moore C, Herich J, et al. Neuroendocrine actions of amylin. In: Poyner D, Marshall I, Brain SD, eds. The CGRP Family: Calcitonin Gene-Related Peptide (CGRP), Amylin, and Adrenomedullin. Georgetown, TX: Landes Bioscience, 2000:91–102.
8. Beaumont K, Kenney MA, Young AA, et al. High affinity amylin binding sites in rat brain. Mol Pharmacol 1993; 44(3):493–7.
9. Gedulin B, Jodka C, Green D, et al. Amylin inhibition of arginine-induced glucagon secretion: comparison with glucagon-like-peptide-1 (7-36)-amide (GLP-1) [abstract 584]. Diabetologia 1996; 39 (Suppl. 1):A154.
10. Gedulin BR, Rink TJ, Young AA. Dose–response for glucagonostatic effect of amylin in rats. Metabolism 1997; 46(1):67–70.
11. Gedulin B, Jodka C, Percy A, et al. Neutralizing antibody and the antagonist AC187 may inhibit glucagon secretion in rats. Diabetes 1997; 40(Suppl. 1):238A.
12. Silvestre RA, Rodriguez-Gallardo J, Jodka C, et al. Selective amylin inhibition of the glucagon response to arginine is extrinsic to the pancreas. Am J Physiol Endocrinol Metab 2001; 280(3):E443–9.
13. Young AA, Gedulin B, Vine W, et al. Gastric emptying is accelerated in diabetic BB rats and is slowed by subcutaneous injections of amylin. Diabetologia 1995; 38(6):642–8.
14. Young AA, Gedulin BR, Rink TJ. Dose–responses for the slowing of gastric emptying in a rodent model by glucagon-like peptide (7-36)NH2, amylin, cholecystokinin, and other possible regulators of nutrient uptake. Metabolism 1996; 45(1):1–3.
15. Rushing PA, Hagan MM, Seeley RJ, et al. Amylin: a novel action in the brain to reduce body weight. Endocrinology 2000; 141(2):850–3.
16. Rushing PA. Central amylin signaling and the regulation of energy homeostasis. Curr Pharm Des 2003; 9(10):819–25.
17. Kruger DF, Gatcomb PM, Owen SK. Clinical implications of amylin and amylin deficiency. Diabetes Educ 1999; 25(3):389–97.
18. Janes S, Gaeta L, Beaumont K, et al. The selection of pramlintide for clinical evaluation. Diabetes 1996; 45(Suppl. 2):235A.
19. Young AA, Vine W, Gedulin BR, et al. Preclinical pharmacology of pramlintide in the rat: comparisons with human and rat amylin. Drug Dev Res 1996; 37(4):231–48.
20. [SYMLIN] Amylin Pharmaceuticals, Inc. 2005. SYMLIN prescribing information [online]. Accessed on 18 July 2006. URL: http://symlin.com/pdf/SYMLIN-pi-combined.pdf.
21. Fineman M, Weyer C, Maggs DG, et al. The human amylin analog, pramlintide, reduces postprandial hyperglucagonemia in patients with type 2 diabetes mellitus. Horm Metab Res 2002; 34:504–8.
22. Nyholm B, Moller N, Gravholt CH, et al. Acute effects of the human amylin analog AC137 on basal and insulin-stimulated euglycemic and hypoglycemic fuel metabolism in patients with insulin-dependent diabetes mellitus. J Clin Endocrinol Metab 1996; 81(3):1083–9.
23. Nowak TV, Johnson CP, Kalbfleisch JH, et al. Highly variable gastric emptying in patients with insulin dependent diabetes mellitus. Gut 1995; 37:23–9.
24. Frank JW, Saslow SB, Camilleri M, Thomforde GM, Dinneen S, Rizza RA. Mechanism of accelerated gastric emptying of liquids and hyperglycemia in patients with type II diabetes mellitus. Gastroenterology 1995; 109:755–65.

25. Schwartz JG, Green GM, Guan D, McMahan CA, Phillips WT. Rapid gastric emptying of a solid pancake meal in type II diabetic patients. Diabetes Care 1996; 19:468–71.
26. Rayner CK, Samsom M, Jones KL, Horowitz M. Relationships of upper gastrointestinal motor and sensory function with glycemic control. Diabetes Care 2001; 24:371–81.
27. Kong MF, King P, Macdonald IA, et al. Infusion of pramlintide, a human amylin analogue, delays gastric emptying in men with IDDM. Diabetologia 1997; 40:82–8.
28. Kong MF, Stubbs TA, King P, et al. The effect of single doses of pramlintide on gastric emptying of two meals in men with IDDM. Diabetologia 1998; 41(5):577–83.
29. Chapman I, Parker B, Doran S, et al. Effect of pramlintide on satiety and food intake in obese subjects and subjects with type 2 diabetes. Diabetologia 2005; 48(5):838–48.
30. Hollander PA, Levy P, Fineman MS, et al. Pramlintide as an adjunct to insulin therapy improves long-term glycemic and weight control in patients with type 2 diabetes: a one-year randomized controlled trial. Diabetes Care 2003; 26(3):784–90.
31. Ratner RE, Want LL, Fineman MS, et al. Adjunctive therapy with the amylin analogue pramlintide leads to a combined improvement in glycemic and weight control in insulin-treated subjects with type 2 diabetes. Diabetes Technol Ther 2002; 4(1):51–61.
32. Thompson RG, Gottlieb A, Organ K, et al. Pramlintide: a human amylin analogue reduced postprandial plasma glucose, insulin and c-peptide concentrations in patients with type II diabetes. Diabetes Technol Ther 2007; 9:191–199.
33. Maggs DG, Fineman M, Kornstein J, et al. Pramlintide reduces postprandial glucose excursions when added to insulin lispro in subjects with type 2 diabetes: a dose-timing study. Diabetes Metab Res Rev 2004; 20:55–60.
34. Purnell JQ, Weyer C. Weight effect of current and experimental drugs for diabetes mellitus. Treat Endocrinol 2003; 2:33–47.
35. Hollander P, Maggs DG, Ruggles JA, et al. Effect of pramlintide on weight in overweight and obese insulin-treated type 2 diabetes patients. Obes Res 2004; 12:661–8.
36. Edelman S, Garg S, Frias J, et al. A double-blind, placebo-controlled trial assessing pramlintide treatment in the setting of intensive insulin therapy in type 1 diabetes. Diabetes Care 2006; 29(10): 2189–95.
37. Karl D, Philis-Tsimikas A, Darsow T, et al. Pramlintide as an adjunct to insulin in patients with type 2 diabetes in a clinical practice setting reduced A1C, postprandial glucose excursions and weight. Diabetes Technol Ther 2007; 9:191–9.
38. Lush C, Strobel S, Zhang B, Frias J. Pramlintide, as an adjunct to long-acting insulin, led to improved A1C and body weight in patients with type 2 diabetes [abstract 521-P]. Diabetes 2006; 55:A124.
39. Frias J, Zhang B, Darsow T. Pramlintide as an adjunct to insulin glargine reduced A1C and body weight in patients with type 2 diabetes [abstract 472-P]. Diabetes 2006; 55:A112.
40. Giugliano D, Ceriello A, Paolisso G. Oxidative stress and diabetic vascular complications. Diabetes Care 1996; 19(3):257–67.
41. Rosen P, Nawroth PP, King G, Moller W, Tritschler HJ, Packer L. The role of oxidative stress in the onset and progression of diabetes and its complications: a summary of a Congress Series sponsored by UNESCO-MCBN, the American Diabetes Association and the German Diabetes Society. Diabetes Metab Res Rev 2001; 17(3):189–212.
42. West IC. Radicals and oxidative stress in diabetes. Diabet Med 2000; 17(3):171–80.
43. Brownlee M. Biochemistry and molecular cell biology of diabetic complications. Nature 2001; 414 (6865):813–20.
44. Ceriello A, Lush C, Piconi L, et al. Pramlintide reduced markers of oxidative stress in the postprandial period in subjects with type 2 diabetes [abstract 447-P]. Diabetes 2006; 55:A106.
45. Weyer C, Fineman MS, Strobel S, et al. Properties of pramlintide and insulin upon mixing. Am J Health Syst Pharm 2005; 62:816–22.

14 | Insulin Therapy in Type 2 Diabetes

Kathleen L. Wyne and Pablo F. Mora
Division of Endocrinology and Metabolism, Department of Internal Medicine, University of Texas Southwestern Medical Center, Dallas, Texas, U.S.A.

Type 2 diabetes mellitus is defined by hyperglycemia, which is the result of an inability of the pancreas to make enough insulin for an individual's insulin resistance. Once this relative deficiency in insulin develops, the ability to produce insulin is no longer balanced with the insulin resistance and hepatic glucose production, thus the sugar begins to rise (1). When this mismatch is present, it is a progressive disease with a relentless decline in insulin secretion (2). The therapeutic armamentarium for the management of type 2 diabetes has widely expanded with the introduction of new oral and injectable agents, but their individual blood glucose-lowering potency is limited (3). In contrast, the blood glucose-lowering potential of insulin is only limited by the dose that one is willing to take. Insulin therapy should no longer be viewed as a "last resort" to be used after long-term oral agent combinations have failed, but, rather, as a therapeutic tool for earlier use in achieving glycemic targets. Simple strategies for starting insulin therapy with low doses in combination with oral agents have been shown to be effective (4–7). Once patients on combination oral therapy are started on insulin replacement, a structured titration regimen may suffice to accomplish glycemic targets. Many people will require an insulin regimen that will include prandial insulin to address postprandial hyperglycemia and to achieve and maintain target A_{1c} levels.

RATIONALE FOR EARLY INSULIN REPLACEMENT IN TYPE 2 DIABETES

The Initial Defect: Beta-Cell Dysfunction

Type 2 diabetes results from two fundamental pathogenic defects: impaired insulin secretion (or β-cell dysfunction) and insulin resistance manifested by increased hepatic glucose production and reduced peripheral glucose uptake (8). These defects are both genetically determined and influenced by environmental factors, such as physical inactivity and obesity (9). Preserved β-cell function to secrete sufficient insulin in response to peripheral resistance has emerged as the pivotal point in determining whether or not a patient progresses towards type 2 diabetes. Studies in young and apparently healthy Caucasian populations with normal glucose tolerance (NGT) or impaired fasting glucose (IFG) demonstrated that the β-cell function varied quantitatively with differences in insulin sensitivity (10,11). Analysis of first degree relatives of patients with type 2 diabetes has shown that the relationship between insulin sensitivity and β-cell function is reciprocal in that changes in one directly affect the other but not in a linear or logarithmic fashion (Fig. 1) (12). The natural history has been extensively studied in the Pima Indians of Arizona who have a high percentage of their adult population developing type 2 diabetes by age 40 (13,14). Further characterization of the β-cell dysfunction have demonstrated that insulin secretion defects are indeed present prior to the progression to hyperglycemia and can predict progression from NGT to IGT to diabetes (DM) (12,13).

A longitudinal study that monitored progression at yearly intervals in patients with initial NGT, found that transition from NGT to IGT was associated with an increase in body weight, a decline in insulin-stimulated glucose disposal, and a decline in the acute insulin secretory response to intravenous glucose ($AIR_{glucose}$), but no change in endogenous glucose output (15). Longitudinal evaluation in the Mexico City study showed that beta cell function and not body weight or IR predicted progression to DM (16).

Similarly, studies in women who have had a history of gestational diabetes shows that the progression to type 2 DM is correlated with the extent of impairment of insulin secretion (17).

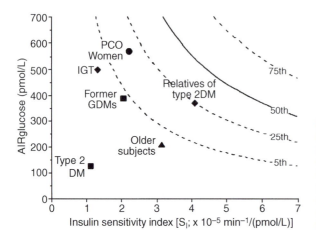

FIGURE 1 Percentile lines for the relationship between insulin sensitivity (SI) and the first-phase insulin response (AIRglucose) based on data from normal subjects with type 2 diabetes, healthy older subjects, women with a history of gestational diabetes (GDM), women with poly-cystic ovarian disease (PCO) and a family history of type 2 diabetes, subjects with IGT, subjects with a first-degree relative with type 2 diabetes.

The role of the progressive nature of the insulin secretory defect was classically demonstrated by the UKPDS in newly diagnosed patients with Type 2 DM. Beta cell function, as measured by the homeostasis model assessment method (HOMA), showed an inexorable decline over time which explains why most patients with type 2 DM will eventually necessitate insulin therapy if glycemic targets were to be achieved (18,19). Although individuals in the UKPDS receiving sulfonylurea therapy demonstrated an early increase in β-cell function from 45% to 78% in year 1 of the study (consistent with a secretagogue effect of the sulfonylurea agent) β-cell function subsequently decreased along the same slope as the diet treated group. This inevitable decline in β-cell function also occurred in the metformin group in which β-cell function initially increased (similar to that in the sulfonylurea group) then declined from 66% to 38% by year 6. These data suggest that a significant amount of beta cell function has typically been lost at the time of diagnosis and it continues to decrease rapidly when treated with traditional monotherapies.

Over time, insulin secretion declines, presumably accelerated by glucotoxicity and lipotoxicity (20–23). Any therapeutic strategy that corrects hyperglycemia and reduces free fatty acid levels can potentially improve insulin action and increase the efficiency of insulin secretion. It is conceivable that earlier intervention with a combination of agents that reduce insulin resistance and also promote insulin secretion may preserve β-cell functional integrity to maintain a durable glycemic response but eventually, supplemental insulin replacement will be needed to achieve near-normoglycemia. Insulin replacement should be considered an option as part of the initial therapy in patients with type 2 diabetes in an attempt to correct the pathogenic defects and effectively reach glycemic targets.

The fact that this inexorable decline could not be altered with our traditional monotherapies suggests that a new approach to diabetes is needed. Given that the hyperglycemia develops because of a relative deficiency of insulin, this raises the question as to why insulin is typically not included in the regimen from the time of diagnosis.

Indeed, short-term intensive insulin therapy in type 2 diabetes has been shown to improve insulin action by reversing glucotoxicity/lipotoxicity and possibly inducing " β-cell rest" that results in improved insulin secretion (24–28). It is tempting to speculate, therefore, that much earlier insulin administration, perhaps from the outset of the disease, might be crucial for preserving β-cell function. Preliminary support for this "β-cell rest" hypothesis is provided by a small study in newly diagnosed hyperglycemic patients with type 2 diabetes subjected to a period of 2 weeks of intensive insulin therapy, resulting in near-normoglycemia (29). Most of the patients subsequently sustained good glycemic control for long periods of time without pharmacologic intervention. These intriguing findings, albeit with small numbers of patients, suggest that insulin treatment in recently diagnosed type 2 diabetes might halt disease progression and permit long-term maintenance of nearly normal blood glucose levels with better response to oral agents or to simpler long-term insulin supplementation.

Insulin Therapy Can Improve Insulin Resistance

Insulin resistance, manifested by increased hepatic glucose production and reduced peripheral glucose disposal is a major pathogenic defect in type 2 diabetes, which correlates with obesity and hyperinsulinemia (30,31). Consequently, concern has been raised that treatment with insulin may worsen insulin resistance. However, short term intensive insulin therapy has been shown to improve insulin resistance (24–26). Peripheral insulin sensitivity, using the glucose-insulin clamp method, has been assessed before and after restoration of near-normoglycemic control in type 2 diabetes patients on intensive insulin treatment. In each case the treatment period was short (2 to 4 weeks) and relatively high insulin dosage was required (>100 U daily). Fig. 2 shows the tissue insulin sensitivity before and after treatment, expressed as a percentage of the mean value for insulin sensitivity of a non-diabetic control group that was matched in age, gender, and weight to the diabetic subjects. The three studies had remarkably similar results, with insulin sensitivity before treatment with insulin reduced by half, compared to the non-diabetic values, indicating marked insulin resistance. After treatment, insulin sensitivity improved toward the non-diabetic values, though some insulin resistance persisted, as would be expected. This improvement is presumably due to the resolution of the hyperglycemia and consequent reduced "glucotoxicity". Whether the improvement of insulin sensitivity persists when insulin treatment is continued for longer periods of time was not tested in these studies. However, these data show that, at least in the short term, successful insulin treatment reduces rather than worsens insulin resistance. Defronzo and colleagues showed that aggressive insulin therapy over 12 weeks that resulted in near-normalization of A_{1cs} (decreased from 10.1–6.6%) improved insulin resistance through improving insulin-stimulated glucose disposal but did not fully corrected the inherent insulin resistance (27).

Insulin Therapy and Potential Cardiovascular Benefits

Insulin resistance and the consequent endogenous hyperinsulinemia are strongly associated with central obesity, hypertension and dyslipidemia, all factors that contribute substantially to cardiovascular (CV) risk and in fact characterize the Metabolic Syndrome (31,32). Epidemiological studies in non-diabetic populations have shown an association between endogenous hyperinsulinemia and atherosclerosis (33) thus physicians have been concerned that initiating insulin therapy would be harmful and may accelerate coronary artery disease. However, the association of hyperinsulinemia and atherosclerosis is mainly an association between endogenous hyperproinsulinemia and atherosclerosis (34). In fact, there is no evidence from animal or human studies that exogenous insulin administration causes accelerated atherosclerosis. The UKPDS actually was very reassuring in demonstrating that the insulin treated patients, who presumably had exogenous hyperinsulinemia, showed no evidence at all of increased atherosclerotic-related events (35).

Furthermore, the 5-year diabetes mellitus insulin-glucose infusion in acute myocardial infarction (DIGAMI) trial showed that insulin infusion therapy during acute MI followed by intensive multiple dose insulin therapy reduced the relative mortality risk by 28% as compared to control (conventional therapy) after an average follow-up of 3.4 years (36,37). The subjects were randomized at the time of myocardial infarction to either control (continued management according to the judgment of their physicians) or to intravenous infusion of

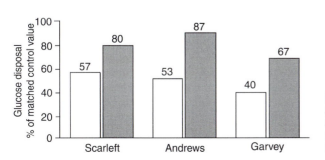

FIGURE 2 Improvement in insulin sensitivity as measured by the glucose clamp technique, at baseline and after intensive insulin treatment. Solid bars, after insulin; open bars, baseline. *Source*: From Refs. 24–26.

insulin and glucose for 48 h followed by a four-injection regimen for as long as 5 years. The rationale underlying the study was the preliminary observations that, in animal experiments and in studies of small numbers of humans, infarct size and outcome were improved by the insulin-glucose-potassium infusion, which is theorized to be related to suppression of otherwise elevated free fatty acid levels in plasma (38–41). Fig. 3 shows the cumulative total mortality rates in the whole population of 620 subjects randomized to the two treatments, as well as the rates for a predefined subgroup of subjects who were judged likely to survive the initial hospitalization and were not previously using insulin (36). The whole population showed an 11% actual and a 28% relative risk reduction in mortality with intensive insulin treatment after 5 years, and the subgroup not previously using insulin showed a 15% actual and a 51% relative risk reduction. Most of the benefit was apparent in the first month of treatment and presumably was partly due to immediate intravenous infusion of insulin; however, the survival curves tended to separate further over time, suggesting an ongoing benefit from intensive insulin treatment. This study suggests that insulin is an entirely appropriate treatment for type 2 diabetes patients with high cardiovascular risk, especially at the time of myocardial infarction. These same investigators then tried to repeat the study but found that the use of insulin had become standard in this patient population thus the DIGAMI 2 study was not able to reproduce the benefits found in DIGAMI (42).

BARRIERS TO INSULIN THERAPY

The major barriers for some physicians to use insulin in the treatment of type 2 diabetes are

- the misconception that insulin therapy may increase the risk of cardiovascular disease
- excessive concerns with weight gain
- the potential risk of hypoglycemia
- the inconvenience of having to instruct and persuade the patients to take injections

Traditionally, insulin therapy has been considered a therapy of last resort in type 2 diabetes due to these concerns and the lack of understanding that insulin deficiency is one of the initial defects that worsen with the progressive nature of the disease (Table 1).

Insulin Therapy and Weight Gain

Initiation of insulin therapy is typically associated with weight gain. The weight gain is most rapid in the first 3 to 6 months of therapy and is correlated with improvements in glycemic

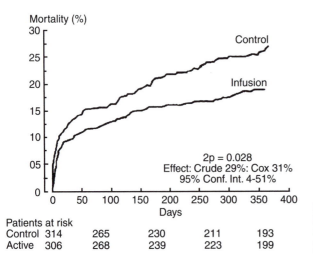

FIGURE 3 Mortality after MI reduced by insulin therapy in the DIGAMI study. Cumulative reinfarction date during the first year of follow-up.

TABLE 1 Major Barriers to Insulin Therapy in Patients with Type 2 Diabetes

Preconceived barriers	Actual effects of insulin therapy
Insulin resistance	Improves insulin sensitivity by reducing glucose toxicity
Cardiovascular (CV) risk	No evidence of atherosclerotic effects; may reduce CV risk
Weight gain	Typically modest
Hypoglycemia	Rarely causes severe events

control. Some simple but partial explanation for the weight gain comes from patients typically maintaining the same prior dietary transgressions but no longer having the caloric loss from glycosuria (43,44). Most studies have shown no change in basal metabolic rate (BMR) with improvement in glycemic control, perhaps due to the fact that the increase in BMR attributable to weight gain offsets the decrease in BMR attributable to improved glucose control (45–51). BMR is typically higher in diabetic subjects than that of non-diabetic subjects matched for BMI. Bogardus and colleagues showed an improvement in resting metabolic rate after improved glucose control in obese Pima Indians with T2DM when weight of the subjects was maintained constant from beginning to end of therapy by decreasing daily calorie intake. Insulin therapy is also known to noticeably lower plasma non-esterified fatty acid concentrations, a change which is associated with a lowering of gluconeogenesis (45). A decrease in non-esterified fatty acid concentrations may also lower heat production by decreasing mitochondrial uncoupling, i.e. the ratio between heat and ATP production. This emphasizes the importance of increasing daily activity and decreasing caloric intake to minimize weight gain. Of note, studies in obese patients with type 2 diabetes treated with insulin therapy have shown that, despite weight gain, CV risks factors such as blood pressure remained unchanged, and lipid patterns (triglycerides, lipoproteins) were generally improved (52–55). These findings challenge the notion that insulin therapy negatively affects blood pressure and lipid profiles through weight gain. Importantly, as previously discussed, intensive insulin therapy has been shown to improve rather than worsen insulin sensitivity by virtue of improving glycemic control, thus reducing and to some degree reversing the toxic effects of hyperglycemia (glucotoxicity).

In the UKPDS, patients in both the main study and the metformin sub study gained weight. In the main study, patients assigned to treatment with a sulfonylurea gained more weight than the conventional group, and those assigned insulin gained more weight than those on a sulfonylurea (35). In the cohort followed for 10 years, as compared to the patients on conventional therapy, those assigned to glyburide gained an excess of 1.7 kg and those on insulin gained an excess of 4.0 kg. In the metformin sub study, which included the more obese subjects in the trial (mean BMI ~31 kg/m^2), the changes of body weight were similar to those in the main study except that the group randomized to metformin showed weight gain similar to the conventionally treated group but lower than the groups treated with insulin or a sulfonylurea (18). Indeed, combination insulin therapy with metformin is an effective strategy to potentiate the effectiveness of the insulin regimen while limiting weight gain, as it will be reviewed later.

The inevitability of weight gain has been challenged by the unexpected observation that improving glucose control with inhaled insulin or with the newest insulin analogues, glulisine and detemir, was associated with weight loss or, at least, reduced weight gain (56–59). These observations have stimulated a renewed interest in the mechanisms of weight gain as glycemic control improves. The commonly believed mechanism has been that patients are storing the calories instead of losing them as glucose in the urine. Metformin has been believed to minimize weight gain by decreasing overall caloric intake. This observation with the newer insulin's has several theories that are currently being studied. One plausible suggestion has been that with the improved predictability in absorption and action compared with other insulin's, the newer insulin analogues are associated with less risk of hypoglycemia, which may reduce the need for eating to minimize the risk of hypoglycemia (60). This possibility is supported by the reduced incidence of hypoglycemic episodes. However, treatment with insulin glargine similarly reduced hypoglycemia, compared with neutral protamine hagedorn (NPH), in the Treat-to-Target study and both were associated with less weight gain than expected over 24 weeks (5).

Although this appears to be the most likely explanation, as the decreased weight gain is consistent across the multiple studies, the question has also been raised as to whether the unique mechanism of absorption of insulin detemir may also have other properties. It is certainly possible that the fatty acid modification of insulin that is unique to insulin detemir may modulate other effects in the liver and brain that do not occur with traditional insulin preparations. While further studies are needed, the important clinical observation is that weight gain is not obligatory and does not need to occur as glucose control improves.

Insulin Therapy and Hypoglycemia

Hypoglycemia is the most important limiting factor for insulin adjustments to improve glycemic control. The risk of hypoglycemia depends on a number of factors including age, weight, degree of insulin resistance, duration of disease, duration of insulin therapy, targeted degree of glycemic control and history of hypoglycemic episodes. Additional causal factors in hypoglycemia include overinsulinization, dietary transgressions, strenuous unplanned exercise, excessive alcohol intake, and unawareness of hypoglycemia. The actual incidence of severe hypoglycemia in type 2 DM patients of <2 to 3% per year as shown by UKPDS is relatively very low (35,61). Indeed, the UKPDS is the largest long-term treatment study using insulin for type 2 diabetes. Hypoglycemic episodes were monitored as a measure of outcome during 10 years of treatment. The groups treated with insulin from the start showed more hypoglycemia, as might be expected, with little difference between the nonobese and the obese groups but most of the hypoglycemia was mild in severity. Severe hypoglycemic events occurred only in 2% to 3% of subjects in this group each year, on average. This rate is certainly not trivial, but it is far less than the rate seen with intensive insulin treatment of type 1 diabetes in the diabetes control and complications trial (DCCT) (62). It is conceivable that in patients with insulin resistance, exogenous insulin and the subsequent fall in glucose concentration into the normal range, leads to a more physiologic endogenous insulin release from the β-cells which may contribute to decreased hypoglycemia (63). However, most interventional insulin studies have failed to achieve target A_{1c} levels and it is possible that hypoglycemia would have become more common if the patients had completely attained near-normoglycemia.

Limitations of Insulin Preparations

Over the years, multiple insulin preparations have been developed with recombinant DNA technology resulting in major improvements in purity but still with significant limitations in pharmacokinetics and pharmacodynamics, after subcutaneous injections (64,65). A comparison of the kinetics of available insulins is listed in Table 2

The time course of action of any insulin may vary between individuals, or at different times in the same individual. Consequently, table data should be considered only as general guidelines. NPH=Neutral Protamine Hagedorn.

Regular human insulin has a slow onset of action with delayed peak concentrations requiring patients to administer their injection 20 to 40 min prior to the meal in an attempt to improve the mismatch with the postprandial hyperglycemic peaks (66). This is inconvenient, is infrequently achieved, and poses the risk of premeal hypoglycemia if the meal is inadvertently delayed. Furthermore, the duration of action of regular insulin is much longer than the normal endogenous insulin peak following meals, typically at least 6 h and up to 12 h when large doses are injected. This persistence of high insulin levels leads to risk of hypoglycemia, which is often countered by between-meal snacks that foster weight gain in type 2 diabetes patients.

The three short-acting insulin analogs, insulin lispro, insulin aspart and insulin glulisine have absorption profiles that more closely match normal mealtime patterns (67–73). Small alterations in their amino acid structure relative to human insulin reduce their tendency to aggregate into dimers or hexamers, thus speeding their absorption after subcutaneous injection. Lispro, aspart and gluclisine have very desirable action profiles at mealtime because they have a rapid onset of action ranging from 5 to 15 min; the peak of action occurs 1 h after injection, and the insulin effect practically vanishes 4 to 5 h after administration. Their quick onset of action matches normal mealtime peaks of plasma insulin better than doe's human regular insulin.

TABLE 2   Pharmacokinetics of Human Insulin and Analogs

	Onset of action(h)	Peak (h)	Duration of action (h)
Human Insulins			
Regular	0.5–1	2–4	6–10
NPH	1–3	5–7	10–20
Lente®	1–3	4–8	10–20
Inhaled insulin	10–20 min	1–2	6
Ultralente®	2–4	Unpredictable	16–20
Insulin Analogs			
Lispro (Humalog®)	5–15 min	1-2	4–6
Aspart (Novolog®)	5–15 min	1-2	4–6
Glulisine (Apidra®)	5–15 min	1-2	4–6
Glargine (Lantus®)	1–2	Minimal peak	up to 24
Detemir (Levemir®)	1–2	Minimal peak	up to 24
Premixed Insulin			
Human 70/30	0.5–1	2–4 & 5–7	10–20
Premixed Insulin Analogs			
Lispro 75/25	5–15 min	2–4 & 5–7	10–20
Lispro 50/50	5–15 min	2–4 & 5–7	10–20
Aspart 70/30	5–15 min	2–4 & 5–7	10–20

Clinical studies have shown that these properties lead to less prominent peaks of glucose after meals and less late postprandial hypoglycemia (74–91). However, rapid waning of the effects of mealtime analogue insulin leads to greater dependency on adequate basal insulin levels between meals and overnight.

The intermediate-acting insulins, NPH and lente, have gradual onset and the peak effects is usually between 4 and 8 h, with a total duration of 10 to 16 h. Human ultralente insulin is somewhat longer acting, but still usually falls short of a 24-h effect. NPH and lente, have pronounced peaks of action and ultralente is thought to have substantial day-to-day variation with erratic peaks. These limitations cause variations of glucose levels and unpredictable hypoglycemia which are the leading factors limiting glycemic control at the present time. Indeed the lack of reproducibility in glucose-lowering effects of conventional basal insulin preparations, including NPH and ultralente, has been a major limitation for most insulin regimens.

There has been a growing need for reliable long-acting basal insulin that would mimic normal pancreatic basal insulin secretion to control hepatic glucose production in the postabsorptive state. Clinical use of the rapid acting insulin analogues (lispro, aspart or glulisine) has directed attention to the properties of extended-release human insulins that have been used to provide basal insulin replacement. Human NPH, lente, and ultralente insulin all have mean durations of action of less than 24 h, precluding them from providing adequate basal insulin replacement for many patients. All three, but especially NPH and lente, have pronounced peaks of action. Ultralente is thought to have substantial day-to-day variation of action. These limitations cause variations of glucose levels and unpredictable hypoglycemia, which are the leading factors limiting glycemic control at the present time. Indeed the lack of reproducibility in glucose-lowering effects of conventional basal insulin preparations, including NPH and ultralente, has been a major limitation for most insulin regimens.

The first insulin analogue with a prolonged duration of action that approaches 24 h, thus possibly dosed once daily, that became available for clinical use is insulin glargine (65). Insulin glargine results from two modifications of human insulin: a substitution of glycine at position A21 and the addition of two positive charges (two arginine molecules) at the C terminal of the B chain. Changes in amino acid content shift the isoelectric point, reducing the aqueous solubility of insulin glargine at physiologic pH and stabilizing the hexamer, delaying its dissociation into monomers. It is released gradually from the injection site and because of the delay in absorption its action is prolonged, allowing a relatively constant basal insulin supply. However, because insulin glargine is formulated as a clear acidic solution, it cannot be mixed with insulin formulated at a neutral pH, such as regular insulin. Studies have demonstrated no variation in absorption rates at various injection sites (arm, leg, abdomen) (92).

Glucose-insulin clamp studies have compared the actions of insulin glargine with those of NPH and ultralente (93–96). These studies have found that insulin glargine, compared with the other insulins provides an essentially flat profile with a longer duration for about 15 to 24 h (Fig. 4). The duration of action of insulin glargine is a function of the dose delivered. When used as a basal insulin in treating type 1 diabetes, because of the low doses required, insulin glargine may not have a long enough duration of action and thus may need to be given in a twice daily regimen (97–99). Clinical trials have shown improvements in glycemic control similar to NPH, with a slightly lower frequency of nocturnal hypoglycemia (100–106). Use of the flat or peakless insulin glargine profile now allows for a more vigorous titration regimen and more patients can reach target A_{1c} levels with considerable less risk of nocturnal hypoglycemia (5).

Insulin Detemir is another long acting analogue that is available for clinical use (65). The principle for the longer duration of acting is based on covalent acylation of the epsilon amino group of Lys B29. This modification promotes reversible binding of insulin to albumin thereby delaying its resorption from subcutaneous tissue and also, possibly because of size, reducing the rate of transendothelial transport (107). The myristoyl fatty acid side chain at the C terminus of the B-chain does not alter aggregation properties of the molecule. NN304 has a slower disappearance rate from subcutaneous tissue and a much flatter time-action profile than NPH (108). The time action profile is very similar to that found with insulin glargine. When used as basal insulin in treating type 1 diabetes, because of the low doses required, insulin detemir may need to be given in a twice daily regimen. However, in the treatment of type 2 diabetes, the doses of basal insulin are typically high enough that both glargine and detemir can usually be dosed once daily.

In a 6-week crossover study, 59 patients with type 1 diabetes who were given NPH once daily before bedtime plus pre-meal soluble human insuli, titrated to achieve equivalent glycemic control, required a two-fold to three-fold higher dose than those given NPH in the same way (109). However, while some studies observe a need for higher doses of "basal" insulin with the use of insulin detemir, it has not been a consistent finding (110–112). In a long-term safety study, where insulin detemir or NPH were used as part of basal-bolus therapy for 252 patients with type 1 diabetes, they found similar improvement in A_{1c}s with comparable rates of hypoglycemia but no weight gain in the group that received detemir (113).

Comparison of the use of twice daily insulin detemir with once daily glargine in 320 subjects with Type 1 diabetes showed that after 26 weeks, the two groups had similar glycemic control with similar weight gain (Fig. 5). The overall risk of hypoglycemia was comparable, whereas the risks of both severe and nocturnal hypoglycemia were significantly lower with insulin detemir (114). Studies in subjects with type 2 diabetes have shown similar decreases in A_{1c} with the addition of insulin detemir or NPH insulin however, with insulin detemir more people achieved an $A_{1c} \leq 7.0\%$, the risk for all hypoglycemia was lower and mean weight gain was lower (110).

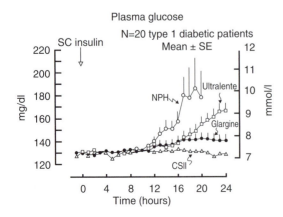

FIGURE 4 Kinetics of insulin glargine. Plasma glucose concentration after subcutaneous injection of glargine, NPH, and ultralente and after continuous subcutaneous infusion of lispro. *Source*: From Ref. 93.

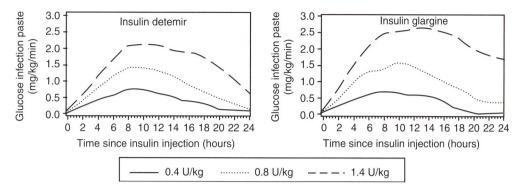

FIGURE 5 Mean GIR-profiles (smoothed with a local regression technique) for 0.4, 0.8, and 1.4 U/kg insulin detemir and insulin glargine.

Insulin detemir has primarily been studied in comparison with NPH insulin thus most of the studies have looked at twice daily dosing. At doses exceeding 0.4 units kg^{-1} day^{-1}, the duration of action approaches 24 h and can then be used as a once daily basal insulin (115). These data show that the addition of either basal insulin can facilitate attaining an A_{1c} below 7%. However, the challenge now is to show that the level of glycemia can be maintained over time. Likely prandial insulin will need to be added to the regimen to prevent the A_{1c} from rising. Another important question is whether the addition of basal insulin to oral agents is sufficient to safely attain a normal A_{1c} (i.e. below 6% in most assays) or whether prandial insulin will also need to be added to the regimen. Studies are now needed to answer these questions.

The Mechanical Barrier

Despite the improvements in insulin kinetics with the new insulin analogues, the need to mix and inject insulin remains a barrier to patients' acceptance and compliance. The introductions of smaller syringes which only draw up 30 or 50 units have improved the accuracy of delivery of low doses of insulin. The pen delivery devices have made it easier for patients to carry their insulin with them and give injections in settings other than their homes (116,117). The syringes and pens now have the option of small needles (i.e. 30–31 gauge) of varying lengths which can make the shots less painful. The introduction of inhaled insulin has also provided an easy way to take prandial insulin. Continuous subcutaneous delivery of insulin using an infusion pump is another method of conveniently providing insulin and having it easily available for all meals.

Inhaled insulin has the potential to dramatically change the way we approach insulin therapy. The barrier of doing injections has been removed. However, the "stigma" of taking insulin remains. The advantage of inhaled insulin is that the insulin is delivered in a non-invasive fashion removing the ultimate barrier of insulin injections. Pharmacokinetic studies have shown rapid peaks of action for inhaled insulin similar to lispro insulin but with slightly longer duration (118,119). Time–action profiles of inhaled insulin compared to subcutaneous regular and lispro insulin were studied using a euglycemic glucose clamp (120). After 120 min, subjects received 6 mg of inhaled insulin, 18 U of subcutaneous regular insulin or 18 U of subcutaneous insulin lispro. Inhaled insulin showed a faster onset of action than subcutaneous regular insulin and even insulin lispro with early $t_{50\%}$ of 32, 48 and 40 min, respectively. The duration of action of inhaled insulin was intermediate between that of lispro and regular insulin (382, 309 and 413 min, respectively). The maximal metabolic action based on glucose infusion rates was comparable for the three groups.

The proof of concept for inhaled insulin, a dry powder aerosol delivery system of human insulin, was initially examined in an early phase II study on 69 patients with type 2 diabetes who were randomized to a 3-month treatment period of either continued oral agents alone (sulfonylurea and/or metformin) or in combination with 1 or 2 puffs of inhaled insulin before meals (121). The inhaled insulin doses were titrated based on glucose testing four times daily. Patients continuing on oral agents alone showed little change in HbA_{1c} at 12 weeks (–0.13%), while those receiving the inhaled insulin in addition to the oral agents exhibited a marked improvement in HbA_{1c} (–2.28%). The decreases in A_{1c} when inhaled insulin is added to oral glucose lowering agents are a function of the baseline A_{1c} such that those with the highest A_{1cs} tend to have the greatest drop in A_{1c} (122,123).

The efficacy of adding preprandial insulin as inhaled pulmonary delivery of dry powder insulin to oral therapy has also been demonstrated in patients with type 2 diabetes who did not maintain an $A_{1c} < 8\%$ on combination oral therapy (secretagogue plus metformin or a glitazone). They were randomized just 3 months of treatment with 136 either inhaled insulin alone, continuing on the oral agents or adding the inhaled insulin to the current doses of oral agents. The group receiving combination therapy oral agents plus inhaled insulin showed the largest decrease in A_{1c} of 1.9% with a decrease of 1.4% with inhaled insulin alone and 0.2% with continuing oral agents. Weight gain and hypoglycemia were comparable in the groups receiving insulin with only one episode of severe hypoglycemia overall. This study shows that adding prandial inhaled insulin results in a can facilitate the lowering of the A_{1c}.

The long-term safety and efficacy of inhaled human insulin has been demonstrated in adult patients with type 1 diabetes. At the end of two years the improvement in glycemic control was sustained with less weight gain and a lower incidence of severe hypoglycemic events in the inhaled insulin group than in the subcutaneous insulin. An important safety evaluation was to monitor the annual rate of decline in pulmonary function (forced expiratory volume in 1 s [FEV1] and carbon monoxide diffusing capacity [DL(CO)]). The changes in lung function that occurred with the inhaled insulin were small, developed within the first three months and did not progress over the 2 years of therapy (58).

As the delivery of insulin has become less invasive, consideration of initiation of insulin therapy must occur earlier than has traditionally been the usual practice.

INSULIN REPLACEMENT STRATEGIES: THE BASAL/BOLUS CONCEPT

Insulin has been used therapeutically for more than 75 years and remains the most powerful diabetes agent with almost unlimited potential to lower plasma glucose levels. Ideally, insulin replacement therapy should be modeled with insulin preparations that can reproduce the physiologic patterns of insulin secretion in response to the 24-h post absorptive and postprandial glucose profiles (Table 3). The basal/bolus insulin concept is a physiologically sound regimen that attempts to mimic the normal insulin patterns to control glucose levels (66). The role of basal insulin is to suppress hepatic glucose production so that the glucose levels remain constantly regulated overnight and also during prolonged periods between meals (124). Basal insulin meets about 50 to 70% of the patient's daily need for insulin and may be sufficient when considerable endogenous insulin remains. Bolus insulin (10–20% of the total daily insulin requirement given at each meal) limits hyperglycemia after meals. Conceptually, each component of insulin replacement therapy should come from a different type of insulin with a specific profile to fit the patient's needs.

TABLE 3 Rationale for Insulin Replacement Therapy. Applying the Basal/Bolus Insulin Concept

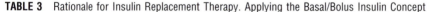

Basal insulin
Nearly constant day-long insulin level
Suppress hepatic glucose production between meals and overnight
Cover 50–70% of daily needs

Bolus insulin (mealtime)
Immediate rise and sharp peak at 1 hour
Limit postmeal hyperglycemia
Cover 10% to 20% of total daily insulin requirement at each meal

Note: Ideally, each component should come from a different insulin, with a specific profile.

The basal/bolus insulin concept has long been used in the management of patients with Type 1 diabetes but can also apply to Type 2 diabetes. Since both fasting and postprandial glucose levels are abnormal in type 2 diabetes and the underlying insulin deficiency typically progresses, most patients will need both basal and mealtime insulin replacement if glycemic targets are not achieved or can not be maintained with basal insulin alone.

Starting Insulin Therapy with Basal Insulin

Rationale for Early Combination Oral Agents Plus Insulin

It has been established that most patients with type 2 diabetes will eventually require insulin – but traditionally is used as a "last resort after maximal combination therapy has failed – 10 to 15 years after disease onset. However, our improved understanding of the natural history of type 2 diabetes suggests that insulin therapy should be started sooner rather than later and that insulin should be viewed as an essential therapeutic tool for achieving disease management goals, at an earlier stage in the natural progression of the disease, rather than a sign of failure on the part of the physician or patient. The oral agents can be divided into two general categories based on their primary mechanism of action: augmenting the supply of insulin by increasing the secretion of insulin into the portal circulation, decreasing hepatic gluconeogenesis and/or enhancing the effectiveness of insulin (3). Injected insulin, in turn, increases insulin in the systemic circulation. Because the mechanisms of action for these classes of oral agents differ, they may have complementary or additive effects and can help meet the individualized needs of patients. Furthermore, where their mechanism of action complements that of insulin, they should be continued when insulin is initiated.

The sulfonylureas and the glitinides are oral agents that augment the supply of portal insulin (125–128). They increase hepatic levels of endogenous insulin and enhance meal-mediated insulin release. Incretin mimetics also act as secretagogues but only augment glucose stimulated insulin release (129). They do have other actions that are not as well characterized, which include augmenting the physiologic suppression of glucagons after meals. Metformin and the thiazolidinediones are oral agents that enhance the effectiveness of insulin. Metformin improves insulin sensitivity reduces hepatic glucose production and appears to have a modest effect on improving insulin sensitivity (47,130–133). The thiazolidinediones improve insulin action in peripheral tissues, enhance glucose uptake and have a modest effect on decreasing hepatic glucose production (134–138). The α-glucosidase inhibitors have a different mechanism of action, decreasing postprandial glucose absorption by inhibiting digestion of complex carbohydrates and disaccharides, thereby retarding gastrointestinal glucose absorption (139–141). The studies utilizing insulin therapy in patients with type 2 diabetes have been based on either the addition of insulin to the oral therapy or switching the oral agent to insulin. Unfortunately these studies usually enroll subjects that are "failing" their oral agent which is very late in the disease process.

The fundamental issue is which regimen will be the most cost effective in achieving the individual target HbA_{1c} of <6% with an amount of hypoglycemia and side effects that will be acceptable to patients and physicians. The question still remains as to how early should insulin therapy be started in type 2 diabetes? Ongoing studies are asking whether starting with early insulin replacement strategies to achieve target glycemic control will prevent progression of the disease process and reduce the development of macrovascular complications.

Practical Advantages of Early Combination of Oral Agents Plus Insulin

Patients who are not at target HbA_{1c} (<6%) or no longer respond adequately to oral agents will benefit from combination therapy that consists of maintaining the use of oral antidiabetic agents together with supplemental insulin therapy (Table 4). Simple strategies of starting with a very low dose and giving the patient an algorithm to increase the insulin based on home glucose monitoring have made it easy to start insulin. Different strategies have been developed starting with once day basal or once daily premixed insulin with similar efficacy. Ultimately, most people will require some from of basal/bolus regimen (whether 2–4 shots daily) to allow physiologic insulin replacement therapy.

TABLE 4   Practical Guidelines: Combination Therapy Regimens

Average patient

Early combination of insulin secretagogue and insulin sensitizers

Most simple and cost-effective with longest experience
Consider starting with a combination of two oral agents with low doses once or twice daily
    Metformin + DPP-4 or SU or Meglitinide
    Metformin + TZD
    Metformin, TZD or SU + AGI
    TZD + DPP-4
Titrate to full-doses of each component of the combination therapy

For marked insulin resistance
Start with a combination of metformin + thiazolidinedione

If target HbA$_{1c}$ < 7% not achieved
    Try triple therapy (ie secretagogue + metformin + thiazolidinedione)
    Add an incretin mimetic to triple oral therapy
    Add basal insulin or low dose premixed insulin while continuing oral therapy

Abbreviation: HbA$_{1c}$, hemoglobin A$_{1c}$.

Starting insulin with a single daily injection has become widely accepted in recent years as practitioners have recognized the need to start insulin earlier than has traditionally been practiced. The advantages of adding once daily basal insulin to prior treatment with oral agents include the following:

(1)   only one insulin injection may be required each day, with no need for mixing different types of insulin
(2)   titration can be accomplished in a slow, safe, simple fashion
(3)   the use of insulin pens can enhance patient acceptance of the treatment
(4)   combination therapy eventually requires a lower total dose of insulin.

The result is effective improvement in glycemic control while causing only limited weight gain. Adding insulin in the evening is a simple and effective strategy that can be regarded as "bridge therapy." It allows patients to overcome their initial resistance to start using insulin, facilitating long-term acceptance and compliance.

Sulfonylurea Plus Once-Daily Insulin
One of the early studies that combined an oral agent with insulin was reported by the Oxford groups in 1987 (142). Fifteen asymptomatic, sulfonylurea-treated type 2 diabetic patients were treated in a randomized crossover study of consecutive 8-week periods. The overnight mean basal plasma glucose level on sulfonylurea therapy was reduced to normal by adding ultralente insulin. Compared to ultralente insulin therapy alone, combining sulfonylurea with ultralente insulin therapy did not show a significant difference in glucose control, but it did significantly lower the required insulin dose for restoring fasting normoglycemia. The authors concluded that in type 2 diabetic patients who continue to have fasting hyperglycemia on maximal sulfonylurea therapy, the addition of a basal insulin supplement can easily result in normoglycemia.

This strategy was then incorporated into the UKPDS in the last eight centers to enter the trial (61). The investigators had recognized that maximal dose sulfonylurea therapy was not maintaining HgbA$_{1c}$ below 7% so they added a protocol that differed from the main study in those eight centers whereby insulin therapy (once daily ultralente insulin) was offered immediately to patients allocated to sulfonylurea therapy if maximal doses did not maintain FPG levels ≤108 mg/dL (Fig. 6). The patients did have the option to refuse. The sulfonylurea therapy was continued unchanged with the starting dose of ultralente based on body weight and administered once daily before the evening meal then increased weekly or biweekly as necessary to maintain FPG ≤108 mg/dL. Human soluble insulin was added before meals if

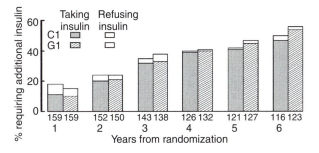

FIGURE 6 Proportions of patients requiring early addition of insulin. Proportions of patients (%) allocated to sulfonylurea requiring early addition of insulin each year because FPG increased to ≥108 mg/dL (6.0 mmol/L) despite maximal sulfonylurea doses. Those requiring but refusing additional insulin are indicated separately. The number below each column is the number of patients per year. There were no significant differences between the chlorpropamide and glyburide groups at any time point. *Source*: From Ref. 61.

preprandial home blood glucose levels remained ≥126 mg/dL. Median A_{1c} over 6 years was significantly lower for those allocated to sulfonylurea + insulin (SI) (6.6% [6.0–7.6]) than insulin alone (7.1[6.2–8.0], $p = 0.0066$). The proportion of patients with $A_{1c} < 7\%$ at 6 years was greater in patients taking SI compared with those taking insulin alone (47 vs. 35%, $p = 0.011$) (Fig. 7). The Glucose Study 2 component of the UKPDS shows that glycemic control can be significantly improved with almost 50% of patients maintaining A_{1c} target of <7% using insulin plus sulfonylurea therapy and without promoting substantial increases in hypoglycemia or weight gain despite the limitations of ultralente insulin.

Combining a sulfonylurea with bedtime intermediate or long acting insulin is an effective strategy to improve glucose control and to overcome secondary sulfonylurea failure. The rationale of combination therapy with sulfonylureas and insulin is based on the assumption that, if bedtime insulin (BI) lowers the fasting glucose concentration to normal, then daytime sulfonylureas (DS) will have a more effective meal-mediated insulin release controlling postprandial hyperglycemia throughout the day (143). In addition, the fasting blood glucose concentration is highly correlated with the degree of hepatic glucose production during the early morning hours (144).

Shank et al., studied 30 subjects with type 2 diabetes in whom sulfonylurea therapy had failed by switching them to the various combinations of BI/DS therapy in a double-blind fashion (145). To confirm sulfonylurea failure, subjects were switched to glipizide for (phase I) and then randomly assigned BI/DS, BI alone, and DS alone. During phase II the BI dose was fixed (20 U/1.732 m^3, low dose) then during phase III the BI dose was titrated up to achieve good control or until further dose increases were prevented by hypoglycemic symptoms. During phase IV, which lasted for 6 months, 25 of the original 30 subjects received open-labeled, high-dose BI/DS. Unlike low-dose BI alone or DS alone, low-dose BI/DS (phase II) markedly reduced FPG, mean 24-h glucose, HbA_{1c} from 8.9% ± 0.7% to 7.6% ± 0.3%, and basal hepatic glucose production. High-dose BI/DS (phase III) further reduced the HbA_{1c} to

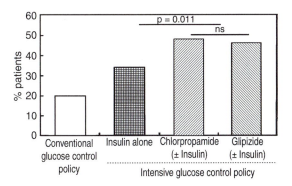

FIGURE 7 Proportions (%) of patients achieving $HbA_{1c} \geq 7\%$ at 6 years. *Source*: From Ref. 61.

7.1%±0.3%. Subjects who received the same dose of insulin without sulfonylurea had no improvement in glycemic control or weight gain. The study showed that combined BI/DS can achieve good long-term glycemic control for up to 1 year.

Riddle et al., added further proof of concept to the BI/DS regimen with a modified strategy in which 145 patients were randomized to receive either glimepiride or placebo in combination with insulin (70/30 at supper) (Fig. 7) (146). Reduction in mean HbA_{1c} values was comparable in the two treatment groups after 24 weeks (9.7–7.6%, glimepiride plus insulin; 9.9–7.9%, placebo plus insulin). The addition of glimepiride produced a much more rapid decrease in FPG levels compared with placebo and demonstrated a significant insulin-sparing effect, with a 38% reduction of insulin requirements allowing for more patients to use only one injection of insulin 70/30 at supper (Fig. 8).

Starting Insulin Therapy with Bolus Insulin

For patients starting insulin therapy, the need for multiple premeal injections makes mealtime insulin supplementation strategy considerably more complex and less attractive than the once-daily evening dose of basal insulin. While the addition of prandial insulin is scientifically very appealing for the management of diabetes, the successful implementation of the addition of prandial insulin, in a pilot study of patients who were already treated with metformin and a glitizone, demonstrated that adding prandial insulin alone can significantly improve glucose control (147). While patients are slow to accept premeal insulin injections, it is possible they will be more open to the addition of premeal inhaled insulin. Perhaps with the availability of inhaled insulin, non injectable premeal insulin replacement may turn into first-line intervention followed by basal insulin supplementation as required. Although this would require a paradigm shift in the management of type 2 diabetes, the fact that we are not reaching A_{1c} goals suggests that we need to change the ways we have traditionally managed hyperglycemia.

Starting Therapy with Basal/Bolus

Traditionally, twice-daily mixtures of NPH and regular insulin have been widely used for type 2 diabetes for many years. However, most patients using this "split-mixed" regimen rarely achieve reasonably good glycemic control by present standards and often experience late morning or nocturnal hypoglycemia because of excessive levels of insulin at these times as well as intermittent hyperglycemia due to insufficient insulin replacement.

Intensive insulin strategies using the twice daily split-mixed regimen were largely unsuccessful until a study by Henry et al. who studied a group of 14 patients with type 2 diabetes to determine whether tight glycemic control can be obtained using conventional insulin therapy in an outpatient setting by aggressively titrating insulin therapy (25). Patients received conventional subcutaneous NPH and regular insulin before breakfast and supper for 6 months, with dose adjustments based on an algorithm built on frequent blood glucose measurements (4–6 times a day). The total dose of required exogenous insulin was 86±13 U at 1 month and 100±24 U at 6 months. One month after initiating intensive insulin therapy,

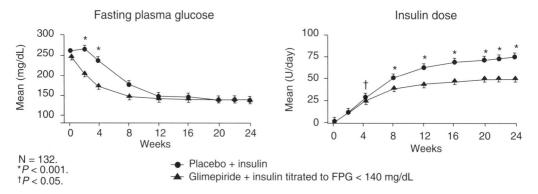

N = 132.
*P < 0.001.
†P < 0.05.

—●— Placebo + insulin
—▲— Glimepiride + insulin titrated to FPG < 140 mg/dL

FIGURE 8   Fasting plasma glucose and insulin dose after addition of glimepiride to insulin. *Source*: From Ref. 146.

day-long glycemia had improved to within normal range and remained at this level through 6 month of therapy. The A_{1c}, which was 7.7%±0.3% at baseline, decreased to 5.1%±0.2% at 6 months. This study underscores the importance of early insulin therapy, when the baseline A_{1c} is only mildly elevated just above 7%, and insulin is aggressively titrated.

However, these results are hardly ever achieved when the split-mixed regimen, which fails to mimic the basal/bolus needs, is used in general practice and insufficient insulin is administered. Often, premixed 70/30 insulin is used but the insulin profiles do not come close to matching the normal endogenous secretory pattern to control fasting and postprandial hyperglycemia. In addition, the rigid premixed preparations have the significant limitation of having no flexibility for insulin adjustments according to the patient's blood glucose profile.

Multiple daily doses of short acting insulin can be added when patients do not attain adequate control. Lindstrom and colleagues showed that this strategy may be effective in normalizing HbA_{1c} but was best accomplished with four injection of regular per day (137). They performed a randomized crossover study of 8 weeks of oral hypoglycemic agents followed by 8 weeks of 2- or 4-dose insulin regimens. Mean blood glucose and free-insulin profiles show that patients taking the oral agents had higher blood glucose and lower postprandial insulin concentrations than those receiving insulin. When patients received the daily 4-dose regimen of preprandial regular insulin and intermediate-acting NPH insulin at 10:00 PM, glycemic control improved. The mean HbA_{1c} was 8.8% during treatment with oral therapy compared with 5.6% on the intensive 4-dose insulin regimen.

Perhaps the best evidence that near-normoglycemia is beneficial and feasible with multiple daily insulin injections in type 2 diabetes is the Kumamoto Study. The 8 year analysis of the Kumamoto Study showed a sustained lowering of A_{1c}s and of microvascular complications in the 99 patients treated with either conventional (once or twice daily intermediate insulin) or multiple injection therapy (short and intermediate-acting insulin with a goal of FBG< 140 mg/dL, 2-h postprandial < 200 mg/dL, an A_{1c} < 7% and a mean amplitude of glycemic excursion < 100 mg/dL).138 They found no worsening of retinopathy or nephropathy in patients whose A_{1c}, FBG and 2-h postprandial blood glucose concentration were below 6.5%, 110 mg/dL, and 180 mg/dL, respectively. The longest study includes 15 patients that have been followed for 110 months while taking insulin after sulfonylurea failure (139). While there was little difference in insulin dosage between the first weeks of insulin treatment and the 27-month examination, the dosage was increased at the 110-month examination from 51.3±5.2 to 79.5±10.8 U. The glycemic control was improved with reduction of HbA_{1c} from 8.9±0.2% during treatment with oral hypoglycemic agents to 7.3±0.3% ($p < 0.001$ vs. baseline) at the 110-month examination. Body weight increased rapidly during the first 4–5 months, but after 12 months there was no significant change.

Adding Oral Agents to Insulin Therapy

Most of the studies reported on the combination insulin plus oral sensitizers have been based on the addition of an oral agent such as metformin or a glitazone to patients already treated with conventional insulin therapy, which is fundamentally a different issue than starting and intensifying insulin replacement strategies to achieve target glycemic control as was discussed extensively above. Nevertheless, the option of adding an insulin sensitizer or even a secretagogue to patients who are already on insulin therapy should be considered if the A_{1c} target is not achieved despite aggressive insulin replacement therapy.

Metformin Plus Insulin

There are several studies that have used metformin as "add-on" therapy to insulin with significant improvements in HbA_{1c}. The addition of metformin to pre-existing insulin therapy was first shown to have efficacy beyond that of continuing insulin alone in a study by Giugliano et al in 1993 (148). Subsequently, several studies have addressed this strategy with decreases in HbA_{1c} between 1 to 2.5% (149–151).

The largest A_{1c} reduction was obtained with maximized intensive insulin therapy in 43 patients with type 2 DM who were randomize to added placebo or metformin (149) (Fig. 9). The goal of this study was to maximally decrease HbA_{1c} with intensive insulin adjustments

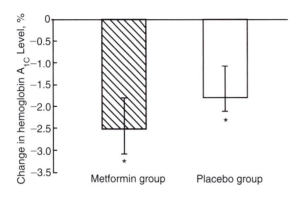

FIGURE 9 Metformin plus insulin. The change in Hemoglobin A_{1c} from baseline to 24 weeks after the addition of metformin to insulin in patients with poorly controlled type 2 diabetes. *Source*: From Ref. 149.

instead of the traditional goal of reducing insulin doses to demonstrate the sensitizer effect. Hemoglobin A_{1c} levels decreased by 2.5% in the metformin group, a significantly greater change than the decrease of 1.6% in the placebo group. Average final HbA_{1c} levels were 6.5% in the metformin group and 7.6% in the placebo group. For patients who received placebo, the insulin dose increased 22.8 units which are 29% more than did the dose for patients who received metformin whose insulin dose decreased slightly. The strategy of adding metformin to insulin can result in significant improvements in HbA_{1c}, especially when insulin dose is not decreased.

Thiazolidinedione Plus Insulin
The clinical availability of the thiazolidinediones introduced the possibility of improvements of insulin sensitivity in muscle, liver and adipose tissue potentiating the effects and reducing the doses of exogenous insulin. The first study to demonstrate the efficacy of this combination was utilizing troglitazone (152) which is no longer available in the United States due to idiosyncratic hepatotoxicity. Subsequently, the addition of either pioglitazone or rosiglitazone to insulin in patients with poorly controlled type 2 diabetes ($A_{1c} \geq 9\%$) showed a dose related decrease in A_{1c} s of 1.2 to 1.3% despite mild reductions of insulin dosages (153,154). The addition of pioglitazone (15 or 30 mg daily) to pre-existing conventional insulin therapy for 16 weeks showed statistically significant decreases in A_{1c} in 566 patients who were poorly controlled on conventional insulin alone (154). Low dose pioglitazone (15 mg) decreased A_{1c} from 9.75% to 8.76% while medium dose (30 mg) decreased A_{1cs} from 9.84% to 8.58% while the insulin doses remain constant. Similarly, the addition of rosiglitazone (4 or 8 mg daily) to pre-existing insulin therapy for 26 weeks showed statistically significant decreases in A_{1c} in 209 patients who were poorly controlled (146). Medium dose rosiglitazone (4 mg) decreased A_{1c} from 9.1 ± 1.3 to $8.5 \pm 1.4\%$ while high dose (8 mg) decreased A_{1cs} from 9.0 ± 1.3 to $7.9 \pm 1.4\%$. Body weight increased by 2.3 to 3.7 kg during 16 weeks treatment with pioglitazone or 4.0 to 5.3 kg during the 26 weeks of treatments with rosiglitazone. The incidence of edema was comparable 15.3% with pioglitazone and 14.7% with rosiglitazone. Safety issues remain a major concern especially fluid retention and the potential risk of developing or worsening congestive heart failure especially in high risk patients with coronary disease with or without preexisting CHF. However, the warning for its use in patients stresses extreme caution in patients with edema, coronary disease and mild forms of CHF (not recommended in NYHA Class III and IV but in our opinion better not to use it in any form of CHF at all). Further studies are ongoing to determine the long term safety effects of the glitazones on fluid retention and especially frequency and severity of CHF. When initiating these agents in any patients it is prudent to carefully evaluate their cardiovascular status and start at a very low dose and increase the dose very slowly (i.e. at 3 to 6 month intervals).

Combination Oral Agents Plus Once-Daily Insulin

The FINFAT study, conducted in four centers in Finland, randomly assigned 96 patients with type 2 diabetes who were inadequately controlled with sulfonylurea therapy alone to receive four different regimens in addition to bedtime NPH insulin: glyburide, metformin, glyburide + metformin, or a second injection of NPH insulin in the morning (155). The patients were instructed to self-adjust the evening insulin dose if their FPG level was elevated. After 12 months of therapy, this study suggested that self-adjustment of the insulin dose and the addition of metformin produced slightly better overall glucose control, less weight gain, and the lowest frequency of hypoglycemic episodes. However, the group receiving metformin alone in addition to the insulin had the highest dropout rate, with 21% of patients not completing the trial. The investigators of this study attributed the improved glycemic control seen across treatment groups to successful patient education regarding adjustment of insulin doses. Although it was expected that patients receiving only one oral drug in addition to bedtime insulin would require greater increases in the insulin doses than those receiving both oral drugs, this was not the case. Patients who received metformin had greater insulin requirements than those who received the sulfonylurea, who had a higher frequency of symptomatic, mild hypoglycemic episodes (Fig. 10).

A current and increasingly used strategy would be to add to the oral agents the peakless long acting analogue, either insulin glargine or insulin detemir, at bedtime. The Treat to Target Study, is a 24-week U.S. multicenter, randomised, parallel-group comparing basal replacement therapy with bedtime insulin glargine (Lantus®) or NPH added to oral combination therapy (70% of patients were on sulfonylurea + metformin and the rest on different combinations of two agents such as sulfonylurea + glitazone or metformin + glitazone with only 10% on monotherapy) in 756 insulin-naive patients. This study confirmed the efficacy of these insulin when administered in a forced titration manner to achieve fasting plasma glucose (FPG) levels of <100 mg/dL and reach HbA$_{1c}$ levels of <7% (100,101). This was the first study to demonstrate that starting insulin therapy with a low dose of 10 units at bedtime followed by a very simple algorithm based on FPGs was successful in achieving remarkable glycemic improvements in the overall study population with rare incidence of severe hypoglycemia, no patterns of serious adverse events, and only a modest increase in body weight. HbA$_{1c}$ values decreased from 8.6% at baseline to 6.9% by the end of the study, with highly significant differences in FPG between baseline and endpoint. Significantly more patients treated with insulin glargine attained an A$_{1c}$ <7% without documented hypoglycemia. Most notably 58% of the patients in both groups achieved the target A$_{1c}$ of <7 % but patients on the insulin glargine group had a 44 to 48% risk reduction in confirmed nocturnal hypoglycemia which is an advantage for the basal insulin, insulin glargine, especially as this strategy has the potential to be applied to large populations of patients with type 2 diabetes managed by general physicians.

Combination Oral Agents Plus Once, Twice or Thrice Daily Premixed Insulin

The strategy of starting insulin therapy with a low dose of 10 to 12 units daily, whether once or twice daily or at bedtime, followed by a very simple titration algorithm based on FPGs has now

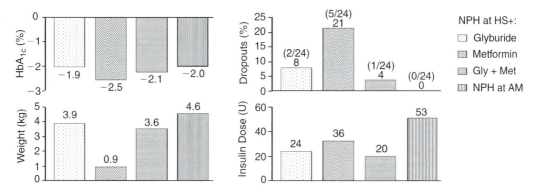

FIGURE 10 Starting with Bedtime Insulin: FINFAT Study. Changes in HgbA$_{1c}$, insulin dose and weight and percent dropout of the patients with type 2 diabetes who were inadequately controlled with sulfonylurea therapy that received four different regimens in addition to bedtime NPH insulin: glyburide, metformin, glyburide + metformin, or a second injection of NPH insulin in the morning. *Source*: From Ref. 155.

been tested in several studies employing different strategies using basal or premixed insulin analogs. The first study, described above, was the Treat-to-Target Study which compared the addition at bedtime of NPH versus Glargine (5). Subsequently, the INITIATE Trial showed that starting 5 to 6 units twice daily of premixed biphasic insulin aspart 70/30 (BIAsp 70/30) was superior to using 10 to 12 units of insulin glargine at bedtime when patients self-titrated the dose to target blood glucose (80–110 mg/dL) by algorithm-directed titration (6). The patient controlled strategy was taken one step further in the 1-2-3 Study which started with a low dose of BIAsp 70/30 prior to the evening meal and every the dose titrated 3 to 4 days to achieve fasting blood glucose of 80 to 110 mg/dL (7). If the A_{1c} was not $\leq 6.5\%$ at 16 weeks then the insulin was increased to twice daily. If the A_{1c} was not $\leq 6.5\%$ at 32 weeks then the insulin was further increased to three times daily. Addition of once-daily BIAsp 70/30 before dinner enabled 41% to achieve an $A_{1c} \leq 7\%$ and 21% of the patients attained an $A_{1c} \leq 6.5\%$. With two daily injections of BIAsp 70/30, these glycemic goals were achieved by 70 and 52% of the subjects. With three daily BIAsp 70/30 injections, 77% achieved an $A_{1c} \leq 7.0\%$ and 60% achieved an $A_{1c} \leq 6.5\%$. Further studies have shown the value of patient controlled titration. The important points are that the insulin can be started at low doses and increased by the patient, based on home blood glucose monitoring, safely with few side effects.

Practical Guidelines for Insulin Replacement Therapy

For physicians managing patients with type 2 diabetes, practical guidelines for pharmacologic interventions are particularly important in view of the major changes over the past 10 years in managing type 2 diabetes and the growing movement toward starting aggressive pharmacotherapy earlier in the course of the disease. There has also been a paradigm shift that involves the increased use of flexible combination therapy with lower doses of any of the insulin secretagogues (whether sulfonylurea, incretin mimetic or DPP-4 inhibitor) plus metformin and a glitazone almost from the initiation of pharmacotherapy. This strategy is embraced by the community of diabetes experts who also view early insulin therapy to supplement oral treatment as an effective tactic to reach a patient's glycemic target.

A practical approach to overcome the complexity of MDI regimens—and perhaps the best and most acceptable way to initiate insulin therapy—is to start with evening basal insulin replacement in patients who are no longer responding to oral agents. Starting basal insulin replacement while maintaining the use of oral agents has considerable advantages: (a) only 1 daily injection may be required without the need of mixing different insulin preparations; (b) titration can be accomplished in a slow, safe, and simple fashion; and (c) a lower total dose of insulin will eventually be required because of the synergy of effects from the oral combination therapy.

When insulin is added to combination oral agent in asymptomatic patients with type 2 diabetes, it can be initiated with a simple regimen with a low dose of 5 to 10 units of insulin daily (Table 5). The patient can then increase the dose weekly according to fasting self monitored blood glucose (SMBG) based on the average of 2 to 5 consecutive days, as long as

TABLE 5   Practical Guidelines: Starting Insulin

Continue oral agent(s) at same dosage (eventually reduce the secretagogue)
Add single, evening insulin dose (around 10 units)
Glargine (morning, noon, evening or bedtime)
NPH (bedtime)
Premixed insulin
Adjust dose according to an average of 2-5 fasting blood glucose monitoring
Increase insulin dose weekly as needed
Increase by 2 units if FBG 100–120 mg/dL
Increase by 4 units if FBG 121–140 mg/dL
Increase by 6 units if FBG 141–180 mg/dL
Increase by 8 units if FBG >180 mg/dL

Abbreviation: NPH, neutral protamine hagedorn.

there is no evidence of nocturnal hypoglycemia with any measurements ≤72 mg/dL (Table 5). Insulin adjustments with appropriate reductions will be required in instances of SMBG <56 mg/dL or with the occurrence of a severe hypoglycemic episode.

Whether the oral agents should be continued once the insulin regimen has been optimized, will depend on the individual patient response. If the secretagogue is stopped then it would need to be switched to prandial insulin. Metformin should be continued to provide weight control as long as there is no evidence of renal impairment or CHF. A glitazone should also be continued to reduce insulin resistance and potentially preserve beta-cell function. Ideally the glitazone would have been added prior to insulin initiation as adding high doses of glitazones to ongoing insulin therapy is associated with substantial weight gain and fluid retention. The use of a DPP-4 inhibitor with insulin has not yet been studied so cannot be addressed here. Similarly, incretin mimetics, such as exenatide, have not yet been studied in combination with insulin.

Over time, the need to intensify insulin regimens arises in response to disease progression. Clinical judgment should prevail to determine when to advance to a more intensive basal/bolus insulin regimen. Clearly, when the target fasting plasma glucose of 80 to 120 mg/dL has been achieved and the HbA$_{1c}$ remains >7% further increments of the evening basal insulin glargine may be attempted but this approach can result in increased risk of hypoglycemia. Therefore, at this point adding pre-prandial fast acting insulin analogues at their main meal or meals will result in subsequent improvements of the A$_{1c}$ levels. Postprandial hyperglycemia can be further improved if patients follow simple algorithms, based on self-monitoring of blood glucose levels to adjust and deliver sufficient premeal insulin doses, using insulin aspart, glulisine, lispro or inhaled insulin independently. This approach provides more flexibility and allows additional doses of supplemental insulin as needed to control postprandial hyperglycemia. MDI regimens are progressively introduced as a further step toward intensifying insulin therapy (Table 6). The use of effective and less troublesome injection devices, such as insulin pens, can facilitate the implementation of the new advances in insulin replacement therapy.

It is conceivable that this practical and simple strategy may have translational implications and benefit large number of patients with type 2 DM when followed by general practitioners. This structured regimen can realistically reach A$_{1c}$ targets in patients who have progressively intensified oral combination therapy by adding evening basal insulin glargine and eventually premeal lispro, aspart or glulisine insulin, or inhaled insulin, to control fasting and postprandial glycemic levels.

Future Insulin Replacement Therapies

Traditionally, the approach to glucose lowering therapy has been that most patients with type 2 diabetes require insulin—but used as a "last resort after maximal combination therapy has failed—10 to 15 years after disease onset. However, our improved understanding of the natural history of type 2 diabetes suggests that insulin therapy should be started sooner rather

TABLE 6   Practical Guidelines: Advancing Basal/Bolus Insulin

Indicated when FBG is acceptable (80–120 mg/dL) but
  HbA$_{1c}$ >6.5%
  and/or
  SBGM before dinner >140–180 mg/dL

Insulin options
  To glargine: add lispro, aspart, glulisine or inhaled insulin at main meal or all meals
  To bedtime NPH: add morning NPH and mealtime lispro, aspart, glulisine or inhaled insulin

Oral agent options
  Continue secretagogue for endogenous insulin secretion?
  Continue metformin for weight control?
  Continue glitazone for glycemic stability?

Abbreviations: FBG, fasting blood glucose; HbA$_{1c}$, hemoglobin A$_{1c}$; NPH, neutral protamine hagedorn; SBGM, self blood-glucose monitoring.

than later and that insulin should be viewed as an essential therapeutic tool for achieving disease management goals, at an earlier stage in the natural progression of the disease, rather than a sign of failure on the part of the physician or patient. New strategies involving insulin analogues with improved pharmacokinetic properties, the new armamentarium of oral agents for type 2 diabetes, and new injectable agents will expand treatment options and combination regimens to facilitate the attainment of specific targeted glycemic levels in a safer and more effective manner.

REFERENCES

1. Cnop M, Vidal J, Hull RL, et al. Progressive loss of {beta}-cell function leads to worsening glucose tolerance in first-degree relatives of subjects with type 2 diabetes. Diabetes Care. March 1, 2007; 30(3):677–82.
2. UK Prospective Diabetes Study Group. Overview of 6 years' therapy of type II diabetes: a progressive disease. UKPDS 16. Diabetes. November 1, 1995; 44(11):1249–58.
3. Inzucchi SE. Oral Antihyperglycemic therapy for type 2 diabetes: scientific review. J Am Med Assoc January 16, 2002; 287(3):360–72.
4. Yki-Jarvinen H. Combination therapies with insulin in type 2 diabetes. Diabetes Care. April 1, 2001; 24(4):758–67.
5. Riddle MC, Rosenstock J, Gerich J. The treat-to-target trial: randomized addition of glargine or human NPH insulin to oral therapy of type 2 diabetic patients. Diabetes Care. November 1, 2003; 26(11):3080–6.
6. Raskin P, Allen E, Hollander P, et al. Initiating insulin therapy in type 2 diabetes: a comparison of biphasic and basal insulin analogs. Diabetes Care. February 1, 2005; 28(2):260–5.
7. Garber AJ, Wahlen J, Wahl T, et al. Attainment of glycaemic goals in type 2 diabetes with once-, twice-, or thrice-daily dosing with biphasic insulin aspart 70/30 (The 1-2-3 study). Diabetes, Obesity and Metabolism. 2006; 8(1):58–66.
8. DeFronzo RA. Pharmacologic therapy for type 2 diabetes mellitus. Ann Intern Med. August 17, 1999; 131(4):281–303.
9. Stern M, Gonzalez C, Mitchell B, Villalpando E, Haffner S, Hazuda H. Genetic and environmental determinants of type II diabetes in Mexico City and San Antonio. Diabetes. April 1, 1992; 41(4): 484–92.
10. Kahn SE, Prigeon RL, Schwartz RS, et al. Obesity, body fat distribution, insulin sensitivity and islet beta-cell function as explanations for metabolic diversity. J Nutr February 1, 2001; 131(2):354S–60.
11. Utzschneider KM, Prigeon RL, Carr DB, et al. Impact of differences in fasting glucose and glucose tolerance on the hyperbolic relationship between insulin sensitivity and insulin responses. Diabetes Care. February 1, 2006; 29(2):356–62.
12. Kahn SE. The relative contributions of insulin resistance and beta-cell dysfunction to the pathophysiology of Type 2 diabetes. Diabetologia January 1, 2003; V46(1):3–19.
13. Saad M, Knowler W, Pettitt D, Nelson R, Mott D, Bennett P. The natural history of impaired glucose tolerance in the Pima Indians. N Engl J Med December 8, 1988; 319(23):1500–6.
14. Weyer C, Bogardus C, Mott DM, Pratley RE. The natural history of insulin secretory dysfunction and insulin resistance in the pathogenesis of type 2 diabetes mellitus. J Clin Invest September 15, 1999; 104(6):787–94.
15. Bogardus C, Tataranni PA. Reduced early insulin secretion in the etiology of type 2 diabetes mellitus in Pima Indians. Diabetes February 1, 2002; 51(90001):S262–4.
16. Ferrannini E, Nannipieri M, Williams K, Gonzales C, Haffner SM, Stern MP. mode of onset of type 2 diabetes from normal or impaired glucose tolerance. Diabetes January 1, 2004; 53(1):160–5.
17. Buchanan TA, Xiang AH, Peters RK, et al. Preservation of pancreatic {beta}-cell function and prevention of type 2 diabetes by pharmacological treatment of insulin resistance in high-risk hispanic women. Diabetes September 1, 2002; 51(9):2796–803.
18. UK Prospective Diabetes Study Group. Effect of intensive blood-glucose control with metformin on complications in overweight patients with type 2 diabetes (UKPDS 34). The Lancet September 12, 1998; 352(9131):854–65.
19. Matthews D, Cull C, Stratton I, Holman R, Turner R. UKPDS 26: sulphonylurea failure in non-insulin-dependent diabetic patients over six years. UK Prospective Diabetes Study (UKPDS) Group. Diabet Med April 1998; 15(4):297–303.
20. Leahy J, Weir G. Evolution of abnormal insulin secretory responses during 48-h in vivo hyperglycemia. Diabetes February 1, 1988; 37(2):217–22.
21. Leibowitz G, Yuli M, Donath M, et al. Beta-cell glucotoxicity in the Psammomys obesus model of type 2 diabetes. Diabetes February 1, 2001; 50(90001):S113–7.
22. McGarry JD. Banting Lecture 2001: dysregulation of fatty acid metabolism in the etiology of type 2 diabetes. Diabetes January 1, 2002; 51(1):7–18.

23. Unger RH, Orci L. Lipoapoptosis: its mechanism and its diseases. Biochimica et Biophysica Acta (BBA) – Molecular and Cell Biology of Lipids. 2002/12/30 2002; 1585(2–3):202–12.

24. Andrews W, Vasquez B, Nagulesparan M, et al. Insulin therapy in obese, non-insulin-dependent diabetes induces improvements in insulin action and secretion that are maintained for two weeks after insulin withdrawal. Diabetes July 1, 1984; 33(7):634–42.

25. Garvey W, Olefsky J, Griffin J, Hamman R, Kolterman O. The effect of insulin treatment on insulin secretion and insulin action in type II diabetes mellitus. Diabetes March 1, 1985; 34(3):222–34.

26. Henry R, Gumbiner B, Ditzler T, Wallace P, Lyon R, Glauber H. Intensive conventional insulin therapy for type II diabetes. Metabolic effects during a 6-mo outpatient trial. Diabetes Care January 1, 1993; 16(1):21–31.

27. Pratipanawatr T, Cusi K, Ngo P, Pratipanawatr W, Mandarino LJ, DeFronzo RA. Normalization of plasma glucose concentration by insulin therapy improves insulin-stimulated glycogen synthesis in type 2 diabetes. Diabetes February 1, 2002; 51(2):462–8.

28. Ilkova H, Glaser B, Tunckale A, Bagriacik N, Cerasi E. Induction of long-term glycemic control in newly diagnosed type 2 diabetic patients by transient intensive insulin treatment. Diabetes Care September 1, 1997; 20(9):1353–6.

29. Carey D, Jenkins A, Campbell L, Freund J, Chisholm D. Abdominal fat and insulin resistance in normal and overweight women: Direct measurements reveal a strong relationship in subjects at both low and high risk of NIDDM. Diabetes May 1, 1996; 45(5):633–8.

30. Fujimoto WY. The importance of insulin resistance in the pathogenesis of type 2 diabetes mellitus. The Am J Med 2000/4/17 2000; 108(6, Supplement 1):9–14.

31. Reaven GM. Banting lecture 1988. Role of insulin resistance in human disease. Diabetes Dec 1988; 37(12):1595–607.

32. Executive summary of the third report of The National Cholesterol Education Program (NCEP) Expert panel on detection, evaluation, and treatment of high blood cholesterol in adults (Adult Treatment Panel III). Jama: the Journal of the American Medical Association. May 2001; 285(19): 2486–97.

33. Pyorala K. Relationship of glucose tolerance and plasma insulin to the incidence of coronary heart disease: results from two population studies in Finland. Diabetes Care March 1, 1979; 2(2):131–41.

34. Haffner SM, Hanley AJG. Do increased proinsulin concentrations explain the excess risk of coronary heart disease in diabetic and prediabetic subjects? Circulation April 30, 2002; 105(17): 2008–9.

35. UK Prospective Diabetes Study Group. Intensive blood-glucose control with sulphonylureas or insulin compared with conventional treatment and risk of complications in patients with type 2 diabetes (UKPDS 33). The Lancet 1998; 352(9131):837–53.

36. Malmberg K, Ryden L, Hamstent A, et al. Effects of insulin treatment on cause-specific one-year mortality and morbidity in diabetic patients with acute myocardial infarction. Eur Heart J September 1, 1996; 17(9):1337–44.

37. Malmberg K, Norhammar A, Wedel H, Ryden L. Glycometabolic state at admission: important risk marker of mortality in conventionally treated patients with diabetes mellitus and acute myocardial infarction: long-term results from the diabetes and insulin-glucose infusion in acute myocardial infarction (DIGAMI) study. Circulation May 25, 1999; 99(20):2626–32.

38. Sodi-Pallares D, Testelli MR, Fishleder BL, et al. Effects of an intravenous infusion of a potassium-glucose-insulin solution on the electrocardiographic signs of myocardial infarction. A preliminary clinical report. Am J Cardiol Feb 1962; 9:166–81.

39. Sodi-Pallares D, Bisteni A, Medrano GA, Testelli MR, De Micheli A. The polarizing treatment of acute myocardial infarction. Possibility of its use in other cardiovascular conditions. Dis Chest Apr 1963; 43:424–32.

40. Oliver MF, Opie LH. Effects of glucose and fatty acids on myocardial ischaemia and arrhythmias. Lancet Jan 15 1994; 343(8890):155–8.

41. Opie L. Proof that glucose-insulin-potassium provides metabolic protection of ischaemic myocardium? The Lancet 1999/3/6 1999; 353(9155):768–9.

42. Malmberg K, Ryden L, Wedel H, et al. Intense metabolic control by means of insulin in patients with diabetes mellitus and acute myocardial infarction (DIGAMI 2): effects on mortality and morbidity. Eur Heart J April 1, 2005; 26(7):650–61.

43. Bogardus C, Taskinen M, Zawadzki J, Lillioja S, Mott D, Howard B. Increased resting metabolic rates in obese subjects with non-insulin-dependent diabetes mellitus and the effect of sulfonylurea therapy. Diabetes January 1, 1986; 35(1):1–5.

44. Jacob AN, Salinas K, Adams-Huet B, Raskin P. Weight gain in type 2 diabetes mellitus. Diabetes, Obesity and Metabolism 2007; 9(3):386–93.

45. Yki-Jarvinen H, Helve E, Sane T, Nurjhan N, Taskinen MR. Insulin inhibition of overnight glucose production and gluconeogenesis from lactate in NIDDM. Am J Physiol Jun 1989; 256(6 Pt 1):E732–9.

46. Franssila-Kallunki A, Groop L. Factors associated with basal metabolic rate in patients with type 2 (non-insulin-dependent) diabetes mellitus. Diabetologia. Oct 1992; 35(10):962–6.

47. Stumvoll M, Nurjhan N, Perriello G, Dailey G, Gerich JE. Metabolic effects of metformin in non-insulin-dependent diabetes mellitus. N Engl J Med Aug 31 1995; 333(9):550–4.

48. Makimattila S, Nikkila K, Yki-Jarvinen H. Causes of weight gain during insulin therapy with and without metformin in patients with Type II diabetes mellitus. Diabetologia Apr 1999; 42(4):406–12.

49. Yki-Jarvinen H, Ryysy L, Kauppila M, et al. Effect of obesity on the response to insulin therapy in noninsulin-dependent diabetes mellitus. J Clin Endocrinol Metab. Dec 1997; 82(12):4037–43.

50. Lee A, Morley JE. Metformin decreases food consumption and induces weight loss in subjects with obesity with type II non-insulin-dependent diabetes. Obes Res. Jan 1998; 6(1):47–53.

51. Yki-Jarvinen H, Juurinen L, Alvarsson M, et al. INITIATE (INITiate Insulin by Aggressive Titration and Education). A randomized study to compare initiation of insulin combination therapy in type 2 diabetic patients individually and in groups. Diabetes Care Mar 23, 2007; 30:1364–69.

52. Billingham MS, Milles JJ, Bailey CJ, Hall RA. Lipoprotein subfraction composition in non-insulin-dependent diabetes treated by diet, sulphonylurea, and insulin. Metabolism Sep 1989; 38(9):850–7.

53. Rivellese AA, Patti L, Romano G, et al. Effect of insulin and sulfonylurea therapy, at the same level of blood glucose control, on low density lipoprotein subfractions in type 2 diabetic patients. J Clin Endocrinol Metab Nov 2000; 85(11):4188–92.

54. Cusi K, Cunningham GR, Comstock JP. Safety and efficacy of normalizing fasting glucose with bedtime NPH insulin alone in NIDDM. Diabetes Care Jun 1995; 18(6):843–51.

55. Emanuele N, Azad N, Abraira C, et al. Effect of intensive glycemic control on fibrinogen, lipids, and lipoproteins: veterans affairs cooperative study in type ii diabetes mellitus. Arch Intern Med Dec 7–21 1998; 158(22):2485–90.

56. De Leeuw I, Vague P, Selam J, et al. Insulin detemir used in basal-bolus therapy in people with type 1 diabetes is associated with a lower risk of nocturnal hypoglycaemia and less weight gain over 12 months in comparison to NPH insulin. Diab Obes Metab 2005; 7:73–82.

57. Dreyer M, Prager R, Robinson A, et al. Efficacy and safety of insulin glulisine in patients with type 1 diabetes. Horm Metab Res Nov 2005; 37(11):702–7.

58. Skyler JS, Jovanovic L, Klioze S, Reis J, Duggan W. Two-year safety and efficacy of inhaled human insulin (Exubera) in adult patients with type 1 diabetes. Diabetes Care Mar 2007; 30(3):579–85.

59. Hollander PA, Blonde L, Rowe R, et al. Efficacy and safety of inhaled insulin (exubera) compared with subcutaneous insulin therapy in patients with type 2 diabetes: results of a 6-month, randomized, comparative trial. Diabetes Care Oct 2004; 27(10):2356–62.

60. Heise T, Nosek L, Ronn BB, et al. Lower Within-subject variability of insulin detemir in comparison to NPH insulin and insulin glargine in people with type 1 diabetes. Diabetes June 1, 2004; 53(6): 1614–20.

61. Wright A, Burden AC, Paisey RB, Cull CA, Holman RR. Sulfonylurea inadequacy: efficacy of addition of insulin over 6 years in patients with type 2 diabetes in the U.K. Prospective Diabetes Study (UKPDS 57). Diabetes Care Feb 2002; 25(2):330–6.

62. The Diabetes Control and Complications Trial Research Group. The effect of intensive treatment of diabetes on the development and progression of long-term complications in insulin-dependent diabetes mellitus. N Engl J Med September 30, 1993; 329(14):977–86.

63. Boyle PJ, Cryer PE. Growth hormone, cortisol, or both are involved in defense against, but are not critical to recovery from, hypoglycemia. Am J Physiol. Mar 1991; 260(3 Pt 1):E395–402.

64. Bolli GB, Di Marchi RD, Park GD, Pramming S, Koivisto VA. Insulin analogues and their potential in the management of diabetes mellitus. Diabetologia Oct 1999; 42(10):1151–67.

65. Owens DR, Zinman B, Bolli GB. Insulins today and beyond. Lancet Sep 1 2001; 358(9283):739–46.

66. Skyler JS. Diabetes Mellitus, Types I and II. Humes HD, ed. Kelley's Textbook of Internal Medicine. 4th ed. Philadelphia: Lippincott Williams & Wilkins; 2000.

67. Becker RH, Frick AD, Burger F, Potgieter JH, Scholtz H. Insulin glulisine, a new rapid-acting insulin analogue, displays a rapid time-action profile in obese non-diabetic subjects. Exp Clin Endocrinol Diabetes Sep 2005; 113(8):435–43.

68. Becker RH, Frick AD, Burger F, Scholtz H, Potgieter JH. A comparison of the steady-state pharmacokinetics and pharmacodynamics of a novel rapid-acting insulin analog, insulin glulisine, and regular human insulin in healthy volunteers using the euglycemic clamp technique. Exp Clin Endocrinol Diabetes May 2005; 113(5):292–7.

69. Howey DC, Bowsher RR, Brunelle RL, Woodworth JR. [Lys(B28), Pro(B29)]-human insulin. A rapidly absorbed analogue of human insulin. Diabetes Mar 1994; 43(3):396–402.

70. Holleman F, Hoekstra JB. Insulin lispro. N Engl J Med Jul 17 1997; 337(3):176–83.

71. Home PD, Barriocanal L, Lindholm A. Comparative pharmacokinetics and pharmacodynamics of the novel rapid-acting insulin analogue, insulin aspart, in healthy volunteers. Eur J Clin Pharmacol May 1999; 55(3):199–203.

72. Gammeltoft S, Hansen BF, Dideriksen L, et al. Insulin aspart: a novel rapid-acting human insulin analogue. Expert Opin Investig Drugs. Sep 1999; 8(9):1431–42.

73. Rakatzi I, Seipke G, Eckel J. [LysB3, GluB29] insulin: a novel insulin analog with enhanced [beta]-cell protective action. Biochemical and Biophysical Research Communications 2003; 310(3):852–9.

74. Anderson JH Jr., Brunelle RL, Koivisto VA, et al. Reduction of postprandial hyperglycemia and frequency of hypoglycemia in IDDM patients on insulin-analog treatment. Multicenter Insulin Lispro Study Group. Diabetes Feb 1997; 46(2):265–70.

75. Raskin P, Guthrie RA, Leiter L, Riis A, Jovanovic L. Use of insulin aspart, a fast-acting insulin analog, as the mealtime insulin in the management of patients with type 1 diabetes. Diabetes Care. May 2000; 23(5):583–8.

76. Tuominen JA, Karonen SL, Melamies L, Bolli G, Koivisto VA. Exercise-induced hypoglycaemia in IDDM patients treated with a short-acting insulin analogue. Diabetologia. Jan 1995; 38(1): 106–11.

77. Torlone E, Pampanelli S, Lalli C, et al. Effects of the short-acting insulin analog [Lys(B28), Pro(B29)] on postprandial blood glucose control in IDDM. Diabetes Care Sep 1996; 19(9):945–52.

78. Del Sindaco P, Ciofetta M, Lalli C, et al. Use of the short-acting insulin analogue lispro in intensive treatment of type 1 diabetes mellitus: importance of appropriate replacement of basal insulin and time-interval injection-meal. Diabet Med Jul 1998; 15(7):592–600.

79. Gale EA. A randomized, controlled trial comparing insulin lispro with human soluble insulin in patients with Type 1 diabetes on intensified insulin therapy. The UK Trial Group. Diabet Med Mar 2000; 17(3):209–14.

80. Brunelle BL, Llewelyn J, Anderson JH Jr, Gale EA, Koivisto VA. Meta-analysis of the effect of insulin lispro on severe hypoglycemia in patients with type 1 diabetes. Diabetes Care Oct 1998; 21 (10):1726–31.

81. Heinemann L. Hypoglycemia and insulin analogues: is there a reduction in the incidence? J Diabetes Complications Mar–Apr 1999; 13(2):105–14.

82. Home PD, Lindholm A, Hylleberg B, Round P. Improved glycemic control with insulin aspart: a multicenter randomized double-blind crossover trial in type 1 diabetic patients. UK Insulin Aspart Study Group. Diabetes Care Nov 1998; 21(11):1904–9.

83. Home PD, Lindholm A, Riis A. Insulin aspart vs. human insulin in the management of long-term blood glucose control in Type 1 diabetes mellitus: a randomized controlled trial. Diabet Med Nov 2000; 17(11):762–70.

84. Heller SR, Amiel SA, Mansell P. Effect of the fast-acting insulin analog lispro on the risk of nocturnal hypoglycemia during intensified insulin therapy. U.K. Lispro Study Group. Diabetes Care Oct 1999; 22(10):1607–11.

85. Lalli C, Ciofetta M, Del Sindaco P, et al. Long-term intensive treatment of type 1 diabetes with the short-acting insulin analog lispro in variable combination with NPH insulin at mealtime. Diabetes Care Mar 1999; 22(3):468–77.

86. Colombel A, Murat A, Krempf M, Kuchly-Anton B, Charbonnel B. Improvement of blood glucose control in Type 1 diabetic patients treated with lispro and multiple NPH injections. Diabet Med Apr 1999; 16(4):319–24.

87. Zinman B, Tildesley H, Chiasson JL, Tsui E, Strack T. Insulin lispro in CSII: results of a double-blind crossover study. Diabetes Mar 1997; 46(3):440–3.

88. Melki V, Renard E, Lassmann-Vague V, et al. Improvement of HbA$_{1c}$ and blood glucose stability in IDDM patients treated with lispro insulin analog in external pumps. Diabetes Care Jun 1998; 21(6): 977–82.

89. Renner R, Pfutzner A, Trautmann M, Harzer O, Sauter K, Landgraf R. Use of insulin lispro in continuous subcutaneous insulin infusion treatment. Results of a multicenter trial. German Humalog-CSII Study Group. Diabetes Care May 1999; 22(5):784–8.

90. Garg SK, Carmain JA, Braddy KC, et al. Pre-meal insulin analogue insulin lispro vs Humulin R insulin treatment in young subjects with type 1 diabetes. Diabet Med Jan 1996; 13(1):47–52.

91. Mortensen HB, Lindholm A, Olsen BS, Hylleberg B. Rapid appearance and onset of action of insulin aspart in paediatric subjects with type 1 diabetes. Eur J Pediatr Jul 2000; 159(7):483–8.

92. Owens DR, Coates PA, Luzio SD, Tinbergen JP, Kurzhals R. Pharmacokinetics of 125I-labeled insulin glargine (HOE 901) in healthy men: comparison with NPH insulin and the influence of different subcutaneous injection sites. Diabetes Care Jun 2000; 23(6):813–9.

93. Lepore M, Pampanelli S, Fanelli C, et al. Pharmacokinetics and pharmacodynamics of subcutaneous injection of long-acting human insulin analog glargine, NPH insulin, and ultralente human insulin and continuous subcutaneous infusion of insulin lispro. Diabetes December 1, 2000; 49(12):2142–8.

94. Heinemann L, Linkeschova R, Rave K, Hompesch B, Sedlak M, Heise T. Time-action profile of the long-acting insulin analog insulin glargine (HOE901) in comparison with those of NPH insulin and placebo. Diabetes Care May 2000; 23(5):644–9.

95. Scholtz HE, Pretorius SG, Wessels DH, Becker RHA. Pharmacokinetic and glucodynamic variability: assessment of insulin glargine, NPH insulin and insulin ultralente in healthy volunteers using a euglycaemic clamp technique. Diabetologia 2005; 48(10):1988–95.

96. Kudva YC, Basu A, Jenkins GD, et al. Randomized controlled clinical trial of glargine versus ultralente insulin in the treatment of type 1 diabetes. Diabetes Care January 1, 2005; 28(1):10–4.

97. Ashwell SG, Gebbie J, Home PD. Optimal timing of injection of once-daily insulin glargine in people with Type 1 diabetes using insulin lispro at meal-times. Diabet Med Jan 2006; 23(1):46–52.
98. Ashwell SG, Gebbie J, Home PD. Twice-daily compared with once-daily insulin glargine in people with Type 1 diabetes using meal-time insulin aspart. Diabet Med Aug 2006; 23(8):879–86.
99. Karaguzel G, Satilmis A, Akcurin S, Bircan I. Comparison of breakfast and bedtime administration of insulin glargine in children and adolescents with Type 1 diabetes. Diabetes Res Clin Pract Oct 2006; 74(1):15–20.
100. Rosenstock J, Park G, Zimmerman J. Basal insulin glargine (HOE 901) versus NPH insulin in patients with type 1 diabetes on multiple daily insulin regimens. U.S. Insulin Glargine (HOE 901) Type 1 Diabetes Investigator Group. Diabetes Care Aug 2000; 23(8):1137–42.
101. Pieber TR, Eugene-Jolchine I, Derobert E. Efficacy and safety of HOE 901 versus NPH insulin in patients with type 1 diabetes. The European Study Group of HOE 901 in type 1 diabetes. Diabetes Care Feb 2000; 23(2):157–62.
102. Ratner RE, Hirsch IB, Neifing JL, Garg SK, Mecca TE, Wilson CA. Less hypoglycemia with insulin glargine in intensive insulin therapy for type 1 diabetes. U.S. Study Group of Insulin Glargine in Type 1 Diabetes. Diabetes Care May 2000; 23(5):639–43.
103. Raskin P, Klaff L, Bergenstal R, Halle JP, Donley D, Mecca T. A 16-week comparison of the novel insulin analog insulin glargine (HOE 901) and NPH human insulin used with insulin lispro in patients with type 1 diabetes. Diabetes Care Nov 2000; 23(11):1666–71.
104. Mohn A, Strang S, Wernicke-Panten K, Lang AM, Edge JA, Dunger DB. Nocturnal glucose control and free insulin levels in children with type 1 diabetes by use of the long-acting insulin HOE 901 as part of a three-injection regimen. Diabetes Care Apr 2000; 23(4):557–9.
105. Yki-Jarvinen H, Dressler A, Ziemen M. Less nocturnal hypoglycemia and better post-dinner glucose control with bedtime insulin glargine compared with bedtime NPH insulin during insulin combination therapy in type 2 diabetes. HOE 901/3002 Study Group. Diabetes Care Aug 2000; 23(8):1130–6.
106. Rosenstock J, Schwartz SL, Clark CM Jr, Park GD, Donley DW, Edwards MB. Basal insulin therapy in type 2 diabetes: 28-week comparison of insulin glargine (HOE 901) and NPH insulin. Diabetes Care Apr 2001; 24(4):631–6.
107. Markussen J, Havelund S, Kurtzhals P, et al. Soluble, fatty acid acylated insulins bind to albumin and show protracted action in pigs. Diabetologia Mar 1996; 39(3):281–8.
108. Heinemann L, Sinha K, Weyer C, Loftager M, Hirschberger S, Heise T. Time-action profile of the soluble, fatty acid acylated, long-acting insulin analogue NN304. Diabet Med Apr 1999; 16(4):332–8.
109. Hermansen K, Madsbad S, Perrild H, Kristensen A, Axelsen M. Comparison of the soluble basal insulin analog insulin detemir with NPH insulin: a randomized open crossover trial in type 1 diabetic subjects on basal-bolus therapy. Diabetes Care Feb 2001; 24(2):296–301.
110. Hermansen K, Davies M, Derezinski T, et al. A 26-week, randomized, parallel, treat-to-target trial comparing insulin detemir with nph insulin as add-on therapy to oral glucose-lowering drugs in insulin-naive people with type 2 diabetes. Diabetes Care June 1, 2006; 29(6):1269–74.
111. Home P, Bartley P, Russell-Jones D, et al. Insulin detemir offers improved glycemic control compared with nph insulin in people with type 1 diabetes: a randomized clinical trial. Diabetes Care May 1, 2004; 27(5):1081–7.
112. Russell-Jones D, Simpson R, Hylleberg B, Draeger E, Bolinder J. Effects of QD insulin detemir or neutral protamine Hagedorn on blood glucose control in patients with type I diabetes mellitus using a basal-bolus regimen. Clin Ther May 2004; 26(5):724–36.
113. Standl E, Lang H, Roberts A. The 12-month efficacy and safety of insulin detemir and NPH insulin in basal-bolus therapy for the treatment of type 1 diabetes. Diabetes Technol Ther Oct 2004; 6(5): 579–88.
114. Pieber TR, Treichel H-C, Hompesch B, et al. Comparison of insulin detemir and insulin glargine in subjects with Type 1 diabetes using intensive insulin therapy. Diabetic Medicine March 22, 2007; 24: 635–42.
115. Klein O, Lynge J, Endahl L, Damholt B, Nosek L, Heise T. Detemir and insulin glargine: similar time-action profiles in subjects with type 2 diabetes. Diabetes 2006; 55(Supplement):325–OR.
116. D'Eliseo P, Blaauw J, Milicevic Z, Wyatt J, Ignaut DA, Malone JK. Patient acceptability of a new 3.0 ml pre-filled insulin pen. Curr Med Res Opin 2000; 16(2):125–33.
117. Gall MA, Mathiesen ER, Skott P, et al. Effect of multiple insulin injections with a pen injector on metabolic control and general well-being in insulin-dependent diabetes mellitus. Diabetes Res Jun 1989; 11(2):97–101.
118. Patton JS, Bukar J, Nagarajan S. Inhaled insulin. Adv Drug Deliv Rev Feb 1 1999; 35(2–3):235–47.
119. Heinemann L, Klappoth W, Rave K, Hompesch B, Linkeschowa R, Heise T. Intra-individual variability of the metabolic effect of inhaled insulin together with an absorption enhancer. Diabetes Care Sep 2000; 23(9):1343–7.
120. Weiss SR, Cheng S-L, Kourides IA, Gelfand RA, Landschulz WH. Inhaled insulin provides improved glycemic control in patients with type 2 diabetes mellitus inadequately controlled

with oral agents: a randomized controlled trial. Arch Intern Med October 27, 2003; 163(19): 2277–82.

121. Hausmann M, Dellweg S, Osborn C, et al. Inhaled insulin as adjunctive therapy in subjects with type 2 diabetes failing oral agents: a controlled proof-of-concept study. Diabetes, Obesity and Metabolism 2006; 8(5):574–80.

122. Barnett AH, Dreyer M, Lange P, Serdarevic-Pehar M, on behalf of the Exubera Phase III Study Group. An open, randomized, parallel-group study to compare the efficacy and safety profile of inhaled human insulin (Exubera) with glibenclamide as adjunctive therapy in patients with type 2 diabetes poorly controlled on metformin. Diabetes Care August 1, 2006; 29(8):1818–25.

123. Rosenstock J, Zinman B, Murphy LJ, et al. Inhaled insulin improves glycemic control when substituted for or added to oral combination therapy in type 2 diabetes: a randomized, controlled trial. Ann Intern Med Oct 18 2005; 143(8):549–58.

124. Cherrington AD. Banting Lecture 1997. Control of glucose uptake and release by the liver in vivo. Diabetes May 1999; 48(5):1198–214.

125. Doar JW, Thompson ME, Wilde CE, Sewell PF. Diet and oral antidiabetic drugs and plasma sugar and insulin levels in patients with maturity-onset diabetes mellitus. Br Med J Feb 28 1976; 1(6008): 498–500.

126. Fuhlendorff J, Rorsman P, Kofod H, et al. Stimulation of insulin release by repaglinide and glibenclamide involves both common and distinct processes. Diabetes Mar 1998; 47(3):345–51.

127. Malaisse WJ. Stimulation of insulin release by non-sulfonylurea hypoglycemic agents: the meglitinide family. Horm Metab Res Jun 1995; 27(6):263–6.

128. Perfetti R, Ahmad A. Novel sulfonylurea and non-sulfonylurea drugs to promote the secretion of insulin. Trends Endocrinol Metab Aug 2000; 11(6):218–23.

129. Drucker DJ, Nauck MA. The incretin system: glucagon-like peptide-1 receptor agonists and dipeptidyl peptidase-4 inhibitors in type 2 diabetes. The Lancet 368(9548):1696–705.

130. Inzucchi SE, Maggs DG, Spollett GR, et al. Efficacy and metabolic effects of metformin and troglitazone in type II diabetes mellitus. N Engl J Med Mar 26 1998; 338(13):867–72.

131. Johansen K. Efficacy of metformin in the treatment of NIDDM. Meta-analysis. Diabetes Care Jan 1999; 22(1):33–7.

132. Kirpichnikov D, McFarlane SI, Sowers JR. Metformin: an update. Ann Intern Med Jul 2 2002; 137(1): 25–33.

133. Musi N, Hirshman MF, Nygren J, et al. Metformin increases AMP-activated protein kinase activity in skeletal muscle of subjects with type 2 diabetes. Diabetes Jul 2002; 51(7):2074–81.

134. Nolan JJ, Ludvik B, Beerdsen P, Joyce M, Olefsky J. Improvement in glucose tolerance and insulin resistance in obese subjects treated with troglitazone. N Engl J Med November 3, 1994; 331(18): 1188–93.

135. Petersen KF, Krssak M, Inzucchi S, Cline GW, Dufour S, Shulman GI. Mechanism of troglitazone action in type 2 diabetes. Diabetes May 2000; 49(5):827–31.

136. Mudaliar S, Henry RR. New oral therapies for type 2 diabetes mellitus: the glitazones or insulin sensitizers. Annu Rev Med 2001; 52:239–57.

137. Frias JP, Yu JG, Kruszynska YT, Olefsky JM. Metabolic effects of troglitazone therapy in type 2 diabetic, obese, and lean normal subjects. Diabetes Care Jan 2000; 23(1):64–9.

138. Maggs DG, Buchanan TA, Burant CF, et al. Metabolic effects of troglitazone monotherapy in type 2 diabetes mellitus. A randomized, double-blind, placebo-controlled trial. Ann Intern Med Feb 1 1998; 128(3):176–85.

139. Goke B, Herrmann-Rinke C. The evolving role of alpha-glucosidase inhibitors. Diabetes Metab Rev Sep 1998; 14 Suppl 1:S31–8.

140. Lebovitz HE. Oral antidiabetic agents. The emergence of alpha-glucosidase inhibitors. Drugs 1992; 44 Suppl 3:21–8.

141. Lebovitz HE. Alpha-glucosidase inhibitors. Endocrinol Metab Clin North Am Sep 1997; 26(3): 539–51.

142. Holman RR, Steemson J, Turner RC. Sulphonylurea failure in type 2 diabetes: treatment with a basal insulin supplement. Diabet Med Sep-Oct 1987; 4(5):457–62.

143. Riddle MC, Hart JS, Bouma DJ, Phillipson BE, Youker G. Efficacy of bedtime NPH insulin with daytime sulfonylurea for subpopulation of type II diabetic subjects. Diabetes Care Oct 1989; 12(9): 623–9.

144. Gastaldelli A, Baldi S, Pettiti M, et al. Influence of obesity and type 2 diabetes on gluconeogenesis and glucose output in humans: a quantitative study. Diabetes Aug 2000; 49(8):1367–73.

145. Shank ML, Del Prato S, DeFronzo RA. Bedtime insulin/daytime glipizide. Effective therapy for sulfonylurea failures in NIDDM. Diabetes Feb 1995; 44(2):165–72.

146. Riddle MC, Schneider J. Beginning insulin treatment of obese patients with evening 70/30 insulin plus glimepiride versus insulin alone. Glimepiride Combination Group. Diabetes Care Jul 1998; 21(7):1052–7.

147. Poulsen MK, Henriksen JE, Hother-Nielsen O, Beck-Nielsen H. The combined effect of triple therapy with rosiglitazone, metformin, and insulin aspart in type 2 diabetic patients. Diabetes Care Dec 2003; 26(12):3273–9.

148. Giugliano D, Quatraro A, Consoli G, et al. Metformin for obese, insulin-treated diabetic patients: improvement in glycaemic control and reduction of metabolic risk factors. Eur J Clin Pharmacol 1993; 44(2):107–12.

149. Aviles-Santa L, Sinding J, Raskin P. Effects of metformin in patients with poorly controlled, insulin-treated type 2 diabetes mellitus. A randomized, double-blind, placebo-controlled trial. Ann Intern Med Aug 3 1999; 131(3):182–8.

150. Relimpio F, Pumar A, Losada F, Mangas MA, Acosta D, Astorga R. Adding metformin versus insulin dose increase in insulin-treated but poorly controlled Type 2 diabetes mellitus: an open-label randomized trial. Diabet Med Dec 1998; 15(12):997–1002.

151. Robinson AC, Burke J, Robinson S, Johnston DG, Elkeles RS. The effects of metformin on glycemic control and serum lipids in insulin-treated NIDDM patients with suboptimal metabolic control. Diabetes Care May 1998; 21(5):701–5.

152. Schwartz S, Raskin P, Fonseca V, Graveline JF. Effect of troglitazone in insulin-treated patients with type II diabetes mellitus. Troglitazone and Exogenous Insulin Study Group. N Engl J Med Mar 26 1998; 338(13):861–6.

153. Raskin P, Rendell M, Riddle MC, Dole JF, Freed MI, Rosenstock J. A randomized trial of rosiglitazone therapy in patients with inadequately controlled insulin-treated type 2 diabetes. Diabetes Care Jul 2001; 24(7):1226–32.

154. Rosenstock J, Einhorn D, Hershon K, Glazer NB, Yu S. Efficacy and safety of pioglitazone in type 2 diabetes: a randomised, placebo-controlled study in patients receiving stable insulin therapy. Int J Clin Pract May 2002; 56(4):251–7.

155. Yki-Jarvinen H, Ryysky L, Nikkila K. Comparison of bedtime insulin regimens in patients with type 2 diabetes mellitus. Ann Intern Med 1999; 130:389–96.

15 | Combination Therapy for Treatment of Type 2 Diabetes

Anthony L. McCall
Center for Diabetes and Hormone Excellence, University of Virginia, Charlottesville, Virginia, U.S.A.

INTRODUCTION

Combinations of oral antihyperglycemic agents or oral agents with insulin are more appropriate for treatment of type 2 diabetes mellitus than for type 1 diabetes. This discussion concentrates on how to match the therapy of type 2 diabetes with the underlying pathophysiologic defects and to rectify specific patterns of hyperglycemia. While currently approved combinations are given most attention, therapeutic combinations that are not yet approved by the U.S. Food and Drug Administration (FDA) are also discussed to the extent that published data about them are available. Although the American Diabetes Association's (ADA) minimal treatment goal (<7% glycosylated hemoglobin [HbA_{1c}] with patients recommended to achieve 6% if possible without undue risk) is assumed as a therapeutic target, intensive insulin therapy, which in some cases is necessary to achieve this goal, is not discussed.

HISTORY OF COMBINATION THERAPY

Monotherapy

Since the development of sulfonylureas, pharmacotherapy for type 2 diabetes was commonly begun with these agents once nutrition therapy and active lifestyle proved insufficient to maintain glycemic control. Until the introduction of biguanides, patients were usually switched to once- or twice-daily insulin administration when therapeutic goals were no longer achieved with sulfonylureas. Sometimes insulin was combined with sulfonylureas, but for years there was little insight into how best to do this, nor clear demonstration of the value of this combination. After metformin came into use in some parts of the world, this agent was used as initial pharmacotherapy for many patients, especially those who were notably obese, until the time of treatment (secondary) failure and initiation of insulin. In some cases, metformin and a sulfonylurea were used together to delay the need for insulin, but when insulin became necessary both oral agents were commonly discontinued.

Delayed Insulin Use

An important aspect of this traditional approach to type 2 diabetes was that initiation of insulin therapy was often delayed until severe hyperglycemia occurred. One reason was the inconvenience and sometimes, fear of injecting insulin. In addition, type 2 diabetes was often considered a mild disorder (1), for which insulin was not necessary or appropriate. This erroneous concept has since been rejected because of evidence of the severe microvascular and macrovascular complications of this form of diabetes. Moreover, better insulins and devices, such as insulin pens for its delivery, have made treatment much less burdensome. However, many physicians continue to use insulin only as a last resort.

This persisting reluctance to begin insulin seems related to several factors, including concern that insulin therapy causes hyperinsulinemia, weight gain, and hypoglycemia and, for these reasons, may lead to poor clinical outcomes. Poor outcomes are assured for any therapy if its use is delayed until the condition is far advanced. In the case of insulin, poor outcomes of patients with type 2 diabetes seem more likely due to delay of treatment than because insulin has any intrinsic toxicity. With this in mind, this chapter proposes simple strategies for initiating and advancing insulin therapy for type 2 diabetes, using the principles of combination therapy.

The UKPDS and the Progression of Therapy

The United Kingdom Prospective Diabetes Study (UKPDS) was a landmark trial that examined the ability of several medications used in the treatment of type 2 diabetes to limit the development of common long-term complications. The principal intervention in the UKPDS was a monotherapy trial of glycemic control. In this "glucose control" study (2), sulfonylurea and insulin monotherapy were assessed for their ability to reduce complications, using an intensive treatment policy in comparison with a conventional policy based on nutrition advice. Glycemic control achieved over a 10-year period, as estimated by median HbA$_{1c}$, was 7% for the intensive policy group and 7.9% for the conventional policy group. The improvement of glycemic control reflected by this 0.9% difference of HbA$_{1c}$ resulted in a reduction of 25% to 35% in microvascular endpoints, such as retinopathy, and a trend toward fewer rather than more cardiovascular events. In a smaller substudy, including patients who were more overweight, and also testing the effects of metformin, a lesser reduction of HbA$_{1c}$ occurred (about 0.6%). This resulted in a trend for microvascular benefits and a significant benefit in some macrovascular endpoints, such as reduced risk of death and myocardial infarction (3). The UKPDS study provided convincing evidence of the benefit of good glycemic control with currently available monotherapies, and largely laid to rest the fear that treatment with either insulin or sulfonylureas increases cardiovascular mortality.

Progressive Insulin Secretory Defect

An important physiological analysis performed by the UKPDS investigators estimated insulin secretion using a homeostasis (HOMA) model (4). Fasting insulin and glucose levels were measured initially and repeated yearly over a 6-year period to determine by a mathematical model the natural history of beta-cell function. As shown in Figure 1 and, in more detail, in Figure 2, beta-cell function in the group assigned to nutrition therapy was initially reduced and then inexorably deteriorated. The groups taking sulfonylureas or metformin showed similar patterns of deteriorating beta-cell function. That is, function was initially impaired and, after a short-term improvement associated with the initiation of pharmacotherapy, deteriorated at the same rate as the nutrition therapy group. Apparently, sulfonylureas did not accelerate the loss of beta-cell function, and metformin did not protect against it, as had been proposed. Thus, the UKPDS gave another important message, that type 2 diabetes is a

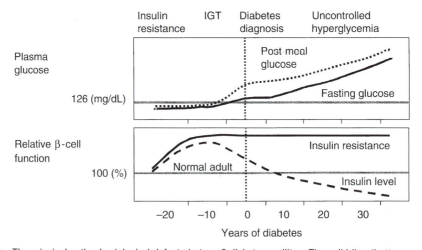

FIGURE 1 The principal pathophysiological defects in type 2 diabetes mellitus. The solid line (bottom panel) shows that insulin resistance starts well before the onset of hyperglycemia and the diagnosis of diabetes. The dashed line in the bottom panel shows that the onset of diabetes is caused by failure of the compensatory hyperinsulinemia that characterizes the metabolic syndrome of insulin resistance, the precursor to diabetes or impaired glucose tolerance (IGT). In the top panel, the dotted line shows that post-meal glucose levels rise as insulin deficiency progresses and that only later does fasting glycemia deteriorate (solid line).

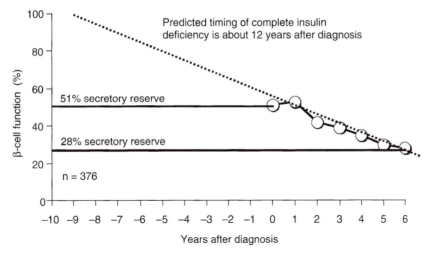

FIGURE 2 Based upon a homeostasis (HOMA) model, residual maximal insulin secretory reserve is depicted at the time of diagnosis and yearly for 6 years in subjects receiving diet only in the U.K. Prospective Diabetes study. This figure illustrates that nearly half of insulin secretion is lost at diagnosis. It also shows the progressive loss of insulin secretory reserve, which predicts essentially complete insulin deficiency in about a dozen years if further loss were linear.

progressive disorder, mainly because of declining insulin secretion over time. It is hoped that current or future therapies, such as thiazolidinediones or glucagon-like peptide-1 (GLP-1) mimetics, may ameliorate this progressive insulin secretory dysfunction. However, rigorous evidence that any therapy has this benefit in humans is still lacking, despite some promising preliminary results.

Progressive Attenuation of the Response to Monotherapy

Presumably linked to the gradual loss of insulin secretory function, there is a decline in the effectiveness of any monotherapy (5). Figure 3 shows a gradual upward climb of HbA_{1c} for patients using either conventional or intensive policy in the UKPDS. The deterioration of metabolic control was not prevented by any of the monotherapy regimens, including injected insulin—although the insulin regimen was not consistently advanced to intensive insulin therapy. The ADOPT study showed a modest benefit of rosiglitazone to slow disease progression in comparison to metformin and glyburide.

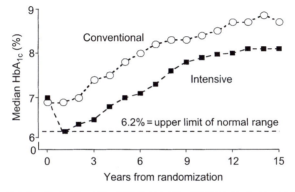

FIGURE 3 This figure, which is adapted from the U.K. Prospective Diabetes study comparing conventional policy to intensive policy with sulfonylureas or insulin, shows the progressive rise of HbA_{1c} that presumably is related to the progressive insulin secretory defect present in untreated type 2 diabetes mellitus.

Thus, type 2 diabetes is a progressive disease caused by progressive beta-cell dysfunction. It is the development of beta-cell dysfunction which initiates the transition from the metabolic syndrome of insulin resistance to impaired glucose tolerance and, ultimately, to diabetes. It appears that this progressive beta-cell dysfunction necessitates progressive therapy, including the use of combinations of agents. This insight is another major contribution from the UKPDS. As shown in Figure 1, type 2 diabetes has two defects that are crucial to the genesis of the disorder. This review, to some degree, simplifies the defects conceptually. Abnormalities of insulin secretion are both quantitative and qualitative, and include abnormal pulsatility, ultradian rhythms and clearance, but the net effect of these abnormalities is the lack of a timely insulin response for adequate compensation of insulin resistance (6). Similarly, insulin resistance is a complex phenomenon, with evidence of tissue-specific abnormalities and complex interactive effects. Again, the net effect is diminished biologic signaling of insulin action at multiple tissues, relative to the availability of insulin at a given moment. The molecular mechanisms underlying these defects still are only partly understood.

A Long Prodrome of Insulin Resistance Relates to Cardiovascular Disease

As indicated in Figure 1, tissue resistance to insulin action takes place long before the development of type 2 diabetes. Indeed, insulin resistance that precedes the development of type 2 diabetes by many years, may contribute greatly to the very high rate of cardiovascular events which account for the deaths of most people with this disorder (7). Haffner et al. have referred to a "ticking clock" hypothesis (8), suggesting that a long prodrome of insulin resistance before diabetes develops, associated with multiple cardiovascular risk factors (mildly abnormal glycemic patterns, dyslipidemia, hypertension, procoagulant and inflammatory state, etc.), sets the stage for the markedly increased risk of cardiovascular disease known to prevail once diabetes has been diagnosed (9). Resistance to the action of insulin occurs both in the traditionally insulin-sensitive tissues of the skeletal muscle and adipose tissue, and in the liver (10). Excessive production of glucose by the liver, despite insulin levels that are not markedly different from those of persons without diabetes and of similar adiposity, is one of the main causes of hyperglycemia in type 2 diabetes. Metformin's main action is to improve the hepatic response to insulin at least partly through its effects upon hepatic adenosine monophosphate kinase, which acts as a fuel sensor and thus controls the excessive hepatic glucose output. Resistance to insulin action at skeletal muscle and adipose tissue also affects glycemic control. An important effect of healthy eating and an active lifestyle is improved sensitivity of these tissues to insulin. Drugs of the thiazolidinedione class reduce peripheral resistance to the actions of insulin.

RATIONALE FOR COMBINATION THERAPY

In the context of two major physiologic defects, insulin resistance and insulin secretory failure, combination treatments with differing actions are entirely logical. Several different advantages of combining agents can be distinguished.

Efficacy

The first rationale for combination therapy (either with oral agents alone or with oral agents and insulin or oral agents with other injectable medicine such as incretin mimetics) is its superior efficacy. One principle that emerges from randomized controlled trials of antidiabetic therapies is that switching from one medication to another does not work as well as combination therapy. Figure 4 shows a classic study of combination oral agent therapy that illustrates this point (11). Patients with inadequate glycemic control on maximal doses of glyburide were randomized to continuation of that monotherapy, to metformin monotherapy gradually titrated to maximal doses (850 mg orally three times a day), or to a combination of glyburide and metformin. Neither monotherapy resulted in any significant improvement in fasting plasma glucose (FPG), but combination therapy with an insulin secretagogue and metformin, showed a dramatic improvement. Similarly, studies with other combination

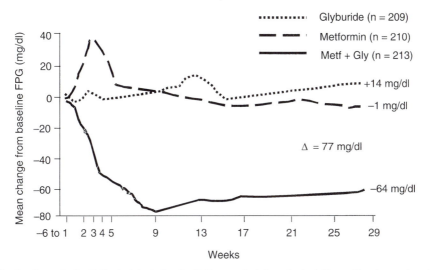

FIGURE 4 As shown in the U.S. pivotal studies by DeFronzo et al. in patients failing sulfonylureas (maximal dose glyburide in the dotted line), continuation of "failing" secretagogue therapy resulted in gradual worsening of glycemia. Similarly, a switch from glyburide to metformin in maximally effective doses showed no significant improvement in glycemic control. In fact, the deterioration of glycemia shown by rise in fasting plasma glucose (FPG) was marked in the metformin group after glyburide had been stopped and before full dose titration of metformin had occurred. Switching makes little sense as the combination of therapy (solid line) showed a substantial improvement in FPG not observed with either drug alone.

therapies showed no benefit of switching to a new agent class, but greater glucose-lowering efficacy through combining it with an agent of a different mechanism.

Tolerability and Convenience

Many side effects of medications are dose related. For example, hypoglycemia is a side effect of insulin or insulin secretagogues, gastrointestinal side effects are common with metformin, and with alpha-glucosidase inhibitors, and fluid retention or weight gain may occur with the thiazolidinediones. These side effects are dose related, and using lower doses of medications and slow titration may minimize them. Combinations of oral agents, therefore, may minimize side effects while achieving equal or better glycemic control. This principle has been tested directly for the combination of glyburide and metformin (12). Combinations of oral agents may seem more complex than monotherapy, but in some cases their convenience can be enhanced. Combining a single dose of a long-acting sulfonylurea, such as glimepiride, with one or two tablets of metformin, may have equal or more benefit than three or four tablets of metformin alone. Metformin–secretagogue (metformin–glyburide, metformin–glipizide) combination pills (Glucovance, Metaglip), have been introduced. Similarly, metformin–thiazolidinedione (metformin–rosiglitazone, metformin–pioglitazone) combination pills (Avandamet, Actosplusmet) are available. Recently, thiazolidinediones–secretagogue (rosiglitazone–glimepiride, pioglitazone–glimepiride) combination pills have become available (Avandaryl, Duetect). This trend will likely increase in the future. Convenient formulations of two agents in a single pill with dual actions may appeal to many patients and practitioners. While separate titration of agents may be desirable for many patients, for others a case can be made for combination preparations. This tactic may prove especially attractive for patients who must take not only two or more agents for glycemic control, but also many other medications for blood pressure, lipid abnormalities, heart disease, and other problems.

Avoiding Insulin

A final aspect of convenience of combined oral agent therapy deserves comment, the convenience of avoiding insulin treatment. As mentioned above, many patients and physicians prefer not to use insulin if it can be avoided. Use of insulin may be frightening and may appear to be a punishment for poor lifestyle choices, and brings the risk of hypoglycemia. It remains to be seen whether combinations of three or even four oral agents will prove equally or better tolerated, and will lead to equal or better outcomes than earlier introduction of insulin. The availability of dry powder inhaled insulin may facilitate earlier insulin use in some patients for whom the barrier of injections is otherwise insurmountable.

Insulin and Oral Agents

The combination of insulin and oral agents can also offer convenience and therapeutic benefits for patients. The use of oral agents can reduce the dosage of insulin required to meet therapeutic goals. This may have the benefit of reducing the weight gain associated with insulin use, and patients taking insulin often perceive lower doses to be an advantage, as minimizing the number of injections and the size of an individual injection can reduce the discomfort and inconvenience of multiple or large injections. This advantage is most evident for patients who are very insulin resistant, requiring more than 100 units (lesser amounts for insulin pens) at a time, thus making a single injection impossible. For some patients who are on pure basal insulin treatment with little or no prandial regulation of glycemia, use of secretagogues or other agents with prandial control (e.g., incretin mimetics) also may reduce the number of insulin injections needed.

Non-Glycemic Effects of Combination Therapy

A final rationale for combination therapy relates to proven or potential benefits other than those resulting from better glycemic control. This concept has been most emphasized for metformin and the thiazolidinediones. Both of these classes of agents have potential non-glycemic effects that may reduce cardiovascular risk. In the UKPDS, metformin use by obese patients reduced cardiovascular events, such as myocardial infarction, relative to the rate seen with diet alone. Statistically significant benefits of this kind were lacking with insulin or sulfonylurea treatment (2,3). Similarly, the thiazolidinediones may have various non-glycemic effects, among them reducing markers for procoagulant and inflammatory states, and normalizing endothelium-dependent vasorelaxation and smooth muscle migration. Some studies have found lipid and blood pressure benefits as well. Ongoing randomized clinical trials which are testing whether thiazolidinedione therapy improves clinical outcomes are just beginning to report results and suggest that there may be some reduction in ischemic cardiovascular events, but raise concerns about congestive heart failure which may mitigate the overall cardiovascular benefit of this drug class (13).

TACTICS FOR ACHIEVING CONTROL WITH COMBINATION THERAPY

Addressing Dual Defects with Dual Therapies

Both insulin deficiency and insulin resistance are present in most patients with type 2 diabetes. As a result, most patients will need treatments that address both physiologic abnormalities and, therefore, combination pharmacotherapy. In some patients with marked insulin resistance, endogenous insulin production may be adequate once insulin resistance has been aggressively counteracted through both lifestyle change and dual pharmacotherapy using metformin and a thiazolidinedione for pre-prandial glycemic control, but post-prandial control may still require secretagogues.

Secretagogues and Insulin-Assisting Agents

Insulin secretagogues that are currently available include several sulfonylureas (first and second generation) and the fast acting, short-duration insulin secretagogues (repaglinide, nateglinide). Insulin-assisting agents that are available include the biguanide metformin and the thiazolidinediones, rosiglitazone and pioglitazone. Not included in either of these groups are the alpha-glucosidase inhibitors acarbose, miglitol and voglibose. Conceptually, they do not neatly address a known physiologic defect of diabetes as do the other classes of agents. By delaying carbohydrate absorption from the small intestine, through inhibition of the breakdown of disaccharides and polysaccharides, they reduce the amount of insulin required to combat meal-related hyperglycemia. Thus, they may be considered another type of insulin-assisting agent. The most widely used forms of oral combination therapy for diabetes pair an insulin secretagogue with an insulin-assisting agent or two insulin-assisting agents together especially in more obese insulin-resistant patients. Incretins are peptide hormones from the gut that enhance insulin secretion with food. Some have other therapeutic effects including slowing gastric motility, reducing glucagon levels and curbing appetite, thus acting as both secretagogue and insulin-assisting agent. These hormones include GLP-1 and gastrointestinal insulinotropic polypeptide (GIP). In type 2 diabetes GLP-1 is deficient, while GIP is present in normal levels, but defective in its tissue action. Incretin agonists are available as the GLP-1 receptor agonists, such as exenatide and liraglutide, which deliver superphysiologic GLP-1 activity, and also GLP-1 enhancers, which include the DPP-IV enzyme inhibitors sitagliptin and vildagliptin, which raise the levels of endogenous GLP-1 and GIP, and thus restores physiologic activity by preventing their rapid proteolytic degradation. While both exenatide and the DPP-IV inhibitors have similar glycemic reduction effects, to date, exenatide is the only incretin agonist that has been associated with sustained weight loss, which likely reflects the superphysiologic activity of the drug. Incretin agonists have been shown to be safe in combination with metformin (14), sulfonylureas (15), both (16), and with thiazolidinediones.

Combining Insulin and Insulin-Assisting Agents

Later in the course of type 2 diabetes, when insulin deficiency is more marked, oral therapy alone fails to maintain control and insulin therapy is needed. Continuation of previously used oral agents while starting insulin is a form of combination therapy that has become increasingly common. This tactic allows insulin to be started with a simple regimen and titrated gradually, giving the patient time to learn the new procedures and gain confidence with insulin therapy. It also avoids the temporary loss of glycemic control that may occur when oral agents are discontinued and the dosage of insulin required is being established. Later, as a more complex insulin regimen combining basal and meal insulin becomes necessary, the benefit of ongoing oral–insulin combination therapy is less obvious, but use of insulin-assisting agents may continue to improve the results of treatment.

ORAL AGENT COMBINATION THERAPY

Secretagogues with Biguanides

This combination has become very widely used in clinical practice and, for this reason, requires few comments. The first published data on oral agent combination in the United States were for glyburide and metformin (11), as illustrated in Figure 4. Drug dosing in this study (20 mg of glyburide and up to 2550 mg of metformin daily) probably exceeded clinically effective maximum doses for both the sulfonylurea and the metformin. Sulfonylureas have hyperbolic dose–response curves. Thus, doses for most patients need not exceed one-half of the approved maximal dose because this conveys most of the long-term glycemic benefit. Although metformin has been used for many decades, dose–response data have been published (17) only in the last decade. This study showed that maximal glucose lowering occurred at 2 g/day, suggesting the most appropriate full dosage regimen should be 1000 mg twice a day. Similar benefit can be gained with combined use of other sulfonylureas or insulin secretagogues with metformin (18). The author tends to favor use of once a day sulfonylureas, such as glimepiride and extended release glipizide, in combination with metformin, because of their convenient once daily dosing and reduced risk of hypoglycemia in comparison with glyburide.

Secretagogues with Thiazolidinediones

Combining insulin secretagogues with insulin-assisting agents such as thiazolidinediones also are effective. One large trial (19) found that adding troglitazone restored glycemic control in patients with secondary failure of glyburide, in a dose-dependent manner. Similarly, a more recent study (20) found that patients failing sulfonylurea therapy had improvement with the addition of 4 mg of rosiglitazone. In addition, this trial (20) showed clearly that titration up of more than half the maximally recommended dose of glipizide failed to improve hyperglycemia over the 6 months of this trial. It is perhaps important to note that the most positive response to the thiazolidinedione in such studies was in the subjects who were obese, with mean body mass index (BMI) of 30kg/m^2 or above. Subjects in combination trials appear to have a better absolute response when their baseline glycemic control is relatively poor (A1c >9%). Thiazolidinediones have a relatively linear dose–response curve within the recommended dose range. This means that if $\geq 2\%$ reduction of HbA_{1c} is needed, maximally approved doses will usually be required to approach the glycemic target. Side effects, such as edema or weight gain may limit their use in a few patients (20). Since it is hard to predict which patients will gain excess weight, tracking weight gain is important. Presumably, maximum doses of other thiazolidinediones will yield similar improvements to those demonstrated by troglitazone combined with sulfonylureas. In the case of rosiglitazone (21), evidence for this comes from a study in which 574 patients were randomized to continue sulfonylureas, or add submaximal doses of rosiglitazone (1 or 2 mg twice daily, compared to the maximal approved 4 mg twice daily dosage) for 26 weeks in a placebo-controlled trial. The higher dose of rosiglitazone reduced HbA_{1c} by 1.0% and FPG by 44 mg/dL (2.44 mmol/L), while the lower dose reduced HbA_{1c} by 0.6% and glucose by 24 mg/dL (1.35 mmol/L). Likewise, in a study of similar size (22), pioglitazone was given at less than the 45 mg maximal dosage(15 and 30 mg), and reduced HbA_{1c} and FPG by 0.9% and 39 mg/dL (2.17 mmol/L) and 1.3% and 58 mg/dL (3.2 mmol/L) in a randomized comparison with placebo. Although studies directly comparing the effects of these agents are few, these findings suggest they have similar therapeutic power when combined at full dosage with sulfonylureas. Short-acting secretagogues, such as repaglinide, can also be used in combination with thiazolidinediones. In a 22-week randomized study (23) of troglitazone (up to 600 mg) and repaglinide (up to 4 mg pre-prandially), combination therapy had a synergistic affect, reducing HbA_{1c} by 1.7% and fasting serum glucose by 80 mg/dL in comparison to monotherapy with repaglinide alone (0.8% and 43 mg/dL) or troglitazone (0.4% and 46 mg/dL). Similar benefits have been seen with repaglinide and pioglitazone or rosiglitazone combination trials.

Secretagogues with Alpha-Glucosidase Inhibitors

Although alpha-glucosidase inhibitors are commonly used in Europe and Japan, they are less often used in the United States. Addition of an alpha-glucosidase inhibitor to an insulin secretagogue may reduce HbA_{1c} by 0.5% to 1%. For example, in a 28-week trial of acarbose added to nutrition therapy or sulfonylurea-treated subjects with inadequate control, the mean HbA_{1c} reduction was 0.66% compared with placebo (24). Much of this effect was due to reduction of postprandial hyperglycemia. The mean 1 hr PPG level declined by 41 mg/dL (2.3 mmol/L) when acarbose was added.

Combinations of Insulin-Assisting Agents

Insulin resistance may occur at multiple sites and several kinds of insulin-assisting agents exist to address these various defects, making several combinations of these agents a plausible therapeutic option. However, the glycemic effect is generally less robust than that seen in studies of combined secretagogue and sensitizer therapy. In one early study (25), 3 months of treatment with metformin reduced fasting and postprandial plasma glucose levels by 20% (58 mg/dL or 3.2 mmol/L) and 25% (87 mg/dL or 4.8 mmol/L). The same duration of troglitazone treatment exerted similar monotherapeutic benefit, with a reduction in fasting and postprandial plasma glucose of 20% (54 mg/dL or 2.9 mmol/L) and 25% (83 mg/dL or 4.6 mmol/L). The combination of these therapies resulted in a further reduction of fasting and postprandial glucose of 18% (41 mg/dL or 2.3 mmol/L) and 21% (54 mg/dL or 3.0 mmol/L) and a reduction of mean HbA_{1c} of 1.2%. Another study showed that addition of 30 mg of pioglitazone to metformin reduced HbA_{1c} by 0.83 over 16 weeks, with further improvement in an open label extension of the trial that permitted higher doses of pioglitazone (26). A third study showed that addition of full-dose (8 mg) rosiglitazone to metformin led to 1.2% reduction of HbA_{1c} over 26 weeks. These studies suggest that combining a thiazolidinedione with metformin is useful for some patients (27), especially those who are very obese and have marked insulin resistance with significant endogenous insulin remaining.

Combinations of Three Oral Agents

Relatively few reports of triple oral agent therapy exist. A retrospective study (28) examined the addition of troglitazone 600 mg daily for patients inadequately controlled on metformin and the sulfonylurea glimepiride. In this study, significant declines in HbA_{1c} occurred at 2 and 6 months (1.6% and 2.5%). In another small, non-randomized, prospective study (29) of patients offered troglitazone 400 mg for 3 months in addition to metformin and a sulfonylurea, about 62% of the patients achieved $\geq 1\%$ decline and of these 68% reached the minimal HbA_{1c} goal of 8%. Increasing the dose to 600 mg and extending the observation to 6 months did little to improve glycemia further. One randomized placebo controlled trial (30) of triple agent oral therapy that has been published found that adding 400 mg of troglitazone for 6 months to patients with poor glycemic control (HbA_{1c} 9.7%), already on a sulfonylurea and metformin, resulted in a mean 1.4% reduction of HbA_{1c}. While this was far superior to placebo, only 43% of patients in this trial reached the minimally acceptable glycemic target of <8% HbA_{1c}. The question should be raised whether use of triple oral agent therapy makes sense from a cost-effectiveness standpoint when compared with injected insulin, the main therapeutic alternative. One study (31) addressed the efficacy of added thiazolidinedione versus basal insulin. In a 24-week trial, 217 patients with HbA_{1c} ranging from 7.5% to 11% already on effective doses of sulfonylurea and metformin received insulin glargine at 10 units/day that was titrated to target an FPG of ≤ 5.5 to 6.7 mmol/L (≤ 100–120 mg/dL). In a parallel arm rosiglitazone was started at 4 mg once daily and then rosiglitazone was increased to 8 mg/day any time after 6 weeks if FPG was >5.5 mmol/L (100 g/dL). In this study reduction in HbA_{1c} was similar for the two arms (–1.7% vs. –1.5% for insulin glargine vs. rosiglitazone, respectively). Nonetheless, when baseline HbA_{1c} was >9.5%, the reduction of HbA_{1c} with insulin glargine was greater than with rosiglitazone ($P < 0.05$). Additionally, insulin glargine was associated with slightly more hypoglycemia but less weight gain, no edema, and beneficial lipid changes at a lower cost of therapy. The studies described above provide support for trying a thiazolidinedione for a few months in patients who are not successful with metformin plus a secretagogue, and have HbA_{1c} levels that are less than 9%, or those for whom using insulin is problematic.

Incretin Therapy Additions to Failing Oral Agents

The recent availability of incretin mimetics, either GLP-1 receptor agonists such as exenatide or DPP-IV inhibitors, has opened up new possibilities in combination therapy. Exenatide is an injectable synthetic analog of the Gila monster (*Heloderma suspectum*) salivary protein exendin-4. This compound has substantial homology with GLP-1 and tightly binds to GLP-1 receptors and thereby mimics the actions of native GLP-1 when given in doses of 5 or 10 mcg twice daily.

Three published trials show the use of exenatide in 30-week long studies with patients with oral agent failure with either sulfonylureas (15), metformin (14) or both (16). The design of the studies was similar. After a 4-week placebo injection run in phase, subjects were randomized to blinded administration of placebo versus exenatide 5 mcg twice daily for 1 month and then continued this dose or followed with 10 mcg twice daily. All subjects continued use of prior oral agents. When exenatide versus placebo was added to metformin, 272 patients completed the study (14). They were middle-aged (53 ± 10 years), obese (34.2 ± 5.9 BMI) and with inadequate glycemic control (HbA_{1c} $8.2 \pm 1.1\%$). At 30 weeks, the HbA_{1c} change from baseline was $-0.78 \pm 0.1\%$ (10 mcg), $-0.4 \pm 0.11\%$ (5 mcg) and $0.08 \pm 0.1\%$ for placebo; $P < 0.002$. Exenatide was associated with weight loss: -2.8 ± 0.5 kg (10 mcg), -1.6 ± 0.4 kg (5 mcg); $P < 0.001$ versus placebo. Gastrointestinal side effects including nausea, vomiting and diarrhea were more common with exenatide but lessened toward the end of the trial. In the 5 and 10 mcg groups, exenatide resulted in a placebo subtracted percentage for nausea of 11% and 22%, for vomiting 7% and 8%, and for diarrhea 4% and 8 % overall during the study. In the sulfonylurea failure study (15), the study population was similar with obese, middle-aged subjects with slightly higher baseline glycemia (HbA$_{1c}$ 8.6$\pm$1.2%). The change from baseline HbA$_{1c}$ at 30 weeks was –0.86$\pm$0.11 (10 mcg), –0.46$\pm$0.12 (5 mcg) and 0.12$\pm$0.09% (placebo); P <0.001. Weight loss was somewhat less with 10 mcg than in the metformin alone study (–1.6 kg). The third trial was for patients inadequately controlled on the combination of effective doses of sulfonylurea and metformin. Similar subjects were studied with middle-aged obese poorly controlled subjects (baseline HbA$_{1c}$ 8.5$\pm$1.0%). The change from baseline HbA$_{1c}$ occurred at 30 weeks was –0.8 + 0.1% (10 mcg), –0.6 + 0.1% (5 mcg) and + 0.2 + 0.1% (placebo); P <0.0001. Weight loss in this study averaged 1.6 kg for the 10 mcg dose group and was like the sulfonylurea alone study. A similar study has been conducted but not yet published showing comparable glycemic benefit in patients in a thiazolidinedione alone to which 5 and 10 mcg doses of exenatide were added for about 11/2 year.

Is it reasonable to choose exenatide as an alternative to basal insulin therapy? Perhaps if patients are not very far from glycemic goal. Heine et al. (32) reported a study of 551 type 2 diabetes subjects who were inadequately controlled. They were randomized to either insulin glargine once a day at bedtime versus 5 mcg for 1 month then 10 mcg of exenatide for the duration of this 26-week long trial. The results showed that baseline HbA$_{1c}$ was 8.2% for patients receiving exenatide and 8.3% for those receiving insulin glargine. By study end exenatide and insulin glargine therapies resulted in identical reduction of HbA$_{1c}$ levels by 1.11%. Exenatide reduced postprandial plasma glucose levels more than insulin glargine, while insulin glargine reduced FPG levels more than exenatide. This is particularly well illustrated in the 7-point self-monitored glucose levels before and after meals and at 3 am performed at study beginning and end (Fig. 6). Body weight decreased 2.3 kg with exenatide and increased 1.8 kg with insulin glargine. Rates of symptomatic hypoglycemia were similar, but nocturnal hypoglycemia occurred less frequently with exenatide (0.9 event/patient-year versus 2.4 events/patient-year). Gastrointestinal symptoms were more common in the exenatide group than in the insulin glargine group, including nausea (57.1% vs. 8.6%), vomiting (17.4% vs. 3.7%) and diarrhea (8.5% vs. 3.0%). The nearly identical lowering of average glycemia is noteworthy in comparison to the marked difference in prandial versus pre-prandial control, suggesting these interventions had different patterns of benefit.

In all of the studies of exenatide in which sulfonylureas were used, an increased risk of hypoglycemia occurred that sometimes required a reduction in sulfonylurea dose to reduce the risk of hypoglycemia symptoms. In patients on sulfonylureas treated with exenatide (and perhaps also with DPP-IV inhibitors), it may be appropriate to preemptively reduce sulfonylurea doses substantially if patients' lowest blood sugars are less than 100 mg/dL since the glucose-dependent insulin secretion with this combination is lost as a result of the sulfonylurea. Taken together, these studies suggest that exenatide may represent a desirable alternative for overweight patients for whom lifestyle intervention alone is insufficient in improving weight and who also need improved glycemia control but are reluctant to use insulin.

DPP-IV Inhibitors

Incretin action can also be provided by inhibiting the rapid degradation of GLP-1 and GIP. Although the levels of GLP-1 probably do not rise to a degree similar to that seen with receptor agonists such as exenatide and liraglutide, nonetheless DPP-IV inhibitors such as sitagliptin and vildagliptin are close to the glycemic lowering efficacy seen with receptor agonists. Vildagliptin (33) 50 mg once daily added to patients inadequately controlled on metformin (baseline HbA$_{1c}$ 7.7%) resulted in a placebo subtracted difference in HbA$_{1c}$ at 52 weeks of –1.0$\pm$0.2%; P <0.001. DPP-IV inhibitors do not cause nausea and vomiting and 1 year studies lack the weight reduction effect (they are weight neutral) seen with the GLP-1 agonists. This is likely due to lower levels of GLP-1 activity. Sitagliptin (34) has recently been FDA approved for use as monotherapy and as additional treatment for those not meeting glycemic goals on either metformin or a thiazolidinedione. In doses of 100 mg for patients with normal renal function in two monotherapy studies of 18 and 24 weeks duration, sitagliptin reduced HbA$_{1c}$

by 0.6% and 0.8%. Added to either metformin or pioglitazone, it further reduced HbA_{1c} by 0.7% in 24-week duration studies. DPP-IV inhibitors are weight neutral, probably due to an appetite effect of raising endogenous GLP-1 levels. Their glycemic effects on peak prandial control appear superior to effects on pre-prandial control. This should complement the primarily pre-prandial effects of metformin or thiazolidinediones.

Incretin drugs appear especially favorable for prandial glycemic control and may be favored also because of positive effects of weight loss or minimal weight gain. Prandial control has been observed by Monnier et al. (35,36) to be important particularly as HbA_{1c} nears goal (Fig. 7). Also if prandial euglycemia contributes to decreased cardiovascular risk through reducing oxidative stress then incretins could have an additional favorable action.

COMBINATION INSULIN AND ORAL AGENT THERAPY: TRANSITION TO INSULIN

Insulin therapy is eventually needed for most patients with type 2 diabetes. An evening insulin strategy is a simple way to begin insulin therapy that will achieve glycemic goals and is easily understood by patients. The rationale for evening insulin has previously been reviewed (37–39). In brief, an evening injection of intermediate or long-acting insulin addresses a fundamental need in management of type 2 diabetes by suppressing overnight endogenous glucose production and thereby preventing hyperglycemia prior to the first meal of the day. This approach is useful for most patients with type 2 diabetes, with the notable exception of patients taking morning glucocorticoid therapy.

There are several versions of this strategy, including the use of intermediate-acting insulin at bedtime, intermediate and quick-acting insulin mixed in a single injection at dinnertime, and insulin glargine or insulin detemir at bedtime. For some patients an alternate timing of glargine may be used earlier in the day; for those using large doses (0.8 units/kg) of detemir this may also be possible. Most of the evidence for these regimens comes from trials of insulin combined with a sulfonylurea alone or with metformin, with the oral agents continued while the insulin dosage is gradually increased until control is re-established.

NPH at Bedtime

Addition of an injection of NPH insulin within an hour of bedtime is usually able to restore adequate glycemic control for patients who are no longer well-controlled with one or more oral agents alone. This tactic may be best employed in leaner patients (BMI ≤ 29), who seem to need short-acting insulin at suppertime less often. A multicenter trial has shown bedtime NPH insulin plus daytime oral agents achieves glycemic control as good as insulin taken in the morning with oral agents, or mixed intermediate and regular insulin twice daily without oral agents. However, there is less weight gain with evening NPH (40). Other trials show better glycemic control with bedtime NPH plus a sulfonylurea than with a single injection of insulin alone (41,42). Evening NPH insulin also reduces free fatty acids to a greater degree than use of daytime insulin (43).

Patients can begin with a low dose of NPH insulin, usually about 10 units. They are instructed to self titrate the dose up by 2 to 4 units every 3 to 7 days based upon the stability of their fasting glycemic response. Stable patients may titrate more quickly, based upon the pattern of response, but there is little reason to hurry because glucose control will steadily improve at any rate of titration so long as the oral agents are continued. The insulin dosage required is frequently in the range of 30 to 50 units daily, or about 0.4 to 0.5 units/kg of body weight. The target for fasting glucose should be individualized and adjusted when hypoglycemia occurs, but often can be the ADA recommended 90–130 mg/dL (5–7.2 mmol/L) value in plasma-referenced home glucose-monitoring systems. Patients need to wake at a reasonably consistent time and eat breakfast consistently. Oral agents are continued, although sulfonylureas are usually given only with the first meal of the day. A randomized trial has examined the choice of daytime therapy accompanying bedtime NPH insulin (44). This study compared four different regimens in a prospective 1-year randomized controlled trial. The four regimens included bedtime insulin combined with morning insulin, glyburide alone, metformin alone, or glyburide combined with metformin. The least weight gain occurred when metformin was the only oral agent, and hypoglycemia was a limiting factor when glyburide was used.

Pre-Mixed Insulin with the Evening Meal

A second form of evening insulin that appears to work better for more obese patients (BMI ≥ 30) is the combination of morning sulfonylureas and suppertime mixed insulin, the latter commonly offered as 70/30 (70% NPH with 30% Regular) insulin. In a multicenter study using the long-acting sulfonylurea glimepiride (45), illustrated in Figure 5, patients achieved a more rapid restoration of glycemic control with self-titration of 70/30 insulin while continuing the oral agent, rather than with insulin alone. Insulin was started at 10 units and titrated weekly, seeking FPG equivalent to 140 mg/dL (7.8 mmol/L, plasma-referenced). Nearly all subjects using the combination regimen reached the titration target rapidly, but 15% of the subjects in the placebo plus insulin group dropped out, mainly due to hyperglycemia during the transition to insulin. The mean HbA$_{1c}$ declined from almost 10% to 7.6% for subjects completing the trial in both groups. The mean dose in the insulin alone group was 78 units and, for the glimepiride plus insulin combination, was 49. More subjects on insulin alone needed doses higher than 100 units daily, and so had to take more than one injection. A smaller study with a more aggressive titration scheme found better glycemic control using 70/30 insulin with the evening meal plus glyburide once daily, than with evening insulin alone (46). Premixed rapid analog mixes [e.g., lispro/neutral protamine lispro (25%/75%) and aspart/ neutral protamine aspart (30%/70%)] similarly may achieve control with somewhat more convenient meal timing of insulin. Use of pens with meals is often desirable especially for those who eat outside the home frequently. These are commonly given twice a day, sometimes more or less frequently. Garber et al. (47) have reported a small observational study using either once, twice or three times daily administration at meal time of the 70/30 aspart mixture in patients inadequately controlled or oral agents with or without basal insulin treatment. In this study, once daily administration at dinner of 70/30 reduced HbA$_{1c}$ by 1.4%, twice daily at breakfast and supper by 1.9% and thrice daily with an added lunch dose by 1.8%.

Insulin Glargine at Bedtime

A study using insulin glargine (48) suggests this agent may offer another option for starting insulin with an evening injection. In this 1-year European study, 426 subjects were randomly assigned to either insulin glargine or NPH insulin at bedtime, while continuing previous oral therapy. The therapeutic target was a fasting blood glucose < 120 mg/dL (6.7 mmol/L), using a method that was probably not plasma-referenced. The insulin dosages used (23 units for

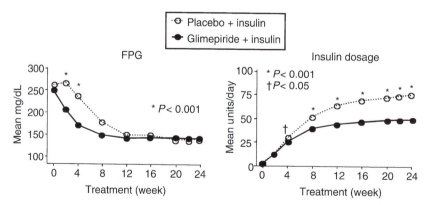

FIGURE 5 A transition strategy of adding insulin for obese patients failing oral agents using morning secretagogue plus a suppertime mixed insulin preparation (70/30 insulin combining NPH and Regular insulin). The titration of insulin dosing based on the fasting glucose achieves more rapid control with combination therapy and does so at lower insulin doses.

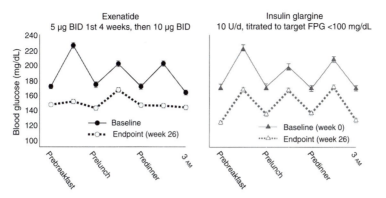

FIGURE 6 A study comparing once daily insulin glargine titrated to achieve fasting glucose control versus exenatide, a GLP-1 mimetic that is injectable twice daily. The average glycemia response is similar in this study with HbA$_{1c}$ reduced by 1.1% from 8.2% to 7.1% in both groups. A striking difference in the preprandial versus the postprandial effects of the two medications is evident.

glargine and 21 for NPH) and HbA$_{1c}$ values achieved (8.3% and 8.2%) were similar with the two insulins, but the rates of hypoglycemia were significantly less for the group using glargine (33% vs. 51% for all symptomatic hypoglycemia), despite similar average insulin doses. Nocturnal hypoglycemia occurred in less than half as many subjects using glargine (13% vs. 28%). Moreover, glucose control was better in the afternoon and evening with glargine, presumably because of its longer duration of action than NPH. The Treat to Target Trial (49) also compared insulin glargine versus NPH insulin at bedtime. Subjects in this study averaged a baseline HbA$_{1c}$ of 8.6%. Both NPH and glargine study groups were instructed to initiate doses of 10 units of insulin at bedtime and each week the dose was raised between 0 and 8 units based upon how close to goal (<5.5 mmol/L; 100 mg/dL). This forced weekly titration of dose based upon fasting glucose concentration with patient self-adjustment according to pattern of therapy response is a key concept in reaching the targeted goal of HbA$_{1c}$ <7% in about 60% of patients in this study on both NPH and glargine insulin. Subjects in this study did not need to achieve the targeted FPG because hypoglycemia would have been too frequent. Hypoglycemia overnight was more common with NPH insulin as might be expected based upon the differences in kinetics of NPH versus glargine with the former having a greater peak effect usually within the first 4 to 8 hours after s.c. administration.

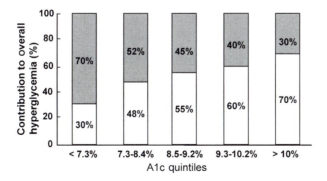

FIGURE 7 The relative contribution of fasting plasma glucose (FPG; show in the open bars) and the postprandial plasma glucose (PPG; shown in the shaded bars) to overall hyperglycemia. An area under the curve analysis suggests that as HbA1c approaches the ADA goal for minimum desirable glycemic control, the PPG makes a greater contribution to overall hyperglycemia. Conversely, as the HbA1c rises far from goal, the contribution of FPG to overall hyperglycemia is greater. For patients with poor hyperglycemia a focus on the fasting glucose thus becomes an important priority. As patient approaches targeted glycemic goals, greater attention should be directed to postprandial glycemia.

Insulin Detemir

Insulin detemir is a new formulation of intermediate to long-acting insulin with a duration of effect in type 1 diabetes single dose studies that is dose dependent. Based upon a common dosage of 0.4 units/kg an average duration of action of about 20 hours is predicted. With higher doses a longer duration approaching 24 hours is achieved (50). In one study (51), twice daily insulin therapy with NPH versus detemir in type 2 diabetes subjects inadequately controlled (HbA_{1c} 8.5% and 8.6% for NPH and detemir, respectively) on therapy (mostly metformin plus secretagogues with some use of glucosidase inhibitors and about 30% of subjects not on oral agents when insulin was used). A total of 475 subjects were randomized to participate in a 24-week study comparing twice daily administration of these two insulins at breakfast and bedtime. Starting with 10 units per injection subjects were instructed to titrate doses every 3 days based upon pre-dinner and pre-breakfast self-monitored glucose averages from 2 up to 10 units per injection. At 24 weeks subjects with insulin detemir decreased HbA_{1c} by 1.8% to an average value of 6.8% while subjects on NPH decreased the HbA_{1c} by 1.9% to an average value of 6.6%. Most subjects (about 70%) achieved HbA_{1c} less than 7% but more subjects on detemir achieved the goal without hypoglycemia. Overall hypoglycemia was significantly less *on* detemir, which by non-inferiority analysis was comparable in overall glycemic lowering efficacy to NPH. Doses of insulin were a bit higher than might have been expected (36.1 units am and 29.5 units pm for detemir; and 25.3 units am and 19.7 pm for NPH given that the average BMI of these patients was a little over 29. Detemir can be administered once in the evening or twice daily. Its desirable features include a lower rate of hypoglycemia, somewhat greater consistency in glycemic response from day to day, and possibly a reduced tendency for weight gain.

Use of Dry Powder Inhaled Insulin

Recently the approval of the first orally inhaled insulin for delivery by pulmonary capillaries to the body has begun to permit patients to choose insulin without concerns about injections. While injection delivery will not represent a barrier for many patients, inhaled insulin may encourage the earlier use of insulin for some reluctant patients and providers. In monotherapy studies with very poorly controlled patients (HbA_{1c} 9.5–9.6%), it can lower HbA_{1c} greater than 2% (52). In studies comparing the addition of inhaled insulin to an oral regimen versus substituting inhaled insulin for dual therapy in poorly controlled subjects, change in HbA_{1c} was −1.67% versus −1.18%, respectively (53). Use of inhaled insulin has substantial meal effects and it is intended for use primarily at meal times. Importantly, however, it also appears to have a significant ability to contribute to fasting glucose lowering, perhaps as a result of a longer duration of action than rapid acting analogs. Thus, one may need to anticipate some caution for avoiding overnight and between-meal hypoglycemia in well controlled patients. It seems unlikely that inhaled insulin will fully replace basal insulin treatment, but, like basal insulin, it may form a bridge from oral agents (with or without incretin mimetics) to more complex insulin regimens.

MULTIPLE INJECTIONS OF INSULIN AND INSULIN-ASSISTING AGENTS

Over time, glycemic control will eventually no longer be maintained by an evening injection of insulin plus oral agents, and additional doses of insulin will be needed. Physicians may choose to begin with more than one injection of insulin and not continue oral agents but, in some cases, this approach may not achieve the desired level of control. In either situation, a decision must be made on the possible value of using (or continuing to use) one or more oral agents along with multiple injections of insulin. Relatively little guidance on this point is provided by published studies.

In general it appears that use of a basal insulin regimen is probably reasonable in patients whose initial HbA_{1c} concentration is less than 9%. However, for those where the glycemic control is significantly worse, it unlikely that they will achieve recommended glycemia goals without use of some meal insulin. For some patient with type 2 diabetes, there are strong advocates of the convenience and use of fixed ratio rapid analog insulin mixtures including those such as 75/25 (neutral protamine lispro/lispro) and 70/30 (neutral protamine aspart/aspart). One study (54) suggests that for patients with HbA_{1c} values in excess of 9.5%, they are superior to a basal insulin-like glargine. Caution should be used however in patients who monitor infrequently or whose schedules and eating habits are inconsistent as these fixed ratio insulins appear to increase the likelihood of hypoglycemia in some studies. The author finds the addition of basal insulin plus insulin at the largest meal of the day may be a strategy that works well for many type 2 diabetes patients who eat little during the day but consume large meals in the evening.

Insulin and Sulfonylureas

Several reviews have examined the evidence regarding the combination of a sulfonylurea with multiple injections of insulin (55–57). The majority of studies show some benefit, presumably based on enhancement of remaining endogenous insulin secretion, but this effect is most apparent at the time of insulin initiation, and the benefit is likely to diminish as endogenous insulin secretion continues to decline. In general, the author discontinues secretagogues once more than one injection of insulin is necessary. Sulfonylureas may be most useful when a pure basal insulin, such as glargine or detemir, is used with metformin and/or thiazolidinediones, as these other agents provide effects primarily on fasting hyperglycemia and their prandial effects depend mostly on their pre-prandial glucose lowering. Although not approved for use with insulin, nor yet studied in this combination, it is possible that GLP-1 mimetics such as exenatide may be combined with basal insulin. One might expect similar complementary fasting and prandial effects with glargine and DPP-IV inhibitors although no studies are yet available showing this.

Insulin with Metformin

A modest number of studies suggest better glycemic control with the combination of insulin and metformin than with insulin alone (57), and it is likely that enhancing the effectiveness of endogenous insulin is not the only benefit. Perhaps the most compelling evidence comes from a small 24-week, placebo-controlled study of the addition of metformin to insulin therapy that was aggressively intensified seeking optimal control (58). Forty-three patients previously taking insulin, but with poor glycemic control, were randomized to receive either a placebo or metformin, while insulin therapy was optimized using two or more injections of NPH and Regular insulin. Metformin-treated patients achieved a 2.5% reduction of HbA_{1c} (from 9.0 to 6.5%), while those taking insulin alone had a smaller 1.6% reduction (9.1% to 7.5%). With combination therapy, a slight reduction of insulin dosage occurred (96 to 92 units daily), but with insulin alone a greater dosage was used (102 to 125 units daily). Moreover, the patients taking insulin alone gained about 3 kg, while little change of weight occurred despite the impressive improvement of control with insulin–metformin combination therapy. Other studies have documented a similar weight-limiting effect of metformin during insulin treatment (44,57), and this may be of great importance, both for assisting glycemic control and minimizing cardiovascular risk.

Insulin with Thiazolidinediones

The now discontinued drug troglitazone showed considerable benefit when added to insulin in a randomized, controlled trial (59). Troglitazone at doses of 200 and 400 mg were compared with placebo over 26 weeks in 350 patients taking >30 units of insulin daily and having suboptimal glycemic control. Mean HbA_{1c} was reduced 0.8% and 1.4%, and fasting serum glucose was reduced 39 mg/dL (1.9 mmol/L) and 45 mg/dL (2.7 mmol/L) with the two doses of troglitazone respectively. This improvement occurred despite a reduction of 11% and 29% in insulin dose for the lower and higher troglitazone doses, respectively. Troglitazone has been withdrawn from the market due to serious liver toxicity, but similar findings are available for rosiglitazone in combination with insulin. A randomized, controlled trial (60) studied 319 subjects with suboptimal glycemic control (HbA_{1c} >7.5%) despite treatment with at least 30 units of insulin daily. After an 8-week period of insulin standardization, subjects were randomized to placebo, 4 mg, or 8 mg of rosiglitazone in addition to insulin. After a 26-week follow-up, the higher dose of rosiglitazone resulted in a 1.2% mean reduction of HbA_{1c} (to 7.9%) and a 45 mg/dL (2.5 mmol/L) reduction of fasting glucose, and there was a 12% mean reduction in daily insulin dose. Data with pioglitazone suggest similar benefits. One feature that distinguishes metformin from the thiazolidinediones is the weight gain associated with the latter class of drugs. On occasion hypoglycemia may occur with the combination of insulin and thiazolidinediones. Although this side effect is absent or not significant for most patients, occasionally marked weight-gain occurs. This is partly due to fluid retention, but increased adipose tissue mass occurs as well. Clinically apparent peripheral edema is common, and there is much concern about the possibility of congestive heart failure in susceptible persons, especially when a thiazolidinedione is used together with insulin. The studies of rosiglitazone or pioglitazone combined with insulin are reasonably reassuring (61). The rates of congestive heart failure occurring during trials, from which patients with severe heart disease were excluded, were in the 1% to 2% range. Some patients using these agents, with (or without) insulin, have dramatic improvements of glycemic control, better information on the risk to benefit ratio remains needed, including more data on the cardioprotective effects independent of improvement of glycemic control and the relative risks of congestive heart failure beyond that from the ProACTive trial (13). A consensus statement from the American Heart Association and the American Diabetes Association suggests caution with the combination of insulin and thiazolidinediones in patients with known risk factors even absent a prior clinical history of heart failure (61). Close monitoring of weight gain and fluid retention and a precautionary reduction or rarely stopping of thiazolidinediones may be warranted in those deemed at risk.

Alpha-glucosidase Inhibitors with Insulin

As with oral agent combination therapy with alpha-glucosidase inhibitors, a modest benefit on glucose-control may be seen when these drugs are combined with insulin (62). However, perhaps because of the effectiveness of short-acting insulin in limiting postprandial hyperglycemia, this combination is not widely used. A point in favor of the combination, however, is the lack of weight-gain accompanying use of this class of oral agents.

Gut Peptides and Their Analogs with Insulin

Analogs of gut peptides, which appear to have important physiologic roles in normal regulation of plasma glucose, are now being used therapeutically. Amylin, a 37 amino acid peptide that is localized to the pancreatic islets and co-secreted with insulin, slows gastric emptying, reduces glucagon secretion, and induces satiety with the latter effect probably mediated in the brain (63). Plasma levels of the beta-cell co-hormone amylin are reduced (or lacking) in patients treated with insulin. Pramlintide is an analog of amylin that is able to mimic its actions and has been tested in therapeutic trials in both type 1 and type 2 diabetes. In a 4-week trial in type 2 diabetes, pramlintide lowered fructosamine and HbA_{1c} when used in doses of 30–60 µg injected three or four times daily (64). While HbA_{1c} was reduced only about 0.5%, this change is both statistically and potentially clinically significant in light of the study's short duration. Longer term studies (65,66) suggest maintained moderate weight loss and A1c improvement usually 0.6% to 0.7%. This agent may have other beneficial effects, notably weight-control, and it may therefore prove useful as an adjunct to insulin therapy in the future.

SUMMARY

Combined oral agent therapy offers superior efficacy and an opportunity to minimize side effects. In selecting oral combinations, an important objective is minimizing the number of tablets needed and their cost, and this practical imperative has led to various formulations, including several with two agents in a single tablet. Early use of combination therapy is recommended in consensus algorithms (67). Combining oral agents even with the addition of incretin mimetics may delay the need for insulin injections, but when insulin is needed it should be promptly started. Continuing oral agents while starting a single evening injection of insulin is a simple and reliable way to make the transition to insulin therapy (68). Use of inhaled insulin and incretin mimetics may represent a reasonable alternative for some patients for a while. Poor glycemic control with a single injection plus a secretagogue, insulin-assisting agents, or both, may signal a decline of endogenous insulin and call for further daily injections often to control prandial hyperglycemia (69); at this point secretagogues are usually stopped. Similarly, poor glycemic control with two or more injections of insulin alone may call for addition of an insulin-assisting agent, such as metformin or a thiazolidinedione. The glycemic and non-glycemic benefits, as well as risks, of combining insulin-assisting agents while intensifying insulin therapy must be better defined. It seems likely that such combinations will be necessary for most patients with type 2 diabetes to achieve the currently recommended minimum glycemic target ($<7\%$ HbA_{1c}), and especially the more ambitious targets that have been proposed ($\leq6.5\%$ or 6% HbA_{1c}). Additional oral or injected agents, such as pramlintide and incretin mimetics, are becoming available and offer further options for combination therapy to achieve the glycemic targets of the future.

REFERENCES

1. Nathan DM, Singer DE, Godine JE, Perlmuter LC. Non-insulin-dependent diabetes in older patients. Complications and risk factors. Am J Med 1986; 81:837–42.
2. United Kingdom Prospective Diabetes Study Group. Intensive blood–glucose control with sulphonylureas or insulin compared with conventional treatment and risk of complications in patients with type 2 diabetes (UKPDS 33). Lancet 1998; 352:837–53.
3. United Kingdom Prospective Diabetes Study Group. Effect of intensive blood–glucose control with metformin on complications in overweight patients with type 2 diabetes (UKPDS 34). Lancet 1998 352:854–65.
4. UKPDS Study Group. Overview of 6 years' therapy of type II diabetes: a progressive disease (UKPDS16). Diabetes 1995; 44:1249–58.
5. Turner RC, Cull CA, Frighi V, Holman RR. Glycemic control with diet, sulfonylurea, metformin, or insulin in patients with type 2 diabetes mellitus: progressive requirement for multiple therapies (UKPDS 49). J Am Med Assoc 1999; 281:2005–12.
6. Polonsky KS, Sturis J, Bell GI. Non-insulin dependent diabetes mellitus: a genetically programmed failure of the beta cell to compensate for insulin resistance. N Engl J Med 1996 334:777–83.
7. Haffner SM, D'Agostino R Jr, Mykkanen L, et al. Insulin sensitivity in subjects with type 2 diabetes. Relationship to cardiovascular risk factors: the Insulin Resistance Atherosclerosis Study. Diabetes Care 1999; 22:562–8.
8. Haffner SM, Stern MP, Hazuda HP, et al. Cardiovascular risk factors in confirmed prediabetic individuals: does the clock for coronary heart disease start ticking before the onset of clinical diabetes? J Am Med Assoc 1990; 263:2893–8.
9. Haffner SM, Lehto S, Ronnemaa T, et al. Mortality from coronary heart disease in subjects with type 2 diabetes and in nondiabetic subjects with and without prior myocardial infarction. N Engl J Med 1998; 339:229–34.
10. DeFronzo RA. Pharmacologic therapy for type 2 diabetes mellitus. Ann Intern Med 1999; 131: 281–303, [Review].
11. DeFronzo RA, Goodman AM. Efficacy of metformin in patients with non-insulin-dependent diabetes mellitus. The Multicenter Metformin Study Group. N Engl J Med 1995; 333:541–9.
12. Hermann LS, Schersten B, Bitzen PO, et al. Therapeutic comparison of metformin and sulfonylurea, alone and in various combinations. A double-blind controlled study. Diabetes Care 1994; 17:1100–9.
13. Dormandy JA, Charbonnel B, Eckland DJA, et al. Secondary prevention of macrovascular events in patients with type 2 diabetes in the PROactive Study (PROspective pioglitAzone Clinical Trial In macroVascular Events): a randomised controlled trial. Lancet 2005; 366(9493):1279–89.
14. DeFronzo RA, Ratner RE, Han J, Kim DD, Fineman MS, Baron AD. Effects of Exenatide (Exendin-4) on glycemic control and weight over 30 weeks in metformin-treated patients with type 2 diabetes. Diabetes Care 2005; 28:1092–100.
15. Buse JB, Henry RR, Han J, Kim DD, Fineman MS, Baron AD. Effects of exenatide (exendin-4) on glycemic control over 30 weeks in sulfonylurea-treated patients with type 2 diabetes. Diabetes Care 2004; 27:2628–35.
16. Kendall DM, Riddle MC, Rosenstock J, et al. Effects of exenatide (exendin-4) on glycemic control over 30 weeks in patients with type 2 diabetes treated with metformin and a sulfonylurea. Diabetes Care 2005; 28:1083–91.
17. Garber AJ, Duncan TG, Goodman AM, et al. Efficacy of metformin in type II diabetes: results of a double-blind, placebo-controlled, dose response trial. Am J Med 1997; 103:491–7.

18. Moses R, Slobodniuk R, Boyages S, et al. Effect of repaglinide addition to metformin monotherapy on glycemic control in patients with type 2 diabetes. Diabetes Care 1999; 22:119–24.
19. Horton ES, Whitehouse F, Ghazzi MN, et al. Troglitazone in combination with sulfonylurea restores glycemic control in patients with type 2 diabetes. The Troglitazone Study Group. Diabetes Care 1998; 21:1462–9.
20. Rosenstock J, Goldstein BJ, Vinik AI, et al. Effect of early addition of rosiglitazone to sulphonylurea therapy in older type 2 diabetes patients (>60 years): the Rosiglitazone Early vs. SULphonylurea Titration (RESULT) study. Diabetes Obes Metab 2006; 8:49–57.
21. Wolffenbuttel BH, Gomis R, Squatrito S, et al Addition of low dose rosiglitazone to sulphonylurea therapy improves glycaemic control in Type 2 diabetic patients. Diabet Med 2000; 17:40–7.
22. Kipnes MS, Krosnick A, Rendell MS, et al. Pioglitazone hydrochloride in combination with sulfonylurea therapy improves glycemic control in patients with type 2 diabetes mellitus: a randomized, placebo-controlled study. Am J Med 2001; 111:10–7.
23. Raskin P, Jovanovic L, Berger S, et al. Repaglinide troglitazone combination therapy: improved glycemic control in type 2 diabetes. Diabetes Care 2000; 23:979–83.
24. Buse J, Hart K, Minasi L. The PROTECT Study: final results of a large multicenter postmarketing study in patients with type 2 diabetes. Precise Resolution of Optimal Titration to Enhance Current Therapies. Clin Ther 1998; 20:257–69.
25. Inzucchi SE, Maggs DG, Spollett GR, et al. Efficacy and metabolic effects of metformin and troglitazone in type II diabetes mellitus. N Engl J Med 1998; 338:867–72.
26. Einhorn D, Rendell M, Rosenzweig J, et al. Pioglitazone hydrochloride in combination with metformin in the treatment of type 2 diabetes mellitus: a randomized, placebo-controlled study. The Pioglitazone 027 Study Group. Clin Ther 2000; 22:1395–409.
27. Rosenstock J, Rood J, Cobitz A, Huang C, Garber A. Improvement in glycaemic control with rosiglitazone/metformin fixed-dose combination therapy in patients with type 2 diabetes with very poor glycaemic control. Diabetes Obes Metab 2006; 8:643–9.
28. Ovalle F, Bell DSH. Triple oral antidiabetic therapy in type 2 diabetes mellitus. Endocr Pract 1998; 4:146–7.
29. Gavin LA, Barth J, Arnold D, Shaw R. Troglitazone add on therapy to a combination of sulfonylureas plus metformin achieved and sustained effective diabetes control. Endocr Pract 2000; 6:305–10.
30. Yale J-F, Valiquett TR, Ghazzi MN, et al. The effect of a thiazolidinedione drug, troglitazone, on glycemia in patients with type 2 diabetes mellitus poorly controlled with sulfonylurea and metformin. A multi-center, randomized, double blind, placebo-controlled trial. Ann Intern Med 2001; 134:737–45.
31. Rosenstock J. Triple therapy in type 2 diabetes: insulin glargine or rosiglitazone added to combination therapy of sulfonylurea plus metformin in insulin-naive patients: response to hamid and simmons. Diabetes Care 2006; 29:23–32.
32. Heine RJ, Van Gaal LF, Johns D, Mihm MJ, Widel MH, Brodows RG, for the GWAA Study Group. Exenatide versus insulin glargine in patients with suboptimally controlled type 2 diabetes: a randomized trial. Ann Intern Med 2005; 143:559–69.
33. Ahren B, Pacini G, Foley JE, Schweizer A. Improved meal-related beta-cell function and insulin sensitivity by the dipeptidyl peptidase-IV inhibitor vildagliptin in metformin-treated patients with type 2 diabetes over 1 year. Diabetes Care 2005; 28:1936–40.
34. Raz I, Hanefeld M, Xu L, et al. Efficacy and safety of the dipeptidyl peptidase-4 inhibitor sitagliptin as monotherapy in patients with type 2 diabetes mellitus. Diabetologia 2006; 49(11):2564–71.
35. Monnier L, Mas E, Ginet C, et al. Activation of oxidative stress by acute glucose fluctuations compared with sustained chronic hyperglycemia in patients with type 2 diabetes. JAMA 2006; 295: 1681–7.
36. Monnier L, Lapinski H, Colette C. Contributions of fasting and postprandial plasma glucose increments to the overall diurnal hyperglycemia of type 2 diabetic patients: variations with increasing levels of HbA(1c). Diabetes Care 2003; 26:881–5.
37. Riddle MC. Evening insulin strategy. Diabetes Care 1990; 13:676–86.
38. Riddle MC. Combined insulin and sulfonylurea therapy for type 2 diabetes mellitus. Diabetes Res Clin Pract 1991; 11:3–8.
39. Riddle MC. Combined therapy with a sulfonylurea plus evening insulin: safe, reliable, and becoming routine. Hormone Metabol Res 1996; 28:430–3 [Review].
40. Yki-Järvinen H, Kauppila M, Kujansuu E, et al. Comparison of insulin regimens in patients with non-insulin-dependent diabetes mellitus. N Engl J Med 1992; 327:1426–33.
41. Riddle MC, Hart JS, Bouma DJ, et al. Efficacy of bedtime NPH insulin with daytime sulfonylurea for subpopulation of type II diabetic subjects. Diabetes Care 1989; 12:623–9.
42. Shank ML, Del Prato S, DeFronzo RA. Bedtime insulin/daytime glipizide. Effective therapy for sulfonylurea failures in NIDDM. Diabetes 1995; 44:165–72.
43. Taskinen MR, Sane T, Helve E, et al. Bedtime insulin for suppression of overnight free-fatty acid, blood glucose, and glucose production in NIDDM. Diabetes 1989; 38:580–8.

44. Yki-Jarvinen H, Ryysy L, Nikkila K, et al Comparison of bedtime insulin regimens in patients with type 2 diabetes mellitus: a randomized, controlled trial. Ann Intern Med 1999; 130:389–96.

45. Riddle MC, Schneider J. Beginning insulin treatment of obese patients with evening 70/30 insulin plus glimepiride versus insulin alone. Glimepiride Combination Group. Diabetes Care 1998; 217:1052–7.

46. Riddle M, Hart J, Bingham P, et al. Combined therapy for obese type 2 diabetes: suppertime mixed insulin with daytime sulfonylurea. Am J Med Sci 1992; 303:151–6.

47. Garber AJ, Wahlen J, Wahl T, et al. Attainment of glycaemic goals in type 2 diabetes with once-, twice-, or thrice-daily dosing with biphasic insulin aspart 70/30 (The 1-2-3 study). Diabet Obes Metab 2006; 8:58–66.

48. Yki-Jarvinen H, Dressler A, Ziemen M, HOE 901/300s Study Group. Less nocturnal hypoglycemia and better post-dinner glucose control with bedtime insulin glargine compared with bedtime NPH insulin during insulin combination therapy in type 2 diabetes. HOE 901/3002 Study Group. Diabetes Care 2000; 23:1130–6.

49. Riddle MC, Rosenstock J, Gerich J. The treat-to-target trial: randomized addition of glargine or human NPH insulin to oral therapy of type 2 diabetic patients. Diabetes Care 2003; 26:3080–6.

50. Plank J, Bodenlenz M, Sinner F, et al. A double-blind, randomized, dose-response study investigating the pharmacodynamic and pharmacokinetic properties of the long-acting insulin analog detemir. Diabetes Care 2005; 28:1107–12.

51. Hermansen K, Davies M, Derezinski T, et al. on behalf of the Levemir Treat-to-Target Study Group. A 26-week, randomized, parallel, treat-to-target trial comparing insulin detemir with NPH insulin as add-on therapy to oral glucose-lowering drugs in insulin-naive people with type 2 diabetes. Diabetes Care 2006; 29:1269–74.

52. DeFronzo RA, Bergenstal RM, Cefalu WT, et al. For the Exubera Phase III Study Group. Efficacy of inhaled insulin in patients with type 2 diabetes not controlled with diet and exercise: a 12-week, randomized, comparative trial. Diabetes Care 2005; 28:1922–8.

53. Rosenstock J, Zinman B, Murphy LJ, et al. Inhaled insulin improves glycemic control when substituted for or added to oral combination therapy in type 2 diabetes: a randomized, controlled trial. Ann Intern Med 2005; 143:549–58.

54. Raskin P, Allen E, Hollander P, et al. For the INITIATE Study Group. Initiating insulin therapy in type 2 diabetes: a comparison of biphasic and basal insulin analogs. Diabetes Care 2005; 28:260–5.

55. Pugh JA, Wagner ML, Sawyer J, et al. Is combination sulfonylurea and insulin therapy useful in NIDDM patients? A meta-analysis. Diabetes Care 1992; 15:953–9.

56. Johnson JL, Wolf SL, Kabadi UM. Efficacy of insulin and sulfonylurea combination therapy in type 2 diabetes. A meta-analysis of the randomized placebo-controlled trials. Arch Intern Med 1996; 156:259–64.

57. Yki-Jarvinen H. Combination therapies with insulin in type 2 diabetes. Diabetes Care 2001; 24:758–67.

58. Aviles-Santa L, Sinding J, Raskin P, et al. Effects of metformin in patients with poorly controlled, insulin-treated type 2 diabetes mellitus. A randomized, double-blind, placebo-controlled trial. Ann Intern Med 2000; 284:472–7.

59. Schwartz S, Raskin P, Fonseca V, Graveline JF. Effect of troglitazone in insulin-treated patients with type II diabetes mellitus. Troglitazone and Exogenous Insulin Study Group. N Engl J Med 1998; 338:861–6.

60. Raskin P, Rendell M, Riddle MC, et al. A randomized trial of rosiglitazone therapy in patients with inadequately controlled insulin-treated type 2 diabetes. Diabetes Care 2001; 24:1226–32.

61. Nesto RW, Bell D, Bonow RO, et al. Thiazolidinedione use, fluid retention, and congestive heart failure: a consensus statement from the American Heart Association and American Diabetes Association. Diabetes Care 2004; 27(1):256–63.

62. Hollander P, Pi-Sunyer X, Coniff RF. Acarbose in the treatment of type I diabetes. Diabetes Care 1997; 20:248–53.

63. Young AA. Amylin's physiology and its role in diabetes. Curr Opin Endocrinol Diabetes 1997; 4:282–90.

64. Thompson RG, Pearson L, Schoenfeld SL, Kolterman OG. Diabetes Care 1998; 21:987–93.

65. Ratner RE, Want LL, Fineman MS, et al. Adjunctive therapy with the amylin analogue pramlintide leads to a combined improvement in glycemic and weight control in insulin-treated subjects with type 2 diabetes. Diabetes Technol Ther 2002; 4:51–61.

66. Hollander PA, Levy P, Fineman MS, et al. Pramlintide as an adjunct to insulin therapy improves long-term glycemic and weight control in patients with type 2 diabetes: a 1-year randomized controlled trial. Diabetes Care 2003; 26:784–90.

67. Nathan DM, Buse JB, Davidson MB, et al. Management of hyperglycemia in type 2 diabetes: a consensus algorithm for the initiation and adjustment of therapy: a consensus statement from the

American Diabetes Association and the European Association for the Study of Diabetes. Diabetes Care 1006; 29:1963–72.

68. Mooradian AD, Bernbaum M, Albert SG. Narrative review: a rational approach to starting insulin therapy. Ann Intern Med 2006; 145:125–34.

69. Karl DM. The use of bolus insulin and advancing insulin therapy in type 2 diabetes. Curr Diab Rep 2004; 4:352–7.

16 | Hypoglycemia in Type 2 Diabetes

Philip E. Cryer
Washington University School of Medicine, St. Louis, Missouri, U.S.A.

HYPOGLYCEMIA: THE LIMITING FACTOR

Comprehensive treatment, including glycemic control, makes a difference for people with diabetes. Glycemic control prevents or delays the microvascular complications—retinopathy, nephropathy and neuropathy—of both type 1 diabetes (1) and type 2 diabetes (2); it may also reduce macrovascular events (3,4). However, because of the imperfections of all current treatment regimens, iatrogenic hypoglycemia is the limiting factor in the glycemic management of diabetes (5). Were it not for the potentially devastating effects of hypoglycemia on the brain—which requires a continuous supply of glucose from the circulation—diabetes would be rather easy to treat. Enough insulin, or any effective drug, to lower plasma glucose concentrations to or below the normal range would eliminate the symptoms of hyperglycemia, prevent acute hyperglycemic complications (ketoacidosis, hyperosmolar syndrome), almost assuredly prevent the long-term microvascular complications (1,2) and likely reduce atherosclerotic risk to baseline (3,4). But the effects of hypoglycemia on the brain are real, and the glycemic management of diabetes is therefore complex.

Iatrogenic hypoglycemia is, in fact, the limiting factor in the glycemic management of diabetes (5). It causes recurrent morbidity in most people with type 1 diabetes and many with type 2 diabetes, and is sometimes fatal. In addition, even asymptomatic episodes compromise defenses against subsequent hypoglycemia by causing hypoglycemia-associated autonomic failure (HAAF)—the syndromes of defective glucose counterregulation and hypoglycemia unawareness—and thus a vicious cycle of recurrent hypoglycemia. Finally, the barrier of hypoglycemia precludes maintenance of euglycemia over a lifetime of diabetes and thus full realization of the vascular benefits of glycemic control. For example, in the Diabetes Control and Complications Trial in type 1 diabetes, retinopathy developed or progressed in 14% of the patients treated intensively (compared with 32% in those treated conventionally) (1). In the UK Prospective Diabetes Study (UKPDS) in type 2 diabetes, any microvascular endpoint was reached in 8% of the patients treated intensively (compared with 11% of those treated conventionally) (2). Similarly, there is a direct relationship between atherosclerotic events and mean glycemia. However, it appears that lower plasma glucose concentrations over time are required to reduce macrovascular complications than to reduce microvascular complications (Fig. 1) (4).

The topic of hypoglycemia, including hypoglycemia in diabetes, has been reviewed in detail (5,6). The focus in this chapter is on iatrogenic hypoglycemia in type 2 diabetes in the context of the larger body of knowledge concerning hypoglycemia in type 1 diabetes.

FREQUENCY OF HYPOGLYCEMIA

Hypoglycemia is a fact of life for most people with established (i.e., C-peptide negative) type 1 diabetes (5,6). Those attempting to achieve some degree of glycemic control suffer untold numbers of episodes of asymptomatic hypoglycemia; plasma glucose concentrations may be <50 mg/dL (2.8 mmol/L) 10% of the time. They suffer an average of two episodes of symptomatic hypoglycemia per week—thousands over a lifetime of diabetes—and episodes of severe, at least temporarily disabling hypoglycemia approximately once a year (Table 1). Indeed, an estimated 2% to 4% of deaths of people with type 1 diabetes have been attributed to hypoglycemia.

Over a lifetime of diabetes, the incidence of iatrogenic hypoglycemia is considerably lower in type 2 diabetes than in type 1 diabetes. As discussed later, this likely reflects intact defenses against falling plasma glucose concentrations early in the course of the disease.

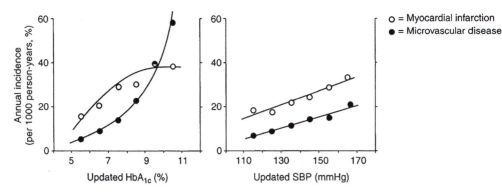

FIGURE 1 Relationship between updated systolic blood pressure (SBP) (*right*) and updated HbA$_{1C}$ (*left*), and the incidence of microvascular complications (closed symbols) and macrovascular, specifically myocardial infarction, complications (open symbols) of type 2 diabetes in the UKPDS. *Source*: From Ref. 4.

Ascertainment of hypoglycemia is a challenge. Asymptomatic episodes will be missed unless they are detected by routine glucose monitoring. Mild to moderate symptomatic episodes may not be recognized. Even if recognized, they are soon forgotten. Episodes of severe hypoglycemia (those requiring the assistance of another person) are more dramatic events that are more likely to be recalled (by the patient or by a witness). Therefore, when based on patient recall, estimates of the severe hypoglycemia event rates are more reliable although they represent only a small fraction of the hypoglycemic experience.

Hypoglycemia occurs in people with type 2 diabetes treated with insulin or with a sulfonylurea or another insulin secretagogue such as repaglinide or nateglinide. Insulin sensitizers (e.g., metformin or a thiazolidinedione), GLP-1 analogues or receptor agonists and DPP-IV inhibitors should not cause hypoglycemia when used as monotherapy, although metformin has been reported to do so (Table 2) (7). In general, insulin secretion decreases appropriately as plasma glucose concentrations decline, and hypoglycemia does not occur, when these drugs are used. However, all of these increase the risk of hypoglycemia when used with an insulin secretagogue or insulin. In that regard, it should be recalled that the majority of people with type 2 diabetes ultimately require treatment with insulin.

Severe hypoglycemia event rates have been reported to range from 62 to 170 episodes per 100 patient-years in type 1 diabetes and from 3 to 73 episodes per 100 patient-years in insulin-treated type 2 diabetes (Table 1). Hypoglycemia event rates in the UKPDS in type 2 diabetes have not been reported, but 11.2% of the patients treated with insulin and 3.3% of

TABLE 1 Severe Hypoglycemia during Aggressive Therapy of Diabetes

	Episodes per 100 patient-years
Type 1 diabetes	
Edinburgh series (*Diabet Med* 1993; 10:238)	170
Utrecht series (*Diabetes Care* 2000; 23:1467)	150
Danish-British multicenter survey (*Diabet Metab Res Rev* 2004; 20:479)	130
Tayside series (*Diabetic Med* 2005; 22:749)	115
Stockholm diabetes intervention study (*Diabetes* 1994; 43:313)	110
Diabetes control and complications trial (*N Engl J Med* 1993; 329:977)	62
Type 2 diabetes	
Edinburgh series (*Diabet Med* 1993; 10:238)	73
Tayside series (*Diabet Med* 2005; 22:749)	35
Veterans affairs pump study[a] (*J Am Med Assoc* 1996; 276:1322)	10
Veterans affairs cooperative study (*Diabetes Care* 1993; 8:1113)	3

[a] Multiple daily insulin injection group.

TABLE 2 Cumulative Incidence of Hypoglycemia in Type 2 Diabetes over 6 years in the UKPDS

Therapy[a]	n	HbA$_{1c}$ (%)	Percent with hypoglycemia	
			Any	Major[b]
Diet	379	8.0	3.0	0.15
Sulfonylurea	922	7.1	45.0	3.3
Insulin	689	7.1	76.0	11.2[c]
Diet	297	8.2	2.8	0.4
Metformin	251	7.4	17,6	2.4

[a] Taking assigned medication.
[b] Requiring medical assistance or admission to hospital.
[c] Compared with severe hypoglycemia (that requiring the assistance of another individual) in 65% of type 1 diabetes over 6.5 years in the DCCT[1].
Abbreviation: UKPDS, U.K. Prospective Diabetes Study.

those treated with a sulfonylurea suffered a hypoglycemic event requiring medical assistance over 6 years (Table 2) (7). Stated differently, the data indicate a relative risk of major hypoglycemia, as defined in the UKPDS, of six during treatment with metformin, 22 during treatment with a sulfonylurea and 75 during treatment with insulin (Table 2).

Population-based data indicate that the severe hypoglycemia event rate in insulin-treated type 2 diabetes is approximately 30% of that in type 1 diabetes (35 vs. 115 per 100 patient-years) (8) and that event rates for hypoglycemia requiring emergency medical treatment in insulin-treated type 2 diabetes range from 40% (9) to 100% (10) of those in type 1 diabetes. Since type 2 diabetes is approximately 20-fold more prevalent than type 1 diabetes, and since more than half of people with type 2 diabetes ultimately require treatment with insulin, most episodes of severe iatrogenic hypoglycemia occur in people with type 2 diabetes.

The frequency of hypoglycemia is highest in type 2 diabetes patients treated with insulin (Table 2) (7). That may well be because of the greater glucose-lowering potency of that drug—given in sufficient doses—relative to that of the other drugs, and its pharmacokinetic imperfections. However, it may also be because many patients who ultimately require treatment with insulin have advanced, insulin-deficient type 2 diabetes with the resulting compromised defenses against falling plasma glucose concentrations (5,6) discussed later in this chapter.

CLINICAL DIAGNOSIS OF HYPOGLYCEMIA

It is not possible to specify a plasma glucose concentration that defines clinical hypoglycemia in people with diabetes because the glycemic thresholds for the manifestations of hypoglycemia shift to higher than normal glucose levels in poorly controlled diabetes and lower than normal glucose levels in well controlled diabetes. The diagnosis is made most convincingly by Whipple's triad: symptoms consistent with hypoglycemia, a low plasma glucose concentration and relief of those symptoms after the plasma glucose concentrations is raised to (or above) normal. Ideally, suggestive symptoms should prompt a monitor-measured glucose level to confirm that those symptoms are indicative of hypoglycemia. However, patients often self-treat on the basis of symptoms alone. On the other hand, low self-monitored glucose levels should not be ignored even in the absence of symptoms. The American Diabetes Association Workgroup on Hypoglycemia (11) recommended that people with diabetes should become concerned, and consider defensive actions, at a plasma glucose concentration ≤70 mg/dL (3.9 mmol/L).

IMPACT OF HYPOGLYCEMIA

There is little published information about the clinical impact of hypoglycemia in type 2 diabetes. While it is reasonable to extrapolate from the experience in type 1 diabetes, there are obvious differences. As noted earlier, episodes of hypoglycemia become familiar events early in the course of type 1 diabetes. They are infrequent early in the course of type 2 diabetes, even during treatment with insulin secretagogues or insulin, but become progressively more frequent as the patient approaches the insulin-deficient end of the spectrum of type 2 diabetes (12,13). Furthermore, while type 2 diabetes occurs in all age groups including children, most affected people are middle aged and older and, therefore, at higher risk of erratic food ingestion and even malnutrition, co-morbid conditions and drug interactions, impaired drug metabolism and renal insufficiency with reduced insulin clearance. They are also more susceptible to macrovascular events because of underlying cardiovascular disease.

Iatrogenic hypoglycemia causes both physical morbidity (and some mortality) and psychosocial morbidity (6). While estimates of hypoglycemic mortality rates in type 2 diabetes are not available, deaths caused by sulfonylurea-induced hypoglycemia (like insulin-induced hypoglycemia) are well documented (14). The mortality of a given episode of severe sulfonylurea-induced hypoglycemia has been reported to be as high as 10% (14,15). The physical morbidity of an episode of hypoglycemia ranges from unpleasant neurogenic (autonomic) symptoms, such as sweating, hunger, palpitations, tremor and anxiety, to neuroglycopenic manifestations. The latter range from cognitive impairments and behavioral changes to seizures and coma (and rarely death). Transient focal neurological deficits occur occasionally. While seemingly complete neurological recovery is the rule following an episode of hypoglycemia, prolonged severe hypoglycemia can cause permanent neurological damage. The extent to which the latter might be more frequent in older individuals with type 2 diabetes is unknown.

At the very least, an episode of hypoglycemia is a nuisance and a distraction; it can be embarrassing and lead to social ostracism. The psychological morbidity includes fear of hypoglycemia, guilt about that rational fear, high levels of anxiety and low levels of overall happiness. Fear of hypoglycemia can be an impediment to glycemic control. Thus, hypoglycemia is often a psychological, as well as a pathophysiological, barrier to glycemic control. The performance of critical tasks, such as driving, is measurably impaired during hypoglycemia, as is judgment. Finally, the demands of the management of diabetes, including the prevention of both hyperglycemia and hypoglycemia, become progressively more obtrusive over time in type 2 diabetes, albeit over a longer time span than in type 1 diabetes.

PATHOPHYSIOLOGY OF GLUCOSE COUNTER-REGULATION

While marked hyperinsulinemia alone can cause hypoglycemia, iatrogenic hypoglycemia is the result of the interplay of relative or absolute insulin excess and compromised physiological and behavioral defenses against falling plasma glucose concentrations in type 1 diabetes and in advanced (i.e., insulin-deficient) type 2 diabetes (Table 3) (5,6). Normally, decrements in insulin are the first physiological defense and increments in glucagon are the second defense against falling plasma glucose concentrations. Increments in epinephrine, the third defense, become critical when glucagon is deficient. Decrements in insulin and increments in glucagon and epinephrine increase endogenous glucose production; epinephrine also limits glucose clearance in insulin-sensitive tissues. The sympathoadrenal response (largely the sympathetic neural response) to hypoglycemia causes neurogenic symptoms and thus prompts the

TABLE 3 Pathophysiology of Glucose Counter-Regulation in Type 1 and Type 2 Diabetes

Glucose		Insulin	Glucagon	Epinephrine
↓	Nondiabetic	↓	↑	↑
↓	T1DM	No↓	No↑	Attenuated ↑
	• Defective glucose counter-regulation			
	• Hypoglycemia unawareness			
↓	T2DM	↓-No↓	↑-No↑	↑-Attenuated ↑

Iatrogenic hypoglycemia is the result of the interplay of absolute or relative insulin excess and compromised glucose counter-regulation in type 1 diabetes and in advanced type 2 diabetes.

behavioral defense, the ingestion of food. All of these defenses are compromised in insulin-deficient diabetes (Table 3) (5,6). In the setting of absent decrements in insulin and absent increments in glucagon, attenuated epinephrine responses cause defective glucose counter-regulation. Attenuated sympathoadrenal, largely sympathetic neural, responses cause hypoglycemia unawareness, loss of the warning symptoms that previously prompted food ingestion.

The concept of HAAF in diabetes (Fig. 2) posits that recent antecedent hypoglycemia causes both defective glucose counterregulation (by reducing the epinephrine response to a given level of subsequent hypoglycemia in the setting of absent decrements in insulin and absent increments in glucagon) and hypoglycemia unawareness (by reducing the sympathoadrenal and the resulting neurogenic symptom responses to a given level of subsequent hypoglycemia) and thus a vicious cycle of recurrent hypoglycemia (5). Sleep and prior exercise have similar effects (5). Developed in type 1 diabetes (16), the concept of HAAF also applies to advanced type 2 diabetes (17). Insulin secretion decreases progressively and hypoglycemia becomes more limiting to glycemic control over time in type 2 diabetes (7). As the patients become absolutely insulin deficient, insulin levels do not decrease and glucagon levels do not increase as plasma glucose concentrations fall in type 2 diabetes (17), as in type 1 diabetes (5,16). Furthermore, recent antecedent hypoglycemia shifts the glycemic thresholds for sympathoadrenal and symptomatic responses to subsequent hypoglycemia to lower plasma glucose concentrations in type 2 diabetes (17), as in type 1 diabetes (5,16). Thus, people with advanced type 2 diabetes are also at risk for HAAF. This may well explain why the frequency of iatrogenic hypoglycemia increases from uncommon early in the course of type 2 diabetes, when glucose counterregulatory defenses are intact, to common as patients approach the insulin-deficient end of the spectrum of type 2 diabetes.

The clinical impact of HAAF is well established, at least in type 1 diabetes (5). Remarkably, as little as 2 to 3 weeks of scrupulous avoidance of iatrogenic hypoglycemia reverses hypoglycemia unawareness and improves the epinephrine response in most affected patients (18–20). On the other hand, the specific mechanisms of HAAF are largely unknown (21).

RISK FACTORS FOR HYPOGLYCEMIA

The conventional risk factors for iatrogenic hypoglycemia (5,6,22) are based on the premise that absolute or relative insulin excess is the sole determinant of risk (Table 4). Absolute or relative insulin excess occurs when:

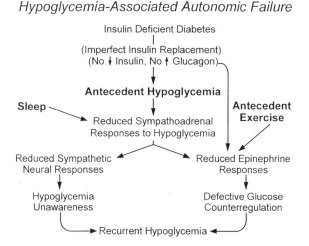

FIGURE 2 Schematic diagram of the concept of hypoglycemia-associated autonomic failure, and the pathogenesis of the syndromes of defective glucose counterregulation and hypoglycemia unawareness, in type 1 diabetes (and in advanced type 2 diabetes). *Source*: From Ref. 5.

TABLE 4   Risk Factors for Iatrogenic Hypoglycemia

Absolute or relative insulin excess
1. Insulin, or insulin secretagogue dose excessive, ill-timed, or of the wrong type
2. Decreased exogenous glucose delivery Missed meals or snacks, overnight fast
3. Decreased endogenous glucose production Alcohol
4. Increased glucose utilization Exercise
5. Increased sensitivity to insulin
       Insulin sensitizer
       Weight loss
       Late after exercise
       Improved fitness
       Middle of the night
       Glycemic control
6. Decreased insulin clearance
       Renal failure

Compromised glucose counterregulation
1. Insulin deficiency
2. History of severe hypoglycemia, hypoglycemia unawareness, or both
3. Aggressive glycemic therapy *per* se
       Lower HbAlc
       Lower glycemic goals

- Insulin or insulin secretagogue doses are excessive, ill-timed or of the wrong type.
- Exogenous glucose delivery is decreased, as following missed meals or snacks, or during an overnight fast.
- Endogenous glucose production is decreased, as following alcohol ingestion.
- Glucose utilization is increased, as during exercise.
- Sensitivity to insulin is increased, as during treatment with an insulin sensitizer, late after exercise, in the middle of the night, or following weight loss, increased fitness or improved glycemic control.
- Insulin clearance is decreased, as in renal failure.

However, while they must be considered carefully, these conventional risk factors explain only a minority of episodes of severe iatrogenic hypoglycemia, at least in type 1 diabetes (23).

As discussed earlier, iatrogenic hypoglycemia is the result of the interplay of absolute or relative insulin excess and compromised physiological and behavioral defenses against falling plasma glucose concentrations (Table 3, Fig. 2) (5,6). Risk factors related to compromised defenses (Table 4) include:

- Insulin deficiency.
- A history of severe hypoglycemia, hypoglycemia unawareness, or both.
- Aggressive glycemic therapy per se, as evidenced by lower HbA_{1C} levels, glycemic goals, or both.

These are clinical surrogates of HAAF (5,6). Insulin deficiency indicates that insulin levels will not decrease, and predicts accurately that glucagon levels will not increase, as glucose levels fall. A history of severe hypoglycemia indicates, and hypoglycemia unawareness or even aggressive glycemic therapy per se implies, recent antecedent hypoglycemia which attenuates sympathoadrenal epinephrine and neurogenic symptom responses to falling glucose levels by shifting the glycemic thresholds for these responses to lower plasma glucose concentrations. Thus, these risk factors are indicative of defective glucose counterregulation and hypoglycemia unawareness, the components of HAAF.

RISK FACTOR REDUCTION

The prevention of iatrogenic hypoglycemia is similar in advanced type 2 diabetes and type 1 diabetes (6,22). Hypoglycemia risk reduction involves:

- Addressing the issue of hypoglycemia in every patient contact.
- Applying the principles of aggressive glycemic therapy—patient education, frequent self-monitoring of blood glucose, flexible insulin (or other drug) regimens, individualized glycemic goals and ongoing professional guidance.
- Considering both the conventional risk factors and those indicative of compromised defenses against hypoglycemia, and adjusting the treatment regimen accordingly.

Given a history of hypoglycemia unawareness, a 2- to 3-week period of scrupulous avoidance of hypoglycemia is advisable since that often restores awareness of hypoglycemia and improves the epinephrine response (18–20). The use of insulin analogues (e.g., glargine or detemir as the basal insulin and lispro, aspart of glulisine as the prandial insulin) reduces the risk at least of nocturnal hypoglycemia (22,24). Despite its theoretical advantages, continuous subcutaneous insulin infusion has not been found to cause less hypoglycemia than a bolus-based insulin regimen with insulin analogues in type 2 diabetes (25). Among patients with type 2 diabetes responsive to a sulfonylurea, hypoglycemia occurs more frequently in those treated with glyburide (glibenclamide) than with glipizide or, particularly, glimepiride.

With these approaches it is possible to improve glycemic control substantially and reduce the risk of hypoglycemia in many patients with type 2 diabetes (22,24,25). Nonetheless, hypoglycemia continues to be a problem for many patients with advanced type 2 diabetes. Ultimately, the problem of hypoglycemia (and hyperglycemia) will likely be solved by therapeutic methods that provide glucose-regulated insulin replacement or secretion.

TREATMENT OF HYPOGLYCEMIA

Obviously, prevention of iatrogenic hypoglycemia, as just discussed, is preferable to treatment of hypoglycemia. Episodes of asymptomatic hypoglycemia (detected by self-monitoring of blood glucose) and most episodes of mild to moderate symptomatic hypoglycemia, are effectively self-treated by ingestion of glucose tablets or carbohydrate in the form of juices, soft drinks, milk, crackers, candy or a meal. A glucose dose of 20 g is reasonable (26). However, in the setting of ongoing hyperinsulinemia, the glycemic response to oral glucose is transient, typically <2 hours (26). Therefore, ingestion of a snack or meal shortly after the glucose level is raised is generally advisable.

Parenteral treatment is necessary when a hypoglycemic patient is unable or unwilling (because of neuroglycopenia) to take carbohydrate orally. While subcutaneous or intramuscular glucagon (1.0 mg in adults) is often used, by family members, to treat hypoglycemia in type 1 diabetes, glucagon is less useful in many patients with type 2 diabetes because it stimulates insulin secretion. Thus, intravenous glucose (25 g initially) is the preferable treatment for severe hypoglycemia in type 2 diabetes. Because sulfonylurea-induced hypoglycemia can persist for hours and even days, prolonged glucose infusion and frequent feedings are often required. This may require hospitalization. Clearly, it is critical that the absence of recurrent hypoglycemia is established unequivocally before the patient is discharged.

SUMMARY AND PERSPECTIVE

Iatrogenic hypoglycemia is the limiting factor in the glycemic management of diabetes, and a barrier to true glycemic control and its established long-term vascular benefits. Hypoglycemia is less frequent overall in type 2 diabetes, compared with type 1 diabetes, because glucose counterregulatory defenses remain intact early in the course of type 2 diabetes. However, iatrogenic hypoglycemia becomes a progressively more frequent problem, ultimately approaching that in type 1 diabetes, as patients approach the insulin-deficient end of the spectrum of type 2 diabetes because of compromised physiological and behavioral defenses against developing hypoglycemia. The syndromes of defective glucose counterregulation and hypoglycemia unawareness, and the concept of HAAF, in advanced (insulin deficient) type 2 diabetes are analogous to those that develop early in the course of type 1 diabetes. By practicing hypoglycemia risk reduction, i.e., addressing the issue, applying the principles of aggressive glycemic therapy, and considering both the conventional risk factors and those indicative of compromised defenses against hypoglycemia, healthcare providers should strive to reduce mean glycemia as much as can be accomplished safely. Clearly, given current treatment limitations, people with diabetes need more physiological approaches to glycemic control, tailored to their degree of insulin deficiency.

Hypoglycemia should not be used, by the provider or the patient, as an excuse for poor glycemic control, particularly in view of the growing array of glucose-lowering drugs that can be used to optimize therapy and achieve the best control possible in a given patient with type 2 diabetes. Nonetheless, better methods—such as those that would provide glucose-regulated insulin replacement or secretion—are clearly needed for people with type 2 diabetes, as well as for those with type 1 diabetes, if we are to maintain euglycemia over a lifetime of diabetes.

ACKNOWLEDGMENTS

The author's work cited in this chapter was supported, in part, by National Institutes of Health grants R37 DK27085, M01 RR00036, P60 DK20579, and T32 DK07120 and a fellowship award from the American Diabetes Association. The assistance of Ms. Penny Casey and Ms. Janet Dedeke in the preparation of this manuscript is gratefully acknowledged.

REFERENCES

1. The Diabetes Control and Complications Trial Research Group. The effect of intensive treatment of diabetes on the development and progression of long-term complications in insulin-dependent diabetes mellitus. N Engl J Med 1993; 329:977–86.
2. The United Kingdom Prospective Diabetes Study Research Group. Intensive blood-glucose control with sulfonylureas or insulin compared with conventional treatment and risk of complications in patients with type 2 diabetes. Lancet 1998; 352:837–53.
3. The Diabetes Control and Complications Trial/Epidemiology of Diabetes Interventions and Complications (DCCT/EDIC) Study Research Group. Intensive diabetes treatment and cardiovascular disease in patients with type 1 diabetes. N Engl J Med 2005; 353:2643–53.
4. Stratton IM, Adler AI, Neil AW, et al. on behalf of the UK Prospective Diabetes Study Group. Association of glycaemia with macrovascular and microvascular complications of type 2 diabetes (UKPDS 35): prospective observational study. BMJ 2000; 321:405–12.
5. Cryer PE. Diverse causes of hypoglycemia-associated autonomic failure in diabetes. N Engl J Med 2004; 350:2272–9.
6. Cryer PE. Glucose homeostasis and hypoglycemia. In: Kronenberg H, Larsen PR, Melmed S, Polonsky K, eds. Williams Textbook of Endocrinology. 11th ed. Philadelphia: Elsevier, in press.
7. The United Kingdom Prospective Diabetes Study Research Group. Overview of 6 years of therapy of type II diabetes: a progressive disease. Diabetes 1995; 44:1249–58.
8. Donnelly LA, Morris AD, Frier BM, et al. Frequency and predictors of hypoglycaemia in Type 1 and insulin-treated Type 2 diabetes: a population based study. Diabet Med 2005; 22:749–55.
9. Holstein A, Plaschke A, Egberts E-H. Clinical characteristics of severe hypoglycemia—a prospective population-based study. Exp Clin Endocrinol Diabetes 2003; 111:364–9.
10. Leese GP, Wang J, Broomhall J, et al. Frequency of severe hypoglycemia requiring emergency treatment in type 1 and type 2 diabetes: a population based study of health service resource use. Diabetes Care 2003; 26:1176–80.
11. American Diabetes Association Workgroup on Hypoglycemia. Defining and reporting hypoglycemia in diabetes. Diabetes Care 2005; 28:1245–9.
12. The United Kingdom Prospective Diabetes Study Research Group. A 6-year, randomized, controlled trial comparing sulfonylurea, insulin and metformin therapy in patients with newly diagnosed type 2 diabetes that could not be controlled with diet therapy. Ann Intern Med 1998; 128:165–75.
13. Hepburn DA, MacLeod KM, Pell ACH, et al. Frequency and symptoms of hypoglycemia experienced by patients with type 2 diabetes treated with insulin. Diabet Med 1993; 10:231–7.

14. Campbell IW. Hypoglycaemia and type 2 diabetes: sulphonylureas. In: Frier BM, Fisher BM, eds. Hypoglycemia and Diabetes. Clinical and Physiological Aspects. London: Edward Arnold, 1993: 387–92.
15. Gerich JE. Oral hypoglycemic agents. N Engl J Med 1989; 321:1231–45.
16. Dagogo-Jack SE, Craft S, Cryer PE. Hypoglycemia-associated autonomic failure in insulin-dependent diabetes mellitus. J Clin Invest 1993; 91:819–28.
17. Segel SA, Paramore DS, Cryer PE. Hypoglycemia-associated autonomic failure in advanced type 2 diabetes. Diabetes 2002; 51:724–33.
18. Fanelli CG, Pampanelli S, Epifano L, et al. Long-term recovery from unawareness, deficient counterregulation and lack of cognitive dysfunction during hypoglycemia following institution of rational intensive therapy in IDDM. Diabetologia 1994; 37:1265–76.
19. Cranston I, Lomas J, Maran A, et al. Restoration of hypoglycemia unawareness in patients with long duration insulin-dependent diabetes mellitus. Lancet 1994; 344:283–7.
20. Dagogo-Jack S, Rattarasarn C, Cryer PE. Reversal of hypoglycemia unawareness, but not defective glucose counterregulation, in IDDM. Diabetes 1994; 43:1426–34.
21. Cryer PE. Mechanisms of hypoglycemia-associated autonomic failure and its component syndromes in diabetes. Diabetes 2005; 54:3592–601.
22. Cryer PE, Davis SN, Shamoon H. Hypoglycemia in diabetes. Diabetes Care 2003; 26:1902–12.
23. The Diabetes Control and Complications Trial Research Group. Epidemiology of severe hypoglycemia in the Diabetes Control and Complications Trial. Am J Med 1991; 90:450–9.
24. Rosenstock J, Dailey G, Massi-Benedetti M, et al. Reduced hypoglycemia risk with insulin glargine. Diabetes Care 2005; 28:950–5.
25. Herman WH, Ilag LL, Johnson SL, et al. A clinical trial of continuous subcutaneous insulin infusion versus multiple daily injections in older adults with type 2 diabetes. Diabetes Care 2005; 28:1568–73.
26. Wiethop BV, Cryer PE. Alanine and terbutaline in the treatment of hypoglycemia in IDDM. Diabetes Care 1993; 16:1131–6.

17 | Diabetic Coma: Current Therapy of Diabetic Ketoacidosis and Non-Ketoacidotic Hyperosmolar Coma

Johannes Hensen
Department of Medicine, Krankenhaus Nordstadt, Klinikum Region Hannover GmbH, Hannover, Germany

INTRODUCTION AND PREVALENCE

This review summarizes the current therapeutic approach to diabetic ketoacidosis and hyperosmolar coma. The focus is on emergency treatment and intensive care management, particularly with regard to volume substitution, insulin therapy and potassium replacement. The basic concepts of low and very low insulin therapy are presented, with special emphasis on the pathogenesis and avoidance of the disequilibrium syndrome. Furthermore, the indications for bicarbonate therapy as well as phosphate and magnesium replacement in diabetic ketoacidosis are discussed.

Until the introduction of substitution therapy with insulin in the 1920s, the diabetic coma was the inevitable cause of death for all patients with type 1 diabetes mellitus and for many patients with type 2 diabetes. During the following decades, high-dose insulin therapy was wide-spread. Today, therapy of diabetic ketoacidosis is differentiated with the combination of low dose of insulin and avoidance of disequilibrium syndrome by limited and controlled reconciliation of electrolytes and fluid.

Katsch (1) gave the first recommendation for a differentiated application of a smaller dose of insulin, which has been the standard therapy in many countries for about the last 30 years (2). The association of the development of early recognition with controlled management has greatly reduced mortality.

In general, one can see the incidence of coma diabeticum as an indicator for the quality of early recognition and quality of diabetes therapy in our countries. In Germany about 5 to 12.5 per 1000 patients with diabetes mellitus (type 1 and type 2) are admitted to the hospital because of coma diabeticum (3).

In a review of more than 100 childrens hospitals in Germany, about 19% of patients had a first manifestation of type 1 diabetes with diabetic ketoacidosis (4). Besides coma as a clinical manifestation of disease, specific situations can be a trigger, which are summarized in Table 1.

PATHOPHYSIOLOGY

Coma diabeticum can appear not only in patients with type 1 diabetes but also in patients with type 2 diabetes. The high concentration of glucose in serum is always associated with an increased serum osmolality. In the untreated patient with type 1 diabetes, the absolute deficiency of insulin leads not only to hyperglycemia, but also to diabetic ketoacidosis. The extent of hyperglycemia in diabetic ketoacidosis is mainly determined by an increased hepatic glucose production; the peripheral insulin resistance plays only a minor role in this situation (5). The blood levels of the insulin antagonizing hormones, like catecholamines, glucagon, cortisol and growth hormone, are in most cases increased in diabetic coma. Because of the complete deficiency of insulin in type 1 diabetes, the missing antilipolytic effect of insulin causes a dramatic increase in free fatty acids from adipose tissue. Metabolic pathways of fatty acids in liver regulate the ratio of insulin and glucagon. A low ratio of insulin to glucagon, as seen in insulin-deficient type 1 diabetes, is associated with low intracellular levels of Malonyl-CoA, a major inhibitor of carnitin palmitoyl transferase and reduced citrate cyclus activity. Free fatty acids are taken up in the liver concentration dependently and are shuttled into mitochondria for β-oxidation and subsequent ketogenesis. Since the ratio of insulin to

TABLE 1 Triggering Situations for Hyperglycemia

Manifestation coma (25%)
Feverish infection (especially gastrointestinal)
Therapy with corticosteroids or catecholamines
Myocardial infarction, critical ischemia in pAVK
Thromboses, pulmonary embolism
Failure to increase insulin dose in situations with higher insulin needs
Erroneous or iatrogenic discontinuation of insulin therapy
Interruption of intravenous insulin supply, e.g., in insulin pump therapy
Repeated vomiting, decreased ingestion, diarrhea
Preexisting acidosis when beginning an intensive physical exercise
Thyrotoxicosis

glucagon in the liver is different in patients with type 2 diabetes, most of them do not develop ketoacidosis although high levels of glucose and decreased insulin action in the periphery are present.

In addition, catabolism of proteins can enhance ketogenesis in the liver via the Cori-cycle. The increase of β-hydoxbutyrate and acetate are the main causes for metabolic acidosis leading to compensatory hyperventilation, hyperkalemia, and hypotension.

Since patients with type 2 diabetes have only relative insulin deficiency, the small residual amount of insulin appears to be sufficient to prevent ketogenesis in the liver. However, mild ketosis may develop in some patients with type 2 diabetes, too.

CLINICAL MANIFESTATION

In clinical practice one speaks of diabetic coma even if the patient has not lost conscious. About 10% of patients with coma diabeticum are really unconscious (6). The causes of these conscious disturbances are cerebral dysfunction in association with severe hypertonic dehydration. The transition from hyperglycemic decompensation with severe ketoacidosis toward coma diabeticum is substantially dependent on the extent of the increase in serum osmolality. The consciousness correlates best with plasma osmolality and less well with the extent of other changes in clinical chemistry, like elevation of blood glucose, ketone concentration, pH value, or the sodium concentration in serum (7).

Primary symptoms of hyperglycemic ketoacidotic decompensation are polyuria, thirst, and loss of weight. Furthermore, these patients complain of weakness, tiredness, headache, lack of appetite, nausea or vomiting. Typical clinical signs of ketoacidosis are the acetonic fetor ex ore and the so-called Kussmaul's respiration. Exsiccosis or hypovolemia manifests clinically as oligo- or anuria (prerenal insufficiency) and hypotension. Further clinical signs of the dehydration are tachycardia, dry tongue, standing skin folds, muscle cramps, and soft bulbi. A special clinical picture is the pseudoperitonitis diabetica, which is a painful tension of the abdominal wall in association with diabetic ketoacidosis. This can be associated with elevated serum-alpha-amylase levels as well as with leukocytosis. It is very important to recognize this clinical picture early and to differentiate it from other causes of an acute abdomen, to avoid unnecessary surgery.

LABORATORY CRITERIA OF COMA DIABETICUM

The criteria in clinical chemistry of a diabetic coma are summarized in Table 2 (8): approximately 15% of patients with diabetic ketoacidosis have glucose concentration in plasma <350 mg/dL. In these cases one speaks of "euglycemic diabetic ketoacidosis." This appears in situations in which gluconeogenesis appears to be disturbed, e.g., liver disease, alcoholism, prolonged fasting or in cases where insulin-independent glucose consumption is very high (i.e., in pregnancy). In cases where blood glucose levels are below <16 mmol/L (240 mg/dL) and there is only mild ketonemia a diabetic cause for an unclear coma is virtually excluded. In these cases one must look for other causes of coma, e.g., intracerebral bleeding, liver failure, intoxication, uremia, and hypoglycemic coma.

TABLE 2 Laboratory Criteria of Diabetic Ketoacidosis and Non-Ketoacidotic Hyperosmolar Coma

Lab criteria	Ketoacidosis	Hyperosmolar corna
Serum glucose (mg/dL)	>250	>600
pH arterial	<7.3	>7.3
HCO_3^-	<15	>15
Blood urea N (mmol/L)	<ca. 14	>ca. 17
Osmolality (mOsm/kg)	<320	>330
Ketone bodies in urine	>+3	Negative or few
Ketone bodies in plasma	Positively >1:2 dilution	Negative or few
Anion gap	>12	<12

Source: From Ref. 8.

DIAGNOSTIC PROCEDURES

The following basic diagnostic steps are needed usually during the first 24 hours: clinical history, physical examination, clinical chemistry including TSH, parameters of sepsis, blood gases, urine status, blood and urine cultures in case of signs of infection, ECG, ultrasound of the abdomen, chest X-ray and eventually echocardiography. Especially in the beginning of the therapy of diabetic ketoacidosis, regular control of capillary blood glucose, potassium, and blood gases is needed. Initially, the blood glucose should be controlled every hour or if needed even more frequently, especially to monitor a gradual decrease of blood glucose. In cases where the individual insulin need of the patient is known and the patient is not anymore in severe danger, the time span of controls can be widened. As long as a continuous insulin infusion is running, an hourly control of blood glucose levels is recommended. In cases where the preceding blood glucose levels are in the stabile target level, one can measure every other hour. Serum concentration of potassium, sodium, venous BGA (pH-value, bicarbonate levels) should be determined every 2 to 3 hours during the first days and then every 4 to 8 hours as needed.

THERAPY OF DIABETIC COMA

The aim of treatment of a severe hyperglycemic decompensation can be summarized as follows:

- Substitution of fluid electrolyte loss
- Re-compensation of normal carbohydrate and lipid metabolism
- Treatment of the underlying cause
- Management of specific complications

The diagnosis of coma diabeticum must lead to an immediate hospitalization of the patient. In severe forms the medical treatments must be performed on an intensive or at least intermediate care unit.

GRADED THERAPY

The treatment of diabetic coma can be subdivided in three stages (Fig. 1 and Table 3) (9): The *first stage* is the one of rapid rehydration. As a consequence of fluid substitution cerebral dysfunction is ameliorated as well as the vital parameters like cardiovascular and renal function. Already by dilution and improvement of renal perfusion by re-hydration, glucose levels can decrease by about 35 to 70 mg/dL per hour (10).

The *second stage* is the one of insulin therapy. Blood glucose levels should be lowered slowly, continuously, and within limits. The optimal rates of decrease to avoid disequilibrium syndrome are estimated to the around 50 mg/dL per hour (3 mmol/L per hour) (11). The careful lowering of the blood glucose helps to prevent cerebral complications like brain edema and cerebral convulsions. Insulin therapy inhibits ketogenesis and thereby reduces metabolic acidosis.

TABLE 3 Three Stages of Treatment for Diabetic Coma

Stages of therapy	Targets
Rapid rehydration	Improvement of cerebral dysfunction and renal function
	Supportive care for cardiovascular system
Insulin therapy	Slow, continuous lowering of the blood sugar (optimal correction rate: 50 mg/dL per hour) Inhibition of ketogenesis
Stabilization and slow adjustment	Stabilization of blood sugar to approx. 200 mg/dL
	Further lowering to near normal values within 2 days
	Avoidance of disequilibrium syndrome

The *third stage* is stabilization of blood glucose levels around 200 mg/dL with a consecutive lowering into the normal range within the next 2 days (9). In cases where blood glucose levels are around 250 mg/dL, the insulin dose is greatly reduced and if needed additional infusion of glucose (5% glucose) is used. In cases where the aim of a slow and a gradual decrease of the glucose weight in stage 2 of approximately 50 mg/dL per hour has been achieved using a very low dose of insulin therapy and there are no clinical indications for a syndrome of disequilibrium, one can reduce blood glucose levels from 250 mg/dL to normoglycemia within a half or whole day. Through close to normal values of blood glucose the course of concomitant diseases or complications like sepsis and infections are decreased (12,13).

GENERAL PROCEDURES OF INTENSIVE MEDICAL CARE

Main procedures of general intensive medical care are to insure respiration and function of the cardiovascular system. Because of elevated concentration of hemoglobin and hematocrit the risk for thrombotic or thromboembolic complications, like myocardial infarction, stroke and infarction of the mesenteries is high. Therefore, a starting dose of low molecular heparin 500 to 1000 IE/hr is recommended. In patients who are not in shock and have an adequate renal function, alternatively also low molecular heparin can be used subcutaneously. Concomitant coma-triggering diseases like infections should be treated early. There should be continuous ECG-monitoring, a gastric tube (specially in diabetic gastroparesis), application of oxygen, and possibly a urinary catheter. A central venous catheter is needed in severely-ill patients to monitor fluid balance as well as the intravenous pressure during volume repletion because there is a danger of volume overload during therapy.

VOLUME AND ELECTROLYTE SUBSTITUTION

The most important step in the therapy is an adequate volume and electrolyte substitution with the aim of improving the cardiovascular situation (Table 4). In most patients with diabetic

TABLE 4 Summary of Indications to Adequate Volume and Electrolyte Substitution

Indication	Infusion solution	Infusion rate
Stage of fast rehydration	Ringer or isotonic saline	With extreme volume deficit:
Ketoacidosis (with intact oxidative metabolism)	Ringer-Lactate (altern. to Ringer)	1000 mL/hr for the first 4 hr
		Without extreme volume deficit:
Hypernatremia (>150 mg/dL)	NaCl 0.45% or hypoosmolar Ringer	500 mL/hr for the first 4 hr
Hyperosmolality (>320 mOsm/L)		250 mL/hr for the next 4 hr
Oligo- or anuria	Isotonic saline	1000 mL/hr for the first hour
Danger of volume overload		Further administration CVP controlled (Table 5)
Rapid lowering of blood sugar under insulin therapy	Ringer and glucose 5% 1:1 (parallel)	50–100 mL/hr

ketoacidosis initial ringer solution or isotonic saline solution 0.9% is preferred. The optimal infusion rate is dependent on the clinical situation of the patient. Patients with extreme volume deficiency need about 1000 mL/hr for the first 4 hours. Patients with less extreme volume deficit can be substituted more carefully, e.g., at a rate of 500 mL/hr for the first 4 hours followed by 250 mL/hr for the next 4 hours (14).

The guidelines of the German diabetes association recommend in patients with high risk for volume overload, e.g., heart failure, especially with concomitant oligo- or anuria, controlling volume therapy by central venous pressure. After primary infusion of saline solution (0.9%), the balance should have a surplus of less than 500 to 1000 mL/hr (Table 5) (3,11). In cases where sodium levels are initially already in the upper limit of normal one should change to an infusion of half isotonic sodium chloride or hyporosmolar electrolyte fluids. This regimen should be used initially, in cases where sodium levels are greater than 150 mmol/L or if severe hyperosmolality (>320 mOsm/L) is present.

As an alternative for saline an isoltonic ringer lactate solution can be used. The precondition is an intact oxidative metabolism. It contains about 130 mmol natrium and 112 mmol chloride per liter and thereby less than 0.9% saline, which contains 150 mmol/L sodium and 150 mmol/L chloride. Lactate blinds hydrogen ions and will be metabolized in cases where the oxidative metabolism is intact. Because of the content of lactate (27 mmol/L) ringer lactate is lightly alkalizing. In cases of metabolic acidosis this can alleviate the bicarbonate-CO_2-buffer system.

To prevent hyperchloremia, especially in cases of oligo- or anuria, an electrolyte substitution with lower chloride concentration such as sodium is recommended (11).

INSULIN THERAPY OF DIABETIC KETOACIDOSIS

The aim of diabetic ketoacidosis therapy is a reconstitution of the normal "milieu interior" without complications. To avoid a disequilibrium syndrome, reduction of glucose in the blood should be slow limited, and controlled, e.g., <3 mmol/L or 54 mg/dL per hour (11,15).

In normal persons, where acute hyperglycemia has been induced by inhibiting insulin production by infusion of somatostatine and glucose, blood glucose lowering after reconstitution of insulin secretion may be up to 500 mg/dL per hour. In cases of hyperglycemic patients with diabetes a comparable insulin dose can reduce plasma glucose by only 65 to 125 mg/mL per hour (16–18). In comparison, this lower decrease in comparison to normal individuals reflects the severe insulin resistance in patients with diabetic coma. Furthermore, substitution of volume alone can lower plasma glucose by about 35 to 70 mg/dL per hour. The reasons are an improvement of renal perfusion with an increase of renal excretion of glucose as well as a decrease of contraregulatory hormones (10,17). From the above, in cases of combined therapy of re-hydration and low-dose insulin one can calculate a glucose decrease between 100 and 200 mg/hr (19). This would already be more than wanted. Since fluid substitution reduces glucose levels followed by a decrease in glucose toxicity on β cells, insulin therapy should only be carefully initiated after initial re-hydration and adapted to insulin doses required to decrease blood glucose level slowly (10,13,20). Since insulin sensitivity is further

TABLE 5 CVP-Controlled Fluid Substitution

Normal urine production Physiological salt solution	Oligo- or anuria Hypotonic electrolyte solution or half isotonic saline
CVP (cmH$_2$0)	Infusion rate (mL/hr)
0	1000
0–3	500
4–8	250
9–12	100
>12	0

Source: From German Diabetes Association 2003.

improved during therapy one can expect that the insulin need is further reduced in the course of treatment.

LOW-DOSE VERSUS VERY-LOW-DOSE INSULIN THERAPY

Usually low-dose insulin therapy is initiated by an infusion of insulin of about 5 to 10 IE/hr. Under this treatment plasma insulin levels reach 75 to 200 U/mL, which is in the upper limit of physiological insulin concentrations in humans. The designation of low-dose insulin therapy relates to a historical point of view, since in former times high-dose insulin therapy used to be 500 IE i.v. followed by 20 to 100 IE/hr (13,20,21). Investigations examining the effect of increasing doses of insulin on glucose metabolism have shown that a very low dose of insulin (1 IE/hr) sufficiently inhibits lipolysis by 100% and suppresses hepatic gluconeogenesis by 50% (22). If a dose of 2 IE/hr is used, the main causes of acidotic hyperglycemia, which are hepatic glucose production and ketone production, are inhibited by 90% and 100%, respectively. The peripheral glucose metabolism is increased to 21 g/hr. Using insulin in a dose of 8 IE/hr hepatic glucose production is completely inhibited and peripheral glucose metabolism is increased to 50 g/hr. However, the increase of the insulin dose is associated with an increase of cellular potassium uptake and therefore an increased risk of hypokalemia. These are the reasons for recommending a very low dose of insulin in the treatment of diabetic ketoacidosis, e.g., to begin with 6 IE/hr and to reduce the dose to a mean of 0.9 IE/hr after 2 hours (21).

INITIAL BOLUS OF INSULIN

The German diabetes association recommends in their latest guideline, to begin the insulin therapy with an intravenous initial bolus of 10 to 20 IE (11,20). The insulin therapy should not be started without concomitant volume substitution, because a rapid decrease in blood glucose without fluid expansion can lead to intracellular edema (17). In accordance with the concept outlined above, it is sensible to choose a lower dose of initial insulin, e.g., 2 to 15 IE (13). The question of if and in which dose the primary doctor outside of the hospital should begin with an insulin therapy depends on several factors.

The adjustment of individual risk and advantages should consider, for example, the extent of the disease, the age of the patient, the time and duration of transport, the degree of insulin resistance, the putative potassium level (is the patient vomiting or not?), and the risk for rapidly developing hypokalemia as well as the potential risk for triggering the syndrome of disequilibrium if insulin substitution is initiated immediately.

Therefore, the initial measure for the primary care doctor is to substitute volume (1 L/hr saline solution i.v.). Volume therapy leads quickly to a significant decrease in glucose concentration. Therefore, in general, early insulin substitution is not recommended but if so only in small amounts, like 2 to 5 IE, which may be repeated. An insulin injection into the muscle appears to be as efficient as an intravenous therapy, when the patient is not in shock (23,24). Subcutaneous application of insulin can also be effective. However this is not a general recommendation, since the subcutaneous blood flow in combination with volume depletion and secondary activation of the sympatho-adrenal system is decreased.

INSULIN PERFUSION

The normal insulin need is about 1 IE/hr and should be adapted to the increased needs depending on the extent of ketoacidosis, sepsis, overweight, activation of counter regulatory hormone systems and eventually therapy with catecholamines or glucocorticoids leading to insulin resistance. The guidelines of the German diabetes association recommend the low-dose insulin therapy with a starting dose of 6 IE/hr (0.1 IE/kg bodyweight) until ketoacidosis is controlled and blood glucose is lowered to 14 mmol/L (250 mg/dL) (11).

The alternative concept of a very low dose of insulin targets an infusion rate of approximately 1 IE/hr. An analysis of 114 consecutive patients ages of 11 to 74 (mean 34 years old) in the ICU is to date the description of the largest patient collective treated with a very-low-dose insulin therapy (15). The therapy was started with fluid substitution of 1000 mL/hr ringer's solution during the first 4 hours. After the values of clinical chemistry were known, the infusion was changed to 0.9% saline or half electrolyte solution. Initially an insulin bolus of 2 to 15 IE was given, followed by a low-dose insulin therapy with the basal insulin infusion rate of 1 IE/hr (0.5–4.0 IE/hr i.v.) titrated to a maximal decrease of blood glucose levels around 50 mg/dL/hr. In cases where the decrease of blood glucose was higher, 100 mg/dL per hour, despite the dose of insulin 5% glucose infusion was given. In addition there was a substitution of potassium (10–20 mmol/hr) and heparin therapy (500–1000 IE/hr i.v.). The mortality rate was very low, so that this concept can be recommended.

BICARBONATE THERAPY

The therapy with bicarbonate is one of the mostly discussed procedures of management in the treatment of diabetic ketoacidosis. In general, acidosis is decreased after adequate rehydration and implementation of insulin treatment. The main indication for bicarbonate is the emergency treatment of serious disturbances of heart rhythm with severe acidosis and hyperkalemia.

In such cases a body weight-adjusted amount of sodium bicarbonate (e.g., 50–100 mL) is infused. Otherwise, bicarbonate therapy should only be used reluctantly, when pH-value is below 7.0 or standard bicarbonate is below 5 mmol/L (11). Usually, one should elevate the pH-value just outside the dangerous range, e.g., 7.15 to 7.20.

A rule of thumb for bicarbonate substitution is body weight × 0.3 × negative base excess, 25% of this in mL (1 mL contains 1 mmol/L).

Potential complications of bicarbonate therapy are sodium overload, development of brain edema, intracellular acidosis, development or exacerbation of hypokalemia, development of "rebound alkalosis" as well as reduced tissue oxygenation by shifting the oxyhemoglobin dissociation curve to the left.

ELECTROLYTE AND WATER LOSS

Diabetic ketoacidosis is associated with severe loss of water and electrolytes. The loss of fluid can be up to 50% of body weight and is associated with a reduction in blood pressure. The total loss of electrolytes can be calculated to about 500 mmol sodium, 500 mmol potassium, 100 mmol phosphate (Table 6) (11). The total loss of electrolytes is not reflected in the levels of potassium and sodium in serum. In many countries the calculation of the anion gap plays a great role in the diagnosis and the therapy of coma diabeticum (AG = $[Na^+]$–$[Cl^-]$–$[HCO_3^-]$ [mmol/L]). The normal anion gap is between 8 and 16 (e.g., 15=140–100–25). In the case of diabetic ketoacidosis the anion gap is elevated, indicating the presence of other anions like ketone bodies (19).

SERUM SODIUM

The loss of sodium in diabetic ketoacidosis is severe. The plasma levels of sodium can be variable, but are low in most cases. Very low sodium levels can be associated with vomiting. Several factors affect the regulation of sodium concentration in diabetic ketoacidosis.

Antidiuretic Hormone

The two most important stimuli of antidiuretic hormone (ADH) secretion are hypovolemia via non-osmotic volume and baroreceptor-mediated stimuli, and hyperosmolality, via osmotic stimuli. Both factors are present in diabetic ketoacidosis, leading to a strong stimulation of ADH secretion. Especially the intracerebral hypertonicity caused by hyperglycemia leads to

TABLE 6 Electrolyte and Water Losses from Intracellular and Extracellular Space in Diabetic Coma

Lab criteria	Deficits per body weight	Total deficit	Compartment
Water	100–150 mL/kg	7–10 L	2/3 ECS, 1/3 ICS
Sodium	5–13 mmol/kg	600 mmol	ECS
Chloride	5–7 mmol/kg	400 mmol	ECS
Potassium	4–10 mmol/kg	500 mmol	ICS
Phosphate	0.5–4 mmol/kg	70 mmol	ICS

Abbreviations: ECS, extracellular space; ICS, intracellular space.

shrinkage of osmosensitive neurons and thereby to osmotic-mediated ADH-stimulation (25). ADH reduces the excretion of free water and enhances the development of hyponatremia.

Fluid Uptake

Excessive thirst and drinking of hypotonic fluids in the presence of high ADH levels may lead to hyponatremia. Only when a fluid uptake is not possible anymore might hypernatremia develop, indicating severe hypertonic dehydration with poor clinical prognosis.

Intra- and Extracellular Fluid Shift

An increase in glucose of 500 mg/dL moves about 1 L of water from intracellular to the extracellular space. Therefore one can calculate that an increase of only 100 mg/dL glucose leads to a decrease of the plasma sodium by about 1.7 mmol/L.

Osmotic Diuresis

Osmotic diuresis leads to loss of electrolytes, mainly sodium and potassium as well as free water. The consequence is an increase in sodium and osmolality in serum, if fluid intake is not increased simultaneously.

Insulin Treatment

The treatment of hyperglycemic patients with insulin lowers osmolality in plasma and consequently water is shifted to the intracellular space. This leads to a swelling of cells on one hand, and to an increase of sodium concentration in serum on the other hand (26). This is a reason why patients with initial normal sodium concentrations in plasma rarely develop hypernatremia. The extent of the expected hypernatremia can be estimated via calculation of the corrected sodium concentration. This is an indication of the sodium concentration, which would appear after insulin therapy (27). The calculation is: [corrected Na$^+$] = [measured Na$^+$] + [delta glucose (mg/dL)/42].

    Example: glucose 600 mg/dL, measured plasma Na$^+$: 130 mmol/L, delta glucose: 600 – 100=500; corrected sodium concentration: 130 mmol/L + 12=142 mmol/L.

    Volume substitution with ringer or isotonic saline solution will adjust sodium losses. To avoid cerebral pontine myelinolysis, plasma sodium concentration should not be increased by more than 12 mmol/L per day. Hypertonic sodium solution (e.g., 3% saline solution) should be avoided even in severe hyponatremia (28). In cases of severe hypernatremia (>150 mmol/L) or hyperosmolality (>320 mOsm/L) volume substitution should be performed with half isotonic saline solution or hyposmolar ringer solution.

POTASSIUM

The losses of potassium via urine are severe in diabetic coma. Despite severe potassium depletion, the concentration of potassium in serum can be normal or even be increased initially. The combination of hyperosmolality, acidosis and insulin deficiency leads to a shift from intracellular potassium to the extracellular space (29). This is accompanied by normal or hyperkalemic values in the laboratory analysis although the patient is kaliopenic. In cases of chronic or acute prerenal insufficiency this discrepancy can be even more evident. After insulin application there is a dramatic decrease of potassium concentration.

The potassium deficit must be counterbalanced by substituting potassium in the infusion solution, e.g., isotonic saline solution with 20 mmol/L potassium. If potassium in serum is below 3.3 mmol/L the amount should be increased to 40 mmol/L. Furthermore, one can provide a continuous infusion of potassium chloride with 10 to 40 mmol/hr under control of heart rhythm by a monitor. Potassium infusion of more than 20 mmol/hr is reserved for severe hypokalemia and needs closely controlled potassium levels. In addition, one should consider that changes in serum pH can lead to shifts of potassium: an increase of the pH-value of 0.1 leads to a decrease of serum potassium by about 0.4 to 1.2 mmol/L.

PHOSPHATE

In diabetic ketoacidosis the excretion of phosphate leads to phosphate depletion, which can, comparable to the situation with potassium, be manifested during rehydration and insulin therapy of diabetic ketoacidosis. Possibly the increased uptake of phosphate by skeletal muscles via carbohydrate assimilation might play a role. Since the concentration within the erythrocytes of 2.3 diphosphoglycerate is lowered in diabetic ketoacidosis this leads to a decrease of tissue oxygenation. This was the reason why there was hope that substitution of phosphate might alleviate the clinical course of diabetic coma. However, most of the studies have shown no significant effect on the clinical course by phosphate substitution in diabetic ketoacidosis with or without coma. In cases of severe hypophoshatemia a low dose of phosphate repletion is recommended, e.g., using sodium glycerol phosphate (20 mL infusion additive contain 20 mmol) in a dose of 10 to 20 mmol/L (without calcium). Higher doses such as 50 mmol phosphate per day can lead to hypocalcemia and hypomagnesemia. A dose of 20 mmol/hr and a total dose of 100 mmol/day should be the limit even in cases of severe phosphate deficiency. The control of calcium and phosphate under therapy is recommended at least every 12 hours (30,31).

MAGNESIUM

The clinical relevance of magnesium replacement is until today unclear. Consciousness is worsened by high magnesium levels. For correction of severe hypomagnesaemia with or without concomitant severe cardiac arrhythmia and heart failure, magnesium can be given as magnesium sulfate in a dose of 0.5 g/hr (2 mmol/hr) for 24 hours laboratory controls should be performed at least every 12 hours. In cases of ventricular tachycardia one can give 1 to 2 f (2–4 mL 50% $MgSO_4$, corresponding to 8–16 mval or 4–8 mmol) in 10 mL glucose 5% for 1 to 2 minutes; in cases of ventricular fibrillation also as bolus. The maximal dose of magnesium corresponds to 50 mmol/day; in cases of renal insufficiency the dose has to be adapted. The antidote to magnesium is calcium gluconate, e.g., 1 g infused slowly in i.v.

MECHANICAL VENTILATION IN DIABETIC KETOACIDOSIS

In diabetic ketoacidosis, very frequently severe hyperventilation with deep respiratory breaths are observed, also called Kussmaul-respiration. This is a compensatory mechanism aiming to get rid of CO_2 in cases of severe metabolic acidosis. The blood gases show severely lowered pCO_2, a relatively high pO_2 with relatively high hemoglobin O_2 saturation as well as low standard bicarbonate. Respiratory compensation by hyperventilation is a compensatory mechanism; this is the reason why medications which can decrease respiratory capacity or compensatory mechanisms, like sedatives, should be avoided as long as possible. The indication for tracheal intubation of a patient with diabetic coma is mainly the potential of aspiration in the case of severe coma and vomiting. In most cases it is sufficient and most sensible to let the patient respirate by himself after intubation with a closed cuff to prevent aspiration. In case the patient has to be ventilated mechanically, one should take care to keep up the high respiratory minute volume by high respiratory volume and frequency. If one does not pay attention to that, pCO_2 can relatively increase to the bicarbonate level which results in severe acidosis, hyperkalemia and cardiovascular insufficiency.

If patients with compensated metabolic acidosis are intubated and ventilated, the rule of thumb is that, a pCO_2-level "1.5-fold of the serum bicarbonate level $+8$" should be the goal. If the bicarbonate level is increased in the course of treatment, the ventilation should be adapted correspondingly (32).

MORTALITY

Mortality is increased with age. Patients below the age of 50 are treated with low-dose insulin therapy approximately 2% to 5%, depending on the patient collective and concomitant diseases. In cases of controlled rehydration and very low insulin therapy mortality in specialized centers is observed around 1% (15). In children, this rate is not higher (9,33). Mortality is higher in elderly patients especially if diabetic ketoacidosis is accompanied by other severe diseases like acute pancreatitis, myocardial infarction, sepsis (34).

In cases of non-ketoacidotic hyperosmolar coma, mortality in patients younger than 50 years is about 20%; in patients above the age of 50 the mortality rate is similar to complicated diabetic ketoacidosis with concomitant disease (approximately 25%) (34).

COMPLICATIONS AND AVOIDABLE MISTAKES IN THERAPY

In the treatment of diabetic coma several potentially avoidable complications can appear (Table 7). In particular, syndrome disequilibrium associated with cerebral edema is caused by an overly rapid fall of osmolality, especially by hypotonic solutions and inadequate bicarbonate therapy. Hypernatremia and hyperchloremia can be induced by excessive infusion of sodium chloride, especially with decreased renal function and infusion of sodium bicarbonate. If there is a lack of monitoring of central venous pressure, volume therapy can lead to pulmonary edema. Over dosage of bicarbonate can induce paradoxical acidosis of the central nervous system. Hypokalemia appears frequently after rapid application of a high insulin dose and inadequate potassium substitution. Phosphate depletion in disturbed renal function and lack of balance can lead to individual problems and hypocalcemia can be the consequence of a high phosphate substitution. High insulin replacement increases the risk of disequilibrium syndrome and hypoglycemia. In addition, complicating factors are thromboembolic events like myocardial, cerebral, and mesenteric infarction. This can be compounded by cardiopulmonary complications with cardiovascular shock and adult respiratory distress syndrome, as well as by severe thyrotoxicosis.

CEREBRAL EDEMA

A severe, but avoidable complication of therapy is cerebral edema (9). Brain edema is observed mostly 3 to 13 hours after beginning of therapy. It must be considered especially in patients below 20 years. In one study in children and young adults a total of 55 death cases were investigated (35). Thirty-six of these patients had a ketoacidosis. A further retrospective study in children investigated searched for risk factors for the development symptomatic brain edema (33). The prevalence of cerebral edema was in this collective 0.9%, of which 42% died or had permanent neurological deficits. The identified risk factors were low anterior pCO_2 and

TABLE 7 Complications of Therapy in Diabetic Coma

Symptom/statement	Cause
Brain edema	Rapid lowering of osmolality, especially by hypotonic solution, bicarbonate
Hypernatremia, hyperchloremia	Excessive NaCl supply and impaired renal function
Hypoglycemia	Insulin excess
CNS acidosis, brain edema	Bicarbonate overdose
Phosphate depletion	Disturbed renal function, inadequate adjustment
Hypocalcemia	High phosphate supply
Mechanic ventilation	Acidosis with inadequate hyperventilation
Thromboses	Missing administration of heparin

the level of urea concentration in serum in the beginning of treatment. Pathogenetically, both factors can be seen as indicators of cerebral hyperperfusion and hypoxia. Hyperventilation and hypocapnia enhance cerebral vasoconstriction in children and young adults. The elevation of urea is an indicator for extreme dehydration with consecutive reduced cerebral perfusion. A further risk factor for cerebral edema was bicarbonate therapy. Animal experiments have indicated that bicarbonate can induce ZNS-hypoxia (36). Also, correction of bicarbonate in the treatment of extracellular acidosis can lead to activation of the sodium hydrogen transport which can lead to potassium influx with cellular swelling. Finally, it was shown that bicarbonate increases even ketogenesis.

Cerebral edema begins with headache followed by neurological deficits (37). Early signs are severe headache, incontinence or lowered mental status. In this situation, an early therapy with hypertonic manitol solution as bolus i.v. in a dose of 0.5 to 2.0 g/kg body weight can be helpful (37). Manitol is an osmotic active plasma expander which reduces blood viscosity and leads to an elevation of peripheral blood flow to induce an increase of cerebral oxygenation. This effect is observed within 15 to 30 minutes after injection of the bolus and can be observed then for approximately 6 hours. Control of plasma osmolality and creatinine are needed. The administration of dexamethasone and hyperventilation are of no evident benefit (38).

TRANSITION FROM INTRAVENOUS TO SUBCUTANEOUS INSULIN THERAPY

The transition from i.v. insulin therapy to subcutaneous insulin and oral nutrition can be initiated in an awake patient when significant improvement and a pH-value of >7.2 have been reached. It is recommended to pursue a primary intensified therapy with pre-prandial applied doses of short acting insulin analogs combination with the prolonged acting insulin two or three times per day, or alternatively very long acting insulin analog once or twice a day. The first dose of long acting insulin should be given about 2 hours after stopping a continuous insulin infusion. The total dose of insulin can be calculated from the current insulin need, thereby the improvement of insulin resistance and the change of eating habits should be considered. Forty percent of the daily insulin dose can be given as a long acting insulin s.c. and about 20% as short acting insulin three times per day pre-prandially. The therapy should be initiated on the intensive care or intermediacy care unit and should include dose algorithm for dose correction.

After control of ketoacidosis or coma diabeticum the education of patients should be initiated to avoid a relapse (39).

SPECIAL FEATURES OF HYPEROSMOLAR NON-KETOTIC COMA

Many properties elucidated above for diabetic ketoacidosis are also true for hyperosmolar non-ketotic diabetic coma and will not be repeated. The hyperosmolar coma corresponds to extreme hyperglycemia with a high level of dehydration and appears very frequently in elderly patients with type 2 diabetes (Table 8) (11). Mortality is higher than in diabetic ketoacidosis. Since there is only relative insulin deficiency, the liver is still "seeing" enough insulin to prevent severe ketoacidosis. However, some patients might develop mild acidosis. Extremely high levels of blood glucose concentrations of sometimes more than 1000 mg/dL are not a rarity. The latter is the main player of elevated plasma osmolality. The fluid deficit may even be more pronounced than in diabetic ketoacidosis.

A hyperosmolar coma diabeticum can have different causes. The triggers mostly are concomitant diseases like infections, e.g., pneumonia pancreatitis, cerebral insult, dialysis, burns and, thyrotoxicosis, which all have a strong influence of mortality. Drugs like diuretics, glucocorticoids and possibly non-selective β-blockers can aggravate decompensation.

Comparably to diabetic ketoacidosis the primary aim of therapy should be the slowly lowering of blood glucose by about 50 mg/dL per hour and the avoidance of osmotic disequilibrium with concomitant brain edema (11). If plasma osmolality can be measured, the rate of lowering should not be higher then 5 mOsm/L per hour. Therapeutically, volume

TABLE 8   Highlights of Hyperosmolar Coma Diabeticum

Elderly patients with type 2 diabetes, insulin resistance and impaired insulin secretion
Often triggered by feverish infection
Relative insulin deficiency, therefore no severe ketoacidosis ("insulinized" liver "diabetic" periphery)
Severe hyperglycemia
Severely increased plasma osmolality
Extreme dehydration
Lethality 20–25%
Infusion therapy most important
Initial administration of insulin can be waived, as long as blood glucose decreases by infusion treatment
Reduce blood glucose slowly by approximately 50 mg/dL/hr
Decrease plasma osmolality by approx 5 mOsm/L

therapy is the first step with ringer-solution or isotonic saline solution in the amount of 1 L/hr. The following volume therapy should be adjusted to central venous pressure. Hypotonic fluid substitution with 0.45% isotonic saline solution or half-half-solution (saline solution vs. glucose 5%) should be considered. An initial insulin therapy can be retarded as long as blood glucose decreases only by fluid replacement. Potassium substitution is necessary as described in ketoacidotic coma. As said before, once a blood glucose of 250 mg/dL is reached, further reduction would be performed very slowly to avoid disequilibrium syndromes (8,11). Many patients with hyperosmolar coma are not really insulin dependent after acute therapy (8,10).

CONCLUSIONS FOR DAILY CLINICAL PRACTICE

The mortality in the treatment of patients with diabetic comas has decreased continuously during the last decades, especially due to the recognition and avoidance of treatment mistakes. The most important therapeutic measure in the acute stadium is volume substitution, whereas ringer solution or isotonic saline solutions are the most suitable. Insulin substitution should be utilized carefully. In most cases a very low dose is sufficient to lower blood glucose level by not more than 50 mg/dL per hour. The therapy includes substitution of potassium and thrombus prophylaxis by heparin. Bicarbonate is indicated in special situations. Use of these therapies leads to a low mortality rate, especially in younger patients.

REFERENCES

1. Katsch G. Insulinbehandlung des diabetischen Komas. Dtsch Ges Wesen 1945; 1:651–5.
2. Menzel R, Jutzi E. Zum Blutzuckerverhalten bei der Rekompensation des Coma diabeticum. Dtsch Ges Wesen 1970; 25:727–32.
3. Waldhausl W, Kleinberger G, Bratusch-Marrain P, Komjati M. Pathophysiology and therapy of diabetic ketoacidosis and of non-ketoacidotic hyperosmolar diabetic coma. Wien Klin Wochenschr 1984; 96:309–19.
4. Kintzel R, Holl R, Haberland H, Grabert M, Dost A. Die diabetische Ketoazidose bei Erkrankungsbeginn im Kindes- und Jugendalter in der Bundesrepublik. Diab Stoffw 2003; 12:8–12.
5. Luzi L, Barrett EJ, Groop LC, Ferrannini E, DeFronzo RA. Metabolic effects of low-dose insulin therapy on glucose metabolism in diabetic ketoacidosis. Diabetes 1988; 37:1470–7.
6. Foster DW, McGarry JD. The metabolic derangements and treatment of diabetic ketoacidosis. N Engl J Med 1983; 309:159–69.
7. Arieff AI, Carroll HJ. Cerebral edema and depression of sensorium in nonketotic hyperosmolar coma. Diabetes 1974; 23:525–31.
8. Delaney MF, Zisman A, Kettyle WM. Diabetic ketoacidosis and hyperglycemic hyperosmolar nonketotic syndrome. Endocrinol Metab Clin North Am 2000; 29:683–705, V.
9. White N. Diabetic ketoacidosis in children. In: Hirsch B, Neil HW, eds. Endocrinology and Metabolism Clinics of North America Acute Complications of Diabetes. Philadelphia, PA: Saunders, 2000:657–82.
10. Waldhausl W, Kleinberger G, Korn A, et al. Severe hyperglycemia: effects of rehydration on endocrine derangements and blood glucose concentration. Diabetes 1979; 28:577–84.

11. Dreyer M, Berger M, Kiess M, et al. Evidenzbasierte Leitlinie—Therapie des *Diabetes mellitus* Typ 1. In: Scherbaum WA, Lauterbach KW, Renner R, eds. Evidenzbasierte Diabetes-Leitlinien DDG: Deutsche Diabetes-Gesellschaft, 2003.

12. Van den Berghe G, Wouters PJ, Bouillon R, et al. Outcome benefit of intensive insulin therapy in the critically ill: Insulin dose versus glycemic control. Crit Care Med 2003; 31:359–66.

13. Van den Berghe G, Wilmer A, Hermans G, et al. Intensive insulin therapy in the medical ICU. N Engl J Med 2006; 354:449–61.

14. Adrogue HJ, Barrero J, Eknoyan G. Salutary effects of modest fluid replacement in the treatment of adults with diabetic ketoacidosis. Use in patients without extreme volume deficit. JAMA 1989; 262: 2108–13.

15. Wagner A, Risse A, Brill HL, et al. Therapy of severe diabetic ketoacidosis. Zero-mortality under very-low-dose insulin application. Diabetes Care 1999; 22:674–7.

16. Brown PM, Tompkins CV, Juul S, Sonksen PH. Mechanism of action of insulin in diabetic patients: a dose-related effect on glucose production and utilisation. Br Med J 1978; 1:1239–42.

17. McCurdy DK. Hyperosmolar hyperglycemic nonketotic diabetic coma. Med Clin North Am 1970; 54: 683–99.

18. Rosenthal NR, Barrett EJ. An assessment of insulin action in hyperosmolar hyperglycemic nonketotic diabetic patients. J Clin Endocrinol Metab 1985; 60:607–10.

19. Rose B, Robertson R. Treatment of diabetic ketoacidosis and nonketotic hyperglycemia. http://www.uptodate.com, 2003.

20. Kitabchi AE, Ayyagari V, Guerra SM. The efficacy of low-dose versus conventional therapy of insulin for treatment of diabetic ketoacidosis. Ann Intern Med 1976; 84:633–8.

21. Kitabchi AE. Low-dose insulin therapy in diabetic ketoacidosis: fact or fiction? Diabetes Metab Rev 1989; 5:337–63.

22. DeFronzo R, Matsuda M, Barrett E. Diabetic ketoacidosis: a combined metabolic-nephrologic approach to therapy. Diabetes Care 1994; 2:209–38.

23. Fisher JN, Shahshahani MN, Kitabchi AE. Diabetic ketoacidosis: low-dose insulin therapy by various routes. N Engl J Med 1977; 297:238–41.

24. Alberti KG, Hockaday TD, Turner RC. Small doses of intramuscular insulin in the treatment of diabetic "coma". Lancet 1973; 2:515–22.

25. Durr JA, Hoffman WH, Hensen J, et al. Osmoregulation of vasopressin in diabetic ketoacidosis. Am J Physiol 1990; 259:E723–8.

26. Daugirdas JT, Kronfol NO, Tzamaloukas AH, Ing TS. Hyperosmolar coma: cellular dehydration and the serum sodium concentration. Ann Intern Med 1989; 110:855–7.

27. Hillier TA, Abbott RD, Barrett EJ. Hyponatremia: evaluating the correction factor for hyperglycemia. Am J Med 1999; 106:399–403.

28. Simon E. Hyponatremia. http://www.emedicine.com/med/topic1130.htm, 2007.

29. Adrogue HJ, Lederer ED, Suki WN, Eknoyan G. Determinants of plasma potassium levels in diabetic ketoacidosis. Medicine (Baltimore) 1986; 65:163–72.

30. Fisher JN, Kitabchi AE. A randomized study of phosphate therapy in the treatment of diabetic ketoacidosis. J Clin Endocrinol Metab 1983; 57:177–80.

31. Zipf WB, Bacon GE, Spencer ML, et al. Hypocalcemia, hypomagnesemia, and transient hypoparathyroidism during therapy with potassium phosphate in diabetic ketoacidosis. Diabetes Care 1979; 2:265–8.

32. Brandis K. http://www.qldanaesthesia.com/Acid-BaseBook/AB8_2B.htm, 2003.

33. Glaser N, Barnett P, McCaslin I, et al. Risk factors for cerebral edema in children with diabetic ketoacidosis. The Pediatric Emergency Medicine Collaborative Research Committee of the American Academy of Pediatrics. N Engl J Med 2001; 344:264–9.

34. Carroll P, Matz R. Uncontrolled diabetes mellitus in adults: experience in treating diabetic ketoacidosis and hyperosmolar nonketotic coma with low-dose insulin and a uniform treatment regimen. Diabetes Care 1983; 6:579–85.

35. Scibilia J, Finegold D, Dorman J, Becker D, Drash A. Why do children with diabetes die? Acta Endocrinol Suppl (Copenh) 1986; 279:326–33.

36. Bureau MA, Begin R, Berthiaume Y, et al. Cerebral hypoxia from bicarbonate infusion in diabetic acidosis. J Pediatr 1980; 96:968–73.

37. Rosenbloom AL. Intracerebral crises during treatment of diabetic ketoacidosis. Diabetes Care 1990; 13:22–33.

38. Lebovitz HE. Diabetic ketoacidosis. Lancet 1995; 345:767–72.

39. Hirsch IB, Farkas-Hirsch R, Skyler JS. Intensive insulin therapy for treatment of type I diabetes. Diabetes Care 1990; 13:1265–83.

18 | Diabetic Retinopathy and Ocular Complications

Brett Rosenblatt
Long Island Vitreoretinal Consultants, Great Neck, New York, U.S.A.

Carl D. Regillo
Department of Ophthalmology, Thomas Jefferson University Hospital and Wills Eye Hospital, Philadelphia, Pennsylvania, U.S.A.

William E. Benson
Retina Service, Wills Eye Hospital, Philadelphia, Pennsylvania, U.S.A.

INTRODUCTION

Ophthalmic complications of type 2 diabetes mellitus include cataract, glaucoma, and cranial nerve palsies, but diabetic retinopathy is by far the most frequent and potentially blinding complication. Nearly three decades ago it was estimated that diabetics are 20 times more likely to be blind than the general population (1). Despite the great strides that have since been made in our understanding and management of diabetes, ocular complications continue to have a major impact on the well-being of patients with this disease. Results from several recent studies have made clear that, with tight metabolic control, vigilant screening and timely well-executed intervention, vision loss due to diabetes can be drastically reduced (2). This chapter describes the ophthalmic complications associated with type 2 diabetes, with particular attention given to their clinical characteristics and management.

EPIDEMIOLOGY

The prevalence of retinopathy increases with duration and severity of diabetes. Patients with type 2 diabetes are more likely to have signs of retinopathy at the time of diagnosis than those with type 1 diabetes. This difference is primarily a result of the frequent delay in diagnosis in older patients with more insidious onset of symptoms. However, over time, the prevalence of retinopathy increases at a slower rate in type 2 diabetics, who tend to have a more manageable disease, in contrast to the more difficult to control type 1 diabetics. The Wisconsin Epidemiologic Study of Diabetic Retinopathy (WESDR), a large population-based study, found a prevalence of retinopathy 10 years after diagnosis of 90% in type 1, compared with 60% in type 2 diabetes (3). In the WESDR, type 2 diabetics requiring insulin had nearly twice the prevalence of retinopathy, in contrast to those who did not need insulin (70% vs. 39%) (4).

The controversy regarding whether or not tight metabolic control prevents the development or progression of retinopathy has been settled by two large randomized studies. The first of these, the Diabetes Control and Complications Trial, proved that tight glucose monitoring and control reduced diabetic complications, including retinopathy, in type 1 diabetes. The intensive-therapy group achieved a median glycosylated hemoglobin (HbA$_{1c}$) of 7.2% (compared with 9.1% in the conventional group), and had a 65% risk reduction for clinically important progression of retinopathy at 10-year follow-up (5). Results of the UK Prospective Diabetes Study (UKPDS) demonstrated that intensive treatment of hyperglycemia benefited type 2 diabetics as well. In the UKPDS over 5000 patients with recently diagnosed type 2 diabetes were randomly assigned to intensive or conventional treatment. Various hypoglycemic agents, including insulin, were used to maintain a fasting blood glucose level near 110 mg/dL in the intensive-treatment group, whereas diet alone was used in the conventional-treatment cohort. The intensive-treatment group achieved a median HbA$_{1c}$ of 7%, compared with the significantly higher 7.9% in the conventional-treatment group. Tighter control was associated with a 21% risk reduction for the progression of diabetic retinopathy at the 12-year follow-up (38% intensive group vs. 48% conventional group) (6). Physicians can now be assured that the current American Diabetes Association recommendation of aiming for an HbA_{1c} of 7.0% is an indispensable aspect of diabetes management (7). Despite the benefits that meticulous control of serum glucose provides, it may not prevent progression in diabetics with very advanced retinopathy (8).

The development and progression of retinopathy most certainly is influenced by many factors, including race, gender, hypertension and other vasculopathic systemic disorders. Epidemiologic studies have been unable to conclusively demonstrate a definitive association between these factors and retinopathy in patients with type 2 diabetes (9–15). Pregnancy, however, has been shown to be a significant risk factor for development and progression of diabetic retinopathy. In women without retinopathy at the start of pregnancy, 10% will show mild retinal changes that resolve after delivery. However, in women with pre-existing retinopathy, up to 25% will progress to proliferative changes during pregnancy (16). Those at greatest risk for severe visual deterioration are those who are rapidly brought under strict control (17). Women should be encouraged to have their eyes examined and their glycemic control optimized prior to becoming pregnant.

CLINICAL FEATURES

Systemic complications of diabetes typically manifest clinically after permanent tissue damage has already occurred. Unlike the changes occurring in other organs, the microvascular alterations responsible for preventable vision loss can be observed directly through a dilated pupil (Fig. 1). Clinicians caring for diabetics should be skilled at recognizing the signs and symptoms of diabetic retinopathy, not only because it minimizes visual sequelae, but also because the status of the retina reflects microvascular complications occurring elsewhere in the body.

Ophthalmologists classify diabetic retinopathy as non-proliferative diabetic retinopathy (NPDR) and proliferative diabetic retinopathy (PDR). The non-proliferative changes are also commonly referred to as background diabetic retinopathy. The ocular changes seen in eyes with NPDR all occur at the level of the retina, in contrast to PDR, which is characterized by the growth of blood vessels and fibrous tissue beyond the surface of the retina. The clinical

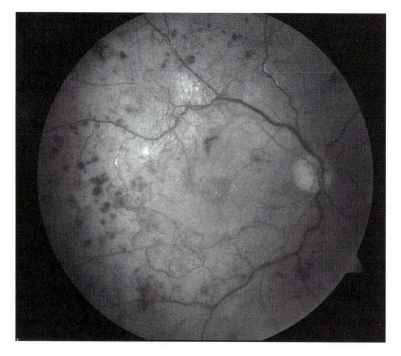

FIGURE 1 Diabetic retinopathy.

features of diabetic retinopathy, including microaneurysms, cotton wool spots (CWS), retinal edema, exudates, venous abnormalities and neovascularization, are all secondary to compromised capillary endothelium, which leads to increased capillary permeability and fragility. Widespread small vessel damage leads to areas of ischemia, which can promote intraocular angiogenesis.

Numerous hypotheses explaining the microvascular complications of diabetes have been investigated, including the role of the polyol pathway, glycosylated end products, growth factors and oxidative stress (18–20). Angiogenic factors, such as growth hormone and vascular endothelial growth factor (VEGF) are being evaluated for their mechanistic and potential therapeutic role in diabetic retinopathy. Increased concentrations, or overexpression of intraocular VEGF has been shown to lead to neovascularization, as well as increased permeability of retinal vasculature. Furthermore, inhibitors of VEGF have been shown to prevent ischemia-induced neovascularization in several animal models (21,22).

Protein kinase C (PKC) activation is required for VEGF to induce its effects on vascular endothelium. Orally ingested inhibitors of PKC, currently in clinical trials, have shown promise as an effective way of preventing many of the diabetes-induced vascular complications. Interest in the interaction between components of blood flow, including blood viscosity and red-cell deformability, has also increased recently. Blood viscosity, a potentially modifiable factor, has been shown in small studies to impact the progression and visual impact of diabetic retinopathy (23,24).

Non-Proliferative Diabetic Retinopathy

Microaneurysms are the most common, and usually the first detectable, signs of retinopathy. These saccular out-pouching of capillaries appear as small discrete red dots within the retina, which tend to increase in number and size with progression of NPDR. Retinal hemorrhages, another early finding, result from ruptured micro aneurysms, capillaries or venules. The morphology of retinal hemorrhages depends on how deep within the retina they lie. The deeper "dot-blot" hemorrhages are round with distinct borders; whereas superficial nerve fiber layer hemorrhages assume a flame or splinter shape (Fig. 2). These early, often subtle,

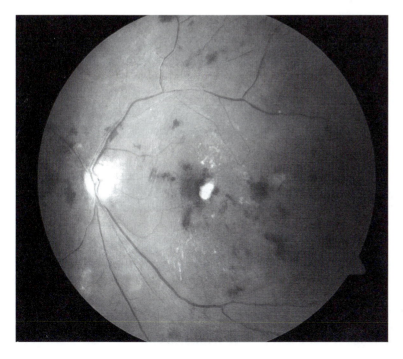

FIGURE 2 Non-proliferative diabetic retinopathy demonstrating retinal hemorrhages.

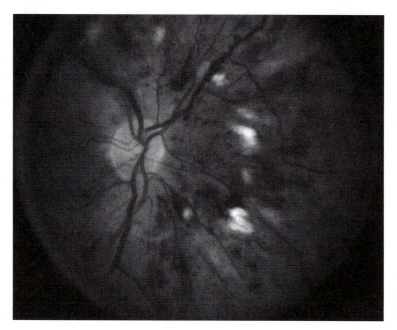

FIGURE 3 Non-proliferative diabetic retinopathy with numerous cotton wool spots.

manifestations of NPDR are important to recognize, because an increasing number of microaneurysms may indicate deterioration of retinopathy (25).

Cotton wool spots are seen ophthalmoscopically as superficial white lesions with feathery margins (Fig. 3). Although they are commonly called "soft exudates," they result from ischemia, not exudation. Local ischemia causes effective obstruction of axoplasmic flow in the normally transparent nerve fiber layer; the subsequent swelling of the nerve fibers gives CWS their characteristic white appearance. CWS are not specific for diabetes, and are commonly seen in association with hypertension, collagen-vascular disease, AIDS, carotid obstruction and cardiac valvular disease. The presence of even a single CWS deserves a systemic evaluation (26).

Hard exudates are extracellular deposits of lipid within the retina. They are sharply demacated yellow "waxy" lesions of varying size and configuration that, unlike CWS, have well-defined borders. This lipid derives from leaky vessels; hard exudates are therefore often associated with areas of retinal edema.

Macular edema, which is defined as thickening of the central retina, is the leading cause of legal blindness in diabetics (27). Clinically significant macula edema (CSME) is edema or hard exudates that involve or threaten the part of the retina which subserves central vision (the fovea) (28). This important sign is often difficult to visualize, because alterations of retinal thickness are subtle. It is best evaluated through the stereoscopic view provided by a contact lens and slit-lamp biomicroscope.

As NPDR advances, signs of retinal ischemia appear. These include increasing CWS, hemorrhages, venous irregularities and intraretinal microvascular abnormalities (IRMA). Venous beading (irregularly dilated venules) and IRMA (telangiectatic capillaries that shunt blood around areas of non-perfusion) often portend progression to proliferative changes. The Early Treatment Diabetic Retinopathy Study found that multiple retinal hemorrhages, venous beading, IRMA and widespread capillary non-perfusion were the clinical signs that best predicted progression to proliferative retinopathy. Eyes that had many of these features in excess have up to a 50% risk of progression to PDR after 1 year (29). Although the macular edema, exudates, and capillary occlusions that occur in NPDR can occasionally cause legal blind ness, affected patients usually maintain at least ambulatory vision. Proliferative diabetic retinopathy, on the other hand, is more likely to result in disabling, severe vision loss.

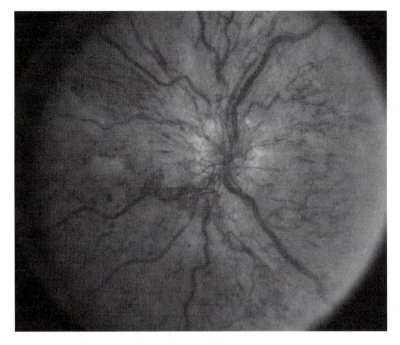

FIGURE 4 Neovascularization of the disc.

Proliferative Diabetic Retinopathy

Proliferative retinopathy is heralded by the growth of neovascular and fibrous tissue. The overall prevalence of PDR in type 2 diabetics is 10%, but the rate is higher in those requiring insulin (14%) compared with those not requiring insulin (3%) (4). Blood vessel growth from the optic nerve is termed neovascularization of the disc (NVD); whereas vessels arising from any other part of the retina is referred to as neovascularization elsewhere (NVE) (Figs. 4 and 5). Neovascular tissue extends into the vitreous—the clear delicate connective tissue that fills the space bounded posteriorly by the retina and anteriorly by the lens. The complications of PDR are related to the propensity for new vessels to bleed (vitreous hemorrhage), as well as

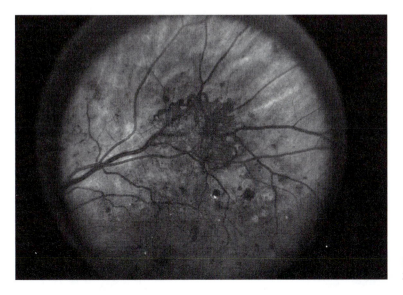

FIGURE 5 Neovascularization elsewhere.

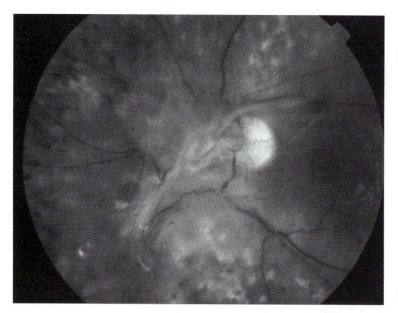

FIGURE 6 Tractional retinal detachment.

the tendency of the vitreous body to shrink and pull the retina forward (traction retinal detachment) (Fig. 6). Bleeding within the vitreous causes sudden painless loss of acuity.

The extent and location of the hemorrhage determine the magnitude of vision loss. Examining eyes with vitreous hemorrhage is difficult because blood in the vitreous obscures retinal details. When necessary, intraocular structures are assessed with ultrasonography. Tractional retinal detachments, the other major complication of PDR, appear as elevations of all or portions of the retina. Tractional retinal detachment occurs when fibrous tissue pulls on the retina, overwhelming the adhesive forces keeping it attached. Patients with detached retinas present with loss of vision corresponding to the part of the retina that has detached. For example, a superior retinal detachment will cause an inferior visual field defect because of the inverted topographic representation of the retina. Vision loss is often preceded by the sensation of flashing lights or floaters. If suspected, prompt referral to an ophthalmologist experienced in the repair of retinal detachments is critical.

MANAGEMENT

Non-Proliferative Diabetic Retinopathy

Management of NPDR relies heavily on patient education, periodic screening and, when necessary, laser treatment. The American College of Physicians/American Academy of Ophthalmology has recommended a schedule for ophthalmic evaluation for patients with diabetes (Table 1). Periodic eye examinations enable ophthalmologists to identify patients who would benefit from prophylactic treatment, before serious complications develop. The potential sight-threatening sequelae associated with diabetic retinopathy and other ocular complications should be stressed to patients with diabetes; they should be made aware that regular eye examinations are integral to their diabetes management. Patients, as well as all clinicians caring for diabetics, should be able to recognize the signs and symptoms of diabetic eye disease.

Clinically significant macula edema, which can occur in non-proliferative or proliferative retinopathy, must be suspected in any patient with diabetes complaining of blurred vision. A delay in referral, or recognition of the signs or symptoms of macular edema, can diminish the success of intervention. Treatment of CSME with laser decreases the rate of moderately severe vision loss at 3-year follow-up from 30% in untreated to 15% in treated eyes (28). Laser energy applied in a grid pattern to the area of retinal thickening facilitates the resorbtion of fluid, allowing the retina to resume its normal thickness and function. Focal laser treatment can also be used to close off the leaking vessels that are causing the edema. This requires

TABLE 1 Suggested Follow-Up and Intervention for Patients with Diabetic Retinopathy

Retinal abnormality	Follow-up	Action
None or minimal NPDR (none or rare microaneurysms)	Annually	Optimize control of serum glucose, hypertension, serum lipids, renal disease
Mild NPDR (few scattered retinal hemorrhages and microaneurysms)	Every 6–12 months	Optimize control of serum glucose, hypertension, serum lipids, renal disease
Moderate NPDR (moderate hemorrhages and microaneurysms; hard exudates or soft exudates may be present)	Every 6–12 months	Optimize control of serum glucose, hypertension, serum lipids, renal disease
Severe or very severe NPDR (widespread retinal hemorrhages, venous abnormalities or IRMA)	Every 1–4 months	Consider early scatter laser treatment as retinopathy progresses
Macular edema (CSME if thickening or hard exudates threaten the fovea)	Every 2–4 months	Treat CSME with focal laser treatment Fluorescein angiogram necessary to locate leaking sources
Proliferative diabetic retinopathy, less than high risk (minimal neovascularization without bleeding)	Every 2–4 months	Consider early scatter laser treatment as retinopathy progresses
Proliferative diabetic retinopathy, high risk (extensive NVD, NVD with hemorrhage, extensive NVE with hemorrhage)	Every 1–4 months	Pan retinal photocoagulation is indicated More than 1500 laser burns, applied to peripheral retina in one or multiple sessions
Vitreous hemorrhage (blood dispersed in the vitreous cavity, poor retinal view)	Every 1–3 months	Serial ultrasonography; Vitrectomy for persistent hemorrhage, for active retinopathy requiring laser (which is prohibited by hemorrhage) or for retinal detachment that threatens the macula
Traction retinal detachment (elevation of part of the retina associated with fibrous tissue)	Every 1–3 months	Vitrectomy if threatening macula; otherwise careful observation

Abbreviations: CSME, clinically significant macula edema; IRMA, intraretinal microvascular abnormalities; NPDR, non-proliferative diabetic retinopathy; NVD, neovascularization of the disc; NVE, neovascularization elsewhere.

precision; the exact location of leaking sources can only be identified by fluorescein angiography. This diagnostic study involves the intravenous injection of a fluorescent dye, which is captured on film or digital media as it passes through the retinal circulation. The proper management of diabetic macular edema relies heavily on the information provided by these detailed images of retinal vasculature (Figs. 7 and 8). Intravitreal corticosteroids are also utilized to treat diabetic macular edema, especially those cases that are refractory to laser treatment. In addition, anti-VEGF agents may also prove to be a valuable treatment for diabetic macular edema. These agents are currently under investigation.

Proliferative Diabetic Retinopathy

The goal of managing PDR is to prevent vitreous hemorrhage and retinal detachments. Pan-retinal photocoagulation (PRP) involves the application of approximately 1500 to 2000, or more, laser burns to the peripheral retina, effectively ablating large areas of ischemic retina. It is believed that this, in turn, reduces the production of angiogenic substances, such as VEGF.

In the Diabetic Retinopathy Study, PRP reduced the rate of severe vision loss from 26% in observed eyes to 11% in treated eyes at 2-year follow-up, a 60% risk reduction (30).

Pan-retinal photocoagulation, although successful in promoting regression of the neovascularization in 72% of patients by 3 weeks, is associated with loss of peripheral vision and, occasionally, with other vision-compromising side effects (31). PRP is typically reserved for patients with high-risk characteristics—eyes that have the most to gain from treatment (Fig. 9).

The use of aspirin deserves special attention because its role in the management in diabetic retinopathy has been extensively debated. Many clinicians have been concerned that the antiplatelet effect of aspirin may promote intraocular bleeding. Others felt that the rheologic alterations induced by aspirin might decrease microvascular complications. However, evidence from a large randomized study revealed that aspirin has no clear beneficial or harmful effect on vision or progression of diabetic retinopathy. More importantly, this study found that those

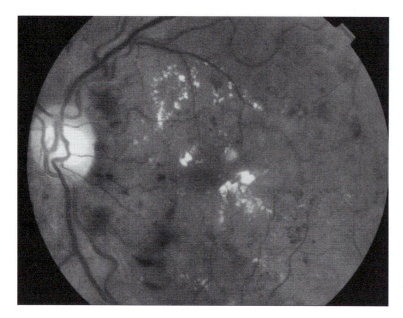

FIGURE 7 Macular edema with associated hard exudates.

receiving aspirin had a 17% decreased risk of morbidity and death from cardiovascular disease (32). Patients with diabetic retinopathy may take an aspirin daily unless otherwise contraindicated.

Vitrectomy, the surgical evacuation of the vitreous cavity, plays a vital role in the management of severe complications of diabetic retinopathy. Removal of the vitreous limits the progression of neovascularization, because it eliminates the collagen fibrils that act as scaffolding upon which new blood vessels grow. Several studies have evaluated whether vitrectomy might improve the visual prognosis by reducing neovascularization and its concomitant complications. Two independent studies of patients with non-clearing vitreous hemorrhage for at least 6 months found that >80% had improvement in vision following vitrectomy (33,34). The surgical complication rate, including retinal detachment and ocular

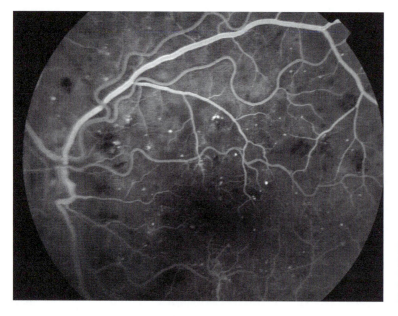

FIGURE 8 Fluorescein angiogram of eye as in Figure 7, showing macular edema. Bright spots localize the focal areas of leakage.

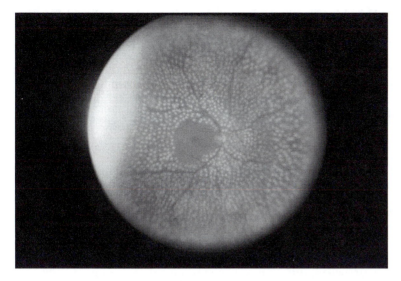

FIGURE 9 Wide-angle view of an eye following PRP.

infections, in these early investigations approached 10% (33). Fortunately, surgical techniques and instrumentation have improved substantially over the last decade, vitrectomy is now an even safer, more effective procedure. The most common indications for vitrectomy in patients with PDR are non-clearing vitreous hemorrhage, or tractional retinal detachment.

OTHER OCULAR COMPLICATIONS

Lens

Diabetes is an important risk factor for the development of cataracts. The incidence of cataracts are two to four times greater in diabetics than in non-diabetics, and may be the most frequent cause of decreased vision in type 2 diabetics (35,36). Cataracts in diabetes, although indistinguishable from typical age-related lens opacities, often require surgical extraction at a much younger age. Diabetics with retinopathy are at higher risk for complications of cataract surgery (37). However, those without retinopathy tend to have excellent results, with 90% to 95% having a final visual acuity of 20/40 or better (38,39). The best-known predictor of postoperative success is the preoperative severity of retinopathy (40).

Reversible changes in the refractive power of the lens associated with poor glycemic control can cause fluctuations in vision. Patients who are unaware that they have diabetes commonly present to ophthalmologists complaining that they need new glasses. Careful examination typically reveals a significant change in their spectacle correction, often without other signs of diabetic eye disease. It is thought that local accumulation of sorbitol, an end-product of glucose metabolism, leads to osmotic swelling of the lens (41). Although the symptoms can be temporarily corrected by prescribing new spectacles, the refractive shift is usually transient. Vision gradually returns to normal following achievement of metabolic control.

Glaucoma

Primary open angle glaucoma (POAG) is common in patients with diabetes, although a cause and effect association is unclear (42,43). POAG is a progressive loss of neural tissue in the optic nerve, associated with loss of peripheral vision. Increasing age, elevated intraocular pressure, black race and family history are other important risk factors for POAG. Current management of POAG relies on early detection and preventing progression. Medical or surgical reduction of the intraocular pressure, the only modifiable risk factor, is believed to slow the loss of vision in patients with POAG. All patients with diabetes should be watched closely for glaucoma, because vision loss is irreversible.

Neovascular glaucoma is a feared complication of PDR. Normal eyes should not have blood vessels visible on the surface of the iris. Neovascularization of the iris and the anterior chamber angle are due to widespread intraocular ischemia. Proliferating blood vessels and fibrous tissue arising from the iris can cause angle closure glaucoma by obstructing the normal outflow of aqueous from the eye. Aqueous that continues to be produced, despite the limited drainage capacity of the eye, results in very high intraocular pressures, rapid loss of vision and pain. Neovascular glaucoma is often refractory to treatment; however, PRP can be effective in reducing neovascularization before it results in angle closure (44,45).

Optic Neuropathy

Diabetes is a risk factor for several optic nerve problems, most important of which is anterior ischemic optic neuropathy (AION). AION presents as sudden, painless monocular loss of vision, associated with a swollen optic nerve and prominent afferent pupillary defect (Marcus Gunn pupil). This condition is common in older diabetics with other vasculopathic risk factors, such as hypertension and hyperlipidemia. Although there is no medical or surgical intervention that has been shown to reverse the damage in AION, reducing other risk factors may minimize the risk to the other eye. Diabetic papillopathy, a less common optic nerve disorder, is characterized by transient unilateral or bilateral optic disc swelling. Despite the alarming appearance, patients typically have minimal loss of vision. The prognosis in diabetic papillopathy, unlike ischemic optic neuropathy, is excellent, as nearly all patients recover 20/50 or better visual acuity (46).

Cranial Neuropathy

Cranial neuropathies involving the oculomotor (CN III), trochlear (CN IV), or abducens (CN VI) nerves occur frequently in elderly type 2 diabetics (47). Extraocular muscles become paretic secondary to focal microangiopathy causing ischemic demyelination of the associated cranial nerve. Patients typically present with binocular double vision, with or without pain. Symptoms characteristically resolve in 1 to 3 months, with little or no sequelae (48). If double vision persists for >3 months, cranial and orbital imaging should be obtained to rule out other pathology. Other indications for further work-up include involvement of multiple cranial nerves, associated neurologic deficits, or young patient age. Persistent double vision can be treated with monocular occlusion, prisms or extraocular muscle surgery.

Orbital Infections

Rhino-orbital mucormycosis is an opportunistic fungal infection that is seen most frequently in poorly controlled diabetes and other immuno-compromised states. It should be suspected in any patient with restricted ocular motility, decreased vision, ptosis, chemosis and proptosis. The black eschar classically seen in the nasal mucosa represents necrotic tissue that typically needs to be debrided. Early diagnosis and aggressive medical and surgical management is crucial. Prior to the availability of effective antifungal agents, mucormycosis was uniformly fatal. Prompt recognition, with aggressive medical and surgical treatment, is the key to managing this potentially devastating infection (49).

CONCLUSION

Ocular complications of diabetes can have a profound impact on the well-being of patients with diabetes. Visual loss often can be prevented, ameliorated, or delayed, but timely referral is a key. Even those who cannot be helped medically or surgically can be assisted in making use of remaining visual function and other remaining senses. Many patients are not screened or referred according to American College of Physicians/American Academy of Ophthalmology guidelines, and thus are not receiving the best possible care. Periodic detailed ophthalmic examinations for retinopathy, and a search for other ocular conditions for which persons with diabetes are at increased risk (especially cataract and glaucoma), are critical. Prompt eye examination should also be performed if symptoms such as ocular pain, redness, reduced vision, double vision, floaters, light flashes, or other unexplained visual symptoms occur.

REFERENCES

1. Kahn HA, Hiller R. Blindness caused by diabetic retinopathy. Am J Ophthalmol 1974; 78:58–67.
2. American Diabetes Association. Screening for diabetic retinopathy. Diabetes Care 1996; 19(Suppl.): 20–2.
3. Klein R, et al. The Wisconsin Epidemiologic Study of diabetic retinopathy. XIV. Ten-year incidence and progression of diabetic retinopathy. Arch Ophthalmol 1994; 112:1217–28.
4. Klein R, et al. The Wisconsin epidemiologic study of diabetes retinopathy. III. Prevalence and risk of diabetic retinopathy when age of diagnosis is 30 or more years. Arch Ophthalmol 1984; 102:527–32.
5. Diabetes Control and Complications Trial Research Group. The effect of intensive diabetes treatment on the progression of diabetic retinopathy in insulin-dependent diabetes mellitus. Arch Ophthalmol 1995; 113:36–51.
6. Group, UKPDS. Intensive blood-glucose control with sulfonylureas or insulin compared with conventional treatment and risk of complications in patients with type 2 diabetes. UKPDS 33. Lancet 1998; 352:837–53.
7. American Diabetes Association. Standards of medical care for patients with diabetes mellitus. Diabetes Care 1998; 21(Suppl.):S23–31.
8. Ramsay RC, Goetz FC, Sutherland DE, et al. Progression of diabetic retinopathy after pancreas transplantation for insulin-dependent diabetes mellitus. N Engl J Med 1988; 318:208–14.
9. Raab MF, Gagliano DA, Sweeney HE. Diabetic retinopathy in blacks. Diabetes Care 1990; 13:1202–6.
10. Arfken CL, Salicrup AE, Meuer SM, et al. Retinopathy in African Americans and whites with insulin-dependent diabetes mellitus. Arch Intern Med 1994; 154:2597–601.
11. Klein R, Klein BE, Moss SE. Is blood pressure a predictor of the incidence or progression of diabetic retinopathy? Arch Intern Med 1989; 149:2427.
12. Klein R, Klein BE. Epidemiology of proliferative diabetic retinopathy. Diabetes Care 1992; 15: 1875–91.
13. Klein R, Klein BE, Moss SE, Davis MD, DeMets DL. The Wisconsin epidemiologic study of diabetic retinopathy. II. Prevalence and risk of diabetic retinopathy when age is less than 30 years. Arch Ophthalmol 1984; 102:520–6.
14. Nelson RG, Wolfe JA, Horton MB, et al. Proliferative retinopathy in NIDDM. Diabetes 1989; 38:435.
15. Janka HU, et al. Risk factors for progression of background retinopathy in long-standing IDDM. Diabetes 1989; 38:460.
16. Klein BEK, Moss SE, Klein R. Effect of pregnancy on progression of diabetic retinopathy. Diabetes Care 1990; 13:34–40.
17. Rosenn B, Miodovnik M, Kranias G, et al. Progression of diabetic retinopathy in pregnancy: association with hypertension in pregnancy. Am J Obstet Gynecol 1992; 166:1214–8.
18. Greene D, Sima A, Stevens M. Aldose reductase inhibitors: an approach to the treatment of diabetic nerve damage. Diabetes Metab Rev 1993; 9:189–217.
19. Brownlee M. The pathologic implications of protein glycolation. Clin Invest Med 1995; 18:275–81.
20. Baynes JW, Thorpe S. Role of oxidative stress in diabetic complications: a new perspective on an old paradigm. Diabetes 1999; 48:1–9.
21. Williams J, Adamis A, Aiello L. Vascular endothelial growth factor in ocular neovascularization and proliferative diabetic retinopathy. Diabetes Metab Rev 1997; 13:37–50.
22. Aiello L. Vascular endothelial growth factor: 20th century mechanisms, 21st-century therapies. Invest Ophthalmol Vis Sci 1997; 38:1647–52.
23. Fujisawa T, Ikegami H, Yamato E, et al. Association of plasma fibrinogen level and blood pressure with diabetic retinopathy, and renal complications associated with proliferative diabetic retinopathy, in Type 2 diabetes mellitus. Diabet Med 1999; 16:522–6.
24. Widder RA, Brunner R, Walter P, et al. Improvement of visual acuity in patients suffering from diabetic retinopathy after membrane differential filtration: a pilot study. Transfus Sci 1999; 21:201–6.
25. Kohner EM, Sleightholm M. Does microaneurysm count reflect severity of early diabetic retinopathy? Ophthalmology 1986; 93:586–9.
26. Brown GC, Brown MM, Hiller T, et al. Cotton-wool spots. Retina 1985; 5:206–14.
27. Patz A, Schatz H, Berkow JW, et al. Macularedema: an overlooked complication of diabetic retinopathy. Trans Am Acad Ophthalmol Otolaryngol 1973; 77:34–42.
28. Early Treatment Diabetic Retinopathy Study Research Group. Photocoagulation for diabetic macular edema: Early Treatment Diabetic Retinopathy Study Report no. 4. Int Ophthalmol Clin 1987; 27: 265–72.

29. Early Treatment Diabetic Retinopathy Study Research Group. Fundus photographic risk factors for progression of diabetic retinopathy. Early Treatment Diabetic Retinopathy Study Report no. 12. Ophthalmology 1991; 98:823–33.

30. Diabetic Retinopathy Study Group. Clinical applications of Diabetic Retinopathy Study (DRS) findings: Diabetic Retinopathy Study Report no. 8. Ophthalmology 1981; 88:583–600.

31. Doft BH, Blankenship GW. Single versus multiple treatment sessions of argon laser panretinal photocoagulation for proliferative diabetic retinopathy. Ophthalmology 1982; 89:772.

32. Early Treatment Diabetic Retinopathy Study Research Group. Effects of aspirin treatment on diabetic retinopathy. Early Treatment Diabetic Retinopathy Study Report no. 8. Ophthalmology 1991; 98: 757–65.

33. Benson WE, Brown GC, Tasman W, McNamara JA. Complications of vitrectomy for non-clearing vitreous hemorrhage in diabetic patients. Ophthalmic Surg 1988; 19:862–5.

34. Thompson JT, de Bustros S, Michels RG, Rice TA. Results and prognostic factors in vitrectomy for diabetic vitreous hemorrhage. Arch Ophthalmol 1987; 105:191–5.

35. Bernth-Peterson P, Bach E. Epidemiologic aspects of cataract surgery. III: Frequencies of diabetes and glaucoma in a cataract population. Acta Ophthalmol 1983; 61:406–16.

36. Klein BEK, Klein R, Moss RE. Prevalence of cataracts in a population-based study of persons with diabetes mellitus. Ophthalmology 1985; 92:1191.

37. Minckler D, Astorino A, Hamilton A. Cataract surgery in patients with diabetes. Ophthalmology 1998; 105:949–50.

38. Krupsky S, Zalish M, Oliver M, Pollack A. Anterior segment complications in diabetic patients following extracapsular cataract extraction and posterior chamber intraocular lens implantation. Ophthalmic Surg 1991; 22:526–30.

39. Straatsma BR, Pettit TH, Wheeler N, Miyamasu W. Diabetes mellitus and intraocular lens implantation. Ophthalmology 1983; 90:336–3.

40. Hykin PG, Gregson RM, Stevens JD, Hamilton PA. Extracapsular cataract extraction in proliferative diabetic retinopathy. Ophthalmology 1993; 100:394–9.

41. Benson WE, Brown GC, Tasman W. Diabetes and Its Ocular Complications. Philadelphia: WB Saunders, 1988:27–34.

42. Tielsch JM, Katz J, Quigley HA, Javitt JC, Sommer A. Diabetes, intraocular pressure, and primary open-angle glaucoma in the Baltimore Eye Survey. Ophthalmology 1995; 102:48–53.

43. Klein B, Klein R, Jensen S. Open-angle glaucoma and older-onset diabetes: the Beaver Dam Eye Study. Ophthalmology 1994; 101:173–7.

44. Little HL, Rosenthal AR, Dellaporta A, Jacobson DR. The effect of panretinal photocoagulation on rubeosis iridis. Am J Ophthalmol 1976; 81:804.

45. Jacobson DR, Murphy RP, Rosenthal AR. The treatment of angle neovascularization with pan retinal photocoagulation. Ophthalmology 1979; 86:1270–5.

46. Regillo CD, Brown GC, Savino PJ, et al. Diabetic papillopathy. Patient characteristics and fundus findings. Arch Ophthalmol 1995; 113:889–95.

47. Watanabe K, Hagura R, Akanuma Y, et al. Characteristics of cranial nerve palsies in diabetic patients. Diabetes Res Clin Pract 1990; 10:19–27.

48. Burde RM. Neuro-ophthalmic associations and complications of diabetes mellitus. Am J Ophthalmol 1992; 114:498–501.

49. Benson WE, Brown GC, Tasman W. Diabetes and Its Ocular Complications. Philadelphia: WB Saunders, 1988:117–8.

19 | Renal Dysfunction and Hypertension

Carl Erik Mogensen
Medical Department, Aarhus Sygehus, Aarhus University Hospital, Aarhus, Denmark

INTRODUCTION

Nephropathy in type 2 diabetes has emerged as a severe clinical problem in diabetes of this type and is now much more frequently seen than advanced renal disease in type 1 diabetes (1,2). However, in the 1970s and 1980s, renal complications due to type 2 diabetes seemed to be rare in the clinic so this new development is surprising. Today, most patients in dialysis units are type 2 diabetics, which raises the following question: Why and how did type 2 diabetes lose its "renal innocence" (3–5)?

There is probably not one single factor responsible for this new problem. In all likelihood, there are more frequent referrals of old and severely ill patients with terminal renal failure than previously. It is also clear that there is a dramatically rising prevalence of type 2 diabetes in the general population. This is partly due to the adoption of new and "less healthy" lifestyles. However, an even more important factor in this context is that survival of patients with type 2 diabetes has improved simply because of better treatment of hypertension, especially coronary heart disease, conditions that previously were quite common in these patients, and which earlier could not or were not treated properly.

There is thus a change in life pattern of these patients—they often live long enough to develop renal disease and even renal failure. The increase in number of patients is thus a result of medical progress (4) where cardiovascular mortality at least to some extent has been replaced by end-stage renal disease (ESRD) as the terminal fate of these patients. Clearly cardiovascular mortality is still overwhelming. It should be noted that the strict classification of type 1 and type 2 diabetes may by no means be completely relevant because there are many patients with ESRD in whom classification is problematic. Also, the pathogenesis and treatment strategy is very similar. Thus, new studies suggest that the clinical course of renal disease is very much the same in the two types of diabetes as far as a fall in glomerular filtration rate (GFR) is concerned (3,5).

Type 2 diabetes is probably a polygenic condition that acts in a complicated interplay of lifestyle and environment. Ironically, our improved living conditions, with more abundant food and less hard physical work, has reappeared as a boomerang, creating new degenerative diseases which are not due to physical burdens and hard work—rather the opposite.

HISTORICAL ASPECTS

In the pre-insulin era, patients who developed complications related to diabetes would be type 2 diabetics because type 1 patients would simply not survive long enough. As early as the 19th century, it was recognized that urine of diabetic patients contained abnormal amounts of coagulable matters, likely to be proteins (6,7).

The French physician Rayer (8) also described in 1839 the characteristic renal hypertrophy that was rediscovered only in the 1970s, and German physicians identified renal involvement in diabetes: when glucosuria would disappear due to a severe decrease in renal function, patients would quite often have heavy proteinuria and edema (6).

Pathologists were also aware of the typical diabetic kidney and quite often Arman Epstein lesions were identified because of lack of treatment (9). However, the understanding of the disease was changed by the observation in 1936 by Kimmelstiel and Wilson (10) who found glomerular lesions in eight patients, all of whom were likely to be type 2 diabetic patients with renal impairment and hypertension. Kimmelstiel and Wilson clearly understood that the renal disease was due to diabetes. However, for many years such complications were still considered rare in type 2 diabetes and the clinical course was not considered malignant (benign diabetes) (11).

In the last few years, there has been a change in treatment strategy, partly because of the UK Prospective Diabetes Study (UKPDS) that clearly negated the concept that glycemic treatment with sulfonylurea (SU) agents and metformin and even insulin, could be deleterious (12,13). The opposite is rather the case although with some reservations (14). Still results from the DART study suggest some problems with SU treatment (15). However, no comparison was done comparing old and new SU. Now recent evidence favors use of newer SU (14,16).

EVALUATION OF DIABETIC RENAL DISEASE AND CLASSIFICATION

It is now widely accepted that patients with type 1 diabetes exhibit a very characteristic evolution of renal changes (Table 1). Initially, there may be hyperfiltration and renal hypertrophy, but normal albumin excretion rate unless the normal are or have been badly controlled with respect to glycemia. The reservation is, however, that many type 2 diabetic patients have had undiagnosed diabetes for several years.

In contrast to type 1 diabetes, patients with type 2 diabetes quite often have hypertension related to abnormalities of obesity and the metabolic syndrome (17). They may also exhibit signs of loss of renal autoregulation meaning that a high blood pressure is inflicted on the glomeruli (18). However, over the years, there is an increasing thickening of the basement membrane and expansion of the mesangium. GFR may even be high because of glycemic dysregulation (19).

Renal structural lesions may be found in patients with type 2 diabetes, but they may be more unspecific due to longstanding hypertension and age-related vascular disease. Therefore, it is not uncommon that many patients have microalbuminuria early on.

The typical course in type 1 and 2 diabetes with incipient nephropathy is microalbuminuria (Table 2), generally found after 5- to 15-year duration of diabetes. The renal excretion of albumin is usually clearly elevated in patients with type 1 diabetes when they exhibit elevated blood pressure. However, quite often blood-pressure is in the so-called upper normal range.

Regarding type 2 diabetes, arterial hypertension is very common and a patient with microalbuminuria who is followed for many years is at an increased risk of overt renal disease and importantly also of cardiovascular mortality (20–22). The observations related to microalbuminuria were done in Europe many years ago and have now been confirmed in

TABLE 1   Characteristics in the Development of Renal Dysfunction and Nephropathy in Type 2 Diabetes

Stage 1: At the clinical diagnosis without pre-diagnostic diabetes	Normal serum creatinine and somewhat elevated GFR (but not to the same extent as in type 1 diabetes). Some patients may have microalbuminuria at clinical diagnosis due to undiagnosed diabetes. Blood pressure may be elevated since essential hypertension may be related to the metabolic syndrome and type 2 diabetes.
Stage 2: Silent stage	After the diagnosis and treatment of hyperglycemia abnormal albuminuria may be found (or it may be reduced if initially increased). In some studies, GFR has been found to be moderately decreased. Blood pressure has a tendency to increase over time.
Stage 3	Microalbuminuria typically develops from normoalbuminuria after some years with diabetes related to blood pressure elevation and glycemic control. Hypertension is quite common in such patients. GFR may still be normal, but tends to decrease progressively.
Stage 4: Overt diabetic nephropathy	Proteinuria typically after 10–20 years with diabetes. GFR declines variably related to metabolic control and blood pressure, even borderline BP-elevation should be carefully treated. Cardiovascular disease is common. On biopsy, these patients typically have lesions, but a few percentages do not show any changes or non-diabetic lesions. Biopsy is, however, generally not indicated. Retinopathy is quite often found, but not necessarily.
Stage 5	The late stage, just before or with renal insufficiency.

Abbreviation: GFR, glomerular filtration rate.

TABLE 2 Albumin Excretion in Microalbuminuria

Range short-term collections	20–200 µg/min
24-hr urines	30–300 mg/24 hr
Albumin creatinine ratio (85) (morning or spot urine)	Men: 2.5–25 mL/mmol creatinine
	Women: 3.5–35 mL/mmol creatinine

a number of subsequent studies (21). Persistent microalbuminuria is a clear ominous sign of both renal involvement and cardiovascular disease (20), and also an indicator for treatment (21–23).

The next stage is the well-known situation with proteinuria, diagnosed by means of old-fashioned methods. GFR starts to fall and correlates to the level of blood pressure and glycemia. Without treatment the fall rate is about 10 mL/min/year if blood pressure is not well regulated and proteinuria increases, correlated again to glycemia (20–22).

High blood pressure is common in type 1 and even more so in type 2 diabetes (Table 3). As shown in two large trials as well as other studies, the decline in GFR in type 2 diabetes is quite rapid. Thus, patients with proteinuria and type 2 diabetes have a very poor prognosis, not only due to renal disease and later ESRD, but also due to the increase in risk of cardiovascular mortality that presently may be better controlled by new agents that control the risk elements (23–25). Antihypertensive treatment encompasses several types of drugs (13) with concomitant beneficial effects. Beta-blockers may control arrhythmia and heart insufficiency while diuretics are useful for fluid overload. Renin–angiotensin system (RAS) blockade controls systemic blood pressure (BP)-elevation as well as increased pressure in the glomeruli. BP-lowering is per se a key element, often using calcium blockers and other antihypertensives (Fig. 1).

PROBLEMATIC ISSUES

There has been some discussion about the significance of non-diabetic renal disease in diabetic patients. In my experience this is quite rare, but selected studies from nephrology departments show that the problem may be more common there. However, it is now generally accepted that non-diabetic renal disease is not more common in diabetic patients than in the background population (4). It has taken many years to reach this understanding. Renal biopsies are very rarely indicated.

The understanding of diabetic renal disease has been distorted by the following hypotheses:

1. It has been claimed that high blood pressure would be essential to maintain renal function—a prevailing concept in the United States for many years (24, 25).
2. It has also been alleged that hyperglycemia is not important in the genesis of diabetic renal disease—clearly an unsound and faulty statement (24).
3. It has also been claimed that genetic factors are decisive in determining renal disease—this has never been adequately substantiated (26).
4. The idea that non-diabetic renal disease like glomerulonephritis was important also hindered our understanding for many years (27).
5. P-pill users may have a greater risk of nephropathy (28, 29), which is of interest in relation to young patients with type 2 diabetes.

It is now clear that normalizing or even "sub-normalizing" blood pressure is essential. The exception seems to be for the patients with advanced renal disease where a U-formed

TABLE 3 Optimal Blood Pressure Level in Diabetic Patients

Without nephropathy	<130/80
With nephropathy	Somewhat lower

Source: From Refs. 22, 24.

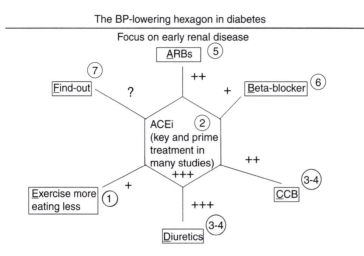

FIGURE 1 The BP-lowering hexagone in diabetes (+) indicates the level of evidence. The numbers indicate sequence of treatment (1–7) (vary from patient to patient). Remember sufficient doses, clinical, and laboratory control.

curve has been documented in the IDNT-study in type 2 diabetes (30). It is also clear that hyperglycemia is a main risk factor in the genesis of diabetic renal disease. Genetic factors have not been identified and there is no reason to believe that genetic factors are decisive although they may modulate the development (26). Combining the effect of high blood pressure and hyperglycemia may be sufficient to explain the development of renal disease. Hall emphasizes that BP-lowering can reduce progression of diabetic renal disease—an observation made more than 25 years ago (25).

DIAGNOSTIC PROCEDURES

It is imperative to ensure the correct diagnosis of diabetic renal disease in patients with type 2 diabetes and, fortunately, the procedures to obtain this are usually very simple.

First of all, it should be ensured that the patients actually have diabetes. This is not difficult based upon the patients' medical history, treatment, blood glucose measurements and HbA_{1c} levels. On this background, the diagnosis is usually certain. There may be cases that are not quite obvious, for instance a patient who has had diabetes, but who has become euglycemic by weight loss; the patient may still have renal lesions derived from diabetes.

In the presence of diabetes, it is always necessary to examine the patient for other diabetic lesions, such as retinopathy, heart and vascular disease, as well as neuropathy. It is perhaps surprising, but retinopathy is not always found in type 2 diabetic patients with microalbuminuria or even proteinuria, but this is a common clinical observation.

Measurements of albuminuria are essential and usually it is necessary to do two or three tests at intervals of some weeks or months to be on solid ground. Normally, early morning urine is used and albumin creatinine ratio is measured in this specimen, which is a very simple and reliable test. If one test is positive, two more tests should be taken to be sure of the degree of renal involvement. One should ensure that glycemic control is satisfactory since there may be a fall in albuminuria levels with better glycemic control. There are several bedside tests for measuring albumin concentrations that are also quite easy to use. Exact measurements such as nephelometry or other immune-related techniques are to be preferred. All patients should be followed longitudinally in the outpatient clinic (31–35).

It should be noted that some patients may have signs of renal disease already at the time of diagnosis and maybe even retinopathy (36). This is due to the fact that some patients may not have been aware of their diabetes because sometimes symptoms are mild or even non-existent. It may be of value to perform renal sonography. In diabetes, the kidney is usually of normal size or larger than normal (with poor glycemic control), at least in the absence of proteinuria.

Regarding measurements of renal function, it is usually sufficient to measure serum creatinine although exact measurements of GFR may be warranted in some cases, e.g., determined as EDTA clearance, or creatinine clearance, but usually this is not needed in the diabetic clinic. It is possible to calculate GFR on the basis of serum creatinine or cystatin C, but this concept is still under evaluation and results may often be incorrect (38).

In rare situations, renal biopsy may be indicated, in particular if the disease has developed very rapidly, but even so, in most cases typical diabetic lesions are found (27). In some situations, the renal biopsy may not show specific diabetic abnormalities, which is by no means a sign of non-diabetic renal disease (and by no means minimal change disease). Structural lesions might also be explained by hypertension (39). Obviously, screening for urinary tract infection that may be more common in diabetic patients due to cystopathy is a very reasonable procedure. Often blood pressure is moderately elevated in these patients so careful measurements of blood pressure are always warranted. BP-elevation is often related to sodium retention (40), therefore, careful clinical examination regarding edema is crucial, but even without edema, there might be sodium retention (40). Diuretic treatment becomes essential, also for BP-lowering.

However, the conclusion is that in the daily clinic and in the follow-up of diabetic patients the diagnosis is not difficult. Usually, patients are followed longitudinally and it is possible to observe the slow increase in albuminuria in these patients, 5% to 20% per year (41) as well as later a change in S-creatinine. These increases are related to glycemic control and blood pressure, and in patients with high blood pressure and poor glycemic control there is often a rapid rate of progression. Measurements of serum lipid levels are also warranted, although this parameter is not decisive in determining the renal treatment for these patients other than the strategy to prevent or delay cardiovascular complications (42–44). Almost all patients should be under statin treatment (43). There may be other clinicians who are more inclined to renal biopsies, but in my opinion this is not necessary. Usually, the treatment strategy is exactly the same, with or without biopsy, and it is extremely rare that the treatment strategy is altered due to a biopsy. Steroid and related treatment may be needed in rare cases of the nephrotic syndrome, and as a consequence glycemic control may deteriorate.

PREVENTION

It has been suggested that there may be a genetic background for the development of renal disease in diabetes (45), but so far this has not been confirmed. There may be a higher risk in certain patients, and some patients may be critically exposed due to clustering of risk factors, but there are neither genetic markers for hypertension nor for adiposity. Hypertension in the family may be a risk factor. So genetics in diabetic renal disease is still considered a "big black hole" (45). Risk factors/markers are indicated in Tables 4 and 5.

It is quite clear, both from experimental studies and human studies, that glucose toxicity is an important factor in the genesis of diabetic vascular disease (46). The mechanistic background for glucose toxicity is not completely clear, but it may well be that advanced glycation end-products play an important role along with the activation of the polyol pathway. Activation of protein kinase C and growth factors are of potential interest, but a detailed discussion of these pathogenetic factors is outside the scope of this chapter.

The UKPDS was important in this respect as in particular the effectiveness of SU agents, insulin and metformin is verified. Combination therapy is quite often used and there is no reason to believe that any of these treatment strategies should be problematic. Unfortunately, the difference between the well-treated and the less well-treated group in the UKPDS was not dramatic; HbA$_{1c}$ levels 7.0 versus 7.9 (12).

Besides optimal glycemic control, it is also clear that antihypertensive treatment is of top priority, as documented in the UKPDS where both beta-blockers and angiotensin-converting enzyme (ACE)-inhibitors together with other types of antihypertensive therapy were effective in preventing all complications, including renal complications. The UKPDS showed that the lower the blood pressure, the better the outcome, and therefore the usual goals for antihypertensive treatment may be lower in diabetics; the goal is 140/90 in non-diabetics and 130/80 in diabetics or even lower (125/80) (47,48).

TABLE 4 Risk Factors/Markers for Development of Diabetic
Renal Disease in Type 2 Patients

Type 2	
Normoalbuminuria (above median)	+
Microalbuminuria	+
Sex	M>F
Familial clustering	+
Predisposition to arterial hypertension	+
Ethnic conditions	+
Glycemic control	+
Prorenin	?
Smoking	+/−
S-cholesterol	+
Presence of retinopathy	+
Protein intake	?

+ , present; ?, scanty or no relevant information; +/−, uncertain.

One should, however, be careful regarding patients who may be at risk for renal arteriostenosis and therefore careful follow-up in such patients is needed. Patients who are generally arteriosclerotic should be followed even more carefully, including patients who are smokers (49). In my view it is not generally indicated to screen for renal arteriostenosis. If serum creatinine increases above about 20% during antihypertensive treatment, further investigations may be relevant.

TREATMENT STRATEGY

The first sign of diabetic renal disease in the clinical setting is the presence of microalbuminuria. The genesis of microalbuminuria is complex and not only related to long-standing diabetes, but also to blood pressure elevation, which is quite common in these patients. Poor glycemic control is a main underlying factor. Loss of renal autoregulation may also be important due to lesions in the vasculature of the kidney and therefore the systemic blood pressure may be transferred unhindered to glomeruli in these patients (18,50). Still, the best possible glycemic control is important in patients with microalbuminuria just as in the prevention situation. However, antihypertensive treatment is a key feature in these patients and blood pressure should probably be much lower in patients with microalbuminuria and overt renal disease, perhaps around 125/80. Several studies show that ACE-inhibitors or angiotensin receptor blockers (ARBs) are effective in the treatment of these patients, but obviously other agents may be used if the goal for antihypertensive treatment is not reached (51–53). Treatment with diuretics is also essential since sodium restriction may be difficult to maintain (40).

TABLE 5 Pathogenesis of Diabetic Nephropathy

Familial/genetic pathways
Metabolic pathways
Glucose itself
Non-enzymatic glycosylation
Increased protein kinase C activity
Abnormal polyol metabolism
Biochemical abnormalities of extracellular matrix
Hemodynamic pathways
Cytokines and growth factors
Endothelial dysfunction

According to the published CALM studies (53,54), it is possible to combine ACE-inhibitors with receptor blockers. It should be mentioned that small doses of ACE-inhibitors (22) are usually not sufficient. Monitoring of renal function by measuring serum creatinine, serum potassium, and albuminuria is obviously imperative in these patients to avoid side effects, especially in patients with arteriotic disease where renal arteriostenosis may exist.

Beta-blockers also have a strong case in treatment. Overriding hypoglycemic unawareness in patients with type 2 diabetes is rare so the counter-indication for beta-blockers is not present in most patients. On the contrary, a number of patients need beta-blockers for cardiac protection against arrhythmia and heart insufficiency. Combination therapy with calcium channel blockers (CCBs) is also useful and most physicians should not start treatment with CCBs, but use them instead as a supplement (Fig. 1).

The goal regarding antihypertensive treatment is stable renal function and stable serum creatinine, and a decline in albuminuria brought about by a pressure. There seems to be no lower limit regarding blood pressure and if patients can manage a level of 120/75, this may be very useful in renal protection. There is only evidence of a so-called J-shaped curve in patients with advanced renal disease and type 2 diabetes (30).

There are only few studies examining the role of low protein diets in diabetic patients. Studies so far performed are not positive in patients with type 2 diabetes (55). Regarding the dietary approach, a low protein diet may not be warranted, but rather it may be useful to use a low sodium diet, especially if the patient does not respond to ordinary therapy. In some cases, restriction of sodium may be useful in achieving the goal for antihypertensive treatment, but diuretic treatment is a useful substitute. Some patients eat excessive amounts of salt.

There is little evidence that treatment of dyslipidemia will protect renal function and the few studies that do exist are conflicting. Obviously, treatment of hyperlipidemia is more important for the prevention of cardiac and vascular disease. However, with very advanced renal disease, statins are not effective (56), and the role of optimal glycemic control is still being discussed. Strict blood glucose control is hardly necessary (and very difficult) (57). Cigarette smoking is also considered a risk factor and all patients should be given advice regarding smoking cessation (49).

NEW META-ANALYSIS ON BP LOWERING

Recently, some major meta-analyses on the effect of blood-pressure lowering on major cardiovascular events and renal outcomes have been published (58–60). The principal messages from these important studies that are based upon randomized trials indicate that the main effect of blood-pressure lowering is in fact the blood-pressure lowering in itself, and not very much the specific method or type of blood pressure lowering. This is clearly the case for major cardiovascular events (58). The studies indicate that the benefits from ACE-inhibition or ARBs on renal outcomes in placebo-controlled trials probably result from an effective blood pressure lowering effect of these agents. The renal meta-analysis concludes (59) that in patients with diabetes, additional renal protection action of these substances beyond blood pressure remains unproven. It is, however, important to point out that lowering of urinary albumin concentration is seen with RAS-inhibition. This is considered as a positive effect seen in patients with diabetes as well as in patients without diabetes. A comparison between ACE-i and ARBs provides similar results in early nephropathy (60).

Regarding risk reduction of ESRD in clinical trials, the positive effect of blocking the RAS is clearly related to blood pressure. If the blood pressure is reduced by in mean 6.8 mmHg, there is a major benefit in using agents that block the RAS. With only a minor reduction of the blood pressure, the effect is almost neutral, suggesting that it is the blood pressure lowering per se associated with RAS inhibition that is important (58–61).

This clearly points to the old observation that increase of blood pressure is a major risk factor for progression of diabetic renal disease and that treatment of blood pressure reduces the later decline in GFR as well as development of ESRD (25). The use of ACE inhibitors and ARBs is thus beneficial by lowering BP. Argument against this concept has recently been discussed, but Casas et al. still argue that their study shows that there is an absence of evidence to support renoprotective effects of renin–angiotensin inhibitors independently of BP lowering; further studies may be needed, but difficult to conduct (59).

Blocking the RAS seems to have a beneficial effect by reducing the risk of type 2 diabetes (62,63). Outside nephropathy, the use of ACE inhibitors is clearly beneficial in diabetic patients with heart disease, commonly seen with nephropathy. However, the Diabetes REduction Approaches with ramipril and rosiglitazone Medications (DREAM) study did not confirm the effect of Ramipril on development of diabetes (64,65).

META-ANALYSIS AND THE EFFECT OF ACE INHIBITORS AND ARBS ON RENAL OUTCOMES AND MORTALITY

It would be of interest to compare ACE-inhibitors with ARBs, because we know that ACE-inhibitors are quite effective in type 1 and type 2 diabetes according to many studies, and an important review article on this issue was recently published in the British Medical Journal. It is an interesting meta-analysis conducted in a very systematic way (60).

The question put forward in this paper was relevant and clear: when considering all papers dealing with ACE-inhibitors and ARBs on renal outcomes and all-cause mortality in patients with diabetic nephropathy—is there a difference? The data sources were solid: Medline, EM-base, and Cochane Central Register for controlled clinical data and contacts to investigators. Patients with all stages of disease were included which may be a drawback.

The data extracted concerned mortality and renal outcomes, which were:

1. Prevention of progression of micro- and macroalbuminuria as well as regression to normoalbuminuria.
2. Doubling of serum creatinine concentration.
3. End-stage renal disease, and the final outcome in all studies: mortality.

All the relevant papers were identified on the date of submission, including about 7500 patients. A major interest in this area is ESRD and renal dysfunction.

Importantly, both agents had similar effect on both renal outcomes, even when confounders were taken into consideration. Comparing ACE-inhibitors directly with ARBs was at that time difficult, but results from a new study [Diabetics Exposed to Telmisartan And enalaprIL (DETAIL)] are now available (66).

The important point here is that ACE-inhibitors had a significant effect on overall mortality, mainly driven by the MICRO-HOPE study (62). The test for the overall effect on mortality had a P-value of 0.04. In contrast, the ARBs had no significant effect on mortality. This is important because patients with renal disease may not die from ESRD (they undergo dialysis), and the cause of death, especially in type 2 diabetes, is primarily cardiac mortality.

The authors (60, 61) finally point out the need for more comparative trials. For instance, the ARB, losartan, was compared positively with an old beta-blocker in hypertensive diabetic (and non-diabetic) patients with left ventricular hypertrophy in the LIFE study (63). In addition, the authors conclude that combination therapy—including the use of diuretics—is important.

PREVENTION OF DIABETES—ACE INHIBITOR AND ARB?

In the treatment of hypertension in non-diabetic individuals, great care should be taken to select agents that do not confer an increased risk for the development of new diabetes. The aim should be to use agents that may at least be neutral or, even better to some extent, protective against the development of glucose intolerance.

A number of studies have thus shown that both ACE-inhibitors and ARBs seem to confer an antidiabetic effect, at least when compared with diuretics and beta-blockers.

However, the issue is not completely settled. First of all, we may need a more definitive study, such as the ongoing DREAM study (64), which will assess the effects of ramipril and rosiglitazone in patients at high risk of developing diabetes. Rosiglitazone reduces blood glucose—not surprising (65). Whether this will reduce long-term incidence of diabetes when treatment is stopped remains an open question (64).

PREVENTING MICROALBUMINURIA IN DIABETES

Prevention of microalbuminuria is the initial step in preventing diabetic kidney disease (23,24). Patients with normoalbuminuria have been examined, first in type 2 diabetes, with an ACE-inhibitor by Ravid et al. (35). The ACE-inhibitor prevented development of micro-albuminuria (35). Kvetny et al. showed the same for type 1 diabetes using perindopril (67). The Bergamo Nephrologic Diabetes Complications Trial (BENEDICT) study was recently published (68). Indeed, it is important to distinguish between normoalbuminuria and microalbuminuria and renal insufficiency, as confirmed in the study by Adler et al. from UKPDS (69). Clearly, patients with normoalbuminuria have the best prognosis and there is evidence to show that preventing progression is associated with a much better prognosis, which was also documented in the recent paper by Gaede et al. from the Steno Diabetes Center (17). They showed that regression to normoalbuminuria is associated with much better preservation of renal function in terms of GFR fall, which is stabilized (70).

Now there seems to be a very good foundation for substantial improvements of the prognosis for patients with type 2 diabetes (22, 25), and early treatment of hypertension leads to better prognosis, as does, but maybe to a lesser extent, improved euglycemic control. Clearly treatment with statins is also important, as documented in many studies, among others the Steno 2 study (17, 70). Now we have apparently completed the paradigm shift: it is essential to normalize glycemia, blood pressure, and dyslipidemia in all patients with type 2 diabetes.

ACE INHIBITORS OR ARBS IN EARLY NEPHROPATHY

Furthermore, while it is evident that both classes of drugs inhibiting the RAS appear to be beneficial, an important question remains: is one class superior for the prevention of the development of cardiovascular and renal disease? This particular issue has now been addressed by the DETAIL trial (66).

DETAIL was a much-needed, long-term study comparing an ACE-inhibitor with an ARB head-to-head in a diabetic population. The 5-year, prospective, multicenter, double-blind study directly compared the ACE-inhibitor, enalapril, with the ARB, telmisartan, in patients with type 2 diabetes, hypertension and evidence of early nephropathy, and in many cases microalbuminuria. DETAIL was also the first study of its kind to monitor the progression of kidney disease by directly measuring the GFR, now recognized as the best indicator of overall kidney function and ESRD. The fall in GFR at 5 years—the main endpoint—was the same in patients treated with either drug.

Blood pressure was lowered to a comparable degree in each treatment group, and cardiovascular mortality was much lower than would be expected at 5 years, with three and five cardiovascular-related deaths in the telmisartan and enalapril groups, respectively. Other adverse event rates were similar between the two groups, since ACE-inhibitor-intolerant patients were excluded from the study. There were no cases of ESRD in either group.

Other shorter studies have indicated that the ACE-inhibitors and ARBs exert similar effects as far as albuminuria and blood pressure are concerned (53,54,71–73). Furthermore, dual blockade using a drug of each class is a possible approach in patients who do not respond well to single blockade, especially in microalbuminuric patients (53, 54).

The strong endpoint studies, namely the Reduction of End-points in NIDDM with the Angiotensin II Antagonist Losartan (RENAAL) and the IDNT, in patients with type 2 diabetes and overt nephropathy, should be considered (74, 75). The results of these studies would favor the use of ARBs, and yet as there are no similar studies comparing ACE-inhibitors with ARBs, is needed further information in this patient group. Indeed, comparison to advanced disease intervention in microalbuminuric patients may prove much more effective (77–80).

REGRESSION OF ALBUMINURIA—IMPORTANT CLINICAL SIGNIFICANCE: A NEW PARADIGM SHIFT BY ACE INHIBITORS AND ARBS AND AHT TREATMENT

It is well known to all diabetologists that patients with "proteinuria" or "albuminuria" carry a poor prognosis. The same is the case for microalbuminuria, but to a lesser extent. Indeed, the higher the level of albuminuria, the greater the risk of renal progression and the risk of all complications including early mortality. These results derive from studies of the so-called natural history of diabetic nephropathy, both in type 1 and type 2. The next question is, of course, to ask whether regression or remission of albuminuria is of clinical relevance. Is it really associated with better prognosis? Blocking the RAS as well as dual blockade should be considered along with several BP-lowering measures.

This question was recently discussed by Hovind et al., who analyzed whether remission of nephrotic-range albuminuria is associated with a better prognosis (76). This, indeed, seems to be the case. It is now clear also from other studies that remission of albuminuria (78–80) signifies a good prognosis, also in microalbuminuric patients. The results from the LIFE study (62), including diabetic patients, and the RENAAL study clearly documents that reduction of albuminuria and microalbuminuria really indicates a better prognosis (75).

Thus, it is obvious that it is important to screen for microalbuminuria, but now also to do a follow-up on the degree of albuminuria. Physicians should look for reduction by means of better blood pressure control, especially ACE-inhibition or other blockade of the RAS.

This is indeed a second paradigm shift. The first paradigm shift was to screen for microalbuminuria, and the next is now to follow up on the level of albuminuria.

It is not difficult to screen for microalbuminuria. In our unit we use the first morning urine sample. This is used for screening using the albumin creatinine ratio, which is a good parameter very well associated with excretion rate, both short-term and 24 hours. They are good and reliable reference values. It could be argued that the classification normo-, macro- and microalbuminuria is somewhat artificial because albuminuria—like many other parameters (glycemic control and blood pressure as well as cholesterol)—is a continuous variable. However, it is practical in the screening process to classify according to these entities. Early studies show that microalbuminuria is not only associated with progression to renal disease, but also to early mortality.

How can it be explained that reduction in albuminuria/microalbuminuria translates into better prognosis? Part of the explanation is reduction of blood pressure and treatment with agents that block the RAS, but this may not be the whole story. Reduction in albuminuria means that the pressure over the glomerular membrane is specifically reduced, and there is good evidence to indicate that pressure-induced damage is an important factor for the deterioration in renal function observed in diabetic patients with proteinuria. Patients with microalbuminuria usually have relatively well-preserved renal function, and thus, by reducing microalbuminuria by better treatment, both glycemic and antihypertensive treatment translate into better preservation of GFR (78, 79), and in this situation, preservation of renal function before the decline in GFR (81–84). With proteinuria there is normally a decline in GFR, which is related to traditional risk factors, namely elevated blood pressure, microalbuminuria, and HbA_{1c}—risk markers that are clearly modifiable (Table 6).

TABLE 6 Inhibition of the RA(A)S in Diabetes

	Prevention of T2 DM	Prevention of micro	Treating micro	Treating macro	LVH	Heart failure
ACEi[a]	++ (63)	+++ BENEDICT (68)	T1 +++ (2) T2 +++ (61)	T1 +++ (22) T2 + (22)		+++
ARBs[a]	++ (63)	Roadmap (85)	T1 – T2 +++ (61)	T1 – T2 +++ (RENAAL) IDNT (74,75)	T2 +++ LIFE (62)	+

[a]most often combined with diuretics
+, some evidence; ++, good evidence; +++, very well established; -, little or no evidence.
Abbreviations: ACEi, ACE inhibitor; ARB, angiotensin receptor blockers; BENEDICT, Bergamo nephrologic diabetes complications trial; IDNT, irbesartan in diabetic nephropathy trial; LIFE, losartan intervention for endpoint reduction in hypertension study; LVH, left ventricular hypertrophy; RENAAL, reduction of endpoints in NIDDM with the angiotensin II antagonist losartan study; ROADMAP, randomized olmesartan and diabetes microalbuminuria prevention study.

It is quite clear that early antihypertensive treatment has improved the prognosis for diabetic patients dramatically, and the prognosis may further improve with early screening for microalbuminuria and follow-up to monitor whether microalbuminuria is reduced. On the other hand, it may seem a paradox that we still have an increase in the number of patients developing end-stage renal failure due to diabetes. However, this is explained by the fact that many more patients develop type 2 diabetes, and that these patients have a longer period of survival because of better cardiovascular management, but further studies are needed.

However, in most parts of the world, especially in the United States, more than 50% of the patients with ESRD have diabetes as the background. It is interesting to note that screening for microalbuminuria is primarily used in Europe. However, this has for several years been proposed in guidelines from the ADA. Indeed, the earlier treatment, the better (77–84).

SUMMARY

Hyperglycemia is an important contributor to complications, including nephropathy. In order to obtain the best possible glycemic control throughout the course of diabetes, it is important to diagnose renal disease early by screening for microalbuminuria, which prevents progression of diabetes. Blood pressure elevation is also an important factor and normalizing blood pressure throughout the course of type 2 diabetes is essential.

Studies show that treatment with ACE-inhibitors can prevent the development of microalbuminuria. Many studies also show that microalbuminuria can be reduced not only by antihypertensive treatment, especially with ACE-inhibitors, but also with other agents. Comparisons between some ACE-inhibitors and ARBs have been performed with similar results.

Thus, ACE-inhibitors seem to be important in preventing cardiovascular disease and mortality, and both ACE-inhibitors and ARBs are important in preventing or postponing ESRD. There may thus be a theoretical case for using a combined blockade or a so-called dual blockade of the RAS.

Patients with diabetic renal disease need long-standing effective antihypertensive treatment on top of ACE-inhibition using diuretic treatment, beta-blocker treatment, and calcium blockers with prolonged action.

Dyslipidemia should be treated carefully, although there are no clinical studies that suggest that the renal outcome is better with statins or other lipid-lowering agents. With advanced renal disease there seems to be no effect of statins on cardiovascular disease. All general risk factors should be treated and patients should be urged to quit smoking, lose weight and maintain a low sodium diet. The role for protein reduction is less clear and it is even weak in patients with other types of renal disease. Multifactorial intervention is a key issue.

REFERENCES

1. Ritz E, Rychlik I (eds.). Nephropathy in Type 2 Diabetes. Oxford: Oxford Press, 1999.
2. Ritz E, Stefanski A. Diabetic nephropathy in type 2 diabetes (in-depth review). Am J Kidney Dis 1996; 27:167–94.
3. Biesenbach G, Janko O, Zazgornik J. Similar rate of progression in the predialysis phase in type 1 and type 2 diabetes mellitus. Nephrol Dial Transplant 1994; 9:1097–102.
4. Ritz E, Orth SR. Nephropathy in patients with type 2 diabetes mellitus. N Engl J Med 1999; 341:1127–33.
5. Ruggenenti P, Remuzzi G. Nephropathy of type 1 and type 2 diabetes: diverse pathophysiology, same treatment? Nephrol Dial Transplant 2000; 15:1900–2.
6. Schmitz R. Über die prognostische Bedeutung und die Ätiologie der Albuminurie bei Diabetes. Berlin Klin Wschr 1891; 28:373–7.
7. Fahr T. Über atypische Befunde aus den Kapiteln des Morbus Brightii nebst anhangsweisen Bemerkungen zur Hypertoniefrage. Virchows Arch Path Anat 1924; 248:323.
8. Rayer P. Traité des maladies des reins et des alterations de la sécrétion urinaire étudiées en elles-mêmes et dans leurs rapports avec les maladies des uretères de la vessie, de la prostate et de l'urètre. Paris: Librairie de l'Académie Royale de Médecine, NB, 1839.
9. Ebstein W. Weiteres über Diabetes, insbesondere über die Complication desselben mit Typhus abdominalis. Dtsch Arch Klein Med 1882; 30:1.

10. Kimmelstiel P, Wilson C. Intercapillary lesions in the glomeruli of the kidney. Am J Pathol 1936; 12: 83–97.

11. Fabre J, Balant LP, Dayer PG, et al. The kidney in maturity onset diabetes mellitus: a clinical study of 510 patients. Kidney Int 1982; 27:167–94.

12. UK Prospective Diabetes Study Group. Intensive blood-glucose control with sulfonylureas or insulin compared with conventional treatment and risk of complications in type 2 diabetes (UKPDS33). Lancet 1998; 352:837–53.

13. UK Prospective Diabetes Study Group. Tight blood pressure control and risk of macrovascular and microvascular complications in type 2 diabetes (UKPDS38). BMJ 1998; 317:703–12.

14. Johnsen SP, Monster TBM, Olsen ML, et al. Risk and short-term prognosis of myocardial infarction among users of antidiabetic drugs. Am J Ther 2006; 13:134–40.

15. Evans MM, Ogston SA, Emslie-Smith A, et al. Risk of mortality and adverse cardiovascular outcomes in type 2 diabetes: a comparison of patients treated with sulfonylureas and metformin. Diabetologia 2006; 49:930–6.

16. Thisted T, Jacobsen R, Thomsen RW. Use of sulphonylureas and mortality after myocardial infarction in diabetic patients: a Danish nationwide population-based study. Diabetologia 2006; 46 (Suppl. 1):57–8.

17. Gaede P, Vedel P, Larsen N, et al. Multifactorial intervention and cardiovascular disease in patients with type 2 diabetes. N Engl J Med 2003; 348(5):383–93.

18. New JP, Marshall SM, Bilous RW. Renal auto-regulation is normal in newly diagnosed normotensive NIDDM patients. Diabetologia 1998; 41:206–11.

19. Vedel P, Obel J, Nielsen FS, et al. Glomerular hyperfiltration in microalbuminuric NIDDM patients. Diabetologia 1996; 39:1584–9.

20. Parving H-H, Lewis JB, Ravid M, et al. Prevalence of risk factors for microalbuminuria in a referred cohort of type II diabetic patients: a global perspective. Kidney Int 2006; 69:2057–63.

21. Basi S, Lewis JB. Microalbuminuria as target to improve cardiovascular and renal outcomes. Am J Kidney Dis 2006; 47(6):927–46.

22. Mogensen CE. Microalbuminuria and hypertension with focus on type 1 and type 2 diabetes. J Intern Med 2003; 254:45–66.

23. De Jong PE, Gansevoort R. Prevention of chronic kidney disease: the next step forward. Nephrology 2006; 11:240–4.

24. Mogensen CE. Diabetic renal disease: the quest for normotension—and beyond. Diabet Med 1995; 12:756–69.

25. Hall PM. Prevention of progression in diabetic nephropathy. Diabetes Spectr 2006; 19:18–24.

26. Bain SC, Chowdhury TA. Genetics of diabetic nephropathy and microalbuminuria. J R Soc Med 2000; 93:62–6.

27. Olsen S, Mogensen CE. How often is NIDDM complicated with non-diabetic renal disease? An analysis of renal biopsies and the literature. Diabetologia 1996; 39:1638–45.

28. Ahmed SB, Hovind P, Parving HH, et al. Oral contraceptive, angiotensin-dependent renal vasoconstriction, and risk of diabetic nephropathy. Diabetes Care 2005; 28:1988–94.

29. Costacou T, Demetrius E, Orchard TJ. Oral contraceptive use and overt nephropathy in women with type 1 diabetes. Diabetes 2006, 26-OR (abstract).

30. Pohl MA, Blumentahl S, Cordonnier DJ, et al. Independent and additive impact of blood pressure control and angiotensin ii receptor blockade on renal outcomes in the Irbesartan Diabetic Nephropathy Trial: clinical implications and limitations. JASN 2005; 16(10):3027–37.

31. Stults B, Jones RE. Management of hypertension in diabetes. Diabetes Spectr 2006; 19:25–31.

32. Mogensen CE. Prediction of clinical diabetic nephropathy in type 1 diabetic patients: alternatives to microalbuminuria? Messages related to the microalbuminuria concept: 1990–2006. Diabetes 1990; 39: 761–7.

33. Gerstein HC, Mann JFE, Qilong Y. Albuminuria and risk of cardiovascular events, death, and heart failure in diabetic and non-diabetic individuals. JAMA 2001; 286:421–6.

34. Rachmani R, Levi Z, Lidar M, et al. Considerations about the threshold value of microalbuminuria in patients with diabetes mellitus: lessons from an 8-year follow-up study of 599 patients. Diabetes Res Clin Pract 2000; 49:187–94.

35. Ravid M, Brosh D, Levi Z, et al. Use of enalapril to attenuate decline in renal function in normotensive, normoalbuminuric patients with type 2 diabetes mellitus. A randomized controlled trial. Ann Intern Med 1998; 128:982–8.

36. Olivarius, Andreasen AH, Keiding N, Mogensen CE. Epidemiology of renal involvement in newly-diagnosed middle-aged and elderly diabetic patients. Cross-sectional data from the population-based study "Diabetes Care in General Practice", Denmark. Diabetologia 1993; 36:1007–16.

37. Froissart M, Rossert, J, Jacquot C, et al. predictive performance of the modification of diet in renal disease and Cockcroft-Gault equations for estimating function. J Am Soc Nephrol 2005; 16:763–73.

38. MacIsaac RJ, Tsalamandris C, Thomas MC, et al. Estimating glomerular filtration rate in diabetes: a comparison of cystatin-C- and creatinine-based methods. Diabetologia 2006; 49:1686–9.

39. Vestra MD, Saller A, Bortoloso E, et al. Structural involvement in type 1 and type 2 diabetic nephropathy. Diabet Metab 2000; 26:8–14.
40. Dodson PM, Beevers M, Hallworth R. Sodium restriction and blood pressure in hypertensive type 2 diabetics: randomised blind controlled and crossover studies of moderate sodium restriction and sodium supplementation. BMJ 1989; 298:227–30.
41. Nielsen S, Schmitz A, Rehling M, Mogensen CE. The clinical course of renal function in NIDDM patients with normo- and microalbuminuria. J Intern Med 1997; 241:133–41.
42. Nielsen S, Schmitz O, Møller N, et al. Renal function and insulin sensitivity during simvastatin treatment in type 2 (non-insulin-dependent) diabetic patients with microalbuminuria. Diabetologia 1993; 36:1079–86.
43. Heart Protection Study Collaborative Group. MRC:BHF heart protection study of cholesterol lowering with simvastatin in 20536 high-risk individuals: a randomised controlled trial. Lancet 2002; 360:7–22.
44. Hommel E, Andersen P, Gall MA, et al. Plasma lipoproteins and renal function during simvastatin treatment in nephropathy. Diabetologia 1992; 35:447–51.
45. Genetics and diabetic renal disease. Still a big black hole [editorial]. Diabetes Care 2003; 26(5):1631–2.
46. Pirart J. Diabetes mellitus and its degenerative complications: a prospective study of 4,400 patients observed between 1947 and 1973. Diabetes Care 1978; 1:168–88.
47. Astrup AS, Tarnow L, Rossing P, et al. Improved prognosis in type 1 diabetic patients with nephropathy: a prospective follow-up study. Kidney Int 2005; 68:1250–7.
48. Stratton IM, Cull CA, Adler AI, et al. Additive effects of glycaemia and blood pressure exposure on risk of complications in type 2 diabetes: a prospective observational study (UKPDS 75). Diabetologia 2006; 49:1761–9.
49. Orth SR, Ritz E, Schrier RW. The renal risks of smoking. Kidney Int 1997; 51:1669–77.
50. Christensen PK, Hansen HP, Parving HH. Impaired autoregulation of GFR in hypertensive non-insulin dependent diabetic patients. Kidney Int 1997; 52:1369–74.
51. Foggensteiner L, Mulroy S, Firth J. Management of diabetic nephropathy. J R Soc Med 2001; 94:210–7.
52. Mann JFE, Gerstein HC, Pogue J, et al. for the HOPE investigators. Renal insufficiency as a predictor of cardiovascular outcomes and the impact of ramipril: the HOPE Randomized Trial. Ann Intern Med 2001; 134:629–36.
53. Mogensen CE, Neldam S, Tikkannen I, et al. for the CALM Study Group. Randomised controlled trial of dual blockade of the renin-angiotensin system in hypertensive, microalbuminuric, non-insulin dependent diabetes: the candesartan and lisinopril microalbuminuria (CALM) study. BMJ 2000; 321:1440–4.
54. Andersen NH, Poulsen PL, Knudsen ST. Long-term dual blockade with candesartan and lisinopril in hypertensive patients with diabetes. Diabetes Care 2005; 28:273–7.
55. Pijls LTJ, de Vries H, Donker AJ, et al. The effect of protein restriction on albuminuria in patients with type 2 diabetes mellitus: a randomised trial. Nephrol Dial Transpl 1999; 14:1445–53.
56. Wanner C, Krane V, Winfried M, et al. Atorvastatin in patients with type 2 diabetes mellitus undergoing hemodialysis. N Engl J Med 2005; 535(3):238–48.
57. Feldt-Rasmussen B. Is there a need to optimize glycemic control in hemodialyzed diabetic patients. Kidney Int 2006; 70:1392–4.
58. Blood Pressure Lowering Treatment Trialists' Collaboration. Effects of different blood pressure-lowering regimens on major cardiovascular events in individuals with and without diabetes mellitus. Arch Intern Med 2005; 165:1410–9.
59. Casas JP, Chua W, Loukogeorgakis S, et al. Effect of inhibitors of the renin–angiotensin system and other antihypertensive drugs on renal outcomes: systematic review and meta-analysis. Lancet 2005; 36:2026–33.
60. Casas JP, Vallance P, Smeeth L, et al. Authors' reply. Lancet 2006; 367:900–1.
61. Strippoli GF, Craig M, Deeks JJ, et al. Effect of angiotensin converting enzyme inhibitors and angiotensin II receptor antagonists on mortality and renal outcomes in diabetic nephropathy: systematic review. Br Med J 2004; 329:828–31.
62. Heart Outcomes Prevention Evaluation Study Investigators. Effects of ramipril on cardiovascular and microvascular outcomes in people with diabetes mellitus: results of the HOPE study and MICRO-HOPE substudy. Lancet 2000; 355:253–9.
63. Ibsen H, Olsen MH, Wachtell K, et al. Does albuminuria predict cardiovascular outcomes on treatment with losartan versus atenolol in patients with diabetes, hypertension, and left ventricular hypertrophy? The LIFE Study. Diabetes Care 2006; 29(3):595–600.
64. The Dream Trial Investigators. Effect of rosiglitazone on the frequency of diabetes in patients with impaired glucose tolerance or impaired fasting glucose: a randomised controlled dial. Lancet 2006; 368:1096–105.
65. Heneghan C, Thompson M, Perera R. Prevention of diabetes. Br Med J 2006; 333(7572):764–5.
66. Barnett AH, Bain SC, Bouter P, et al. Angiotensin-receptor blockade versus converting-enzyme inhibition in type 2 diabetes and nephropathy. N Engl J Med 2004; 351:1952–61.

67. Kvetny J, Gregersen G, Pedersen RS. Randomized placebo-controlled trial of perindopril in normotensive, normoalbuminuric patients with type 1 diabetes mellitus. Q J Med 2001; 94(2): 89–94.

68. Ruggenenti P, Fassi A, et al. Preventing microalbuminuria in type 2 diabetes. N Engl J Med 2004; 351 (19):1941–51.

69. Adler AI, Stevens RJ, et al. Development and progression of nephropathy in type 2 diabetes: the United Kingdom Prospective Diabetes Study. Kidney Int 2003; 63:225–32.

70. Gæde P, et al. Remission to normoalbuminuria during multifactorial treatment preserves kidney function in patients with type 2 diabetes and microalbuminuria. Nephrol Dial Transplant 2004; 19(11):2784–8.

71. Lacourcière Y, Bélanger A, Godin C, et al. Long-term comparison of losartan and enalapril on kidney function in hypertensive type 2 diabetics with early nephropathy. Kidney Int 2000; 58:762–9.

72. Derosa G, Cicero AFG, Ciccareeli L, Fogari R. A randomized, double-blind, controlled parallel-group comparison of perindopril and candesartan in hypertensive patients with type 2 diabetes mellitus. Clin Ther 2003; 25(7):2006–21.

73. Muirhead N, Feagan BF, Mahon J, et al. The effects of valsartan and captopril on reducing microalbuminuria in patients with type 2 diabetes mellitus: a placebo-controlled trial. Curr Ther Res 1999; 60:650–60.

74. Lewis EJ, et al. Renoprotective effect of the angiotensin-receptor antagonist irbesartan in patients with nephropathy due to type 2 diabetes. N Engl J Med 2001; 345:851–60.

75. Brenner BM, Cooper ME, de Zeeuw D, et al. for the Reduction of End-points in NIDDM with the Angiotensin II Antagonist Losartan (RENAAL) Study Investigators. Effects of losartan on renal and cardiovascular outcomes in patients with type 2 diabetes and nephropathy. N Engl J Med 2001; 345: 861–9.

76. Hoving P, Tarnow L, et al. Improved survival in patients obtaining remission of nephrotic range albuminuria in diabetic nephropathy. Kidney Int 2004; 66:1180–6.

77. Rossing P. Prediction, progression and prevention of diabetic nephropathy. Diabetologia 2005; 49:1.

78. Yuyun MF, Dinnesen SF, et al. Absolute level and rate of change of albuminuria over 1 year independently predict mortality and cardiovascular events in patients with diabetic nephropathy. Diabet Med 2003; 20:277–82.

79. Spoelstra-de Man AM, Brouwer CB, et al. Rapid progression of albumin excretion is an independent predictor of cardiovascular mortality in patients with type 2 diabetes and microalbuminuria. Diabetes Care 2001; 24:2097–101.

80. Mogensen CE. Prediction of clinical diabetic nephropathy in type 1 diabetic patients: alternatives to microalbuminuria? In: Robertson PR, ed. Commentaries on Perspectives in Diabetes, Vol. 1 (1988–1992). Alexandria, Virginia, USA: American Diabetes Association, 2006:113–5.

81. Amin R, Turner C, Van Aken S, et al. The relationship between microalbuminuria and glomerular filtration rate in young type 1 diabetic subjects. The Oxford Regional Prospective Study. Kidney Int 2005; 68:1740–9.

82. Steinke JM, Sinaiko AR, Kramer MS, et al. The early natural history of nephropathy in type 1 diabetes. III. Predictors of 5-year urinary albumin excretion rate patterns in initially normoalbuminuric patients. Diabetes 2005; 54(7):2164–71.

83. Premaratue E, MacIsaac RS, Tsalakandris C, et al. Renal hyperfiltration in type 2 diabetes: effect of age-related decline in glomerular filtration rate. Diabetologia 2005; 48:2486–93.

84. Parving HH, Lehnert H, Bröchner-Mortensen J, et al. The effect of Irbesartan on the development of diabetic nephropathy in patients with type 2 diabetes, N Engl J Med 2001; 34:870–8.

85. Haller H, Viberti CG, Mimran, et al. Preventing microalbuminuria in patients with diabetes—rationale and design of the Randomised Olmesartan and Diabetes Microalbuminuria Prevention study. J Hypertens 2006; 24:403–8.

20 | Diabetic Peripheral Neuropathy and Sexual Dysfunction

Dan Ziegler

Institute of Clinical Diabetes Research, German Diabetes Center, Leibniz Center for Diabetes Research, Heinrich Heine University, Düsseldorf, Germany

CLASSIFICATION, EPIDEMIOLOGY, AND CLINICAL IMPACT OF DIABETIC NEUROPATHY

Diabetic neuropathy has been defined as a demonstrable disorder, either clinically evident or subclinical, that occurs in the setting of diabetes mellitus without other causes for peripheral neuropathy. It includes manifestations in the somatic and/or autonomic parts of the peripheral nervous system (1), which are classified along with clinical criteria. However, due to the variety of the clinical syndromes with possible overlaps there is no universally accepted classification. The most widely used classification of diabetic neuropathy, proposed by Thomas (2), has recently been modified (3). This proposal differentiates between rapidly reversible, persistent symmetric polyneuropathies, and focal or multifocal neuropathies (Table 1). The distal symmetric sensory or sensorimotor polyneuropathy (DSP) represents the most relevant clinical manifestation affecting approximately 30% of the hospital-based population and 20% of community-based samples of diabetic patients (4). The incidence of DSP is approximately 2% per year. The most important etiological factors that have been associated with DSP are poor glycemic control, visceral obesity, diabetes duration and height, with possible roles for hypertension, age, smoking, hypoinsulinemia, and dyslipidemia (4). Moreover, DSP is related to both lower-extremity impairments such as diminished position sense and functional limitations such as walking ability (5). There is accumulating evidence suggesting that not only surrogate markers of microangiopathy such as albuminuria but also those used for polyneuropathy such as nerve conduction velocity (NCV) and vibration perception threshold (VPT) may predict mortality in diabetic patients (6,7). Elevated VPT also predicts the development of neuropathic foot ulceration, one of the most common causes for hospital admission and lower limb amputations among diabetic patients (8). Pain associated with diabetic neuropathy exerts a substantial impact on the quality of life, particularly by causing considerable interference in sleep and enjoyment of life (9). Chronic neuropathic pain is present in 16% to 26% of diabetic patients (10,11). Pain is a subjective symptom of major clinical importance as it is often this complaint that motivates patients to seek health care. However, in a recent survey from the United Kingdom only 65% of diabetic patients received treatment for their neuropathic pain, although 96% had reported the pain to their physician (10). Pain treatment consisted of antidepressants in 43.5% of the cases, anticonvulsants in 17.4%, opiates in 39%, and alternative treatments in 30%. While 77% of the patients reported persistent pain over 5 years, 23% were pain free over at least 1 year (10). Thus, neuropathic pain persists in the majority of diabetic patients over periods of several years.

CLINICAL MANIFESTATIONS

Distal Symmetric Polyneuropathy

The term "hyperglycemic neuropathy" is being used to describe sensory symptoms in poorly controlled diabetic patients that are rapidly reversible following institution of near-normoglycemia (3). The most frequent form is the DSP commonly associated with autonomic involvement. The onset is insidious, and, in the absence of intervention, the course is chronic and progressive. It seems that the longer axons to the lower limbs are more vulnerable toward the nerve lesions induced by diabetes (length-related distribution). This notion is supported by the correlation found between the presence of DSP and height. DSP typically develops as a

TABLE 1 Classification of Diabetic Neuropathies

Rapidly reversible
Hyperglycemic neuropathy
Persistent symmetric polyneuropathies
Distal somatic sensory/motor polyneuropathies
involving predominantly large fibers
Autonomic neuropathies
Small fiber neuropathies
Focal/multifocal neuropathies
Cranial neuropathies
Thoracoabdominal radiculopathies
Focal limb neuropathies
Proximal neuropathies
Compression and entrapment neuropathies

Source: From Ref. 3.

dying-back neuropathy, affecting the most distal extremities (toes) first. The neuropathic process then extends proximally up the limbs and later it may also affect the anterior abdominal wall and then spread laterally around the trunk. Occasionally are the upper limbs involved with the fingertips being affected first (glove-and-stocking distribution). Variants including painful small-fiber or pseudosyringomyelic syndromes and an atactic syndrome (diabetic pseudotabes) have been described. Small-fiber unmyelinated (C) and thinly myelinated (Aδ) fibers as well as large-fiber myelinated (Aα, Aβ) neurons are typically involved. However, it is as yet uncertain whether the various fiber type damage develops following a regular sequence, with small fibers being affected first, followed by larger fibers, or whether the small-fiber or large-fiber involvement reflects either side of a continuous spectrum of fiber damage. However, there is evidence suggesting that small fiber neuropathy may occur early, often presenting with pain and hyperalgesia before sensory deficits or nerve conduction slowing can be detected (3). The reduction or loss of small fiber-mediated sensation results in loss of pain sensation (heat pain, pin-prick) and temperature perception to cold (Aδ) and warm (C) stimuli. Large-fiber involvement leads to nerve conduction slowing and reduction or loss of touch, pressure, two-point discrimination, and vibration sensation which may lead to sensory ataxia (atactic gait) in severe cases. Sensory fiber involvement causes "positive" symptoms such as paresthesiae, dysesthesiae (hypersensitivity), and pain as well as "negative" symptoms such as numbness.

Persistent or episodic pain that typically may worsen at night and improve during walking is localized predominantly in the feet. The pain is often described as a deep-seated aching but there may be superimposed lancinating stabs or it may have a burning thermal quality (12). In a clinical survey including 105 patients with painful polyneuropathy the following locations of pain were most frequent: 96% feet, 69% balls of feet, 67% toes, 54% dorsum of foot, 39% hands, 37% plantum of foot, 37% calves, and 32% heels. The pain was most often described by the patients as "burning/hot," "electric," "sharp," "achy," and "tingling," was worse at night time and when tired or stressed (9). The average pain intensity was moderate, approximately 5.75/10 on a 0 to 10 scale, with the "least" and "most" pain 3.6 and 6.9/10, respectively. Allodynia (pain due to a stimulus which does not normally cause pain, e.g. stroking) may occur. The symptoms may be accompanied by sensory loss, but patients with severe pain may have few clinical signs. Pain may persist over several years (13) causing considerable disability and impaired quality of life in some patients (9), whereas it remits partially or completely in others (14,15), despite further deterioration in small fiber function (15). Pain remission tends to be associated with sudden metabolic change, short duration of pain or diabetes, preceding weight loss, and less severe sensory loss (14,15).

Compared to the sensory deficits, motor involvement is usually less prominent and restricted to the distal lower limbs resulting in muscle atrophy and weakness at the toes and foot. Ankle reflexes are frequently reduced or absent. At the foot level, the loss of the protective sensation (painless feet), motor dysfunction, and reduced sweat production due to autonomic involvement result in a markedly increased risk of callus and foot ulcers. Thus, the neuropathic patient is a high-risk patient to develop severe and potentially life-threatening foot complications such as ulceration, osteoarthropathy (Charcot foot), and osteomyelitis as well as medial arterial calcification and neuropathic edema. Because DSP is the major contributory factor for diabetic foot ulcers and the lower limb amputation rates in diabetic subjects are 15 times higher than in the non-diabetic population, an early detection of DSP by screening is of paramount importance (8). This is even more imperative due to the fact that many patients with DSP are asymptomatic or have only mild symptoms. In view of these causation pathways the majority of amputations should be potentially preventable if appropriate screening and preventative measures were adopted.

Acute Painful Neuropathy

Acute painful neuropathy has been described as a separate clinical entity (16). It is encountered infrequently in both type 1 and type 2 diabetic patients presenting with continuous burning pain particularly in the soles ("like walking on burning sand") with nocturnal exacerbation. A characteristic feature is a cutaneous contact discomfort to clothes and sheet which can be objectified as hypersensitivity to tactile (allodynia) and painful stimuli (hyperalgesia). Motor function is preserved, and sensory loss may be only slight, being greater for thermal than for vibration sensation. The onset is associated with and preceded by precipitous and severe weight loss. Depression and impotence are constant features. The weight loss has been shown to respond to adequate glycemic control, and the severe manifestations subsided within 10 months in all cases. No recurrences were observed after follow-up periods of up to 6 years (16). The syndrome of acute painful neuropathy seems to be equivalent to "diabetic cachexia" as described by Ellenberg (17). It has also been described in girls with anorexia nervosa and diabetes in association with weight loss (18).

The term *insulin neuritis* was used by Caravati (19) to describe a case with precipitation of acute painful neuropathy several weeks following the institution of insulin treatment. Sural nerve biopsy shows signs of chronic neuropathy with prominent regenerative activity (20) as well as epineurial arterio-venous shunting and a fine network of vessels, resembling the new vessels of the retina, which may lead to a steal effect rendering the endoneurium ischemic (21). This may happen in analogy to the transient deterioration of a preexisting retinopathy following rapid improvement in glycemic control.

Focal and Multifocal Neuropathies

Most of the focal and multifocal neuropathies tend to occur in long-term diabetic patients of middle age or older. The outlook for most of them is for recovery, either partial or complete, and for eventual resolution of the pain that frequently accompanies them. With this in mind, physicians should always maintain an optimistic outlook in dealing with patients with these afflictions (22).

Cranial Neuropathy

Palsies of the third cranial nerve (diabetic ophthalmoplegia) are painful in about 50% of the cases (23). The onset is usually abrupt. The pain is felt behind and above the eye, and at times precedes the ptosis and diplopia (with sparing of pupillary function) by several days. Oculomotor findings reach their nadir within a day or at most a few days, persist for several weeks, and then begin gradually to improve. Full resolution is the rule and generally takes place within 3 to 5 months (22). The fourth, sixth, and seventh cranial nerves are next in frequency.

Mononeuropathy of the Limbs

Focal lesions affecting the limb nerves, most commonly the ulnar, median, radial, and peroneal may be painful, particularly if of acute onset, as may entrapment neuropathies such as the carpal tunnel syndrome which is associated with painful paresthesias (12).

Diabetic Truncal Neuropathy

Mononeuropathy of the trunk (thoracoabdominal neuropathy or radiculopathy) presents with an abrupt onset, with pain or dysesthesias being the heralding feature sometimes accompanied by cutaneous sensory impairment or hyperesthesia. Pain has been described as deep, aching, or boring, but also the descriptors of jabbing, burning, sensitive skin, or tearing have been used. The neuropathy is almost always unilateral or predominantly so. As a result, the pain felt in the chest or the abdomen may be confused with pain of pulmonary, cardiac, or gastrointestinal origin. Sometimes it may have a radicular or girdling quality, half encircling the trunk in a root-like distribution. Pain may be felt in one or several dermatomal distributions, and, almost universally, it is worst at night. Rarely, abdominal muscle herniation may occur predominantly in middle-aged men, involving three to five adjacent nerve roots between T6 and T12 (24). The time from first symptom to the peak of the pain syndrome is often just a few days, although occasionally spread of the pain to adjacent dermatomes may continue for weeks or even months. Weight loss of 15 to 40 pounds occurs in >50% of the cases. The course of truncal neuropathy is favorable, and pain subsides within months with a maximum of 1.5 to 2 years (22).

Diabetic Amyotrophy

Asymmetric or symmetric proximal muscle weakness and muscle wasting (iliopsoas, obturator, and adductor muscles) are easily recognized clinically in the syndrome of lower limb proximal motor neuropathy (synonyms: Bruns–Garland syndrome, diabetic amyotrophy, proximal diabetic neuropathy, diabetic lumbosacral plexopathy, ischemic mononeuropathy multiplex, femoral-sciatic neuropathy, femoral neuropathy). Pain is nearly universal in this syndrome. Characteristically, it is deep, aching, constant, and severe, invariably worse at night, and may have a burning, raw quality. It is usually not frankly dysesthetic and cutaneous. Frequently, pain is first experienced in the lower back or buttock on the affected side, or may be felt as extending from hip to knee. Although severe and tenacious, the pain of proximal motor neuropathy has a good prognosis. Concurrent distal sensory polyneuropathy is frequently present. Weight loss is also a frequently associated feature and may be as much as 35 to 40 pounds. The weight is generally regained during the recovery phase (22).

Patients with proximal or multifocal diabetic neuropathy show marked ischemic nerve lesions with vasculitis and inflammatory infiltration of mononuclear cells (25,26) and T cells of the CD8+ cell type (27). Activated endoneurial lymphocytes express immunoreactive cytokines and major histocompatibility class II antigens (27). To classify these changes Krendel (28) coined the term diabetic inflammatory vasculopathy which he describes as a "multifocal axonal neuropathy" caused by inflammatory vasculopathy, predominantly encountered in type 2 diabetic patients, indistinguishable from diabetic proximal neuropathy or mononeuritis multiplex. Separated from this form is the "demyelinating neuropathy" without vascular inflammation, predominantly encountered in type 1 diabetic patients, indistinguishable from chronic inflammatory demyelinating polyneuropathy (29). These findings suggest that immunological mechanisms may be implicated in the pathogenesis of these neuropathies.

Central Nervous System Dysfunction

Relatively little attention has been directed toward impairment of the central nervous system (CNS) in diabetic patients with DSP. Previous autopsy studies in diabetic patients have demonstrated diffuse degenerative lesions in the CNS including demyelination and loss of axon cylinders in the posterior columns (30,31), degeneration of cortical neurons (32), and abnormalities in the midbrain and cerebellum (32,33) which have been described as "diabetic myelopathy" (31) and "diabetic encephalopathy" (32,34).

Studies that evaluated CNS function in diabetic patients using evoked potentials in response to stimulation of peripheral nerves, event-related potentials, and neuropsychological tests have yielded variable results as to the existence of spinal or supraspinal (central) conduction deficits or cognitive dysfunction. However, we have shown that the degree of dysfunction along the somatosensory afferent pathways in type 1 diabetic patients depends on the stage of peripheral neuropathy, is not related to the duration of diabetes or glycemic control, and can be characterized by an alteration of the cortical sensory complex and peripheral rather than spinal or supraspinal conduction deficits (35). We also demonstrated evidence of cognitive dysfunction with increasing degree of DSP in diabetic patients using event-related potentials (P300 latency) and neuropsychological tests. The P300 latency as an electrophysiological index of cognitive dysfunction was normal in diabetic patients without DSP but was significantly prolonged in those with stage 1 (asymptomatic) and stage 2 (symptomatic) DSP (36). Dejgaard et al. (37) using magnetic resonance imaging, have found an increased frequency of subcortical and brainstem lesions in type 1 diabetic patients with peripheral neuropathy. Using positron emission tomography and [^{18}F]-2-deoxy-2-fluoro-D-glucose we have shown reduced cerebral glucose metabolism in type 1 diabetic patients with DSP as compared with newly diagnosed diabetic patients and healthy subjects (38). Eaton et al. (39) found a smaller cross-sectional chord area at C4/5 and T3/4 as assessed magnetic resonance imaging in patients with DSP as compared to those without DSP and controls. Thus, there is accumulating evidence suggesting that neuropathic involvement at central and spinal levels is a feature of DSP. However, it is not clear whether these are primary or secondary events in DSP.

PATHOGENETIC MECHANISMS

Recent experimental studies suggest a multifactorial pathogenesis of diabetic neuropathy. Most data have been generated in the diabetic rat model, on the basis of which two approaches have been chosen to contribute to the clarification of the pathogenesis of diabetic neuropathy. Firstly, it has been attempted to characterize the pathophysiological, pathobiochemical, and structural abnormalities that result in experimental diabetic neuropathy. Secondly, specific therapeutic interventions have been employed to prevent the development of these alterations, to halt their progression, or to induce their regression despite concomitant hyperglycemia. At present, the following six pathogenetic mechanisms are being discussed which, however, in contrast to previous years are no longer regarded as separate hypotheses but in the first place as a complex interplay with multiple interactions between metabolic and vascular factors:

1. Increased flux through the polyol pathway that leads to accumulation of sorbitol and fructose, *myo*-inositol depletion, and reduction in Na$^+$,K$^+$-ATPase activity.
2. Disturbances in n-6 essential fatty acid and prostaglandin metabolism which result in alterations of nerve membrane structure and microvascular and hemorrheologic abnormalities.
3. Endoneural microvascular deficits with subsequent ischemia and hypoxia, generation of reactive oxygen species (oxidative stress), activation of the redox-sensitive transcription factor NF-κB, and increased activity of protein kinase C (PKC).
4. Deficits in neurotrophism leading to reduced expression and depletion of neurotrophic factors such as nerve growth factor (NGF), neurotrophin-3, and insulin-like growth factor and alterations in axonal transport.
5. Accumulation of non-enzymatic advanced glycation end products (AGEs) on nerve and/or vessel proteins.
6. Immunological processes with autoantibodies to vagal nerve, sympathetic ganglia, and adrenal medulla as well as inflammatory changes.

From the clinical point of view it is important to note that, based on these pathogenetic mechanisms, therapeutic approaches could be derived, some of which have been evaluated in randomized clinical trials (see Treatment section).

DIAGNOSIS

Due to the increasing recognition of diabetic neuropathy as a major contributor to morbidity and the recent burst of clinical trials in this field on one hand, but the lack of agreement on the definition and diagnostic assessment of neuropathy on the other hand, several consensus conferences were convened to overcome the current problems.

Diagnostic Assessment

The Consensus Development Conference on Standardized Measures in Diabetic Neuropathy (40) recommended the following five measures to be employed in the diagnosis of diabetic neuropathy:

1. clinical measures,
2. morphological and biochemical analyses,
3. electrodiagnostic assessment,
4. quantitative sensory testing (QST),
5. autonomic nervous system testing.

Clinical Measures

Clinical measures include:

1. general medical history and neurological history,
2. neurological examination, which consists of
    a.   sensory (pain, light touch, vibration, position)
    b.   motor [graded as normal = 0, weak = 1–4 (25–100%)]
    c.   reflex (present or absent)
    d.   autonomic examination (simple bedside tests including heart rate variation during deep breathing and postural blood pressure response) (40).

Both the severity of symptoms and the degree of neuropathic deficits should be assessed using scores such as the Neuropathy Symptom Score (NSS) and Neuropathy Disability or Impairment Score (NDS, NIS), which appear to be sufficiently reproducible (41). For routine clinical and epidemiological purposes the simplified versions of the NSS and NDS for assessment of DSP suggested by Young et al. (42) can be used (Table 2 and Table 3). Minimum criteria for diagnosis of neuropathy according to the NSS and NDS are:

1. moderate signs with or without symptoms, and
2. mild signs with moderate symptoms.

TABLE 2   Neuropathy Symptom Score (NSS)

- Burning, numbness or tingling = 2
- Fatigue, cramping or aching = 1
- Distribution:
   Feet = 2
   Calves = 1
   Elsewhere = 0
- Nocturnal exacerbation = 2
   Day and night = 1
   Daytime alone = 0
- Woken from sleep = 1
- Reduction by:
   Walking = 2
   Standing = 1
   Sitting or lying down = 0

NSS score:
   3–4 = mild symptoms
   5–6 = moderate symptoms
   7–9 = severe symptoms

Source: From Ref. 43.

TABLE 3 Neuropathy Disability Score (NDS)

- Ankle reflexes
- Vibration perception threshold
- Pin-prick sensation
- Temperature sensation (cold tuning fork)
- Reflexes:
  Normal = 0
  Present with reinforcement = 1
  Absent = 2 at each side
- Sensory
  Present = 0
- Modalities:
  Reduced or absent = 1 at each side
NDS score:
  3–5 = mild signs
  6–8 = moderate signs
  9–10 = severe signs of neuropathy

Source: From Ref. 43.

Clinical measures are used to

1. establish the presence or absence of neurological dysfunction in diabetes,
2. exclude non-neuropathic causes of neurological dysfunction,
3. eliminate non-diabetic causes of neuropathy,
4. distinguish and classify the different forms of diabetic neuropathy, and
5. to monitor progression and provide a clinical correlate of outcome in trials.

The limitations to clinical measures include:

1. lack of sensitivity to change once they become abnormal,
2. limited reliability and reproducibility, and
3. positive symptoms that may reflect different pathophysiology than deficits, i.e., pain or paresthesiae may be related to the degree of compensatory regeneration rather than to the degree of nerve fiber damage. Hence, it has been suggested that symptom or pain scores should not be used to evaluate overall presence or progression of diabetic neuropathy but only to assess pain severity (40).

Sural Nerve Biopsy

Sural nerve biopsy does not represent a routine method in the diagnosis of diabetic neuropathy. It may be used to

1. study the role of various pathogenetic mechanisms,
2. enhance our understanding of the natural history of diabetic neuropathy,
3. examine drug levels in nerve tissue and to assess the structural effects of treatment (controversial issue), and
4. establish the diagnosis when the etiology of the neuropathy is in doubt.
   The limitations to this technique are derived from the fact that the information from the biopsy is of no direct benefit to the patient and that the procedure is associated with a certain morbidity and may result in complications (40).

Skin Biopsy

Skin biopsy has become a widely used tool to investigate small caliber sensory nerves including somatic unmyelinated intraepidermal nerve fibers (IENF), dermal myelinated nerve fibers, and autonomic nerve fibers in peripheral neuropathies and other conditions. Different techniques for tissue processing and nerve fiber evaluation have been used. A Task Force of the

European Federation of Neurological Societies recently developed guidelines on the use of skin biopsy in the diagnosis of peripheral neuropathies. For diagnostic purposes in peripheral neuropathies, the guideline recommends performing a 3-mm punch skin biopsy at the distal leg and quantifying the linear density of IENF in at least three 50-μm thick sections per biopsy, fixed in 2% paraformaldehyde- lysine-periodete (PLP) or Zamboni's solution, by bright-field immunohistochemistry or immunofluorescence with anti-protein gene product 9.5 antibodies (level A recommendation). Quantification of IENF density closely correlated with warm and heat-pain threshold, and appeared more sensitive than sensory nerve conduction study and sural nerve biopsy in diagnosing small-fiber sensory neuropathy. Diagnostic efficiency and predictive values of this technique were very high (level A recommendation). Longitudinal studies of IENF density and regeneration rate are warranted to correlate neuropathologic changes with progression of neuropathy and to assess the potential usefulness of skin biopsy as an outcome measure in peripheral neuropathy trials (level B recommendation). In conclusion, punch skin biopsy is a safe and reliable technique (level A recommendation) (43).

Electrodiagnostic Measures

Electrophysiological techniques have the advantage of being the most objective, sensitive, specific, and reproducible methods which are available in many neurophysiological laboratories worldwide.

Electrodiagnostic measures also have limitations as they

1.   measure only function in the largest, fastest conducting myelinated fibers,
2.   have relatively low specificity in detecting diabetic neuropathy,
3.   show relatively high intra-individual variability for certain parameters (amplitudes),
4.   are vulnerable to external factors such as electrode locations or limb temperature, and
5.   provide only indirect information about symptoms and deficits (40).

Quantitative Sensory Testing

Quantitative sensory testing is the "determination of the absolute sensory threshold, defined as the minimal energy reliably detected for a particular modality." The Peripheral Nerve Society has recommended that detection thresholds of touch-pressure, vibration, coolness, warmth, heat pain, cold pain, and mechanical pain be used to characterize cutaneous sensation (44).

The procedures that are being used for QST include

1.   the method of limits (continuous increase or decrease in intensity to appearance or disappearance threshold),
2.   threshold tracking (combination of appearance or disappearance threshold),
3.   titration method (graded steps to appearance and disappearance threshold),
4.   the two-alternative forced-choice method (pairs of stimulus and null-stimulus phases) (44).

The advantages of QST techniques are that they

1.   are highly sensitive, relatively simple, non-invasive, and non-aversive,
2.   afford precise control over stimulus intensity and testing algorithms,
3.   contribute to differentiation of the relative deficit in small versus large fibers,
4.   are particularly valuable in screening large populations or in longitudinal trials (40).

The limitations to QST procedures include that they

1.   constitute psychophysical methods vulnerable to the effects of alertness, mood, concentration, ambient noise, etc.,
2.   show a relatively high intra-individual variability,
3.   have not been adequately standardized,

4. may be time-consuming (forced-choice methods), which may lead to a decline in concentration or boredom in the person tested and thereby result in diagnostic errors.

The method of limits has been criticized, because it may be associated with a response delay due to reaction time which may vary between subjects. However, it has been demonstrated that this approach yields a degree of sensitivity and reliability that is similar to the forced-choice techniques. The reproducibility of the QST indices is less favorable than that of nerve conduction but still in an acceptable range.

Staging

A staging approach has been suggested by Dyck (41) using the following criteria for polyneuropathy:

1. neuropathic symptoms (NSS)
2. neuropathic deficits (NDS)
3. motor/sensory nerve conduction velocity (M/SNCV)
4. quantitative sensory examination (QSE: VDT or CDT)
5. quantitative autonomic examination (QAE: DB or VAL)

The minimal criteria for the diagnosis of polyneuropathy required ≥2 abnormalities among criteria 1 to 5 with at least one being 3 or 5. The following staging approach was used:

- No neuropathy (N0): minimal criteria unfulfilled
- Asymptomatic neuropathy (N1):
  - N1a: minimal criteria fulfilled, NSS = 0, normal ankle dorsiflection
  - N1b: minimal criteria fulfilled, NSS = 0, abnormal ankle dorsiflection
- Symptomatic neuropathy (N2):
  - N2a: minimal criteria fulfilled, NSS ≥1, normal ankle dorsiflection
  - N2b: minimal criteria fulfilled, NSS ≥1, abnormal ankle dorsiflection
- Disabling neuropathy (N3): minimal criteria fulfilled, disabling features

Distal polyneuropathy was diagnosed if

1. neuropathic symptoms and findings were due to diabetes,
2. symptoms and signs predominated in the distal segments of lower limbs,
3. findings were symmetric (NDS < 10±3; NDS ≥ 10±25%), or
4. two abnormalities among NSS, NDS, NCV, QSE, or QAE were present.

TREATMENT

Role of Intensive Diabetes Therapy in Treatment and Prevention of Diabetic Neuropathy

Seven long-term prospective studies that assessed the effects of intensive diabetes therapy on the prevention and progression of chronic diabetic complications have been published (Table 4). The large randomized trials such as the Diabetes Control and Complications Trial (DCCT) and UK Prospective Diabetes Study (UKPDS) were not designed to evaluate the effects of intensive diabetes therapy on DSP, but rather to study the influence of such treatment on the development and progression of the chronic diabetic complications (45,46) Thus, only a minority of the patients enrolled in these studies had symptomatic polyneuropathy at entry. In type 1 diabetic patients these studies show that intensive diabetes therapy retards but not completely prevents the development of polyneuropathy and autonomic neuropathy. In type 1 diabetic patients these studies show that intensive diabetes therapy retards but not completely prevents the development of polyneuropathy and autonomic neuropathy. In the EDIC study the benefits of 6.5 years of intensive therapy on neuropathy status extended for at least 8 years beyond the end

TABLE 4 Effects of Randomized Clinical Trials of Intensive Diabetes Therapy in Prevention and Treatment of Diabetic Polyneuropathy

Trail	n	Duration (yr)	HbA$_{1c}$ (%) CT versus IT	Neuropathy outcome Clinical	NCV	VPT	HRV
Type 1 diabetes							
DCCT	1441	Up to 9	9.1 vs. 7.2	+	+	n.a.	+
Stockholm Study	91	10	8.3 vs. 7.2	+	+	n.a.	n.a.
Oslo Study	45	8	n.a.	n.a.	+	n.a.	n.a.
Type 2 diabetes							
UKPDS	3867	Up to 15	7.9 vs. 7.0	−	n.a.	+[a]	−
Kumamoto Study	110	6	9.4 vs. 7.1	n.a.	+[b]	+[c]	−
Steno Type 2 Study	160	7.8	9.0 vs. 7.7	n.a.	n.a.	−	+[d]
VA CSDM	153	2	9.5 vs. 7.4	−	n.a.	−	−

[a] Only $n = 217$ patients available after 15 years out of $n = 3.836$ at baseline.
[b] Only NCV in the upper but not lower limbs available.
[c] Significant difference between CT and IT for VPT on the hand but not foot.
[d] Effects of ACE inhibitors, antioxidants, and statins not discernible from those of glycemic control.
Abbreviations: +, benefit; −, no effect; n.a., not available; CT, conventional treatment; IT, intensive treatment; NCV, nerve conduction velocity; VPT, vibration perception threshold; HRV, heart rate variability.

of the DCCT despite equal HbA$_{1c}$ levels, similar to the findings described for diabetic retinopathy and nephropathy (47). In contrast, in type 2 diabetic patients, who represent the vast majority of people with diabetes, the results were variable. Intensive diabetes therapy either had no effect or only partially slowed the progression of polyneuropathy, and the effect on autonomic neuropathy was largely negative. Moreover, improved glycemic control was achieved at the expense of increased risk of hypoglycemia and weight gain.

Only a few smaller studies have evaluated the effects of intensive diabetes therapy on established polyneuropathy in type 1 diabetic patients. They indicate that improved glycemic control may improve some parameters of diabetic neuropathy, but imperfect study designs and methodology hamper the validity of most of these small-sample size trials. At more advanced stages improvement is still possible for some nerve function parameters such as MNCV but less likely for autonomic dysfunction. This may be due to the fact that true normoglycemia could not be achieved in many patients. A large-sample randomized controlled trial to specifically show favorable effects of intensive diabetes therapy on diabetic polyneuropathy is not available. In type 1 patients with most advanced stages of peripheral neuropathy the progression of nerve conduction deficits is halted after 3 to 4 years of normoglycemia following pancreatic transplantation, but no effect is seen in autonomic neuropathy. However, successful pancreas transplantation results in long-term normoglycemia. Hence, the effect on nerve function that can be achieved with this method cannot be extrapolated to the widely used current methods of intensive diabetes therapy. Using these methods the majority of diabetic patients do not achieve sustained normoglycemia due to various reasons. Although observational studies suggested a glycemic threshold for the development and progression of the long-term complications in type 1 diabetes, the DCCT data do not support such an assumption. Thus, attempts to achieve optimal glycemic control should not aim at a certain HbA$_{1c}$ threshold within the diabetic range but follow "the goal of achieving normal glycemia as early as possible in as many type 1 patients as is safely possible." In general, intensive diabetes therapy is associated with a moderately increased risk of weight gain and hypoglycemia.

Treatment Based on Pathogenetic Concepts

Recent experimental studies suggest a multifactorial pathogenesis of diabetic neuropathy. From the clinical point of view it is important to note that, based on the various pathogenetic mechanisms, therapeutic approaches could be derived, some of which have been evaluated in randomized clinical trials (Table 5). These drugs have been designed to favorably influence the underlying neuropathic process rather than for symptomatic pain treatment. For clinical use α-lipoic acid is licensed and used for treatment of symptomatic DSP in several countries worldwide, while epalrestat is marketed in Japan. Since in the foreseeable future normoglycemia will not be achievable in the majority of diabetic patients, the advantage of the aforementioned treatment approaches is that they may exert their effects despite prevailing hyperglycemia. Experimental studies of low-dose combined drug treatment suggest enhanced drug efficacy mediated by facilitatory interactions between drugs. In the future, combinations of drugs that produce synergistic effects could be a therapeutic option.

Aldose Reductase Inhibitors

An increased flux through the polyol pathway resulting in multiple biochemical abnormalities in the diabetic nerve is thought to play a major role in the pathogenesis of diabetic neuropathy. Aldose reductase inhibitors (ARI) block the increased activity of aldose reductase, the rate-limiting enzyme that converts glucose to sorbitol (Table 5). The first trials of ARI in diabetic neuropathy were published 20 years ago. The various compounds that have been evaluated are alrestatin, sorbinil, ponalrestat, tolrestat, epalrestat, zopolrestat, zenarestat, and fidarestat. Except for epalrestat which is marketed in Japan, none of these agents could be permanently licensed due to serious adverse events (sorbinil, tolrestat, zenarestat) or lack of efficacy (ponalrestat, zopolrestat). A meta-analysis of 13 clinical trials with ARI revealed a marginal effect on peroneal MNCV of 1.24 m/sec and an even weaker effect on median MNCV of 0.69 m/sec after 1 year (48). Data of 738 subjects from three trials of tolrestat showed a benefit equal to 1 m/sec in a pooled analysis of NCV in all the nerves studied. The following degrees of changes in motor and sensory NCV that are associated with a change in the NIS of 2 points have been considered to be clinically meaningful in controlled clinical trials: median MNCV 2.5 m/sec, ulnar MNCV: 4.6 m/sec, peroneal MNCV: 2.2 m/sec, median SNCV: 1.9 m/sec, and sural SNCV: 5.6 m/sec (49). According to this suggestion the changes in NCV obtained from

TABLE 5 Treatment of Diabetic Neuropathy Based on the Putative Pathogenetic Mechanisms

Abnormality treatment	Compound	Aim of treatment	Status of RCTs
Polyol pathway ↑	Aldose reductase inhibitors	Nerve sorbitol↓	
	Sorbinil		Withdrawn (AE)
	Tolrestat		Withdrawn (AE)
	Ponalrestat		Ineffective
	Zopolrestat		Withdrawn (marginal effects)
	Zenarestat		Withdrawn (AE)
	Lidorestat		Withdrawn (AE)
	Fidarestat		Effective in phase II trials
	Ranirestat		Effective in phase II trial
	Epalrestat		Marketed in Japan
Myo-Inositol ↑	*Myo*-Inositol	Nerve *myo*-inositol ↑	Equivocal
GLA synthesis ↓	γ-Linolenic acid (GLA)	EFA metabolism↑	Withdrawn (effective: deficits)
Oxidative stress↑	α-Lipoic acid	Oxygen free radicals ↓	Effective in RCTs
	Vitamin E	Oxygen free radicals ↓	Effective in 1 RCT
Nerve hypoxia ↑	Vasodilators	NBF ↑	
	ACE inhibitors		Effective in phase II trial
	Prostaglandin analogs		Effective in phase II trial
	PhVEGF$_{165}$ gene transfer	Angiogenesis ↑	Phase III trial ongoing
Protein kinase C ↑	PKC β inhibitor (ruboxistaurin)	NBF ↑	Phase III trial ongoing
C-peptide ↓	C-peptide	NBF ↑	Effective in phase II trials
Neurotrophism ↓	Nerve growth factor (NGF)	Nerve regeneration, growth ↑	Ineffective
	BDNF	Nerve regeneration, growth ↑	Ineffective
LCFA metabolism ↓	Acetyl-L-carnitine	LCFA accumulation ↓	Ineffective
NEG ↑	Aminoguanidine	AGE accumulation ↓	Withdrawn

Abbreviations: AE, adverse events; AGE, advanced glycation end products; BDNF, brain-derived neurotrophic factor; EFA, essential fatty acids; LCFA, long-chain fatty acids; NBF, nerve blood flow; NEG, non-enzymatic glycation; RCTs, randomized clinical trials.

the ARI trials so far do not appear to reflect a meaningful magnitude of a treatment effect. In a recent 1-year phase II trial of zenarestat including 208 patients with diabetic polyneuropathy a dose-dependent improvement in small myelinated fiber loss and peroneal NCV was observed, but subsequent large phase III trials of zenarestat had to be prematurely terminated due to a significant deterioration in renal function in some patients.

A 52-week controlled multicenter trial of fidarestat (1 mg/day) including 279 patients with diabetic polyneuropathy showed an improvement in F-wave conduction velocity and reduction in neuropathic symptoms. No significant adverse reactions to fidarestat were observed in this trial (50). However, no phase III trials are available for this compound.

In an open randomized multicenter study 289 diabetic patients with DSP were treated with epalrestat (150 mg/day), while 305 patients served as untreated controls. After 3 years epalrestat treatment prevented deterioration in median sensory NCV, MFWL, and VPT. Numbness, sensory deficits, and crampi were also improved. However, this study was biased by its uncontrolled design, i.e., control group without treatment (51).

Ranirestat, a novel ARI was evaluated in a phase II study over 60 weeks. Peroneal MNCV, sural sensory NCV, and VPT were improved during treatment with ranirestat (20 mg/day), without any relevant adverse events (52). These data require confirmation in phase III trials.

γ-Linolenic Acid

Two multicenter trials have demonstrated improvement in neuropathic deficits and NCV after 1 year of treatment with γ-linolenic acid (GLA) in diabetic peripheral neuropathy (53). However, since GLA could not be licensed on the basis of these data in the UK, no further trials have been initiated.

α-Lipoic Acid (Thioctic Acid)

There is accumulating evidence suggesting that free radical-mediated oxidative stress is implicated in the pathogenesis of diabetic neuropathy by inducing neurovascular defects that result in endoneurial hypoxia and subsequent nerve dysfunction. Antioxidant treatment with α-lipoic acid has been shown to prevent these abnormalities in experimental diabetes, thus providing a rationale for a potential therapeutic value in diabetic patients (Table 6). In Germany, α-lipoic acid is licensed and used for treatment of symptomatic diabetic neuropathy since more than 40 years. According to a meta-analysis comprising 1258 patients infusions of α-lipoic acid (600 mg i.v./day) ameliorated neuropathic symptoms and deficits after 3 weeks, while the ALADIN III Study showed oral treatment with 600 mg t.i.d. resulted in a favorable effect on neuropathic deficits after 6 months (54,55). Moreover, the SYDNEY 2 Trial suggests that treatment for 5 weeks using 600 mg of α-lipoic acid orally q.d. reduces the chief symptoms of diabetic polyneuropathy including pain, paresthesias, and numbness to a clinically meaningful degree (56). In a multicenter, randomized, double-masked, parallel-group clinical trial (NATHAN 1) including 460 diabetic patients with stage 1 or stage 2a DSP were randomly assigned to oral treatment with α-lipoic acid 600 mg q.d. ($n = 233$) or placebo ($n = 227$) for 4 years. After 4 years some neuropathic deficits and symptoms, but not NCV were improved, and the drug was well tolerated throughout the trial (57). Clinical and postmarketing surveillance studies have revealed a highly favorable safety profile of this drug.

Vasodilators

Microvascular changes of the vasa nervorum and reduced endoneurial blood flow resulting in hypoxia are thought to be important factors in the pathogenesis of diabetic neuropathy. Thus, there is solid theoretical background to support treatment with vasodilating drugs (Table 5). In a 1-year trial including 41 normotensive patients with mild neuropathy several attributes of NCV, but not neuropathic symptoms and deficits were improved after 1 year of treatment with the ACE inhibitor trandolapril (58). Further studies are clearly needed to define the therapeutic role of ACE inhibitors in diabetic neuropathy.

Several open-label trials from Japan reported pain relief after treatment with vasodilating agents such as the prostacyclin (PGI$_2$) analogs iloprost or beraprost and the prostaglandin derivative PGE$_1$. αCD reported relief of pain or dysesthetic symptoms after 2,

TABLE 6 Randomized Double-Blind Placebo-Controlled Trials of α-Lipoic Acid (Thioctic Acid) in Diabetic Peripheral and Cardiac Autonomic Neuropathy

Trial	Number (*n*)	Dose (mg)	Duration	Effects	Safety
ALADIN	328	100/600/1200/placebo	3 wk i.v.	TSS+ NDS+ HPAL+	Good
ALADIN II	65[a]	600/1200/placebo	2 yr orally	Sural SNCV+ Sural SNAP+ Tibial MNCV+ Tibial DML– NDS–	Good
ALADIN III	508	600 i.v./1800 orally/placebo	3 wk i.v./ 6 mo orally	TSS–/– NIS+/(+) NIS[LL](+)/(+)	Good
DEKAN	73	800/placebo	4 mo orally	HRV+	Good
ORPIL	24	1800/placebo	3 wk orally	TSS+ HPAL(+) NDS+	Good
SYDNEY	120	600/placebo	3 wk i.v.	TSS+ NIS+ NIS[LL]plus7+	Good
SYDNEY 2	181	600/1200/1800/placebo	5 wk orally	TSS+ NSC+ NIS+/(+) NIS[LL]+/(+)	Good for 600 mg/day
NATHAN 1	460	600/placebo	4 years orally	NIS[LL]plus7– NIS+ NIS[LL]+ NCV–	Good

[a] *n* = 299 randomized.

Abbreviations: DML, distal motor latency; HPAL, Hamburg Pain Adjective List; HRV, heart rate variability; MNCV, motor nerve conduction velocity; NDS, Neuropathy Disability Score; NIS[LL], Neuropathy Impairment Score [lower limbs]; NSC, Neuropathy Symptoms and Change. +, improvement vs. placebo; SNAP, sensory nerve action potential; SNCV, sensory nerve conduction velocity; TSS, Total Symptom Score; (+), trend towards improvement vs. placebo; –, no effect; good, no significant adverse reactions versus placebo.

12, and 4 weeks, respectively. Due to the uncontrolled study designs these effects are uninterpretable. However, a large controlled multicenter trial including 170 patients with symptomatic polyneuropathy or foot ulcers showed a >50% improvement in pain or other neuropathic symptoms in 56% of the patients treated with an i.v. infusion of PGE_1 incorporated in lipid microspheres (lipo-PGE_1) for 4 weeks compared to 28% on placebo. In a second trial comparing lipo-PGE_1 with PGE_1-CD in 194 patients the corresponding rates were 51% and 35%. Side effects were observed in 7% of the patients treated with lipo-PGE_1 (59). Further studies are needed to confirm these findings.

Nerve Growth Factor

Nerve growth factor selectively promotes the survival, differentiation, and maintenance of small fiber sensory and sympathetic neurons in the peripheral nervous system (Table 5). It is expressed in the skin and other target tissues of its responsive neuronal populations, binds to its high-affinity receptor (trk A) on nerve terminals, and exerts its trophic effects after being retrogradely transported back to the neuronal perikaryon. A 6-month phase II trial including 250 patients with symptomatic diabetic neuropathy showed an improvement of the sensory component of the neurologic examination and both cooling detection and heat as pain threshold, but no effect on neuropathic symptoms could be observed following treatment with recombinant human NGF. In contrast, a subsequent large 12-month phase III trial failed to demonstrate a favorable effect of rhNGF on subjective and objective variables of diabetic neuropathy (60). The reasons for the latter disappointing result could be the following: (i) the DSP did not progress during the trial in the placebo group, (ii) the dose chosen may have been below the threshold to produce an effect, (iii) the most distal testing site (big toe) was selected for assessment, where the most advanced neuropathic changes are expected which are less susceptible to intervention than more proximal sites, (iv) the primary outcome measure NIS at the lower limbs (NIS-LL) is not sensitive to small fiber sensory dysfunction, (v) the drug did not get to the target tissue, and (vi) the manufacturing process for NGF has been altered after the phase II trial prior to the phase III trial leaving the possibility that the drug was not identical (60).

PKC-β Inhibitors

Increased activity of PKC, a family of serine-threonine kinases that regulate various vascular functions, including contractility, hemodynamics, and cellular proliferation, has been implicated in the pathogenesis of diabetic complications including neuropathy (Table 5). Treatment with a PKC-β-selective inhibitor, ruboxistaurin, ameliorated several neuropathic deficits in experimental diabetic neuropathy. However, following some encouraging results from a phase II study (61), phase III clinical trials using this agent over 1 and 3 years, respectively, could not demonstrate a clinically relevant effect on the various nerve function parameters measured.

C-Peptide

Recent studies suggest that C-peptide shows specific binding to cell membrane binding sites and augments skin microcirculation in type 1 diabetic patients possibly via an increase in both nitric oxide (NO) production and Na^+/K^+-ATPase activity. In experimental diabetic neuropathy C-peptide administration prevented the NCV deficit, axonal atrophy, and paranodal swelling and demyelination and produced an increase in Na^+/K^+-ATPase activity and phosphorylation of the insulin receptor (Table 5). Several smaller-size studies showed an improvement in small fiber sensory and autonomic function in type 1 diabetic patients (62,63). In a recent randomized, controlled trial including 139 type 1 diabetic patients C-peptide (1.5 mg/day, given s.c. four times a day) or a threefold higher dose (4.5 mg/day) an improvement in sural SNCV, clinical score, and VPT was observed after 6 months (64). Phase III trials in diabetic neuropathy are needed to confirm these data.

Vascular Endothelial Growth Factor

Based on the experimental concept of endoneurial microvascular abnormalities and reduced nerve blood flow resulting in ischemia and hypoxia, it has recently been hypothesized that destruction of the vasa nervorum can be reversed by administration of vascular endothelial growth factor (VEGF), an endothelial cell mitogen that promotes angiogenesis in several animal models and in humans (Table 5). Intramuscular gene transfer of plasmid DNA encoding VEGF-1 or VEGF-2 reversed experimental neuropathy after 4 weeks in diabetic rats (65). Preliminary data in patients with chronic ischemic neuropathy and critical limb ischemia indicate neurologic improvement in four out of six diabetic patients after 6 months following intramuscular phVEGF165 gene transfer (66). However, caution has been expressed regarding possible adverse effects of VEGF such as retinal neovascularization and increased retinal vascular permeability, induction of peripheral edema, activation of the PKC pathway, and the possible mitogenic effects in tumor development. Thus, provided that VEGF will be evaluated in larger-scale clinical trials a close monitoring of these and other possible consequences will be mandatory.

Symptomatic Treatment of Painful Neuropathy

Painful symptoms in diabetic polyneuropathy may constitute a considerable management problem. The efficacy of a single therapeutic agent is not the rule, and simple analgesics are usually inadequate to control the pain. Therefore, various therapeutic schemes have been previously proposed, but none of them has been validated. Nonetheless, there is agreement that patients should be offered the available therapies in a stepwise fashion. Effective pain treatment considers a favorable balance between pain relief and side effects without implying a maximum effect (67,68).

The various causal and symptomatic treatment options are summarized in Table 7. The advantages and disadvantages of the various drugs and drug classes used for treatment of painful diabetic neuropathy under consideration of the various comorbidities and complications associated with diabetes are summarized in Table 8. Prior to any decision regarding the appropriate treatment, the diagnosis of the underlying neuropathic manifestation allowing to estimate its natural history should be established (67). In contrast to the agents that have been derived from the pathogenetic mechanisms of diabetic neuropathy, those used for symptomatic therapy were designed to modulate the pain, without favorably influencing the underlying neuropathy (68). A number of trials have been conducted to evaluate the efficacy and safety of these drugs, but only a few of them included large patient samples.

The relative benefit of an active treatment over a control in clinical trials is usually expressed as the relative risk, the relative risk reduction, or the odds ratio. However, to estimate the extent of a therapeutic effect (i.e., pain relief) that can be translated into clinical practice, it is useful to apply a simple measure that serves the physician to select the appropriate treatment for the individual patient. Such a practical measure is the "number needed to treat" (NNT), i.e., the number of patients that need to be treated with a particular therapy to observe a clinically relevant effect or adverse event in one patient. This measure is expressed as the reciprocal of the absolute risk reduction, i.e., the difference between the proportion of events in the control group (Pc) and the proportion of events in the intervention group (Pi): $NNT = 1/(Pc - Pi)$. The 95% confidence interval (CI) of NNT can be obtained from the reciprocal value of the 95% CI for the absolute risk reduction. The NNT and number needed to harm (NNH) for the individual agents used in the treatment of painful diabetic neuropathy are given in Table 7.

Tricyclic Antidepressants

Psychotropic agents, among which tricyclic antidepressants (TCAs) have been evaluated most extensively, constitute an important component in the treatment of chronic pain syndromes since more than 30 years. Putative mechanisms of pain relief by antidepressants include the inhibition of norepinephrine and/or serotonin reuptake at synapses of central descending pain control systems and the antagonism of N-methyl-D-aspartate receptor that mediate hyperalgesia and allodynia. Imipramine, amitriptyline, and clomipramine induce a balanced reuptake inhibition of both norepinephrine and serotonin, while desipramine is a relatively selective norepinephrine inhibitor. The NNT (CI) for a ≥50% pain relief by TCA is 2.4 (2.0–3.0) (69). The NNH is 2.8 for minor adverse events and 19 for major adverse events (Table 7). Thus, among 100 diabetic patients with neuropathic pain who are treated with antidepressants, 30 will experience pain relief by ≥50%, 30 will have mild adverse events, and five will discontinue treatment due to severe adverse events. The mean NNT for drugs with balanced reuptake inhibition is 2.2, while it is 3.6 for the noradrenergic agents (69).

The most frequent adverse events of TCAs include tiredness and dry mouth. The starting dose should be 25 mg (10 mg in frail patients) and taken as a single night-time dose 1 hour before sleep. It should be increased by 25 mg at weekly intervals until pain relief is achieved or adverse events occur. The maximum dose is usually 150 mg/day. Amitriptyline is frequently the drug of first choice, but alternatively desipramine may be chosen due to its less pronounced sedative und anticholinergic effects. The effect is comparable in patients with and without depression and is independent of a concomitant improvement in mood. The onset of efficacy is more rapid (within 2 weeks) than in the treatment of depression. The median dose for amitriptyline is 75 mg/day, and there is a clear dose–response relationship. In two studies of imipramine, the dose was adjusted to obtain the optimal plasma concentration of 400 to 500 nmol/L to ensure maximum effect. The target concentration could be attained in 57% of the patients (69).

Whether combined treatment with antidepressants and phenothiazines offers any advantage is not known. Nortriptyline has been evaluated in combination with fluphenazine compared to placebo and carbamazepine. This combination resulted in significant pain relief with an NNT of 1.6 against placebo and both pain reduction and rates of adverse events similar to carbamazepine.

TABLE 7   Treatment Options for Painful Diabetic Neuropathy

Approach	Compound/measure	Dose per day	Remarks	NNT
Optimal diabetes control	Diet, OAD, insulin	Individual adaptation	Aim: HbA_{1c}<7.0%	–
Pathogenetically oriented treatment	α-Lipoic acid (thioctic acid)[a]	600 mg i.v. infusion 1200–1800 mg orally	Duration: 3 wk Excellent safety profile	6.3[b]
Symptomatic treatment	*Tricyclic antidepressants (TCA)*			
	Amitriptyline	(10–)25–150 mg	NNMH: 15	2.1
	Desipramine	(10–)25–150 mg	NNMH: 24	2.2/3.2
	Imipramine	(10–)25–150 mg	CRR	1.3/2.4/3.0
	Clomipramine	(10–)25–150 mg	NNMH: 8.7	2.1
	Nortriptyline	(10–)25–150 mg	plus Fluphenazine	1.2[c]
	SSRI			
	Citalopram	40 mg	Small sample	7.7 (ns)
	Paroxetine	40 mg	Small sample, CRR	2.9
	SNRI			
	Venlafaxine	150–220 mg	Not licensed	6.9
	Duloxetine[d]	60–120 mg	NNT 120 mg, 60 mg	5.3, 4.9
	Calcium channel modulators			
	Gabapentin	900–3600 mg	High dose	3.8/4.0
	Pregabalin[e]	300–600 mg	NNT 600 mg, 300 mg	5.9, 4.2
	Weak opioids			
	Tramadol	50–400 mg	NNMH: 7.8	3.1/4.3
	Local treatment			
	Capsaicin (0.025%) cream	q.i.d. topically	Max. duration: 8 wk	8.1
Pain resistant to standard pharmacotherapy	*Strong opioids*			
	Oxycodone		Add-on treatment	2.6
	Electrical spinal cord stimulation (ESCS)		Invasive, complications	
Non-pharmacological therapy	TENS, medical gymnastics,		No AE	
	Balneotherapy, relaxation therapy		No AE	
	Acupuncture		Uncontrolled study	
	Psychological support			

[a] Available only in some countries.
[b] 50% symptom relief after 3 wk.
[c] Combined with fluphenazine.
[d] Licensed in U.S. and E.U.
[e] Analgesic effectiveness as ascertained by the physician.
Abbreviations: AE, adverse events; CRR, concentration–response relationship; NNMH, number needed for major harm; Ns, not significant; OAD, oral antidiabetic drugs; SNRI, serotonin norepinephrine reuptake inhibitors; SSRI, selective serotonin reuptake inhibitors; TENS, transcutaneous electrical nerve stimulation.

The notion that the character of the neuropathic pain is predictive of response, so that burning pain should be treated with antidepressants and shooting pain with anticonvulsants, is obviously unfounded, since both pain qualities respond to TCAs. Most evidence of efficacy of antidepressants comes from studies that have been conducted over only several weeks. However, many patients continue to achieve pain relief for months to years, although this is not true for everybody. Tricyclic antidepressants should be used with caution in patients with

TABLE 8 Differential Treatment of Painful Diabetic Neuropathy Considering Diabetes Comorbidities

	Duloxetine	Pregabalin	Tricyclics	Opioids	α-Lipoic acid
Depression	+[a]	n[a]	+	n	n
Obesity	n	–	–	n	n
Sleep disturbances	+	+	+	+	ne
Coronary heart disease	n	n	–	n	n
Autonomic neuropathy	ne	ne	–	–	+

[a] Anxiolytic effect in generalized anxiety disorder.
Effect: +, favorable; –, unfavorable; n, neutral; ne, not evaluated.

orthostatic hypotension and are contraindicated in patients with unstable angina, recent (<6 months) myocardial infarction, heart failure, history of ventricular arrhythmias, significant conduction system disease, and long QT syndrome. Several authors consider TCAs to be the drug treatment of choice for neuropathic pain. However, their use is limited by relative high rates of adverse events and several contraindications. Thus, there is a need for agents that exert efficacy equal to or better than that achieved with TCAs but have a more favorable side-effect profile.

Selective Serotonin Reuptake Inhibitors (SSRI)
Because of the relative high rates of adverse effects and several contraindications of TCA, it has been reasoned whether patients who do not tolerate them due to adverse events could alternatively be treated with SSRI. SSRI specifically inhibit presynaptic reuptake of serotonin but not norepinephrine, and unlike the tricyclics they lack the postsynaptic receptor blocking effects and quinidine-like membrane stabilization. Three studies showed that treatment with paroxetine and citalopram, but not fluoxetine resulted in significant pain reduction. Paroxetine appeared to influence both steady and lancinating pain qualities (69). The therapeutic effect was observed within 1 week and was dependent on the plasma levels, being maximal at concentrations of 300 to 400 nmol/L. Besides the relatively low rates of adverse events the advantage of SSRI compared to the tricyclic compounds is the markedly lower risk of mortality due to overdose. However, a recent case–control study suggested that SSRI moderately increased the risk of upper gastrointestinal bleeding to a degree about equivalent to low-dose ibuprofen. The concurrent use of non-steroidal anti-inflammatory drugs or aspirin greatly increases this risk. Because of these limited efficacy data, SSRI have not been licensed for the treatment of neuropathic pain.

Serotonin–Norepinephrine Reuptake Inhibitor (SNRI)
Because SSRI have been found to be less effective than TCAs, recent interest has focused on antidepressants with dual selective inhibition of serotonin and norepinephrine (SNRI) such as duloxetine and venlafaxine. The efficacy and safety of duloxetine was evaluated in three controlled studies using a dose of 60 and 120 mg/Tag over 12 weeks (29,30). In all three studies the average 24-hour pain intensity was significantly reduced with both doses as compared to placebo treatment, the difference between active and placebo being achieving statistical significance after 1 week. The response rates defined as ≥50% pain reduction were 48.2% (120 mg/day), 47.2% (60 mg/day) and 27.9% (Placebo), giving an NNT of 4.9 (95% CI: 3.6–7.6) for 120 mg/day and 5.3 (3.8–8.3) for 60 mg/day (70–72). Pain severity but not variables related to diabetes or neuropathy predicts the effects of duloxetine in diabetic peripheral neuropathic pain. Patients with higher pain intensity tend to respond better than those with lower pain levels (73). The most frequent side effects of duloxetine (60/120 mg/day) include nausea (16.7/27.4%), somnolence (20.2/28.3%), dizziness (9.6/23%), constipation 14.9/10.6%), dry mouth (7.1/15%), and reduced appetite (2.6/12.4%). These adverse events are usually mild to moderate and transient. To minimize them the starting dose should be 30 mg/day for 4 to 5 days. In contrast to TCAs and some anticonvulsants duloxetine does not cause weight gain, but a small increase in fasting blood glucose may occur (74).

In a 6-week trial comprising 244 patients the analgesic response rates were 56%, 39%, and 34% in patients given 150 to 225 mg venlafaxine, 75 mg venlafaxine, and placebo, respectively. Because patients with depression were excluded, the effect of venlafaxin (150–225 mg) was attributed to an analgesic, rather than antidepressant, effect. The most common adverse events were tiredness and nausea (75). Duloxetine but not venlafaxine has been licensed for the treatment of painful diabetic neuropathy.

Anticonvulsants

Calcium Channel Modulators. Gabapentin is an anticonvulsant structurally related to γ-aminobutyric acid (GABA), a neurotransmitter that plays a role in pain transmission and modulation. The exact mechanisms of action of this drug in neuropathic pain are not fully elucidated. Among others, they involve an interaction with the system L-amino acid transporter and high affinity binding to the α2-subunit of voltage-activated calcium channels. In an 8-week multicenter dose-escalation trial including 165 diabetic patients with painful neuropathy 60% of the patients on gabapentin (3600 mg/day achieved in 67%) had at least moderate pain relief compared to 33% on placebo. Dizziness and somnolence were the most frequent adverse events in about 23% of the patients each (76). Pregabalin is a more specific α2-δ ligand with a sixfold higher binding affinity than gabapentin. The efficacy and safety of pregabalin was reported in a pooled analysis of six studies over 5 to 11 weeks in 1346 diabetic patients with painful neuropathy. The response rates defined as ≥50% pain reduction were 46% (600 mg/day), 39% (300 mg/day), 27% (150 mg/day) and 22% (Placebo), giving an NNT of 4.2, 5.9, and 20.0 (33). The most frequent side effects for 150 to 600 mg/day are dizziness (22.0%), somnolence (12.1%), peripheral edema (10.0%), headache (7.2%) and weight gain (5.4%) (77). The evidence supporting a favorable effect in painful diabetic neuropathy is more solid and dose titration is considerably easier for pregabalin than gabapentin.

Sodium Channel Blockers. Although carbamazepine has been widely used for treating neuropathic pain, it cannot be recommended in painful diabetic neuropathy due to very limited data. Its successor drug, oxcarbazepine (78,79), as well as other sodium channel blockers such as topiramate (80) and lamotrigine (81) showed only marginal efficacy and presumably will not be licensed for the treatment of painful diabetic neuropathy.

A single i.v. infusion of lidocaine (5 mg/kg body weight over 30 min during continuous ECG monitoring) resulted in a significant pain relief after 1 and 8 days in a controlled study including 15 diabetic patients with chronic painful neuropathy. The individual effect was sustained for 3 to 21 days. The NNT for a pain reduction of >30% after 3 days was 2.2. The onset of the analgesic effect during the i.v. infusion (500 mg in 60 min) is abrupt over a narrow dosage and concentration range (82). Potential adverse systemic effects associated with i.v. lidocaine have led to the development of a newer and potentially safer agent, the topical lidocaine patch 5% (Lidoderm), a targeted peripheral analgesic. In patients with postherpetic neuralgia, the lidocaine patch 5% has demonstrated relief of pain and tactile allodynia with a minimal risk of systemic adverse effects or drug–drug interactions (83). Studies in patients with DSP are underway.

Topical Capsaicin

Capsaicin (trans-8-methyl-N-vanillyl-6-nonenamide) is an alkaloid and the most pungent ingredient in the red pepper. It depletes tissues of substance P and reduces neurogenic plasma extravasation, the flare response and chemically induced pain. Substance P is present in afferent neurons innervating skin, mainly in polymodal nociceptors, and is considered the primary neurotransmitter of painful stimuli from the periphery to the CNS. Several studies have demonstrated significant pain reduction and improvement in quality of life in diabetic patients with painful neuropathy after 8 weeks of treatment with capsaicin cream (0.075%). On the basis of a meta-analysis of four controlled trials (84) the NNT for capsaicin is 4.2 for analgesic effectiveness as ascertained by the physician. However, a 12-week trial in painful neuropathy of different etiologies failed to demonstrate pain relief by capsaicin, and no effect on thermal perception was noted. It has been criticized that a double-blind design is not feasible for topical capsaicin due the transient local hyperalgesia (usually mild burning sensation >50% of the cases) it may produce as a typical adverse event. Treatment should be restricted to a maximum of 8 weeks, as during this period no adverse effects on sensory function (due to the mechanism of action) were noted in diabetic patients. However, a skin blister study in healthy subjects showed that there is a 74% decrease in the number of nerve fibers as early as 3 days following topical capsaicin application, suggesting that degeneration of epidermal nerve fibers may contribute to the analgesia induced by the drug (85). This finding questioning the safety of capsaicin in the context of an insensitive diabetic foot limits its use.

Opioids

Tramadol acts directly via opioid receptors and indirectly via monoaminergic receptor systems. Because the development of tolerance and dependence during long-term tramadol treatment is uncommon and its abuse liability appears to be low, it is an alternative to strong opioids in neuropathic pain. In painful diabetic neuropathy tramadol (up to 400 mg/day orally, mean dose: 210 mg/day orally) has been studied in a 6-week multicenter trial including 131 patients (86). Pain relief was 44% on tramadol vs. 12% on placebo. The most frequent adverse events were nausea and constipation. The NNH of 7.8 for drop-outs due to adverse events was relatively low, indicating significant toxicity. In a 4-week study including patients with painful neuropathy of different origins, one-third of which being diabetes, tramadol significantly relieved pain [NNT: 4.3 (2.4–20)] and mechanical allodynia. One conceivable mechanism for the favorable effect of tramadol could be a hyperpolarization of postsynaptic neurons via postsynaptic opioid receptors. Alternatively, the reduction in central hyperexcitability by tramadol could be due to a monoaminergic or a combined opioid and monoaminergic effect.

Most severe pain requires administration of strong opioids such as oxycodone. Although there is little data available on combination treatment, combinations of different substance classes have to be used in patients with pain resistant to monotherapy. Two trials over 4 and 6 weeks have demonstrated significant pain relief and improvement in quality of life following treatment with controlled-release oxycodone, a pure μ-agonist, in a dose range of 10 to 100 mg (mean 40 mg/day) in patients with painful diabetic neuropathy whose pain was not adequately controlled on standard treatment with antidepressants and anticonvulsants which were not discontinued throughout the trial (87,88). As expected, adverse events were frequent and typical of opioid-related side effects. A recent study examined the maximum tolerable dose of a combination treatment of gabapentin and morphine as compared to monotherapy of each drug. The maximum tolerable dose was significantly lower and efficacy was better during combination therapy than with monotherapy, suggesting an additive interaction between the two drugs (89). The results of these studies suggest that opioids should be included among the therapeutic options for painful diabetic neuropathy, provided that careful selection of patients unresponsive to standard treatments, regular monitoring, appropriate dose titration, and management of side effects are ensured. Combination therapy using antidepressants and anticonvulsants may also be useful, particularly if monotherapy is not tolerated due to side effects.

NewDrugs in Phase III Trials

Lacosamide

Lacosamide is a novel anticonvulsant which selectively enhances the slow inactivation of voltage-dependent sodium channels, but in contrast to the aforementioned sodium channel blockers, does not influence the fast sodium channel inactivation. Its second putative mechanism is an interaction with a neuronal cytosolic protein, the collapsin response mediator protein 2 which plays an important role in nerve sprouting and excitotoxicity.

Lacosamide has been evaluated in several studies in painful diabetic neuropathy, one of which has recently been published (90). In this controlled trial lacosamide ($n = 60$) (100–400 mg/day or maximal tolerated dose) was compared with placebo treatment ($n = 59$). The pain relief on the Likert scale was –1.21 points with lacosamide and –0.87 points on placebo ($P = 0.039$). Most frequent side effects versus placebo were headache (18% vs. 22%), vertigo (15% vs. 8%), and nausea (12% vs. 7%). It is possible that the drug will be licensed for painful DSP in 2008.

Non-Pharmacological Treatment
Because there is no entirely satisfactory pharmacotherapy of painful diabetic neuropathy, non-pharmacological treatment options should always be considered. As for the pharmacological treatment, considerable efforts must also be made to develop effective non-pharmacological approaches.

Psychological Support
A psychological component to pain should not be underestimated. Hence, an explanation to the patient that even severe pain may remit, particularly in poorly controlled patients with acute painful neuropathy or in those painful symptoms precipitated by intensive insulin treatment. Thus, the emphatic approach addressing the concerns and anxieties of patients with neuropathic pain is essential for their successful management (91).

Physical Measures
The temperature of the painful neuropathic foot may be increased due to arterio-venous shunting. Cold water immersion may reduce shunt flow and relieve pain. Allodynia may be relieved by wearing silk pyjamas or the use of a bed cradle. Patients who describe painful symptoms on walking likened to walking on pebbles may benefit from the use of comfortable footwear (91).

Acupuncture
In a 10-week uncontrolled study in diabetic patients on standard pain therapy 77% showed significant pain relief after up to six courses of traditional Chinese acupuncture without any side effects. During a follow up period of 18 to 52 weeks 67% were able to stop or significantly reduce their medications and only 24% required further acupuncture treatment (92). Controlled studies using placebo needles should be performed to confirm these findings.

Transcutaneous Electrical Nerve Stimulation
Transcutaneous electrical nerve stimulation (TENS) influences neuronal afferent transmission and conduction velocity, increases the nociceptive flexion reflex threshold, and changes the somatosensory-evoked potentials. In a 4-week study of TENS applied to the lower limbs, each for 30 min daily, pain relief was noted in 83% of the patients compared to 38% of a sham-treated group. In patients who only marginally responded to amitriptyline, pain reduction was significantly greater following TENS given for 12 weeks as compared with sham treatment. Thus, TENS may be used as an adjunctive modality combined with pharmacotherapy to augment pain relief (93).

Extended Muscle Stimulation
We recently showed a better effect of external muscle stimulation than TENS on neuropathic symptoms after 3 days (94).

Frequency-Modulated Electromagnetic Nerve Stimulation
Frequency-modulated electromagnetic nerve stimulation applied during 10 sessions over 3 weeks resulted in a significant pain reduction as compared to placebo stimulation (95). A larger-scale multicenter study is currently ongoing.

Monochromatic Infrared Energy
Monochromatic infrared energy (MIRE) has been shown to reduce neuropathic symptoms and signs in diabetic patients in uncontrolled studies (96). However, 30 min of active MIRE applied 3 days per week for 4 weeks was no more effective than placebo in increasing sensation in subjects with diabetic peripheral neuropathy (97), emphasizing the need for controlled studies in this area to allow an evidence-based treatment decision.

Electrical Spinal Cord Stimulation
It is generally agreed that electrical stimulation is effective in neurogenic forms of pain. Experiments indicate that electrical stimulation is followed by a decrease in the excitatory

amino acids glutamate and aspartate in the dorsal horn. This effect is mediated by a GABAergic mechanism. In diabetic painful neuropathy that was unresponsive to drug treatment, electrical spinal cord stimulation (ESCS) with electrodes implanted between T9 and T11 resulted in a pain relief >50% in 8 of 10 patients. In addition, exercise tolerance was significantly improved. Complications of ESCS included superficial wound infection in two patients, lead migration requiring reinsertion in two patients, and "late failure" after 4 months in a patient who had initial pain relief (98). This invasive treatment option should be reserved for patients who do not respond to drug treatment.

Surgical Decompression

Surgical decompression at the site of anatomic narrowing has been promoted as an alternative treatment for patients with symptomatic DSP. Systematic review of the literature revealed only Class IV studies concerning the utility of this therapeutic approach. Given the current evidence available, this treatment alternative should be considered unproven (Level U). Prospective randomized controlled trials with standard definitions and outcome measures are necessary to determine the value of this therapeutic intervention (99).

CONCLUSIONS ON TREATMENT

Although considerable improvement in the quality of controlled trials has recently been achieved, no major breakthrough in slowing the progression of diabetic neuropathy in the long run has been achieved with drugs used on the basis of present pathogenetic concepts. Some of the newer drugs have shown promising results in phase II trials which require confirmation from large phase III trials. It is conceivable that drugs interfering with the pathogenesis of diabetic neuropathy may be most effective in terms of prevention, rather than intervention. Although several novel analgesic drugs have recently been introduced into clinical practice, the pharmacologic treatment of chronic painful diabetic neuropathy remains a challenge for the physician. Individual tolerability remains a major aspect in any treatment decision. Almost no information is available from controlled trials on long-term analgesic efficacy and only a few studies have used drug combinations. Combination drug use or the addition of a new drug to a therapeutic regimen may lead to increased efficacy. In future, drug combinations may also include those aimed at symptomatic pain relief and quality of life on the one hand, and improvement or slowing of the progression of the underlying neuropathic process on the other hand.

Erectile Dysfunction and Female Sexual Dysfunction

Erectile Dysfunction

Epidemiology

Erectile dysfunction (ED), defined as "the consistent or recurrent inability of a man to attain and/or maintain a penile erection sufficient for sexual activity" (100), is one of the most common sexual dysfunctions in men. ED is more common with advancing age, and since the aged population will increase, its prevalence will continue to rise (101). Diabetes mellitus is the most frequent organic cause for ED, the onset of which starts about 15 years earlier in the diabetic than in the non-diabetic population. In the Massachusetts Male Aging Study (MMAS), the age-adjusted prevalence of minimal, moderate, or complete ED was 17%, 25%, and 10% among 1238 non-diabetic men and 8%, 30%, and 25% among 52 treated diabetic men, respectively (102). Thus, although the number of diabetic subjects in the MMAS was low, this population-based study showed an increased prevalence particularly of complete ED among men with diabetes. In the Cologne Male Survey (103) the prevalence of ED was threefold increased, reaching 60% among diabetic men compared to only 19% in the general population. The presence of diabetes was associated with an increased odds ratio for ED by 3.95 (2.98–5.23). The prevalence of ED in the younger age groups (40–60 years) with diabetes was as high as in the older groups of non-diabetic subjects (60–80 years). Thus, in presence of diabetes the development of ED starts around 20 years earlier than in the non-diabetic population. The crude incidence rate of ED in the MMAS was 26 cases/1000 person-years in 847 men aged 40 to 69 without ED at baseline who were followed for an average of 8.8 years (104).

Population projections for men in this age group suggest an estimate of 617,715 new cases of ED per year for the United States. The age-adjusted risk of ED was higher for men with lower education, diabetes, heart disease, and hypertension. The incidence rate of ED in diabetic men was twofold increased, with 50 cases/1000 person-years. In a population-based study from southern Wisconsin the prevalence of ED among 365 type 1 diabetic patients increased with increasing age from 1.1% in those aged 21 to 30 years to 47.1% in those 43 years of age or older and with increasing duration of diabetes (105). In a study from Italy including 9868 men with diabetes, 45.5% of those aged >59 years reported ED. Risk factors and clinical correlates included the following [OR (95% CI)]: autonomic neuropathy [5.0 (3.9–6.4)], diabetic foot [4.0 (2.9–5.5)], peripheral neuropathy [3.3 (2.9–3.8)], peripheral arterial disease [2.8 (2.4–3.3)], nephropathy [(2.3 (1.9–2.8)], poor glycemic control [2.3 (2.0–2.6)], retinopathy [2.2 (2.0–2.4)], hypertension [2.1 (1.6–2.9)], and diabetes duration [2.0 (1.8–2.2)] (106). In another survey from Italy the combination of diabetes and hypertension was the major risk factor for ED, giving an OR (95% CI) of 8.1 (1.2–55.0) as compared with diabetes without hypertension: 4.6 (1.6–13.7), hypertension without diabetes: 1.4 (0.7–3.2), current smoking: 1.7 (1.2–2.4), and ex-smoking: 1.6 (1.1–2.3) (107). However, even when neuropathic complications are present, psychiatric illness such as generalized anxiety disorder or depression may be important contributors to ED in men with diabetes (108). Thus, a psychogenic component must not be overlooked in many patients.

Physiology and Pathophysiology
Penile erection is a neurovascular event modulated by psychological factors and hormonal status depending on appropriate trabecular smooth muscle and arterial relaxation in the corpus cavernosum (Fig. 1). On sexual stimulation, nerve impulses cause the release of cholinergic and non-adrenergic non-cholinergic (NANC) neurotransmitters that mediate erectile function by relaxing the smooth muscle of the corpus cavernosum. A principal neural mediator of erection is NO which activates guanil cyclase to form intracellular cyclic guanosine monophosphate (GMP), a potent second messenger for smooth muscle relaxation. Cyclic GMP in turn activates a specific protein kinase, which phosphorylates certain proteins and ion channels, resulting in a drop of cytosolic calcium concentrations and relaxation of the smooth muscle. During the return to the flaccid state, cyclic GMP is hydrolyzed GMP by phosphodiesterase (PDE) type 5. In the corpus cavernosum four PDE isoforms have been

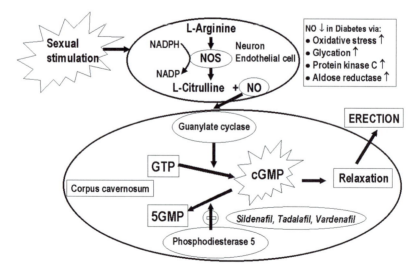

FIGURE 1   Mechanisms of erection mediated by cavernosal smooth muscle relaxation including the generation of nitric oxide (NO) by nitric oxide synthase (NOS), which is impaired in diabetes.

identified (types 2, 3, 4, and 5), but PDE-5 is the predominant isoform, while the others do not appear to have an important role in erection (109).

The pathogenesis of ED in diabetes is thought to be multifactorial as it may be linked to neuropathy, accelerated atherosclerosis, and alterations in the corporal erectile tissue. Such alterations may include smooth muscle degeneration, abnormal collagen deposition, and endothelial cell dysfunction (110). If irreversible, these corporal degenerative changes can limit the success of any pharmacotherapy. AGEs have been shown to quench NO and to be elevated in human diabetic penile tissue. It has been hypothesized that AGEs may mediate ED via upregulation of inducible nitric oxide synthase and downregulation of endothelial NOS (eNOS) (111). Furthermore, PKC activation by diabetes may reduce NOS activity (112).

In vivo studies of isolated corpus cavernosum tissue from diabetic men have shown functional impairment in neurogenic and endothelium-dependent relaxation of corpus cavernosum smooth muscle (113). In diabetic rats endothelium-dependent NO-mediated relaxation to acetylcholine and NANC stimulation are reduced by 40% after 4 to 8 weeks (114). These alterations were prevented by administration of the anti-oxidant α-lipoic acid, suggesting an involvement of increased oxidative stress. In contrast, endothelium-independent relaxation to the NO donor sodium nitroprusside is not impaired by diabetes (114). Increased penile endothelial and total NOS activity was found after 2 to 3 months in diabetic rats (115). After 4 to 8 months, however, reduced penile total (endothelial and neuronal) NOS activity and neuronal NOS levels were observed in type 1 and type 2 diabetic rats. (116). Thus, diabetes-induced changes in NOS activity may be biphasic, with an initial increase followed by a decrease. Because RhoA/Rho-kinase may suppress eNOS, RhoA/Rho-kinase could contribute to diabetes-related ED and downregulation of eNOS. Colocalization of Rho-kinase and eNOS protein is present in the endothelium of the corpus cavernosum. Diabetic rats transfected with an adeno-associated virus encoding the dominant-negative RhoA mutant (AAVTCMV19NRhoA) had a reduction in RhoA/Rho-kinase and MYPT-1 phosphorylation at a time when cavernosal eNOS protein, constitutive NOS activity, and cGMP levels were restored to levels found in control rats. AAVT19NRhoA gene transfer improved erectile responses in the diabetic rats to values similar to controls. Thus, activation of the RhoA/Rho-kinase pathway may represent one important mechanism for the downregulation of penile eNOS in diabetes, implying that inhibition of RhoA/Rho-kinase improves eNOS protein content and activity and thereby restores erectile function in diabetes (117).

Diagnosis

A good clinical history and physical examination are the basis of assessment. It is important to establish the nature of the erectile problem and to distinguish it from other forms of sexual difficulty such as penile curvature or premature ejaculation. An interview with the partner is advisable and will confirm the problem but may also reveal other causes of the difficulties, e.g., vaginal dryness. The relative importance of psychological and organic factors may be determined from the history. Drugs which may be associated with ED include tranquillizers (phenothiazines, benzodiazepines), antidepressants (tricyclics, SSRI), and antihypertensives (β-blockers, vasodilators, central sympathomimetics, ganglion blockers, diuretics, ACE inhibitors) (100). In most patients sophisticated investigation is not indicated. A three-step diagnostic approach is shown in Table 9. A detailed history is most important, and for many patients examination can be limited to the regular monitoring of diabetes and its risk factors and complications as well as examination of the genitalia. Patients should be informed about

TABLE 9   Practical Three-step Algorithm for Diagnosis of Erectile Dysfunction

Step 1
General sexual history
Clinical examination; relevant laboratory parameters
Information about treatment options
Step 2
Therapeutic trial with PDE-5 inhibitor
Step 3
Intracavernous pharmacotesting: color Doppler or duplex ultrasound of penile arteries

the advantages and disadvantages of each treatment and given advice on treatment outcome and ease of use. Even if the cause is organic, almost all men with ED will be affected psychologically. Sexual counseling is an important aspect of any treatment, and it is preferable to also involve the partner.

The second Princeton consensus on sexual dysfunction and cardiac risk issued new guidelines for sexual medicine emphasizing that ED is an early symptom or harbinger of cardiovascular disease, due to the common risk factors and pathophysiology mediated through endothelial dysfunction. Major comorbidities include diabetes, hypertension, hyperlipidemia and heart disease. Any asymptomatic man who presents with ED that does not have an obvious cause (e.g., trauma) should be screened for vascular disease and have blood glucose, lipids, and blood pressure measurements. Ideally, all patients at risk but asymptomatic for coronary disease should undergo an elective exercise electrocardiogram to facilitate risk stratification. Thus, the recognition of ED as a warning sign of silent vascular disease has led to the concept that a man with ED and no cardiac symptoms is a cardiac (or vascular) patient until proven otherwise (118).

Management

Lifestyle Modification. A stepwise therapeutic approach for ED is shown in Table 10. An algorithm for treatment of ED has been suggested by the Second International Consultation on Erectile and Sexual Dysfunctions (Fig. 2) (100). The initial management should advise the patient to reduce or treat possible risk factors such as obesity, hypertension, hyperlipidemia, or smoking and to optimize glycemic control. However, no studies are available to show that improvement in glycemic control will exert a favorable effect on ED. In fact, the VA CSDM Study could not demonstrate an effect of intensive diabetes therapy maintained for 2 years on ED in type 2 diabetic men (119). Healthy lifestyle factors are associated with maintenance of erectile function in men. A controlled study evaluated the effect of weight loss and increased physical activity on erectile and endothelial functions in obese men. Men randomly assigned to the intervention group received detailed advice about how to achieve a loss of 10% or more in their total body weight by reducing caloric intake and increasing their level of physical activity. Men in the control group were given general information about healthy food choices and exercise. After 2 years the mean International Index of Erectile Function (IIEF) score improved in the intervention group from 13.9 to 17 points, but not in the control group. In multivariate analyses, changes in body mass index (BMI), physical activity, and C-reactive

TABLE 10 Stepwise Algorithm for Treatment of Erectile Dysfunction

General management	Control of risk factors and diabetes; sexual counseling
	First-line therapy
Pharmacological treatment	Sildenafil (Viagra®), 50–100 mg
	Vardenafil (Levitra®), 10–20 mg
	Tadalafil (Cialis®), 10–20 mg
	Oral therapy inappropriate
	Transurethral alprostadil (MUSE), 500–1000 μg
	Intracavernosal injection therapy:
	Alprostadil (Caverject®), 5–20 μg
	Papaverine/Phentolamine (Androskat®)
	Thymoxamine (Erecnos®), 10–20 mg
	VIP/Phentolamine (Invicorp®)
	Papaverine/phentolamine/alprostadil (Trimix®)
Surgery and mechanical treatments	Pharmacological therapy inappropriate
	Vacuum devices
	Arterial/venous surgery
	Penile prostheses

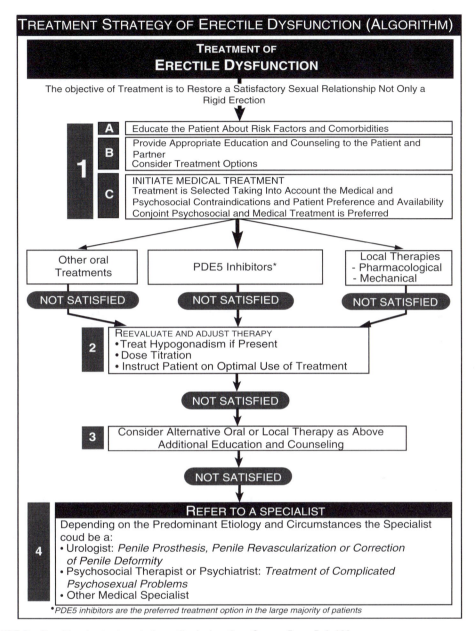

FIGURE 2　Algorithm for treatment of erectile dysfunction. *Source*: From Ref. 100.

protein were independently associated with changes in IIEF score. Thus, lifestyle changes are associated with improvement in sexual function in obese men with ED (120).

A second study from the same group evaluated the effect of a Mediterranean-style diet on ED in men with the metabolic syndrome. After 2 years, men on the Mediterranean diet ($n = 35$) consumed more fruits, vegetables, nuts, whole grain, and olive oil as compared with men on the control diet ($n = 30$). Endothelial function score and inflammatory markers (C-reactive protein) improved in the intervention group, but remained stable in the control group. There were 13 men in the intervention group and two in the control group ($P = 0.015$) that reported an IIEF score of ≥ 22 (121). Thus, Mediterranean-style diet might be effective per se in improving ED in men with the metabolic syndrome.

Oral Agents

CENTRAL INITIATORS. Yohimbine was the first drug officially listed for this indication. Yohimbine acts via central alpha-2-receptor blockade and thus increases the centrally initiated efferences of the erectogenic axis. Although its effectivity is often debated due to insufficient historic data, it showed a significant effect in a recent double-blind prospective study compared to placebo. Its side effect profile is benign including palpitations, tremor, hypertension, and anxiety. The pro-erectile effect usually starts after about 2 weeks (122). In a meta-analysis yohimbine has been found to be more effective than placebo for all types of ED combined, but the effect was most prominent in non-organic ED (123). Because of its marginal effect on organic ED, yohimbine cannot be generally recommended for treatment of ED in diabetic men.

Apomorphine is a potent emetic agent that acts via central dopaminergic (D1 or D2) receptors as well as central μ-, δ-, and κ-receptors. In the hypothalamus, it increases the centrally initiated efferences of the erectogenic axis thus improving the erectile response in a patient with erectile failure (124). The FDA concluded from the available evidence data that even though the 4 mg dose and the combined analysis showed statistical significance, the clinical significance is questionable due to the relatively modest benefits noted over placebo (125). Indeed, the NNT for the 4 mg dose based on the aforementioned results is relatively high, i.e., 10 patients need to be treated in order to achieve an erection firm enough for intercourse in one of these patients. The rates of nausea, the most prominent adverse effect of apomorphine, were 21.2%, 12.9%, and 1.0% for 4 mg, 5 mg, and placebo, respectively. The corresponding rates of vomiting were 6.7%, 1.0%, and 0%, respectively. Moreover, three syncopal events and three episodes of significant hypotension were reported in patients taking apomorphine (125).

Peripheral Conditioners

PHOSPHODIESTERASE 5 INHIBITORS

Sildenafil (Viagra®). To understand the mode of action of Sildenafil, a drug believed to act predominantly via PDE-5 inhibition, the basic physiology is briefly explained: cAMP and cGMP are synthesized from the corresponding nucleoside triphosphates by their respective membrane bound or soluble adenylate or guanylate cyclases. cAMP and cGMP are inactivated by PDE by hydrolytic cleavage of the 3'-ribose-phosphate bond (Fig. 1). Because the distribution and functional role of PDE isoenzymes varies in different tissues, selective inhibitors have the potential to exert at least partially specific tissue effects. Currently, over 40 PDE isoenzymes and isoforms are known (126). The functional assays revealed a predominant functional role for PDE 3 and 5 (127). There was no difference in PDE expression in diabetic compared to non-diabetic patients with ED.

Sildenafil acts as conditioner on the cavernous smooth muscle side by blocking PDE5. It is taken 60 minutes before anticipated sexual activity and its effects last approximately 4 hours. The drug is available in three doses (25, 50, or 100 mg). It does not stimulate the sexual desire and provoke an erection as such, but enhances the continued relaxation of the cavernous smooth muscle initiated by the release of endogenous NO with an improved quality of erection (Fig. 1).

In a controlled, flexible-dose US multicenter trial including a mixed group of 268 type 1 and type 2 diabetic men the rates of those with improved erections after 12 weeks of treatment with 25 to 100 mg sildenafil were 56% as compared with 10% in the placebo group (128). In a 12-week European multicenter trial including 219 type 2 diabetic men the response rate was even higher achieving 64.6% on sildenafil versus 10.5% on placebo (129). The estimated percentages of intercourse attempts that were successful significantly improved from baseline to end of treatment in patients receiving sildenafil (14.4–58.8%) compared with those receiving placebo (13.2–14.4%). Three quarters of the patients required the 100 mg sildenafil dose. The response rates were independent of the baseline HbA_{1c} levels and number of chronic complications, suggesting that sildenafil is effective in improving ED even in cases with poor glycemic control and in presence of angiopathy and neuropathy. In a combined analysis of 11 controlled trials of sildenafil (25–100 mg) the percentages of the maximum score for the six questions in the erectile function domain of the IIEF were 61.3% among 69 type 1 and 60.8%

among 399 type 1 diabetic men on sildenafil as compared to 39.3% among 452 diabetic men on placebo (130).

Side effects consist mainly of headache (18%), facial flushing (15%), and dyspepsia (2%). A mild and transient disturbance of color vision and also increased sensitivity to light or blurred vision has been found in 4.5% of diabetic men (129). Concerns have been expressed regarding an increased number of deaths associated with sildenafil as compared with other treatments for ED (131). However, after an average follow-up of 6 months the Prescription Event Monitoring Study including 5601 sildenafil users from England showed an expected mortality rate of 28.9 per 1000/year for ischemic heart disease/myocardial infarctions. The comparison rate in the general population of England in 1998 was 73.9 per 1000/year (132). The prevalence of diabetes in the cohort was 15%, which is similar to the rate of 16% included in the clinical trials of sildenafil, but much higher than the rate of 3.3% of men with diabetes in England in 1998. Although these results are reassuring, further follow-up of this study and other pharmacoepidemiological research is needed for confirmation. In men with severe stenosis of at least one coronary artery acute administration of sildenafil (100 mg) did not result in adverse hemodynamic effects on coronary blood flow or vascular resistance, but coronary flow reserve was improved (133).

Apart from its effect on ED, favorable effects of sildenafil have recently been reported in studies of various disorders including primary pulmonary hypertension, achalasia, and endothelial dysfunction (134).

According to the recommendations of the American Heart Association sildenafil is contraindicated in men taking nitrates due to the risk of hypotension and those with severe cardiovascular disease. Before sildenafil is prescribed, treadmill testing may be indicated in men with heart disease to assess the risk of cardiac ischemia during sexual intercourse. Initial monitoring of blood pressure after the administration of sildenafil may be indicated in men with congestive heart disease who have borderline low blood pressure and low volume status and men being treated with complicated, multidrug antihypertensive regimens (134).

Because some men do not respond to sildenafil treatment, attempts have been undertaken to characterize these non-responders. A recent penile biopsy study identified severe vascular lesions and atrophy of cavernous smooth muscle to represent the main factors that determined the lacking response to 100 mg sildenafil in men with ED aged from 28 to 74 years. The age, diabetes and low testosterone level were not related to the response failures (135).

Tadalafil (Cialis®). In a 12-week multicenter trial including 216 diabetic men (type 2: 91%), but excluding sildenafil non-responders, the rates of men with improved erections were 64% with 20 mg tadalafil, 56% with 10 mg tadalafil, and 25% on placebo (136). Both tadalafil 10 and 20 mg were superior to placebo in improving penetration ability (IIEF question 3) and ability to maintain an erection during intercourse. Thus, although non-responders to sildenafil were excluded, the effect of tadalafil was not superior to that of sildenafil. Treatment-related adverse events (>5%) on 20 mg, 10 mg, and placebo were dyspepsia (8.3%, 11.0%, and 0%) and headache (6.9%, 8.2%, and 1.4%). Despite more severe baseline ED in men with diabetes as compared to the non-diabetic population of men with ED, tadalafil was efficacious and well tolerated. As reported for other phosphodiesterase 5 inhibitors, the response to tadalafil was slightly lower in men with diabetes than in men without diabetes (137). The pharmacokinetic profile of tadalafil differs from that of sildenafil and vardenafil in that it has a much longer half-life (Fig. 3). This means that the effect of tadalafil may last over 24 hours or even longer, while the duration of action for the other two drugs is around 4 to 5 hours. Such a longer "window of opportunity" may be preferable by some men, but in the same way possible side effects may also be prolonged.

So far trials of PDE-5 inhibitors in men with ED assessed exclusively on-demand treatment. In contrast, two recent studies evaluated once-a-day dosing of tadalafil (2.5–10 mg/day) over 12 and 24 weeks, respectively. Both trials have demonstrated that once-daily tadalafil improves erectile function in men with ED and is well tolerated (138,139). Against the background of potential favorable effects on endothelial function a daily administration of PDE-5 inhibitors appears an attractive option. However, the pros and cons of such a long-term treatment are unknown. One advantage could be the lower dose required for daily dosing, but the cost of this approach would obviously be high.

Parameter	Vardenafil 20 mg	Sildenafil 100 mg	Tadalafil 20 mg
Tmax (min)	40	70	120 (30 - 720)
T1/2 (h)	4 - 4,8	3,8	17,5

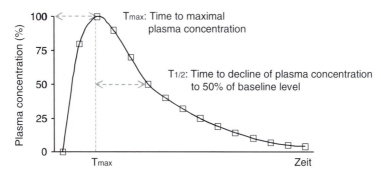

FIGURE 3   Pharmacokinetics of PDE-5 inhibitors.

Vardenafil (Levitra®).   In a large 12-week multicenter trial including 439 diabetic men (type 2: 88%) that excluded sildenafil non-responders, the rates of men with improved erections were 72% with 20 mg vardenafil, 57% with 10 mg vardenafil, and 13% on placebo (140). Both vardenafil 10 and 20 mg were superior to placebo in improving the IIEF erectile function domain score (questions 1–5, 15). Similar to tadalafil, despite the exclusion of non-responders to sildenafil the effect of vardenafil was comparable to that reported previously for sildenafil. Treatment-related adverse events (>5%) on 20 mg, 10 mg, and placebo were headache (10%, 9%, and 2%), flushing (10%, 9%, and <1%), and headache (6%, 3%, and 0%).

In a multicenter, double-blind, placebo-controlled clinical trial, PDE-5 inhibitor-naive type 1 diabetic patients were randomized to receive placebo ($n = 149$) or flexible-dose (5–20 mg) ($n = 153$) vardenafil. Vardenafil significantly improved mean success rates for Sexual Encounter Profile 2 and 3 compared with baseline and placebo at 4, 8, and 12 weeks. These rates were unaffected by stratification into distinct subsets according to the level of HbA(1c) (HbA(1c) < 7%, good glycemic control; HbA(1c) >7 to ≥8%, moderate glycemic control; and HbA(1c) >8%, poor glycemic control). The most commonly reported treatment-emergent adverse events were headache (3.1%) and flushing (2.5%), which were mild to moderate and transient in nature. These data suggest that vardenafil significantly improves erectile function in men with type 1 diabetes and is well tolerated, regardless of the level of glycemic control (141).

Data from head-to-head clinical trials of PDE-5 inhibitors are scarce. One recent randomized, double-blind, crossover head-to-head clinical trial compared patient preference, efficacy, and safety of vardenafil and sildenafil in men with ED and diabetes, hypertension, and/or hyperlipidemia. Prospective analysis was performed on two studies in which 1057 men were randomized to vardenafil 20 mg ($n = 530$) or sildenafil 100 mg (2 x 50 mg encapsulated tablets) ($n = 527$) for 4 weeks. Following a 1-week washout, patients switched treatment for 4 weeks. Non-inferiority of vardenafil over sildenafil was achieved for overall preference (vardenafil 38.9%; sildenafil 34.5%; and no preference 26.6%). Additionally, the change from baseline in the EF domain score of the IIEF achieved nominal significance for vardenafil over sildenafil (10.00 vs. 9.40; $P = 0.0052$). Patients also had a higher percentage of positive responses for vardenafil for SEP2, SEP3, GAQ, and 12 of 19 questions on the TSS. However, several sources of potential bias such as the sildenafil formulation, pooled analysis of two studies, and sponsorship of the study by the manufacturer of vardenafil have to be considered when interpreting these data (142).

A recent systematic review assessed the overall effect of PDE-5 inhibitors on the management of ED in diabetic men. The weighted mean difference (WMD) for the IIEF questions 3 and 4 (frequency of penetration during and maintaining erection to completion of intercourse) was 0.9 (95% CI 0.8–1.1) and 1.1 (95% CI 1.0–1.2) at the end of the study period, in favor of the intervention group. The WMD for the IIEF ED domain at the end of the study period was 6.6 (95% CI 5.2–7.9) in favor of the PDE-5 inhibitors arm. The relative risk for answering "yes" to a global efficacy question ("did the treatment improve your erections?") was 3.8 (95% CI 3.1–4.5) in the PDE-5 inhibitors compared with the control arm. The WMD between the percentage of successful attempts in the PDE-5 inhibitors and in the control arm was 26.7 (95% CI 23.1–30.3). The overall risk ratio for developing any adverse reaction was 4.8 (95% CI 3.74–6.16) in the PDE-5 inhibitors arm as compared to the control. Thus, sufficient evidence exists that PDE-5 inhibitors form a care that improves ED in diabetic men (143).

Vacuum Devices

These have the merit of being non-invasive and may be effective in all men. They create a vacuum around the penis and blood is drawn into the corporal spaces. A band is slipped off the plastic cylinder around the base of the penis to maintain penile tumescence without rigidity in the crura. The disadvantages are that they require some degree of dexterity in handling them, and some time spent in application of the device. They should only be used for 30 minutes at a time, and require the willing cooperation of the partner. There are few side effects although there is some degree of discomfort and the penis feels cold. Ejaculation is usually blocked and some men find this makes orgasm less satisfactory. Bruising can occur in 10% to 15% of men. Vacuum devices are particularly useful in older men in stable relationships and when other treatment options are ineffective. They may also be used to augment the result of pharmacotherapy. Some men find that the constrictive ring is a useful aid in itself for maintaining the erection without the use of a vacuum device (144). However, the long-term drop-out rates among users of vacuum constriction devices are relatively high. A recent study showed an overall drop-out rate over 3 years for the ErecAid system of 65%, i.e., 100% in men with mild ED, 56% in those with moderate ED, and 70% in those with complete ED. The main reasons for stopping use were that the device was ineffective (57%), too cumbersome (24%), and too painful (20%) (144).

Transurethral Alprostadil

Alprostadil was first licensed for the treatment of ED by intracavernous injection. Alprostadil, the synthetic preparation of the naturally occurring prostaglandin E1 acts by initiating the erection. In contrast to sildenafil it initiates the relaxation of cavernous smooth muscle to bring about erection. This drug has been incorporated into a pellet that can be given by intraurethral application [Medical Urethral System for Erection (MUSE)]. Patients need to be instructed in the use of MUSE which is introduced into the urethra with a disposable applicator. The patient first passes urine to act as a lubricant to facilitate the passage of the applicator and the absorption of the drug. Absorption of the drug is also facilitated by the patient rolling his penis between the palms of his hands. Some patients find that a constrictive ring around the base of the penis enhances the efficacy. The erection takes about 10 minutes to develop and the dose range varies between 125 and 1000 μg although the majority of patients require 500 or 1000 μg. The use of MUSE is contraindicated without a condom when the partner is pregnant or likely to conceive (145).

In the United States and European multicenter trials about 65% of men with different causes of ED who tried MUSE had erections sufficient for intercourse during in-clinic testing (145,146). About one half of the treatments at home were successful, but the drop-out rate after 15 months was 75%, the main reason being lack of efficacy (146). The most common side effects are penile pain (30%), urethral burning (12%) or minor urethral bleeding (5%) (65). Systemic side effects (such as hypotension or even syncope) were usually uncommon but help to highlight the role of the physician in administering the first supervised dose. Disappointing results have been reported in a study conducted in a urology practice setting, in which an adequate rigidity score was achieved in only 13% and 30% of the patients using 500 and 1000 μg, respectively. Pain, discomfort, or burning in the penis were observed in 18%, but orthostatic hypotension (defined as a decrease in systolic/diastolic blood pressure by 20/10 mmHg or orthostatic symptoms) was present in 41% of the patients. The discontinuation rate was very high, achieving 81% after 2 to 3 months (148).

Intracavernosal Injection Therapy

Intracavernosal therapy requires some specialist knowledge and the ability to treat priapism should it occur. Many specialists used to regard this as the standard treatment and use it for both diagnostic and therapeutic reasons although its role as first-line therapy has been replaced by less invasive treatment modalities. Patients need to be taught how to perform self-injection and the dose needs to be chosen carefully to avoid prolonged erections or priapism. Some patients find it helpful to use one of the many autoinjector devices available. The erection occurs after 10 minutes and may be enhanced by sexual stimulation. The incidence of complications varies with the different pharmacological agents. Some pain is not uncommon but long-term problems are limited to priapism or penile fibrosis.

Alprostadil is the most widely used agent (149,150). It is effective in more than 80% of patients with different etiologies of ED and has a low incidence of side effects. In a recent comparative study of intracavernosal versus intraurethral administration of alprostadil the rates of erections sufficient for sexual intercourse were 82.5% versus 53.0%, respectively (150). Patient and partner satisfaction was higher with intracavernosal injection, and more patients preferred this therapy. Penile pain occurs in 15% to 50% of patients but is often not troublesome. The dose range is 5 to 20 µg but some physicians will increase it further or use a combination with papaverine and phentolamine. Priapism occurs in about 1% of patients. The cumulative incidence of penile fibrosis was 11.7% after a period of 4 years, and the risk of irreversible fibrotic alterations was 5% (151). About half of the cases with fibrosis resolved spontaneously. Other less frequently used agents include thymoxamine [moxisylyte hydrocholoride (Erecnos)], papaverine/phentolamine mixtures, (Androskat), papaverine/phentolamine/alprostadil mixtures (Trimix), and VIP/Phentolamine (Invicorp).

Penile Prostheses and Surgery

This type of treatment is carried out only after careful patient selection and a trial of the less invasive options. There are a number of different devices ranging from the simple malleable prosthesis to more complex hydraulic prostheses. The choice of prosthesis is very much dependent upon the wishes of the patient and is often cost-related. A prosthesis does not restore a normal erection but makes the penis rigid enough for sexual intercourse. The hydraulic prostheses have the advantage of flaccidity and are now mechanically reliable with revision rates of less than 5% per annum. Infection remains a major complication in approximately 3% to 5% of cases with different causes of ED and usually leads to removal of the device.

Arterial reconstruction is associated with complication rates of more than 30% and remains an experimental procedure which cannot be generally recommended to diabetic patients with ED.

Other Sexual Problems in Diabetic Men

Diminished or absent testicular pain has been described as an early sign of autonomic neuropathy. Retrograde ejaculation from the prostatic urethra into the bladder may occur occasionally and follows loss of sympathetic innervation of the internal sphincter which normally contracts during ejaculation. Complete loss of ejaculation probably indicates widespread pelvic sympathetic involvement and, like retrograde ejaculation, causes infertility which may be treated by insemination (152).

Female Sexual Dysfunction

Female sexual dysfunctions (FSD) include persistent or recurrent disorders of sexual interest/desire, disorders of subjective and genital arousal, orgasm disorder, pain and difficulty with attempted or completed intercourse. The scientific knowledge on sexual dysfunction in women with diabetes is rudimentary. Sexual dysfunction was observed in 27% of type 1 diabetic women. FSD was not related to age, BMI, HbA$_{1c}$, duration of diabetes, and diabetic complications. However, FSD was related to depression and the quality of the partner relationship (153). Recently, the prevalence of FSD in premenopausal women with the metabolic syndrome was compared to the general female population. Women with the metabolic syndrome had reduced mean full Female Sexual Function Index (FSFI) score, reduced satisfaction rate, and higher circulating levels of C-reactive protein. There was an inverse relation between CRP levels and FSFI score (154).

Problems affecting sexuality in diabetic women are fatigue, changes in perimenstrual blood glucose control, vaginitis, decreased sexual desire, decreased vaginal lubrication, and an increased time to reach orgasm. Even minor episodes of depression which is twice more frequent than in men can result in a loss of libido. To which degree these symptoms are related to autonomic neuropathy has also been examined in a few studies, the results of which are at variance (155). The examination for a diabetic woman with sexual dysfunction should include the duration of symptoms, psychological state, concomitant, medications, presence of vaginitis, cystitis, and other infections, frequency of intercourse, blood pressure, BMI, retinal status, pelvic examination, presence of discharge, and glycemic control (156).

There is evidence to suggest that in men with diabetes, sexual dysfunction is related to somatic and psychological factors, whereas in women with diabetes, psychological factors are more predominant (153). The effect of diabetes on women's sexual function is complex: the most consistent finding is a correlation between sexual dysfunction and depression. More research on the sexual effects of abnormal adrenal and thyroid function, hyperprolactinemia, and metabolic syndrome in women should be prioritized (157). Solid data are available on local management of the genital consequences of estrogen lack, but there is need to better understand the potential role of systemic estrogen supplementation from menopause onwards in sexually symptomatic women.

REFERENCES

1. Consensus statement. Report and recommendations of the San Antonio conference on diabetic neuropathy. Diabetes Care 1988; 11:592–7.
2. Thomas PK. Metabolic neuropathy. J Roy Coll Phys Lond 1973; 7:154.
3. Sima AAF, Thomas PK, Ishii D, Vinik A. Diabetic neuropathies. Diabetologia 1997; 40:B74–7.
4. Shaw JE, Zimmet PZ. The epidemiology of diabetic neuropathy. Diabetes Rev 1999; 7:245–52.
5. Resnick HE, Vinik AI, Schwartz AV, et al. Independent effects of peripheral nerve dysfunction on lower-extremity physical function in old age. The Women's Health and Aging Study. Diabetes Care 2000; 23:1642–7.
6. Forsblom CM, Sane T, Groop PH, et al. Risk factors for mortality in Type II (non-insulin-dependent) diabetes: evidence of a role for neuropathy and a protective effect of HLA-DR4. *Diabetologia* 1998; 4: 1253–62.
7. Coppini DV, Bowtell PA, Weng C, Young PJ, Sönksen PH. Showing neuropathy is related to increased mortality in diabetic patients—a survival analysis using an accelerated failure time model. J Clin Epidemiol 2000; 53:519–23.
8. Abbott CA, Vileikyte L, Williamson S, Carrington AL, Boulton AJM. Multicenter study of the incidence of and predictive risk factors for diabetic neuropathic foot ulceration. Diabetes Care 1998; 21:1071–5.
9. Galer BS, Gianas A, Jensen MP. Painful diabetic neuropathy: epidemiology, pain description, and quality of life. Diabetes Res Clin Pract 2000; 47:123–8.
10. Daousi C, Benbow SJ, Woodward A, MacFarlane IA. The natural history of chronic painful peripheral neuropathy in a community diabetes population. Diabet Med 2006; 23:1021–4.
11. Davies M, Brophy S, Williams R, Taylor A. The prevalence, severity, and impact of painful diabetic peripheral neuropathy in type 2 diabetes. Diabetes Care 2006; 29:1518–22.
12. Thomas PK. Painful diabetic neuropathy: mechanisms and treatment. Diabetes Nutr Metab 1994; 7: 359–68.
13. Boulton AJM, Scarpello JHB, Armstrong WD, Ward JD. The natural history of painful diabetic neuropathy—a 4-year study. Postgrad Med J 1983; 59:556–9.
14. Young RJ, Ewing DJ, Clarke BF. Chronic and remitting painful diabetic neuropathy. Diabetes Care 1988; 11:34–40.
15. Benbow SJ, Chan AW, Bowsher D, MacFarlane IA, Williams G. A prospective study of painful symptoms, small-fibre function and peripheral vascular disease in chronic painful diabetic neuropathy. Diabet Med 1993; 11:17–21.
16. Archer AG, Watkins PJ, Thomas PK, Sharma AK, Payan J. The natural history of acute painful neuropathy in diabetes mellitus. J Neurol Neurosurg Psychiatry 1983; 46:491–9.
17. Ellenberg M. Diabetic neuropathic cachexia. Diabetes 1974; 23, 418–23.
18. Steele JM, Young RJ, Lloyd GG, Clarke BF. Clinically apparent eating disorders in young diabetic women: associations with painful neuropathy and other complications. Br Med J 1987; 294:859–66.
19. Caravati CM. Insulin neuritis: a case report. Va Med Mon 1933; 59:745–6.

20. Llewelyn JG, Thomas PK, Fonseca V, King RHM, Dandona P. Acute painful diabetic neuropathy precipitated by strict glycaemic control. Acta Neuropathol 1986; 72:157–63.

21. Tesfaye S, Malik R, Harris N, et al. Arterio-venous shunting and proliferating new vessels in acute painful neuropathy of rapid glycaemic control (insulin neuritis). Diabetologia 1996; 39:329–35.

22. Asbury AK. Focal and multifocal neuropathies of diabetes. In: Dyck PJ, Thomas PK, Asbury AK, Winegrad AI, Porte D, eds. Diabetic Neuropathy. Philadelphia: Saunders, 1987:45–55.

23. Zorilla E, Kozak GP. Ophthalmoplegia in diabetes mellitus. Ann Intern Med 1967; 67:968–74.

24. Chaudhuri KR, Wren DR, Werring D, Watkins PJ. Unilateral abdominal muscle herniation with pain: a distinctive variant of diabetic radiculopathy. Diabet Med 1997; 14:803–7.

25. Said G, Goulon-Goeau C, Lacroix C, Moulonguet A. Nerve biopsy findings in different patterns of proximal diabetic neuropathy. Ann Neurol 1994; 35:559–69.

26. Said G, Elgrably F, Lacroix C, et al. Painful proximal diabetic neuropathy: inflammatory nerve lesions and spontaneous favorable outcome. Ann Neurol 1997; 41:762–70.

27. Younger DS, Rosoklija G, Hays AP, Trojaborg W, Latov N. Diabetic peripheral neuropathy: a clinicopathologic and immunohistochemical analysis of sural nerve biopsies. Muscle Nerve 1996; 19:722–7.

28. Krendel DA. Diabetic inflammatory vasculopathy. Muscle Nerve 1997; 20:520.

29. Krendel DA, Costigan DA, Hopkins LC. Successful treatment of neuropathies in patients with diabetes mellitus. Arch Neurol 1995; 52:1053–61.

30. Reske-Nielsen E, Lundbaek K. Pathological changes in the central and peripheral nervous system of young long-term diabetics. II. The spinal cord and peripheral nerves. Diabetologia 1968; 4:34–43.

31. Slager U. Diabetic myelopathy. Arch Pathol Lab Med 1978; 102:467–9.

32. Olsson Y, Säve-Söderbergh J, Sourander P, Angervall L. A patho-anatomical study of the central and peripheral nervous system in diabetics of early onset and long duration. Pathol Eur 1968; 3:62–79.

33. Reske-Nielsen E, Lundbaek K, Rafaelsen OJ. Pathological changes in the central and peripheral nervous system of young long-term diabetics. I. Diabetic encephalopathy. Diabetologia 1965; 1:233–41.

34. DeJong RN. The nervous system complications in diabetes mellitus with special reference to cerebrovascular changes. J Nerv Ment Dis 1950; 111:181–206.

35. Ziegler D, Mühlen H, Dannehl K, Gries FA. Tibial nerve somatosensory evoked potentials at various stages of peripheral neuropathy in Type 1 diabetic patients. J Neurol Neurosurg Psychiatry 1993; 56:58–64.

36. Ziegler D, Seemann-Monteiro M, Mühlen H, Gries FA. The degree of cognitive dysfunction is associated with the stage of peripheral neuropathy in Type 1 diabetic patients. Diabetologia 1993; 36(Suppl. 1):A185.

37. Dejgaard A, Gade A, Larsson H, Balle V, Parving A, Parving H-H. Evidence for diabetic encephalopathy. Diabetic Med 1991; 8:162–167.

38. Ziegler D, Langen K-J, Herzog H, et al. Cerebral glucose metabolism in Type 1 diabetic patients. Diabet Med 1994; 11:205–9.

39. Eaton SE, Harris ND, Rajbhandari SM, et al. Spinal-chord involvement in diabetic peripheral neuropathy. Lancet 2001; 358:35–6.

40. American Diabetes Association Proceedings of a consensus development conference on standardized measures in diabetic neuropathy. Diabetes Care 1992; 15(Suppl. 3):1080–107.

41. Dyck PJ. Detection, characterization, and staging of polyneuropathy: assessed in diabetics. Muscle Nerve 1988; 11:21–32.

42. Young MJ, Boulton AJM, Macleod AF, Williams DRR, Sonksen PH. A multicentre study of the prevalence of diabetic peripheral neuropathy in the United Kingdom hospital clinic population. Diabetologia 1993; 36:150–4.

43. Lauria G, Cornblath DR, Johansson O, et al. European Federation of Neurological Societies. EFNS guidelines on the use of skin biopsy in the diagnosis of peripheral neuropathy. Eur J Neurol 2005; 12:747–58.

44. Peripheral Neuropathy Association Quantitative sensory testing: a consensus report. Neurology 1993; 43:1050–2.

45. The Diabetes Control and Complications Trial Research Group. The effect of intensive treatment of diabetes on the development and progression of long-term complications in insulin-dependent diabetes mellitus. N Engl J Med 1993; 329:977–86.

46. UK Prospective Diabetes Study (UKPDS) Group. Intensive blood-glucose control with sulphony-lureas or insulin compared with conventional treatment and risk of complications in patients with type 2 diabetes (UKPDS 33). Lancet 1998; 352:837–53.

47. Martin CL, Albers J, Herman WH, et al. DCCT/EDIC Research Group. Neuropathy among the diabetes control and complications trial cohort 8 years after trial completion. Diabetes Care 2006; 29:340–4.

48. Nicolucci A, Carinci F, Cavaliere D, et al. on behalf of the Italian study group for the implementation of the St. Vincent Declaration. A meta-analysis of trials on aldose reductase inhibitors in diabetic peripheral neuropathy. Diabet Med 1996; 13:1017–26.

49. Dyck PJ, O'Brien PC. Meaningful degrees of prevention or improvement of nerve conduction in controlled clinical trials of diabetic neuropathy. Diabetes Care 1989; 12:649–52.

50. Hotta N, Toyota T, Matsuoka K, et al. SNK-860 Diabetic Neuropathy Study Group. Clinical efficacy of fidarestat, a novel aldose reductase inhibitor, for diabetic peripheral neuropathy: a 52-week multicenter placebo-controlled double-blind parallel group study. Diabetes Care 2001; 24:1776–82.

51. Hotta N, Akanuma Y, Kawamori R, et al. Long-term clinical effects of epalrestat, an aldose reductase inhibitor, on diabetic peripheral neuropathy: the 3-year, multicenter, comparative Aldose Reductase Inhibitor-Diabetes Complications Trial. Diabetes Care 2006; 29:1538–44.

52. Bril V, Buchanan RA. Long-term effects of Ranirestat (AS-3201) on peripheral nerve function in patients with diabetic sensorimotor polyneuropathy. Diabetes Care 2006; 29:68–72.

53. The γ-Linolenic Acid Multicenter Trial Group. Treatment of diabetic neuropathy with γ-linolenic acid. Diabetes Care 1993; 16:8–15.

54. Ziegler D, Nowak H, Kempler P, Vargha P, Low PA. Treatment of symptomatic diabetic polyneuropathy with the antioxidant α-lipoic acid: a meta-analysis. Diabet Med 2004; 21:114–21.

55. Ziegler D. Thioctic acid for patients with symptomatic diabetic neuropathy. A critical review. Treat Endocrinol 2004; 3:1–17.

56. Ziegler D, Ametov A, Barinov A, et al. Oral treatment with alpha-lipoic acid improves symptomatic diabetic polyneuropathy: the SYDNEY 2 trial. Diabetes Care 2006; 29:2365–70.

57. Ziegler D, Low PA, Boulton AJM, et al. Effect of 4-year antioxidant treatment with α-lipoic acid in diabetic polyneuropathy: the NATHAN 1 trial. Diabetes 2007; 56(Suppl.).

58. Malik RA, Williamson S, Abbott C, et al. Effect of angiotensin-converting-enzyme (ACE) inhibitor trandolapril on human diabetic neuropathy: randomised double blind placebo controlled trial. Lancet 1998; 352:1978–81.

59. Toyota T, Hirata Y, Ikeda Y, Matsuoka K, Sakuma A, Mizushima Y. Lipo-PGE1, a new lipid-encapsulated preparation of prostaglandin E1: placebo- and prostaglandin E1-controlled multi-center trials in patients with diabetic neuropathy and leg ulcers. Prostaglandins 1993; 46:453–68.

60. Apfel SC, Schwartz S, Adornato BT, et al. Efficacy and safety of recombinant human nerve growth factor in patients with diabetic polyneuropathy. JAMA 2000; 284:2215–21.

61. Vinik AI, Bril V, Kempler P, et al. the MBBQ Study Group. Treatment of symptomatic diabetic peripheral neuropathy with the protein kinase C beta-inhibitor ruboxistaurin mesylate during a 1-year, randomized, placebo-controlled, double-blind clinical trial. Clin Ther 2005; 27:1164–80.

62. Johansson B-L, Borg K, Fernqvist-Forbes E, Kernell A, Odergren T, Wahren J. Beneficial effects of C-peptide on incipient nephropathy and neuropathy in patients with Type 1 diabetes mellitus. Diabet Med 2000; 17:181–9.

63. Ekberg K, Brismar T, Johansson BL, Jonsson B, Lindstrom P, Wahren J. Amelioration of sensory nerve dysfunction by C-Peptide in patients with type 1 diabetes. Diabetes. 2003; 52(2):536–41.

64. Ekberg K, Brismar T, Johansson BL, et al. C-Peptide replacement therapy and sensory nerve function in type 1 diabetic neuropathy. Diabetes Care 2007; 30:71–6.

65. Schratzberger P, Walter DH, Rittig K, et al. Reversal of experimental diabetic neuropathy by VEGF gene transfer. J Clin Invest 2001; 107:1083–92.

66. Simovic D, Isner JM, Ropper AH, Pieczek A, Weinberg DH. Improvement in chronic ischemic neuropathy after intramuscular phVEGF165 gene transfer in patients with critical limb ischemia. Arch Neurol 2001; 58:761–8.

67. Jensen TS, Backonja MM, Hernandez Jimenez S, Tesfaye S, Valensi P, Ziegler D. New perspectives on the management of diabetic peripheral neuropathic pain. Diab Vasc Dis Res 2006; 3:108–19.

68. Boulton AJ, Vinik AI, Arezzo JC, et al. Diabetic neuropathies: a statement by the American Diabetes Association. Diabetes Care 2005; 28:956–62.

69. Finnerup NB, Otto M, McQuay HJ, Jensen TS, Sindrup SH. Algorithm for neuropathic pain treatment: An evidence based proposal. Pain 2005; 118:289–305.

70. Wernicke JF, Pritchett YL, D'Souza DN, et al. A randomized controlled trial of duloxetine in diabetic peripheral neuropathic pain. Neurology 2006; 67:1411–20.

71. Goldstein DJ, Lu Y, Detke MJ, Lee TC, Iyengar S. Duloxetine vs. placebo in patients with painful diabetic neuropathy. Pain 2005; 116:109–18.

72. Raskin J, Pritchett YL, Wang F, et al. A double-blind, randomized multicenter trial comparing duloxetine with placebo in the management of diabetic peripheral neuropathic pain. Pain Med 2005; 6:346–56.

73. Ziegler D, Pritchett YL, Wang F, et al. Impact of disease characteristics on the efficacy of duloxetine in diabetic peripheral neuropathic pain. Diabetes Care 2007; 30:664–9.

74. Hardy T, Sachson R, Shen S, Armbruster M, Boulton AJ. Does treatment with duloxetine for neuropathic pain impact glycemic control? Diabetes Care 2007; 30:21–6.

75. Rowbotham MC, Goli V, Kunz NR, Lei D. Venlafaxine extended release in the treatment of painful diabetic neuropathy: a double-blind, placebo-controlled study. Pain 2004; 110:697–706.

76. Backonja M, Beydoun A, Edwards KR, et al. Gabapentin for the symptomatic treatment of painful neuropathy in patients with diabetes mellitus. JAMA 1998; 280:1831–6.

77. Griesing T, Freeman R, Rosenstock J, et al. Efficacy, safety, and tolerability of pregabalin treatment for diabetic peripheral neuropathy: findings from 6 randomized controlled trials. Diabetologia 2005; 48(Suppl. 1):A351.

78. Grosskopf J, Mazzola J, Wan Y, Hopwood M. A randomized, placebo-controlled study of oxcarbazepine in painful diabetic neuropathy. Acta Neurol Scand 2006; 114:177–80.

79. Beydoun A, Shaibani A, Hopwood M, Wan Y. Oxcarbazepine in painful diabetic neuropathy: results of a dose-ranging study. Acta Neurol Scand 2006; 113:395–404.

80. Thienel U, Neto W, Schwabe SK, Vijapurkar U; Topiramate Diabetic Neuropathic Pain Study Group. Topiramate in painful diabetic polyneuropathy: findings from three double-blind placebo-controlled trials. Acta Neurol Scand 2004; 110:221–31.

81. Vinik AII, Tuchman M, Safirstein B, et al. Lamotrigine for treatment of pain associated with diabetic neuropathy: results of two randomized, double-blind, placebo-controlled studies. Pain 2007; 128: 169–79.

82. Mo J, Chen LL. Systemic lidocaine for neuropathic pain relief. Pain 2000; 87:7–17.

83. Davies PS, Galer BS. Review of lidocaine patch 5% studies in the treatment of postherpetic neuralgia. Drugs 2004; 64:937–47.

84. Zhang WY, Li Wan Po A. The effectiveness of topically applied capsaicin. A meta-analysis. Eur J Clin Pharmacol 1994; 46:517–22.

85. Nolano M, Simone DA, Wendelschafer-Crabb G, Johnson T, Hazen E, Kennedy WR. Topical capsaicin in humans: parallel loss of epidermal nerve fibers and pain sensation. Pain 1999; 81:135–45.

86. Harati Y, Gooch C, Swenson M, et al. Double-blind randomized trial of tramadol for the treatment of the pain of diabetic neuropathy. Neurology 1998; 50:1842–6.

87. Watson CP, Moulin D, Watt-Watson J, Gordon A, Eisenhoffer J. Controlled-release oxycodone relieves neuropathic pain: a randomized controlled trial in painful diabetic neuropathy. Pain 2003; 105:71–8.

88. Gimbel JS, Richards P, Portenoy RK. Controlled-release oxycodone for pain in diabetic neuropathy: a randomized controlled trial. Neurology 2003; 60:927–34.

89. Gilron I, Bailey JM, Tu D, Holden RR, Weaver DF, Houlden RL. Morphine, gabapentin, or their combination for neuropathic pain. N Engl J Med 2005; 31(352):1324–34.

90. Rauck RL, Shaibani A, Biton V, Simpson J, Koch B. Lacosamide in painful diabetic peripheral neuropathy: a phase 2 double-blind placebo-controlled study. Clin J Pain 2007; 23:150–8.

91. Tesfaye S. Painful diabetic neuropathy. Aetiology and nonpharmacological treatment. In: Veves A, ed. Clinical Management of Diabetic Neuropathy. Totowa, NJ: Humana Press, 1998:133–46.

92. Abuaisha BB, Costanzi, Boulton AJM. Acupuncture for the treatment of chronic painful peripheral diabetic neuropathy: a long-term study. Diabetes Res Clin Pract 1998; 39:115–21.

93. Kumar D, Alvaro MS, Julka IS, Marshall HJ. Diabetic peripheral neuropathy. Effectiveness of electrotherapy and amitriptyline for symptomatic relief. Diabetes Care 1998; 21:1322–5.

94. Reichstein L, Labrenz S, Ziegler D, Martin S. Effective treatment of symptomatic diabetic polyneuropathy by high-frequency external muscle stimulation. Diabetologia 2005; 48:824–8.

95. Bosi E, Conti M, Vermigli C, et al. Effectiveness of frequency-modulated electromagnetic neural stimulation in the treatment of painful diabetic neuropathy. Diabetologia 2005; 48:817–23.

96. Powell MW, Carnegie DH, Burke TJ. Reversal of diabetic peripheral neuropathy with phototherapy (MIRE^{TM}) decreases falls and the fear of falling and improves activities of daily living in seniors. Age Ageing 2006; 35:11–6.

97. Clifft JK, Kasser RJ, Newton TS, Bush AJ. The effect of monochromatic infrared energy on sensation in patients with diabetic peripheral neuropathy: a double-blind, placebo-controlled study. Diabetes Care 2005; 28:2896–900.

98. Tesfaye S, Watt J, Benbow SJ, Pang KA, Miles J, MacFarlane IA. Electrical spinal-cord stimulation for painful diabetic peripheral neuropathy. Lancet 1996; 348:1696–701.

99. Therapeutics and Technology Assessment Subcommittee of the American Academy of Neurology, Chaudhry V, Stevens JC, Kincaid J, So YT. Practice Advisory: utility of surgical decompression for treatment of diabetic neuropathy: report of the Therapeutics and Technology Assessment Subcommittee of the American Academy of Neurology. Neurology 2006; 66:1805–8.

100. Lue TF, Giuliano F, Montorsi F, et al. Summary of the recommendations on sexual dysfunctions in men. J Sex Med 2004; 1:6–23.

101. Wagner G, Saenz de Tejada I. Update on male erectile dysfunction. Br Med J 1998; 316:678–82.

102. Feldman HA, Goldstein I, Hatzichristou DG, Krane RJ, McKinlay JB. Impotence and its medical and psychosocial correlates: results of the Massachusetts male ageing study. J Urol 1994; 151:54–61.

103. Braun M, Wassmer G, Klotz T, Reifenrath B, Mathers M, Engelmann U. Epidemiology of erectile dysfunction: results of the 'Cologne Male Survey'. Int J Impot Res 2000; 12:305–11.

104. Johannes CB, Araujo AB, Feldman HA, Derby CA, Kleinman KP, McKinlay JB: Incidence of erectile dysfunction in men 40 to 69 years old: longitudinal results from the Massachusetts male aging study. J Urol 2000; 163:460–3.
105. Klein R, Klein BE, Lee KE, Moss SE, Cruickshanks KJ. Prevalence of self-reported erectile dysfunction in people with long-term IDDM. Diabetes Care 1996; 19:135–41.
106. Fedele D, Coscelli C, Santeusanio F, et al. Erectile dysfunction in diabetic subjects in Italy. Diabetes Care 1998; 21:1973–7.
107. Parazzini F, Menchini FF, Bortolotti A, et al. Frequency and determinants of erectile dysfunction in Italy. Eur Urol 2000; 37:43–9.
108. Lustman PJ, Clouse RE. Relationship of psychiatric illness to impotence in men with diabetes. Diabetes Care 1990; 13:893–5.
109. Lue TF. Erectile dysfunction. N Engl J Med 2000; 342:1802–13.
110. Saenz de Tejada I, Goldstein I. Diabetic penile neuropathy. Urol Clin North Am 1988; 15:17–22.
111. Seftel AD, Vaziri ND, Ni Z, et al. Advanced glycation end products in human penis: elevation in diabetic tissue, site of deposition, and possible effect through iNOS or eNOS. Urology 1997; 50:1016–26.
112. Hirata K, Kuroda R, Sakoda T, et al. Inhibition of endothelial nitric oxide synthase activity by protein kinase C. Hypertension 1995; 25:180–5.
113. Saenz de Tejada I, Goldstein I, Azadzoi K, Krane RJ, Cohen RA. Impaired neurogenic and endothelium-mediated relaxation of penile smooth muscle from diabetic men with impotence. N Engl J Med 1989; 320:1025–30.
114. Keegan A, Cotter MA, Cameron NE. Effects of diabetes and treatment with the antioxidant α-lipoic acid on endothelial and neurogenic responses of corpus cavernosum in rats. Diabetologia 1999; 42:343–50.
115. Elabbady AA, Gagnon C, Hassouna MM, Begin LR, Elhilali MM. Diabetes mellitus increases nitric oxide synthase in penises but not in major pelvic ganglia of rats. Br J Urol 1995; 76:196–202.
116. Vernet D, Cai L, Garban H, et al. Reduction of penile nitric oxide synthase in diabetic BB/WORdp (type I) and BBZ/WORdp (type II) rats with erectile dysfunction. Endocrinology 1995; 136:5709–17.
117. Bivalacqua TJ, Champion HC, Usta MF, et al. RhoA/Rho-kinase suppresses endothelial nitric oxide synthase in the penis: a mechanism for diabetes-associated erectile dysfunction. Proc Natl Acad Sci U S A 2004; 101:9121–6.
118. Jackson G, Rosen RC, Kloner RA, Kostis JB. The Second Princeton Consensus on Sexual Dysfunction and Cardiac Risk: new guidelines for sexual medicine. J Sex Med 2006; 3:28–36.
119. Azad N, Emanuele NV, Abraira C, et al. the VA CSDM Group. The effects of intensive glycemic control on neuropathy in the VA Cooperative Study on Type II diabetes mellitus. TJ Diabetes Complications 2000; 13:307–13.
120. Esposito K, Giugliano F, Di Palo C, et al. Effect of lifestyle changes on erectile dysfunction in obese men: a randomized controlled trial. JAMA 2004; 291:2978–84.
121. Esposito K, Giugliano F, De Sio M, et al. Dietary factors in erectile dysfunction. Int J Impot Res 2006; 18:370–4.
122. Vogt HJ, Brandl P, Kockott G, et al. Double-blind, placebo-controlled safety and efficacy trial with yohimbine hydrochloride in the treatment of nonorganic erectile dysfunction. Int J Impot Res 1997; 9(3):155–61.
123. Ernst E, Pittler MH. Yohimbine for erectile dysfunction: a systematic review and meta-analysis of randomized clinical trials. J Urol 1998; 159:433–6.
124. Rampin O, Bernabe J, Guilano F. Spinal control of penile erection. World J Urol 1997; 15:2–13.
125. Reproductive Health Drugs Advisory Committee. Urology Subcommittee. FDA Briefing Package, April 10, 2000:42–110.
126. Küthe A, Wiedentoth A, Stief C, Mägert H, Forssmann W, Jonas U. Identification of 13 PDE isoforms in human cavernous tissue. Eur Urol 1999; 35:404.
127. Taher A, Stief CG, Raida M, Jonas U, Forssmann WG. Cyclic nucleotide phosphodiesterase activity in human cavernous smooth muscle and the effect of various selective inhibitors. Int J Impotence Res 1992; 4(Suppl. 2):P11.
128. Rendell MS, Rajfer J, Wicker PA, Smith MD: Sildenafil for treatment of erectile dysfunction in men with diabetes: a randomized controlled trial. Sildenafil Diabetes Study Group. JAMA 1999; 281: 421–6.
129. Boulton AJM, Selam J-L, Sweeney M, Ziegler D. Sildenafil citrate for the treatment of erectile dysfunction in men with type II diabetes mellitus. Diabetologia 2001; 44:1296–301.
130. Sellam R, Ziegler D, Boulton AJM. Sildenafil citrate is effective and well tolerated for the treatment of erectile dysfunction in men with Type 1 or Type 2 diabetes mellitus. Diabetologia 2000; 43(Suppl. 1):A253.
131. Mitka M. Some men who take Viagra die—Why? JAMA 2000; 283:590–3.
132. Shakir SAW, Wilton LV, Boshier A, Layton D, Heeley E. Cardiovascular events in users of sildenafil: results from first phase of prescription event monitoring in England. Br Med J 2001; 322:651–2.

133. Herrmann HC, Chang G, Klugherz BD, Mahoney PD: Hemodynamic effects of sildenafil in men with severe coronary artery disease. N Engl J Med 2000; 342:1622–6.

134. Cheitlin MD, Hutter AM, Brindis RG, et al. Use of sildenafil (Viagra) in patients with cardiovascular disease. Circulation 1999; 99:168–77.

135. Wespes E, Rammal A, Garbar C. Sildenafil non-responders: haemodynamic and morphometric studies. Eur Urol 2005; 48:136–9.

136. Saenz de Tejada I, Anglin G, Knight JR, Emmick JT. Effects of tadalafil on erectile dysfunction in men with diabetes. Diabetes Care 2002; 25:2159–64.

137. Fonseca V, Seftel A, Denne J, Fredlund P. Impact of diabetes mellitus on the severity of erectile dysfunction and response to treatment: analysis of data from tadalafil clinical trials. Diabetologia 2004; 47:1914–23.

138. Porst H, Giuliano F, Glina S, et al. Evaluation of the efficacy and safety of once-a-day dosing of tadalafil 5 mg and 10 mg in the treatment of erectile dysfunction: results of a multicenter, randomized, double-blind, placebo-controlled trial. Eur Urol 2006; 50:351–9.

139. Rajfer J, Aliotta PJ, Steidle CP, Fitch WP 3rd, Zhao Y, Yu A. Tadalafil dosed once a day in men with erectile dysfunction: a randomized, double-blind, placebo-controlled study in the US. Int J Impot Res 2007; 19:95–103.

140. Goldstein I, Young JM, Fischer J, Bangerter K, Segerson T, Taylor T; Vardenafil Diabetes Study Group. Vardenafil, a new phosphodiesterase type 5 inhibitor, in the treatment of erectile dysfunction in men with diabetes: a multicenter double-blind placebo-controlled fixed-dose study. Diabetes Care 2003; 26:777–783.

141. Ziegler D, Merfort F, van Ahlen H, Yassin A, Reblin T, Neureither M. Efficacy and safety of flexible-dose vardenafil in men with type 1 diabetes and erectile dysfunction. J Sex Med 2006; 3:883–891.

142. Rubio-Aurioles E, Porst H, Eardley I, Goldstein I; Vardenafil-Sildenafil Comparator Study Group. Comparing vardenafil and sildenafil in the treatment of men with erectile dysfunction and risk factors for cardiovascular disease: a randomized, double-blind, pooled crossover study. J Sex Med 2006; 3:1037–49.

143. Vardi M, Nini A. Phosphodiesterase inhibitors for erectile dysfunction in patients with diabetes mellitus. Cochrane Database Syst Rev 2007; 24(1):CD002187.

144. Dutta TC, Eid JF: Vacuum constriction devices for erectile dysfunction: a long-term, prospective study of patients with mild, moderate, and severe dysfunction. Urology 1999; 54:891–3.

145. Padma-Nathan H, Hellstrom WJ, Kaiser FE, et al. Treatment of men with erectile dysfunction with transurethral alprostadil. Medicated Urethral System for Erection (MUSE) Study Group. N Engl J Med 1997; 336:1–7.

146. Porst H. Transurethrale Alprostadilapplikation mit MUSE™ ("medicated urethral system for erection"). Urologe [A] 1998; 37:410–6.

147. Spivack AP, Peterson CA, Cowley C, et al. VIVUS-MUSE Study Group. Long-term safety profile of transurethral alprostadil for the treatment of erectile dysfunction. J Urol 1997; 157(Suppl.):203.

148. Fulgham PF, Cochran JS, Denman JL, Feagins BA, Gross MB, Kadesky KT, Kadesky MC, Clark AR, Roehrborn CG: Disappointing initial results with transurethral alprostadil for erectile dysfunction in a urology practice setting. J Urol 1998; 160:2041–6.

149. Linet OI, Ogrinc FG. Efficacy and safety of intracavernosal alprostadil in men with erectile dysfunction. The Alprostadil Study Group. N Engl J Med 1996; 334:873–7.

150. Shabsigh R, Padma-Nathan H, Gittleman M, McMurray J, Kaufman J, Goldstein I. Intracavernous alprostadil alfadex is more efficacious, better tolerated, and preferred over intraurethral alprostadil plus optional actis: a comparative, randomized, crossover, multicenter study. Urology 2000; 55:109–13.

151. Porst H, Buvat J, Meuleman EJH, Michal V, Wagner G. Final results of a prospective multi-center study with self-injection therapy with PGE$_1$ after 4 years of follow-up. Int J Impot Res 1996; 6:151, D118.

152. Ewing DJ, Clarke BF: Diabetic autonomic neuropathy: present insights and future prospects. Diabetes Care 1986; 9:648–65.

153. Enzlin P, Mathieu C, Van Den Bruel A, Vanderschueren D, Demyttenaere K. Prevalence and predictors of sexual dysfunction in patients with type 1 diabetes. Diabetes Care 2003; 26:409–14.

154. Esposito K, Ciotola M, Marfella R, Di Tommaso D, Cobellis L, Giugliano D. The metabolic syndrome: a cause of sexual dysfunction in women. Int J Impot Res 2005; 17:224–6.

155. Enzlin P, Mathieu C, Vanderschueren D, Demyttenaere K. Diabetes mellitus and female sexuality: a review of 25 years' research. Diabet Med 1998; 15:809–15.

156. Jovanovic L. Sex and the woman with diabetes: desire versus dysfunction. IDF Bull 1998; 43:23–8.

157. Bhasin S, Enzlin P, Coviello A, Basson R. Sexual dysfunction in men and women with endocrine disorders. Lancet 2007; 369:597–611.

21 | Diabetic Foot Ulcers

Michael Edmonds
Diabetic Foot Clinic, Kings College Hospital, Denmark Hill, London, U.K.

INTRODUCTION

At some time in their life, 15% of people with diabetes develop foot ulcers, which are highly susceptible to infection (1). These may spread rapidly leading to overwhelming tissue destruction and amputation. Eighty-five percent of amputations are preceded by an ulcer (2) and there is an amputation every 30 seconds throughout the world (3). However, major advances have taken place. Evidence-based protocols for diabetic foot ulcers have been developed (4). Diabetic foot programs that have promoted a multidisciplinary approach to heal foot ulcers with aggressive management of infection and ischemia have achieved a substantial decrease in amputation rates (5,6). Furthermore, a reduction in amputations has been reported nationwide in diabetic patients throughout the Netherlands (7). Recently, a decrease in major amputation incidence has been reported in diabetic as well as in nondiabetic patients in Helsinki (8).

The aim of this chapter is to help practitioners treat diabetic foot ulcers by developing a clear understanding of the overall natural history of the diabetic foot and by recognizing a definite framework of crucial stages or milestones that demand appropriate treatment.

THE NATURAL HISTORY OF THE DIABETIC FOOT

The natural history can be divided into the following stages (9):

1. Normal foot. The foot is normal and does not have the risk factors of ulceration namely neuropathy, ischemia, deformity, callus and edema.
2. At-risk foot. The patient has developed one or more risk factors noted in stage 1.
3. Foot with ulcer. There are two main types of diabetic foot, which have characteristic ulceration: ulceration in the neuropathic foot develops at the sites of high mechanical pressure on the plantar surface. In contrast, ulcers in the foot with both neuropathy and ischemia (neuroischemic foot) occur on the margins of the foot and toes, at sites of prolonged low pressure usually from poorly fitting shoes. Recent studies have shown that ischemic ulcers make up approximately 50% of the total number of ulcers (10,11).
4. Foot with cellulitis. The ulcer has developed infection with the presence of cellulitis, which can complicate both the neuropathic and the neuroischemic foot.
5. Foot with necrosis. In the neuropathic foot, infection is usually the cause; in the neuroischemic foot infection is still the most common reason for tissue destruction although ischemia contributes.

The foot with extensive necrosis cannot be saved and comes to major amputation. Every diabetic patient can be placed into one of these stages, which demand appropriate multidisciplinary management, addressing various aspects of wound, microbiological, mechanical, vascular, metabolic and educational care. Metabolic management is similar for all stages. Thus, tight control of blood glucose is extremely important to preserve neurological function and treatment of blood pressure and lipids to maintain cardiovascular function. Advice should be given to stop smoking.

Stage 1: Normal Foot

Diagnosis
All diabetic patients should be screened annually to detect risk factors for foot ulcers, namely, neuropathy, ischemia, deformity, callus, and swelling. Their absence confirms a normal foot and their presence shows a foot that is at risk.

Neuropathy

A simple technique to assess pressure sensation is to use a nylon monofilament, which, when applied perpendicular to the foot, buckles at a given force of 10 g. If the patient does not detect the filament, then protective pain sensation is lost (12). Alternatively, vibration perception threshold can be measured using a neurothesiometer although this is more suitable for research purposes. A vibration threshold greater than 25 V is strongly predictive of foot ulceration (13). Recently, the vibration perception threshold has been shown to be more sensitive than the 10 g monofilament for the assessment of individuals at risk for foot ulcers (14).

Ischemia

If either dorsalis pedis or posterior tibial pulse can be felt, then it is highly unlikely that there is significant ischemia. However, the American Diabetes Association has recommended that the ankle-brachial pressure should be measured in all diabetic patients above 50 years of age (15). Indeed, a recent study showed a 21% prevalence of peripheral arterial disease as indicated by a low ankle-brachial pressure index in newly diagnosed diabetic patients (16). However, many diabetic patients have medial arterial calcification, giving an artificially elevated systolic pressure, even in the presence of ischemia.

Deformity

Deformity often leads to bony prominences, which are associated with high mechanical pressures on the overlying skin. This leads to ulceration, particularly in the absence of protective pain sensation and when shoes are unsuitable. Common deformities that should be noted include claw toes, pes cavus, hallux valgus, hallux rigidus, hammer toe, Charcot foot and nail deformities.

Callus

This is a thickened area of epidermis that develops at sites of high pressure and friction. It should not be allowed to become excessive, as this can be a forerunner of ulceration (usually in the presence of neuropathy).

Edema

Edema is a major factor predisposing to ulceration, and often exacerbates a tight fit inside poorly fitting shoes. It also impedes healing of established ulcers.

Management

Advice on basic foot care including nail-cutting techniques, the treatment of minor injuries and the purchase of shoes should be given to the patient and caregivers. Nails should be cut after a bath or shower when they are softer. It is unwise to try to cut the whole nail in one piece. The patient should never try to cut out the corner of the nail or dig down the sides. Sensible shoes should be made of soft leather and have broad rounded or square toes, with a high toe box. The heels should be low to avoid excessive toe pressure on the forefoot and they should be either fitted with laces, Velcro, or buckle straps to prevent movement within the shoe.

Stage 2: At-Risk Foot

Diagnosis

If, on annual review, one or more risk factors for ulceration are detected, then the patient enters Stage 2. One of the most important deformities to diagnose is the Charcot foot.

Management

Neuropathy

Patients who have lost protective pain sensation need to protect their feet from mechanical, thermal and chemical trauma. They should compensate for lack of protective pain sensation by establishing a habit of regular inspection of the feet so that problems can be detected quickly and help sought sufficiently early. It is important to educate Stage 2 patients to avoid trauma as far as possible. Patients who go away on holiday are particularly prone to develop foot problems and need special advice. Dry skin resulting from neuropathy should be treated with an emollient such as E45 cream or Calmurid cream.

Ischemia

Patients with absent foot pulses should have the pressure index measured to confirm ischemia and to provide a baseline, so that subsequent deterioration can be detected. When the pulses are not palpable and the pressure index is >1, a reduced Doppler arterial waveform usually indicates ischemia. The main advantage in detecting peripheral vascular disease at this stage is that it is a sign of systemic atheroscerosis and treatment should be started with aspirin and statins and other risk factors for arterial disease such as hypertension and smoking should be addressed. If the patient has rest pain, disabling claudication, or the pressure index is below 0.5, further investigations of the peripheral arterial circulation should be carried out as described below under Stage 3.

Deformity (Including the Charcot Foot)

Ideally, deformity should be recognized early and accommodated in properly fitting shoes before ulceration occurs. Footwear can be divided into three broad types:

- Sensible shoes (from high street shops) for patients with only minimal sensory loss.
- Ready made stock (off the shelf) shoes, suitable for neuroischemic feet that need protection along the margins of the foot but that are not greatly deformed.
- Customized or bespoke (made to measure) shoes containing cushioned insoles that redistribute areas of high plantar pressure.

With regard to the prevention of ulcers, most studies have examined the effect of therapeutic shoes on ulcer recurrence. The majority have been positive, but not all. In a recent review of studies, assessing the association between therapeutic footwear and re-ulceration, risk ratios in all of them were below 1.0, suggesting some protective footwear benefit (17). One study ($N = 69$) found that therapeutic shoes with custom-made insoles could reduce ulcers in people at high risk (18). The relapse or new ulcer rate at 1 year was 28% in the intervention group compared with 58% among those who continued to wear their own shoes ($P < 0.01$). However, in the most rigorous experimental study, no statistically significant benefit was observed between control patients wearing their own footwear and intervention patients wearing study footwear (19). However, in patients with severe foot deformity or prior toe or ray amputation, observational studies suggested a significant protective benefit from therapeutic shoes. However, this issue remains contentious (20).

The Charcot foot refers to bone and joint destruction that occurs in the neuropathic foot (21). It is important to diagnose it early so as to prevent severe deformity. The foot presents with unilateral erythema, warmth and edema. There may be a history of minor trauma. About 30% of patients complain of pain or discomfort. X-ray at this time may be normal. However, a technetium-99 m diphosphonate bone scan will detect early evidence of bony destruction, which in this particular situation, is indicative of a Charcot foot. Early diagnosis is essential. Cellulitis, gout and deep vein thrombosis may masquerade as a Charcot foot.

Initially the foot is immobilized in a cast to prevent bone destruction and deformity that on X-ray is shown as fragmentation, fracture, new bone formation, subluxation and dislocation. Immobilization is continued until there is no longer evidence on X-ray of continuing bone destruction and the foot temperature is within 2°C of the contralateral foot. The patient can now progress from a cast to an orthotic walker, fitted with cradled moulded insoles. Bisphosphonates may be helpful in the initial treatment of the Charcot foot (22).

Callus

Patients should never cut their callus off or use callus removers. Instead, the callus should be removed regularly by the podiatrist to prevent ulceration.

Edema

The main cause will be impaired cardiac and renal function, which should be assessed and then treated accordingly. Venous insufficiency can cause swelling and should be investigated with duplex scanning, treated with compression hose if there is no peripheral arterial disease and considered for surgery if there is significant venous reflux.

Overall Management in Stage 2

Recent studies have demonstrated the value of foot protection programmes including education and footwear intervention. A large randomized controlled trial (RCT) demonstrated that amputation rates among people at high risk of ulcers could be significantly reduced by a foot protection program, and is cost effective (23). Patients with foot deformities, history of foot ulceration, significant vascular or neuropathic disease were randomized to the intervention, weekly clinics providing chiropody hygiene, hosiery, protective shoes and education or usual care. At 2 years the ulcer rate in the intervention group was nonsignificantly reduced, to 2.4% compared with 3.5% in the usual care group ($p = 0.14$). Amputations, however, were reduced threefold with 7 in the intervention group and 23 among controls ($p < 0.04$).

Education and podiatry may improve knowledge of foot care and in some studies have led to improvements in the condition of the feet (24). A recent review of the role of patient education in preventing diabetic foot ulceration concluded that there was poor methodology and conflicting results (25). *In a prospective, randomized study (43), it was shown that the incidence of foot ulcers and amputations could be considerably reduced by use of a simple 1-hour educational program.* However, weak evidence suggests that education may have positive but short-lived effects on foot care and upon the knowledge and behaviour of patients in the short term.

Risk Stratification

The foot risk classification system of the International Working Group divided patients into four groups: subjects without neuropathy, patients with neuropathy but without deformity or peripheral vascular disease, patients with neuropathy and deformity or peripheral vascular disease, and patients with a history of foot ulceration or a lower extremity amputation. This system has recently been shown to be effective in predicting clinical outcomes of ulceration and amputation (26).

Stage 3: The Ulcerated Foot

Diagnosis

Ulceration in the neuropathic foot develops at the sites of high mechanical pressure and shear forces on the plantar surface of the toes (27). In contrast, neuroischemic ulcers develop on the margins of the foot and apices of the toes, on sites that are vulnerable to trauma and pressure from poorly fitting shoes.

Management

Multidisciplinary management is urgently required from a foot ulcer care team with specialized control of mechanical, wound, microbiological and vascular aspects.

Mechanical Control

In the neuropathic foot, the ulcer is managed by off-loading, by which means there is a redistribution of load bearing on the plantar surface of the foot. The most efficient way is by the immediate application of some form of cast, including the removable cast walker such as the Aircast Walker, the Scotchcast boot and the total contact cast (21). The Aircast is a removable bi-valved cast. It is lined with four air cells, which can be inflated with a hand pump to ensure a close fit. The Scotchcast boot is a simple removable boot made of stockinet, felt and fibreglass tape. The total contact cast is a close fitting plaster cast applied over minimum padding. It should be reserved for plantar ulcers that have not responded to other casting treatments (28). It is also useful in patients with recurrent foot ulceration (29). Nonremovable fibreglass casts have been also used (30).

Recently, standard removable cast walkers have been modified by wrapping plaster around them to make them nonremovable and to increase patient compliance. This is just as successful in healing diabetic foot ulcers as the total contact cast (31). If casting techniques are not available, accommodative sandals such as half shoes can off load the site of ulceration. A recent study showed that total contact cast healed a higher proportion of wounds in a shorter time than the removable cast and the half shoe (32).

In the neuroischemic foot, a high street shoe that is sufficiently long, broad and deep and fastens with a lace or strap high on the foot to reduce frictional forces on the vulnerable margins of the foot may be sufficient. Alternatively, a ready-made stock shoe, which is wide fitting, may be suitable.

Heel ulcers can be off-loaded by a foam wedge or pressure relief ankle-foot orthosis (PRAFO), which suspends the heel to protect against further breakdown and allow the ulcer to drain. The PRAFO has a washable fleece liner with an aluminium and polyproprylene adjustable frame and a nonslip walking neoprene base (33).

Wound Control

Wound control includes debridement, dressings, advanced wound healing products, vacuum-assisted closure (VAC), ultrasound, hyperbaric oxygen and skin grafting.

Debridement. Debridement is the most important part of wound control and is best carried out with a scalpel. It allows removal of callus and devitalized tissue and enables the true dimensions of the ulcer to be perceived. It reduces the bacterial load of the ulcer even in the absence of overt infection, restores chronic wounds to acute wounds and releases growth factors to aid the healing process (34). It also enables a deep swab to be taken for culture. The larvae of the green bottle fly are sometimes used to debride ulcers (35) especially in the neuroischemic foot (36). Maggot debridement therapy has recently been shown to reduce short-term morbidity in nonambulatory patients with diabetic foot wounds, decreasing antibiotic use and risk of amputation (37).

Dressings. Although moist wound healing is generally carried out in the management of chronic wounds, the situation with diabetic foot ulcers is more complex (38). Indeed, a fine balance is needed to avoid maceration of tissues whilst, on the other hand encouraging conditions that prevent eschar formation and assist cell migration within the wound (39).

There is no firm evidence that any dressing is better or worse than any other. A review that assessed 10 randomized trials and two controlled trials concluded that there was no evidence to support the effectiveness of any one type of protective dressing over any other for treating diabetic foot ulcers (10). Sterile, nonadherent dressings should cover all ulcers to protect them from trauma, absorb exudate, reduce infection and promote healing. Wounds should be inspected frequently to ensure that problems or complications are detected quickly, especially in-patients who lack protective pain sensation.

The following dressing properties are essential for the diabetic foot: ease and speed of lifting, the ability to be walked on without suffering disintegration and good exudate control. Dressings should be lifted every day to ensure that problems or complications are detected quickly, especially in patients who lack protective pain sensation.

Advanced Wound Healing Products. When ulcers do not respond to basic treatment, advanced products to stimulate wound healing may have to be put into practice (40). These are expensive treatments and should only be used when basic treatments have failed. Clinical decisions about when to use advanced or more experimental therapies may be based on healing rates. Studies in venous and diabetic ulcers suggest that advancement of more than 0.7 mm per week is 80% sensitive and specific for eventual wound closure (41). Advanced wound healing products include:

- Growth factors
- Skin substitutes
- Extracellular matrix proteins
- Protease inhibitors
- Vaso-active compounds

GROWTH FACTORS.   Platelet derived growth factor (Regranex), stimulates fibroblasts and other connective tissue cells located in the skin and is beneficial in enhancing wound healing processes of cell growth and repair. Four placebo-controlled trials of PDGF-BB in neuropathic ulcers have been carried out. The pivotal study of 382 patients demonstrated that Regranex gel (100 mcg/g) healed 50% of chronic diabetic ulcers, which was significantly greater than the 35% healed with a placebo gel (42). Recombinant human epidermal growth factor (hEGF) had a positive effect on healing in a small double-blind randomized controlled study.

SKIN SUBSTITUTES.   Dermagraft is an artificial human dermis manufactured through the process of tissue engineering. Human fibroblast cells obtained from neonatal foreskin are cultivated on a three-dimensional polyglactin scaffold. This results in a metabolically active dermal tissue with the structure of a papillary dermis of newborn skin. A randomized controlled multicenter study of 281 patients with neuropathic foot ulcers demonstrated that at 12 weeks, 50.8% of the Dermagraft group experienced complete wound closure that was significantly greater than in the controls, of whom 31.7% healed (43). In another 12-week randomized study with living foreskin fibroblasts in a vicryl mesh, incidence of complete wound closure of neuropathic foot ulcers was 30% in the active group and 18% in the control group (44).

Apligraf consists of a collagen gel seeded with fibroblasts and covered by a surface layer of keratinocytes (45). In a randomized 12-week trial of 208 patients with neuropathic ulcers, the bilayered construct, Apligraf, led to complete wound closure in 56% of patients, compared with 38% in controls ($P = 0.0042$). There was a reduced the time to complete closure (65 days vs 90 days, $P = 0.0026$).

Bilayered Cellular Matrix (BCM) is a porous collagen sponge containing cocultured allogeneic keratinocytes and fibroblasts harvested from human neonatal foreskin. Patients with chronic, diabetic, neuropathic foot ulcers were randomized a multicenter, randomized, controlled, parallel-group pilot study to receive either standard care (moist saline gauze cover for up to 12 weeks ($n = 20$)) or to active treatment ($n = 20$) of standard care plus an application of BCM at each weekly visit for up to six total applications, followed by standard care alone for an additional six weeks or until complete healing. By 12 weeks, 7 of 20 wounds (35%) treated with BCM showed complete healing compared with 4 of 20 wounds (20%) treated with standard care (46).

EXTRACELLULAR MATRIX PROTEINS.   There has also been considerable interest in the application of extracellular matrix proteins to accelerate healing of diabetic foot ulcers, including hyaluronic acid and collagen.

Hyaff is an ester of hyaluronic acid, which is a major component of the extracellular matrix Hyaff-based autologous grafts both dermal and epidermal have been used to treat two groups of diabetic foot ulcers: plantar ulcers and postoperative wounds located on the dorsum of the foot. Patients in both groups had offloading, which was total contact casting for plantar ulcers and a rigid-sole shoe for dorsal ulcers. After 11 weeks there was no difference in the rate of healing in patients with plantar ulcers but in the dorsal ulcers, the autologous bioengineered graft showed increased rate of ulcer healing compared with control group (67% vs 31%, $p = 0.049$) (47).

OASIS wound matrix (Cook Biotech, Lafayette, IN) is derived from the pig small intestine submucosa. This consists of a natural collagenous, three-dimensional extracellular matrix that act as a framework for cytokines and cell adhesion molecules for tissue growth. A recent study has compared the healing rates at 12 weeks for full-thickness diabetic foot ulcers treated with OASIS Wound Matrix, an acellular wound care product, vs Regranex Gel. This study reported that complete wound closure after 12 weeks of treatment was observed in 49% of the OASIS-treated patients ($n = 18$), compared with only 28% of the Regranex-treated group ($n = 10$), $p = 0.055$ (48).

PROTEASE INHIBITORS.   Promogran is a protease inhibitor that consists of oxidized regenerated cellulose and collagen. It inhibits proteases in the wound and protects endogenous growth factor. In a 12 week study, of 184 patients, 37% of Promogran treated patients healed compared with 28% of saline gauze treated patients, a nonsignificant difference (49).

VASO-ACTIVE COMPOUNDS. The effect on dalteparin on ulcer outcome in diabetic patients with peripheral arterial occlusive disease has been investigated in a prospective, randomized, double-blind, placebo-controlled trial. A total of 87 patients were randomized to treatment with subcutaneous injection of 5000 units dalteparin (Fragmin, Pharmacia Corporation; $n = 44$) or an equivalent volume of physiological saline ($n = 43$) once daily until ulcer healing or for a maximum of 6 months. There was a better ulcer outcome ($p = 0.042$) and a greater number of patients healed with intact skin or decreased the ulcer area $\geq 50\%$ in the Dalteparin group compared with the placebo group (50).

Chrysalin(R) a thrombin peptide, in saline or saline alone was applied topically, twice weekly, to diabetic ulcers with standardized care and offloading. A dose-dependent effect was seen in the per-protocol population where 1 and 10 mug Chrysalin(R) treatment resulted in 45% and 72% more subjects with complete healing than placebo treatment. Chrysalin(R) more than doubled the incidence of complete healing ($p < 0.05$), increased mean closure rate approximately 80% ($p < 0.05$), and decreased the median time to 100% closure by approximately 40% ($p < 0.05$).

Vacuum-assisted Closure (VAC). In this technique, the VAC pump applies gentle negative pressure to the ulcer through a tube and foam sponge that are applied to the ulcer over a dressing and sealed in place with a plastic film to create a vacuum. Exudate from the wound is sucked along the tube to a disposable collecting chamber. The negative pressure improves the vascularity and stimulates granulation of the wound. In a recent study, 162 patients with postoperative wounds, following partial foot amputation, were enrolled into a 16-week, 18-center, randomized clinical trial in the USA. More patients were healed in the VAC pump group than in the control group (43 [56%] vs 33 [39%], $p = 0.040$). The rate of wound healing, based on the time to complete closure, was faster in the VAC pump group than in controls ($p = 0.005$) (51). A recent consensus statement on negative pressure wound therapy (VAC Therapy) for the management of diabetic foot wounds has recently been published and summarizes current clinical evidence (52)

Hyperbaric Oxygen. Adjunctive systemic hyperbaric oxygen therapy has been shown to reduce the number of major amputations in ischemic diabetic feet (53). Studies involving relatively small groups of patients have shown that hyperbaric oxygen accelerates the healing of ischemic diabetic foot ulcers. It is reasonable to use hyperbaric oxygen as an adjunctive in severe or life threatening wounds (54). A recent Cochrane review concluded that hyperbaric oxygen significantly reduced the risk of major amputation and may improve the chance of healing of foot ulcers at 1 year. Although this should be regarded cautiously because of modest number of patients, methodological shortcomings in previous studies (55).

Skin Grafting. To speed healing of ulcers that have a clean granulating wound bed, a split skin graft may be harvested and applied to the ulcer. If chosen from within the distribution of sensory neuropathy, the donor site will be less painful.

Microbiological Control
When the skin of the foot is broken, the patient is at great risk of infection as there is a clear portal of entry for invading bacteria. At every patient visit, the foot should be examined for local signs of infection, cellulitis or osteomyelitis. If these are found, antibiotic therapy is indicated However, in the presence of neuropathy and ischemia, the inflammatory response is impaired. Furthermore, there may be a failure of vasodilation due to an impaired axon reflex (56). Also, the patient lacks protective pain sensation, which would otherwise automatically force him to rest.

Topical anti-microbials may be used (57). Iodine is effective against a wide spectrum of organisms. At high concentrations it can be toxic to human cells, but bacteria are more sensitive to these effects than human cells such as the fibreblast. Povidone-iodine is effective in anti-bacterial prophylaxis in burn patients. Cadexomer-iodine consists of microspheres, formed from a three dimension lattice of cross linked starch chains and has been used with success in diabetic foot ulcers. Silver compounds are also widely used in anti-bacterial prophylaxis (58). Mupirocin is active against gram positive bacteria, including methicillin resistant staphylococcus aureus (MRSA).

It is important to maintain close surveillance of the ulcer to detect signs of infection that would be an indication for antibiotic therapy. A controlled trial was conducted in patients with neuropathic ulcers who were randomized to oral amoxicillin plus clavulinic acid or matched placebo. At 20 days follow-up, there was no significant difference in outcome (59). In a small RCT, antibiotic therapy of uninfected ulcers reduced the incidence of clinical infection and hospital admission and amputation and increased the prospects of healing (64). In this study, 32 patients with new foot ulcers were treated with oral antibiotics and 32 patients without antibiotics. In the group with no antibiotics, 15 patients developed clinical infection compared with none in the antibiotic group ($P < 0.001$). Seven patients in the nonantibiotic group needed hospital admission and three patients came to amputation (one major and 2 minor). Seventeen patients healed in the nonantibiotic group compared with 27 in the antibiotic group ($p < 0.02$). When the 15 patients who developed clinical infection were compared to 17 patients who did not, there were significantly more ischemic patients in the infected group. Furthermore, out of the 15 patients who became clinically infected, eleven had positive ulcer swabs at the start of the study compared with only one patient out of 17 in the noninfected group ($p < 0.01$). From this study, it was concluded that diabetic patients with clean ulcers associated with peripheral vascular disease and positive ulcer swabs should be considered for early antibiotic treatment.

Vascular Control
If an ulcer has not responded to optimum treatment within two weeks and ankle brachial pressure index is less than 0.5 and the Doppler waveform is damped, then angiography should ideally be carried out. Angiography can be performed by a Duplex examination, which combines the features of Doppler waveform analysis with ultrasound imaging to produce a picture of arterial flow dynamics and morphology. Alternatively, magnetic resonance angiography can be carried out. In contrast to conventional arteriography, this can be performed, without the need for intra-arterial catheter and potentially nephrotoxic contrast. Severe ischemia can also be confirmed by a transcutaneous oxygen on the dorsum of the foot of less than 30 mmHg or a toe pressure of less than 30 mmHg.

Angioplasty is a valuable treatment to improve arterial flow in the presence of ischemic ulcers and is indicated for the treatment of isolated or multiple stenoses as well as short segment occlusions less than l0 cm in length (60). Endovascular procedures have been shown to be feasible and successful in the tibial and peroneal arteries of the diabetic patient (61). and subintimal angioplasty has also been used to recanalize long arterial occlusions in the tibial arteries (62). Angioplasty must be applied early when tissue loss is not extensive and when arterial stenoses and occlusions are still suitable for this procedure (63). If lesions are too widespread for angioplasty, then arterial bypass may be considered. However, this is a major, sometimes lengthy, operation, not without risk, and is more commonly reserved to treat the foot with severe tissue destruction that cannot be managed without the restoration of pulsatile blood flow.

Stage 4: Foot with Infection

Diagnosis
Ulcers are often complicated by infection, caused by organisms from the surrounding skin. The following signs indicate that an ulcer has become infected: the base of ulcer changes from healthy pink granulations to yellowish or grey tissue, purulent discharge, unpleasant smell, sinuses develop in an ulcer, edges may become undermined, bone or tendon becomes exposed.

Cellulitis presents as localized erythema, warmth and swelling. In severe infection, there is an intense widespread erythema and swelling. Lymphangitis, regional lymphadenitis, malaise, "flu-like" symptoms fever and rigors may be present. Often there is a generalized sloughing of subcutaneous tissues, which eventually liquefy and disintegrate. Infection can also present as a blue purple discoloration when there is an inadequate supply of oxygen to the soft tissues. In severe infection, blue discoloration can occur in neuroischemic foot, particularly in the toes and must not be automatically attributed to worsening ischemia. It is important to remember that classical signs of infection may not be present because of neuropathy and ischemia. Only 50% of episodes of severe cellulitis will provoke a fever or leucocytosis (64).

Osteomyelitis is usually associated with ulceration and cellulitis. In the initial stages, X-ray may be normal but MRI can detect early changes (65). Clinically, it can be diagnosed if a sterile probe inserted into the ulcer penetrates to bone. Also, this test has a sensitivity of 66%, a specificity of 85% and a positive predictive value of 89% (66). Although a recent study reported a lower positive predictive value of 33% (67).

The microbiology of diabetic foot infections is unique and gram positive, gram negative and anaerobes can be responsible. Staphylococci and streptococci are the most common pathogens. However, infection due to gram negative and anaerobic organisms occur in approximately 50% of patients and often infection is polymicrobial. Staphylococcus aureus is the most common organism although MRSA is increasingly found in infected ulcers (68). There is a poor immune response of the diabetic patient to sepsis and even bacteria regarded as skin commensals, may cause severe tissue damage. This includes gram negative organisms such as Citrobacter, Serratia, Pseudomonas and Acinetobacter. It is advisable to send swabs or preferably tissue for culture after initial debridement in all Stage 4 patients (69,70). In osteomyelitis, superficial swab cultures may not reliably identify bone bacteria and percutaneous bone biopsy seems to be safe for patients with diabetic foot osteomyelitis (71).

Management

The development of infection constitutes a foot care emergency, which requires referral to a specialized foot-care team within 24 h. The underlying principle is to detect the bacteria responsible and treat aggressively.

Mild Infections

Mild infections with limited cellulitis can generally be treated with oral antibiotics on an outpatient basis. Several antibiotics have been shown to be effective in clinical trials including cephalexin, clindamycin, ciprofloxacin. ofloxacin, levofloxacin, clindamycin, pexiganan, and linezolid. However, no single drug or combination of agents appears to be better than others. If MRSA is grown and there are no local or systemic signs of infection, topical mupirocin 2% ointment (if sensitive) may be used. If MRSA is grown and accompanied by local signs of infection, oral therapy with two of the following should be considered: sodium fusidate, rifampicin, trimethoprim and doxycycline, according to sensitivities, together with topical mupirocin 2% ointment.

Antibiotics should be consistent with local antibiotic policies and initially, commonly used first line antibiotics should be prescribed and new broad spectrum antibiotics reserved for later use for resistant organisms.

Severe Infections

Severe deep infections need urgent admission to hospital for wide spectrum intravenous antibiotics. Indications for urgent surgical intervention are infected sloughy tissue, localized fluctuance and expression of pus, crepitus with gas in the soft tissues on x-ray and purplish discoloration of the skin indicating subcutaneous necrosis. Infected tissue should be sent for culture after debridement. Clinical and microbiological response rates have been similar in trials of various antibiotics and no single agent or combination has emerged as most effective. Recently, clinical and microbiological outcomes for patients treated with ertapenem were equivalent to those for patients treated with piperacillin/tazobactam, in a randomized, double-blinded, multicenter trial in adults ($n = 586$) with diabetes and a foot infection classified as moderate-to-severe and requiring intravenous antibiotics (72). In an open-label, randomized study comparing efficacy and safety of intravenous piperacillin/tazobactam (P/T) and ampicillin/sulbactam (A/S). clinical efficacy rates (cure or improvement) were statistically equivalent overall (81% for P/T vs 83.1% for A/S), and median duration of treatment was similar in the clinically evaluable populations (9 days for P/T, 10 days for A/S) (73).

It is important to have a practical approach to the treatment of severe infections reserving complex new antibiotics for resistant organisms, as described in the approach to mild infections. Ideally, the diabetic patient with severe cellulitis needs admission for intravenous antibiotics. If admission is not possible, then ceftriaxone may be given intramuscularly together with metronidazole orally. Ceftriaxone has been demonstrated to be just as efficacious as ticarcillin/clavulanate (74). On review as an outpatient, if cellulitis is controlled, ceftriaxone intra-muscularly and metronidazole orally should be continued and the patient reviewed 1 week later.

If cellulitis is increasing, then the patient should be admitted for intravenous antibiotics. Quadruple therapy may be used including amoxycillin, flucloxacillin, metronidazole and ceftazidime. REF If patient is allergic to penicillin, amoxycillin and flucloxacillin should be replaced with erythromycin or vancomycin (with doses adjusted according to serum levels). On admission the foot should be urgently assessed as to the need for surgical debridement. On follow-up, the infected foot should inspected daily to gauge the initial response to antibiotic therapy. Appropriate antibiotics should be selected when sensitivities are available. If MRSA is isolated, then vancomycin (dosage to be adjusted according to serum levels) or teicoplanin should be given. These antibiotics may need to be accompanied by a further appropriate oral antibiotic such as sodium fusidate or rifampicin. When the signs of cellulitis have resolved. intravenous antibiotic therapy can be changed to the appropriate oral therapy usually two of sodium fusidate, rifampicin trimethoprim or doxycycline.

Osteomyelitis

Classically, the treatment of osteomyelitis is surgical removal of bone. But long-term suppressive antibiotic therapy is also used. As osteomyelitis is usually associated with an infected ulcer and cellulitis, wide spectrum antibiotics should be initially given. On review, antibiotic selection is guided by the results of cultures. Ideally percutaneous bone biopsy should be carried out but this is not always practical especially in ischemic feet. Bone fragments in the base of the wound should be removed as in "office" debridement and then be sent for culture. It is useful to choose antibiotics with good bone penetration such as sodium fusidate, rifampicin clindamycin and ciprofloxacin. Antibiotics should be given for at least 12 weeks. Such therapy is often successful with resolution of cellulitis and healing of the ulcer (75). A recent report noted that diabetic foot osteomyelitis was effectively managed with oral antimicrobial therapy with or without limited "office" debridement in most patients (76). However, if after 6 month's treatment, it is still possible to probe to bone, then operative resection may be necessary.

Vascular Control

It is important to explore the possibility of revascularization of the infected neuroischemic foot as improvement of perfusion will help to control infection as well as to promote healing of the ulcer and wounds if operative debridement is carried out. Revascularization may be carried out by angioplasty or arterial bypass. When there is considerable tissue destruction it is necessary to restore pulsatile blood flow (77). In these circumstances, distal arterial bypass, in particular to the dorsalis pedis artery, which may be relatively spared, has been established as a valuable procedure in conjunction with surgical debridement, adjunctive plastic surgery and antibiotic therapy (78).

Stage 5: The Necrotic Foot

Diagnosis

Necrosis has very grave implications, threatening the loss of the limb and is caused by infection or ischemia or by both together. It is classified as either wet or dry, each with its specific management. In the neuropathic foot, necrosis is invariably wet initially and is nearly always due to a septic arteritis secondary to soft tissue infection complicating a digital or metatarsal ulcer. The arterial lumen is often occluded by a septic thrombus. Both wet and dry necrosis can occur in the neuroischemic foot. The commonest cause of a black toe is again septic arteritis, exacerbated by large vessel disease in the leg. Dry necrosis can also develop in the neuroischemic foot and is secondary to a severe reduction in arterial perfusion.

Management

In the neuropathic foot, operative debridement is nearly always indicated for wet necrosis. There is a good arterial circulation and the wound usually heals as long as infection is controlled. In the neuroischemic foot, wet necrosis should also be removed when it is associated with severe spreading sepsis. This should be done whether pus is present or not. In cases when the limb is not immediately threatened, and the necrosis is limited to one or two toes, it may be possible to control infection with intravenous antibiotics and proceed to urgent revascularization and at the same operation, perform digital or ray amputation, which should subsequently heal. Some patients may not be suitable for revascularization. Wet necrosis should be allowed to convert to dry necrosis with antibiotics and then autoamputate.

The microbiological principles of managing wet necrosis are similar to that of the management of infection in Stage 4. When the patient presents, deep wound swabs and tissue should be sent for culture and wide spectrum antibiotic therapy commenced to be adjusted when results of cultures are available.

When necrosis occurs in the background of severe arterial disease, revascularization is usually necessary to maintain the viability of the limb. In some patients, increased perfusion following angioplasty may be useful, but many patients with necrosis will need arterial bypass to restore pulsatile blood flow to the foot. After operative debridement of wet necrosis, revascularization is necessary to heal the tissue deficit. Distal bypass is now established as successful treatment in the diabetic lower limb. Diabetic ischemic foot patients with end-stage renal disease are the most difficult to treat because of the presence of diffuse disease, greater involvement of the distal and pedal vessels, and extensive tissue necrosis. However, bypass can be performed safely and effectively in patients who have undergone renal transplantation and in a dialysis-dependent patient population (79,80).

CONCLUSION

This chapter has defined five specific stages in the natural history of the diabetic foot. In Stages 1 and 2, the emphasis is on prevention of ulceration. Stage 3 describes the management of foot ulceration. Finally, Stages 4 and 5 deal with the complications of foot ulceration, namely, cellulitis and necrosis. It has described a simple plan of management for each stage, which requires a well-organized multidisciplinary approach that should be available to all diabetic patients.

REFERENCES

1. Reiber GE. Epidemiology of foot ulcers and amputations in the diabetic foot. In: Bowker JH, Pfeifer MA, eds. Levin and O'Neal's The Diabetic Foot, 6th Edition. St Louis: Mosby, 2001:13–32.
2. Pecoraro RE, Reiber GE, Burgess EM. Pathways to diabetic limb amputation. Diabetes Care 1990; 13 (5):513–21.
3. Bakker K, Foster AVM, van Houtoum WH, Riley P, eds. International Diabetes Federation and International Working Group of the Diabetic Foot. Time to act. The Netherlands, 2005.
4. Brem H, Sheehan P, Rosenberg HJ, Schneider JS, Boulton AJ. Evidence-based protocol for diabetic foot ulcers. Plast Reconstr Surg 2006; 117(7 Sppl):193S–209S.
5. Driver VR, Madsen J, Goodman RA. Reducing amputation rates in patients with diabetes at a military medical center: the limb preservation service model. Diabetes Care 2005; 28(2):248–53.
6. Edmonds M, Foster AVM. Reduction of major amputations in the diabetic ischemic foot: a strategy to "take control" with conservative care as well as revascularisation. VASA 2001; 58(Suppl): 6–14.
7. van Houtum WH, Rauwerda JA, Ruwaard D, Schaper NC, Bakker K. Reduction in diabetes-related lower-extremity amputations in The Netherlands: 1991–2000. Diabetes Care 2004; 27:1042–6.
8. Eskelinen E, Eskelinen A, Alback A, Lepantalo M. Major amputation incidence decreases both in non-diabetic and in diabetic patients in Helsinki. Scand J Surg 2006; 95(3):185–9.
9. Edmonds M, Foster AVM and Sanders LJ. A practical manual of diabetic foot care Blackwell Science, Oxford 2004.
10. Jeffcoate WJ, Chipchase SY, Ince P, Game FL. Assessing the outcome of the management of diabetic foot ulcers using ulcer-related and person-related measures. Diabetes Care 2006; 29(8):
11. Prompers L, Huijberts M, Apelqvist J et al. High prevalence of ischaemia, infection and serious comorbidity in patients with diabetic foot disease in Europe. Baseline results from the Eurodiale study. Diabetologia 2007; 50(1):18–25.
12. Rith-Najarian SJ, Stolusky T, Godhes DM. Identifying diabetic patients at risk for lower extremity amputation in a primary healthcare setting. Diabetes Care 1992; 15:1386–9.
13. Abbott CA, Vileikyte L, Williamson S, et al. Multicenter Study of the Incidence of and Predictive Risk Factors for Diabetic Neuropathic Foot Ulceration. Diabetes Care July 1998; 21(7):1071–5.

14. Miranda-Palma B, Sosenko JM, Bowker JH, Mizel MS, Boulton AJ. A comparison of the monofilament with other testing modalities for foot ulcer susceptibility. Diabetes Res Clin Pract 2005; 70(1):8–12.
15. American Diabetes Association. Peripheral arterial disease in people with diabetes. Diabetes Care 2003; 26(12):3333–41.
16. Faglia E, Caravaggi C, Marchetti R, et al.. SCAR (SCreening for ARteriopathy) Study Group. Screening for peripheral arterial disease by means of the ankle-brachial index in newly diagnosed Type 2 diabetic patients. Diabet Med 2005; 22(10):1310–14.
17. Maciejewski ML, Reiber GL, Smith DG et al.. Effectiveness of diabetic therapeutic footwear in preventing reulceration. *Diabetes Care* 2004; 27:1774–82.
18. Uccioli L, Aldeghi A, Faglia E, et al. Manufactured shoes in the prevention of diabetic foot ulcers. Diabetes Care 1995; 18:1376–8.
19. Reiber GE, Smith DG, Wallace C, et al. Effect of therapeutic footwear on foot reulceration in patients with diabetes: a randomized controlled trial. JAMA 2002; 15;287(19):2552–8.
20. Boulton AJ, Jude EB. Therapeutic footwear in diabetes: the good, the bad, and the ugly? Diabetes Care 2004; 27(7):1832–3.
21. Sanders LJ, Frykberg RG. Charcot neuroarthropathy of the foot. In: Bowker JH, Pfeifer MA, eds. Levin and O'Neal's The Diabetic Foot, 6th Edition. St Louis: Mosby 2000: 467–82.
22. Jude EB, Selby PL, Burgess J, et al. Boulton Bisphosphonates in the treatment of Charcot neuroarthropathy: a double-blind RCT. Diabetologia 2001; 44(11):2032–7.
23. McCabe CJ, Stevenson RC, Dolan AM. Evalutation of a diabetic foot screening and protection programme. Diabetic Medicine 1998; 15: 80–84.
24. McGill M, Molyneaux L, Yue DK. Which diabetic patients should receive podiatry care? An objective analysis. Int Med J 2005; 35(8):451–6.
25. Valk GD, Kriegsman DMW, Assendelft WJJ. Patient education for preventing diabetic foot ulceration (Cochrane Review). In: The Cochrane Library, Issue 3, 2003. Oxford.
26. Peters EJG, Lavery LA. Effectiveness of the diabetic foot risk classification system of the International working group on the diabetic foot. Diabetes Care 2001; 24:1442–7.
27. Boulton AJ. The diabetic foot: from art to science: The 18th Camillo Golgi lecture. Diabetologia 2004; 47(8): 1343–53. Epub 2004 July 28 (Review).
28. Nabuurs-Franssen MH, Sleegers R, Huijberts MS, et al. Total contact casting of the diabetic foot in daily practice: a prospective follow-up study. Diabetes Care 2005; 28(2):243–7.
29. Nabuurs-Franssen MH, Huijberts MS, Sleegers R, et al. Casting of recurrent diabetic foot ulcers: effective and safe? Diabetes Care 2005; 28(6): 1493.
30. Caravaggi C, Faglia E, De Giglio R, et al. Effectiveness and safety of a non-removable fibreglass oo-bearing cast versus a therapeutic shoe in the treatment of neuropathic foot ulcers: a randomised study. Diabetes Care 2000; 23:1746–51.
31. Ira A Katz, Anthony Harlan, Bresta Miranda-Palma, Luz Prieto-Sanchez, et al. A Randomized trial of two irremovable off-loading devices in the management of plantar neuropathic diabetic foot ulcers. Diabetes Care 2005; 28(3):555 (5 pp.).
32. Armstrong DG, Nguyen HC, Lavery LA, et al. Off loading the diabetic foot wound. Diabetes Care 2001; 24:1019–22.
33. Edmonds ME, Foster AVM. Managing the Diabetic Foot. Oxford: Blackwell Science 2005.
34. Steed DL. Foundations of good ulcer care. Am J Surg 1998; 176(Suppl 2a): 20S–5S.
35. Wolff H, Hansson C. Larval therapy – an effective method of ulcer debridement. Clin Exp Dermatol 2003; 28(2):134–7.
36. Rayman A, Stansfield G, Woollard T, et al. Use of larvae in the treatment of the diabetic necrotic foot. Diabetic Foot 1998; 1:7–13.
37. Armstrong DG, Salas P, Short B, et al.. J Am Podiatr Med Assoc 2005; 95(3):254–7. Maggot therapy in "lower-extremity hospice" wound care: fewer amputations and more antibiotic-free day.
38. Falanga V. Wound healing and its impairment in the diabetic foot. Lancet 2005 12; 366(9498):1736–43. (review).
39. Hilton JR, Williams DT, Beuker B, et al.. Wound dressings in diabetic foot disease. Clin Infect Dis 2004; 39(Suppl 2):S100–3.
40. Edmonds M, Bates M, Doxford M, et al.. New treatments in ulcer healing and wound infection. Diabetes/Metabolism Research and Reviews 2000; 16(Suppl 1):S51–4.
41. Falanga V, Sabolinski ML. Prognostic factors for healing of venous and diabetic ulcers. Wounds 2000; 12:42A–6A.
42. Wieman TJ, Smiell JM, Su Y. Efficacy and safety of a topical gel formulation of recombinant human platelet derived growth factor – BB (Becaplermin) in patients with non healing diabetic ulcers: a phase III, randomized, placebo-controlled, double-blind study. Diabetes Care 1998; 21: 822–7.
43. Naughton G, Mansbridge J, Gentzkow G. A metabolically active human dermal replacement for the treatment of diabetic foot ulcers. Artifical Organs 1997; 21: 1203–10.

44. Marston WA, Hanft J, Norwood P, et al. Dermagraft Diabetic Foot Ulcer Study Group. The efficacy and safety of Dermagraft in improving the healing of chronic diabetic foot ulcers: results of a prospective randomized trial. Diabetes Care 2003; 26(6):1701–5.

45. Veves A, Falanga V, Armstrong DG, et al. Graftskin, a human skin equivalent, is effective in the management of noninfected neuropathic diabetic foot ulcers: a prospective randomized multicenter clinical trial. Diabetes Care 2001; 24(2):290–5.

46. Lipkin S, Chaikof E, Isseroff Z, Silverstein P. Effectiveness of Bilayered Cellular Matrix in Healing of Neuropathic Diabetic Foot Ulcers: Results of a Multicenter Pilot Trial. Wounds 2003; 15 (7):230–6.

47. Caravaggi C, De Giglio R, Pritelli C, et al. HYAFF 11-based autologous dermal and epidermal grafts in the treatment of noninfected diabetic plantar and dorsal foot ulcers: a prospective, multicenter, controlled, randomized clinical trial. Diabetes Care 2003; 26(10):2853–9.

48. Niezgoda JA, Van Gils, CC, Frykberg RG, et al. Randomized Clinical Trial Comparing OASIS Wound Matrix to Regranex Gel for Diabetic Ulcers. Adv Skin Wound Care 2005; 18(5):258–66.

49. Veves A, Sheehan P, Pham HT. A randomized, controlled trial of Promogran (a collagen/oxidized regenerated cellulose dressing) vs standard treatment in the management of diabetic foot ulcers. Arch Surg 2002; 137(7):822–7.

50. Kalani M, Apelqvist J, Blombäck M, et al. Effect of Dalteparin on Healing of Chronic Foot Ulcers in Diabetic Patients With Peripheral Arterial Occlusive Disease. Diabetes Care 2003; 26:2575–80.

51. Armstrong DG, Lavery LA. Diabetic Foot Study Consortium. Negative pressure wound therapy after partial diabetic foot amputation: a multicentre, RCT. Lancet 2005; 366(9498):1704–10.

52. Andros G, Armstrong DG, Attinger CE, et al. Consensus statement on negative pressure wound therapy (VAC Therapy) for the management of diabetic foot wounds. Ostomy Wound Manage 2006; Suppl:1–32.

53. Faglia E, Favales F, Aldeghi A, et al. Adjunctive systemic hyperbaric oxygen therapy in treatment of severe prevalently ischemic diabetic foot ulcer. A randomized study. Diabetes Care 1996;19(12): 1338–43.

54. Wunderlich RP, Peters EJ, Lavery LA. Systemic hyperbaric oxygen therapy: lower-extremity wound healing and the diabetic foot. Diabetes Care 2000; 23(10):1551.

55. Kranke P, Bennett M, Roeckl-Wiedmann I, Debus S. Hyperbaric oxygen therapy for chronic wounds. Cochrane Database Syst Rev. 2004;(2):CD004123.

56. Edmonds M, Foster A. The use of antibiotics in the diabetic foot. Am J Surg 2004; 187(5A):25S–8S.

57. Cavanagh PR, Lipsky BA, Bradbury AW, Botek G. Treatment for diabetic foot ulcers. Lancet 2005; 366(9498):1725–35.(review).

58. Rayman G, Rayman A, Baker NR, et al. Sustained silver-releasing dressing in the treatment of diabetic foot ulcers. Br J Nurs 2005; 14(2):109–14.

59. Chantelau E, Tanudjaja T, Altenhofer F et al.. Antibiotic treatment for uncomplicated neuropathic forefoot ulcers in diabetes: a controlled trial. Diabetic Med 1996; 13: 156–9.

60. Edmonds ME, Walters H. Angioplasty and the diabetic foot. Vasc Med Rev 1995; 6:205–14.

61. Faglia E, Dalla Paola L, et al. Peripheral angioplasty as the first-choice revascularization procedure in diabetic patients with critical limb ischemia: prospective study of 993 consecutive patients hospitalized and followed between 1999 and 2003. Eur J Vasc Endovasc Surg 2005; 29(6): 620–7.

62. Lazaris AM, Tsiamis AC, Fishwick G, et al. Clinical outcome of primary infrainguinal subintimal angioplasty in diabetic patients with critical lower limb ischemia. J Endovasc Ther 2004; 11(4): 447–53.

63. Sigala F, Menenakos Ch, Sigalas P, et al. Transluminal angioplasty of isolated crural arterial lesions in diabetics with critical limb ischemia. Vasa 2005; 34(3):186–91.

64. Eneroth M, Apelqvist J, Stenstrom A. Clinical characteristics and outcome in 223 diabetic patients with deep foot infections. Foot Ankle Int 1997; 18: 716–22.

65. Morrison WB, Schweitzer ME, Batte WG, et al. Osteomyelitis of the foot: relative importance of primary and secondary MR imaging signs. Radiology 1998; 207(3):625–32.

66. Grayson ML. Diabetic foot infections: Antimicrobial therapy. In: Eliopoulos GM, ed., Infectious Disease Clinics of North America. Philadelphia, PA: WB Saunders Company 1995: pp. 143–62.

67. Lavery LA, Armstrong DG, Peters EJ, Lipsky BA. Probe-to-Bone Test for Diagnosing Diabetic Foot Osteomyelitis: Reliable or relic? Diabetes Care 2007; 30(2):270–4.

68. Tentolouris N, Petrikkos G, Vallianou N, et al.. Prevalence of methicillin-resistant Staphylococcus aureus in infected and uninfected diabetic foot ulcers. N Clin Microbiol Infect 2006; 12(2):186–9.

69. Pellizzer G, Strazzabosco M, Presi S, et al. Deep tissue biopsy vs superficial swab culture monitoring in the microbiological assessment of limb-threatening diabetic foot infection. Diabet Med 2001; 18: 822–7.

70. Slater RA, Lazarovitch T, Boldur I, Ramot Y, Buchs A, Weiss M, Hindi A, Rapoport MJ. Swab cultures accurately identify bacterial pathogens in diabetic foot wounds not involving bone. Diabet Med 2004; 21(7):705–9.

71. Senneville E, Melliez H, Beltrand E, et al. Culture of percutaneous bone biopsy specimens for diagnosis of diabetic foot osteomyelitis: concordance with ulcer swab cultures. Clin Infect Dis 2006; 42(1):57–62. Epub 2005 November 21.

72. Lipsky BA, Armstrong DG, Citron DM, et al.. Ertapenem versus piperacillin/tazobactam for diabetic foot infections (SIDESTEP): prospective, randomised, controlled, double-blinded, multicentre trial. Lipsky 2005 Lancet 2005; 366(9498):1695–703.

73. Harkless L, Boghossian J, Pollak R, et al. An open-label, randomized study comparing efficacy and safety of intravenous piperacillin/tazobactam and ampicillin/sulbactam for infected diabetic foot ulcers. Surg Infect (Larchmt). 2005; 6(1):27–40.

74. Clay PG, Graham MR, Lindsey CC, et al. Clinical efficacy, tolerability, and cost savings associated with the use of open-label metronidazole plus ceftriaxone once daily compared with every 6 hours as empiric treatment for diabetic lower-extremity infections in older males. Am J Geriatr Pharmacother 2004 2(3):181–9.

75. Vekatesan P, Lawn S, Macfarlane RM, et al. Conservative management of osteomyelitis in the feet of diabetic patients. Diab Med 1997; 14: 487–90.

76. Embil JM, Rose G, Trepman E, Math MC, et al. Oral antimicrobial therapy for diabetic foot osteomyelitis. Foot Ankle Int 2006; 27(10):771–9.

77. Lioupis C. The role of distal arterial reconstruction in patients with diabetic foot ischemia. Int J Low Extrem Wounds 2005; 4(1):45–9.

78. Pomposelli FB, Kansal N, Hamdan AD, et al. A decade of experience with dorsalis pedis artery bypass: analysis of outcome in more than 1000 cases. J Vasc Surg 2003; 37(2):307–15.

79. McArthur CS, Sheahan MG, Pomposelli FB Jr, et al. Infrainguinal revascularization after renal transplantation. J Vasc Surg 2003; 37(6):1181–5.

80. Ramdev P, Rayan SS, Sheahan M, et al. A decade experience with infrainguinal revascularization in a dialysis-dependent patient population. J Vasc Surg 2002; 36(5):969–74.

22 | Gastrointestinal and Autonomic Complications of Diabetes Mellitus

Adrian Vella
Endocrine Research Unit, Division of Endocrinology, Mayo Clinic, Rochester, Minnesota, U.S.A.

Michael Camilleri
Enteric Neuroscience Program, Mayo Foundation, Rochester, Minnesota, U.S.A.

INTRODUCTION

Gastrointestinal (GI) function is controlled by the extrinsic and intrinsic nervous systems. Extrinsic neural control is exerted by the parasympathetic and sympathetic nervous components of the autonomic nervous system. Intrinsic control is imposed by the enteric plexuses (the "little brain" in the digestive tract) (Fig. 1). Experimental models of gut motor function suggest a predominant modulatory role for the extrinsic nervous system, and primary control through the (intrinsic) enteric nervous system (1). Thus, derangements of the extrinsic nerves at any level may result in alteration of GI motility and secretion (2).

Intrinsic control can occur quite independently of the extrinsic control. The enteric nervous system consists of 100 million neurons that are organized in distinct ganglionated plexi including the submucous plexus (involved in absorption and secretion), the myenteric plexus (involved in motility), and the plexus of Cajal (which serves pacemaking functions). As with the somatic and autonomic nerves elsewhere, the gut's autonomic and enteric nervous system can be affected in diabetes mellitus.

The GI tract symptoms are common in patients with diabetes seen at *tertiary referral centers*. In the absence of structural lesions in the gut, such patients are commonly assumed to have autonomic neuropathy. This is not unreasonable since autonomic neuropathy is a common complication of diabetes. Although microvascular complications are less frequent in type 2 diabetes, as compared to people with type 1 diabetes, the prevalence of autonomic neuropathy among type 2 diabetics is still significant. The degree of glycemic control affects the incidence and progression of neuropathic complications including GI neuropathy. Moreover, since the rate of gastric emptying and the nature of the ingested meal are important determinants of postprandial glucose concentrations, altered gastric emptying may impact on the ability to achieve good glycemic control in people with diabetes.

The GI involvement is frequently associated with autonomic dysregulation of the eyes, blood pressure, heart and peripheral vessels and the urinary bladder and sexual organs. In this chapter, we aim to focus on the GI manifestations of diabetes mellitus, advances in understanding the mechanism and role of autonomic, enteric and hormonal dysfunctions, the autonomic symptoms and tests that are indicative of autonomic denervation, and management of GI manifestations of diabetes.

DEFINITIONS: DIABETIC ENTEROPATHY, GASTROPARESIS, DYSPEPSIA, DIARRHEA, INCONTINENCE

The GI symptoms that are frequently encountered in patients with diabetes mellitus are outlined in Figure 2. Diabetic enteropathy refers to all the GI complications of diabetes and may result in dysphagia, heartburn, nausea and vomiting, abdominal pain, constipation, diarrhea and fecal incontinence (3). Feldman and Schiller reported that 76% of referrals to a diabetic clinic had at least one GI symptom (3). Clouse also reported that GI symptoms were present in a high proportion (20%) of diabetic patients on the registry of a General Clinical Research Center (4). A third study from a tertiary care center reported an increased incidence of GI symptoms in patients with diabetes as compared with control subjects (5). However, in the Rochester Diabetic Neuropathy Study (6), only 1% of patients had symptoms of

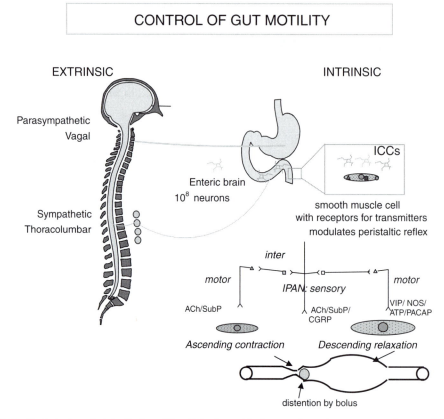

FIGURE 1 Control of gastrointestinal motility. Note the extrinsic or autonomic nervous system modulates the function of the enteric nervous system, which controls smooth muscle cells through transmitters. *Source*: From Ref. 72.

gastroparesis and only 0.6% had nocturnal diarrhea. This discrepancy has been addressed in other community-based epidemiological studies, which are discussed below.

Kassender recognized *asymptomatic* gastric retention in diabetics in 1958 (7) and coined the term "gastroparesis diabeticorum". Since the original report, the term gastroparesis has been used to reflect symptomatic as well as asymptomatic gastric retention. However, the presence of GI symptoms in people with diabetic autonomic neuropathy is not necessarily related solely to delayed gastric emptying. More recently, the term "diabetic dyspepsia" was used to reflect the spectrum of postprandial symptoms in diabetics that are attributable to upper GI dysfunction, including those associated with delayed gastric emptying (8). Thus, while nausea, vomiting and early satiation after meals were the classical symptoms of gastroparesis, the term *diabetic dyspepsia* reflects in addition bloating, fullness and pain in the upper abdomen (8).

Constipation among diabetic patients reflects the common etiologies: impaired rectal evacuation, slow transit or normal transit constipation (9). The extrinsic parasympathetic supply to the colon forms the ascending intracolonic nerves and is a major excitatory mechanism inducing transit of stool in the colon.

The pathogenesis of *chronic diarrhea* in patients with diabetes is incompletely understood. Several mechanisms may contribute to the development of the condition including anorectal dysfunction, intestinal dysmotility, abnormal intestinal secretion, bacterial overgrowth, bile acid diarrhea and exocrine pancreatic insufficiency (10). Celiac disease, which has been reported with increased frequency in type 1 diabetes, may also contribute to diarrhea.

The term "diabetic diarrhea" was first coined in 1936 by Bargen (11) at the Mayo Clinic to describe unexplained diarrhea associated with severe diabetes. Typically, patients with

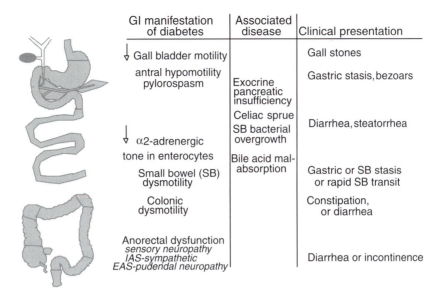

GI manifestation of diabetes	Associated disease	Clinical presentation
↓ Gall bladder motility		Gall stones
antral hypomotility pylorospasm	Exocrine pancreatic insufficiency	Gastric stasis, bezoars
↓ α2-adrenergic tone in enterocytes	Celiac sprue SB bacterial overgrowth	Diarrhea, steatorrhea
Small bowel (SB) dysmotility	Bile acid mal-absorption	Gastric or SB stasis or rapid SB transit
Colonic dysmotility		Constipation, or diarrhea
Anorectal dysfunction *sensory neuropathy* *IAS-sympathetic* *EAS-pudendal neuropathy*		Diarrhea or incontinence

FIGURE 2   Gastrointestinal manifestations of diabetes mellitus. *Source*: From Ref. 73.

diabetic diarrhea have poorly controlled diabetes and evidence of diabetic neuropathy, usually peripheral neuropathy and frequently autonomic neuropathy Diarrhea is often nocturnal and may be associated with anal incontinence. Episodes of diarrhea may be alternate with constipation or normal bowel movements. Symptoms of delayed gastric emptying such as early satiety, nausea and vomiting are often experienced by such patients with diarrhea.

Fecal incontinence is experienced by a substantial percentage of patients with chronic diabetes mellitus referred to tertiary referral centers. This does not necessarily correlate with the presence of diarrhea, although patients may sometimes describe fecal incontinence as "diarrhea". Fecal continence is maintained by the internal and external anal sphincters and the puborectalis sling, which maintains the rectoanal angulation. Anorectal sensation and reflex contractions of the sphincter mechanisms are essential for continence. Wald et al. (12) and Schiller et al. (13) have demonstrated that patients with diabetes and incontinence have a higher threshold (that is reduced sensation) for rectal perception of balloon distention when compared to continent diabetics and healthy controls. Patients with diabetes and incontinence also exhibit decreased resting anal sphincter pressure when compared to continent patients with diabetes. This reflects loss of sympathetic nerve supply to internal anal sphincter. Daytime fecal incontinence aggravated by urgency or raised intra-abdominal pressure is suggestive of external sphincter weakness and pudendal neuropathy.

In summary, diabetic *constipation*, *diarrhea* and *incontinence* refer to the occurrence of these symptoms in the absence of any disorder other than diabetes or neuropathy. For example, in patients with "diabetic diarrhea", associated conditions such as celiac sprue and bacterial overgrowth are excluded. These disturbances of lower bowel function are closely linked with autonomic neuropathy. For example, colonic transit delay may result in constipation secondary to loss of extrinsic or intrinsic neural control of the colon, and diarrhea may result from loss of α adrenergic "tone" in enterocytes. Incontinence may result from loss of sensation, impaired sympathetic supply to the internal anal sphincter, or loss of pudendal innervation of the external sphincter.

EPIDEMIOLOGY OF GI SYMPTOMS IN DIABETES

The first *community-based epidemiological studies* of symptoms in diabetics were performed in Germany and Finland by the groups of Enck et al. (5) and Janatuinen et al. (14). These studies provided the surprising information that the only GI problems with higher prevalence in diabetics than in controls were constipation, use of laxatives, and history of gall bladder surgery. The main findings were confirmed by a questionnaire-based study in Olmsted County, Minnesota (15). This showed that only constipation and use of laxatives were more prevalent in type 1 (not type 2 diabetics) diabetics than in controls matched for age and gender (Table 1) (15).

The high prevalence of functional gastrointestinal disorders such as irritable bowel syndrome, constipation, and functional dyspepsia in Western civilizations confounds any estimates of the prevalence of diabetic enteropathy based on symptoms alone. Prevalence figures do not assess the impact or severity of the upper GI symptoms suggestive of dyspepsia or gastroparesis. Thus, although Maleki et al. identified nausea, vomiting or dyspepsia in ~11% of type 1 diabetics and ~6% of controls, these prevalence figures were not significantly different from age- and gender-matched nondiabetic community controls. A significant number of diabetics experienced impaired sweating, a marker of autonomic neuropathy relative to community controls (15).

Paradoxically, this study demonstrated a lower prevalence of heartburn among the participants with type 1 diabetes (15). Factors that may contribute to this finding are the possibility of vagal neuropathy reducing the sensation of heartburn and the strong recommendation by diabetologists to patients to avoid nonsteroidal anti-inflammatory medications to protect their renal function.

A more recent questionnaire-based community study in South Eastern Australia reported more diarrhea, fecal incontinence, dysphagia and postprandial fullness among diabetics (16). In contrast to the three prior studies (4–6), which included at least 10% type 1 diabetics, in the study from Australia, 95% of the cohort were type 2 diabetics. Constipation (other than the symptom of "anal blockage") was not significantly more prevalent in diabetics, in contrast to the three other epidemiological studies. The odds ratio for nausea was close to significant (OR 0.98–2.35). The nature of these symptoms suggests that they may result from motor and sensory abnormalities of the GI tract. Epidemiological studies attempted to identify risk factors for developing GI symptoms among diabetics. In two Australian studies (16,17), a community evaluation found an association between self-reported poor glycemic control and GI symptom complexes (16). A clinic questionnaire-based study showed GI symptoms were associated with diabetic complications, but not with current glycemic control (as reflected by blood glucose and HbA_{1c} (17)).

Reports of increased mortality among patients with diabetic autonomic neuropathy (18) and the association of diabetic gastroparesis with autonomic neuropathy in some (19,20) but not all (21) studies has led to the expectation of a poor prognosis for diabetic patients with severe GI symptoms. Longitudinal studies of gastric emptying and upper GI symptoms in patients with diabetes mellitus are lacking in number and indeed the few published studies have reported data from relatively small numbers of patients. Natural history studies are limited by relatively small numbers, potential referral bias, or short follow-up. Gastric emptying parameters and symptoms are not markedly different after 12 years' follow up (21). Among 86 outpatients with diabetes (60 type 1) followed for at least 9 years, 21 (24%) had died. However, there was no evidence that gastroparesis was associated with mortality after adjusting for other morbidity (22). While prevalence figures suggest that gastroparesis is rare and of limited mortality, they do not assess the severity of symptoms, nutritional compromise, complications of worse diabetes control, and impact on quality of life. This impact is independent of age, gender, smoking, alcohol use, and type of diabetes (23).

MECHANISM OF GI COMPLICATIONS IN DIABETES

The presence of GI symptoms in patients with diabetes does not correlate with glycemic control (assessed by measurement of HbA_{1c}) at the time of presentation. Good glycemic control at the time of presentation may reflect poor caloric intake secondary to gastroparesis or malabsorption secondary to diarrhea. However, a history of poor glycemic control seems to be more closely associated with GI symptoms than does the presence of diabetic complications such as peripheral or autonomic neuropathy (assessed by tests of cardiovascular autonomic function). It is also important to consider the role of psychological factors in the perception of

TABLE 1 Prevalence (%) of Gastrointestinal and Neurological Symptoms among Diabetic Residents of Olmsted County, Minnesota, Compared to Their Respective Community Controls

	IDDM		NIDDM	
	Patients	Controls	Patients	Controls
Symptoms/syndrome	(n = 138)	(n = 170)	(n = 217)	(n = 218)
Irritable bowel syndrome				
Rome criteria	10.6	7.9	5.1	8.3
Manning criteria	8.0	8.8	5.5	7.8
Constipation				
Symptoms only	16.7	13.5	10.1	11.5
Symptoms and/or laxatives	27.0	19.0	17.0	15.0
Dyschezia	2.9	3.5	2.3	2.3
Diarrhea	0	0	0	0
Fecal incontinence	0.7	1.2	4.6	1.8
Nausea/vomiting	11.6	10.6	6.0	5.5
Dyspepsia	18.8	20.6	13.4	17.4
Heartburn				
Symptoms only	11.6[*]	22.9	19.8	24.3
Symptoms and/or antacids	18.8[*]	36.5	24.0	36.2
P neurosymptoms (overall)	50.0	47.1	65.9[*]	50.5
Numbness	34.8	28.2	41.5[*]	21.6
Muscular weakness	33.3	31.2	54.4[*]	43.6
A neuro symptoms (overall)	9.4	5.9	7.8	7.3
Insufficient sweating	6.5*	1.8	5.5	5.5
Gustatory sweating	3.6	4.1	2.3	2.8

[a] $p \leq 0.05$ (univariate association, diabetes subgroup vs. corresponding controls).
Note: People with insulin-dependent diabetes mellitus (IDDM) have increased prevalence of constipation and/or use of laxatives and decreased prevalence of heartburn. Prevalence of dyspepsia is not greater in diabetics than in controls.
Abbreviations: A Neuro = autonomic neuropathy; IDDM = insulin-dependent diabetes mellitus; NIDDM = noninsulin-dependent diabetes mellitus; P Neuro = peripheral neuropathy.
Source: Reproduced from Ref. 5.

GI symptoms. The Psychosomatic Symptom Checklist score is significantly associated with the reporting of GI tract symptoms (15). Several mechanisms interact to produce disordered gastrointestinal function in diabetes. These are best documented in the function of the stomach; hence the following section addresses the mechanisms that are relevant in diabetic gastroparesis.

Hyperglycemia

Acute hyperglycemia reversibly influences upper-gut motor and sensory function. In situations where postprandial insulin release is defective (type 2 diabetes) or absent (type 1 diabetes), the rate of gastric emptying is a major determinant of postprandial blood glucose concentrations. Therefore, altered gastric emptying can contribute to GI symptoms as well as poor glycemic control (24). Patients with type 2 diabetes mellitus and without neuropathic complications have been shown to exhibit accelerated gastric emptying of liquids when compared to healthy control subjects (25).

In patients with type 1 or type 2 diabetes, and in healthy subjects, acute hyperglycemia slows emptying of both solids and caloric liquids when compared with euglycemia (26,27). This effect is also observed in patients with autonomic neuropathy. In patients with type 2 diabetes, emptying of liquids is related to the blood glucose concentration (28). Conversely, hypoglycemia will lead to marked acceleration of gastric emptying when compared to euglycemia. Hyperglycemia interferes with the prokinetic effect of intravenous erythromycin on gastric emptying in healthy subjects and patients with diabetes (29). Extreme hyperglycemia (>20 mmol/L) may contribute to the acute gastric dilatation sometimes observed at presentation of diabetic ketoacidosis.

Extrinsic Neural Control

Extrinsic Neuropathy

Extrinsic neuropathy results in impaired GI contractility or abnormal myoelectrical control. The syndrome is typically seen in patients with type 1 or insulin-dependent diabetes mellitus (IDDM). Peripheral neuropathy is present in the majority of patients with enteropathy, and other forms of autonomic neuropathy (e.g., orthostatic hypotension) are common. Previous work has attributed these motility disorders mainly to vagal nerve dysfunction (3,30). Motor abnormalities of the small intestine observed in symptomatic diabetic patients (31,32) are often indistinguishable from those seen in patients with other syndromes affecting postganglionic sympathetic function (33). Vagal dysfunction is probably critical in gastric stasis of solid food. Electrolyte imbalances due to diabetic ketoacidosis (e.g., hypokalemia) and uremia may further aggravate impaired motor function in diabetic patients.

Vagal neuropathy is likely to impair normal gastric accommodation and compliance in diabetics (34). However, patients with diabetes and cardio-vagal neuropathy exhibit normal postprandial change in gastric volume as measured using SPECT imaging (Fig. 3) (35). This is consistent with the normalization of gastric accommodation in rats and humans after vagotomy (36). This adaptation in rats is inhibited by treatment with tetrodotoxin, suggesting that enteric neurons are involved in the adaptation to chronic vagal denervation (36).

Intrinsic Neural Control

The importance of nitric oxide (NO) as an intestinal neurotransmitter regulating gastropyloric function is increasingly recognized. Mice with a targeted genomic deletion of neuronal nitric oxide synthase (nNOS) develop pyloric hypertrophy and gastric dilatation. Similarly, loss of pyloric nNOS is associated with infantile hypertrophic pyloric stenosis. This is supported by the observation that exogenous NO reduces the number and amplitude of isolated pyloric pressure waves in normal humans.

Abnormalities of nNOS have been observed in animal models of diabetes. Stomachs of spontaneously diabetic rats and rats with streptozotocin-induced diabetes exhibit decreased NO-mediated relaxation of gastric muscle strips and decreased expression of nNOS. Watkins et al. (33) have subsequently demonstrated that nNOS protein and mRNA are depleted in the pyloric myenteric neurons of diabetic mice. Insulin treatment restores pyloric nNOS protein and reverses the delay in gastric emptying observed in such mice. Sildenafil, a cGMP phosphodiesterase inhibitor augments NO signaling and also reverses delayed gastric

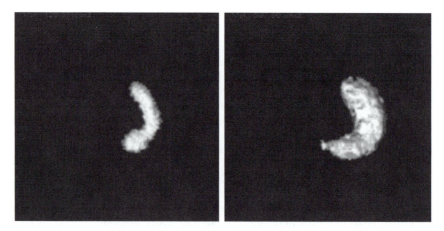

FIGURE 3   Measurement of changes in gastric volume using single photo emission computed tomography after labeling of the stomach wall with intravenous ^{99m}Tc pertechnetate. *Source*: From ref. 35.

emptying in diabetic mice. These data suggest that reversible down regulation of NOS may play an important role in the pathogenesis of diabetic gastropathy.

Neuronal nitric oxide synthase (nNOS)-derived NO acts as a smooth muscle cell relaxant by binding to and activating smooth muscle cell guanylate cyclase (37). The expression of nNOS is particularly high in the pyloric sphincter (38) and nNOS mice exhibit pyloric hypertrophy, gastric dilatation and delayed gastric emptying (39). In humans, inhibition of NOS decreases gastric emptying time and fundic volume (40). Similarly, in murine models of diabetes, NOS expression and activity is decreased but is restored by insulin administration (41).

Peptidergic and serotonergic (42,43) innervation is abnormal in animal models of diabetes.

The interstitial cells of Cajal (ICC) play an important role in the regulation of GI motility. ICC are distributed throughout the GI tract, interspersed in the circular and longitudinal muscle layers and, in the murine and human small intestine and form a dense plexus at the level of the neuronal myenteric plexus ICCs generate the electrical slow wave, required for normal GI motility.

Defects of ICC have been associated with several human gut motility diseases including slow transit constipation, hypertrophic pyloric stenosis, Hirschsprung's disease and pseudo-obstruction. Ordog et al. (44) demonstrated that "spontaneously diabetic mice" develop delayed gastric emptying, impaired electrical slow waves, and reduced motor neurotransmission. They also observed greatly reduced ICCs in the distal stomach. Moreover, the association of the ICC and enteric nerve cells was disrupted.

Loss of ICC has been reported in a patient with type 1 diabetes (45) who underwent full-thickness jejunal biopsy. However, it remains to be ascertained whether defects of ICC are consistently present in patients with GI dysmotility due to diabetes. Altered ICC networks have also been implicated in chronic intestinal pseudoobstruction (46) and idiopathic slow transit constipation (47), underscoring the importance of ICC in health and disease. Diabetes may alter GI function by causing structural, numerical or functional changes in ICC.

Carbon Monoxide (CO) is an important regulator of neurotransmission, smooth muscle tone and response to cellular injury. Two heme oxygenase enzymes (HO1 and HO2) catalyze the formation of CO from heme. Neurons express high concentrations of HO2 (48), and HO1 expression is induced by injury or inflammation (49). Induction of HO1 ameliorates tissue injury in animal models of tissue injury/ileus and therefore modulation of this pathway may be a therapeutic target in the treatment of diabetic enteropathy. A polymorphism in *HMOX-1* (the gene that codes for HO1) is associated with predisposition to diseases in which oxidative damage is central to pathogenesis (50,51). CO is a hyperpolarizing factor in the GI muscle layers. CO production and heme oxygenase activity mirror the smooth muscle membrane potential present across the muscle layers. Since the degree of polarization of smooth muscle determines recruitment of muscle in response to a stimulus, CO is likely to be important in controlling intestinal contractility. Of relevance to this discussion is the fact that nonadrenergic, noncholinergic neurotransmission is nearly abolished in HO-2 knockout mice and this can be restored by addition of exogenous CO.

Hormonal Control

Numerous peptide hormones play a role in the regulation of intestinal motility and gastric emptying and also directly, or indirectly, in the control of satiety and caloric intake. Some of these peptides are also involved in glycemic control. These hormones may also influence the neural control of gut motility.

Glucagon-like peptide-1 (GLP-1) arises from the differential post-transcriptional processing of the proglucagon gene that occurs in the intestinal L cells and in the hypothalamus. It is an incretin hormone because of its potentiation of glucose-induced insulin secretion. When infused in pharmacological concentrations it markedly delays gastric emptying while increasing insulin and suppressing glucagon secretion in response to meal ingestion. Because of these actions, GLP-1 can prevent postprandial hyperglycemia. These actions have led to the development of GLP-1-based therapy for type 2 diabetes. The infusion of GLP-1 in healthy subjects delays gastric emptying and increases gastric accommodation. The increase in abdominal volume is not accompanied by an increased perception of satiety suggesting that GLP-1 alters gastric compliance or the central perception of gastric distention. These actions are accompanied by the suppression of human pancreatic polypeptide (HPP) suggesting that the effects of GLP-1 on the stomach are at least partly dependent on inhibition of vagal cholinergic function (52). Indeed in people with type 2 diabetes and documented cardio-vagal neuropathy GLP-1 does not alter accommodation of the stomach in response to meal ingestion lending further support to the supposition that GLP-1 actions on the stomach are mediated by the vagus. It is interesting to note that the effects of GLP-1 on the stomach are dose-dependent and circulating concentrations encountered in the absence of GLP-1 infusion or after inhibition of its breakdown by dipeptidyl peptidase-4 (DPP-4) have no direct effect on gastric emptying or GI symptoms (53,54).

Since the intestinal L cells are dispersed in the lower small intestine and colon and GLP-1 levels rise markedly in response to nutrient ingestion, it has been hypothesized that GLP-1 may contribute to the ileal brake effect, that is, the inhibition of upper GI motility due to the presence of (unabsorbed) nutrients in the distal small intestine.

Amylin is a 37 amino-acid polypeptide that is co-secreted with insulin by the pancreatic beta cells in response to nutrient stimuli. Human studies have shown that the plasma concentrations of amylin and insulin rise and fall in parallel in both the fasted and fed states. Amylin secretion mirrors the abnormalities of insulin secretion observed in diabetes. People with type 1 diabetes typically do not have detectable amylin in the circulation during the fasting and fed states. Consequently, type 1 diabetes is a state of amylin as well as insulin deficiency. In contrast, amylin concentrations are more variable in people with type 2 diabetes. Amylin concentrations are elevated in early type 2 diabetes, but are decreased in the later stages as insulin secretion wanes.

Infusion of pharmacological concentrations of amylin or the more stable analog, pramlintide in both animals and humans has established that amylin can inhibit gastric emptying (55) and decrease glucagon secretion. The effects of amylin on gastric emptying are similar in type 1 and type 2 diabetes (56).

Studies in rats and, more recently, in humans suggest that like GLP-1, the effects of pramlintide may be centrally mediated. Pramlintide inhibits meal-induced secretion of pancreatic polypeptide a well-established marker of intestinal vagal activity (55,56). The inhibition of gastric emptying produced by pramlintide is avoided during insulin-induced hypoglycemia which is associated with vagal stimulation (57). Pramlintide is now available for clinical use to delay gastric emptying and consequently decrease postprandial hyperglycemia in people with diabetes.

Psychological Factors

Lustman, Clouse et al. (4,58) have provided evidence that symptoms in diabetics are significantly influenced by psychological factors.

CLINICAL EVALUATION OF PATIENTS WITH SUSPECTED DIABETIC ENTEROPATHY

The evaluation of upper GI symptoms in patients with diabetes by means of *esophagogastroduodenoscopy* may document the presence of intercurrent conditions such as peptic ulceration, peptic stricture or Mallory–Weiss tears (a result of repeated retching and vomiting). The presence of bezoars suggests delayed gastric emptying.

Confirmation of the diagnosis of gastroparesis requires documentation of *delayed gastric emptying*. Scintigraphic transit studies are typically used to measure gastric emptying. However, it is important to emphasize measurements using labeled liquid meals are of limited value because gastric emptying may be normal even in the presence of significant symptoms. Assessment of solid emptying by means of a radiolabel that tags the solid phase of the meal is a more sensitive test with a well-defined normal range. The proportion of radioisotope retained in the stomach at 2 and 4 h distinguishes normal function from gastroparesis with a sensitivity of 90% and a specificity of 70% (59).

Another useful test for the measurement of solid phase gastric emptying utilizes a standardized meal with biscuit enriched with ^{13}C, a substrate containing the stable isotope.

When metabolized, the proteins, carbohydrates and lipids of the *S. platensis* or the medium chain triglyceride octanoate give rise to respiratory CO2 that is enriched in ^{13}C. Measurement of $^{13}CO_2$ breath content (a reflection of the amount of biscuit remaining in the stomach) by isotope ratio mass spectrometry allows estimation of gastric emptying $t_{1/2}$ (60).

Gastropyloroduodenal manometry is a specialized technique that allows assessment of the pressure profiles in the stomach and small bowel. Hypomotility of the gastric antrum is an important cause of motor dysfunction and impaired emptying in diabetes. Patients with selective abnormalities of gastric function may be able to tolerate enteral feeding (delivered directly into the small bowel) whereas patients with a more generalized motility disorder may not be able to tolerate enteral feeding.

Gastric accommodation in response to meal ingestion may be impaired in diabetes. This may contribute to the GI symptoms of nausea, bloating and early satiety. Imaging of the stomach wall using ^{99m}Tc pertechnetate allows measurement of gastric volume after meal ingestion (Fig. 3) (61).

Diarrhea and fecal incontinence are often due the effects of diabetes on the GI tract. However, features suggestive of malabsorption such as anemia, macrocytosis or steatorrhea should lead to a consideration of underlying small bowel or pancreatic pathology. Celiac disease or bacterial overgrowth of the small intestine should be actively excluded (10).

Intestinal motor function can be evaluated by measurement of intestinal transit or rarely by small bowel manometry. Abnormal patterns of motility, however, are not reliable indicators of rapid or delayed intestinal transit. Scintigraphic methods that can simultaneously measure gastric, small bowel and colonic transit are accurate, noninvasive and relatively inexpensive.

Anorectal function can be evaluated by anorectal manometry that allows measurement of sphincter strength at rest (sympathetic function) and during squeeze (pudendal nerve function), testing of sensation to balloon distention. Anorectal ultrasound may help identify defects in the anal sphincter while a defecating proctogram allows evaluation of pelvic floor dysfunction or the functional significance of rectoceles or intussusception. However, most of these abnormalities can be successfully evaluated by careful rectal examination.

EVALUATING THE PATIENT FOR AUTONOMIC SYMPTOMS AND SIGNS

Evaluation of patients for autonomic dysfunction should start with a careful review of symptoms. Several symptoms are useful indicators of the possibility of autonomic nervous dysfunction. These symptoms include postural dizziness, lack of sweating, failure of erection or ejaculation, difficulty with emptying the urinary bladder or recurrent urinary tract infections, and dryness of the eyes, mouth or vagina. Table 2 shows the implications for sympathetic and parasympathetic dysfunction in such patients. An infrequently sought symptom in patients with diabetic autonomic neuropathy is gustatory sweating of the face, which reflects parasympathetic denervation. Postprandial hypotension is unlikely to occur except in severe autonomic neuropathies. It results from pooling of blood in the viscera and is aggravated by abrupt standing after meals.

TABLE 2 Symptoms and Signs Suggestive of Autonomic Dysfunction

Sympathetic	Parasympathetic
Failure of pupils to dilate in the dark	Fixed dilated pupils
Fainting, orthostatic dizziness	Lack of pupillary accommodation
Constant heart rate with orthostatic hypotension	Sweating during mastication of certain foods
Absent piloerection	Decreased gut motility
Absent sweating	Dry eyes and mouth
Impaired ejaculation	Dry vagina
Paralysis of dartos muscle	Impaired erection
	Difficulty with emptying urinary bladder
	Recurrent urinary tract infections

Source: From Ref. 2.

AUTONOMIC FUNCTION TESTS IN DIABETICS WITH ENTEROPATHY

While general autonomic reflex tests (62) are useful to assess the function of the autonomic control of the viscera (Table 3), tests that are specific for gut autonomic innervation are:

(A) Pancreatic polypeptide response to hypoglycemia or to modified sham feeding by the "chew and spit" technique: Pancreatic polypeptide concentrations rise after meal ingestion and delivery of nutrients to the duodenum (63). Atropine or vagotomy abolish this response. Normally, pancreatic polypeptide concentrations should increase by at least 25 pg/ml during sham feeding. The modified sham feeding test seems to be a more sensitive means of detecting vagal dysfunction than the postprandial response of plasma pancreatic polypeptide. The coexistence of antral hypomotility with abnormal pancreatic polypeptide responses to sham feeding further supports the presence of vagal dysfunction or impaired gastric emptying of solids in these situations.

(B) R-R interval response to deep breathing: This is a test of cardiovagal reflexes. However, Buyschaert et al. (64) showed that this is a good surrogate for the testing of abdominal vagal function, consistent with the concept that vagal denervation, as with most forms of diabetic neuropathy commences caudally and progresses in a cranial direction.

(C) Mesenteric flow in response to tilt-table tasting (65): Splanchnic blood flow is under baroreflex control, and appropriate regulation is important in the maintenance of postural normotension. Evaluation of mesenteric flow in response to eating and head-up tilt provides important information on intra-abdominal sympathetic adrenergic function, and the ability of the patient to cope with orthostatic stress. Superior mesenteric artery flow in response to perturbations such as tilting and meal ingestion assesses sympathetic adrenergic function in the abdomen. While useful, this technique requires considerable expertise and is not widely available.

PRINCIPLES OF TREATMENT OF DIABETIC ENTEROPATHY

General principles in the management of diabetic enteropathy include optimal control of blood glucose, restoration of hydration, nutrition, and normal intestinal propulsion.

GASTROPARESIS AND DYSPEPSIA

Patients with severe exacerbation of symptoms should be hospitalized and may require nasogastric suction. Intravenous fluids should be provided, and metabolic derangements (ketoacidosis, uremia, hypo/hyperglycemia) corrected. Parenteral nutrition may become necessary in cases of malnutrition. Bezoars may be mechanically disrupted during endoscopy, followed by gastric decompression to drain residual nondigestible particles. *Erythromycin* at a dose of 3 mg/kg body weight intravenously every 8 h appears to be effective in accelerating gastric emptying (56). A week's treatment with oral erythromycin, 250 mg, t.i.d., is worthwhile once patients start to tolerate oral intake of food. Since both liquids and homogenized solids are more readily emptied from the stomach than solids, liquid or blenderized food will be better tolerated. Frequent monitoring of blood glucose levels is essential during this phase. Rarely, it is necessary to bypass the stomach with a jejunal feeding tube if the motor dysfunction is limited to the stomach and there is no response to prokinetic therapy. This procedure should be preceded by a trial for a few days of nasojejunal feeding with infusion rates of at least 60 ml iso-osmolar nutrient per hour. Jejunal tubes are best placed by laparoscopy or mini laparotomy rather than via percutaneous endoscopic gastrostomy tubes. Such tubes allow restoration of normal nutritional status but they are not without adverse effects. There is no evidence to suggest that gastrectomy relieves symptoms or enhances quality of life. Patients with gastroparesis often have concomitant small intestinal denervation which is likely to cause persistent symptoms after gastrectomy (32,66).

If the patient remains symptomatic, other prokinetic agents may be considered as adjuncts. In the USA, the only available medication is metoclopramide, a peripheral cholinergic and antidopaminergic agent. During acute administration, it initially enhances gastric emptying of liquids in patients with diabetic gastroparesis, but its symptomatic efficacy is probably related with its central antiemetic effects. However, its long term use is restricted by a decline in efficacy and by a troubling incidence of central nervous system side effects.

TABLE 3   Commonly Performed Autonomic Tests

Test	Physiologic functions tested	Rationale	Comments/pitfalls
Sympathetic function			
1. *Thermoregulatory sweat test* (% surface area of anhidrosis)	Preganglionic and postganglionic cholinergic	Stimulation of hypothalamic temp. control centers	Cumbersome, whole body test
2. *Quantitative sudomotor axon reflex test* (sweat output latency)	Postganglionic cholinergic	Antidromic stimulation of peripheral fiber by axonal reflex	Needs specialized facilities
3. *Heart rate and blood pressure responses*			
Orthostatic tilt test	Adrenergic	Baroreceptor reflex	Impaired responses if intra-vascular volume is reduced
Postural adjustment ratio	Adrenergic	Baroreceptor reflex	Impaired responses if intra-vascular volume is reduced
Cold pressor test	Adrenergic	Baroreceptor reflex	Impaired responses if intra-vascular volume is reduced
Sustained hand grip	Adrenergic	Baroreceptor reflex	Impaired responses if intra-vascular volume is reduced
4. *Plasma norepinephrine response to*:			
Postural changes	Postganglionic adrenergic	Baroreceptor stimulation	Moderate sensitivity, impaired response if intravascular volume is reduced
Intravenous edrophonium	Postganglionic adrenergic	Anticholinesterase "stimulates" postganglionic fiber at prevertebral ganglia	False-negatives caused by contributions to plasma norepinephrine from many organs
Parasympathetic Function			
1. *Heart rate (RR) variation with deep breathing*	Parasympathetic	Vagal afferents stimulated by lung stretch	Best cardiovagal test available, but not a test of abdominal vagus
2. *Supine/erect heart rate*	Parasympathetic	Vagal stimulation by change in central blood volume	Cardiovagal test
3. *Valsalva ratio* (heart rate, max./min.)	Parasympathetic	vagal Stimulation of by change in central blood volume	Cardiovagal test
4. *Gastric acid secretory* or *plasma pancreatic polypeptide response to modified sham feeding or hypoglycemia*	Parasympathetic	stimulation of Vagal nuclei by sham feeding or hypoglycemia	Abdominal vagal test, critically dependent on avoidance of swallowing food during test
5. *Nocturnal penile tumescence*	Pelvic parasympathetic	Integrity of S_{2-4}	Plethysmographic technique requiring special facilities
6. *Cystometrographic to bethanechol*	Pelvic parasympathetic	Increase in intra-vesical pressure suggests denervation supersensitivity	Tests parasympathetica supply to response bladder, not bowel

Source: From Ref. 74.

"Botulinum toxin" has been injected into the pylorus in several uncontrolled studies which suggested benefit of the intervention (67). However, this has not been borne out by controlled clinical trials (68).

"Gastric electrical stimulation" is still controversial despite approval by the Food and Drug Administration as a humanitarian use device after a controlled study showed decreased vomiting frequency in diabetic gastroparesis when the stimulator was switched on. Gastric emptying was not altered in this study and the mechanism of symptomatic benefit is unclear (69).

"Diabetic diarrhea" is treated symptomatically with loperamide, 2-8 mg per day. Second line approaches are clonidine, 0.1 mg orally (70) or by patch in patients who do not experience significant postural hypotension, and subcutaneous octreotide, 25–50 µg subcutaneously 5–10 min before meals (71).

"Constipation" is typically treated with osmotic and stimulant laxatives. One should avoid lactulose because of potential impact on glycemic control, and magnesium compounds in patients with impaired renal function because of risk of magnesium retention. Polyethylene glycol osmotic laxatives are useful (up to 17 g in 8 ounces of water per day) though care needs to be taken to avoid dehydration or sodium overload in patients requiring regular dosing. Pelvic floor disorders should be excluded before embarking on long-term polyethylene glycol therapy.

"Incontinence" may require physical medicine and biofeedback approaches to enhance rectal sensation, and to strengthen the external anal sphincter. In the presence of a significant pudendal neuropathy or sensory loss, biofeedback may not work and the patient may have a better quality of life with a descending colostomy.

ACKNOWLEDGMENTS

This study was supported in part by grants RO1-DK54681 (MC) and K24-DK02638 (MC) from National Institutes of Health. We wish to thank Mrs. Cindy Stanislav for excellent secretarial assistance.

REFERENCES

1. Wood JD. Enteric neurophysiology. Am J Physiol 1984; 247:G585–98.
2. Camilleri M. Disorders of gastrointestinal motility in neurologic diseases. Mayo Clin Proc 1990; 65: 825–46.
3. Feldman M, Schiller LR. Disorders of gastrointestinal motility associated with diabetes mellitus. Ann Int Med 1983; 98:378–84.
4. Clouse RE, Lustman PJ. Gastrointestinal symptoms in diabetic patients: lack of association with neuropathy. Am J Gastroenterol 1989; 84:868–72.
5. Enck P, Rathmann W, Spiekermann M et al. Prevalence of gastrointestinal symptoms in diabetic patients and non-diabetic subjects. Z Gastroenterol 1994; 32:637–41.
6. Dyck PJ, Karnes JL, O'Brien PC et al. The Rochester Diabetic Neuropathy Study: reassessment of tests and criteria for diagnosis and staged severity. Neurology 1992; 42:1164–70.
7. Kassander P. Asymptomatic gastric retention in diabetics (gastroparesis diabeticorum). Ann Intern Med 1958; 48:797–812.
8. Mearin F, Malagelada JR. Gastroparesis and dyspepsia in patients with diabetes mellitus. Eur J Gastroenterol Hepatol 1995; 7:717–23.
9. Maleki D, Camilleri M, Burton DD, et al. Pilot study of pathophysiology of constipation among community diabetics. Dig Dis Sci 1998; 43:2373–78.
10. Valdovinos MA, Camilleri M, Zimmerman BR. Chronic diarrhea in diabetes mellitus: mechanisms and an approach to diagnosis and treatment. Mayo Clin Proc 1993; 68:691–702.
11. Bargen JAB, Keppler, E.J. The "diarrhea of diabetes" and steatorrhea of pancreatic insufficiency. Mayo Clin Proc 1936; 11:737–42.
12. Wald A, Tunuguntla AK. Anorectal sensorimotor dysfunction in fecal incontinence and diabetes mellitus. Modification with biofeedback therapy. N Engl J Med 1984; 310:1282–7.
13. Schiller LR, Santa Ana CA, Schmulen AC, et al. Pathogenesis of fecal incontinence in diabetes mellitus: evidence for internal-anal-sphincter dysfunction. N Engl J Med 1982; 307:1666–71.
14. Janatuinen E, Pikkarainen P, Laakso M, et al. Gastrointestinal symptoms in middle-aged diabetic patients. Scand J Gastroenterol 1993; 28:427–32.
15. Maleki D, Locke III, GR, Camilleri M, et al. Gastrointestinal tract symptoms among persons with diabetes mellitus in the community. Arch Int Med 2000; 160:2808–16.
16. Bytzer P, Talley NJ, Leemon M, et al. Prevalence of gastrointestinal symptoms associated with diabetes mellitus: a population-based survey of 15,000 adults. Arch Intern Med 2001; 161:1989–96.
17. Bytzer P, Talley NJ, Hammer J, et al. GI symptoms in diabetes mellitus are associated with both poor glycemic control and diabetic complications. Am J Gastroenterol 2002; 97:604–11.
18. Coppini DV, Bowtell PA, Weng C, et al. Showing neuropathy is related to increased mortality in diabetic patients – a survival analysis using an accelerated failure time model. J Clin Epidemiol 2000; 53:519–23.
19. Rundles RW: Diabetic neuropathy. Bull N Y Acad Med 1950; 26:598–616.
20. Stacher G, Lenglinger J, Bergmann H, et al. Impaired gastric emptying and altered intragastric meal distribution in diabetes mellitus related to autonomic neuropathy? Dig Dis Sci 2003; 48:1027–34.
21. Jones KL, Russo A, Berry MK, et al. A longitudinal study of gastric emptying and upper gastrointestinal symptoms in patients with diabetes mellitus. Am J Med 2002; 113:449–55.

22. Kong MF, Horowitz M, Jones KL, et al. Natural history of diabetic gastroparesis. Diabetes Care 1999; 22:503–7.
23. Talley NJ, Young L, Bytzer P, et al. Impact of chronic gastrointestinal symptoms in diabetes mellitus on health-related quality of life. Am J Gastroenterol 2001; 96:71–76.
24. Rayner CK, Samsom M, Jones KL, et al. Relationships of upper gastrointestinal motor and sensory function with glycemic control. Diabetes Care 2001; 24:371–81.
25. Frank JW, Saslow SB, Camilleri M, et al. Mechanism of accelerated gastric emptying of liquids and hyperglycemia in patients with type II diabetes mellitus. Gastroenterology 1995; 109:755–65.
26. Horowitz M, Harding PE, Maddox AF, et al. Gastric and oesophageal emptying in patients with type 2 (non-insulin-dependent) diabetes mellitus. Diabetologia 1989; 32:151–9.
27. Fraser RJ, Horowitz M, Maddox AF, et al. Hyperglycaemia slows gastric emptying in type 1 (insulin-dependent) diabetes mellitus. Diabetologia 1990; 33:675–80.
28. Schvarcz E, Palmer M, Aman J, et al. Physiological hyperglycemia slows gastric emptying in normal subjects and patients with insulin-dependent diabetes mellitus. Gastroenterology 1997; 113:60–66.
29. Samsom M, Jebbink RJ, Akkermans LM, et al. Effects of oral erythromycin on fasting and postprandial antroduodenal motility in patients with type I diabetes, measured with an ambulatory manometric technique. Diabetes Care 1997; 20:129–34.
30. Feldman M, Corbett DB, Ramsey EJ, et al. Abnormal gastric function in longstanding, insulin-dependent diabetic patients. Gastroenterology 1979; 77:12–17.
31. Samsom M, Jebbink RJ, Akkermans LM, et al. Abnormalities of antroduodenal motility in type I diabetes. Diabetes Care 1996; 19:21–27.
32. Camilleri M, Malagelada JR. Abnormal intestinal motility in diabetics with the gastroparesis syndrome. Eur J Clin Invest 1984; 14:420–7.
33. Camilleri M, Malagelada JR, Stanghellini V, et al. Gastrointestinal motility disturbances in patients with orthostatic hypotension. Gastroenterology 1985; 88:1852–59.
34. Samsom M, Salet GA, Roelofs JM, et al. Compliance of the proximal stomach and dyspeptic symptoms in patients with type I diabetes mellitus. Dig Dis Sci 1995; 40:2037–42.
35. Delgado-Aros S, Vella A, Camilleri M, et al. Effects of glucagon-like peptide-1 and feeding on gastric volumes in diabetes mellitus with cardio-vagal dysfunction. Neurogastroenterol Motil 2003; 15:435–43.
36. Takahashi T, Owyang C: Characterization of vagal pathways mediating gastric accommodation reflex in rats. J Physiol 1997; 504(Pt2):479–88.
37. Shah V, Lyford G, Gores G, Farrugia G. Nitric oxide in gastrointestinal health and disease. Gastroenterology 2004; 126:903–13.
38. Chakder S, Bandyopadhyay A, Rattan S: Neuronal NOS gene expression in gastrointestinal myenteric neurons and smooth muscle cells. Am J Physiol 1997; 273:C1868–75.
39. Mashimo H, Kjellin A, Goyal RK. Gastric stasis in neuronal nitric oxide synthase-deficient knockout mice. Gastroenterology 2000; 119:766–73.
40. Tack J, Demedts I, Meulemans A, et al. Role of nitric oxide in the gastric accommodation reflex and in meal induced satiety in humans. Gut 2002; 51:219–24.
41. Watkins CC, Sawa A, Jaffrey S, Blackshaw S, Barrow RK, Snyder SH, Ferris CD: Insulin restores neuronal nitric oxide synthase expression and function that is lost in diabetic gastropathy. J Clin Invest 2000; 106:373–84.
42. Belai A, Lincoln J, Milner P, Burnstock G: Progressive changes in adrenergic, serotonergic, and peptidergic nerves in proximal colon of streptozotocin-diabetic rats. Gastroenterology 1988; 95:1234–41.
43. Belai A, Burnstock G: Changes in adrenergic and peptidergic nerves in the submucous plexus of streptozotocin-diabetic rat ileum. Gastroenterology 1990; 98:1427–36.
44. Ordog T, Takayama I, Cheung WK, Ward SM, Sanders KM: Remodeling of networks of interstitial cells of Cajal in a murine model of diabetic gastroparesis. Diabetes 2000; 49:1731–39.
45. He CL, Soffer EE, Ferris CD, Walsh RM, Szurszewski JH, Farrugia G: Loss of interstitial cells of cajal and inhibitory innervation in insulin-dependent diabetes. Gastroenterology 2001; 121:427–34.
46. Feldstein AE, Miller SM, El-Youssef M, Rodeberg D, Lindor NM, Burgart LJ, Szurszewski JH, Farrugia G: Chronic intestinal pseudoobstruction associated with altered interstitial cells of cajal networks. J Pediatr Gastroenterol Nutr 2003; 36:492–97.
47. Lyford GL, He CL, Soffer E, et al. Pan-colonic decrease in interstitial cells of Cajal in patients with slow transit constipation. Gut 2002; 51:496–501.
48. Ny L, Alm P, Larsson B, Andersson KE: Morphological relations between haem oxygenases, NO-synthase and VIP in the canine and feline gastrointestinal tracts. J Auton Nerv Syst 1997; 65:49–56.
49. Foresti R, Motterlini R: The heme oxygenase pathway and its interaction with nitric oxide in the control of cellular homeostasis. Free Radic Res 1999; 31:459–75.
50. Yamada N, Yamaya M, Okinaga S, et al. Microsatellite polymorphism in the heme oxygenase-1 gene promoter is associated with susceptibility to emphysema. Am J Hum Genet 2000; 66:187–95.
51. Chen YH, Lin SJ, Lin MW, et al. Microsatellite polymorphism in promoter of heme oxygenase-1 gene is associated with susceptibility to coronary artery disease in type 2 diabetic patients. Hum Genet 2002; 111:1–8.

52. Delgado-Aros S, Kim DY, Burton DD, et al. Effect of GLP-1 on gastric volume, emptying, maximum volume ingested, and postprandial symptoms in humans. Am J Physiol Gastrointest Liver Physiol 2002; 282:G424–31.

53. Meier JJ, Gallwitz B, Salmen S, et al. Normalization of glucose concentrations and deceleration of gastric emptying after solid meals during intravenous glucagon-like peptide 1 in patients with type 2 diabetes. J Clin Endocrinol Metab 2003; 88:2719–25.

54. Holst JJ, Deacon CF: Glucagon-like peptide-1 mediates the therapeutic actions of DPP-IV inhibitors. Diabetologia 2005; 48:612–5.

55. Samsom M, Szarka LA, Camilleri M, et al. Pramlintide, an amylin analog, selectively delays gastric emptying: potential role of vagal inhibition. Am J Physiol Gastrointest Liver Physiol 2000; 278:G946–51.

56. Vella A, Lee JS, Camilleri M, et al. Effects of pramlintide, an amylin analogue, on gastric emptying in type 1 and 2 diabetes mellitus. Neurogastroenterol Motil 2002; 14:123–131.

57. Gedulin BR, Young AA. Hypoglycemia overrides amylin-mediated regulation of gastric emptying in rats. Diabetes 1998; 47:93–97.

58. Lustman PJ, Anderson RJ, Freedland KE, et al. Depression and poor glycemic control: a meta-analytic review of the literature. Diabetes Care 2000; 23:934–42.

59. Camilleri M, Zinsmeister AR, Greydanus MP, et al. Towards a less costly but accurate test of gastric emptying and small bowel transit. Dig Dis Sci 1991; 36:609–15.

60. Lee JS, Camilleri M, Zinsmeister AR, et al. A valid, accurate, office based non-radioactive test for gastric emptying of solids. Gut 2000; 46:768–73.

61. Kuiken SD, Samsom M, Camilleri M, et al. Development of a test to measure gastric accommodation in humans. Am J Physiol 1999; 277:G1217–21.

62. Low PA: Composite autonomic scoring scale for laboratory quantification of generalized autonomic failure. Mayo Clin Proc 1993; 68:748–52.

63. Taylor IL, Feldman M, Richardson CT, et al. Gastric and cephalic stimulation of human pancreatic polypeptide release. Gastroenterology 1978; 75:432–37.

64. Buysschaert M, Donckier J, Dive A, et al. Gastric acid and pancreatic polypeptide responses to sham feeding are impaired in diabetic subjects with autonomic neuropathy. Diabetes 1985; 34:1181–1185.

65. Chaudhuri KR, Thomaides T, Mathias CJ: Abnormality of superior mesenteric artery blood flow responses in human sympathetic failure. J Physiol 1992; 457:477–89.

66. Jones MP, Maganti K. A systematic review of surgical therapy for gastroparesis. Am J Gastroenterol 2003; 98:2122–29.

67. Park MI, Camilleri M: Gastroparesis: clinical update. Am J Gastroenterol 2006; 101:1129–39.

68. Arts J, van Gool S, Caenepeel P, et al. Influence of intrapyloric botulinum toxin injection on gastric emptying and meal-related symptoms in gastroparesis patients. Aliment Pharmacol Ther 2006; 24: 661–7.

69. Abell T, McCallum R, Hocking M, et al. Gastric electrical stimulation for medically refractory gastroparesis. Gastroenterology 2003; 125:421–8.

70. Fedorak RN, Field M, Chang EB. Treatment of diabetic diarrhea with clonidine. Ann Intern Med 1985; 102:197–199.

71. Mourad FH, Gorard D, Thillainayagam AV, et al. Effective treatment of diabetic diarrhoea with somatostatin analogue, octreotide. Gut 1992; 33:1578–80.

72. Camilleri M, Phillips SF. Disorders of small intestinal motility. IN: Gastroenterol Clin NA, Vol. 18. Ouyang A, Ed. Philadelphia: WB Saunders, 1989, pp. 405–424.

73. Camilleri M. Gastrointestinal problems in diabetes. IN: Endocrinology and Metabolism Clin NA, Vol. 25. Brownlee MA, King GL, Eds. Philadelphia: WB Saunders, 1996: 361–378.

74. Camilleri M, Ford MJ. Functional gastrointestinal disease and the autonomic nervous system: a way ahead? Gastroenterology 1994; 106:1114–1118.

23 Gestational Diabetes

Asha Thomas-Geevarghese and Robert E. Ratner
MedStar Research Institute, Washington, D.C., U.S.A.

INTRODUCTION

Gestational diabetes mellitus (GDM) is defined as glucose intolerance first recognized during pregnancy (1). This definition applies regardless of treatment regimens and does not distinguish between those unrecognized cases of diabetes that may have preceded pregnancy. GDM occurs in 0.5% to 12.3% of pregnancies depending on the criteria used and the population being tested (2,3). In the United States, prevalence rates are higher in African, Hispanic, Native American, and Asian women than in white women (4–6).

GDM conveys both short–and long–term risk to both mother and offspring. During the index pregnancy, women with GDM suffer from an increased prevalence of pregnancy-induced hypertension, toxemia, polyhydramnios, fetal macrosomia, birth trauma, neonatal metabolic complications (hypoglycemia, hyperbilirubinemia, hypocalcemia) and the need for primary Caesarian section delivery (7). Although most women revert to normal glucose tolerance postpartum, approximately 20% have impaired glucose tolerance (IGT) in the immediate postpartum phase (8,9). The lifetime risk of development of type 2 diabetes exceeds 50% (10–15).

Maternal glucose values have been directly correlated with neonatal mortality (16–18). Furthermore, fasting plasma glucose (FPG) showed an odds ratio (OR) of two for the development of macrosomia. For every 18 mg/dL increase in fasting glucose, the likelihood of developing macrosomia doubles (19). At delivery, GDM is associated with fetal macrosomia, with resultant shoulder dystocia and neonatal hypoglycemia. Long-term complications for infants of diabetic mothers include obesity and increased risk of abnormal glucose tolerance by adolescence.

PATHOPHYSIOLOGY

A thorough review of the pathophysiology of GDM is found in other sources (20–26) and is beyond the scope of this chapter. A brief review of the normal adaptations in glucose homeostasis and the maladaptations seen in GDM follows.

In normal pregnancy, glucose homeostasis changes in order to meet and maintain the demands of the growing fetus. Maternal adaptations ensure that there is an adequate nutrient supply of glucose and amino acids to the fetus, even at the expense of maternal glucose homeostasis. Pregnancy is characterized by hyperplasia of the pancreatic beta cells, increased insulin secretion, and an early increase in insulin sensitivity followed by progressive insulin resistance (23). Yet fasting glucose concentrations are 20% lower during pregnancy due to increased storage of tissue glycogen, increased peripheral glucose utilization, decreased hepatic glucose production, and glucose consumption by the fetus in late pregnancy (23). Increased levels of estrogen, human placental lactogen, growth hormone, corticotropin-releasing hormone and progesterone characterize the hormonal milieu during pregnancy(27) and these hormones play a major role in mobilizing maternal fuels either directly or indirectly increasing maternal insulin resistance. Subsequently, insulin requirements increase 1.5 to 2.5-fold in normal pregnancy over the nonpregnant state (28).

Overcoming the normal insulin resistance of pregnancy requires a compensatory increase in insulin secretion to maintain maternal glucose concentrations within the normal range. When pancreatic beta cells are unable to compensate for the normal insulin resistance of pregnancy, GDM ensues. Individuals with GDM have both decreased insulin sensitivity and decreased insulin secretion. Although patients with GDM have insulin responses similar to those seen in normal pregnancy, their baseline glucose levels are higher indicating a diminished beta-cell response to glucose. In GDM, the insulin response to a glycemic stimulus is about half that of normal pregnancy (29). Euglycemic clamp studies demonstrate diminished insulin secretion in women with GDM, despite the same or greater insulin resistance than that seen in pregnant women without GDM. Thus, failure of appropriate beta-cell compensation characterizes the onset of GDM (20). The mechanism of insulin resistance is unclear. Studies suggest that the GLUT4 transporter may play a role in insulin resistance (30,31). GLUT4 content is normal in skeletal muscle in women with GDM; however, in adipocytes, there is a decrease in number and sub-cellular distribution (30). Fifty percent of women with GDM have significant decreases in GLUT4 concentration, with glucose transporter function depressed by 60% (31).

DIAGNOSTIC ISSUES

Since its first recognition, there has been considerable controversy and lack of consensus in the diagnosis of GDM. There remains no universal standard regarding screening and diagnosis of GDM. Although the 100 g oral glucose-tolerance test (oGTT) is preferred in the USA, much of the world uses the 75 g oGTT for diagnostic purposes.

Who Should be Screened

Prior to the Fourth International Workshop on Gestational Diabetes, universal screening for GDM was recommended (32). The recommendations of the 5th International Workshop on Gestational Diabetes will be soon forthcoming. However, the Workshop and subsequent ADA recommendations advise screening only those women at high risk for GDM (33). The risk factors associated with GDM include:

- Age >25 years
- Elevated pre-pregnancy weight (greater than 110% IBW)
- Family history of diabetes, especially in a first degree relative
- History of macrosomia in prior pregnancy
- History of abnormal glucose tolerance
- History of poor obstetric outcome, or
- Member of minority populations at increased risk for type 2 diabetes

The ADA position statement suggests that it is not cost-effective to screen women at low risk, and recommends screening only be done in the presence of one or more risk factors (34,35). This change in recommendation has been challenged, however, as universal screening appears to improve detection of as many as 10% of all cases of GDM (36).

Screening and diagnosis

Several different methods can be used to diagnose GDM. In the USA, the recommended approach to screening is taken in two steps. Pregnant women without a history of carbohydrate intolerance are screened with a randomly timed 50 g glucose challenge between 24 and 28 weeks of gestation. Those with elevated plasma glucose ≥140 mg/dL are subsequently referred for 100 g oGTT. Although the 50 g glucose challenge test can be done without regard to fasting, in the fed state the sensitivity is improved if the cut-off value is lowered to 130 mg/dL (37).

The 100 g oGTT is used for diagnostic purposes in most areas throughout the USA. This test is performed after 3 days of unlimited carbohydrate intake and 8 h to 14 h of fasting. Evidence to support the use of the 100 g oGTT, includes the classic study by O'Sullivan and Mahan (14). In this study, 752 pregnant women were evaluated with a 3H oGTT. The mean blood glucose values were determined at each time-point. Using two standard deviations (SD) as normal, diagnostic criteria were set (Table 1). These criteria not only predict future diabetes in the mother, but also reveal a four-fold increase in perinatal mortality in untreated GDM compared with control (38). These original criteria for GDM were subsequently modified (3,39) due to changes in assay technique (Table 1). However, these changes were merely mathematical, and are based on criteria that define subsequent diabetes in the mother.

The 75 g oGTT in pregnancy is used in much of the world, and the data supporting its use is even more controversial than that for the 100 g oGTT. The Fourth International

TABLE 1 Historical Evolution of O'Sullivan-Mahan Criteria for the Diagnosis of Gestational Diabetes

O'Sullivan-Mahan criteria (14)	National diabetes data group (39)	Carpenter-Coustan modification (3)
Fasting 5.0 (90)[a]	5.83 (105)	5.28 (95)
1h 9.17(165)	10.56 (190)	10.0 (180)
2h 8.06(145)	9.17 (165)	8.61 (155)
3h 6.94(125)	8.06 (145)	7.78 (140)

[a] Values in brackets give mM (mg dL^{-1}) whole blood.

Workshop on Gestational Diabetes defined cut-off values for the 75 g oGTT in pregnancy as an FPG of 95 mg/dL and a 2 h plasma glucose of 155 mg/dL. These values were arbitrarily defined, based on the mean plus 1.5 SD of the oGTT values in a study of over 3500 patients (40). However, the 2 h value was raised to 155 mg/dL to be more consistent with the 2 h value recommended for the 100 g oGTT (3) and the values of the European Association for the Study of Diabetes (162 mg/dL) (41).

Contrary to the Fourth International Workshop on Gestational Diabetes, the World Health Organization (WHO) defines GDM based on the 75 g oGTT in the same fashion as in the nonpregnant state, with a fasting level ≥ 126 and $2 h \geq 200$. However, they compensate by recommending treatment of those with IGT based on a 2 h glucose ≥ 140 but ≤ 200 (42). Moses et al. (43) suggest lowering the glucose cutoff values to a fasting value of 90 mg/dL and the 2 h value to 140 mg/dL, to significantly reduce the rate of large–for–gestational–age infants, and the need for obstetric interventions. In support of the 75 g oGTT, Pettitt found an increased perinatal mortality rate proportional to the height of the 2 h glucose response to 75 g in Pima Indians (44).

Aside from the debate concerning the appropriate oGTT criteria to be used for the diagnosis of GDM, there is evidence to suggest that a single abnormal value on oGTT may better predict the occurrence of perinatal morbidity. Tallarigo et al. (45) examined the neonatal outcome in 249 women failing to meet O'Sullivan–Mahan criteria for GDM. They found that the 2 h plasma glucose concentration after a 100 g oGTT significantly correlated with the infant's birth weight; the higher the 2 h plasma glucose concentration, the greater the incidence of macrosomia, toxemia, and the need for cesarean section delivery. A significant increase was noted as 2 h plasma glucose concentrations exceeded 140 mg/dL compared with the 165 mg/dL cut–off level noted in traditional O'Sullivan–Mahan criteria. Lindsay et al. (46) found both maternal and fetal morbidity increased in women with only a single abnormal value on GTT. Toxemia was increased in the affected group, with an OR = 2.51, and macrosomia in the infants and subsequent shoulder dystocia were found to have OR of 2.18 and 2.97, respectively. Berkus and Langer (47) found the incidence of large-for-gestational-age infants among women with a single abnormal glucose value during the oGTT to be twice that of mothers in whom the oGTT was entirely normal.

The controversies over which oGTT to perform are further compounded by problems with poor reproducibility (48). In studies performed during pregnancy in which high-risk pregnant women underwent two sequential oGTT 1 week apart, 24% were found to have discordant test results on the two examinations (49). Surprisingly, the majority (80%) of the tests reverted from abnormal to normal glucose tolerance at the second examination.

There are studies ongoing to assess the effects of milder glucose abnormalities on infant and maternal outcomes. Notable is the Hyperglycemia and Adverse Pregnancy Outcome (HAPO) Study. HAPO is a 5-year prospective observational study that will recruit approximately 25,000 pregnant women (50). Glucose tolerance is assessed at 24 to 32 weeks' gestation. Glucose measurement is performed at 34 to 37 weeks or if symptoms suggest hyperglycemia. The investigators, obstetricians and subjects are blinded to the results. Maternal blood is obtained for measurement of serum C-peptide and hemoglobin A_{1c} (HbA$_{1c}$), cord blood for serum c-peptide and plasma glucose, and a capillary specimen is taken for neonatal plasma glucose. Neonatal anthropometrics are obtained, and follow-up data are collected at 4 to 6 weeks post-delivery. The primary outcomes are cesarean delivery, increased fetal size, neonatal morbidity and fetal hyperinsulinism (50). This study hopes to redefine GDM based on the more immediate concern of perinatal morbidity.

TREATMENT

Goals of Therapy

The goals of therapy in GDM are to decrease both maternal and fetal morbidity and mortality attributed to the disease. In particular, to limit macrosomia, intrauterine demise and neonatal morbidity. Preventing macrosomia has been found to decrease birth trauma, and cesarean-section rate (51).

Maternal hyperglycemia conclusively poses a threat to the well-being of the fetus. Fasting hyperglycemia (FPG > 105 mg/dL) is associated with increased risk of fetal death (17,18). Higher postprandial glucose values during weeks 29 to 32 are associated with fetal macrosomia (52). One hour postprandial glucose is a strong predictor of infant birth weight and fetal macrosomia (53). The risk of macrosomia is a continuum that increases further if 1 h postprandial glucose is > 120 mg/dL whole blood capillary glucose (plasma glucose of approximately 140 mg/dL). Despite aggressive treatment with diet, exercise and insulin therapy, which may normalize glycosylated hemoglobin (HbA$_{1c}$), neonatal morbidities persist. The relative risk of neonatal hypoglycemia remains elevated at 5.7, macrosomia risk is elevated 3.2-fold, and polycythemia, hypocalcemia, and hyperbilirubinemia are increased 2.0-fold (7).

Attaining good glycemic control is the cornerstone of therapy. Treatment is aimed at maintaining normoglycemia, and limiting maternal ketosis. Controlling blood sugars using postprandial glucose monitoring goals (1 h postprandial whole blood glucose <140 mg/dL) in combination with fasting blood glucose measurement (fasting blood glucose 60–90 mg/dL) can optimize glycemic control and significantly improve pregnancy outcomes, by decreasing neonatal hypoglycemia, macrosomia and cesarean-section rates (54). Recent assessments of obstetrician gynecologists by self report noted that 96% routinely screen for GDM, nearly all by using a 50-g glucose 1-h oral test. With medical nutrition therapy (MNT), almost 75% of respondents recommend exercise for patients with GDM. When MNT is ineffective for their patients with GDM, 82% of respondents initially prescribe insulin, whereas 13% begin with glyburide. Nearly 75% of respondents routinely perform a postpartum evaluation of glucose tolerance in the patient with GDM. The targets for blood glucose results were fasting mean 97.3 mg/dL; preprandial mean 103.6 mg/dL; 1-h postprandial mean 134.6 mg/dL; 2-h postprandial mean 122.1 mg/dL (55). This shows a significant improvement in adherence to practice guidelines compared to similar previous survey studies (55).

When to Initiate Self-Monitoring of Blood Glucose

Self blood-glucose monitoring (SBGM) should be instituted as soon as possible after diagnosis. Studies using fetal ultrasound (56,57) have shown that accelerated growth begins early in the third trimester so, to avoid fetal consequences, glycemic control should be obtained as soon as possible. In order to attain targeted goals, home SBGM is necessary. Initial therapy, MNT, requires blood-glucose monitoring four times daily, while women treated with insulin typically need to monitor at least six times per day. Care should be taken to give appropriate goals of therapy, since some reflectance meters are calibrated to plasma glucose values, while others reflect whole blood-glucose values.

The importance of SBGM is supported by a study of 153 women with GDM. These women were treated with intensive diet therapy and SBGM, with insulin therapy added only if therapeutic goals were not obtained. There was no difference in the birth weight or incidence of macrosomia between groups, showing that intensive dietary therapy with monitoring and insulin as needed can reduce macrosomia (58).

Medical Nutrition Therapy

MNT is the mainstay of treatment for women with GDM. The optimal diet should provide adequate nutrition and contribute to fetal well-being without causing postprandial hyperglycemia or fasting ketosis. Approximately 70% to 80% of patients can achieve adequate glycemic control when MNT is aggressively applied. Meal plans vary with the practitioner, but often include three meals and one to two snacks per day. Caloric restriction is often necessary in obese women, to prevent hyperglycemia. Since insulin resistance is highest in the morning, carbohydrate intake at breakfast is usually limited. Caloric intake, allotment and distribution need to be taken into consideration.

Optimum weight at delivery is 120% ideal body weight. Recommended weight gain is 12.5 kg to 18 kg if the body mass index (BMI) is $<$19.8 kg/m^2, 11.5 kg to 16 kg when BMI is 19.9 kg/m^2 to 26 kg/m^2, 7 kg to 11.5 kg for BMI 26 kg/m^2 to 29 kg/m^{2}and only 6 kg if BMI is $>$ 35 kg/m^2(59–61). Women with the least amount of weight gain typically have the best glycemic control and pregnancy outcome. However, caloric restriction must be done with caution. Protein malnutrition and ketosis should be avoided. A small study of 22 obese pregnant women demonstrated that moderate caloric restriction, not less than 25 kcal/kg, in obese women is acceptable and does not result in ketonuria (62). When obese women with GDM are subjected to caloric deprivation during late pregnancy there is a greater fall in plasma glucose compared with normal pregnant women, without a greater propensity to ketosis. This suggests that brief periods of fasting are well-tolerated and longer spacing can occur between meals (63).

Caloric restriction is limited by the occurrence of ketosis, when the carbohydrate intake is insufficient. Early studies suggested that ketosis is associated with lower IQ scores in adolescents (64,65). There are no large randomized trials of optimum dietary therapy in GDM. Studies suggest that intensive dietary therapy should be tailored to postprandial glucose. A small study of 14 overweight women with GDM between 32 and 36 weeks gestation looked at the effect of carbohydrate intake on postprandial glucose (66). All women were treated without insulin and received 24 kcal/kg/day. The calories were distributed such that they received 12.5% at breakfast, 28% at lunch, 28% at dinner, and the remainder in snacks. In order to maintain 1 h postprandial capillary whole blood glucose levels $<$ 140 mg/dL, carbohydrate intake needed to be $<$45% at breakfast, $<$55% at lunch and $<$50% at dinner. Aggressive MNT, with $<$33% carbohydrates at breakfast, $<$45% at lunch and $<$40% at dinner succeeded in achieving a blood glucose $<$120 mg/dL (66). This suggests that postprandial glucose is directly dependent on the carbohydrate content consumed during a meal.

Original recommendations from the American Diabetes Association suggested a diet that consisted of 35 kcal/kg pregnant weight, with 50% to 60% of those calories coming from carbohydrates. This caused excessive weight gain and postprandial hyperglycemia. Fifty percent of women on this diet ultimately required insulin therapy (67). A few small studies have looked at caloric restriction as a treatment for obese patients with GDM. Magee and colleagues (68) studied 12 patients. The women were all placed on 2400 kcal diets for 1 week. At the end of the first week, five were randomized to caloric restriction (1200 kcal/day), the remainder continued on the 2400 kcal/day diet. After 1 week, average glucose levels and fasting insulin levels were markedly reduced in the restricted group. Fasting and postprandial glucose challenges were not different. However, ketonuria and ketonemia developed in those patients who received caloric restriction. When women were placed on a 1600 kcal diet, ketonuria did not occur, but there remained marked improvement in glycemic control (68). In a nonrandomized trial of women treated for GDM, restriction of carbohydrates to 35% to 42 % compared with carbohydrate intake $>$45% resulted in improved maternal postprandial glucose with decreased need for insulin, fewer large-for-gestational-age infants and less need for cesarean sections (69). Current dietary recommendations range from 24 kcal/kg for normal pregnant weight, to 12 kcal/kg for morbidly obese, with $<$40% calories coming from carbohydrate (68,70–71).

These general guidelines will help to promote a healthy weight during pregnancy.

Exercise

Exercise serves as an adjunct therapy to medical nutrition in patients with diabetes (72,73) and can be helpful in the primary prevention of GDM (74). Exercise enhances insulin sensitivity and improves hepatic glucose production. However, little data is available on the use of exercise in treatment of GDM. Exercise should be monitored and should not increase fetal distress, lower infant birth weight, cause uterine contractions or maternal hypertension.

Safe exercise programs for pregnancy have been developed, and include the recumbent bicycle, arm ergonomics and brisk walking. In one randomized trial of 19 patients with GDM, six weeks of a cardiovascular fitness program using arm ergometry three times a week for 20 to 30 min per session resulted in normalization of glucose tolerance (75). The 1-h plasma glucose challenge result was 187.5 ± 12.9 mg/dL versus 105.9 ± 18.9 mg/dL for the exercise group, $p < 0.001$. The mean fasting blood glucose concentration fell to 55 mg/dL to 65 mg/dL (75). Similar results were seen in a study using a recumbent bicycle for the mode of exercise (76).

Contraindications to exercise include: pregnancy-induced hypertension, rupture of membranes, pre-term labor, bleeding, incompetent cervix, and intrauterine growth retardation. There are no data to indicate that pregnant women should limit exercise intensity and lower target heart-rates to avoid potential adverse events (77).

Initiation of Pharmacologic Therapy

Success of MNT is measured by weight gain and glycemic control. Blood glucose levels drop rapidly and dramatically in response to MNT. A 2 week trial to obtain and maintain fasting blood glucose < 95 mg/dL and postprandial blood glucose < 120 mg/dL is reasonable. Women with FPG level < 95 mg/dL have significantly higher levels of insulin production than those with glucose > 95 mg/dL. This suggests that women with fasting glucose > 95 mg/dL may not have adequate insulin secretion(78). Fasting glucose > 95 mg/dL, together with increased body weight, predicts failure of diet therapy and, therefore, a more limited trial (1 week) of diet therapy may be indicated (79). MNT is limited by the occurrence of starvation ketosis, and when MNT fails to attain normoglycemia in the absence of ketonuria in an adequate time-frame, pharmacologic therapy becomes necessary. The guideline for the indications for insulin use in GDM varies slightly from differing governing bodies.

The Fourth International Workshop on Gestational Diabetes recommends insulin as follows (80):

> Fasting whole blood glucose
> ≤95 mg/dL (5.3 mmol/L)
> Fasting plasma glucose
> ≤105 mg/dL(5.8 mmol/L)
> or
> 1-h postprandial whole blood glucose
> 2-h postprandial whole blood glucose
> ≤120 mg/dL (6.7 mmol/L)
> or
> 2-h postprandial plasma glucose
> ≤130 mg/dL(7.2 mmol/L)
> ≤140 mg/dL (7.8 mmol/L)
>
> 1-h postprandial plasma glucose
> ≤155 mg/dL (8.6 mmol/L)

The American College of Obstetrics and Gynecology (81) recommends insulin when:
Fasting glucose concentration ≥95 mg/dL (5.3 mmol/L) or
One hour postprandial glucose > 130 to 140 mg/dL (7.2 to 7.8 mmol/L) or
Two hour postprandial blood concentration ≥120 mg/dL (6.7 mmol/L)

The American Diabetes Association (82) recommends administration of insulin when:
Fasting plasma glucose concentration > 105 mg/dL (5.8 mmol/L) or
One hour postprandial plasma glucose > 155 mg/dL (8.6 mmol/L) or
Two hour-postprandial plasma glucose > 130 mg/dL (7.2 mmol/L)

When glucose levels are above the recommended levels with MNT, the goals of pharmacologic therapy are to minimize macrosomnia and the resultant increased risk of shoulder dystocia and birth trauma.

An argument can also be made for the use of third trimester fetal ultrasound in assessing the need for initiating insulin therapy. Seventy-three subjects with GDM treated with MNT, who obtained adequate glycemic control and had a fetal abdominal circumference (AC) by ultrasound >75 percentile, were randomized to continue MNT or begin insulin therapy (83). Treatment with insulin reduced macrosomia, without an increased risk of hypoglycemia, suggesting that ultrasound can be useful in determining treatment strategies in pregnancies complicated by GDM (83). Similarly, ultrasound can be used to identify those at low risk for macrosomia and perinatal complications. In a study using monthly ultrasound to measure fetal AC, participants were randomized to standard therapy or monitoring with ultrasound and glycemic control (84). In the experimental group, insulin was only begun if the fetal AC exceeded the 70th percentile for gestational age, or FPG was >120 mg/dL (84). Of those randomized to the experimental group 38% did not require insulin therapy. Using the study guidelines, there were no differences in birth weight, incidence of macrosomia, duration of insulin therapy or pregnancy-induced hypertension. There was a slight increase in cesarean sections in the experimental group, which was not explained by birth weight. In the experimental group, birth weights were lower in those women who did not receive insulin therapy (84). In women with GDM and fasting hyperglycemia, glucose plus fetal AC measurements identified pregnancies at low risk for macrosomia and resulted in the avoidance of insulin therapy in 38% of patients without increasing rates of neonatal morbidity (84).

Insulin Therapy

If MNT does not achieve the desired goals, insulin is the recommended mode of treatment in the United States. Approximately 15% of women with GDM are placed on insulin therapy. The type and amount of insulin therapy should be individualized, based on blood glucose levels. Patients should be instructed on signs and symptoms of hypoglycemia and given appropriate adjustment algorithms for home use. Close contact with the physician and educator throughout pregnancy is needed. Adjustments in insulin therapy every 3 to 4 days can achieve targeted glycemic control in an optimum time-frame. There are a wide variety of management algorithms used by various practitioners, which require frequent home SMBG.

More frequent injections better mimic pancreatic function. Increasing the number of injections from 2 to 4 per day results in improved glycemic control and perinatal outcomes without increasing the risk of maternal hypoglycemia, pre-term labor or cesarean section rates (85). Insulin requirements increase throughout pregnancy, as a result of increasing hormones of pregnancy and subsequent increasing insulin resistance (86).

Starting doses of insulin in massively obese women are typically 1.5 to 2 U/kg. Twin gestations frequently need twice these requirements. Aggressive use of insulin, with frequent monitoring (6 times per day) and appropriate titration of insulin, decreased macrosomia in one clinic from 18% to 7% (87). No insulin is currently FDA approved for use in pregnancy and only human insulin is recommended. Regular insulin and NPH insulin have long been used in treatment of diabetes in pregnancy, but insulin lispro has been used with increasing frequency in pregnancy since its approval in 1996. Insulin lispro and other rapid-acting analogs offer the benefit of closely controlling post-prandial glucose excursion, without causing late-postprandial or pre-prandial hypoglycemia. Retrospective studies have not shown any significant difference between insulin lispro and regular insulin, however, in regard to either fetal or maternal outcomes (88). To demonstrate that insulin lispro provided better postprandial glucose control than human regular insulin, (42) women with GDM who failed control with diet alone were randomized to NPH and Regular human insulin or NPH and insulin lispro. The group that received insulin lispro had significantly lower glucose levels after meals without an increase in hypoglycemia (89).

One complication of insulin therapy during pregnancy has been the development of insulin antibodies. The presence of insulin antibodies has been associated with macrosomia in the infant, independent of maternal glucose concentration(90). For this reason, animal source insulins such as beef and pork insulins are contraindicated in pregnancy. Human insulin preparations with low antigenicity will minimize transplacental transport of insulin antibodies. Lispro, aspart and glulisine, three rapid acting insulin analogs, are comparable to human insulin in terms of immunogenicity. Only lispro and aspart have been studied in pregnancy. They have minimal transplacental transfer and no reported teratogenesis. Antibodies have not been found in cord blood in patients receiving insulin lispro (89,91–95). Insulin aspart is associated with the development of insulin antibodies initially after treatment. This is a theoretical concern with insulin aspart, since it takes approximately 3 months for antibodies to form, at which point parturition has occurred and GDM has resolved. More data is needed to further assess insulin aspart. The use of the long-acting insulin analog, insulin glargine, is not recommended in pregnancy. Insulin glargine is associated with increased IGF–1 receptor binding. This carries theoretical risks and studies of IGF-1–receptor binding indicated that there was an increase in both IGF-1–receptor affinity and mitogenic potency in a cell-culture model that used human osteosarcoma cells (96). There are theoretical toxicologic effects of these changes, including development of mammary, ovarian, and bone tumors in addition to the development of diabetic retinopathy (88). This preparation, as well as the insulin detemir, are considered category C by the Food and Drug Administration.

Oral Hypoglycemic Agents

Oral hypoglycemic agents are not approved or recommended in the US for treatment of GDM. Older sulfonylureas, such as tolbutamide and chlorpropramide, cross the placenta and cause fetal hyperinsulinemia and macrosomia. They also have the potential to cause prolonged neonatal hypoglycemia. Minimal amounts of glyburide, however, cross the placenta (97). In a study of 404 women with mild GDM randomly assigned to receive either glyburide or insulin, the results demonstrated that the groups achieved similar glycemic control, with no differences in the frequency of macrosomia, neonatal hypoglycemia, and neonatal morbidity, or cord insulin concentration levels, between groups (98,99). The mean blood glucose was 105 mg/dL in both groups. A number of other studies have described the use of glyburide in pregnancy (100–105). Though the results have been promising, more safety and efficacy data are needed before further recommendations can be made.

Although not approved, women with GDM have also been treated with metformin (106–111). To date there are no published randomized trials evaluating metformin in GDM. There is favorable observational data in pregestational diabetics (107–111), but more data in GDM is anticipated. Currently, studies are underway to elucidate the safety and efficacy of metformin in GDM.

Two preliminary studies have suggested efficacy in reducing postprandial glucose excursions in GDM using acarbose, an alpha glucosidase inhibitor. It is poorly absorbed from the gastrointestinal tract resulting in an increased incidence of abdominal cramping. Since a small proportion of this drug may be absorbed systemically, further study should evaluate potential transplacental passage. There are no controlled data available in pregnancy with the use of thiazolidinediones, glinides, dipeptidyl peptidase-4 (DPP-4) inhibitors, or GLP-1 agonists. One study reported that rosiglitazone crossed the human placenta at 12 weeks gestation, fetal tissue levels were about half of maternal serum levels (112). These agents are considered experimental in pregnancy.

TIMING AND NATURE OF DELIVERY

Contemporary efforts to maintain normoglycemia during pregnancy with diet, exercise, and aggressive insulin therapy may result in normalization of HbA1c and near-normal glucose profiles throughout the day by SMBG. Despite this degree of near-normalization of glycemia, neonatal morbidity persists (7).

The optimum timing of delivery is controversial. Most experts agree that women with GDM should be delivered at term. GDM is not an indication for elective cesarean delivery or for delivery prior to 38 weeks in the absence of fetal compromise (1). Most deliveries in patients with GDM, however, occur at 38 to 39 weeks, with a resulting 30% cesarean section rate, without any outcome data to support this practice (113). The Toronto Tri-Hospital study found that making the diagnosis of GDM alone increased cesarean delivery rates, without apparent explanation (114). Similar results were seen by Buchanan, when women with GDM randomized to receive insulin had a higher cesarean section rate, despite reduction in the percentage of large-for-gestational-age babies, compared with those who did not receive insulin therapy (83).

Nevertheless, indications for early delivery include macrosomia (estimated weight >4000 g) or large-for-gestational-age infants, poor maternal compliance, history of previous stillbirth, and presence of vasculopathy or hypertension. During labor and delivery, insulin is usually not indicated. An infusion of normal saline is usually sufficient to maintain normoglycemia. To decrease the risk of adverse outcomes (hypoglycemia, hyperbilirubinemia, hypocalcemia, erythremia) during labor, maternal hyperglycemia should be avoided. The recommended maternal blood glucose concentration should be maintained between 70 and 90 mg/dL.

POST-NATAL CARE AND FUTURE RISK

With delivery, insulin resistance markedly declines as the hormones of pregnancy decline; insulin sensitivity returns within a few hours of delivery of the placenta. Most women with GDM no longer require insulin. Nearly all women (>90%) with GDM are normoglycemic after delivery. However, they are at risk for recurrent GDM, IGT, and overt diabetes. Up to two-thirds of women with GDM will have GDM in a subsequent pregnancy (115–117). The recurrence rate of GDM is reported as 30% to 70% depending on the study cited (118–121) and has been associated with infant birth weight in the index pregnancy, maternal fat intake (122), and maternal pre-pregnancy weight of the subsequent pregnancy. Women who have a recurrence tend to be older, with a greater increase in weight between their pregnancies than women without a recurrence (116).

The lifetime risk of developing type 2 diabetes remains high. The risk of progression to diabetes within 5 years approaches 50% (120) and is associated with gestational age at diagnosis, impairment of beta-cell function, severity of GDM, obesity and subsequent pregnancy. Up to 20% of women with GDM have IGT during the early postpartum period (118–124). Risk factors for IGT and future diabetes are the presence of autoantibodies including glutamic acid decarboxylase, gestational requirement for insulin, maternal obesity, high fasting blood glucose concentrations during pregnancy and early postpartum, and early gestational age at the time of diagnosis (118). Kim, et al. reported the cumulative incidence of future diabetes ranging from 2.6% to 70% (15). The greatest increase in risk was during the first five years after a pregnancy with GDM with a plateau after ten years. In one study, type 2 diabetes occurred in 12% of women with normal glucose tolerance 4 to 16 weeks after delivery versus 84% of women with IGT at that time (121). Early postpartum insulin resistance is correlated with future diabetes risk.

The Diabetes Prevention Program (DPP) sought involvement of women with a history of GDM and IGT to participate in a long-term diabetes prevention study (125). Three hundred and fifty women provided a history of GDM with a mean of 12 years since the index GDM pregnancy. The women with a history of GDM in the placebo group had a 74% increased hazard for developing diabetes compared to their nonGDM controls (17.1%/year compared to 9.8%/year over 3 years, respectively) (125). The data suggest that GDM confers a markedly increased risk for developing diabetes even when compared to a comparably glucose intolerant population (125).

Blood glucose should be measured on the day after delivery to ensure that the mother no longer has hyperglycemia, using criteria established for nonpregnant individuals. A woman with GDM will be able to resume a regular diet postpartum. She should continue to measure blood glucose intermittently at home for a few weeks after discharge from the hospital and report any high values to her physician, especially if she was diagnosed early in gestation or required insulin during the pregnancy.

The ADA recommends that an oGTT be repeated 6 weeks postpartum to ensure resolution of normal carbohydrate handling, and regular postpartum surveillance and annual assessment for diabetes (1). All subsequent pregnancies carry a risk for GDM; therefore patients should be counseled about planning pregnancies with appropriate pre-pregnancy counseling and evaluation. FPG should be measured annually.

A number of studies are addressing the possibility of drug intervention to prevent the onset of diabetes in patients with GDM. The Troglitazone in Prevention of Diabetes (TRIPOD) and Pioglitazone in Prevention of Diabetes (PIPOD) studies were conducted in Hispanic-American women with recent gestational diabetes. TRIPOD is a randomized, placebo-controlled trial in which demonstrated a 55% reduction in the incidence of diabetes during a median of 30 months on troglitazone (126,127). There was a close association between reduction in insulin output during IVGTTs at three months on trial (β-cell rest) and protection from diabetes, persistent protection from diabetes 8 months post-drug, and stable glucose and β-cell function for 4.5 years in women who did not get diabetes during troglitazone treatment (126,127). The PIPOD study is an open-label treatment with pioglitazone, in women who completed TRIPOD. The annual diabetes rate was 4.6%. Multivariate analysis revealed two independent predictors of diabetes: oGTT glucose area at baseline and change in IVGTT total insulin area at one year (128). Together, the TRIPOD and PIPOD studies demonstrate that prevention of type 2 diabetes is possible through β-cell rest.

SUMMARY

GDM affects approximately 1% to 13% of all pregnancies and results from insulin resistance in the setting of limited β-cell reserve. Early universal screening and detection are important to optimize maternal and fetal outcomes. Screening should be performed at 24 to 28 weeks of gestation and earlier if there is a clinical concern of undiagnosed pregestational diabetes. The 50-g oGTT is used for screening. A 3-hour oral 100-g oGTT is used in women who screen positive, but a 75-g 2-h oral glucose tolerance test is also acceptable. Currently, the criteria proposed by the Fourth International Workshop-Conference on Gestational Diabetes are used to diagnose gestational diabetes with >2 of the following noted:

- Fasting serum glucose concentration >95 mg/dL
- One-hour serum glucose concentration >180 mg/dL
- Two-hour serum glucose concentration >155 mg/dL
- Three-hour serum glucose concentration >140 mg/dL

The results of HAPO are anticipated for definitive diagnostic criteria. Achieving the desired weight and glycemic goals require aggressive management. MNT is the first line of treatment and is successful for the majority of women. Failure to achieve the desired goals of therapy within a short period of time is an indication for insulin therapy. Small studies have been done in women using oral agents, but more data is needed before recommending the use of oral agents globally. Although most women revert to normal glucose-tolerance postpartum, the lifetime risk of developing type 2 diabetes remains high and close surveillance of these women is indicated.

REFERENCES

1. Metzger BE, Coustan DR., The Organizing Committee. Summary and recommendations of the fourth international workshop–conference on gestational diabetes mellitus. Diabetes Care 1998; 21 (Suppl 2):B161–7.
2. Dabelea D, Snell-Bergeon JK, Hartsfield CL, et al. Increasing prevalence of gestational diabetes mellitus (GDM) over time and by birth cohort: Kaiser Permanente of Colorado GDM Screening Program. Diabetes Care 2005; 28:579.
3. Carpenter MW, Coustan DR, Criteria for screening tests for gestational diabetes. Am J Obstet Gynecol 1982; 144:768–72.
4. Nicholson WK, Fox HE, Cooper LA, Strobino D, Witter F, Powe NR. Maternal race, procedures, and infant birth weight in type 2 and gestational diabetes. Obstet Gynecol. 2006; 108(3 Pt 1):626–34.
5. Silva JK, Kaholokula JK, Ratner R, Mau M. Ethnic differences in perinatal outcome of gestational diabetes mellitus. Diabetes Care 2006; 29(9):2058–63.

6. Centers for Disease Control. Prenatal care and pregnancies complicated by diabetes. US reporting areas, 1989. MMWR CDC Surveill Summ 1993; 42:119.
7. Hod M, Merlob P, Freidman S, et al. Gestational diabetes mellitus a survey of perinatal complication in the 1980s. Diabetes 1991; (Suppl 2):74.
8. Kjos SL, Buchanan TA, Greenspoon JS, et al. Gestational diabetes mellitus: the prevalence of glucose intolerance and diabetes mellitus in the first two months post partum. Am J Obstet Gynecol 1990; 163:93–8.
9. Catalano PM, Vargo KM, Bernstein IM, et al. Incidence and risk factors associated with abnormal postpartum glucose tolerance in women with gestational diabetes. Am J Obstet Gynecol 1991; 165:914.
10. Kjos SL, Peters RK, Xiang A, et al. Predicting future diabetes in Latino women with gestational diabetes. Diabetes 1995; 44:586.
11. Metzger BE, Cho NH, Roston SM, et al. Prepregnancy weight and antepartum insulin secretion predict glucose tolerance 5 years after gestational diabetes mellitus. Diabetes 1993; 16:1598.
12. O'Sullivan JB. Diabetes mellitus after GDM. Diabetes 1991; 40:131.
13. O'Sullivan JB. Body weight and subsequent diabetes mellitus. J Am Med Assoc 1982; 248:949.
14. O'Sullivan JB, Mahan CM. Criteria for the oral glucose tolerance test in pregnancy. Diabetes 1964; 13:278–85.
15. Kim C, Newton KM, Knopp RH. Gestational Diabetes and the Incidence of Type 2 Diabetes: A systematic review. Diabetes Care 2002; 25:1862.
16. Langer O, Levy J, Brustman L, et al. Glycemic control in gestational diabetes mellitus: how tight is tight enough: small for gestational age versus large for gestational age? Am J Obstet Gynecol 1989; 161:646–53.
17. Sermer M, Naylor CD, Gare DJ, et al. Impact of increasing carbohydrate intolerance on material fetal outcomes in 3637 women without gestation diabetes: the Toronto Tri-Hospital Gestational Diabetes Project. Am J Obstet Gynecol 1995; 173:146–56.
18. Jang HC, Cho NH, Min Y-K, et al. Increased macrosomia and perinatal morbidity independent of maternal obesity and advanced age in Korean women with GDM. Diabetes Care 1997; 20: 1582–8.
19. Pettitt DJ, Bennett PH, Hanson RL, et al. Comparison of World Health Organization and National Diabetes Data Group procedures to detect abormalities of glucose tolerance during pregnancy. Diabetes Care 1994; 17:1264–8.
20. Catalano PM, Tyzbir ED, Wolfe RR, et al. Carbohydrate metabolism during pregnancy in control subjects and women with gestational diabetes. Am J Physiol 1993; 264:E60–7.
21. Ciraldi TP, Kettel M, el-Roeil A, et al. Mechanisms of cellular insulin resistance in human pregnancy. Am J Obstet Gynecol 1994; 170:635–41.
22. Kuhl C. Aetiology of gestational diabetes. Baillere's Clin Obstet Gynecol 1991; 5:279.
23. Butte NF. Carbohydrate and lipid metabolism in pregnancy: normal compared with gestational diabetes mellitus. Am J Clin Nutr 2000; 71:1256S.
24. Homko CJ, Sivan E, Reece EA, Boden G. Fuel metabolism during pregnancy. Semin Reprod Endocrinol 1999; 17:119.
25. Yamashita H, Shao J, Friedman JE. Physiologic and molecular alterations in carbohydrate metabolism during pregnancy and gestational diabetes mellitus. Clin Obstet Gynecol 2000; 43:87.
26. Catalano PM, Kirwan JP, Haugel-de Mouzon S, King J. Gestational diabetes and insulin resistance: role in short- and long-term implications for mother and fetus. J Nutr 2003; 133:1674S.
27. Freinkel N. Effects of the conceptus on maternal metabolism. In Leibel BS, Wrenshall GA, editors. Amsterdam: Excerpta Medica, 1964: 675–91.
28. Freinkel N. The Banting Lecture 1980: of pregnancy and progeny. Diabetes 1980; 29:1023–35.
29. Hormes PJ, Kuhl C, Lauritsa KB. Gastro-enteral-pancreatic hormone in gestational diabetes: a response to protein rich meal. Horm Metab Res 1982; 14:335–8.
30. Garvey WT, Maianu L, Hancock JA. Amsterdam Gene expression of GLUT 4 in skeletal muscle from insulin resistant patients with obesity, IGT, GDM and NIDDM. Diabetes 1992; 41: 465–75.
31. Garvey WT, Maianu L, Zhu JH, et al. Multiple defects in the adipocyte glucose transport system cause cellular insulin resistance in gestational diabetes. Diabetes 1993; 42:1773–85.
32. Metzgar BE, Coustan DR. The Organizing Committee. Summary and recommendations of the Fourth International Workshop Conference on Gestational Diabetes Mellitus. Diabetes Care 1998; 21(Suppl. 2):B61.
33. Report on the expert committee on the diagnosis and classification of diabetes mellitus. Diabetes Care 1997; 20:1183–97.
34. American Diabetes Association. Gestational diabetes mellitus. Diabetes Care 2002; 25(Suppl. 1): S94–6.
35. Solomon CG, Willett WC, Carey VJ, et al. A prospective study of pregravid determinants of gestational diabetes mellitus. J Am Med Assoc 1997; 278:1078.

36. Moses RG, Davis WS. Gestational diabetes: do lean young Caucasian women need to be tested? Diabetes Care 1998; 21:1803–6.
37. Coustan DR, Widness JA, Marshall W, et al. Should the fifty-gram, one-hour plasma glucose screening test for gestational diabetes be administered in the fasting for fed state? Am J Obstet Gynecol 1986; 154:1031–5.
38. O'Sullivan JB, Charles D, Mahan CM, et al. Gestational diabetes and perinatal mortality rate. Am J Obstet Gynecol 1973; 116:901.
39. National Diabetes Data Group. Classification and diagnosis of diabetes mellitus and other categories of glucose intolerance. Diabetes 1979; 28:1039.
40. Sacks DA, Greenspoon JS, Abu-Fadil S, et al. Toward universal criteria for gestational diabetes: The 75-gram glucose tolerance test in pregnancy. Am J Obstet Gynecol 1995; 172:607.
41. Lind T, Phillips PR. The DPSG of the EASD. Influence of pregnancy on the 75 g OGTT: a prospective multicenter study. Diabetes 1991; 40(Suppl 2):8.
42. World Health Organization. Diabetes mellitus: report of a WHO study group. Technical Report Series. Geneva: World Health Organization, 1985. Report No.: 727.
43. Moses RG, Moses M, Russell KG, Schier GM. The 75 g glucose tolerance test in pregnancy: a reference range determined on a low-risk population and related to selected pregnancy outcomes. Diabetes Care 1998; 21:1807–11.
44. Pettitt DJ, Knowler WC, Baird HR, Bennett PH. Gestational diabetes: infant and maternal complications of pregnancy in relation to third-trimester glucose tolerance in Pima Indians. Diabetes Care 1980; 3:458–64.
45. Tallarigo L, Giampietro O, Penno G, et al. Relation of glucose tolerance test to complications of pregnancy in nondiabetic women. N Engl J Med 1986; 315:989.
46. Lindsay MK, W. G, Klein L. The relationship of one abnormal glucose tolerance test value in pregnancy complications. Obstet Gynecol 1989; 73:103–6.
47. Berkus MD, Langer O. Glucose tolerance test: degree of glucose abnormality correlates with neonatal outcome. Obstet Gynecol 1993; 81:344.
48. Freeman H, Looney JM, Hoskins RG. Spontaneous variability of oral glucose tolerance. J Clin Endocrinol 1942; 2:431.
49. Catalano PM, Avallone D, Drago NM, Amini SV. Reproducibility of the oral glucose tolerance test in pregnant women. Am J Obstet Gynecol 1993; 169:874.
50. HAPO Study Cooperative Research Group. The Hyperglycemia and Adverse Pregnancy Outcome (HAPO) Study. International Journal of Gynecology & Obstetrics 2002; 78:69–77.
51. Coustan DR, Imarah J. Prophylactic insulin treatment of gestational diabetes reduces the incidence of macrosomia, operative delivery and birth trauma. Am J Obstet Gynecol 1984; 150: 846–42.
52. Combs CA, Gunderson E, Kitzmiller JL, et al. Relationship of fetal macrosomia to maternal postprandial glucose control during pregnancy. Diabetes Care 1992; 15:1251–7.
53. Jovanovic-Peterson L, Peterson CM, Reed GF, et al. Maternal postprandial glucose levels predict infant birth weight: the diabetes in early pregnancy study. Am J Obstet Gynecol 1991; 164:103–11.
54. DeVeciana M, Major CA, Morgan MA, et al. Postprandial versus preprandial blood glucose monitoring in women with gestational diabetes mellitus requiring insulin therapy. N Engl J Med 1995; 333:1237.
55. Gabbe S, Gregory RP, Power ML, et al. Management of Diabetes Mellitus by Obstetrician–Gynecologists. Obstetrics and Gynecology 2004; 103:1229–34.
56. Ogata ES, Sabbagha R, Metzgar BE, et al. Serial ultrasonography to assess evolving fetal macrosomia. J Am Med Assoc 1980; 243:2405–8.
57. Langer O, Kozlowski S, Brustman L. Abnormal growth patterns in diabetes in pregnancy: a longitudinal study. Israel J Med Sci 1991; 243:2405–8.
58. Wechter D J, Kaufmann RC, Amankwah KS, et al. Prevention of neonatal macrosomia in gestational diabetes by the use of intensive dietary therapy and home glucose monitoring. Am J Perinatol 1994; 8:131–4.
59. King J, Allen H. Nutrition during pregnancy. National Academy of Science 1990. Washington, DC: National Academy Press, 1990.
60. Ratner RE, Hamner LH, Isada NB. Effects of gestational weight gain in morbidly obese women. I. Maternal morbidity. Am J Perinatal 1991; 8:21–4.
61. Ratner RE, Hamner LH, Isada NB. Effects of gestational weight gain in morbidly obese women: II. Fetal effects. Am J Perinatal 1990; 7:295–9.
62. Algert A, Shragg P, Hollingsworth DR. Moderate caloric restriction in obese women with gestational diabetes. Obstet Gynecol 1985; 65:487–91.
63. Buchanan TA, Metzger BE, Freinkel N. Accelerated starvation in late pregnancy: A comparison between obese women with and without gestational diabetes mellitus. Am J Obstet Gynecol 1990; 162:1015–20.

64. Churchill JA, Berrendes HW, Nemore J. Neuropsychological deficits in children of diabetic mothers: a report for the Collaborative Study of Cerebral Palsy. Am J Obstet Gynecol 1969; 105: 257–68.

65. Rizzo T, Metzger BE, Burns WJ, Burns K. Correlations between antepartum maternal metabolism and child intelligence. N Engl J Med 1991; 325:911–6.

66. Peterson CM, Jovanovic-Peterson L. Percentage of carbohydrate and glycemic response to breakfast, lunch and dinner in women with gestational diabetes. Diabetes 1991; 40(Suppl 2):172–4.

67. Jovanovic-Peterson L, Peterson CM Dietary manipulation as the primary treatment strategy for pregnancies complicated by diabetes. J Am Coll Nutr 1990; 9:320.

68. Magee MS, Knopp RH, Benedetti TJ. Metabolic effects of 1,200–kcal diet in obese pregnant women with gestational diabetes. Diabetes 1990; 39:234–40.

69. Major CA, Henry MJ, DeVeciana M, Morgan MS. The effects of carbohydrate restriction in patients with diet-controlled gestational diabetes. Obstet Gynecol 1998; 91:600–4.

70. Jovanovic-Peterson L, Peterson CM. Nutritional management of the obese gestational diabetic woman. J Am Coll Nutr 1996; 11:246–50.

71. Diabetes and pregnancy. Technical bulletin. American College of Obstetricians and Gynecologists 1994: Report No.: 200.

72. Jovanovic-Peterson L, Peterson CM. Exercise and the nutritional management of diabetes during pregnancy. Obstet Gynecol Clin North Am 1996; 23:75–86.

73. Bung P, Artal R. Gestational diabetes and exercise: a survey. Semin Perinatal 1996; 20:328–33.

74. Dye TD, Knox KL, Artal R, et al. Physical activity, obesity and diabetes in pregnancy. Am J Epidemiol 1997; 146:961–5.

75. Jovanovic-Peterson L, Durak EP, Peterson CM. Randomized trial of diet versus diet plus cardiovascular conditioning on glucose levels in gestational diabetes. Am J Obstet Gynecol 1989; 161(2):415–9.

76. Bung P, Artal R, Khodiguian N, Kjos S. Exercise in gestational diabetes. An optional therapeutic approach? Diabetes 1991 40; Suppl 2:182–5.

77. Exercise during pregnancy and the postpartum period. American College of Obstetrics and Gynecology committee opinion. No 267. Obstet Gynecol 2002; 99:171–3.

78. Langer O, Hod M. Management of gestational diabetes mellitus. Obstet Gynecol Clin N Am 1996; 23:137–59.

79. McFarland MR, Langer O, Conway DL, Berkus MD. Dietary therapy for gestational diabetes: how long is long enough? Obstet Gynecol 1999; 93:978–82.

80. The 4th International Workshop on Gestational Diabetes. Diabetes Care 2003; 26:S103–5.

81. American College of Obstetricians and Gynecologists. Gestational Diabetes. ACOG practice bulletin #30, American College of Obstetricians and Gynecologists, Washington, DC, 2001.

82. Gestational diabetes mellitus. Diabetes Care 2004; 27(Suppl 1):S88.

83. Buchanan TA, Kjos SL, Montoro MN, et al. Use of fetal ultrasound to select metabolic therapy for pregnancies complicated by mild gestational diabetes. Diabetes Care 1994; 17:275–83.

84. Kjos SL, Schaefer-Graf U, Sardesi S, et al. A randomized controlled trial using glycemic plus fetal ultrasound parameters versus glycemic parameters to determine insulin therapy in gestational diabetes with fasting hyperglycemia Diabetes Care 2001; 24:1904–10.

85. Nachum A, Ben-Shlomo I, Weiner E, Shalev E. Twice versus four times daily insulin dose regimens for diabetes in pregnancy: randomized controlled trial. Br Med J 1999; 319:1223–7.

86. Jovanovic L, Druzen M, Peterson CM. Effects of euglycemia on the outcome of pregnancy in inuslin-dependant diabetic women as compared with normal control subjects. Am J Med 1981; 71:921–7.

87. Jovanovic-Peterson L, Bevier W, Petersen CM. The Santa Barbara County Health Services Program: birthweight change concomitant with screening for and treatment of glucose intolerance of pregnancy: a potential cost-effective intervention. Am J Perinatal 1997; 14:221–8.

88. Hirsch IB. Insulin analogues. N Engl J Med 2005; 352:174–183.

89. Jovanovic L, Ilic S, Pettitt D, et al. The metabolic and immunologic effects of insulin lispro. Diabetes Care 1999; 22:1422–7.

90. Menon RK, Cohen RM, Sperling MA, et al. Transplacental passage of insulin in pregnant women with insulin-dependent diabetes mellitus. Its role in fetal macrosomia. N Engl J Med 1990; 323: 309–15.

91. Boskovic R, Feig DS, Derewlany L, Knie B, Portnoi G, Koren G. Transfer of insulin lispro across the human placenta: in vitro perfusion studies. Diabetes Care 2003; 26:1390–4.

92. Di Cianni G, Volpe L, Lencioni C, et al. Use of Insulin Glargine During the First Weeks of Pregnancy in Five Type 1 Diabetic Women. Diabetes Care 2005; 28:982–3.

93. Bhattacharyya A, Brown S, Hughes S, Vice PA. Insulin lispro and regular insulin in pregnancy. QJM 2001; 94:255–60.

94. Masson EA, Patmore JE, Brash PD, et al. Pregnancy outcome in Type 1 diabetes mellitus treated with insulin lispro (Humalog). Diabet Med 2003; 20:46–50.

95. Gabbe SG, Graves CR. Management of diabetes mellitus complicating pregnancy. Obstet Gynecol 2003; 102:857–68.

96. Kurtzhals P, Schäffer L, Sørensen A, et al. Correlations of receptor binding and metabolic and mitogenic potencies of insulin analogs designed for clinical use. Diabetes 2000; 49:999–1005.

97. Elliot BD, Langer O, Shenker S, Johnson RF. Insignificant transfer of glyburide occurs in the human placenta. Am J Obstet Gynecol 1991; 165:807.

98. Langer O, Conway DL, Berkus MD, et al. A comparison of glyburide and insulin in women with gestational diabetes mellitus. N Engl J Med 2000; 343:1134–8.

99. Langer O, Yogev Y, Xenakis EM, Rosenn B. Insulin and glyburide therapy: dosage, severity level of gestational diabetes, and pregnancy outcome. Am J Obstet Gynecol 2005; 192:134.

100. Kremer CJ, Duff P. Glyburide for the treatment of gestational diabetes. Am J Obstet Gynecol 2004; 190:1438.

101. Yogev Y, Ben-Haroush A, Chen R, et al. Undiagnosed asymptomatic hypoglycemia: diet, insulin, and glyburide for gestational diabetic pregnancy. Obstet Gynecol 2004; 104:88.

102. Jacobson GF, Ramos GA, Ching JY, et al. Comparison of glyburide and insulin in the management of gestational diabetes in a large managed care organization. Am Obstet Gynecol 2005; 193:118.

103. Gabbe SG, Graves CR. Management of diabetes mellitus complicating pregnancy. Obstet Gynecol 2003; 102:857.

104. Saade G. Gestational diabetes mellitus: a pill or a shot? Obstet Gynecol 2005; 105:456.

105. Conway DL, Gonzales O, Skiver D. Use of glyburide for the treatment of gestational diabetes: the San Antonio experience. J Matern Fetal Neonatal Med 2004; 15:51.

106. Coetzee EJ, Jackson WPU. Metformin in management of pregnant insulin-dependent diabetics. Diabetologia 1979; 16:241–5.

107. Coetzee EJ, Jackson WPU. Diabetes newly diagnosed during pregnancy. A 4-year study at Groote Schur Hospital. S Afr Med J 1979; 56:467–75.

108. Hellmuth E, Damm P, Molsted-Pedersen L. Oral hypoglycaemic agents in 188 diabetic pregnancies. Diabet Med 2000; 7:507–11.

109. Coetzee EJ, Jackson WP. Oral hypoglycaemics in the first trimester and fetal outcome. S Afr Med J 1984; 65:635.

110. Glueck CJ, Wang P, Kobayashi S, et al. Metformin therapy throughout pregnancy reduces the development of gestational diabetes in women with polycystic ovary syndrome. Fertil Steril 2002; 77:520.

111. Glueck CJ, Goldenberg N, Pranikoff J, et al. Height, weight, and motor-social development during the first 18 months of life in 126 infants born to 109 mothers with polycystic ovary syndrome who conceived on and continued metformin through pregnancy. Hum Reprod 2004; 19:1323.

112. Chan LY, Yeung JH, Lau TK. Placental transfer of rosiglitazone in the first trimester of human pregnancy. Fertil Steril 2005; 83:955.

113. Langer O, Rodrigues SA, Xenakis EM-J, et al. Intensified versus conventional management of gestational diabetes. Am J Obstet Gynecol 1994; 170:1036–47.

114. Naylor CD, Sermer M, Chen E, Sykora K. Cesarean delivery in relation to birth weight and gestational glucose tolerance. J Am Med Assoc 1996; 275:1165–70.

115. Philipson EH, Super DM. Gestational diabetes mellitus: does it recur in subsequent pregnancy? Am J Obstet Gynecol 1989; 160:1324.

116. Moses RG. The recurrence rate of gestational diabetes in subsequent pregnancies. Diabetes Care 1996; 19:1348.

117. MacNeill S, Dodds L, Hamilton DC, et al. Rates and risk factors for recurrence of gestational diabetes. Diabetes Care 2001; 24:659.

118. Moses RG. The recurrence rate of gestational diabetes in subsequent pregnancies. Diabetes Care 1996; 19:1348–50.

119. Major CA, DeVicianna M, Weeks J, Morgan MA. Recurrence of gestational diabetes: who is at risk? Am J Obstet Gynecol 1998; 179:1038–42.

120. Phillipson EH, Super DM. Gestational diabetes mellitus: Does it reoccur in subsequent pregnancy? Am J Obstet Gynecol 1989; 160:1324.

121. MacNeill S, Dodds L, Hamilton DC, et al. Rates and risk factors for recurrence of gestational diabetes. Diabetes Care 2001; 24:659–62.

122. Moses RG, Shand JL, Tapsell LC. The recurrence of gestational diabetes: could dietary differences in fat intake be an explanation? Diabetes Care 1997; 20:1647–50.

123. Lobner K, Knopff A, Baumgarten A, et al. Predictors of postpartum diabetes in women with gestational diabetes mellitus. Diabetes 2006; 55(3):792–7.

124. Kjos SL, Peters RK, Xiang A, et al. Predicting future diabetes in Latino women with gestational diabetes: Utility of early postpartum glucose tolerance testing. Diabetes 1995; 44:586.

125. Ratner RE, et al. Prevention of type 2 diabetes in women with previous gestational diabetes mellitus: the diabetes preventions program. Accepted in Diabetes Care 2007; 30:S242–S245.

126. Azen SP, Berkowitz K, Kjos S, Peters R, Xiang A, Buchanan TA: TRIPOD: a randomized placebo-controlled trial of troglitazone in women with prior gestational diabetes mellitus. Controlled Clinical Trials 1998; 19:217–231.
127. Buchanan TA, Xiang AH, Peters RK, et al. Preservation of pancreatic beta-cell function and prevention of type 2 diabetes by pharmacological treatment of insulin resistance in high-risk hispanic women. Diabetes 2002; 51(9):2796–803.
128. Xiang AH, Peters RK, Kjos SL, et al. Effect of pioglitazone on pancreatic beta-cell function and diabetes risk in Hispanic women with prior gestational diabetes. Diabetes 2006; 55(2):517–22.

24 | Epidemiology of Type 2 Diabetes in Children and Adolescents

Arlan L. Rosenbloom
Department of Pediatrics, Division of Endocrinology, University of Florida College of Medicine, Gainesville, Florida, U.S.A.

In 1971, Harvey Knowles made the prescient observation that,

A second type of diabetes in young persons closely resembles that of the stable middle-aged onset type. Herein the patients as a rule have no symptoms, are overweight, can secrete insulin, and respond to sulfonylurea therapy. Often the diagnosis is made serendipitously. In the Juvenile Diabetic Clinic at the Cincinnati General Hospital 11 of these patients have been followed along with 300 patients with the unstable insulin deficient type of diabetes. The age of these 11 patients at diagnosis ranged from 11 to 17 years. The prevalence of this type of diabetes very likely is higher than presently appreciated, because of lack of symptoms or signs leading to suspicion of diabetes. (1)

Twenty-five years later, one-third of all new cases of diabetes in patients age 10 to 19 years in the Cincinnati clinic were type 2 diabetes; the estimated age-specific incidence was 7.2/100,000, approximately one-half the incidence rate for type 1 diabetes in the childhood population. This was a tenfold increase from 1982 to 1994. The proportion of new cases of diabetes in children diagnosed as type 2 went from 2% to 4% before 1992, unchanged from Knowles' 1971 prevalence figure of 3.7%, to 16% by 1994 (2).

Between the 1970s and the 1990s, prevalence of type 2 diabetes increased more than fivefold in young Pima Indians, from 9/1000 15- to 24-year olds to 51/1000 15- to 19-year olds, and the disease emerged in the 10 to 14 year age group with a prevalence of 22/1000 (3,4). Type 2 diabetes is also frequent among First Nations people in Canada (5). Affected females outnumber males 4 to 6 to 1 in the North American Indian populations (6).

African Americans accounted for 70% to 75% of type 2 diabetes patients in the Cincinnati report (2), and in studies from Arkansas (7). In a largely Mexican American clinic population, 31% under the age of 17 with diabetes had type 2 diabetes (8). The sex ratio in the African-American and Mexican-American groups with type 2 diabetes averages 1.5:1, far less distorted than in Native Americans (6).

In a study of 5- to 19-year-old diabetes patients diagnosed between January 1, 1994, and December 31, 1998, at the three University diabetes centers in Florida, 86% of 682 subjects were type 1 and 14% type 2. Females accounted for 63% of type 2 diabetes, but only 47% of type 1 diabetes. In contrast to the studies from Cincinnati and Arkansas, only 46% of type 2 diabetes were African-American, 22% were Hispanic, and the rest nonHispanic whites. For African Americans, the risk of developing type 2 diabetes was threefold that of whites; for Hispanics the relative risk was 3.5. The percentage of newly-diagnosed diabetes that was type 2 increased over the 5-year period from 8.7 to 19, ($p = 0.004$) (9).

Reports over the past decade from Libya, Hong Kong, Japan, Bangladesh, Australia (Aborigines), New Zealand (Maoris), and England (South Asians and Arabs) have indicated that the emergence of type 2 diabetes in young persons is a worldwide phenomenon with ethnic specificities (Table 1) (10–16). In the Tokyo prefecture in Japan, annual urine testing followed by oral glucose tolerance testing when indicated, documented a tenfold increase in type 2 diabetes incidence, from 0.2 to 2/100,000 in primary school children and a doubling among junior high school children, from 7.3 to 13.9/100,000, between 1976–80 and 1991–95, paralleling increasing obesity rates (12).

As in Japan and the US, increasing frequency of type 2 diabetes in children and adolescents in other parts of Asia and Europe is associated with the obesity epidemic (17). The US National

TABLE 1 Estimates of the Frequency of Type 2 Diabetes in Children and Adolescents

Location	Race/ethnicity	Year	Age (yrs)	Incidence per10^5	Prevalence per10^3	% of all DM	Ref.
Arizona	Pima Indian	1979	<15	0	0		
			15–24		9		3
		1996	10–14		22.3		
			15–19		50.9		4
Manitoba	First Nation		5–14		1		5
Ontario	First Nation		<16		2.3		5
Cincinnati	White, African American	1971	0–19			3.5	1
		1994	0–19			16	
			10–19	7.2		33	2
California	Mexican American	1994	0–17			45	8
Libya	Arab	1990	10–14	1.8		22	
			15–19	5.9		39	10
Tokyo	Japanese	1980	6–11	0.2			
			12–15	7.2			
		1995	6–11	2.0			
			12–15	13.9			12
Bangladesh	Asian Indian	1997	15–19		0.6		13

Abbreviation: DM, diabetes mellitus.

Health and Nutrition Examination Survey [1988–1994] identified 20% of children 12–17 years of age with BMI > 85th percentile for age and sex, the definition of overweight, and that depending on ethnicity, 8% to 17% were obese, defined as BMI > 95th percentile. Since 1980, there had been both a doubling in prevalence and an increase in the severity of obesity (18).

The Bogalusa Heart Study found a mean weight increase of 0.2 kg per year and increasing skinfold thickness from 1973 to 1994 in 11,564 5- to 24-year olds living in a biracial community in Louisiana. Overweight increased from 15 to 30%, and obesity from 5% to 11% in 5- to 14-year olds and from 5% to 15% in 15- to 17-year olds. The increases in the second 10 years of the study were 50% greater than those in the first 10 years (19). In the National Longitudinal Survey of Youth, a prospective cohort study of 8270 children aged 4 to 12 years, there was a significant increase in overweight and obesity between 1986 and 1998. In 1998, 38% of African Americans and Hispanics and 26% of whites were overweight, while 22% of African Americans and Hispanics and 12% of whites were obese (20). In Russia, 6% of ~7000 6- to 18-year olds examined in 1992 were obese and 10% were overweight, using US BMI reference data (21). A report from China indicated that 27.7% of boys and 14.1% of girls were overweight in 2003 (22). In 1996, in the United Kingdom, 22% of 6-year olds were overweight, and 10% were obese; by age 15, 31% were overweight and 17% obese (16). Numerous studies in Europe have indicated that the highest rates of childhood obesity occur in Eastern European countries, particularly Hungary, and in the southern European countries of Italy, Spain, and Greece (23,24).

CLASSIFICATION AND DIAGNOSIS OF NON–TYPE 1 DIABETES IN CHILDREN AND ADOLESCENTS

Classification

Type 2 diabetes accounts for most of the nontype 1 or nonautoimmune diabetes in children. Less commonly, other types occur, specifically maturity onset diabetes of the young (MODY) (25) and what has been termed atypical diabetes mellitus (ADM) in African-American youngsters (26). Of these three forms of nontype 1 diabetes, there is only evidence for increasing incidence in the pediatric population for type 2 diabetes.

Diagnostic Criteria

Criteria for the diagnosis of diabetes, recently revised by the American Diabetes Association, are given in Table 2 (27). Earlier criteria differed between children and adults, but the rationale for this difference was never clear (28). The new criteria were based on epidemiologic evidence of risk thresholds for the long-term complications among several populations including Pima Indians, other Americans participating in the National Health and Nutrition Survey (NHANES) and Egyptians. These risk relationships should also apply to a largely adolescent population developing type 2 diabetes.

Diagnostic Strategy

Islet cell autoantibody testing is not always reliable, and the results are not immediately available. Thus, the physician must depend on clinical judgment in classifying new-onset diabetes patients. The pathways in bold in the decision trees provided in Figure 1 indicate the most likely outcomes. Classification may only be possible after months or longer of follow-up.

In African American children with new, acute-onset diabetes, islet autoantibody testing can identify many of the children who have type 1 diabetes. If islet autoantibody studies are negative, a family history of early-onset diabetes in 3 or more generations suggests ADM. In the absence of such a family history, the absence of obesity suggests type 1 diabetes. Some children with new-onset type 1 diabetes, however, are overweight, because of the increasing prevalence of obesity in the society as a whole. Ketoacidosis or ketosis is not useful for distinguishing between type 1 diabetes, ADM, and type 2 diabetes, because as many as 25% of children with type 2 diabetes are initially seen with DKA and 40% with ketonuria (29,30). Obese children with insidious onset diabetes, commonly detected incidentally, most likely have type 2 diabetes. A family history of diabetes affecting at least one parent is found in 50% to 80%, and 75% to 100% have a first or second degree relative with type 2 diabetes (30).

The presence of islet cell autoantibodies strongly argues in favor of type 1 diabetes. Specific autoantibodies to insulin, to glutamic acid dehydrogenase (GAD), or to the tyrosine phosphatase insulinoma antibody (IA)-2 and IA-2β, are seen at the time of diagnosis in 85% to 98% of patients with immune-mediated type 1 diabetes (31). Because MODY is rare, there is no routine value in testing for HNF-4 alpha, glucokinase, HNF-1 alpha, 1PF-1, or HNF-1 beta mutations (26). Mitochondrial mutations account for < 2% of clinical type 2 diabetes in adults; therefore, studies of the mitochondrial genome and identification of genetic defects responsible for MODY remain primarily research tools (6,25).

The Florida experience noted earlier provides a perspective on the difficulty of initial classification in a relatively small subset of patients and the importance of follow-up observation with reconsideration of classification. Of the 723 patients newly diagnosed during the five-year study period, 605 were classified as type 1 and 77 as type 2; 41 were considered either atypical or remained of uncertain classification. Of those initially diagnosed as type 1 diabetes, 17 (2.8%) were subsequently reclassified as type 2 diabetes, and 6 (8%) of those initially diagnosed as type 2 diabetes were reclassified as type 1 diabetes. Most of the 17 reclassified as type 2 had been diagnosed in DKA or with ketosis (9).

TABLE 2 Criteria for the Diagnosis of Diabetes Mellitus[a]

Symptoms of diabetes plus random plasma glucose concentration ≥ 200 mg/dL (ll.l mmol/L). Casual is defined as any time of day without regard to time since last meal. Typical symptoms of diabetes include polyuria, polydipsia, and unexplained weight loss.
or
FPG ≥ 126 mg/dL (7.0 mmol/L). Fasting is defined as no caloric intake for at least 8 h.
or
2-h PG ≥ 200 mg/dL (ll.l mmol/L) during an OGTT. The test should be performed using a glucose load containing the equivalent of 75-g anhydrous glucose dissolved in water for those weighing > 43 kg and 1.75 g/kg for those weighing <43 kg.

[a] In the absence of unequivocal hyperglycemia with acute metabolic decompensation, these criteria should be confirmed by repeat testing on a different day. The third measure (OGTT) is not recommended for routine clinical use.
Abbreviations: FPG, fasting plasma glucose; OGTT, oral glucose tolerance test.
Source: From Ref. 1.

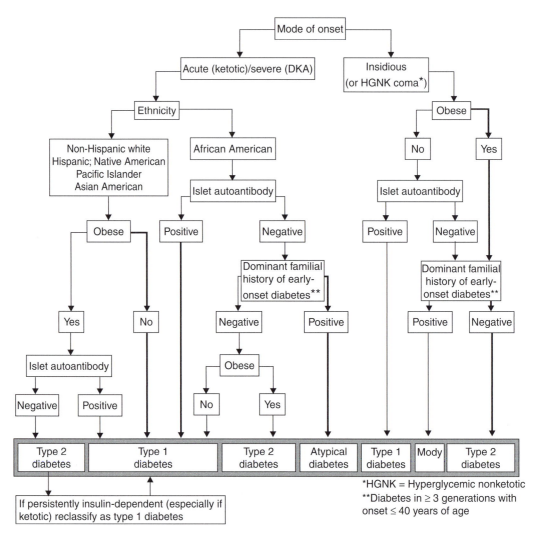

FIGURE 1   Decision tree for the clinical classification of diabetes in children.

PATHOPHYSIOLOGY

The epidemic of obesity, and the difficulty in losing accumulated weight suggest that there may have been an advantage to this metabolic phenotype during human evolution. The development of type 2 diabetes in susceptible individuals would not have been a disadvantage in the absence of opportunities to become obese.

The "thrifty" *genotype* hypothesis was first advanced by JV Neel (24) nearly 40 years ago and recently updated (32,33). This hypothesis explains the insulin resistance and relative beta cell insufficiency associated with the development of type 2 diabetes as an adaptation to conserve energy in times of famine. Changes in gene frequency or in the genetic pool cannot explain the rapid increases in type 2 diabetes prevalence within one or two generations in some populations, emphasizing the importance of environmental factors operating on this genetic background (Fig. 2).

The Role of Fetal and Childhood Nutrition

When it was noted that impaired glucose tolerance (IGT) or type 2 diabetes occurred in adults who had lower birth weight, smaller head circumference, and were thinner at birth, it was thought to indicate *in utero* programming that limited β-cell capacity and induced insulin

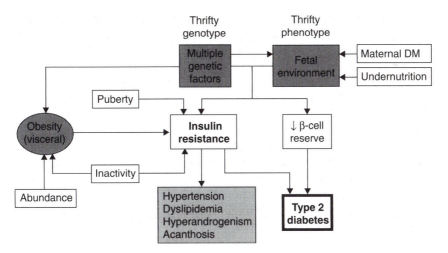

FIGURE 2   Factors in the development of type 2 diabetes in children.

resistance in peripheral tissues. Maternal malnutrition was considered the cause of islet cell hypoplasia (34,35). Later study demonstrated that the glycemic response to insulin was also reduced in individuals who had been thin at birth (44). Large studies in Sweden and the US have confirmed the association of fetal undernutrition with later type 2 diabetes risk (36,37). The adult offspring of women who had starved during the last trimester of pregnancy during the Dutch famine at the end of World War II have also been found to have increased risk for IGT (38). Underweight for gestational age has been associated with increased cortisol axis activity in urbanized South African 20-year olds who were not obese. They also had IGT compared to normal birth weight controls (39).

Two studies in young subjects from high-risk populations support findings in older subjects on the effect of fetal nutrition on the risk for development of the insulin resistance syndrome (type 2 diabetes, hypertension, hyperlipidemia) in adulthood. The relationships between birthweight, present weight, fasting and post-load glucose and insulin concentrations were examined by multiple regression analysis in 3061 Pima Indians aged 5 to 29 years. Their current weight correlated with their birthweight. A U-shaped relationship was noted between two-hour glucose concentrations and birthweight in those over 10 years of age, unrelated to present weight. When adjustment was made for height and weight, negative correlations were found between birthweight and insulin concentrations at baseline and two hours, and insulin resistance in the 2272 subjects without diabetes. These observations supported the hypothesis that insulin resistance has a survival advantage for low birthweight babies (40). In a study of 477 8-year old Indian children, the cardiovascular risk factors of insulin resistance and plasma total and LDL cholesterol concentrations were strongly related to current weight. With adjustment for current weight, age, and sex, lower birthweight was associated with elevated systolic BP, fasting plasma insulin and 32-33 split proinsulin concentrations, glucose and insulin concentrations 30 minutes after glucose, and plasma lipids. Lower birthweight was also associated with increased calculated insulin resistance. Children who had low birthweight but high-fat mass at 8 years had the highest risk for insulin resistance syndrome variables and hyperlipidemia (41).

The *thrifty phenotype* hypothesis has been developed to explain how low birthweight, reflecting fetal undernutrition, is a risk factor for the later development of the insulin resistance syndrome. Poor nutrition in fetal and early infant life would restrict the development and function of the beta cells and insulin sensitive tissues, primarily muscle, leading to insulin resistance. Obesity in later life, with the attendant insulin resistance, would overcome the limited beta cell capacity, leading to type 2 diabetes. These findings could, however, be interpreted as a reflection of the *thrifty genotype*, that genetically determined defective insulin action *in utero* results in decreased fetal growth and obesity-induced IGT in later childhood or adulthood (42).

Racial and Familial Influences

A number of studies comparing African-American and European American children suggest a genetic basis for the apparently greater susceptibility to type 2 diabetes in certain racial/ethnic groups. African Americans had greater insulin responses to oral glucose then European-Americans after adjustment for weight, age, ponderal (obesity) index, and pubertal stage, in a study of 377 children aged 5 to 17 years (43). In another study of nearly 1200 11- to 18-year olds, African Americans had higher insulin levels and lower glucose-to-insulin ratios than did European Americans, after correction for ponderal index, further indicating reduced insulin sensitivity in African-American youngsters (44). African-American prepubertal and pubertal youngsters have higher fasting and stimulated insulin concentrations during glucose clamp studies than do European-American youngsters (45). Rates of lipolysis have also been found to be significantly lower in African-American than in European-American children, further suggesting an energy conservation phenotype that would be detrimental with a surfeit of nutrition (46).

Prepubertal healthy children with a family history of type 2 diabetes ($n=9$) matched for age, pubertal status, total body adiposity determined by dual energy X-ray absorptiometry, abdominal obesity determined by computed tomography scan, and physical fitness measured by $VO_{2max}$with those without such history ($n=13$) had three hour hyperinsulinemic clamp studies to assess insulin sensitivity. Those with a family history of type 2 diabetes had lower insulin stimulated glucose disposal and nonoxidative glucose disposal; there were no differences in glucose oxidation, fat oxidation, or FFA suppression (47). These data indicate that family history of type 2 diabetes is a risk factor for insulin resistance.

The familial clustering of type 2 diabetes can indicate environmental rather than genetic causation. In a study of physical, behavioral, and environmental characteristics of 42 parents and siblings in 11 families of adolescents with type 2 diabetes, 5 mothers and 4 fathers had diabetes before the study and it was diagnosed in 3 of the remaining fathers during the study. All 42 relatives had BMI >85th percentile and skin fold measurements >90th percentile. Fat intake was high and fiber intake low; physical activity was nil to low. Eating disorders were common and diabetes control poor (48).

Maternal Diabetes

Fetal beta cell function was assessed by amniotic fluid insulin (AFI) concentration at 32 to 38 weeks gestation in 88 pregnancies with pre-gestational or gestational diabetes, The offspring had oral glucose tolerance testing annually from 18 months of age. At <5 years of age IGT was present in 1.2%, in 5.4% at 5 to 9 years, and in 19.3% at 10 to 16 years of age. There was no association between IGT and the type of maternal diabetes or macrosomia at birth. One-third of those with elevated AFI had IGT at adolescence in contrast to only one of 27 with normal AFI (49). Studies in the Pima Indian population have also indicated that the diabetic intrauterine environment is an important contributor to the risk of type 2 diabetes. The prevalence of diabetes in the offspring of Pima women with diabetes during pregnancy is significantly greater than in nondiabetic mothers or those who develop diabetes after delivery (50). These studies of the effect of diabetic pregnancy on altered β-cell function and glucoregulation later in life are of great concern because of the possible cumulative effect from generation to generation.

Insulin Resistance in Children

Puberty

The mean age at diagnosis in all studies of type 2 diabetes in children, including the Florida series, is approximately 13.5 years, corresponding to the time of peak adolescent growth and development (9,51). Puberty is a time of relative insulin resistance, with normally a 2- to 3-fold increase in peak insulin response to oral glucose and for those with type 1 diabetes, substantial increase in insulin dose (52). Insulin mediated glucose disposal averages 30% less in adolescents compared to prepubertal children or to young adults (53). This physiologic insulin resistance of puberty is readily countered by increased insulin secretion in the absence of predisposition to type 2 diabetes and the additional stress of obesity. Increased activity of the GH-IGF axis is the likely cause of this physiologic insulin resistance of puberty, because it is transitory and coincident (30).

Obesity

Approximately 55% of the variance in insulin sensitivity can be explained by total adiposity. Obese children have hyperinsulinism and 40% decrease in insulin stimulated glucose metabolism compared to the nonobese (53). There is a direct correlation between the amount of visceral fat in obese adolescents and basal and glucose stimulated insulinemia and an inverse correlation with insulin sensitivity. Body mass index increase results in decrease of insulin stimulated glucose metabolism and increase of fasting insulinemia. This inverse relationship between insulin sensitivity and abdominal fat is greater for visceral than abdominal subcutaneous fat (53).

Ovarian Hyperandrogenism and Premature Adrenarche

Polycystic ovarian syndrome (PCOS) is being increasingly recognized in adolescents, often as part of the metabolic or insulin resistance syndrome. The syndrome includes, in addition to obesity and hyperinsulinism, hypertension, hyperuricemia, PCOS, acanthosis nigricans, dyslipidemia, and elevated plasminogen activator inhibitor-1 (54). Adolescents with PCOS have an approximate 40% reduction in insulin stimulated glucose disposal in comparison to body composition matched nonhyperandrogenic control subjects (55,56). Girls with premature adrenarche are at increased risk for ovarian hyperandrogenism and PCOS (57).

It is of considerable interest that children born small for gestational age are at increased risk for premature adrenarche, similar to the increased risk for insulin resistance from intrauterine undernutrition (58–60). This link between premature adrenarche and insulin resistance has been further explored by examining 60 first-degree adult relatives of girls with precocious adrenarche. Seven of the relatives (11.6%) had type 2 diabetes and another 14 (23.3%) had glucose intolerance, compared to the reported figures for the population of the same age of 2.5% and 7.5%, respectively. At least two abnormal lipid levels were found in 40% of subjects. Gestational diabetes was common and female relatives had lower steroid hormone binding globulin levels than did population controls (61).

CASE FINDING

Epidemiologic Criteria

Screening is testing applied to a group of individuals to separate those who are well from those who have an undiagnosed disease or defect, or who are at high risk. Considerations of testing for type 2 diabetes in children begin with the assumption that this will be done in obese youngsters. Thus, determination of obesity is the screening test. Case finding, the more appropriate designation than 'screening' for testing obese children for type 2 diabetes, is defined as diagnostic testing in a population at risk (62).

Case finding is justified if the condition tested for is sufficiently *common* to justify the investment and type 2 diabetes is sufficiently common in obese children and youth to justify testing such youngsters, especially those with high-risk ethnicity or family history. Another criterion for case finding is that the condition tested for be *serious* in terms of morbidity and mortality, which is unquestionably true of type 2 diabetes in children because of the association with increased cardiovascular risk factors of hypertension and dyslipidemia, hyperandrogenism/infertility, and early onset of microvascular disease. The condition tested for should have a prolonged *latency* period without symptoms, during which abnormality can be detected. Type 2 diabetes in children is often detected in the asymptomatic state, and albuminuria may already be present at the time of diagnosis, indicative of a prolonged latency (63).

Further requirements for case finding include the availability of a test that is *sensitive* (few false negatives) and accurate with acceptable *specificity* for the test (minimal number of false positives). The fasting plasma glucose (FPG) and two-hour plasma glucose (2HPG) have been applied to risk populations and are acceptably *sensitive* and *specific*, depending on criteria selected. There must also be an *intervention* able to prevent or delay disease onset or more effectively treat the condition detected in the latency phase (63). Intervention to reverse hyperglycemia and associated dyslipidemia, or to prevent the development of overt disease in those with IGT involves the daunting challenge of changing lifestyle in asymptomatic individuals, who are at an age when long-term health goals are not on their agenda.

Testing Recommendations

A consensus panel of the American Diabetes Association recommended that individuals overweight as defined in Table 3, and with any two of the other risk factors indicated in the table should be tested every two years starting at age 10 or at the onset of puberty if that begins earlier (30). In the absence of data making definitive recommendations possible, the consensus panel considered it appropriate for the individual physician to test a specific child with any of the risk factors noted. Most instances of type 2 diabetes in children have occurred in the 10 to 19 year age group, although patients have been reported as young as five years. The FPG and the oral glucose tolerance test (FPG + 2HPG) were both considered suitable means of testing and the FPG was thought preferable by the ADA consensus panel because of lower cost and greater convenience (30). If one is testing for glucose intolerance in those at risk, however, the 2HPG will be elevated before the FPG. If necessary for convenience, PG can be measured in individuals who have taken food or drink shortly before testing. A random PG concentration ≥ 140 mg/dL (7.8 mmol/L) is considered an indication for further testing, requiring FPG or 2HPG for confirmation on a different day (27).

The first U.S. population-based study outside the native North American population has recently been reported, involving ~1500 subjects without diabetes aged 12 to 19 years from the National Health and Nutrition Examination Survey of 1999 to 2002 (64). Applying the contemporary criteria for IFG, 11% were abnormal with 95% confidence intervals of 8% to 14%; as expected, there was a significant association between glucose levels and BMI, HbA$_{1c}$, insulin, and C-peptide levels. This surprisingly high frequency of IFG in the random population not selected on the basis of risk factors might raise questions about the specificity of the IFG criterion. This criterion, however, was based on sophisticated epidemiologic analysis, as noted above. Recent studies have emphasized that FPG, similar to other biologic measures such as blood pressure and lipidemia, exists on a continuum from absolutely normal to absolutely abnormal, with predictive value for the eventual development of disease increasing as one moves toward the abnormal end of the spectrum. In a long-term follow-up of 13,000 Israeli Defense Forces recruits aged 26 to 55 years, those with normal FPG levels of < 100 mg/dL (5.6 mmol/L), but in the upper range of 91–99 mg/dL (5.1–5.5 mmol/L) were at much greater risk of developing type 2 diabetes during the years of follow-up than those with lower levels and this risk was heightened by greater BMI and serum triglyceride levels > 150 mg/dL (8.3 mmol/L) (65).

TABLE 3   Testing for Type 2 Diabetes in Children

Criteria
Overweight (BMI 85th percentile for age and sex, weight for height ≥ 85th percentile, or weight > 120% of ideal for height)
PLUS any two of the following risk factors:
Family history of type 2 diabetes in first or second degree relative
Race/Ethnicity (American Indian, African American, Hispanic, Asian/Pacific Islander)
Signs of insulin resistance or conditions associated with insulin resistance (acanthosis nigricans, hypertension, dyslipidemia, PCOS)
Age of initiation: age 10 or at onset of puberty, if puberty occurs at a younger age
Frequency: every two years
Preferred test: fasting plasma glucose

Note: Clinical judgment should be used to test for diabetes in high-risk patients who do not meet these criteria.

More extensive screening programs for investigational purposes are needed. Such studies could establish the strength and risk level of various factors that might influence the development of type 2 diabetes (blood pressure, BMI, fat distribution (waist circumference, skinfold thickness), acanthosis nigricans, family history, race/ethnicity, socioeconomic status). They would also provide useful information about the testing tools, including FPG, 2HPG, random glucose, and HbA$_{1c}$. These school based studies should be carried out in populations with sufficient numbers of high-risk youth and must be ongoing for several years, in order to track subjects with IGT, as well as those with risk factors who test normal, and to establish the predictability of various concentrations of PG and HbA$_{1c}$ (30).

PREVENTION

The long-term global public health implications of the obesity epidemic, increasing the risk of problems associated with insulin resistance and the long-term complications of diabetes, as well as respiratory and orthopedic problems with diminished performance in school and work, are ominous (66,67). That there does not appear to be any reduction in the incidence of diabetes in the Pima population despite extensive involvement of investigators and health workers for over 40 years, is of grave concern.

Prevention of the emergence of type 2 diabetes and other complications of hyperinsulinism that comprise the metabolic syndrome requires lifestyle changes, decreased caloric intake and increased physical activity, that are as basic as they are difficult. This active eucaloric lifestyle is a challenge in a culture that promotes a hypercaloric diet, excessive TV watching, video game playing, and Internet surfing combined with lack of attractive opportunities for vigorous activity in many places.

Because type 2 diabetes has been recognized in Native American youth for >15 years, summer camps and school-based education and prevention programs have been carried out in Canada and the U.S. school-based programs attempt to modify food supply in school meals, provide classroom education, and create a school environment that promotes health and physical activity. Programs for children in Headstart and kindergarten through sixth grade encourage family involvement, whereas high school based programs use social networks and peer pressure to promote behavior change and reduce risk factors. Thus far, these programs have been successful in promoting short-term behavioral change, but long-term studies are needed to determine whether persistent behavior change and reduction in the risk for type 2 diabetes occurs (5,68–70). A large longitudinal, multicenter randomized trial designed to assess the efficacy of school-based intervention on obesity and type 2 diabetes prevention has been undertaken in the United States with National Institutes of Health funding (STOPPT2DM).

Culturally relevant programs for diabetes prevention require careful analysis of the health beliefs and behaviors and the level of knowledge about the disease in the community (6). For example, a study of American Indian youth with family members having diabetes found that they did not relate the complications of retinopathy or amputation, despite their presence in the community, to diabetes. Over half of the youth thought that diabetes was contagious or caused by bad blood, and more than one-third attributed it to "weakness" (71).

The use of pharmacologic agents to reduce weight is not indicated in children until more safety and efficacy data become available (72). Orlistat, which interferes with with fat absorption, has been approved for use in children but is an unpopular choice because it causes flatulence and fecal soilage (73). Metformin has been tested in a six-month randomized placebo-controlled study of 29 black and white adolescents 12 to 19 years of age who had BMI >30 kg/m^2, type 2 diabetes family history, elevated fasting insulin and no biochemical evidence of diabetes (74). In this small study, there was less increase of BMI in those taking metformin, with a decrease in FPG and insulin levels. In adults, lifestyle intervention has been more effective than metformin in preventing progression from IGT to diabetes (75). Sibutramine, a central appetite regulator, while popular for weight control treatment of adults, has not been tested in children, nor have long-term studies assessed the effects on mortality and cardiovascular morbidity (76). Other potential pharmacologic therapies for obesity include topiramate, PYY, magnesium, and rimonabant (77). Topiramate is an anticonvulsant with effects on weight loss which are promising, but the CNS-related side effects, including memory and concentration problems and depression, preclude its use in children (78). Peptide YY3-36 (PYY) is a gut-derived peptide which modulates appetite circuits in the hypothalamus and is present in reduced concentrations in obese individuals (79). Rimonabant is an endocannabinoid inhibitor that decreases appetite and weight in overweight adults. One study showed that 39% of individuals treated with this medication lost 10% of their body weight at one year and 32% of those individuals were able to maintain their weight loss for 2 years (80). Pharmacologic manipulation of other gut-derived hormones and peptides related to hunger and satiety is being investigated. Magnesium deficiency has been associated with insulin resistance and increased risk for type 2 diabetes (81). Magnesium supplementation may, therefore, be indicated for preventing type 2 diabetes in obese children who are magnesium deficient.

Surgery is becoming increasingly popular for adult patients with significant obesity-related morbidities, including type 2 diabetes, and failure of lifestyle modification and medication. Bariatric surgery is being done for adolescents with obesity-related comorbidities in several centers (82). Gastric bypass, the traditional surgical procedure for weight loss, can result in nutrient malabsorption and death. Newer techniques, which appear to be safer, include gastric banding and vagal nerve stimulators. Long-term safety and efficacy of these procedures have not been evaluated in the pediatric population.

The prevention of type 2 diabetes can be considered as a public health approach directed to the general population, promoting improved dietary and physical activity behavior for all children and their families. At the next level, those children who are already at risk because of obesity, regardless of race/ethnicity need to be identified, tested for diabetes and, if they are normal or have IGT, a lifestyle modification program undertaken for prevention of diabetes (30).

TREATMENT

Treatment Goals

The goals of therapy are weight loss, normalization of glycemia and HbA$_{1c}$, and control of hypertension and hyperlipidemia (30,83). Pharmacologic therapy is directed at decreasing insulin resistance, increasing insulin secretion, or slowing postprandial glucose absorption.

Biguanides

The biguanides decrease blood glucose levels by acting on insulin target cells in the liver, muscle and fat. Hepatic glucose production is reduced by decreasing gluconeogenesis and insulin stimulated glucose uptake in peripheral tissues, particularly muscle, contributes to decreasing blood glucose levels (84). The biguanides also have an anorectic effect which may promote weight loss. Long-term use of biguanides has resulted in 1% to 2% reduction in plasma HbA$_{1c}$ with side effects being transient abdominal pain, diarrhea, and nausea. The major risk is the potential for lactic acidosis if the drug is given to patients with renal impairment, hepatic disease, cardiac or respiratory insufficiency, or not stopped with the administration of radiographic contrast materials.

Metformin is the only oral hypoglycemic agent currently approved by the US food and drug administration for use in children. This approval was based on a study of 80 newly diagnosed 8- to 16-year olds randomized to placebo or metformin. By the time of the interim analysis at 8 weeks, few placebo cases remained, having been rescued according to protocol. At week 16, the last double-blind visit before rescue, placebo subjects had increased their mean FPG 20 mg/dL, while metformin subjects had decreased theirs by 44 mg/dL with mean corresponding HbA$_{1c}$ 8.6% versus 7.5%. Lipid profiles improved and there were no serious adverse effects (85).

Metformin may cause gastrointestinal upset interfering with compliance, but the newer extended release formulation has fewer side effects and thus is better tolerated (86). Treatment is begun with 500 mg/day and can be increased to a maximum of 2000 mg/day. If metformin is not having an effect, an in-depth history of medication intake, including refill history from

TABLE 4 Drug Treatement of Type 2 Diabetes

Drug type	Action	Effect on BG	Risk of low BG	Weight ↑	Lipid ↓
Biguanides (metformin)	↑ hepatic glucose output; ↑ hepatic insulin sensitivity	++	0	0	+
Sulfonylureas	↑ insulin secretion and sensitivity	+++	+	+	0
Meglitinide (repaglinide, nateglinide)	short-term ↑ insulin secretion	+++	+	+	0
Glucosidase inhibitors (acarbose, miglitol)	slow hydrolysis and absorption of complex CHO	+	0	0	+
Thiazolidinediones (rosi-, pio-glitazone)	↑ insulin sensitivity in muscle and fat tissue	++	0	+	+
Insulin	↓ hepatic glucose output; overcome insulin resistance	+++	+	++	+

Abbreviation: BG, blood glucose.

the pharmacy, may demonstrate that it is simply not being taken. It is also important to be aware that metformin may normalize ovulation in girls with PCOS or ovarian hyperandrogenism, increasing pregnancy risk.

Sulfonylureas and Meglitinide

Sulfonylureas increase insulin secretion and are most useful when there is partial beta cell failure. When plasma glucose levels rise, there is rapid phosphorylation of glucose to glucose-6-phosphate which is metabolized to convert ADP to ATP. When the ATP:ADP ratio increases, K+ channels close, resulting in depolarization of the adjacent cell membrane with opening of the calcium channels. The secretion of insulin is controlled by the intracellular concentration of calcium. The higher the plasma glucose level, the greater the number of K+ channels that close, resulting in more Ca++ channels opening with increased insulin release. Sulfonylureas bind to receptors on the K+/ATP channel complex. A separate site on the K+/ATP channel complex binds meglitinide. Activation of ATP, sulfonylurea, or meglitinide binding sites causes K+ channels to close. The ATP binding sites equilibrate very rapidly, sulfonylurea sites equilibrate slowly and binding persists for prolonged periods; meglitinide has an intermediate time of equilibration. Thus, the traditional sulfonylureas have prolonged effects whereas the newer metiglinides, result in brief increases in insulin secretion (87). The major adverse effects of the traditional sulfonylureas are hypoglycemia and weight gain. Glimepramide, a third-generation sulfonylurea, has been compared with metformin in pediatric type 2 diabetes, with comparable safety and efficacy (88).

Thiazolidinediones

Thiazolidinediones (TZDs) bind to nuclear proteins, activating peroxisome proliferator activator receptors (PPAR), orphan steroid receptors found primarily in adipocytes. Once activated by a TZD, PPAR forms a heterodimer with a retinoid X receptor, enabling it to bind to the promoter region of target genes, resulting in increased formation of proteins involved in nuclear-based actions of insulin, including cell growth and adipose cell differentiation, regulation of insulin receptor activity and glucose transport into the cell. This action increases insulin sensitivity in the liver, muscle, and adipose tissue and decreases hepatic glucose output (89). During long-term therapy with TZD in adults, a reduction in HbA_{1c} levels of 0.5% to 1.3% has been shown. The major side effects are edema, weight gain, anemia, and, in approximately 1% of subjects, liver enzyme elevations. The latter problem led to sufficient numbers of fatalities in adults taking the first available drug of this group, troglitazone, that it was withdrawn from the US market. Newer thiazolidinediones, rosi- and pio-glitazone promise to be safer. Rosiglitazone was compared with metformin in a 24 week double-blind study with 195 pediatric patients with type 2 diabetes; reduction in HbA_{1c} was comparable in the two groups and there were no safety problems. Weight gain, however, occurred in those taking rosiglitazone, as is seen in adults (90).

Alpha Glucosidase Inhibitors

Alpha glucosidase inhibitors (acarbose, miglitol) reduce the absorption of carbohydrates in the upper small intestine by inhibiting the breakdown of oligosaccharides, resulting in their delayed absorption in the lower small intestine. This delay reduces the postprandial rise of plasma glucose. A reduction in HbA_{1c} levels of approximately 0.5% to 1% is expected during long term therapy with acarbose (91). The most frequent side effect is flatulence, making these agents unacceptable to most children and adolescents.

Insulin

There is a greater readiness to use insulin in the treatment of type 2 diabetes in children and adolescents than in adults, which may be related to the greater experience of pediatric practitioners with insulin than with oral agents. In the United Kingdom Prospective Diabetes Study (UKPDS), adults with type 2 diabetes had already lost 50% of their beta cell function at the time of diagnosis, and by 6 or 7 years afterwards had little or no reserve, consistent with the failure of all oral hypoglycemic regimens to maintain early gains in control of HbA_{1c} (92). There is evidence that the deterioration in pancreatic reserve in youth with type 2 diabetes may be more rapid. Glucose clamp studies have shown that young people with type 2 diabetes have first phase insulin secretion ~74% lower and second phase insulin secretion ~53% lower than obese controls without diabetes, along with 50% less insulin sensitivity and greater hepatic glucose output (93). These findings might reflect irreversible deficiency of insulin secretory capacity or reflect deleterious effects of poor glycemic control on insulin secretion (glucotoxicity). A single case report demonstrated a 15% yearly decline in beta cell function in an adolescent with type 2 diabetes followed over 6 years for a cumulative 90% loss, without any change in insulin sensitivity (94), similar to what has been described in the UKPDS (92).

Incretins

Incretins are gut-derived factors secreted in the small and large intestine soon after food ingestion. Glucagon-like peptide 1 (GLP-1) and glucose-dependent insulinotropic polypeptide (GIP) stimulate glucose dependent insulin biosynthesis and GLP-1 also suppresses glucagon release, delays gastric emptying, and increases satiety. GLP-1 exerts its effects by binding to receptors on the beta cells. In type 2 diabetes it is able to restore first phase insulin release, decrease glucagon secretion, and slow gastric emptying (95). A GLP-1 mimetic, Exenatide, is being used for the treatment of type 2 diabetes in adults (96). Given as a twice a day injection, it is unlikely to be acceptable treatment for children and adolescents with type 2 diabetes. In any case, safety and efficacy have not been established for young patients.

A promising development that could be important for treatment of pediatric type 2 diabetes is an oral agent that inhibits dipeptidyl peptidase-4 (DPP-4), the enzyme responsible for rapid degradation of incretin hormones. In 58 adult patients with type 2 diabetes who were not on oral hypoglycemic agents, a single oral dose of this inhibitor (Sitagliptin) markedly reduced plasma DPP-4 activity over 24 h, enhanced GLP-1 and GIP levels, increased insulin and C-peptide concentrations, decreased glucagon levels, and reduced glycemia following oral glucose tolerance testing (97).

Treatment Approaches

The UKPDS demonstrated that intensive treatment of adults with type 2 diabetes resulted in improved metabolic control and this, in turn, resulted in decreased risk of microvascular disease (98). The HbA_{1c} goal inferred from the UKPDS data is <7%. This study further demonstrated that aggressive treatment of blood pressure resulted in even greater reduction in the risk of both microvascular and macrovascular disease over 8-1/2 years with a 37% reduction in microvascular disease, 44% reduction in stroke, and 56% reduction in heart failure (98).

There is evidence that the microvascular complications of diabetes are extraordinarily aggressive in type 2 diabetes in youth and it is, therefore, essential to strive for normal blood glucose levels (99,100). Among 100 Pima Indian children and adolescents at the time of

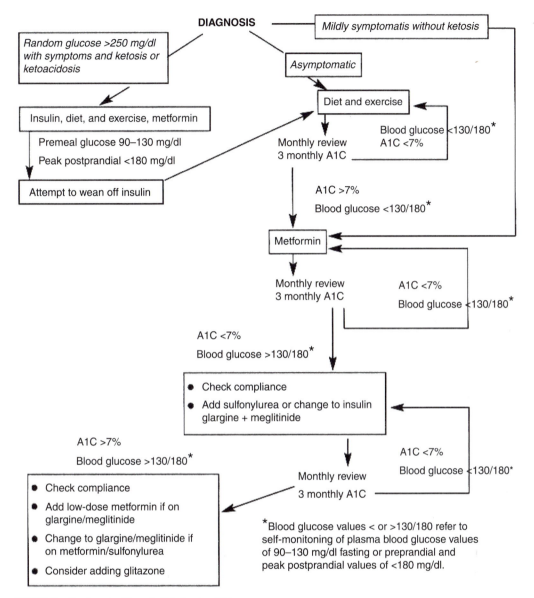

FIGURE 3 Treatment of type 2 diabetes in children.

diagnosis of type 2 diabetes mellitus, 7% had hypercholesterolemia, 18% hypertension, and 22% microalbuminuria. Ten years after diagnosis, the mean HbA_{1c} level was 12%; 60% had microalbuminuria and 17% had macroalbuminuria (100).

Initial therapy is determined by symptoms at diagnosis (Fig. 3). Children who are asymptomatic, diagnosed following a routine physical exam in a doctor's office or by community or family testing, can be treated by nonpharmacologic means. These children need basic education about diabetes and its risks and must be taught to monitor blood glucose levels, be given dietary counseling, and be encouraged to exercise daily.

The essentials of therapy are improved eating habits and increased physical activity, requiring behavior modification. Therefore, a psychologist is an important part of the treatment team along with a dietitian, and, if possible, an exercise specialist. The involvement of the parents and extended family is critical. The entire family should adopt the same healthy eating patterns and exercise either together or individually. Physical activity does not need to be organized sports, but may involve walking to school, not using the elevator, bicycling, etc. Patients should exercise at least 30 minutes daily.

Patients who have not achieved glycemic goals or whose blood glucose and HbA_{1c} values are not improving after three months of an exercise/diet modification program should be started on oral hypoglycemic agents. In the UKPDS, only 3% of patients were able to achieve treatment goals with diet and exercise alone; diet plus metformin resulted in reductions in HbA_{1c} levels comparable to those resulting from sulfonylureas or insulin, but without the weight gain and with fewer episodes of hypoglycemia than observed with the other therapies (92).

There can be an anorectic effect of metformin with weight loss in some people, resulting in increased insulin sensitivity with consequent improved metabolic control. Intensive glycemic control with metformin as a single mode of therapy in the UKPDS trial was associated with a significant reduction in risk of long-term diabetes complications. The magnitude of this reduction was 32%, greater than that seen with sulfonylureas or insulin alone, which reduced the diabetes related endpoints by only 12% (92). In addition, metformin has very few side effects other than transient abdominal discomfort and diarrhea, which has become far less of a problem with the extended release formulation. Because metformin increases insulin sensitivity, it is not associated with the risk of hypoglycemia that is attendant on the use of sulfonylureas, insulin, and benzoic acid derivatives (meglitinide).

If monotherapy with metformin is not successful over a period of 3 to 6 months, sulfonylureas or meglitinide may be added to the regimen. Until more is known about the newer TZDs it may be prudent to avoid their use in children. Insulin is added if oral agents are not able to achieve treatment goals.

Survey respondents from 130 pediatric endocrine practices in the US and Canada reported that a mean 12% of their diabetes patients had type 2 diabetes and that approximately 48% of them were being treated with insulin, 44% with oral hypoglycemic agents. Those children with type 2 diabetes taking insulin were generally treated with two injections per day. Most children being treated with oral hypoglycemic agents received metformin (71%), with 46% using sulfonylureas, 9% TZDs and 4% meglitinide (83). In the Florida diabetes centers study, 50% of the children with type 2 diabetes were being treated with oral hypoglycemic agents, 23% received insulin alone, 9% were treated with combination oral hypoglycemic/ insulin and 11% with diet and exercise alone (9).

Patients who are mildly symptomatic at onset but who have blood glucose levels < 250 mg/dL (14 mM/L) can usually be started on oral hypoglycemic agents. Patients who have substantial ketosis, ketoacidosis, or markedly elevated blood glucose levels are begun on insulin, usually twice a day, until blood glucose control is established and symptoms subside. Metformin is added while the insulin dose is gradually reduced and stopped.

Patients receiving insulin should have blood glucose (BG) checked before meals and at bedtime. Patients treated with exercise/diet or oral hypoglycemics are asked to monitor fasting BG levels and 2 h post prandial levels after dinner daily. Once target BG levels are achieved, fasting BG and 2 h post prandial dinner BG should be monitored three times a week. Assessments of HbA_{1c} should be done at least twice a year or more frequently if metabolic control is unsatisfactory and requires treatment adjustment.

Treatment of Comorbidities

The major goal of therapy is to reduce the risk of microvascular and macrovascular complications. The coexistence of type 2 diabetes with obesity, hypertension and hyperlipidemia place these patients at great risk for development of early cardiovascular disease. Lipid lowering agents have been shown to reduce the risk of number of coronary events in patients with coronary heart disease and diabetes (101). Hypertension is also an independent risk factor for the development of albuminuria and retinopathy (98). Therefore, both blood pressure control (UKPDS) and blood glucose control are important for decreasing the frequency and severity of the late complications of diabetes. Patients should have lipid levels and urine albumin checked annually. Dilated eye examination should also be performed annually in adolescents with type 2 diabetes. Unlike in children with type 1 diabetes, these examinations should begin at the time of diagnosis rather than after 3 to 5 years of disease (30).

Blood pressure should be monitored and treated aggressively with angiotensin converting enzyme (ACE) inhibitors if either the systolic or diastolic pressures are above the child's usual percentile or above the 85th percentile for age and sex. Children with type 2 diabetes may have hyperlipidemia as an indication of insulin resistance, which will improve with exercise, weight loss, and glycemic control. Nutritional changes are made with initiation of a reduced fat diet, consistent with step 1 American Heart Association guidelines. Should such attempts to normalize lipids fail after 2 to 3 months of intensive efforts, however, lipid lowering medications are appropriate. The most commonly used lipid lowering agents are the HMG CoA reductase inhibitors. They are contraindicated in pregnancy or if there is a risk of pregnancy.

TZD binding to PPARγ receptors is ubiquitous, and includes arterial wall smooth muscle, inhibiting growth and migration in response to growth factors. This effect may be important in reducing the enhanced risk of macrovascular disease associated with type 2 diabetes (102).

REFERENCES

1. Knowles HC. Diabetes mellitus in childhood and adolescence. Med Clin N Amer 1971; 55:975–87.
2. Pinhas-Hamiel O, Dolan LM, Daniels SR, et al. Increased incidence of non-insulin-dependent diabetes mellitus among adolescents. J Pediatr 1996; 128:608–15.
3. Savage PJ, Bennett PH, Senter RG, Miller M. High prevalence of diabetes in young Pima Indians. Diabetes 1979; 28:937–42.
4. Dabelea D, Hanson RL, Bennett PH, et al. Increasing prevalence of type 2 diabetes in American Indian children. Diabetologia 1998; 41:904–10.
5. Dean HJ. NIDDM-Y in First Nation children in Canada. Clin Pediatr 1998; 39:89–96.
6. Rosenbloom AL, Joe JR, Young RS, Winter WE: The emerging epidemic of type 2 diabetes mellitus in youth. Diabetes Care 1999; 22:345–54.
7. Scott CR, Smith JM, Cradock MM, Pihoker C. Characteristics of youth-onset noninsulin-dependent diabetes mellitus and insulin-dependent diabetes mellitus at diagnosis. Pediatrics 1997; 100:84–91.
8. Neufeld ND, Raffal LF, Landon C, et al. Early presentation of type 2 diabetes in Mexican-American youth. Diabetes Care 1998; 21:80–6.
9. Macaluso CJ, Bauer UE, Deeb LC, et al. Type 2 diabetes mellitus among Florida children and adolescents, 1994 through 1998. Public Health Reports 2002; 117:373–9.
10. Kadiki OA, Reddy MR, Marzouk AA. Incidence of insulin-dependent diabetes (IDDM) and non-insulin-dependent diabetes (NIDDM) (0–34 years at onset) in Benghazi, Libya. Diabetes Res Clin Pract 1996; 32:165–73.
11. Chan JCN, Cheung CK, Swaminathan R, et al. Obesity, albuminuria, and hypertension among Hong Kong Chinese with non-insulin-dependent diabetes mellitus (NIDDM). Postgrad Med J 1993; 69:204–10.
12. Kitagawa T, Owada M, Urakami T, Yamauchi K. Increased incidence of non-insulin dependent diabetes mellitus among Japanese schoolchildren correlates with an increased intake of animal protein and fat. Clin Pediatr 1998; 37:111–5.
13. Sayeed MA, Hussain MZ, Banu A, et al. Prevalence of diabetes in a suburban population of Bangladesh. Diabetes Res Clin Pract 1997; 34:149–55.
14. Braun B, Zimmerman MB, Kretchmer N, et al. Risk factors for diabetes and cardiovascular disease in young Australian aborigines. A 5-year follow-up study. Diabetes Care 1996; 19:472–9.
15. McGrath NM, Parker GN, Dawson P. Early presentation of type 2 diabetes mellitus in young New Zealand Maori. Diabetes Res Clin Pract 1999; 43:205–9.
16. Ehtisham S, Barrett TG, Shawl NJ. Type 2 diabetes mellitus in UK children – an emerging problem. Diabetic Med 2000; 17:867–71.
17. Pinhas-Hamiel O, Zeitler P. The global spread of type 2 diabetes mellitus in children and adolescents. J Pediatr 2005; 146:693–700.
18. Troiano RP, Flegal KM. Overweight children and adolescents: description, epidemiology, and demographics. Pediatrics 1998; 101:497–504.
19. Freedman DS, Srinivasan SR, Valdez RA, Williamson DF, Berenson GS. Secular increases in relative weight and obesity among children over two decades: the Bogalusa Heart Study. Pediatrics 1997; 99:420–6.
20. Strauss RS, Pollack HA. Epidemic increase in childhood overweight, 1986–1998. JAMA 2001; 286: 2845–8.
21. Wang Y. Cross-national comparison of childhood obesity: the epidemic and the relationship between obesity and socioeconomic status. Int J Epidemiology 2001; 30:1129–36.

22. Cheng TO. Childhood obesity in China. Health and Place 2004; 10:395–6.
23. Livingstone B. Epidemiology of childhood obesity in Europe. Eur J Pediatr 2000; 159(Suppl 1): S14–34.
24. Malecka-Tendera E, Mazur A. Childhood obesity: a pandemic of the twenty-first century. Int J Obes (Lond) 2006;30(Suppl 2):S1–3.
25. Winter WE. Molecular and biochemical analysis of the MODY syndromes. Pediatr Diabetes 2000; 1:88–117.
26. Winter WE, Maclaren NK, Riley WJ, et al. Maturity onset diabetes of youth in black Americans. N Engl J Med 1987; 316:285–91.
27. The Expert Committee on the Diagnosis and Classification of Diabetes Mellitus. Report of the Expert Committee on the Diagnosis and Classification of Diabetes Mellitus. Diabetes Care 2001; 24: S5–20.
28. Rosenbloom AL, Kohrman A, Sperling M. Classification and diagnosis of diabetes mellitus in children and adolescents. J Pediatr 1981; 98:320–3.
29. Pinhas-Hamiel O, Dolan LM, Zeitler PS. Diabetic ketoacidosis among obese African American adolescents with NIDDM. Diabetes Care 1997; 28:484–6.
30. American Diabetes Association. Type 2 diabetes in children and adolescents: Consensus conference report. Diabetes Care 2000; 23:381–9.
31. Feeney SJ, Myers MA, Mackay IR, et al. Evaluation of ICA512As in combination with other islet cell autoantibodies at the onset of IDDM. Diabetes Care 1997; 20:1403–7.
32. Neel JV. Diabetes mellitus: a "thrifty" genotype rendered detrimental by "progress"? Am J Hum Genet 1962; 14:353–62.
33. Lev-Ran A. Thrifty genotype: how applicable is it to obesity and type 2 diabetes? Diabetes Reviews 1999; 7:1–22.
34. Phipps K, Barker DJP. Fetal growth and impaired glucose tolerance in men and women. Diabetologia 1993; 36:225–8.
35. Philips DIW, Barker DJP, Hales CN, et al. Thinness at birth and insulin resistance in adult life. Diabetologia 1994; 37:150–4.
36. Lithell HO, McKeigue PM, Gerglund L, et al. Relation at birth to non-insulin-dependent diabetes and insulin concentrations in men aged 50-60 years. Brit Med J 1996; 312:406–10.
37. Curhan GC, Willett WC, Rimm EB, et al. Birth weight and adult hypertension, diabetes mellitus, and obesity in US men. Circulation 1996; 94:3246–50.
38. Ravelli AC, van der Meulen JH, Michels RP, et al. Glucose tolerance in adults after prenatal exposure to famine. Lancet 1998; 351:173–7.
39. Levitt NS, Lambert EV, Woods D, et al. Impaired glucose tolerance and elevated blood pressure in low birth weight, nonobese, young South African adults: early programming of cortisol axis. J Clin Endocrinol Metab 2000; 85:4611–8.
40. Dabelea D, Pettitt DJ, Hanson RL, et al. Birthweight, type 2 diabetes, and insulin resistance in Pima Indian children and young adults. Diabetes Care 1999; 22:944–50.
41. Bavdekar A, Yajnik CS, Fall CHD, et al. Insulin resistance syndrome in 8-year-old Indian children. Small at birth, big at 8 years, or both? Diabetes 1999; 48:2422–9.
42. Rosenbloom AL. Fetal nutrition and insulin sensitivity: the genetic and environmental aspects of "thrift". J Pediatr 2002; 141:459–62.
43. Svec F, Nastasi K, Hilton C, et al. Black-white contrasts and insulin levels during pubertal development: the Bogalusa Heart Study. Diabetes 1992; 41:313–7.
44. Jiang X, Srinivasan SR, Radhakrishnamurthy B, et al. Racial (black-white) differences in insulin secretion and clearance in adolescents: the Bogalusa heart study. Pediatrics 1996; 97:357–60.
45. Arslanian S. Insulin secretion and sensitivity in healthy African-American vs. American-white children. Clin Pediatr 1998; 37:81–8.
46. Danadian K, Lewy V, Janosky JJ, Arslanian S. Lipolysis in African-American children: is it a metabolic risk factor predisposing to obesity? J Clin Endocrinol Metab 2001; 86:3022–6.
47. Danadian K, Balasekaran G, Lewy V, et al. Insulin sensitivity in African-American children with and without a family history of type 2 diabetes. Diabetes Care 1999; 22:1325–9.
48. Pinhas-Hamiel O, Standiford D, Hamiel D, et al. The type 2 family. A setting for development and treatment of adolescent type 2 diabetes mellitus. Arch Pediatr Adolesc Med 1999; 153:1063–7.
49. Silverman BL, Metzger BE, Cho NH, Loeb CA. Impaired glucose tolerance in adolescent offspring of diabetic mothers. Relationship to fetal hyperinsulinism. Diabetes Care 1995; 18:611–7.
50. Pettitt DJ, Aleck KA, Baird HR, et al. Congenital susceptibility to NIDDM: Role of intrauterine environment. Diabetes 1988; 37:622–8.
51. Fagot-Campagna A, Pettitt DJ, Engelgau MM, et al. Type 2 diabetes among North American children and adolescents: An epidemiological review and a public health perspective. J Pediat 2000; 136:664–72.

52. Rosenbloom AL, Wheeler L, Bianchi R, et al. Age adjusted analysis of insulin responses during normal and abnormal oral glucose tolerance tests in children and adolescents. Diabetes 1975; 24: 820–8.
53. Caprio S, Tamborlane WV. Metabolic impact of obesity in childhood. Endocrinol Metab Clin North Am 1999; 28:731–47.
54. Legro RS, Kunselman AR, Dodson WC, Dunaif A. Prevalence and predictors of risk for type 2 diabetes mellitus and impaired glucose tolerance in polycystic ovary syndrome: a prospective, controlled study in 254 affected women. J Clin Endocrinol Metab 1999; 84:165–169.
55. Lewy V, Danadian K, Arslanian SA. Early metabolic abnormalities in adolescents with polycystic ovarian syndrome (PCOS). Ped Res 1999; 45:93A.
56. Lewy V, Danadian K, Arslanian SA. Roles of insulin resistance and B-cell dysfunction in the pathogenesis of glucose intolerance in adolescents with polycystic ovary syndrome. Diabetes 1999; 48:A292.
57. Banerjee S, Raghavan S, Wasserman EJ, et al. Hormonal findings in African-American and Caribbean Hispanic girls with premature adrenarche: implications for polycystic ovarian syndrome. Pediatrics 1998; 102:E36.
58. Vuguin P, Linder B, Rosenfeld RG, et al. The roles of insulin sensitivity, insulin-like growth factor I (IGF-I), and IGF-binding protein-1 and-3 in the hyperandrogenism of African American and Caribbean Hispanic girls with premature adrenarche. J Clin Endocrinol Metab 1999; 84: 2037–42.
59. Ibañez L, Potau N, Marcos MV, deZegher F. Exaggerated adrenarche and hyperinsulinism in adolescent girls born small for gestational age. J Clin Endocrinol Metab 1999; 84:4739–41.
60. Bennett F, Watson-Brown C, Thame M, et al. Shortness at birth is associated with insulin resistance in prepubertal Jamaican children. Eur J Clin Nutr 2002; 56:506–11.
61. Ibañez L, Castell C, Tresserras R, Potau N. Increased prevalence of type 2 diabetes mellitus and impaired glucose tolerance in first-degree relatives of girls with a history of precocious pubarche. Clin Endocrinol 1999; 51:395–401.
62. Fletcher RH, Fletcher SW, Wagner EH. Clinical Epidemiology, the essentials. 2nd edn. Williams and Wilkins, Baltimore, 1988.
63. Sackett DL, Holland WW. Controversy in detection of disease. Lancet 1965; 2:357–9.
64. Duncan GE. Prevalence of diabetes and impaired fasting glucose among US adolescents: 1999–2002 National Health and Nutrition Examination Survey. Arch Pediatr Adolesc Med 2006; 160:523–8.
65. Tirosh A, Shai I, Tekes-Manova D, Israeli E, et al., for the Israeli Diabetes Research Group. Normal fasting plasma glucose levels and type 2 diabetes in young men. N Engl J Med 2005; 353:1454–62.
66. Troiano RP, Flegal KM. Overweight children and adolescents: description, epidemiology, and demographics. Pediatrics 1998; 101(suppl):497–504.
67. Reilly JJ, Dorosty AR. Epidemic of obesity in UK children. Lancet 1999; 354:1874–5.
68. Cook VV, Hurley JS. Prevention of type 2 diabetes in childhood. Clin Pediat 1998; 37:123–9.
69. Teufel NI, Ritenbaugh CK. Development of a primary prevention program: insight gained in the Zuni Diabetes Prevention Program. Clin Pediat 1998; 37:131–41.
70. Macaulay AC, Paradis G, Potvin L, et al. The Kahnawake Schools Diabetes Prevention Project: intervention, evaluation and baseline results of a diabetes primary prevention program with a native community in Canada. Preventive Medicine 1997; 26:779–90.
71. Joe JR. Perceptions of diabetes by Indian adolescents. In: Joe JR, Young RS, eds. Diabetes as a disease of civilization: the impact of culture change on indigenous peoples. Mouton de Gruyter: Berlin, 1994: pp. 329–56.
72. Daniels S. Pharmacological treatment of obesity in paediatric patients. Paediatr Drugs 2001; 3: 405–10.
73. Chanoine JP, Hampl S, Jensen C, Boldrin M, Hauptman, J. Effect of orlistat on weight and body composition in obese adolescents: a randomized controlled trial. JAMA 2005; 293:2873–83.
74. Freemark M, Bursey D. The effects of metformin on body mass index and glucose tolerance in obese adolescents with fasting hyperinsulinemia and a family history of type 2 diabetes. Pediatrics 2001; 107:E55.
75. Diabetes Prevention Program Research Group. Reduction in the incidence of type 2 diabetes with lifestyle intervention or metformin. New Engl J Med 2002; 346:393–403.
76. Leung WY, Neil Thomas G, Chan JC, Tomlinson B. Weight management and current options in pharmacotherapy: orlistat and sibutramine. Clin Ther 2003; 25:58–80.
77. Thearle M, Aronne LJ. Obesity and pharmacologic therapy. Endocrinol Metab Clin North Am 2003; 32:1005–24.
78. Bray GA, Hollander P, Klein S, Kushner R, Levy B, Fitchet M, Perry BH. A 6–month randomized, placebo-controlled, dose-ranging trial of topiramate for weight loss in obesity. Obes Res 2003; 11: 722–33.
79. Batterham RL, Cohen MA, Ellis SM, Le Roux CW, Withers DJ, Frost GS, Ghatei MA, Bloom SR. Inhibition of food intake in obese subjects by peptide YY3-36. N Engl J Med 2003; 349:941–8.

80. Esposito K, Giugliano D. Effect of rimonabant on weight reduction and cardiovascular risk. Lancet 2005; 366:367–8; author reply 369–70.
81. Huerta MG, Roemmich JN, Kington ML, et al. Magnesium deficiency is associated with insulin resistance in obese children. Diabetes Care 2005; 28:1175–81.
82. Inge TH, Zeller M, Garcia VF, Daniels SR. Surgical approach to adolescent obesity. Adolesc Med Clin 2004; 15:429–53.
83. Silverstein JH, Rosenbloom AL. Treatment of type 2 diabetes in children and adolescents. J Ped Endocrinol Metab 2000; 13:1403–9.
84. DeFronzo RA, Goodman AM. Efficacy of metformin in patients with non-insulin dependent diabetes mellitus. The multicenter metformin study group. N Engl J Med 1995; 333:541–9.
85. Jones K, Arslanian S, McVie R, et al. Metformin improves glycemic control in children with type 2 diabetes. Diabetes Care 2002; 25:89–94.
86. Timmins P, Donahue S, Meeker J, Marathe P. Steady-state pharmacokinetics of a novel extended-release metformin formulation. Clin Pharmacokinet 2005; 44:721–9.
87. Lebovitz HE. Insulin secretagogues, old and new. Diabetes Reviews 1999; 7:139–52.
88. Gottschalk M, Danne T, Cara J, Vlajinic A, Izza M. Glimepramide (GLIM) vs metformin (MET) as monotherapy in pediatric subjects with T2DM: a single blind comparison study. Pediatric Diabetes 2005; 6(suppl 3):24–5 (abstract SP-18).
89. Schwartz S, Raskin P, Fonseca V, Graveline JF. Effect of troglitazone a in insulin treated patients with type 2 diabetes. N Engl J Med 1998; 338:861–6.
90. Dabiri G, Jones K, Krebs J, et al. Benefits of rosiglitazone in children with T2DM. American Diabetes Association 2005; abstract 1904-P.
91. Chiasson J, Josse R, Hunt J, et al. The efficacy of acarbose in the treatment of patients with non-insulin-dependent diabetes mellitus. A multicenter controlled clinical trial. Ann Int Med 1994; 121: 928–35.
92. UKPDS Group. Intensive blood glucose control with sulphonylureas or insulin compared with conventional treatment and risk of complications in patients with type 2 diabetes (UKPDS 33). Lancet 1998; 352:837–53.
93. Gungor N, Bacha F, Saad R, et al. Youth type 2 diabetes: insulin resistance, beta-cell failure, or both? Diabetes Care 2005; 28:638–44.
94. Gungor N, Arslanian S. Progressive beta cell failure in type 2 diabetes mellitus of youth. J Pediatr 2004; 144:656–9.
95. Leon DD, Crutchlow MF, Ham JY, Stoffers DA. Role of glucagon-like peptide-1 in the pathogenesis and treatment of diabetes mellitus. Int J Biochem Cell Biol 2006; 38:845–59.
96. Aston-Mourney K, Proietto J, Andrikopoulos S. Investigational agents that protect pancreatic islet beta-cells from failure. Expert Opin Invest Drugs 2005; 14:1241–50.
97. Herman GA, Bergman A, Stevens C, et al. Effect of single oral doses of sitagliptin, a, dipeptidyl peptidase-4 inhibitor, on incretin and plasma glucose levels following an oral glucose tolerance test in patients with type 2 diabetes. J Clin Endocrinol Metab 2006; doi:10.1210/jc.2006–1009.
98. UKPDS Group. Tight blood pressure control and risk of macrovascular and microvascular complications in type 2 diabetes: UKPDS 38. Br Med J 1998; 317:703–13.
99. Yokoyama H, Okudaira M, Otani T, et al. High incidence of diabetic nephropathy in early-onset Japanese NIDDM patients. Risk analysis. Diabetes Care 1998; 21:1080–5.
100. Fagot-Campagna A, Knowler WC, Pettitt DJ. Type 2 diabetes in Pima Indian Children: Cardiovascular risk factors at diagnosis and 10 years later. Diabetes 1998; 47 (Suppl 1):A155.
101. Haffner SM, Alexander CM, Cook TJ, et al., for the Scandinavian Simvastatin Survival Study Group. Reduced coronary events in Simvastatin treated patients with coronary heart disease and diabetes or impaired fasting glucose levels. Arch Int Med 1999; 59:2661–7.
102. Law RE, GoeTze S, Xi X-P, et al. Expression and function of PPARγ in rat and human vascular smooth muscle cells. Circulation 2000; 101:1311–8.

25 | Insulin Resistance Syndrome and Its Vascular Complications

Tina K. Thethi, Christina Bratcher, Tilak Mallik, and Vivian Fonseca
Department of Medicine, Section of Endocrinology, Tulane University Health Sciences Center, New Orleans, Louisiana, U.S.A.

INTRODUCTION

The insulin resistance syndrome (IRS), also known as the metabolic syndrome, is a "cluster" of cardiovascular (CV) risk factors that are frequently, but not always, associated with obesity. This grouping of risk factors has been known by several other synonyms including Syndrome X, deadly quartet, and cardiometabolic syndrome. Because insulin resistance describes the underlying pathophysiologic basis of the "syndrome," it is the term used for this chapter. Reaven first drew attention to the association of insulin resistance and obesity, type 2 diabetes, high plasma triglycerides and low plasma HDL cholesterol (HDL) and hypertension (1). Since its original description there has been much experimental, clinical, and epidemiological data to support the association of this syndrome with cardiovascular disease (CVD) (2)[2]. Additionally, other "nontraditional" CV risk factors have been frequently included in the description of the syndrome. These include inflammation, abnormal fibrinolysis, and endothelial dysfunction and microalbuminuria (3–5). Figure 1 summarizes the relationship of these risk factors and their link with CVD. It remains unclear to what extent the components of this syndrome develop independently of each other or spring from "common soil" genetic abnormalities (6). In either case, the frequency of these coexisting abnormalities are increasing at an alarming rate, paralleling the obesity and diabetes epidemics. This is now a major clinical and public health problem—NHANES 1999–2000 estimates the prevalence of metabolic syndrome at 26.7% of US adults (7). The IRS is present in approximately 80% of persons with an established diagnosis of type 2 diabetes (8,9).

Historically, research studies have used complex experimental techniques to quantify insulin sensitivity/resistance (Table 1). Epidemiological studies utilize hyperinsulinemia to define insulin resistance. Since plasma insulin concentrations are a reflection of both ambient glucose and pancreatic β cell function (which decreases even before the onset of type 2 diabetes), it is a poor marker of insulin resistance. Furthermore, lack of standardization of the insulin assay makes interpretation of plasma insulin concentration difficult. Therefore, in order to provide a clinically useful framework, several groups have defined and updated criteria for diagnosis of the metabolic syndrome. The World Health Organization (WHO), the National Cholesterol Education Program Adult Treatment Panel III (NCEP-ATP III) and the International Diabetes Federation (IDF) have set forth measurements and values of individual components as shown (see Table 2 and NCEP ATP III at www.nhlbi.nih.gov/guidelines/cholesterol/atp_iii.htm). Subjects identified using these clinical definitions have been shown to be at increased risk of CVD. Recently, there has been much controversy regarding the use of the term the metabolic syndrome and its diagnostic criteria (10–12). Several organizations have suggested that the term not be used until further research is done. Is metabolic syndrome the same as the IRS.

Insulin resistance in the context of type 2 diabetes is discussed elsewhere in this book. In this chapter we will discuss (1) the relationship of the syndrome, and its components to CVD and its associated risk factors; (2) the pathophysiology of the syndrome; and (3) its clinical evaluation and treatment.

ETIOLOGY AND CV CONSEQUENCES OF THE IRS

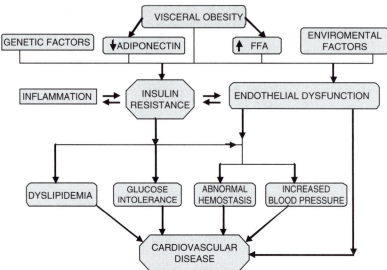

FIGURE 1   Potential links between insulin resistance and cardiovascular disease.

THE IRS AS RISK FACTOR FOR CVD

Prospective studies, now a decade old first suggested that hyperinsulinemia may be an important risk factor for ischemic heart disease. The Quebec Heart Study studied men who were 45 to 76 years of age and who did not have ischemia heart disease (13). A first ischemic event occurred in 114 men who were then matched for age, body mass index (BMI), smoking habits, and alcohol consumption with a control selected from among the 1989 men who remained free of ischemic heart disease during follow-up. Fasting insulin concentrations at base line were 18% higher in the case patients than in the controls. High fasting insulin concentrations were an independent predictor of ischemic heart disease in these men after adjustment for systolic blood pressure, family history of ischemic heart disease, plasma triglyceride, apolipoprotein B, low-density lipoprotein cholesterol, and high-density lipoprotein cholesterol concentrations. Similarly, hyperinsulinemia was associated with increased all-cause and CV mortality in Helsinki policemen independent of other risk factors (14). Because correlations of insulin with other risk factors makes interpretation difficult, factor analysis to study the clustering of risk factors in the baseline data of the Helsinki Policemen Study was carried out. Factor analysis including only risk factor variables proposed to be central components of IRS predicted the risk of coronary heart disease and stroke independently of other risk factors (15). Other population studies as well as a recent meta-analysis have supported these studies (16–18) When adding the metabolic syndrome to models with established risk factors for CVD (smoking, diabetes, hypertension, and serum cholesterol) at

TABLE 1   Laboratory Methods of Measuring Insulin Sensitivity/Resistance

Hyperinsulinemic-euglycemic clamp
Fasting insulin and insulin/glucose ratio[a]
Oral glucose tolerance test with plasma glucose and insulin measured[a]
Intravenous glucose tolerance test with minimal model analysis
Homeostatic model assessment (HOMA-IR)
Constant infusion of glucose with model assessment

[a] Several formulae based on these measurements have been proposed and validated against the euglycemic hyperinsulinemic clamp.

TABLE 2 Criteria for the Diagnosis of the Insulin Resistance Syndrome

WHO	IDF	NCEP ATP III
(1) HYPERTENSION on antihypertensive medication and/or BP> 160/90	(1)HYPERTENSION Systolic BP> 130 or diastolic BP> 85mm Hg or treatment of previously diagnosed hypertension	(1) HYPERTENSION BP> 130/85 or drug treatment for elevated blood pressure
(2) DYSLIPIDEMIA- Plasma triglycerides> 1.7 mmol/L and/or HDL cholesterol< 0.9 mmol/L in men and < 1.0 mmol/L in women	(2) DYSPLIPIDEMIA raised TG level > 150 mg/dL(1.7 mmol/L)or specific treatment for this lipid abnormality reduced HDL cholesterol < 40 mg/dL (1.03 mmol/L)in males and <50 mg/ dL(1.29 mmol/L) in females or specific treatment for this lipid abnormality	(2) DYSLIPIDEMIA Plasma Triglycerides> 150 mg/dL or drug treatment for elevated triglycerides HDL cholesterol< 40 mg/dL (0.9 mmol/L) in men and < 50 mg/dL (1.1 mmol/L) in women. Or drug treatment for reduced HDL-C
(3) OBESITY- BMI> 30 and/or elevated WHR(> 0.90 in males, 0.85 in females)	(3)CENTRAL OBESITY Waist circumference > 94 cm for Europid men and > 80 cm for Europid women (see ethnic specific values)	(3) OBESITY Waist circumference > 40 in(102 cm) in males and > 35 in (88 cm) in females
(4) Microalbuminuria (overnight urinary albumin excretion rate> 20 μg/min	(4) Raised fasting plasma glucose (FPG) > 100 mg/dL (5.6 mmol/L) or previously diagnosed type 2 diabetes	(4) Fasting blood sugar > 100 mg/dL or drug treatment
WHO requires a person to have Type 2 diabetes or impaired glucose tolerance and any TWO of the above criteria. A person with normal glucose tolerance must demonstrate insulin resistance (see Table 1).	IDF requires central obesity plus any two of the other four factors	NCEP requires any THREE of the above criteria to be met.

Abbreviations: WHO, World Health Organization; NCEP ATP III, National Cholesterol Education Program, Adult Treatment Panel; IDF, International Diabetes Federation Ethnic specific values for waist circumference.
Source: Refs. 128–130.

age 50, presence of the metabolic syndrome as defined in the NCEP significantly predicted total and CV mortality (Cox proportional hazard ratios 1.36, 95% confidence interval 1.17 to 1.58; and 1.59, 1.29 to 1.95, respectively). The metabolic syndrome added prognostic information to that of the established risk factors for CVD (likelihood ratio tests, $P < 0.0001$ for both outcomes). Similar results were obtained in a sub sample without diabetes or manifest CVD (19). These studies confirm that components of the syndrome are present for several years before the onset of type 2 diabetes and support the adage that the "clock for coronary heart disease start ticking before the onset of clinical diabetes" (17).

Though it is generally agreed that the clustered risk factors taken in combination are associated with an elevated risk of CVD, IRS is not without controversy and debate as to how it should be employed clinically. More recently, the metabolic syndrome as defined by ATP III was shown to be significantly predictive of vascular events after adjustment for type 2 diabetes but was dependent on the lipid traits of high triglycerides and low HDL cholesterol (20).

Country/Ethnic group	Waist circumference	
	Male	Female
Europids	>94 cm	>80 cm
South Asians	>90 cm	>80 cm
Chinese	>90 cm	>80 cm
Japanese	>85 cm	>90 cm
Ethnic South and Central Americans	Use South Asian recommendations until more specific data are available	
Sub-Saharan Africans	Use European data	
Eastern Mediterranean and Middle Eastern (Arab) populations	Use European data	

ASSOCIATION OF INSULIN RESISTANCE WITH OTHER CV RISK FACTORS

In addition to being a precursor of type 2 diabetes and an independent risk factor for CVD, insulin resistance is also closely associated with several other CV risk factors. The interrelatedness of insulin resistance with the other factors is discussed below.

Obesity

Obesity is frequently associated with several of the components of the IRS and may be critical for the development of the syndrome. The contemporary view is now centered on visceral adiposity Several mechanisms have been proposed for the link between obesity and the IRS (21) CV morbidity and mortality are increased in obese individuals independently of other risk factors. Insulin resistance is very common in obese individuals. However, some nonobese individuals demonstrate hyperinsulinemia and the other features of the IRS (22). Thus, obesity may not be essential for the expression of the syndrome but the presence of obesity or weight gain may accentuate the pathophysiological changes associated with the syndrome.

Body fat distribution rather than body mass may actually be a better predictor of insulin resistance and CV risk (23). Insulin resistance, type 2 diabetes and hypertension are more closely associated with a central distribution of adiposity than with general increases in fat mass. Waist circumference serves as a clinical surrogate of intra-abdominal fat.

Dyslipidemia

One of the earliest relationships between insulin resistance and a CV risk factor is with "diabetic dyslipidemia". The hallmark of the syndrome is hypertriglyceridemia and low plasma HDL cholesterol concentration. Plasma LDL cholesterol concentrations in insulin resistant subjects are no different from those in insulin sensitive subjects. However, there are qualitative changes in LDL cholesterol resulting in "pattern B" distribution of LDL particles-which consists of smaller LDL particles that are more susceptible to oxidation and thus potentially more atherogenic (24).

Several hypotheses have been proposed for the mechanism of the association between insulin resistance and dyslipidemia. Insulin resistance at the level of adipose tissue may result in increased activity of hormone sensitive lipase and therefore increased breakdown of stored triglycerides. Free fatty acids (FFA) released from adipocytes, particularly intra-abdominal adipocytes, can be transported to the liver where they stimulate synthesis of triglycerides and assembly and secretion of very low density lipoprotein (VLDL). Increased plasma VLDL triglycerides exchange with cholesterol esters from HDL, resulting in a lower plasma HDL cholesterol. On the other hand, an increase in circulating FFA has been proposed as having an etiological role in the development of IR (25).

FFAs released from adipose tissue play a pivotal role in insulin resistance. In the skeletal muscle of lean, healthy subjects, a progressive increase in plasma FFA causes a dose-dependent inhibition of insulin-medicated glucose disposal and insulin signaling. The inhibitory effect of plasma FFA develops at concentrations that are well within the physiological range (i.e., at plasma FFA levels observed in obesity and type 2 diabetes).

Boden et al. (26) studied mechanisms by which FFAs cause hepatic insulin resistance by using euglycemic-hyperinsulinemic clamps with and without the infusion of lipid/heparin (to raise or lower FFAs) in alert male rats. FFA-induced hepatic insulin resistance was associated with increased hepatic diacylglycerol content ($+210\%$), increased activation of the proinflammatory nuclear NF-kappa B pathway, increased activities of two serine/threonine kinases, and increased expression of inflammatory cytokines (TNF-α, Interleukin-1beta).

In subjects with insulin resistance, elevated circulating FFA levels precede the onset of glucose metabolism abnormalities. Inappropriate insulin signaling, especially in peripheral tissues such as adipose cells, results in abnormal lipid metabolism. Impaired insulin signaling leads to loss of suppression of Lipolysis (27)and perhaps defects in storage of fatty acids in the adipocytes (28)from the review). The excess amount of lipid from various sources (circulating FFAs originating in the fat, endocytosis of triglyceride-rich lipoproteins, and de novo lipogenesis) leads to the posttranslational stabilization of aopB, the major apolipoprotein of

VLDL, which enhances the assembly and secretion of VLDL particles (29). Insulin signaling, through P13K-dependent pathways, also promotes the degradation of apoB. Thus, a combination of excess delivery of fatty acids and limited degradation of apoB explains the hypertriglyceridemia characteristic of insulin resistance. Insulin resistance also decreases the lipoprotein lipase activity, the major mediator of VLDL clearance.

Hypertension

Although it is well established that essential hypertension is frequently associated with insulin resistance, the impact of this abnormality on blood pressure homeostasis is still a matter of debate. Fasting plasma insulin is frequently higher in hypertensive subjects and glucose disposal during an euglycemic clamp is decreased. The association between hypertension and insulin resistance is more convincing in obese subjects. Significant decreases in blood pressure have been observed in obese subjects, who lose modest amounts of weight, correlating closely with the decline in fasting plasma insulin concentrations. Plasma insulin concentrations are higher and insulin-mediated total-body glucose disposal is reduced in young, normal weight individuals with essential hypertension (2). The impairment in insulin-mediated glucose disposal was closely related to the increase in blood pressure. Multiple potential mechanisms by which IR may cause hypertension have been proposed (30), These include resistance to insulin mediated vasodilatation, impaired endothelial function, sympathetic nervous system over-activity, sodium retention, increased vascular sensitivity to the vasoconstrictor effect of pressor amines and enhanced growth factor activity leading to proliferation of smooth muscle walls. However, some studies do not support the association of metabolic insulin resistance with essential hypertension. Clearly, hypertension is itself a complex disorder with many etiologies, and not all subjects with essential hypertension are insulin resistant.

Prothrombotic State

Factors contributing to a prothrombotic state in diabetes are summarized in Table 3. The endogenous fibrinolytic system represents equilibrium between activators of plasminogen (primarily tissue type plasminogen activator-tPA) and inhibitors of these activators (such as plasminogen activator inhibitor type 1- PAI 1) (31). Coagulation is a continuous process and the fibrinolytic system maintains fluidity of blood. Excessive inhibition of fibrinolysis will lead to coagulation and thrombosis, a critical process in CV events (31). Impaired fibrinolytic function in diabetes correlates with severity of vascular disease in diabetes and is a risk factor for myocardial infarction in both diabetic and nondiabetic subjects.

Impaired fibrinolysis is now recognized as being an important component of the IRS and probably contributes considerably to the increased risk of CV events (17). Plasma PAI 1 antigen and activity are elevated in a wide variety of insulin resistant subjects including obese subjects with and without diabetes and women with the polycystic ovarian syndrome. Immuno-histochemical analysis of coronary lesions from patients with coronary

TABLE 3 Potential Impact of Insulin Resistance and Diabetes on Thrombosis and Fibrinolysis

Factors predisposing to thrombosis
  ↑Platelet hyperaggregability
  ↑Platelet cAMP and cGMP
  ↑Thromboxane synthesis
Elevated concentrations of procoagulants
  ↑Fibrinogen
  ↑Von Willebrand factor and procoagulant activity
  ↑Thrombin activity
Decreased concentration and activity of antithrombotic factors
  ↓Antithrombin III activity
Factors attenuating fibrinolysis
  Decreased t-PA activity
  Increased PAI-1 synthesis and activity
Increased blood viscosity

artery disease has demonstrated an imbalance of the local fibrinolytic system with increased coronary artery tissue PAI-1 in patients with type 2 diabetes. Many studies have attempted to elucidate the mechanistic link between insulin resistance and abnormal fibrinolysis. Insulin, proinsulin, abnormal cholesterol and various cytokines regulate PAI-1 synthesis and release. The greatest elevations in PAI-1 occur when there is a combination of hyperinsulinemia, hyperglycemia and increased FFAs, in obese insulin resistant subjects (32).

Other factors predisposing to thrombosis associated with insulin resistance, include increased platelet hyper-aggregation, elevated concentrations of pro-coagulants particularly fibrinogen and Von Willebrand factor and a decrease in anti-thrombotic factors such as anti thrombin III (31). Many of these abnormalities are nonspecific and the association of insulin resistance with coagulation abnormalities with is less robust than that with abnormal fibrinolysis.

Endothelial Function and Vascular Abnormalities

The importance of the endothelium in maintaining vascular health has been widely recognized. The endothelium is a critical determinant of vascular tone, reactivity, inflammation, vascular remodeling, maintenance of vascular patency and blood fluidity (33). Many of these functions of the endothelium are maintained through regulatory substances secreted from endothelial cells, which may often have opposing actions. For example, nitric oxide (NO) is the most potent known vasodilator, is secreted by endothelial cells, having being synthesized from arginine by nitric oxide synthase (NOS). Endothelial cells also secrete other important vasodilators such as prostacyclin. The vasodilatory actions are opposed by secretion of potent vasoconstrictors such as Endothelin 1. Similarly these and others endothelial products are involved in maintaining the balance between smooth muscle cell growth, promotion and inhibition, thrombosis and fibrinolysis, inflammation and cell adhesion.

Endothelial dysfunction is now recognized as being an early abnormality in the natural history of CVD may be a good predictor of CV events. Abnormalities in production of NO, increased inactivation of NO along with increased activation of angiotensin converting enzyme and local mediators of inflammation, may be key precursors of clinical events in the IRS.

The ability of blood vessels to dilate in response to stimuli, including ischemia is called vascular reactivity, or flow mediated dilatation (FMD). Brachial artery vascular reactivity is a noninvasive method of assessing arterial endothelial function in vivo. Since endothelial injury is an early event in atherogenesis, it has been suggested that abnormal flow-mediated dilatation may precede the development of structural changes in the vessel wall. Abnormal flow-mediated dilatation has been shown in several insulin resistant states and is present in relatives of patient with type 2 diabetes who have normal glucose tolerance. In a study done in healthy subjects across a wide range of BMI (18.6 to 73.1 kg/m2), markers of total body fat/fat distribution, inflammation, metabolism, and blood pressure have been shown to coorelate with FMD (34). The markers of total body fat/fat distribution measured were waist circumference, BMI and waist hip ratio (WHR), while the markers of inflammation measured were interleukin-6 (IL-6), C-reactive protein, and tumor necrosis factor alpha (TNF-α) R2. The parameters of metabolism that were measured were fasting insulin, HDL, LDL and triglycerides. Of all the markers WHR was the only independent predictor of FMD (r2 = 0.30); $p = 0.0001$. It has even been proposed that endothelial dysfunction may be a precursor of the IRS (35). Figure 2 summarizes this hypothesis and illustrates the various determinants and consequences of insulin resistance. Table 4 lists various endothelial abnormalities associated with insulin resistance.

Insulin itself has vasodilatory actions via a NO dependent mechanism (21). In healthy subjects, insulin dilates arterioles supplying skeletal muscle probably through enhancement of NO production. Some in vitro studies have documented that insulin regulates NOS and that this action maybe impaired in insulin resistant subjects- an abnormality that might be attributable to either impairment in the ability of the endothelium to produce NO or enhanced inactivation of NO (36). Since NO plays a critical role in the maintenance of vascular health

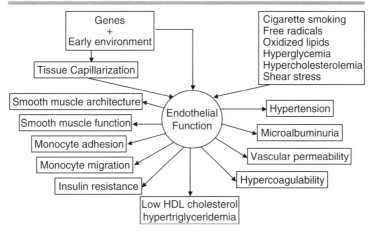

FIGURE 2 Determinants and consequences of endothelial function. *Source*: Ref. 35.

(33) this abnormality may explain much of the increased CVD in the IRS. Impairment of insulin action on glucose metabolism assessed by glucose clamp parallels impairment of insulin action on the vasculature (Fig. 3). Thus obesity and type 2 diabetes are associated with resistance to insulin's vascular effects.

Finally insulin resistance is associated with increased carotid intima-media thickness (IMT) (37), This finding is compatible with the possible effect of hyperinsulinemia on growth of vascular smooth muscle cells and extracellular matrix (38). Carotid IMT is increased in newly diagnosed patients with type 2 diabetes without overt CVD (39). This finding is important since IMT represents a structural abnormality in the arterial wall and is a good predictor of subsequent CV risk (40).

Microalbuminuria

Microalbuminuria is recognized as a complication of diabetes due to changes in the kidney secondary to hyperglycemia. Recent data suggests that it may occur even in nondiabetics and be a precursor of CVD and may be related to insulin resistance (41). It is possible that in individuals who are insulin resistant, microalbuminuria may be a manifestation of endothelial dysfunction, indicating endothelial permeability and is also related to increased carotid IMT (42). Microalbuminuria is included in the criteria used by the WHO to define the IRS.

PATHOGENESIS OF THE IRS

Physical Activity

Habitual physical activity is an important determinant of insulin resistance. Epidemiological studies have shown a strong correlation between a sedentary lifestyle and type 2 diabetes,

TABLE 4 Alterations in the Vascular Endothelium Associated with Diabetes Mellitus and Insulin Resistance

Abnormality	Significance
↓Release of and responsiveness to NO	Impaired endothelial function and reactivity
↑Expression, synthesis, and plasma levels of endothelin-1	Vasoconstriction and hypertension
↓Prostacyclin release	Impaired vasodilatation
↑Adhesion-molecule expression	Increased monocyte adhesion to vessel wall
↑Adhesion of platelets and monocytes	Foam cell formation, thrombosis and inflammation
↑Pro-coagulant activity	Thrombosis
↑Advanced glycosylated end products	Increased stiffness of arterial wall
Impaired fibrinolytic activity	Decreased clot breakdown

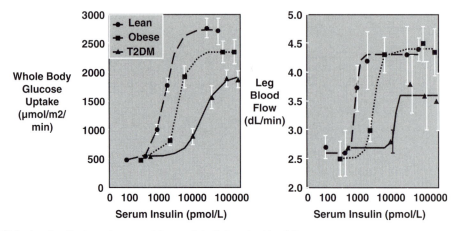

FIGURE 3   Insulin effect on glucose uptake parallels that on leg blood flow.

hypertension and CVD (43–45). Furthermore, exercise has been shown to have significant therapeutic value in treating most of the components of the IRS (see below).

Cytokines and Inflammation

Several studies have suggested a role for inflammation in the etiology of the IRS and its complications. Observations suggest that cytokines arising from adipose tissue may be partly responsible for the metabolic, hemodynamic and hemostatic abnormalities associated with insulin resistance. Studies show a close relationship between obesity and circulating C-reactive protein (CRP), TNF-α and IL-6. Plasma CRP is elevated in obese subjects who have other features of the IRS (46). It has been recently recognized that some of these cytokines are predictors of CVD. Thus inflammation originating from excess adipose tissue cytokine production may contribute not only to the development of the IRS but also the associated CVD.

Increased expression of TNF-α in adipose tissue has been reported in obese subjects. TNF-α inhibits the action of lipoprotein lipase and stimulates lipolysis. It also impairs the function of the insulin-signaling pathway by effects on phosphorylation of both the insulin receptor and insulin-receptor substrate (IRS)-1 (IL-6) may also induce endothelial expression of cytokines thereby contributing to endothelial dysfunction.

Adipose tissue is a major site of energy storage and is important for energy homeostasis. During state of nutritional abundance it functions to store energy in the form of triglycerides and during nutritional deprivation, it releases the energy as FFAs (47–49).

Adipose tissue has been increasingly recognized as an important endocrine organ that secretes a number of biologically active "adipokines" (50–54). Some of these adipokines have been shown to directly or indirectly affect insulin sensitivity through modulation of insulin signaling and the molecules involved in glucose and lipid metabolism (55). Adiponectin is one of the adipokines that has attracted much attention due to its antidiabetic and antiatherogenic properties (56). The adiponectin gene encodes a secreted protein expressed exclusively in both WAT and brown adipose tissue (47). Adiponectin expression is reduced in obese, insulin-resistant rodent models (57) and in obese rhesus monkey model that frequently develop type 2 diabetes (58). In these animals, the onset of diabetes is preceded by the decrease in plasma adiponectin levels in parallel with the observation of decreased insulin sensitivity (58). Plasma adiponectin levels have indeed been reported to be reduced in obese humans, particularly in those with visceral obesity. They correlate inversely with insulin resistance (58–62). Longitudinal and prospective studies (62–67) have shown that lower adiponectin levels are associated with a higher incidence of diabetes. Adiponectin is also significantly related to the development of type 2 diabetes in Pima Indians (65). Hypoadiponectinemia has been independently associated with the metabolic syndrome (68). Reduced plasma adiponectin levels are also commonly observed in various states associated with insulin resistance, such as CVD (69,70) and hypertension(71,72).

Dietary factors such as soy protein (73), fish oils (74), and linoleic acid (75) have been suggested to increase plasma adiponectin level, whiel a carbohydrate-rich diet appears to decrease plasma adiponectin level (76). The insulin sensitizing effect of adiponectin was first identified in 2001 (77–79). Schrere and colleagues (47) have reported that an acute increase in the level of circulating adiponectin triggers a transient decrease in basal glucose level by inhibiting both the expression of hepatic gluconeogenic enzymes and the rate of endogenous glucose production in both wild type and type 2 diabetic mice (77).

Decreased insulin-stimulated glucose transport (Glut 4) (80)activity contributes to decreased insulin-stimulated skeletal muscle glycogen synthesis in insulin resistance. This defect appears to be a result of intracellular lipid-induced inhibition of insulin-stimulated IRS-1 tyrosine phosphorylation resulting in reduced IRS-1 associated phosphatidyl inositol 3 kinase activity. Therefore, insulin resistance could be taken to be a result of accumulation of intracellular lipid metabolites (e.g., fatty acyl CoAs, diacylglycerol) in skeletal muscle and hepatocytes. Furthermore, in patients with type 2 diabetes who undergo weight loss have an increase in hepatic insulin sensitivity. This is accompanied by significant reduction in intrahepatic fat without any changes in circulating adipocytokines. Reduced mitochondrial activity may also lead to increased intramyocellular lipid content and therefore to insulin resistance in skeletal muscles. Intra-islet fat also adversely affects beta cell function and number (beta cell apoptosis) (81).

Mitochondrial Dysfunction

The common etiology of the relationship between insulin resistance and atherosclerosis may be organelle stress in response to nutrient excess occurring in mitochondria, the nucleus and the endoplasmic reticulum (82). Mitochondria are the major source of ATP production in animals. Within the inner mitochondrial membrane, occurs the process of respiration. During this reaction, reactive oxygen species are generated. These reactive oxygen species have been implicated in atherosclerosis. Additionally, the mitochondrial genome may be particularly susceptible to oxidative damage due to its lack of histones and a deficient mismatch repair system. Mitochondrial dysfunction may be involved in skeletal muscle insulin resistance. Decrease in the expression of genes essential for mitochondrial function, such as the gene encoding PGC-1α is decreased in subjects with insulin resistance (83). This is accompainied by impaired energy production in the muscles of insulin resistant subjects (84). As discussed above, insulin resistance causes an increase in circulating fatty acids. Increased fatty acid oxidation by aortic endothelial cells has recently been reported to accelerate the production of supreoxide by the mitochondrial election transport chain (85). This effect is associated with proatherogenic vascular effects thus consistent with the evidence for the role of mitochondrial metabolism in vascular disease.

Alteration of the DNA structure or function is termed genomic stress. Oxidative modifications are frequently responsible for the genomic stress which is another likely contributor to both insulin resistance and atherosclerosis (82). Saturated fatty acids may also induce endoplasmic reticulum stress (86). Both dietary and genetic models of obesity disrupt normal protein folding in the endoplasmic reticulum, leading to stress signals mediated in part by JNK (87). Deficiency of the insulin receptor in macrophages has been shown to increase the endoplasmic reticulum stress response and apoptosis in a mouse model of atherosclerosis (88). Thus, mitochondrial dysfunction plays a key molecular role in insulin resistance.

Abnormal Insulin Signaling, Hyperinsulinemia, and the Vasculature

As outlined above, IR with resultant hyperinsulinemia is an independent risk factor for CVD. However, the specific role of insulin in the pathogenesis of atherosclerosis remains unclear. Several mechanistic hypotheses have been proposed to explain this association (2,89). Firstly, insulin is a growth factor that stimulates vascular cell growth and synthesis of matrix proteins. Secondly, the insulin signaling pathway thought to be responsible for abnormalities in glucose metabolism is also involved in NO production. Thus, the abnormal intracellular signaling that causes hyperglycemia may also be responsible for vascular disease due to loss of insulin's anti-atherogenic properties, while hyperinsulinemia continues to stimulate growth promoting enzymes such as MAP kinase (89) Although some controversy remains, this hypothesis (Fig. 4) has been supported by many studies. In addition, imbalances in insulin homeostasis are associated with abnormalities in expression and action of various peptides, growth factors and cytokines. These include angiotensin II, endothelin –1and insulin –like growth factor –1 (89).

While the exact role of peroxisome proliferator-activated receptors in the pathogenesis of this syndrome is unclear, several studies support the concept that they may have a role in the development of not only insulin resistance but also atherosclerosis (90). For example, these receptors are present in vascular tissue, heterozygous mutations in the ligand-binding domain of PPAR gamma are occasionally associated with insulin resistance, and agonists of these receptors have a significant impact on the syndrome. Thus it is possible that PPARs play a role in the pathogenesis of the complete syndrome that is the subject of much current research.

Drug Induced

Several classes of drugs have been associated with insulin resistance. These include corticosteroids, which frequently cause insulin resistance and type 2 diabetes. Recent data with protease inhibitors, used for the treatment of human immunodeficiency virus infection, frequently cause several manifestations of the IRS (91). Hypertriglyceridemia appears to be an early manifestation of protease inhibitor induced lipodystrophy and is associated with changes in body fat distribution and marked insulin resistance. The long-term effects of these drugs on CVD are unknown.

Intrauterine/Postpartum Growth and Development

Some data have suggested that a low birth weight and/or rapid gain of weight in the early life are associated with the later development of multiple features of the IRS including, type 2 diabetes and other risk factors for CVD (92–94). The mechanisms by which fetal under nutrition and hence, low birth weight increase the risk of developing these diseases are unclear. Animal experiments (94) have been done with a rat model of under nutrition, involving an overall reduction in maternal food intake. In this study, intrauterine growth retardation (IUGR) have a decreased beta cell mass, which persists into adulthood. Maternal under nutrition also causes elevations in glucocorticoid concentrations, which in turn have been implicated in causing reduction of the beta cell mass. A prospective study done in

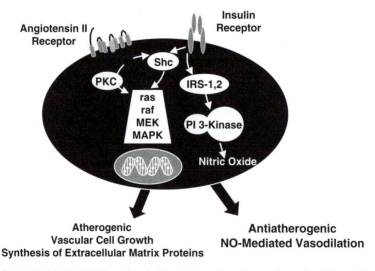

FIGURE 4 Insulin: potential atherogenic and antiatherogenic actions in vascular cells. *Abbreviations*: IRS, insulin receptor substrate; JRS-1,2, insulin receptor substrate; MAPK, mitogen activated protein kinase; MEK, MAP kinase-kinase; PI-3-Kinase, phosphatidylinositol-3-kinase; PKC, protein kinase C. *Source*: From Ref. 89.

630 children (95) has shown that maternal gestational diabetes mellitus results in adiposity and higher glucose and insulin concentrations in female offsprings at 5 years. Metabolic abnormalities persist in adulthood as well as demonstrated by a study done in adults who were born with IUGR (96). Using peripheral glucose uptake and monitoring FFA concentrations under euglycemic hyperinsulinemic clamp, subjects who were born with IUGR, were shown to have decreased insulin-stimulated glucose uptake as early as 25 years of age without major impairment of insulin secretion. Low glucose uptake is associated with a lesser degree of FFA suppression in adipose tissue, which suggests a role of adipose tissue at an early stage of insulin resistance in these subjects. It has also been shown that Large for Gestational Age (LGA) offsprings of mothers with diabetes were at significant risk of developing the metabolic syndrome in childhood when compared to appropriate-for-age (AGA) children (97). Low birth weight is also important. The Bogalusa heart study supports the relationship between low birth weight and the later development of important CV risk factors in African Americans and white individuals. This relationship tends to be stronger in African Americans than in whites, except for systolic blood pressure (98). A study done among children with low birth weight in India supports this relationship between low birth weight and subsequent development of insulin resistance (99). Thus, it has become increasingly evident that impaired intrauterine growth plays a decisive role in the future physiology and function of many organs and body systems.

MANAGEMENT OF THE IRS

The use of insulin sensitizers and lifestyle modifications to improve insulin resistance in the treatment of type 2 diabetes is discussed elsewhere in the book. Any therapeutic maneuver that improves insulin sensitivity should also have beneficial effects on all the metabolic and CV abnormalities associated with the IRS. In this section we will concentrate on management of the syndrome as a whole particularly its link with CVD.

Lifestyle Changes

Since obesity and physical activity are important precursors of the syndrome, lifestyle change may be critical in its prevention and treatment. The NCEP has strongly endorsed the concept of "total lifestyle change" in the prevention of CVD due to the syndrome. Recent clinical trials have demonstrated that modest reductions in calorie and fat intake and a small increase in physical activity can prevent the development of type 2 diabetes (100). While a reduction in CV events has not yet been documented, lifestyle changes significantly improve CV risk factors such as HDL, LDL and blood pressure.

Since many individuals with the metabolic syndrome are overweight, dietary treatment should be primarily focused on weight reduction. While the effect of weight reduction on the components of the IRS are widely accepted, there remains some controversy about specific diets to achieve weight loss.

Insulin sensitivity can also be influenced by diet composition (101,102). There is evidence that a higher saturated fat intake is associated with impaired insulin action, some of which may be mediated by changes in body weight. In contrast, a high-monounsaturated-fat diet significantly improves insulin sensitivity compared to a high-saturated-fat diet. Independent of its effects on insulin sensitivity, diet composition can influence the factors clustering in the metabolic syndrome. Dietary carbohydrate increases blood glucose levels, particularly in the post-prandial period, and consequently also insulin levels and plasma triglycerides. The detrimental effects of a high-carbohydrate diet on plasma glucose/insulin, triglyceride/HDL or fibrinolysis occur only when carbohydrate foods with a high glycemic index are consumed, while they are abolished if the diet is based largely on fiber-rich, low-glycemic-index foods. Mono-unsaturated fats and ω-3 fatty acids can reduce plasma triglycerides. Such diets may also improve endothelial function.

Moderate physical activity (brisk walking for at least 30 min/day) should be feasible for most patients. One of the major anticipated benefits of an active lifestyle is a reduction in CV mortality. Exercise improves insulin sensitivity and glucose tolerance rapidly and independently of weight loss. Exercise training results in preferential loss of fat stores from central regions of the body (103). Aerobic exercise training has been shown to lower systolic and diastolic blood pressure, and plasma triglycerides and increase HDL cholesterol.

Pharmacological Therapy

Unfortunately, no clinical trial data is available to show a reduction in CV events with pharmacological treatment of the IRS per se. However, current pharmacological strategies for established risk factors such as hyperglycemia, hypertension, dyslipidemia and platelet aggregation have been shown to mitigate many of the consequences of the syndrome. Nevertheless, this leads to the prescription of complex multidrug regimens and there is a need for therapy that will directly treat the syndrome. Insulin sensitizers are approved for treatment of hyperglycemia in type 2 diabetes (discussed elsewhere). We will consider their role in the IRS and its vascular complications. The effects of pharmacological therapy on some components of the IRS are summarized in Table 5.

Metformin

Metformin is a biguanide that has been approved for the treatment of type 2 diabetes and has also been shown to prevent diabetes in obese subjects with impaired glucose tolerance. The primary glucose lowering effect of metformin results from a decrease in hepatic gluco-neogenesis with some effect on peripheral glucose disposal (104). The mechanism of action is different from and complementary to that of the thiazolidinediones (TZDs).

Obese patients in the United Kingdom Prospective Diabetes Study (UKPDS) treated with metformin had a 36% lower risk of all cause mortality and a 39% lower risk of myocardial infarction (105). Since there was no difference in glycemic control in subjects treated with Metformin compared to that achieved with other treatment modalities, it is possible that other effects of the drug, including its effects on the IRS may have decreased CV events. Most importantly, patients in the UKPDS gained less weight compared to those treated with other agents (105). Potential mechanisms by which metformin may decrease CV events, include reduced plasma triglycerides, LDL cholesterol concentration, postprandial lipemia, and plasma free fatty acid concentration (106,107) In addition metformin has a favorable effect on several nontraditional CV risk factors including plasminogen activator inhibitor-1, fibrinogen and endothelial function (106,107) (Table 5).

Thiazolidinediones

TZDs are oral anti-diabetic agents developed to improve insulin sensitivity. TZDs primarily exert their insulin sensitizing effect by increasing peripheral uptake of glucose especially at the skeletal muscles (108). Drugs of this class act as ligands for PPARγ, which functions as a transcription factor involved in the regulation of genes involved in glucose homeostasis and lipid metabolism. These receptors have several potential effects in different tissues, including the vasculature. Since PPARγ plays a role endothelial and vascular smooth muscle cells, ligands of these receptors, such as TZDs may play a role in atherosclerosis. For example, the TZDs inhibit vascular smooth muscle cell proliferation and migration (90).

TZDs have been shown to have many other effects other than reduction of hyperglycemia, some of which are summarized in Table 5 (109) They decrease plasma free fatty acid concentrations and the associated inhibition of free fatty acid oxidation. They decrease the release of cytokines and peptides such as TNF-α from adipose tissue that are associated with insulin resistance and vascular inflammation. TZDs have been shown to improve endothelial function and inflammation and have been shown to have an inhibitory effect on carotid artery IMT in patients with type 2 diabetes (110). However, TZDs cause weight gain, although a decrease in visceral fat may help explain the concomitant decrease in insulin resistance (109). They also increase plasma LDL concentration although studies suggest that they change LDL particle size to the less atherogenic large buoyant LDL cholesterol (109). Thus, TZDs may have beneficial effects against CVD, although reductions in CV events have not yet been demonstrated. Clinical trials are in progress to determine whether they will prevent CV events.

TABLE 5 Effect of Pharmacological Therapy on CV Risk Factors and Markers in the Insulin Resistance Syndrome

Drug type	Drug class	Body weight	Blood pressure	HDL	LDL	Tg	PAI-1	Endothelial function	Plasma Insulin
Diabetes treatments	SFU/meglitidnide	↑	—	—	—	→	—	—	←
	TZD	↑	→	←	↑[a]	→	→	—	—
	Metformin	—	→	←	→	→	→	—	→
	Acarbose	—	—	—	—	→	—	—	→
	Insulin	←	—	—	—	→	→	—	→
Lipid lowering	HMGCoA	—	→	→	→	→	—	—	—
Anti-hypertensive	ACE I	—	→	—	→	—	—	—	→
Weight reduction	Orlistat	→	—	—	→	→	—	—	→
	Sibutramine	→	←	←	—	→	—	—	→

[a] decreases LDL particle size and decreases LDL oxidation.
Abbreviations: (—) indicates no change or insufficient data; Tg, plasma triglycerides.

Other Hypoglycemics

Insulin secretagogues such as sulfonylureas and meglitinides do not directly improve insulin sensitivity. However, by reducing glucose concentrations they reduce the effect of "glucose toxicity" on insulin sensitivity. They have very little impact on the components of the metabolic syndrome (107). In addition they cause weight gain, which may explain some of the differences between the effects of this class of agents and Metformin on CV events in the UKPDS. Exogenous insulin has similar effects, but in addition may have a more potent effect on lowering plasma triglycerides and PAI-1.

Alpha glucosidase inhibitors have significant lipid lowering effects especially on triglycerides. Some small studies have also suggested that they may improve insulin sensitivity (Table 5). The clinical benefits of these effects on CV disease are unclear.

Anti-obesity Agents

For individuals who do not respond to lifestyle modification, anti-obesity drugs probably improve insulin resistance through weight loss or decreased food intake, rather than a direct effect on insulin sensitivity. Due to the weight loss these drugs have a significant effect on various components of the syndrome (111). Sibutramine, a serotonin receptor inhibitor, improves glycemic control and the lipid profile (112). Orlistat is a lipase inhibitor that decreases the absorption of dietary fat. Even modest weight loss with Orlistat results in a significant improvement in glucose tolerance, plasma insulin, LDL and HDL cholesterol concentrations (111).

The serotonin, norepinephrine, dopamine and endocannibinoid systems are among some of the systems that mediate hunger and satiety signals (113). Rimonabant is a selective cannabinoid-1 receptor blocker. It has been shown to reduce body weight and improve cardiometabolic risk factors in patients who are obese and overweight (114,115). In a randomized, double-blind, placebo-controlled trial of 3045 obese (BMI ≥ 30) or overweight (BMI >27) and untreated or treated hypertension or dyslipidemia adults rimonabant in the dose of 20 mg once daily produced greater mean reductions in weight, circumference, and level of triglycerides and increase in the level of high-density lipoprotein cholesterol (114). Thus, rimonabant has been shown to reduce body weight and improve CV risk factors in obese and overweight (115).

Other Drugs Affecting Insulin Resistance

Several studies with many pharmacological agents impact different components of the syndrome but very few have been shown to have an effect on the syndrome as a whole. Most intriguing among these are Angiotensin-converting enzyme (ACE) inhibitors and HMG-Co-A reductase inhibitors (statins). ACE inhibitors are antihypertensive agents, that inhibit the conversion of angiotensin I to angiotensin II. Several studies have demonstrated a small but statistically significant reduction in insulin resistance by ACE inhibitors. Furthermore, ACE inhibitors have been shown to decrease the incidence of new onset type 2 diabetes in addition to preventing CV events (116). The mechanism is unclear but may be related to vasodilatory effects on vessels supplying skeletal muscle as well as improving insulin sensitivity.

As discussed above, recent studies suggest a state of chronic, subacute inflammation, mediated specifically by the IKKβ/NF-kB pathway might be involved in the pathogenesis of insulin resistance (117–120). Findings with anti inflammatory salicylates, which inhibit IKKβ and NF-kB have added new impetus to the field. Salicylate has a distinct mechanism of action. At doses of 3 to 7 gm/day, salicylates inhibit NF-kB (121), apparently by binding IKKβ and inhibiting IkB phosphorylation (122). In addition to the molecular rationale for using salicylates to target inflammation in the treatment of insulin resistance, there is historical clinical experience that supports the use of salicylates in treatment of diabetes dating as back as 1875 (123–125). These studies (126,127) clearly demonstrated that high doses (4–7 gm/day) of salicylates, including aspirin dramatically improved glycemic control. TINSAL-2D (Targeting Inflammation using SALsalate for Type 2 Diabetes) (www.clinicaltrials.gov) underway to determine whether salicylates represent a new pharmacologic option in the management of diabetes.

SUMMARY AND CONCLUSIONS

The IRS is a major public health problem contributing to considerable morbidity related to diabetes and CVD. Consensus-based definition of the syndrome should lead to greater recognition in clinical practice. Several components of the syndrome are routinely evaluated in practice and frequently cluster in patients.

Our understanding of the pathophysiological processes that are involved has improved considerably. This has resulted in the development of new treatments directly targeting insulin resistance that has significant benefits on several aspects of the syndrome. Current research is focused on improving our understanding of the etiology of the syndrome and finding new therapeutic interventions.

REFERENCES

1. Reaven GM. Banting lecture 1988. Role of insulin resistance in human disease. *Diabetes* 1988; 37: 1595–1607.
2. McFarlane SI, Banerji M, Sowers JR. Insulin resistance and cardiovascular disease. *J Clin Endocrinol Metab* 2001; 86:713–718.
3. Amann K, Wanner C, Ritz E. Cross-talk between the kidney and the cardiovascular system. *J Am Soc Nephrol* 2006; 17:2112–9.
4. Locatelli F, Pozzoni P, Del VL. Renal manifestations in the metabolic syndrome. *J Am Soc Nephrol* 2006; 17:S81–5.
5. Fonseca VA. Risk factors for coronary heart disease in diabetes. *Ann Int Med* 2000; 133:154–6.
6. Stern MP. Diabetes and cardiovascular disease. The "common soil" hypothesis. *Diabetes* 1995; 44: 369–74.
7. Ford ES, Giles WH, Mokdad AH. Increasing prevalence of the metabolic syndrome among U.S. adults. *Diabetes Care*. 2004; 27:2444–9.
8. Haffner SM, D'Agostino Jr R, Mykkanen L, et al. Insulin sensitivity in subjects with type 2 diabetes. Relationship to cardiovascular risk factors: the Insulin Resistance Atherosclerosis Study. *Diabetes Care* 1999; 22:562–8.
9. Isomaa B, Almgren P, Tuomi T, et al. Cardiovascular morbidity and mortality associated with the metabolic syndrome. *Diabetes Care* 2001; 24:683–9.
10. Gale EA. The myth of the metabolic syndrome. *Diabetologia* 2005; 48:1679–83.
11. Kahn R, Buse J, Ferrannini E, Stern M. The metabolic syndrome: time for a critical appraisal: joint statement from the American Diabetes Association and the European Association for the Study of Diabetes. *Diabetes Care* 2005; 28:2289–304.
12. Kahn R. The metabolic syndrome (emperor) wears no clothes. *Diabetes Care* 2006; 29:1693–6.
13. Despres JP, Lamarche B, Mauriege P, et al. Hyperinsulinemia as an independent risk factor for ischemic heart disease 1. *N Engl J Med* 1996; 334:952–7.
14. Pyorala M, Miettinen H, Laakso M, Pyorala K. Plasma insulin and all-cause, cardiovascular, and noncardiovascular mortality: the 22-year follow-up results of the Helsinki Policemen Study. *Diabetes Care* 2000; 23:1097–102.
15. Pyorala M, Miettinen H, Halonen P, et al. Insulin resistance syndrome predicts the risk of coronary heart disease and stroke in healthy middle-aged men: the 22-year follow-up results of the Helsinki Policemen Study. *Arterioscler Thromb Vasc Biol* 2000; 20:538–44.
16. Folsom AR, Szklo M, Stevens J, et al. A prospective study of coronary heart disease in relation to fasting insulin, glucose, and diabetes. The Atherosclerosis Risk in Communities (ARIC) Study. *Diabetes Care* 1997; 20:935–42.
17. Haffner SM, Stern MP, Hazuda HP, et al. Cardiovascular risk factors in confirmed prediabetic individuals. Does the clock for coronary heart disease start ticking before the onset of clinical diabetes? *JAMA* 1990; 263:2893–8.
18. Ruige JB, Assendelft WJ, Dekker JM, et al. Insulin and risk of cardiovascular disease: a meta-analysis. *Circulation* 1998; 97:996–1001.
19. Sundstrom J, Riserus U, Byberg L, et al. Clinical value of the metabolic syndrome for long term prediction of total and cardiovascular mortality: prospective, population based cohort study. *BMJ* 2006; 332:878–82.
20. Saely CH, Koch L, Schmid F, et al. Adult Treatment Panel III 2001 but not International Diabetes Federation 2005 criteria of the metabolic syndrome predict clinical cardiovascular events in subjects who underwent coronary angiography. *Diabetes Care* 2006; 29:901–7.
21. Kahn BB, Flier JS. Obesity and insulin resistance. *J Clin Invest* 2000; 106:473–81.
22. Ruderman N, Chisholm D, Pi-Sunyer X, et al. The metabolically obese, normal-weight individual revisited. *Diabetes* 1998; 47:699–713.

23. Abate N, Garg A, Peshock RM, et al. Relationship of generalized and regional adiposity to insulin sensitivity in men with NIDDM. *Diabetes* 1996; 45:1684–93.

24. Reaven GM, Chen YD, Jeppesen J, et al. Insulin resistance and hyperinsulinemia in individuals with small, dense low density lipoprotein particles. *J Clin Invest* 1993; 92:141–6.

25. Boden G, Lebed B, Schatz M, et al. Effects of acute changes of plasma free fatty acids on intramyocellular fat content and insulin resistance in healthy subjects. *Diabetes* 2001; 50:1612–17.

26. Boden G, She P, Mozzoli M, et al. Free fatty acids produce insulin resistance and activate the proinflammatory nuclear factor-kappaB pathway in rat liver. *Diabetes* 2005; 54:3458–65.

27. Villena JA, Roy S, Sarkadi-Nagy E, et al. Desnutrin, an adipocyte gene encoding a novel patatin domain-containing protein, is induced by fasting and glucocorticoids: ectopic expression of desnutrin increases triglyceride hydrolysis. *J Biol Chem* 2004; 279:47066–75.

28. Foley JE. Rationale and application of fatty acid oxidation inhibitors in treatment of diabetes mellitus. *Diabetes Care* 1992; 15:773–84.

29. Ginsberg HN. Efficacy and mechanisms of action of statins in the treatment of diabetic dyslipidemia. *J Clin Endocrinol Metab* 2006; 91:383–92 (review).

30. DeFronzo RA, Ferrannini E. Insulin resistance. A multifaceted syndrome responsible for NIDDM, obesity, hypertension, dyslipidemia, and atherosclerotic cardiovascular disease. *Diabetes Care* 1991; 14:173–94.

31. Sobel BE. Insulin resistance and thrombosis: a cardiologist's view. *Am J Cardiol.* 1999; 84:37J–41J.

32. Calles-Escandon J, Mirza SA, Sobel BE, Schneider DJ. Induction of hyperinsulinemia combined with hyperglycemia and hypertriglyceridemia increases plasminogen activator inhibitor 1 in blood in normal human subjects. *Diabetes* 1998; 47:290–93.

33. Calles-Escandon J, Cipolla M. Diabetes and endothelial dysfunction: a clinical perspective. *Endocr Rev* 2001; 22:36–52.

34. Williams IL, Chowienczyk PJ, Wheatcroft SB, et al. Effect of fat distribution on endothelial-dependent and endothelial-independent vasodilatation in healthy humans. *Diabetes Obes Metab* 2006; 8:296–301.

35. Pinkney JH, Stehouwer CD, Coppack SW, Yudkin JS. Endothelial dysfunction: cause of the insulin resistance syndrome. *Diabetes* 1997; 46(Suppl 2):S9–13.

36. Baron AD. Hemodynamic actions of insulin. *Am J Physiol* 1994; 267:E187–202.

37. Howard G, O'Leary DH, Zaccaro D, et al. Insulin sensitivity and atherosclerosis. The Insulin Resistance Atherosclerosis Study (IRAS). Investigators. *Circulation* 1996; 93:1809–17.

38. Hsueh WA, Law RE. Insulin signaling in the arterial wall. *Am J Cardiol* 1999; 84:21J–24J.

39. Wagenknecht LE, D'Agostino Jr R, Savage PJ, et al. Duration of diabetes and carotid wall thickness. The Insulin Resistance Atherosclerosis Study IRAS. *Stroke* 1997; 28:999–1005.

40. O'Leary DH, Polak JF, Kronmal RA, et al. Carotid-artery intima and media thickness as a risk factor for myocardial infarction and stroke in older adults. Cardiovascular Health Study Collaborative Research Group. *N Engl J Med.* 1999; 340:14–22.

41. Pinkney JH, Denver AE, Mohamed-Ali V, et al. Insulin resistance in non-insulin-dependent diabetes mellitus is associated with microalbuminuria independently of ambulatory blood pressure. *J Diabetes Complications* 1995; 9:230–33.

42. Agewall S, Wikstrand J, Ljungman S, Fagerberg B. Urinary albumin excretion is associated with the intima-media thickness of the carotid artery in hypertensive males with non-insulin-dependent diabetes mellitus. *J Hypertens* 1995; 13:463–9.

43. Folsom AR, Kushi LH, Hong CP. Physical activity and incident diabetes mellitus in postmenopausal women. *Am J Public Health* 2000; 90:134–8.

44. Hu FB, Stampfer MJ, Solomon C, et al. Physical activity and risk for cardiovascular events in diabetic women. *Ann Intern Med* 2001; 134:96–105.

45. Kronenberg F, Pereira MA, Schmitz MK, et al. Influence of leisure time physical activity and television watching on atherosclerosis risk factors in the NHLBI Family Heart Study. *Atherosclerosis* 2000; 153:433–43.

46. Festa A, D'Agostino Jr R, Howard G, et al. Chronic subclinical inflammation as part of the insulin resistance syndrome: the Insulin Resistance Atherosclerosis Study (IRAS). *Circulation* 2000; 102: 42–7.

47. Kadowaki T, Yamauchi T, Kubota N, Hara K, Ueki K, Tobe K. Adiponectin and adiponectin receptors in insulin resistance, diabetes, and the metabolic syndrome. *J Clin Invest* 2006; 116: 1784–92.

48. Kahn CR. Triglycerides and toggling the tummy. *Nat Genet* 2000; 25:6–7.

49. Spiegelman BM, Flier JS. Obesity and the regulation of energy balance. *Cell.* 2001; 104:531–43.

50. Hotamisligil GS, Shargill NS, Spiegelman BM. Adipose expression of tumor necrosis factor-alpha: direct role in obesity-linked insulin resistance. *Science* 1993; 259:87–91.

51. Lazar MA. The humoral side of insulin resistance. *Nat Med* 2006; 12:43–44.

52. Steppan CM, Bailey ST, Bhat S, et al. The hormone resistin links obesity to diabetes. *Nature* 2001; 409:307–12.

53. Yang Q, Graham TE, Mody N, et al. Serum retinol binding protein 4 contributes to insulin resistance in obesity and type 2 diabetes. *Nature*. 2005; 436:356–62.
54. Zhang Y, Proenca R, Maffei M, et al. Positional cloning of the mouse obese gene and its human homologue. *Nature* 1994; 372:425–32.
55. Kershaw EE, Flier JS. Adipose tissue as an endocrine organ. *J Clin Endocrinol Metab* 2004; 89: 2548–56.
56. Kadowaki T, Yamauchi T. Adiponectin and adiponectin receptors. *Endocr Rev* 2005; 26:439–51.
57. Hu E, Liang P, Spiegelman BM. AdipoQ is a novel adipose-specific gene dysregulated in obesity. *J Biol Chem* 1996; 271:10697–703.
58. Hotta K, Funahashi T, Bodkin NL, et al. Circulating concentrations of the adipocyte protein adiponectin are decreased in parallel with reduced insulin sensitivity during the progression to type 2 diabetes in rhesus monkeys 2. *Diabetes* 2001; 50:1126–33.
59. Arita Y, Kihara S, Ouchi N, et al. Paradoxical decrease of an adipose-specific protein, adiponectin, in obesity. *Biochem Biophys Res Commun* 1999; 257:79–83.
60. Ryo M, Nakamura T, Kihara S, et al. Adiponectin as a biomarker of the metabolic syndrome. *Circ J* 2004; 68:975–81.
61. Yamamoto Y, Hirose H, Saito I, et al. Adiponectin, an adipocyte-derived protein, predicts future insulin resistance: two-year follow-up study in Japanese population. *J Clin Endocrinol Metab* 2004; 89:87–90.
62. Yatagai T, Nagasaka S, Taniguchi A, et al. Hypoadiponectinemia is associated with visceral fat accumulation and insulin resistance in Japanese men with type 2 diabetes mellitus. *Metabolism* 2003; 52:1274–78.
63. Daimon M, Oizumi T, Saitoh T, et al. Decreased serum levels of adiponectin are a risk factor for the progression to type 2 diabetes in the Japanese Population: the Funagata study. *Diabetes Care* 2003; 26:2015–20.
64. Duncan BB, Schmidt MI, Pankow JS, et al. Adiponectin and the development of type 2 diabetes: the atherosclerosis risk in communities study. *Diabetes* 2004; 53:2473–8.
65. Krakoff J, Funahashi T, Stehouwer CD, et al. Inflammatory markers, adiponectin, and risk of type 2 diabetes in the Pima Indian. *Diabetes Care* 2003; 26:1745–51.
66. Lindsay RS, Funahashi T, Hanson RL, et al. Adiponectin and development of type 2 diabetes in the Pima Indian population. *Lancet* 2002; 360:57–8.
67. Snehalatha C, Mukesh B, Simon M, et al. Plasma adiponectin is an independent predictor of type 2 diabetes in Asian indians. *Diabetes Care* 2003; 26:3226–9.
68. Matsushita K, Yatsuya H, Tamakoshi K, et al. Comparison of circulating adiponectin and proinflammatory markers regarding their association with metabolic syndrome in Japanese men. *Arterioscler Thromb Vasc Biol* 2006; 26:871–6.
69. Kumada M, Kihara S, Sumitsuji S, et al. Association of hypoadiponectinemia with coronary artery disease in men. *Arterioscler Thromb Vasc Biol* 2003; 23:85–9.
70. Pischon T, Girman CJ, Hotamisligil GS, et al. Plasma adiponectin levels and risk of myocardial infarction in men. *JAMA* 2004; 291:1730–7.
71. Adamczak M, Wiecek A, Funahashi T, et al. Decreased plasma adiponectin concentration in patients with essential hypertension. *Am J Hypertens* 2003; 16:72–5.
72. Ouchi N, Ohishi M, Kihara S, et al. Association of hypoadiponectinemia with impaired vasoreactivity. *Hypertension* 2003; 42:231–4.
73. Nagasawa A, Fukui K, Funahashi T, et al. Effects of soy protein diet on the expression of adipose genes and plasma adiponectin. *Horm Metab Res* 2002; 34:635–9.
74. Flachs P, Mohamed-Ali V, Horakova O, et al. Polyunsaturated fatty acids of marine origin induce adiponectin in mice fed a high-fat diet. *Diabetologia* 2006; 49:394–7.
75. Nagao K, Inoue N, Wang YM, Yanagita T. Conjugated linoleic acid enhances plasma adiponectin level and alleviates hyperinsulinemia and hypertension in Zucker diabetic fatty (fa/fa) rats. *Biochem Biophys Res Commun* 2003; 310:562–6.
76. Pischon T, Girman CJ, Rifai N, et al. Association between dietary factors and plasma adiponectin concentrations in men. *Am J Clin Nutr* 2005; 81:780–6.
77. Berg AH, Combs TP, Du X, et al. The adipocyte-secreted protein Acrp30 enhances hepatic insulin action. *Nat Med* 2001; 7:947–53.
78. Fruebis J, Tsao TS, Javorschi S, et al. Proteolytic cleavage product of 30-kDa adipocyte complement-related protein increases fatty acid oxidation in muscle and causes weight loss in mice. *Proc Natl Acad Sci USA* 2001; 98:2005–10.
79. Yamauchi T, Kamon J, Waki H, et al. The fat-derived hormone adiponectin reverses insulin resistance associated with both lipoatrophy and obesity. *Nat Med* 2001; 7:941–6.
80. Petersen KF, Shulman GI. Etiology of insulin resistance. *Am J Med* 2006; 119:S10–6.
81. Rattarasarn C. Physiological and pathophysiological regulation of regional adipose tissue in the development of insulin resistance and type 2 diabetes. *Acta Physiol (Oxford)* 2006; 186:87–101.
82. Semenkovich CF. Insulin resistance and atherosclerosis. *J Clin Invest* 2006; 116:1813–22.

83. Patti ME, Butte AJ, Crunkhorn S, et al. Coordinated reduction of genes of oxidative metabolism in humans with insulin resistance and diabetes: potential role of PGC1 and NRF1. *Proc Natl Acad Sci USA* 2003; 100:8466–71.

84. Petersen KF, Dufour S, Befroy D, et al. Impaired mitochondrial activity in the insulin-resistant offspring of patients with type 2 diabetes. *N Engl J Med* 2004; 350:664–71.

85. Du X, Edelstein D, Obici S, et al. Insulin resistance reduces arterial prostacyclin synthase and eNOS activities by increasing endothelial fatty acid oxidation. *J Clin Invest* 2006; 116:1071–80.

86. Wang D, Wei Y, Pagliassotti MJ. Saturated fatty acids promote endoplasmic reticulum stress and liver injury in rats with hepatic steatosis. *Endocrinology* 2006; 147:943–51.

87. Ozcan U, Cao Q, Yilmaz E, et al. Endoplasmic reticulum stress links obesity, insulin action, and type 2 diabetes. *Science.* 2004; 306:457–61.

88. Han S, Liang CP, Vries-Seimon T, et al. Macrophage insulin receptor deficiency increases ER stress-induced apoptosis and necrotic core formation in advanced atherosclerotic lesions 2. *Cell Metab* 2006; 3:257–66.

89. Feener EP, King GL. Vascular dysfunction in diabetes mellitus. *Lancet* 1997; 350(Suppl 1):SI9–13.

90. Hsueh WA, Jackson S, Law RE. Control of vascular cell proliferation and migration by PPAR-gamma: a new approach to the macrovascular complications of diabetes. *Diabetes Care* 2001; 24: 392–7.

91. Gan SK, Samaras K, Carr A, Chisholm D. Anti-retroviral therapy, insulin resistance and lipodystrophy. *Diabetes Obes Metab* 2001; 3:67–71.

92. Godfrey KM, Barker DJ. Fetal nutrition and adult disease. *Am J Clin Nutr* 2000; 71:1344S–52S.

93. Osmond C, Barker DJ. Fetal, infant, and childhood growth are predictors of coronary heart disease, diabetes, and hypertension in adult men and women. *Environ Health Perspect* 2000; 108(Suppl 3): 545–53.

94. Breant B, Gesina E, Blondeau B. Nutrition, glucocorticoids and pancreas development. *Horm Res* 2006; 65(Suppl 3):98–104.

95. Krishnaveni GV, Hill JC, Leary SD, et al. Anthropometry, glucose tolerance, and insulin concentrations in Indian children: relationships to maternal glucose and insulin concentrations during pregnancy. *Diabetes Care* 2005; 28:2919–25.

96. Jaquet D, Gaboriau A, Czernichow P, Levy-Marchal C. Insulin resistance early in adulthood in subjects born with intrauterine growth retardation. *J Clin Endocrinol Metab* 2000; 85:1401–6.

97. Boney CM, Verma A, Tucker R, Vohr BR. Metabolic syndrome in childhood: association with birth weight, maternal obesity, and gestational diabetes mellitus. *Pediatrics* 2005; 115:e290–6.

98. Mzayek F, Sherwin R, Fonseca V, et al. Differential association of birth weight with cardiovascular risk variables in African-Americans and Whites: the Bogalusa heart study. *Ann Epidemiol* 2004; 14: 258–64.

99. Bavdekar A, Yajnik CS, Fall CH, et al. Insulin resistance syndrome in 8-year-old Indian children: small at birth, big at 8 years, or both?. *Diabetes* 1999; 48:2422–29.

100. Tuomilehto J, Lindstrom J, Eriksson JG, et al. Prevention of type 2 diabetes mellitus by changes in lifestyle among subjects with impaired glucose tolerance. *N Engl J Med* 2001; 344:1343–50.

101. Reaven GM. Diet and Syndrome X. *Curr Atheroscler Rep* 2000; 2:503–7.

102. Riccardi G, Rivellese AA. Dietary treatment of the metabolic syndrome – the optimal diet. *Br J Nutr* 2000; 83(Suppl 1):S143–8.

103. Ross R, Dagnone D, Jones PJ, et al. Reduction in obesity and related comorbid conditions after diet-induced weight loss or exercise-induced weight loss in men. A randomized, controlled trial. *Ann Int Med* 2000; 133:92–103.

104. Stumvoll M, Nurjhan N, Perriello G, et al. Metabolic effects of metformin in non-insulin-dependent diabetes mellitus. *N Engl J Med* 1995; 333:550–4.

105. Turner RC. The UK Prospective Diabetes Study. A review. *Diabetes Care* 1998; 21(Suppl 3):C35–8.

106. Bailey CJ, Turner RC. Metformin. *N Engl J Med* 1996; 334:574–9.

107. Lebovitz HE. Effects of oral antihyperglycemic agents in modifying macrovascular risk factors in type 2 diabetes. *Diabetes Care* 1999; 22(Suppl 3):C41–4.

108. Saltiel AR, Olefsky JM. Thiazolidinediones in the treatment of insulin resistance and type II diabetes. *Diabetes* 1996; 45:1661–69.

109. Parulkar AA, Pendergrass ML, Granda-Ayala R, et al. Nonhypoglycemic effects of thiazolidine-diones. *Ann Int Med* 2001; 134:61–71.

110. Koshiyama H, Shimono D, Kuwamura N, et al. Rapid communication: inhibitory effect of pioglitazone on carotid arterial wall thickness in type 2 diabetes. *J Clin Endocrinol Metab* 2001; 86: 3452–6.

111. Jones PH. Diet and pharmacologic therapy of obesity to modify atherosclerosis. *Curr Atheroscler Rep* 2000; 2:314–20.

112. Fujioka K, Seaton TB, Rowe E, et al. Weight loss with sibutramine improves glycaemic control and other metabolic parameters in obese patients with type 2 diabetes mellitus. *Diabetes Obes Metab* 2000; 2:175–87.

113. Jensen MD. Potential role of new therapies in modifying cardiovascular risk in overweight patients with metabolic risk factors. *Obesity (Silver Spring)* 2006; 14(Suppl 3):143S–9S.

114. Pi-Sunyer FX, Aronne LJ, Heshmati HM, et al. Effect of rimonabant, a cannabinoid-1 receptor blocker, on weight and cardiometabolic risk factors in overweight or obese patients: RIO-North America: a randomized controlled trial. *JAMA* 2006; 295:761–75.

115. Despres JP, Golay A, Sjostrom L. Effects of rimonabant on metabolic risk factors in overweight patients with dyslipidemia. *N Engl J Med* 2005; 353:2121–34.

116. Yusuf S, Sleight P, Pogue J, et al. Effects of an angiotensin-converting-enzyme inhibitor, ramipril, on cardiovascular events in high-risk patients. The Heart Outcomes Prevention Evaluation Study Investigators. *N Engl J Med* 2000; 342:145–53.

117. Cai D, Frantz JD, Tawa Jr NE, et al. IKKbeta/NF-kappaB activation causes severe muscle wasting in mice. *Cell* 2004;119:285–98.

118. Cai D, Yuan M, Frantz DF, et al. Local and systemic insulin resistance resulting from hepatic activation of IKK-beta and NF-kappaB. *Nat Med* 2005; 11:183–90.

119. Kim JK, Kim YJ, Fillmore JJ, et al. Prevention of fat-induced insulin resistance by salicylate. *J Clin Invest* 2001; 108:437–46.

120. Yuan M, Konstantopoulos N, Lee J, et al. Reversal of obesity- and diet-induced insulin resistance with salicylates or targeted disruption of Ikkbeta. *Science* 2001; 293:1673–77.

121. Kopp E, Ghosh S. Inhibition of NF-kappa B by sodium salicylate and aspirin. *Science* 1994; 265: 956–9.

122. Yin MJ, Yamamoto Y, Gaynor RB. The anti-inflammatory agents aspirin and salicylate inhibit the activity of I(kappa)B kinase-beta. *Nature* 1998; 396:77–80.

123. Shoelson S. Invited comment on W. Ebstein: on the therapy of diabetes mellitus, in particular on the application of sodium salicylate. J Mol Med 2002; 80:618–9.

124. Williamson RT. On the treatment of glycosuria and diabetes mellitus with sodium salicylate. Br Med J 1901; 1:760–2.

125. Ebstein W. Zur therapie des diabetes mellitus, insbesondere uber die anwendeng der salicylauren natron bei demselben. Berliner Klinische Wochnschrift 1876; 13:337–40.

126. Gilgore SG. The influence of salicylate on hyperglycemia. Diabetes 1960; 9:392–3.

127. Reid J, MacDougall AI, Andrews MM. Aspirin and diabetes mellitus. *Br Med J* 1957; 1071–4.

128. Alberti KG, Zimmet PZ. Definition, diagnosis and classification of diabetes mellitus and its complications. Part 1: Diagnosis and classification of diabetes mellitus provisional report of a WHO consultation 6. *Diabet Med* 1998; 15:539–53.

129. Executive Summary of The Third Report of The National Cholesterol Education Program (NCEP) Expert Panel on Detection, Evaluation, And Treatment of High Blood Cholesterol In Adults (Adult Treatment Panel III). *JAMA* 2001; 285:2486–97.

130. Alberti KG, Zimmet P, Shaw J. Metabolic syndrome – a new world-wide definition. A Consensus Statement from the International Diabetes Federation. *Diabet Med* 2006; 23:469–80.

26 | Obesity: Influence on Diabetes and Management

Hans Hauner
German Diabetes Research Institute, Heinrich-Heine Universität, Düsseldorf, Germany

INTRODUCTION

Obesity is recognized as a common chronic disorder characterized by excessive body fat. This condition increases the risk of developing a variety of adverse consequences to human health ranging from metabolic disturbances including type 2 diabetes and cardiovascular complications to disorders of the locomotor system, among others. In addition, obesity impairs the subjective quality of life in affected people and is known to reduce life expectancy (1).

The diagnosis of obesity is based on the body mass index (BMI). This simple anthropometric index can be calculated from body weight and height (BMI = weight in kg/ (height in m)^2), is rather independent of body height and correlates reasonably well with body fat mass ($r = 0.4$–0.7). The current classification of body weight according to the World Health Organization is based on BMI as shown in Table 1.

EPIDEMIOLOGY OF OBESITY

Obesity has become a global epidemic that exists not only in the industrialized world but also in most developing countries. At present, the prevalence of obesity (BMI ≥ 30 kg/m^2) ranges between 15% and 30% in the adult populations of Europe and North America, with an unequivocal trend toward further increase. The most dramatic rise in these regions is currently observed in children and adolescents as well as young adults. In addition, there is a particularly alarming increase in the number of affected people in many developing countries (1).

Obesity as a Risk Factor for Type 2 Diabetes

There is a large body of clinical data demonstrating a close relationship between body fat mass and the risk of diabetes. In contrast to other obesity-associated metabolic disturbances, the risk of diabetes increases already in the upper normal range of BMI. In the Nurses' Health Study, women in the upper normal range with a BMI between 23.0 and 24.9 kg/m^2 had a four- to fivefold increased risk of developing diabetes over a 14-year observation period compared to women with a BMI < 22 kg/m^2 (2). In those with a BMI between 29.0 and 30.9 kg/m^2 the risk of diabetes was 27.6-fold higher than in the lean reference group. Almost two-thirds of newly diagnosed women with type 2 diabetes were obese at the time of diagnosis (2). Similar observations were reported for males in the Health Professionals' Study (3). Interestingly, a change in body weight strongly predicts the risk of diabetes. Weight gain from the age of 18 between 11.0 and 19.9 kg, which is the average range of weight change between adolescence and menopause for women in the industrialized countries, was found to be correlated with a 5.5-fold higher risk of diabetes compared to weight-stable women, whereas weight reduction of the same extent reduced the risk of diabetes by almost 80% (2). Similar data were reported for men (3). Another important aspect is that the duration of obesity has a strong impact on the development of type 2 diabetes.

The health risks of obesity, particularly the risk of developing diabetes, depends not only on the extent and duration of obesity, but is also potently influenced by the pattern of fat distribution. Enlarged visceral fat depots, which can be easily assessed by measuring the waist circumference, are closely associated with metabolic disturbances. In a previous study in men, an abdominal pattern of fat distribution was found to be an independent risk factor for type 2 diabetes (4). Subsequent studies confirmed this observation. Particularly at low degrees of overweight, the fat distribution pattern strongly predicts the risk for diabetes and the

TABLE 1 Classification of Human Obesity Based on BMI

Classification	BMI (kg/m^2)
Underweight	<18.5
Normal weight	18.5–24.9
Overweight	≥25.0
Obesity grade I	30–34.9
Grade II	35–39.9
Grade III	≥40

Source: From Ref. 1.

metabolic syndrome. It is now accepted for Caucasians that a waist circumference >80 and >88 cm, respectively, in women and >94 and >102 cm, respectively, in men is associated with a moderately and highly elevated risk of metabolic complications (1). Therefore, waist circumference should be routinely assessed when estimating the risk of diabetes. Other more precise measures of the visceral fat mass are computed tomography, nuclear magnetic resonance imaging and, with some limitations, dual energy X-ray absorptiometry (DEXA) (5).

GENETIC PREDISPOSITION FOR TYPE 2 DIABETES

Despite the major role of body fat as a risk factor for diabetes there is clear evidence that type 2 diabetes has a strong genetic basis. According to family studies every third offspring of a parent with diabetes is expected to develop this disease later in life. If both parents suffer from diabetes this risk is over 50% and the concordance for type 2 diabetes in monozygotic twins is close to 100%. For this reason, it is currently assumed that only those obese subjects will develop the disease who have a genetic failure of the pancreas to compensate for insulin resistance (6). Among severely obese subjects (BMI ≥ 40 kg/m^2) only 30% to 50% will develop diabetes throughout life.

Pathophysiology

Type 2 diabetes is characterized by an impaired insulin action or a defective secretion of insulin or both. Both defects are thought to be required for the manifestation of the disease, both augment each other and both are present many years prior to the clinical onset of the disease (6). The mechanisms by which obesity affects these two central processes is far from being understood but there is agreement that obesity promotes and aggravates insulin resistance. One of the earliest hypotheses to explain the relationship between obesity and diabetes is the "glucose–fatty acid cycle," which is based on the observation of a competition between glucose and fatty acid oxidation in the heart muscle (7). The higher the supply of fatty acids from hypertrophic fat cells and expanded adipose tissue depots the more fatty acids are used as fuel in muscle, the main organ of glucose utilization. As a consequence, the rate of glucose oxidation is reduced. In addition, mechanisms have been described how elevated free fatty acids can impair insulin action. Elevated free fatty acids were found to reduce insulin-stimulated glucose uptake and to decrease muscle glycogen synthesis. Finally, it is well-known that fatty acids promote hepatic glucose production, another key disturbance leading to glucose intolerance (8). Recent studies suggest that obese and type 2 diabetic subjects have a high intramyocellular lipid accumulation, which interferes with muscle glucose metabolism and could play an important role in the pathogenesis of type 2 diabetes (9). There are also studies in beta-cells indicating that long-chain fatty acids may exert an adverse effect on insulin secretion via overproduction of ceramide (10). A new observation is that over-expression of uncoupling protein 2 (UCP2) in the beta-cell, possibly due to elevated fatty acids, may contribute to the development of obesity-linked diabetes by decreasing mitochondrial coupling and impairing insulin secretion (11).

    A recent hypothesis is that secretory products from enlarged adipose tissue depots and fat cells may directly contribute to insulin resistance. Tabel 2 summarizes currently discussed

TABLE 2 Secretory Factors from Adipocytes Possibly Involved in the Pathophysiology of Obesity-Associated Insulin Resistance

Free fatty acids
Tumor necrosis factor-α
Leptin
Resistin
Interleukin-6
Angiotensin II
Monocyte chemotactic protein-1
Adiponectin

factors released from fat cells that have been related to the pathophysiology of insulin resistance. Among these candidates most data have been collected for a mediator role of tumor necrosis factor-α (TNF-α). TNF-α is a multifunctional cytokine that has been shown to exert a variety of catabolic effects in adipose tissue. It has been demonstrated by several groups that TNF-α and its two receptor subtypes are overexpressed in adipose tissue of obese subjects (12–14). The upregulated TNF-α induces multiple effects at the local level such as inhibition of glucose uptake due to an impairment of insulin signaling and suppression of GLUT4 expression, a reduction of lipoprotein lipase expression and activity, and an increase in lipolysis. Taken together, all these catabolic effects of TNF-α promote a state of insulin resistance (15,16). However, it is not yet clarified as to whether adipose overexpression of TNF-α also contributes to muscle insulin resistance in humans. There is no clear evidence from cross-sectional clinical studies for elevated circulating levels of the cytokine (17). Infusion of a soluble TNF-α antibody and neutralization of the cytokine had no effect on insulin sensitivity in subjects with type 2 diabetes (18,19). However, in a recent study in patients with rheumatoid arthritis chronic treatment with infliximab, an antibody against TNF-α, resulted in a significant improvement in insulin resistance (20).

Using an in vitro coculture system of human adipocytes and muscle cells we were recently unable to demonstrate a role of TNF-α secreted from adipocytes for the development of muscle insulin resistance, although the presence of adipocytes induced a state of insulin resistance indicating a role of fat cell secretory products (21). It turned out in a subsequent study that the impairment of insulin signaling in human muscle cells under these conditions can be prevented and overcome by the presence of adiponectin, which represents a recently identified abundantly expressed fat cell hormone with many antidiabetic and antiatherosclerotic properties (22). Another recent study indicated that monocyte chemotactic protein-1 (MCP-1), which is also overproduced in adipose tissue from obese subjects impairs insulin signaling in muscle and may represent a molecular link between obesity and insulin resistance (23). Taken together, many interesting new data on the relationship between fat cell function and muscular insulin resistance have been collected over recent years and may provide a more and more convincing explanation for the unfavorable effect of excess fat mass on systemic insulin action.

ANTIDIABETIC DRUGS AND BODY WEIGHT

It has long been recognized that antidiabetic drugs can promote weight gain in subjects with type 2 diabetes. The strongest weight-promoting effect is exerted by insulin. In the diabetes control and complications trial (DCCT), intensified insulin treatment was associated with substantial weight gain that resulted in unfavorable changes of lipid levels and blood pressure similar to those seen in the insulin resistance syndrome (24). In the UKPDS, insulin treatment caused a mean weight gain of approximately 7 kg over 12 years of treatment in newly diagnosed subjects with type 2 diabetes (25). In addition, sulfonylureas are known to promote weight gain due to their insulin-secretory action. In the UKPDS, the average weight gain under glibenclamide treatment amounted to about 5 kg (25). It was repeatedly reported that PRARγ-agonists lead to weight gain. However, this weight gain occurs mainly in the subcutaneous depots, but not in the visceral depot that may have less deleterious metabolic consequences (26). In the recently published ADOPT study treatment with rosiglitazone over 5 years was followed by a mean body weight increase of 4.8 kg. This weight gain was not associated with an increase in the waist/hip ratio indicating that the expansion of adipose tissue occurred largely in the subcutaneous depots (27). In the same trial, monotherapy with glibenclamide resulted in a mean weight gain of 1.6 kg. In contrast, metformin and α-glucosidase inhibitors have a modest weight-lowering potential (27,28).

OBESITY AND GLYCEMIC CONTROL

It is noteworthy that BMI is the most important predictor of deterioration in glycemic control, regardless of the treatment regimen, according to a study from Finland (25). Moreover, in this study, there was significantly greater decrease in HbA_{1c} levels in patients whose baseline weight was below the mean BMI of 28.1 kg/m^2 than in those whose weight was above this cutoff value (1.7 vs. 0.5 %, $p < 0.01$). For this reason, there is now agreement that prevention of weight gain is an important target when drug treatment is initiated in obese subjects with type 2 diabetes (29). This aspect is particularly significant in insulin-treated patients independent of the type of diabetes.

Management of Obesity in Subjects with Type 2 Diabetes

The management of obesity represents a central component in the treatment strategy for type 2 diabetes, as obesity is not only a major predisposing factor of the disease and its accompanying disorders, but also aggravates the achievement of a good metabolic control. Moreover, it was repeatedly shown that reducing excessive body weight in individuals with type 2 diabetes improves metabolic control and prolongs life (30–33). However, currently available weight reduction programs for patients suffering from diabetes turned out to have only limited success, particularly in the long run. An essential prerequisite for successful treatment are realistic goals. This is particularly important for this group as treatment of obese subjects with type 2 diabetes is usually more difficult than treating obese subjects without diabetes for several reasons. Type 2 diabetic subjects are usually older than nondiabetic obese subjects, which means a smaller weight loss as energy expenditure is decreasing with age. Another reason is that subjects with diabetes are focusing more on blood glucose control, which could result in the neglect of other health problems. Finally, the weight increasing and weight loss preventing potential of antidiabetic agents has to be considered. Irrespective of these specific considerations, the indications, goals and principles of treatment are the same in obese subjects with and without type 2 diabetes (Tabels 3 and 4). Table 5 summarizes in a flowchart current evidence-based therapeutic approaches for the prevention and treatment of obesity depending on the degree of overweight and the presence of comorbidities, which are also valid for overweight/obese subjects with type 2 diabetes.

NONPHARMACOLOGICAL THERAPY

The cornerstones of every weight reduction program are a moderately hypocaloric diet, an increase in physical activity and behavior modification. There are numerous studies that applied and examined such concepts but most of them were short-term and had disappointing long-term results (30–33). Weight loss strategies in overweight patients with type 2 diabetes using lifestyle modification measures produced only small improvements in body weight. The greatest effects were observed for multicomponent interventions including very-low-calorie and low-calorie diets (31).

TABLE 3 Treatment Targets in the Management of Obese Individuals with Type 2 Diabetes

Weight loss of 3 to 10 kg (depending on weight, age, and gender) and maintenance of reduced body weight
Improvement of cardiovascular risk factors
Healthy lifestyle (healthy eating, regular physical activity)
High quality of life

TABLE 4 Treatment Principles for Weight
Management in Obese Individuals with Type 2 Diabetes

Dietary therapy
Low-calorie diet (energy deficit: 500 to 1000 kcal/day)
Very low-calorie diet
Low-fat, carbohydrate ad libitum diet
Increase in physical activity
Behavior modification
Adjuvant drug treatment
Surgical treatment

DIETARY APPROACHES

The gold standard in the dietary treatment of obese patients with type 2 diabetes is a balanced moderately energy-restricted diet. The energy deficit is between 500 and 800 kcal/day. The most important single measure is the reduction in fat intake, particularly in saturated fatty acids. It is generally recommended to prefer a high-carbohydrate low-fat diet. As shown

TABLE 5 Obesity Prevention and Treatment Flowchart

Health status	Treatment goals	Treatment steps
Normal weight (BMI 18.5–24.9)	Weight maintenance	Consider periodic weight monitoring
Normal weight (BMI 18.5–24.9) plus risk factors(s) and/or comorbidity(ies)	Weight maintenance. Prevention of a >3 kg weight gain. Risk factor management, e.g. smoking cessation, healthy lifestyle	Weight monitoring, risk-factor management, treatment of comorbidities, advice for a healthy lifestyle
Pre-obesity (BMI 25–29.9)	Prevention of further weight gain or, preferably, induction of modest weight loss	Best practice program[a]
Pre-obesity (BMI 25–29.9) plus risk factors(s) and/or comorbidity(ies)	5–10% weight reduction in 3-6 months (especially if success in controlling risk factors is only moderate after 3 months) and weight maintenance thereafter	Best practice program[a], risk-factor management, treatment of comorbidities
Obesity Class I (BMI 30–34.9)	5–10% sustained weight reduction	Best practice program[a]
Obesity Class I (BMI 30–34.9) plus risk factors (s) and/or comorbidity(ies)	5–10% sustained weight reduction	Best practice program[a], risk-factor management, treatment of comorbidities If not successful, consider additional drug therapy no earlier than after 12 weeks
Obesity Class II (BMI 35–39.9)	≥10% sustained weight reduction	Best practice program[a]
Obesity Class II (BMI 35–39.9) plus risk factors (s) and/or comorbidity(ies)	10–20% sustained weight reduction	Best practice program[a], risk-factor management, treatment of comorbidities If not successful, consider additional drug therapy no earlier than 12 weeks If conservative treatment is not successful, consider surgical treatment
Obesity Class III (BMI >40)	10–30% sustained weight reduction	Best practice program[a], risk factor management, treatment of comorbidities If conservative treatment is not successful, consider surgical treatment

[a] The best practice program consists of a combination of dietary therapy, increased physical activity, and behavioral modification.
Source: From Ref. 26.

recently, a diet rich in fiber and complex carbohydrates has some beneficial effects on parameters of glucose and lipid metabolism but these effects may be small and possibly of limited clinical importance (34). The concept of a high-carbohydrate, low-fat diet was, however, challenged by clinical studies showing that replacement of saturated fat by monounsaturated fat compared to high-carbohydrate intake is equally favorable or has even some minor advantages with regard to glycemic response and lipids (35). For these reasons, there is convincing evidence that energy content rather than nutrient composition is the major determinant of weight reduction in obese subjects with type 2 diabetes.

From a practical point of view it is extremely important to carefully assess the habitual diet of a patient with type 2 diabetes and to focus counselling on punctual changes of his/her eating habits in order to get close to current dietary recommendations (36,37). It should be stressed that all efforts for dietary changes should be made as simple as possible for the patients as they are burdened by many requirements to manage their diabetes (28). For obese subjects with type 2 diabetes the frequent recommendation to distribute their allowed calories over 5 to 6 meals is difficult to be met and may even hinder weight loss without being of any advantage for metabolic control (38). Therefore, in most cases 3 to 4 meals a day may be more appropriate to reach the individual dietary goals.

Another possible dietary approach is the use of a very-low-calorie diet (VLCD) for initial weight loss. This option may be particularly valuable for patients with poor metabolic control and/or "dietary failure." Usually, there is a rapid improvement of insulin resistance and glycemic control after even short periods of VLCD. However, this approach can only be applied for a limited number of weeks and requires intense medical care. Nevertheless, a recent review concluded with the statement that the long-term results of VLCD are better than those of conventional diets (39). There is certainly a need for new sophisticated solutions such as intermittent VLCD in combination with conventional hypocaloric diets to obtain better long-term results (40). Another potentially promising strategy is to establish a long-term meal-replacement concept, which substitutes 1 or 2 meals daily by balanced formula diets of reduced calorie content, as recently demonstrated in a 4-year clinical study in nondiabetic obese subjects (41). In a recent study in obese type 2 diabetic patients, percentage weight loss by meal replacement was significantly greater than under the diet recommended by the American Diabetes Association (4.57% vs. 2.25%, $p < 0.05$) including a greater reduction of fasting plasma glucose and HbA_{1c} and a greater reduction in the use and dosage of oral hypoglycemic agents (42). Further progress in this field can also be expected from the ongoing Look AHEAD study which is aiming at substantial weight loss in obese diabetic subjects to reduce the high cardiovascular risk of these patients (43). There is no doubt that more research is urgently required to develop strategies that may help to provide better individual solutions and to manage the weight problem of many patients more efficiently.

INCREASE OF PHYSICAL ACTIVITY

Current concepts to increase physical activity in patients with obesity and type 2 diabetes have shown only small efficiency. As most patients are completely sedentary or immobilized due to other health problems such as osteoarthritis regular physical activity is difficult to be established on a regular basis. There is no doubt that most obese type 2 diabetic subjects would benefit from at least some level of physical activity. As almost all of these patients have low physical fitness as assessed by VO_{2max} only low-intensity training is possible and appropriate. Among the low-intensity activities, which should be recommended are walking at a self-selected speed, swimming, or gymnastics/aerobics. There are sufficient data available to demonstrate an improvement of insulin resistance by low-to-moderate physical activity in men and women with and without type 2 diabetes (44). Although there is still some debate how much low-intensity activities are needed to have a detectable impact on metabolic parameters and body weight, there is compelling evidence that even moderate physical activity is beneficial for glycemic control and blood lipids despite little effect on body weight (45).

WEIGHT-LOWERING DRUGS

Another component in the treatment of obesity is the adjunct administration of weight-lowering drugs. As limited experience is available drug treatment is only recommended if the nonpharmacological treatment program is not sufficiently successful and if the benefit/risk ratio justifies drug administration (46). At present, only few compounds are available, which have demonstrated efficacy and safety in obese subjects with and without type 2 diabetes.

Orlistat is a gastric and pancreatic lipase inhibitor that impairs the intestinal absorption of ingested fat. In a 1-year study in obese type 2 diabetic subjects orlistat treatment produced a greater weight loss compared to placebo treatment (6.2% vs. 4.3%, $p<0.001$). In addition, orlistat-treated patients had a small improvement in HbA_{1c} compared to controls (-0.28% vs. $+0.18$%, $p<0.001$). Furthermore, the average dose of sulfonylureas decreased more in the orlistat than in the placebo group (-23 vs. -9%, $p=0.002$) (47). This study as well as other indicates that adjunct treatment of obese type 2 diabetic patients by orlistat provides modest additional weight loss together with small improvements in glycemic control and other risk factors (48).

Sibutramine is a selective serotonin- and noradrenaline-reuptake inhibitor that enhances satiety and slightly increases thermogenesis. There are data from several controlled studies with a duration between 3 and 12 months, which showed an additional average weight loss of 5.1 kg as well as modest decrease in HbA_{1c} (48). However, as sibutramine is well known to increase sympathetic nerve activity this drug should not be used in diabetic patients with uncontrolled hypertension and/or coronary artery disease, which are both frequent comorbidities and its long-term safety is still uncertain.

Rimonabant is a recently approved weight-lowering drug, which acts as a selective blocker of central and peripheral CB1 receptors. In the RIO diabetes study, administration of 20 mg rimonabant in overweight and obese type 2 diabetic patients was associated with a significantly greater reduction in body weight (5.3 vs. 1.4 kg, $p<0.001$) and HbA_{1c} levels (-0.6% vs. $+0.1$%, $p<0.001$) (49). Although rimonabant appears to be well tolerated and to have beneficial metabolic effects beyond weight loss, further studies are needed to fully define its profile including benefit and safety in patients with type diabetes.

BARIATRIC SURGERY

Bariatric surgery is now an established method to reduce body weight in subjects with extreme obesity (≥ 40 kg/m^2), and there is growing consensus that this method can also be applied in subjects with type 2 diabetes at a BMI≥ 35 kg/m^2 (33). In this group of patients surgery is by far the most effective treatment mode with excellent long-term results compared to all other methods. In the Swedish Obese Subjects (SOS) study, a large prospective trial comparing bariatric surgery with conventional dietary treatment, sustained weight loss ≥ 20 kg was exclusively achieved in the operated subjects with practically no significant weight change in the control group. Analysis of the data revealed that the 10-year cumulative incidence of diabetes and of other cardiovascular risk factors with the exception of hypertension was reduced by up to 80% in the operated group compared to the control group (50). Other studies have shown that bariatric surgery of extremely obese subjects with clinical diabetes is associated with a dramatic improvement in glycemic control. In up to 80% of the operated patients insulin treatment was no longer required after substantial weight loss and all other medications for diabetes and other cardiovascular risk factors could be considerably reduced or discontinued (51). In another analysis from the same group, sustained weight reduction in obese type 2 diabetic subjects was associated with a remarkable lower mortality and healthcare utilization compared to patients on the waiting list (52).

IMPACT OF WEIGHT LOSS ON TYPE 2 DIABETES

Numerous studies investigated the consequences of short-term and long-term weight reduction on health. Meta-analyses of the available literature clearly suggest that intentional weight loss using appropriate methods is beneficial. A 5% to 10% weight loss appears to be sufficient to obtain significant health effects (53). Nevertheless, the favorable effects depend on the methods applied for weight reduction and, most importantly, on the degree of weight loss (30,54). In the Finnish Diabetes Prevention Study, a comprehensive lifestyle modification program proved to be highly effective in preventing the development of type 2 diabetes in subjects with impaired glucose tolerance. The beneficial effect was positively influenced by the concomitant weight loss of 4 kg on average (55). Concerning the prognosis of obese individuals with type 2 diabetes weight loss has been shown to reduce the risk of death from comorbid diabetes. Each loss of 1 kg was estimated to add between 3 and 4 months to life expectancy in newly diagnosed subjects with type 2 diabetes (56). In a recent prospective analysis of a subgroup of overweight individuals with diabetes from the American Cancer Society's Cancer Prevention Study I intentional weight loss was associated with a 25% reduction in total mortality and a 28% reduction in coronary heart disease and diabetes mortality (32). These positive changes in the risk factor profile and mortality along with weight loss should encourage efforts to look for more effective strategies for weight reduction in obese diabetic subjects, as currently being done in the Look AHEAD study (43).

LONG-TERM WEIGHT STABILIZATION

The long-term result of any weight management program is critically dependent on the long-term strategy. Since a hypocaloric diet causes a decrease in energy expenditure, a return to previous eating habits will rapidly result in weight regain. Therefore, the patient has to recognize that long-term weight loss is only possible if a new energy balance is achieved at a lower level. To maintain a weight loss of about 10 kg a long-term reduction in energy intake of about 500 kcal/day is required to compensate for the reduction in total energy expenditure (57). To support weight stabilization and to prevent weight relapse the following strategies have proven useful: a low-fat diet rich in complex carbohydrates, an increase in physical activity, social support from family and friends, group support and continued contact with trusted medical care professionals (28,33).

CONCLUSION

Most patients with type 2 diabetes are overweight or obese. Therefore, weight management should be a central component of any treatment strategy, as weight loss has been convincingly shown to provide a marked improvement in metabolic control. However, as conventional concepts combining an energy-reduced diet and an increase in physical activity frequently have poor long-term results, more effective weight loss strategies should be developed and applied. Such components with additional benefit are VLCD, weight-lowering drugs, and bariatric surgery, the latter particularly for severely obese subjects. Long-term studies are urgently needed to obtain more precise information on the relative success of the various strategies in the management of obese diabetic patients.

REFERENCES

1. World Health Organization. Obesity: preventing and managing the global epidemic. Report of a WHO consultation. WHO Technical Report Series 894. Geneva: World Health Organization, 2000.
2. Colditz GA, Willett WC, Rotnitzky A, Manson JE. Weight gain as a risk factor for clinical diabetes in women. Ann Intern Med 1995; 122:481–6.
3. Chan JM, Rimm EB, Colditz GA, Stampfer MJ, Willett WC. Obesity, fat distribution, and weight gain as risk factors for clinical diabetes in men. Diabetes Care 1994; 17:961–9.
4. Ohlson LO, Larsson B, Svärdsudd K, et al. The influence of body fat distribution on the incidence of diabetes mellitus. 13.5 years of follow-up of the participants in the study of men born in 1913. Diabetes 1985; 34:1055–8.
5. Jebb SA, Elia M. Techniques for the measurement of body composition: a practical guide. Int J Obes Rel Metab Dis 1993; 17:611–21.
6. Polonsky KS, Sturis SJ, Bell GI. Non-insulin-dependent diabetes mellitus—a genetically programmed failure of the beta cell to compensate for insulin resistance. N Engl J Med 1996; 334: 777–83.

7. Randle P, Garland P, Hales C, Newsholme E. The glucose-fatty acid cycle. Its role in insulin sensitivity and the metabolic disturbances of diabetes mellitus. Lancet 1963; I:785–9.
8. Boden G. Role of fatty acids in the pathogenesis of insulin resistance and NIDDM. Diabetes 1997; 45: 3–10.
9. Storlien LH, Kriketos AD, Jenkins AB, et al. Does dietary fat influence insulin action. Ann NY Acad Sci 1997; 827:287–301.
10. Shimabukuro M, Higa M, Zhou YT, et al. Lipoapoptosis in beta-cells of obese prediabetic fa/fa rats. Role of serine palmitoyltransferase overexpression. J Biol Chem 1998; 273:32487–90.
11. Langin D. Diabetes, insulin secretion, and the pancreatic beta-cell mitochondrion. N Engl J Med 2001; 345:1772–4.
12. Hotamisligil GS, Arner P, Caro JF, et al.: Increased adipose tissue expression of tumor necrosis factor-α in human obesity and insulin resistance. J Clin Invest 1995; 95:2409–15.
13. Kern PA, Saghizadeh M, Ong JM, et al. The expression of tumor necrosis factor in human adipose tissue. Regulation by obesity, weight loss and relationship to lipoprotein lipase. J Clin Invest 1995; 95: 2111–99.
14. Hube F, Birgel M, Lee Y-M, Hauner H. Expression pattern of tumour necrosis factor receptors in subcutaneous and omental human adipose tissue: role of obesity and non-insulin-dependent diabetes mellitus. Eur J Clin Invest 1999; 29:672–8.
15. Hauner H, Petruschke T, Russ M, Röhrig K, Eckel J. Effects of tumor necrosis factor-alpha (TNF) on glucose transport and lipid metabolism of newly differentiated human fat cells in culture. Diabetologia 1995; 38:764–71.
16. Hube F, Hauner H. The role of TNF-α in human adipose tissue. Prevention of weight gain at the expense of insulin resistance? Horm Metab Res 1999; 31:626–31.
17. Hauner H, Bender M, Haastert B, Hube F. Plasma concentrations of soluble TNF-alpha receptors in obese humans. Int J Obes 1998; 22:1239–43.
18. Ofei F, Hurel S, Newkirk J, Sopwith M, Taylor R. Effects of an engineered human anti-TNF-α antibody (CDP571) on insulin sensitivity and glycemic control in patients with NIDDM. Diabetes 1996; 45:881–5.
19. Paquot N, Castillo MJ, Lefebvre PJ, Scheen AJ. No increased insulin sensitivity after a single intravenous administration of a recombinant human tumor necrosis factor receptor: Fc fusion protein in obese insulin-resistant patients. J Clin Endocrinol Metab 2000; 85:1316–9.
20. Gonzalez-Gay MA, de Matias JM, Gonzalez-Juanatey C, et al. Anti-tumor necrosis factor-α blockade improves insulin resistance in patients with rheumatoid arthritis. Clin Exp Rheumatol 2006; 24:83–6.
21. Dietze D, Koenen M, Röhrig K, et al. Impairment of insulin signaling in human skeletal muscle cells by co-culture with human adipocytes. Diabetes 2002; 51:2369–76.
22. Dietze-Schröder D, Sell H, Uhlig M, et al. Autocrine action of adiponectin on human fat cells prevents the release of insulin resistance-inducing factors. Diabetes 2005; 54:2003–11.
23. Sell H, Dietze-Schröder D, Kaiser U, Eckel J. Monocyte chemotactic protein-1 is a potential player in the negative cross-talk between adipose tissue and skeletal muscle. Endocrinology 2006; 147: 2458–67.
24. Purnell JQ, Hokanson JE, Marcovina SM, et al. Effect of excessive weight gain with intensive therapy of type 1 diabetes on lipid levels and blood pressure. Results from the DCCT. JAMA 1998; 280:140–6.
25. UKPDS. Intensive blood-glucose control with sulphonylureas or insulin compared with conventional treatment and risk of complications in patients with type 2 diabetes (UKPDS 33). Lancet 1998; 12:837–52.
26. Despres JP, Lemieux I, Prud'homme D. Treatment of obesity: need to focus on high risk abdominally obese patients. Br Med J 2001; 322:716–20.
27. Kahn SE, Haffner SM, Heise MA, et al. Glycemic durability of rosiglitazone, metformin, or glyburide monotherapy. N Engl J Med 2006; 355:2427–43.
28. Hauner H. Managing type 2 diabetes mellitus in patients with obesity. Treat Endocrinol 2004; 3: 223–32.
29. Yki-Järvinen H, Ryysy L, Kauppila M, et al. Effect of obesity on the response to insulin therapy in non-insulin-dependent diabetes mellitus. J Clin Endocrinol Metab 1997; 82:4037–43.
30. Brown SA, Upchurch S, Anding R, et al. Promoting weight loss in type II diabetes. Diabetes Care 1996; 19:613–24.
31. Norris SL, Zhang X, Averell A, et al. Long-term non-pharmacological weight loss intervention for adults with type 2 diabetes. Cochrane Database Syst Rev 2005; CD004095.
32. Williamson DF, Thompson TJ, Thun M, et al. Intentional weight loss and mortality among overweight individuals with diabetes. Diabetes Care 2000; 23:1499–504.
33. Expert Panel on the Identification, Evaluation, and Treatment of Overweight and Obesity in Adults. Clinical guidelines on the identification, evaluation, and treatment of overweight and obesity in adults. The evidence report. National Institute of Health National Heart, Lung and Blood Institute, Bethesda, 1998.

34. Chandalia M, Grag A, Lutjohann D, et al. Beneficial effects of high fiber intake in patients with type 2 diabetes mellitus. N Engl J Med 2000; 342:1392–8.

35. Garg A, Bonanome A, Grundy SM, et al. Comparison of a high-carbohydrate diet with high-monounsaturated-fat diet in patients with non-insulin-dependent diabetes mellitus. N Engl J Med 1988; 319:829–34.

36. Mann JI, De Leeuw I, Hermansen K, et al. Evidence-based nutritional approaches to the treatment and prevention of diabetes mellitus. Nutr Metab Cardiovasc Dis 2004; 14:373–94.

37. American Diabetes Association. Nutrition principles and recommendations in diabetes. Diabetes Care 2004; 27(Suppl. 1):S36–44.

38. Arnold L, Mann JI, Ball MJ. Metabolic effects of alterations in meal frequency in type 2 diabetes. Diabetes Care 1997; 20:1651–4.

39. Anderson JW, Konz EC, Frederich RC, Wood CL. Long-term weight-loss maintenance: a meta-analysis of US studies. Am J Clin Nutr 2001; 74:579–84.

40. Ditschuneit HH, Flechtner-Mors M, Johnson TD, Adler G. Metabolic and weight-loss effects of long-term dietary intervention in obese patients. Am J Clin Nutr 1999; 69:198–204.

41. Williams KV, Mullen ML, Kelly DE, Wing RR. The effect of short periods of caloric restriction on weight loss and glycemic control in type 2 diabetes. Diabetes Care 1998; 21:2–8.

42. Li Z, Hong K, Saltsman P, et al. Long-term efficacy of soy-based meal replacements vs. an individualized diet plan in obese type II DM patients: relative effects on weight loss, metabolic parameters, and C-reactive protein. Eur J Clin Nutr 2005; 59:411–8.

43. Look AHEAD Research Group. The Look AHEAD study: a description of the lifestyle intervention and the evidence suggesting it. Obesity 2006; 14:737–52.

44. Mayer-Davis EJ, D'Agostino R, Karter AJ, et al. Intensity and amount of physical activity in relation to insulin sensitivity. The insulin resistance atherosclerosis study. JAMA 1998; 279:669–74.

45. Thomas DE, Elliott EJ, Naughton GA. Exercise for type 2 diabetes mellitus. Cochrane Database Syst Rev 2006; CD002968.

46. National Task Force on the Prevention and Treatment of Obesity. Long-term pharmacotherapy in the management of obesity. JAMA 1996; 276:1907–15.

47. Hollander PA, Elbein SC, Hirsch IB, et al. Role of orlistat in the treatment of obese patients with type 2 diabetes. Diabetes Care 1998; 21:1288–98.

48. Norris SL, Zhang X, Averell A, et al. Pharmacotherapy for weight loss in adults with type 2 diabetes mellitus. Cochrane Database Syst Rev 2005; CD004096.

49. Scheen AJ, Finer N, Hollander P, et al. Efficacy and tolerability of rimonabant in overweight or obese patients with type 2 diabetes: a randomised controlled study. Lancet 2006; 368:1660–72.

50. Sjöström L, Lindroos AK, Peltonen M, et al. Lifestyle, diabetes, and cardiovascular risk factors 10 years after bariatric surgery. N Engl J Med 2004; 351:2683–93.

51. Pories WJ, MacDonald KG, Morgan EJ, et al. Surgical treatment of obesity and its effect on diabetes: 10-y follow-up. Am J Clin Nutr 1992; 55:582S–5.

52. MacDonald KG, Long SD, Swanson MS, et al. The gastric bypass operation reduces the progression and mortality of non-insulin-dependent diabetes mellitus. J Gastrointest Surg 1997; 1:213–20.

53. Goldstein DJ. Beneficial health effects of modest weight loss. Int J Obes Relat Metab Disord 1991; 16: 397–415.

54. Wing RR, Koeske R, Epstein LH, et al. Long-term effects of modest weight loss in type II diabetic patients. Arch Intern Med 1987; 147:1749–53.

55. Tuomilehto J, Lindström J, Eriksson JG, et al. Prevention of type 2 diabetes mellitus by changes in lifestyle among subjects with impaired glucose tolerance. N Engl J Med 2001; 344:1343–9.

56. Lean ME, Powrie JK, Anderson AS, Garthwaite PH. Obesity, weight loss, and prognosis in type 2 diabetes. Diab Med 1990; 7:228–33.

57. Leibel RL, Rosenbaum M, Hirsch J. Changes in energy expenditure resulting from altered body weight. N Engl J Med 1995; 332:621–8.

27 | Dyslipidemia and Diabetes

Ioanna Gouni-Berthold
Department of Internal Medicine, University of Cologne, Cologne, Germany

David John Betteridge and Wilhelm Krone
Department of Medicine, University College Hospital, London, U.K.

INTRODUCTION

Disorders of lipid and lipoprotein metabolism in individuals with insulin resistance or diabetes mellitus type 2 increase cardiovascular risks. The most common characteristics of lipid disorders in insulin-resistant individuals are elevations of triglycerides and low levels of high-density lipoprotein (HDL)-cholesterol. Accordingly, the American Diabetes Association recommends searching for underlying glucose intolerance in individuals with dyslipidemia (HDL cholesterol <0.90 mmol/L, [<35 mg/dL] and/or a triglyceride level ≥2.82 mmol/L [≥250 mg/dL]) with an oral glucose tolerance test (1).

The epidemiology linking dyslipidemia to coronary heart disease (CHD) risk has long been recognized to fulfill the criteria for a causal relationship. However, until relatively recently there has been dispute concerning the overall benefits of lipid lowering and the possible non-cardiovascular adverse events of low plasma cholesterol and cholesterol lowering. The advent of the statins (HMG-CoA reductase inhibitors), which are highly effective and well-tolerated, enabled definitive end-point trials to be performed in populations with and without established CHD. These trials (2–6) have provided a huge evidence base for clinical practice, and national and international bodies have proposed various guidelines and treatment algorithms to enable the results of research to be translated into clinical practice for patients at high risk for vascular events.

Diabetes mellitus, particularly type 2 diabetes, is associated with a markedly increased risk of cardiovascular events mainly due to premature and extensive atherosclerosis. This is not fully explained by the known major CHD risk factors. CHD is increased two- to three-fold and accounts for three-quarters of all cardiovascular deaths among patients with type 2 diabetes. Interestingly, recent data suggest that not all patients with diabetes are at "high risk," such as young (<40 years of age) patients with no additional risk factors (7, 8).

Patients with diabetes who develop CHD have a much worse prognosis than non-diabetic patients and are more likely to die acutely with the first myocardial infarction (MI) (9). In the GUSTO-I trial (Global Utilization of Streptokinase and Tissue Plasminogen Activator for Occluded Coronary Arteries) diabetes remained an independent determinant of 30-day mortality after adjustment for both clinical and angiographic variables (10). In the longer term, the outlook is also poor – the 5-year mortality in a Swedish study was 55% in patients with diabetes compared to 30% in non-diabetics (11).

The incidence of diabetes mellitus type 2 is expected to increase dramatically over the next decade. By 2010, it is estimated that approximately 221 million people worldwide will have this condition, representing a 45% increase over just 10 years (12).

This massive burden of morbidity and mortality from the development of CHD, together with the poor outcome associated with large increases in the risk of cerebrovascular and peripheral vascular disease, provides a huge challenge to the physician caring for patients with diabetes. This short review discusses the diabetic dyslipidemia in relation to CHD risk.

EPIDEMIOLOGY OF DYSLIPIDEMIA IN TYPE 2 DIABETES

Given the predicted increase in the prevalence of diabetes worldwide and the progressive Westernization of lifestyles in developing countries, cardiovascular disease, which is increased two to five times in people with diabetes, has and will continue to have major implications for health and healthcare provision. Although the development of atherosclerosis and clinical vascular disease is multifactorial, dyslipidemia is a major contributing risk factor.

Dyslipidemia is common in patients with type 2 diabetes; it is present at the time of diagnosis, and even in the pre-diabetic phase. It persists despite usual hypoglycemic therapy and its expression will be affected by genetic and lifestyle characteristics, such as gender, obesity, exercise levels, diet, alcohol intake, poor glycemic control, smoking, hypothyroidism, as well as renal and hepatic function. It is also affected by concomitant drugs and the presence of primary dyslipidemia, such as familial combined hyperlipidemia.

The hallmarks of diabetic dyslipidemia are moderate hypertriglyceridemia (usually 1.5 to 3-fold increased) and reduced HDL cholesterol (approximately 10–20%); total and low-density lipoprotein (LDL) cholesterol are generally not different quantitatively from non-diabetics. For example, in the prospective cardiovascular munster (PROCAM) study in the North of Germany 39% of patients with diabetes had triglyceride concentrations >200 mg/dL (>2.3 mmol/L), versus 21% in non-diabetics, and 27% had low HDL cholesterol i.e. <35 mg/dL (<0.9 mmol/L), compared with 16% in non-diabetics (13).

Qualitative changes in the LDL of patients with diabetes, however, suggest increased atherogenicity. In specific, LDL apoprotein B is susceptible to glycation and this decreases its affinity for the LDL receptor and increases its susceptibility to oxidative modification. In addition, the LDL subfraction distribution is altered in patients with diabetes. In specific, LDL is smaller and denser, a form more susceptible to oxidation and therefore more atherogenic (14).

Of the 347 978 men screened for participation in the multiple risk factor intervention trial (MRFIT) (15), 5163 were identified as having diabetes through reporting of medication. In the 12-year follow-up of this cohort, the absolute risk of cardiovascular death was increased three-fold in patients with diabetes after adjustment for age, race, income, serum cholesterol, systolic blood pressure and cigarette smoking. With increasing serum cholesterol cardiovascular deaths increased both in men with and without diabetes; however, for given cholesterol level, men with diabetes had a two- to three-fold excess risk of cardiovascular disease. This was also true for two other major risk factors, cigarette smoking and hypertension, and for the three factors combined. These findings supported the notion that in diabetes rigorous intervention to control risk factors, including cholesterol levels, is needed.

In the UK prospective diabetes study (UKPDS), LDL cholesterol was the major determinant for CHD (16). Triglycerides and CHD have been the subjects of much debate over the last two decades particularly in relation to the independence of their relationship. In both, the PROCAM population (17) and the Helsinki Heart Study (18), hypertriglyceridemia was associated with CHD risk in individuals with an LDL:HDL cholesterol ratio >5. This clustering of lipid abnormalities is often referred to as the atherogenic lipoprotein profile.

Hypertriglyceridemia is associated with several important atherogenic mechanisms in type 2 diabetes. Some triglyceride-rich particles that are directly atherogenic, namely the remnant particles, accumulate in patients with diabetes (19). These cholesterol-rich particles, containing apoproteins B and C-III also accumulate in the rare Type III dyslipidemia (remnant particle disease or broad beta disease), which is associated with premature and extensive atherosclerosis. Hypertriglyceridemia is also associated with significant abnormalities in thrombosis and coagulation, particularly increased levels of plasminogen activator inhibitor-1, and prolonged as well as elevated postprandial lipemia. Haffner et al. (20) investigated 1734 individuals prospectively over 7 years in the San Antonio Heart Study. They found that the 195 individuals who developed type 2 diabetes had a higher body mass index (BMI), as well as waist-to-hip ratio, higher blood pressure, elevated plasma triglycerides and lower HDL-cholesterol levels.

Couillard et al. (19) has shown that high triglyceride levels and low HDL-cholesterol concentrations are associated with postprandial hyperlipidemia. Sixty-three men with low (<0.9 mmol/L, <35 mg/dL) fasting HDL-cholesterol and either low (<2 mmol/L, <176 mg/dL) or high (>2 mmol/L, >176 mg/dL) triglyceride levels were investigated. A significant relation between postprandial triglyceride increase and HDL-cholesterol levels in the fasting state was shown. Normolipidemic controls and men with low HDL-cholesterol as well as low triglyceride levels showed a comparable postprandial lipid increase and no signs of insulin resistance. Individuals with low HDL-cholesterol and high triglyceride levels had a greater increase in postprandial lipemia associated with visceral obesity and insulin resistance.

LIPID AND LIPOPROTEIN METABOLISM IN INSULIN RESISTANT STATES

Insulin resistance is central to the dyslipidemia of type 2 diabetes (21). A simplified overview of the mechanisms of the dyslipidemia of diabetes is shown in Fig. 1. In the presence of insulin resistance there is an increased flux of free fatty acids from adipose tissue to the liver, as a result of decreased inhibition of the hormone-sensitive lipase. Fatty acids stimulate increased hepatic production and secretion of very low-density lipoprotein (VLDL), which is also increased by insulin resistance and hyperinsulinemia. Increased hepatic output of VLDL continues in the postprandial state and competes with exogenously-derived triglyceride carried in chylomicrons for the enzyme lipoprotein lipase. As a result, there is accumulation of triglyceride-rich lipoproteins and prolonged postprandial lipemia. The lipemia stimulates increased lipid transfer via cholesterol ester transfer protein (CETP) exchanging triglyceride for cholesterol ester between triglyceride-rich lipoproteins and lipoproteins of higher density. As a result, LDL and HDL are enriched in triglycerides and become substrates for hepatic lipase (HL), which hydrolyses triglyceride, producing small dense LDL and small dense HDL. The importance of small dense LDL has been discussed above in relation to atherogenesis. Small dense HDL is more rapidly catabolized than other HDL species, leading to lower plasma HDL concentrations (22). Low HDL cholesterol concentrations are a strong predictor of vascular risk in diabetes, as in the general population (9). Furthermore, small dense HDL cannot pick up cholesterol from tissues and deliver it to the liver as efficiently as larger HDL (23).

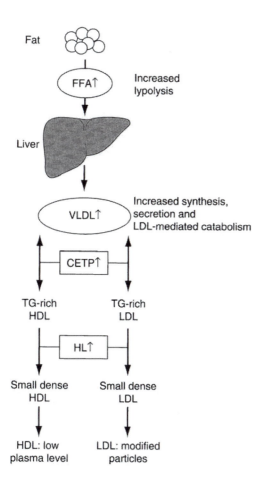

FIGURE 1 Essential steps in the development of diabetic dyslipidemia. Cholesteryl ester transfer protein (CETP) is synthesized in the liver and circulates primarily bound to HDL. It transfers triglycerides from VLDL to HDL and LDL for the exchange of cholesterol, thereby generating triglyceride-rich HDL and LDL particles. These particles are substrate for hepatic lipase (HL), which cleaves triglycerides and leaves small dense HDL and LDL.

IMPACT OF LIPID-LOWERING ON CARDIOVASCULAR ENDPOINTS

Cardiovascular disease (CVD) is a major cause of morbidity and mortality in patients with diabetes, and their risk is similar to that of non-diabetics with prior myocardial infarction (MI) (24). Improved glycemic control alone seems not to be sufficient to improve the CVD risk profile of patients with diabetes. In this regard, in the UKPDS, more intensive hypoglycemic therapy was associated with a 25% risk reduction in microvascular end points compared with conventional therapy (p=0.01), whereas risk reductions in fatal or nonfatal MI did not reach significance (fatal MI, 6% risk reduction, p=0.94; nonfatal MI, 21% risk reduction, p= 0.06) (25).

Following is a brief review the available evidence of cardiovascular benefit of lipid-lowering therapy in patients with diabetes.

Statin Treatment for Patients With Diabetes

There are sufficient numbers of patients with diabetes in the major secondary prevention trials with statins to allow meaningful subgroup analyses. In the Scandinavian Simvastatin Survival Study (4S) (26) an initial analysis described the impact of simvastatin (20–40 mg/day) on 202 patients with diabetes out of a total of 4444 patients with established CHD and raised cholesterol concentrations (212–309 mg/dL, 5.5–8.0 mmol/L). In the diabetic subgroup, simvastatin produced similar effects on serum lipid and lipoprotein concentrations over the course of the trial as in non-diabetics, with reductions in total and LDL cholesterol of 24% and 34%, respectively, an 8% increase in HDL and a 9% reduction in triglyceride. It should be pointed out that the entry criteria for 4S stipulated total serum triglycerides 220 mg/dL ($\leq$2.5 mmol/L). These changes were associated with a significant reduction in major coronary events – relative risk (RR) reduction 0.45 (p=0.002). The reduction in the primary end-point of 4S – all-cause mortality – was not significant, given the small numbers, but did approach significance. RR reduction was 0.57 (p=0.087). A further analysis of 4S data using the new diagnostic criterion for diabetes from the American Diabetes Association, i.e. a fasting plasma venous glucose of $\geq$126 mg/dL (7 mmol/L) revealed 483 patients with diabetes (27). In this larger group, the RR reduction for major coronary events was 0.58 (p=0.001), with a highly significant reduction in revascularisations. Total and coronary mortality were also reduced, but these reductions did not reach statistical significance due to the small sample sizes. In 678 patients with impaired fasting glucose (110–125mg/dL, 6.0–6.9 mmol/L) there was a significant reduction in coronary events (RR=0.62; p=0.003) and total mortality (RR=0.57; p=0.02). These results have been analysed with regard to cost-effectiveness and resource utilisation, and have been found to be highly cost-effective (28).

Subgroup analysis of 586 patients with diabetes included in the Cholesterol and Recurrent Events (CARE) trial provided additional evidence of the benefit of statin therapy (29). Pravastatin 40 mg/day was associated with a RR reduction in major coronary events of 25% (p=0.05). Further evidence of the benefit of pravastatin therapy in patients with diabetes comes from the subgroup analysis of 782 patients with diabetes in the long-term intervention with pravastatin in ischemic disease (LIPID) trial (5).

Furthermore, patients with diabetes have been shown to have CHD risk reductions similar to those of non-diabetics, as shown in many primary and secondary CHD trials (Table 1).

For example the heart protection study (HPS) randomized 20,536 patients at risk of occlusive arterial disease to either simvastatin 40 mg/day or placebo (30). This patient population included a subgroup of 5963 patients with known diabetes (31). At the end of the 5-year treatment period, patients in the overall population treated with statin experienced a 24% reduction in major vascular events (i.e. CHD death, nonfatal MI, stroke and revascularization) compared with patients given placebo. The risk reduction was similar in the subgroup with diabetes (22%). Additional data from HPS demonstrated the impact of low HDL cholesterol on CVD risk in patients with diabetes. In the diabetic subgroup, a greater risk for vascular events was observed in placebo-treated patients with low baseline HDL cholesterol levels (31.1%) than in placebo-treated patients with high baseline LDL cholesterol levels (27.9%), suggesting that strategies targeting low levels of HDL cholesterol may result in benefit in addition to those that target high LDL cholesterol concentrations.

TABLE 1 Coronary Heart Disease (CHD) Prevention Trials with Statins in Subgroup Analyses of Patients with Diabetes Mellitus

Trial	Statin	Patients with diabetes (n)	Overall CHD risk reduction (%)	CHD risk reduction in patients with diabetes (%)	P value
Primary prevention					
AFCAPS/TexCAPS (2)	Lovastatin	155	37	43	NS
HPS (31)	Simvastatin	2.913	24	20	<0.0001
ASCOT-LLA (60)	Atorvastatin	2.532	36	16	NS
Secondary prevention					
CARE (3)	Pravastatin	586	23	25	0.05
4S (26)	Simvastatin	202	32	55	0.002
LIPID (5)	Pravastatin	782	24	19	NS
4S Reanalysis (27)	Simvastatin	483	32	42	0.001
HPS (31)	Simvastatin	3.050	24	18.4	<0.001
Primary/secondary prevention					
ALLHAT (61)	Pravastatin	3.648	9	11	NS

The results from two other recent studies also support a strategy of intensive lipid lowering with statins in patients with diabetes. In specific, the treating to new targets (TNT) trial compared the effects of 10 vs. 80 mg atorvastatin over 5 years (32). A total of 10,001 patients with stable CHD and LDL cholesterol <130 mg/dL (3.3 mmol/L) were randomly assigned to the two aforementioned atorvastatin doses. The primary endpoint was the occurrence of a first major cardiovascular event (death from CHD, nonfatal-non-procedure-related MI, and resuscitation after cardiac arrest, fatal or nonfatal stroke). A primary event occurred in 8.7% of the subjects receiving 80 mg of atorvastatin and in 10.9% of those receiving 10 mg, representing a significant 22% relative risk reduction ($p<0.001$). A total of 1501 patients had diabetes. In this group a primary event occurred in 17.9% of the patients receiving atorvastatin 10 mg compared with 13.8% receiving atorvastatin 80 mg (=0.026). In specific, intensive therapy with atorvastatin 80 mg in patients with diabetes and CHD significantly reduced the rate of major cardiovascular events by 25% compared with atorvastatin 10 mg. End-of-treatment mean LDL cholesterol levels were 2 mmol/L (77 mg/dL) and 2.5 mmol/L (98.6 mg/dL), respectively (33).

Another comparative statin trial in high risk patients was the pravastatin or atorvastatin evaluation and infection therapy-thrombolysis in myocardial infarction 22 trial (PROVE IT-TIMI 22) (34). This trial randomized 4162 patients who had been hospitalized for an acute coronary syndrome to either pravastatin 40 mg d^{-1} or atorvastatin 80 mg d^{-1} 18% of all patients had diabetes. The primary end point was death from any cause, MI, unstable angina requiring rehospitalisation, revascularisation, and stroke. After a mean follow-up of 2 years, atorvastatin therapy was associated with a 16% reduction in risk for the primary end point compared with pravastatin with a similar reduction (17%) seen in the subgroup of patients with diabetes.

While the aforementioned evidence from subgroup post-hoc analyses of major statin trials suggested a benefit from statin therapy in patients with diabetes there are only two statin trials investigating this question in a hypothesis-based prospective fashion thus specifically recruiting patients with diabetes. These are the collaborative atorvastatin diabetes study (CARDS) (35) and the atorvastatin study for prevention of coronary heart disease endpoints in non-insulin-dependent diabetes mellitus (ASPEN) (36). In CARDS the patients had relatively low LDL cholesterol (≤160 mg/dL, 4.14 mmol/L), serum triglycerides ≤600 mg/dL, (6.78 mmol/L), no history of CVD, but ≥1 risk factor for CHD in addition to diabetes. At entry, patients were 40 to 75 years old. A total of 2838 patients were randomized in a double-blind fashion to receive placebo or atorvastatin 10 mg/day. The combined primary endpoint was an acute CHD event, coronary revascularisation and stroke. The trial was originally planned for 5 years, but was terminated at 3.9 years, because of a substantial reduction in the incidence of cardiovascular events observed in the atorvastatin group (37% reduction compared to placebo). All cause mortality was reduced by 27%, although this finding achieved only borderline statistical significance ($p=0.059$). In order to prevent one major CVD event, 27 patients with diabetes would need to be treated for four years. When the parameters of the primary endpoint were assessed separately, atorvastatin therapy was associated with a 36% reduction in coronary events, a 31% reduction in coronary revascularisation procedures and a 48% reduction in stroke compared with placebo. There was also no evidence of heterogeneity by age, gender, baseline systolic blood pressure, retinopathy, albuminuria or smoking. Moreover these effects were independent from the baseline LDL cholesterol, HDL cholesterol or triglyceride concentrations. The authors of CARDS concluded that the question should not be whether all patients with type 2 diabetes warrant statin therapy, but if there are any patients at sufficiently low risk for this treatment to be withheld.

The just recently published ASPEN trial (36), however, failed to reproduce these findings. This combined primary and secondary prevention trial was a 4-year double-blind study involving 2410 patients with type 2 diabetes, which compared the effects of 10 mg/day atorvastatin to placebo. The composite primary endpoint was similar to that of CARDS (cardiovascular death, nonfatal MI, nonfatal stroke, recanalization, coronary artery bypass surgery, resuscitated cardiac arrest and worsening or unstable angina requiring hospitaliza-tion). There was no difference found in the primary end point between the placebo and the atorvastatin group, a result that could be attributed, at least in part, to the high statin drop-in rate (26.9%) in the placebo group.

Fibrate Treatment for Patients With Diabetes

While there is considerable amount of evidence to support that the use of statins reduces LDL cholesterol in patients with diabetes and provides cardiovascular benefit, there is much less persuasive evidence regarding potential beneficial effects of fibrates.

The veterans affairs high-density lipoprotein intervention trial (VA-HIT) (37) was a secondary intervention trial in 2531 men younger than 74 years of age who had an established diagnosis of CHD with low HDL cholesterol levels of ≤40 mg/dL (1 mmol/L) and LDL cholesterol of ≤140 mg/dL (3.6 mmol/L). The subjects were randomized to receive gemfibrozil (1200 mg/day) or placebo. The primary outcome was death due to coronary causes or non fatal MI. Treatment with gemfibrozil resulted in a 22% reduction in the primary endpoint ($p=0.006$) for a mean follow-up period of 5.1 years. In a subgroup analysis, it was revealed that gemfibrozil induced a smaller increase in HDL cholesterol and a smaller decrease in TG in subjects with diabetes compared to non-diabetics (5% vs. 8% and 20% vs. 29%, respectively) (38). Interestingly, despite of the more limited improvement in the lipid profile in patients with diabetes, gemfibrozil use was associated with a greater risk reduction in the combined end points in the subjects with diabetes compared to the non-diabetic patients (32% vs. 18%, respectively). The reduction in CHD death was 41% and in stroke 40%. Moreover, among the non-diabetic patients, gemfibrozil was most effective in reducing major cardiovascular events in individuals having insulin values within the highest fasting plasma insulin (FPI) quartile, in specific 39 μU ml^{-1} (risk reduction 35%, $p=0.04$). In short, this study showed that in men with CHD and low HDL-C levels gemfibrozil significantly reduces the risk of major cardiovascular events.

In a subsequent analysis of VA-HIT data it was shown that the occurrence of new cardiovascular events and the benefit of fibrate therapy was much less dependent on the levels of HDL cholesterol or triglycerides than on the presence or absence of insulin resistance (39).

The St. Mary's Ealing, Northwick park diabetes cardiovascular disease prevention (SENDCAP) study (40) was a double-blind placebo-controlled primary prevention trial of 164 patients (117 men, 47 women) with diabetes and a mean age of 50.9 years, randomized to receive bezafibrate (400 mg daily) or placebo for a minimum of 3 years. No significant differences between the two groups were found in the progress of arterial disease measured by carotid and femoral artery ultrasound. However, those treated with bezafibrate had a significant reduction ($p=0.01$) in the combined incidence of ischemic changes on the resting ECG and documented MI.

The Diabetes atherosclerosis intervention study (DAIS) (41), a combined primary and secondary prevention trial, was designed to examine whether treatment with micronized fenofibrate (200 mg/day) would decrease the rate of progression of CHD in patients with diabetes. The study included 418 men and women between 40 and 65 years of age, in relatively good glycemic control (mean hemoglobin A_{1c} 7.5%), with mild lipoprotein abnormalities (the total cholesterol to HDL cholesterol ratio had to be four or higher) and at least one visible coronary lesion on angiography. Approximately 50% had a previous history of clinical CHD and 33% had previously undergone coronary interventions the primary endpoint was progression or regression of CHD on quantitative angiography. The subjects were randomly assigned to fenofibrate ($n=207$) or placebo ($n=211$) with an average follow-up period of 3.5 years. Serum triglycerides decreased by 29% and HDL cholesterol increased by 6% in the fenofibrate group during the study. The Fenofibrate treatment was associated with 40% less progression in minimum lumen diameter ($p=0.029$), 42% less progression in percentage diameter stenosis ($p=0.2$), and 25% less progression in mean segment diameter, but this change was not significant. The trial was not powered to examine clinical endpoints, but fewer endpoints were observed in the fenofibrate compared to the placebo group (38 vs. 50, respectively). The correlation between plasma lipids and angiographic changes was weak, suggesting the presence of lipid-independent effects of fenofibrate.

The Fenofibrate intervention and event lowering in diabetes (FIELD) (42) study was a multinational, randomized controlled trial with 9.795 participants aged 50 to 75 years, with type 2 diabetes and not taking statin therapy at study entry. After a placebo and a fenofibrate run-in phase, the patients (2131 with previous cardiovascular diseases and 7664 without) with a total cholesterol concentration of 115 mg/dL (3 mmol/L) to 250 mg/dL (6.5 mmol/L) and a total cholesterol to HDL cholesterol ratio of 4.0 or more or plasma triglycerides of 88–442 mg/dL (1.5–5 mmol/L) were randomly assigned to micronized fenofibrate 200 mg daily ($n=4.895$) or placebo ($n=4.900$). The primary outcome was coronary events (CHD death or non-fatal MI); the outcome for prespecified subgroup analyses was total cardiovascular events (the composite of cardiovascular death, MI, stroke and coronary and carotid revascularisation). Over the 5 years duration of the study similar proportions in each group discontinued study medication (10% placebo vs. 11% fenofibrate) and more patients taking placebo (17%) than fenofibrate (8%, $p<0.0001$) started other lipid treatments, predominantly statins. 5.9% of patients on placebo and 5.2% of those on fenofibrate had a coronary event (relative reduction of 11%, HR 0.89, 95% CI 0.75–1.05, $p=0.16$). This finding corresponds to a significant 24% reduction in non-fatal MI (HR 0.76, 0.62–0.94, $p=0.010$) and a non-significant increase in CHD mortality (HR 1.19, 0.90–1.57, $p=0.22$). Total cardiovascular disease events were significantly reduced from 13.9% to 12.5% (HR 0.89, 0.80–0.99, $p=0.035$). This finding included a 21% reduction in coronary revascularisation (0.79, 0.68–0.93, $p=0.003$). Total mortality was 6.6% in the placebo group and 7.3% in the fenofibrate group ($p=0.18$). Fenofibrate was associated with less albuminuria progression ($p=0.002$), and less retinopathy needing laser treatment (5.2% vs. 3.6% $p=0.003$). There was a slight increase in pancreatitis (0.5% vs. 0.8%, $p=0.031$) and pulmonary embolism (0.7% vs. 1.1%, $p=0.022$) but no significant other adverse effects. The authors concluded that fenofibrate does not significantly reduce the risk of the primary outcome of coronary events. It reduces, however, total cardiovascular events, mainly due to fewer non-fatal MIs and revascularisations. In summary, there was an overall non-significant 11% reduction in the primary end point of CHD events (a 25% reduction in those without previous cardiovascular disease and a non-significant 8% increase in those with previous CVD) and a significant 11% reduction in total cardiovascular disease events, mainly because of reductions in non-fatal MI and coronary revascularisations (total cardiovascular events fell by 19% in those without a history of cardiovascular disease and there was no effect in those with previous CVD). These differences in treatment effects between cardiovascular disease subgroups were of borderline significance ($p=0.05$ for CHD, $p=0.03$ for cardiovascular disease) and might be due to chance. Although there was a significant 24% reduction in non-fatal MI, there was a 19% increase (non-significant) in cardiac mortality, largely reflecting an increase in sudden cardiac deaths. Considering that the fenofibrate group also had a significant increase in pulmonary emboli, this increase in sudden deaths might be a matter of concern. While the higher rate of starting statin therapy in patients' allocated placebo might have masked a larger treatment benefit the FIELD trial does not give clear answers on the efficacy and safety of fenofibrate.

Eagerly awaited are the results of the Action to control cardiovascular risk in diabetes (ACCORD) trial (www.accordtrial.org/public/frames.cfm), a multicenter randomized trial in 10.000 patients with diabetes, 40 to 79 years of age. The subjects will be randomized for the purpose of assessing the prevention of major cardiovascular events (nonfatal MI, cardiovascular death and stroke) using a complex factorial design that includes intensive glycemic, lipid and blood pressure control and insulin resistance-lowering therapy. The lipid part of the study ($n=5.800$) will assess whether decreasing triglycerides and increasing HDL cholesterol reduces cardiovascular risk beyond the current strategy of optimal LDL cholesterol and glycemic control. The study is expected to be completed in June 2009.

In summary, statin trials in patients with diabetes provide much more convincing evidence of a substantial benefit than those with fibrates. The available evidence does not justify a recommendation for increased fibrate use in patients with diabetes, and do not support a benefit of fibrate therapy in patients already at target serum LDL cholesterol levels. However, fibrates may have a role in the treatment of diabetic patients with high triglycerides and low HDL cholesterol. If a fibrate is to be combined with a statin, fenofibrate should be preferred, since gemfibrozil seems to inhibit the glucuronidation (43) and therefore the elimination of statins, thus increasing the risk of myopathy (44).

Other Treatments

All patients should have medical nutrition therapy and dietary modification focused on reducing saturated fats and cholesterol intake. Weight loss and increased physical activity could also improve diabetic dyslipidemia (45).

Nicotinic acid increases HDL and decreases triglycerides, small dense LDL and Lp(a) (46), therefore it could represent an attractive treatment for diabetic dyslipidemia. However, because of early reports associating nicotinic acid with decreased insulin sensitivity (47), it has not been widely used in patients with diabetes. Subsequent studies showed that modest doses of nicotinic acid (750–2500 mg/day) have minimal effects on glycemia (48,49). Most of the data on the efficacy of nicotinic acid come from a trial carried out in the 1970s, the Coronary Drug Project, in men with established CHD. In that study, acute coronary events were reduced by 28% and total mortality by 11%. The study excluded patients on insulin but included 251 with fasting glucose levels in the diabetic range. There was no significant difference in the event rate reduction by baseline glucose level (50). The safety and efficacy of the combination of niacin with statins has been shown both for simvastatin (51) and atorvastatin (52).

The new cholesterol lowering drug, ezetimibe, is a cholesterol absorption inhibitor that, when used as monotherapy, decreases LDL cholesterol by about 20%. Recent studies have shown the that its combination with statins (53), fibrates (54) and niacin (55) in patients with diabetes seems to be efficacious and safe.

DYSLIPIDEMIA IN TYPE 1 DIABETES

Current recommendations for the use of lipid lowering drugs in type 1 diabetes are based on their known elevated CVD risk which is identical to that of patients with type 2 diabetes. The only clinical trial evidence of statin therapy in patients with type 1 diabetes comes from the HPS (31), which included 615 patients with type 1 diabetes. There was a 27% reduction in major coronary events which was not though statistically significant, probably because of the small number of patients.

GOALS OF THERAPY AND MANAGEMENT CONSIDERATIONS

Diabetic dyslipidemia plays an important role in the increased cardiovascular mortality and morbidity seen in patients with diabetes. There is robust evidence, coming from landmark secondary prevention trials described above as well as from recent meta-analyses (56), that LDL lowering is associated with significant reduction in cardiovascular risk in patients with diabetes. The optimal treatment strategy for such patients remains controversial. There are a number of guidelines on lipid lowering in diabetes, which are, for the most part, in agreement, but have some differences (Table 2). Both ADA (1) and ATP III (8) guidelines have identified LDL cholesterol as the first priority of lipid lowering, and the optimal level was set at <100 mg/dL (2.6 mmol/L). Furthermore, ATP III and the American Heart Association have designated most of the patients with diabetes at high-risk and recommended risk factor

TABLE 2 Guideline Target Levels for LDL Cholesterol, HDL Cholesterol, and Triglycerides for Patients with Diabetes

	LDL cholesterol[a,b]	HDL cholesterol	Triglycerides[c]
European Joint Societies (62)	<100 mg/dL (<2.5 mmol/L)	Not a goal	Not a goal
international Atherosclerosis Society (57)	<100 mg/dL (<2.6 mmol/L)	Not a goal	Not a goal
ADA (1)	<100 mg/dL (<2.6 mmol/L)	>40mg/dL (1.1 mmol/L)[d]	<150 mg/dL (<1.7 mmol/L)

[a] Goal of 70 mg/dL (1.8 mmol/L) is considered a therapeutic option in those with established CVD.
[b] According to some authorities if the patient with diabetes has an estimated 10-year risk for CHD <20%, an LDL-C goal <130 mg/dL (3.3 mmol/L) is acceptable.
[c] Current NCEP/ATP III guidelines suggest that in patients with triglycerides ≥200 mg/dL (2.2 mmol/L), the "non-HDL cholesterol" (total cholesterol minus HDL) be utilized. The goal is ≤130 mg/dL.
[d] For women it has been suggested that the HDL goal be increased by 10 mg/dL.
Source: From Refs. 1,8,57.

management similar to that given to patients with established CAD and suggest an LDL cholesterol goal of 70 mg/dL (1.8 mmol/L) if there is a very high risk for CHD (8). Other therapeutic targets identified by ADA (1) are achieving optimal concentrations of plasma triglycerides of <150 mg/dL (1.7 mmol/L) and HDL >40 mg/dL (1.1 mmol/L) (for women > 50 mg/dL, >1.3 mmol/L). Ongoing clinical trials, such as the ACCORD, will help clarify the question whether increasing HDL- cholesterol and decreasing triglycerides offers a further benefit than treatment that brings LDL cholesterol at target levels alone.

It has been also pointed out that not all patients with diabetes have a 10-year risk >20% (8). A portion of them can be considered to be only at moderately high risk because of young age (<40 years) or lack of other risk factors (such patients were not studied in HPS). This assumption is supported by recent studies showing that patients with diabetes age 40 or younger do not seem to be at high risk of CVD (7). For these patients an LDL-lowering drug therapy might not be initiated unless LDL cholesterol is ≥130 mg/dL (3.3 mmol/L) (8). This is also supported by the International Atherosclerosis Society Guidelines on Prevention of Atherosclerotic Vascular disease (57).

Unfortunately however, despite the overwhelming evidence of the significant cardiovascular benefits of lipid-lowering, patients with diabetes remain, in their vast majority, undertreated both in Europe (58) and the United States (59). Physicians caring for diabetic patients should ensure that their patients receive high-quality evidence-based care, with the aim to substantially reduce the risk of cardiovascular disease.

Moreover, although data from numerous studies convincingly show that patients with diabetes gain the same or greater (56) benefit from statins as other high-risk patients several large controlled trials, such as HPS, have shown that cardiovascular events still continue to occur in two thirds of the patients, especially in those with diabetes. New candidate targets are therefore emerging for cardiovascular risk reduction such as Lp(a), HDL-C and CRP. In order to successfully address the problem of this "forgotten majority" we must continue to stress the importance of lifestyle changes, optimize control of other risk factors such as blood pressure and develop and evaluate new pharmacologic strategies beyond statins.

REFERENCES

1. American Diabetes Association. Standards of medical care in diabetes–2006. Diabetes Care 2006; 29: S4-S34.
2. Downs JR, Clearfeld M, Weis S, et al. Primary prevention of acute coronary events with lovastatin in men and women with average cholesterol levels. Results of the AFCAPS/TexCAPs. J Am Med Assoc 1998; 279:1615–22.
3. Sacks F, Pfeffer MA, Moye LA, et al. The effect of pravastatin on coronary events after myocardial infarction in patients with average cholesterol levels. N Engl J Med 1996; 335:1001–9.
4. Scandinavian Simvastatin Survival Study Group. Randomized trial of cholesterol lowering in 4444 patients with coronary heart disease: the Scandinavian Simvastatin survival Study (4S). Lancet 1994; 344:1383–89.

5. The Long-Term Intervention with Pravastatin in Ischaemic Disease (LIPID) Study Group. Prevention of cardiovascular events and death with pravastatin in patients with coronary heart disease and a broad range of initial cholesterol levels. N Engl J Med 1998; 339:1349–57.

6. The West of Scotland Coronary Prevention Study Group. Prevention of coronary heart disease with pravastatin in men with hypercholesterolemia. N Engl J Med 1995; 20:1301–07.

7. Booth GL, Kapral MK, Fung K, Tu JV. Relation between age and cardiovascular disease in men and women with diabetes compared with non-diabetic people: a population-based retrospective cohort study. Lancet 2006; 368:29–36.

8. Grundy S, Cleeman JI, Bairey MerzC, et al. Implications of recent clinical trials for the National Cholesterol Education Program Adult Treatment Panel III Guidelines. Circulation 2004; 110: 227–39.

9. Aronson D, Rayfield EJ, Chesebro JH. Mechanisms determining course and outcome of diabetic patients who have had acute myocardial infarction. Ann Intern Med 1997; 126:296–306.

10. Woodfield SL, Lundergan CF, Reiner JS, et al. Angiographic findings and outcome in diabetic patients treated with thrombolytic therapy for acute myocardial infarction: the GUSTO-I experience. J Am Coll Cardiol 1996; 28:1699–701.

11. Herlitz J, Malmberg K, Karlson BW, Ryden L, Hjalmarson A. Mortality and morbidity during a five-year follow-up of diabetics with myocardial infarction. Acta Med Scand 1988; 224:31–8.

12. Amos AF, McCarty DJ, Zimmer P. The rising global burden of diabetes and its complications: estimates and projections to the year 2010. Diabet Med 1997; 14:S1–S85.

13. Assmann SM, Schulte H. The prospective cardiocvascular Munster (PROCAM) study: prevalence of hyperlipidemia in persons with hypertension and/or diabetes mellitus and the relationship to coronary heart disease. Am Heart J 1988; 116:1713–24.

14. Betteridge DJ. LDL heterogeneity: implications for atherogenicity in insulin resistance and NIDDM. Diabetologia 1997; 40:S149–S51.

15. The Multiple Risk Factor Intervention Trial Research Group. Diabetes, other risk factors and 12 year cardiovascular mortality for men screened in the Multiple Risk Factor Intervention Trial. Diabetes Care 1993; 16:434–4.

16. Turner RC, Millns H, Neil HA, et al. Risk factors for coronary artery disease in non-insulin dependent diabetes mellitus: United Kingdom Prospective Diabetes Study (UKPDS:23). Br Med J 1998; 316:823–28.

17. Assmann E, Schulte H. Relation of high-density lipoprotein cholesterol and triglycerides to incidence of atherosclerotic coronary artery disease (the PROCAM experience). Am J Cardiol 1992; 70:733–7.

18. Manninen V, Tenkanen H, Koskinen P, et al. Joint effects of triglycerides and LDL cholesterol and HDL cholesterol concentrations on coronary heart disease risk in the Helsinki Heart Study. Circulation 1992; 85:37–45.

19. Couillard C, Bergeron N, Bergeron J, et al. Metabolic heterogeneity underlying postprandial lipemia among men with low fasting high density lipoprotein cholesterol concentrations. J Clin Endocrinol Metab 2000; 85:4575–82.

20. Haffner SM, Mykkanen L, Festa A, et al. Insulin-resistant prediabetic subjects have more atherogenic risk factors than insulin-sensitive prediabetic subjects: implications for preventing coronary heart disease during the prediabetic state. Circulation 2000; 101:975–80.

21. Ginsberg HN. Insulin resistance and cardiovascular disease. J Clin Invest 2000; 106:453–8.

22. Rashid S, Watanabe T, Sakaue T, Lewis GF. Mechanisms of HDL lowering in insulin resistant, hypertriglyceridemic states: the combined effect of HDL, triglyceride enrichment and elevated hepatic lipase activity. Clin Biochem 2003; 36:421–9.

23. Sheperd J. Does statin monotherapy address the multiple lipid abnormalities in type 2 diabetes? Atherosclerosis 2005; 6:15–9.

24. Haffner SM, Lehto K, Ronnemaa T, Pyorala K, Laakso M. Mortality from coronary heart disease in subjects with type 2 diabetes and in nondiabetic subjects with and without prior myocardial infarction. N Engl J Med 1998; 339:21.

25. UK Prospective Diabetes Study (UKPDS) Group. Intensive blood-glucose control with sulphonylur-eas or insulin compared with conventional treatment and risk of complications in patients with type 2 diabetes. Lancet 1998; 352:837–53.

26. Pyorala K, Pedersen TR, Kjekshus J, Faergemann O, Olsson AG, Thorgeirsson G. Cholesterol lowering with simvastatin improves prognosis of diabetic patients with coronary heart disease: a subgroup analysis of the Scandinavian Simvastatin survival Study (4S). Diabetes Care 1997; 20: 614–20.

27. The Scandinavian Simvastatin Survival Study Group. Reduced coronary events in simvastatin-treated patients with coronary heart disease and diabetes or impaired fasting glucose levels. Arch Intern Med 1999; 159:2661–7.

28. Jonsson B, Cook JR, Pedersen TR. The cost-effectiveness of lipid lowering in patients with diabetes: results from the 4S trial. Diabetologia 1999; 42:1293–301.

29. Goldberg R, Mellies MJ, Sacks F, et al. Cardiovascular events and their reduction with pravastatin in diabetic and glucose-intolerant myocardial infarction survivors with average cholesterol levels: subgroup analyses in the cholesterol and recurrent events (CARE) trial. Circulation 1998; 98:2513–9.
30. Heart Protection Study Collaborative Group. MRC/BHF Heart Protection Study of cholesterol lowering with simvastatin in 20,536 high-risk individuals: a randomised placebo-controlled trial. Lancet 2002; 360:7–22.
31. Collins R, Armitage J, Parish S, Sleigh P, Peto R. MRC/BHF Heart Protection Study of cholesterol-lowering with simvastatin in 5.963 people with diabetes: a randomized placebo-controlled trial. Lancet 2003; 361:2005–16.
32. LaRosa JC, Grundy SM, Waters DD, et al. Intensive lipid lowering with atorvastatin in patients with stable coronary disease. N Engl J Med 2005; 352:1425–35.
33. Sheperd J, Barter P, Carmena R, et al. Effect of lowering LDL cholesterol substantially below currently recommended levels in patients with coronary heart disease and diabetes. Diabetes Care 2006; 29:1220–6.
34. Cannon CP, Braunwald E, McCabe CH, et al. Intensive versus moderate lipid lowering with statins after acute coronary syndromes. N Engl J Med 2004; 350:1495–504.
35. Colhoun H, Betteridge DJ, Durrington PN, et al. Primary prevention of cardiovascular disease with atorvastatin in type 2 diabetes in the Collaborative Atorvastatin Diabetes Study (CARDS): multicentre randomised placebo-controlled trial. Lancet 2004; 364:685–96.
36. Knopp RH, D'Emden M, Smilde JG, Pocock SJ. Efficacy and safety of atorvastatin in the prevention of cardiovascular endpoints in subjects with type 2 diabetes. Diabetes Care 2006; 29:1478–85.
37. Rubins HB, Robins SJ, Collins D, et al. Gemfibrozil for the secondary prevention of coronary heart disease in men with low levels of high-density liporotein cholesterol: Veterans Affairs High-Density Lipoprotein Cholesterol Intervention Trial Study Group. N Engl J Med 1999; 341:410–8.
38. Rubins HB, Robins SJ, Collins D, et al. Diabetes, plasma insulin, and cardiovascular disease: Subgroup analysis from the Department of Veterans Affairs High-density lipoprotein Intervention Trial (VA-HIT). Arch Intern Med 2002; 162:2597–604.
39. Robins SJ, Bloomfield-Rubins H, Faas FH, et al. Insulin resistance and cardiovascular events with low HDL cholesterol. Diabetes Care 2003; 26:1513–7.
40. Elkeles RS, Diamond JR, Poulter C, et al. Cardiovascular outcomes in type 2 diabetes: a double-blind placebo-controlled study of bezafibrate: the St. Mary's Ealing, Northwick Park Diabetes Cardiovascular Disease Prevention (SENDCAP) study. Diabetes Care 1998; 21:641–8.
41. Diabetes Atherosclerosis Intervention Study Investigators. Effect of fenofibrate on progression of coronary-artery disease in type 2 diabetes: the Diabetes Atherosclerosis Intervention Study, a randomized study. Lancet 2001; 357:905–10.
42. The FIELD study investigators. Effects of long-term fenofibrate therapy on cardiovascular events in 9795 people with type 2 diabetes mellitus (the FIELD study): randomised controlled trial. Lancet 2005; 366:1849–61.
43. Prueksaritanont T, Tang C, Qiu Y, Mu L, Subramanian R, Lih JH. Effects of fibrates on metabolism of statins in human hepatocytes. Drug Metab Dispos 2002; 30:1280–7.
44. Davidson MH. Combination therapy for dsylipidemia: safety and regulatory considerations. Am J Cardiol 2002; 90:50K–60K.
45. Colhoun H, Betteridge DJ. Treatment of lipid disorders in patients with diabetes. Curr Treat Options Cardiovasc Med 2006; 8:37–45.
46. Pan J, Lin M, Kesala R, Van J, Charles M. Niacin treatment of the atherogenic lipid profile and Lp(a) in diabetes. Diab Obes Metab 2002; 4:255–61.
47. Garg A, Grundy SM. Nicotinic acid as therapy for dyslipidemia in non insulin dependent diabetes mellitus. J Am Med Assoc 1990; 264:723–6.
48. Elam MB, Hunninghake DB, Davis KB, et al. Effect of niacin on lipid and lipoprotein levels and glycemic control in patients with diabetes and peripheral arterial disease. The ADMIT study: a randomized trial. J Am Med Assoc 2000; 284:1263–70.
49. Grundy SM, Vega GL, McGovern ME, et al. Efficacy, safety and tolerability of once daily niacin for the treatment of dyslipidemia associated with type 2 diabetes; results of the assessment of diabetes control and evaluation of the efficacy of Niaspan trial. Arch Intern Med 2002; 162:1568–76.
50. Canner PL, Furberg CD, Terrin ML, McGovern ME. Benefits of niacin by glycemic status in patients with healed myocardial infarction (from the coronary drug Project). Am J Cardiol 2005; 95:254–7.
51. Brown BG, Zhao XQ, Chait A, et al. Simvastatin and niacin, antioxidant vitamins or the combination for the prevention of coronary disease. N Engl J Med 2001; 345:1583–92.
52. Van JT, Pan J, Wasty T, Chan E, Wu X, Charles A. Comparison of extended-release niacin and atorvastatin monotherapies and combination treatmentof the atherogenic lipid profile in diabetes mellitus. Am J Cardiol 2002; 89:1306–8.
53. Gaudiani LM, Lewin A, Meneghini I, Plotkin D, Mitchel Y, Shah S. Efficacy and safety of ezetimibe co-administered with simvastatin in thiazolidinedione-treated type 2 diabetic patients. Diab Obes Metab 2005; 7:88–97.

54. Farnier M, Freman MW, Macdonell G, et al. Efficacy and safety of the coadministration of ezetimibe with fenofibrate in patients with mixed hyperlipidemia. Eur Heart J 2005; 26:897–905.

55. Jelesoff NE, Ballantyne CM, Xylakis AM, Chiou P, Jones PH, Guyton JR. Effectiveness and tolerability of adding ezetimibe to niacin-based regimens for treatment of primary hyperlipidemia. Endocr Pract 2006; 12:159–64.

56. Costa J, Borges M, David C, Vaz Carneiro A. Efficacy of lipid lowering drug treatment for diabetic and non-diabetic patients: meta-analysis of randomized controlled trials. Br Med J 2006; 332:1115–24.

57. International Atherosclerosis Society. Harmonized guidelines on prevention of atherosclerotic vascular disease. Available at http://www athero org 2003.

58. Tonstad S, Rosvold EO, Furu K, Skurtveit S. Undertreatment and overtreatment with statins: the Oslo Health Study 2000–2001. J Intern Med 2004; 255:494–502.

59. Saydah SH, Fradkin J, Cowie CC. Poor control of risk factors for vascular disease among adults with previously diagnosed diabetes. J Am Med Assoc 2004; 291:335–42.

60. Sever PS, Dahlof B, Poulter NR, et al. Prevention of coronary and stroke events with atorvastatin in hypertensive patients who have average or lower-than-average cholesterol concentrations, in the Anglo-Scandinavian Cardiac Outcomes Trial-Lipid Lowering Arm (ASCOT-LLA): a multicentre randomized controlled trial. Lancet 2003; 361:1149–58.

61. ALLHAT Officers and Coordinators for the ALLHAT Collaborative Research Group. Major outcomes in high-risk hypertensive patients randomized to angiotensin-converting enzyme inhibitor or calcium channel blocker vs diuretic: The Antihypertensive and Lipid-Lowering Treatment to Prevent Heart Attack Trial (ALLHAT). J Am Med Assoc 2002; 288:2981–97.

62. Third Joint Task force of European and other Societies on Cardiovascular Disease Prevention in Clinical Practice. European guidelines on cardiovascular disease prevention in clinical practice. Eur Heart J 2003; 24:1601–10.

28 | Hypertension and Diabetes: Need for Combination Therapy

Guntram Schernthaner
Department of Medicine I, Rudolfstiftung Hospital, Vienna, Austria

Gerit-Holger Schernthaner
Department of Medicine II, Medical University of Vienna, Vienna, Austria

HYPERTENSION AND DIABETES: NEED FOR COMBINATION THERAPY

Hypertension is an extremely common comorbidity in patients with diabetes, affecting approximately 20–60% of patients, depending on type of diabetes, age, ethnicity, and body weight (1). The development of hypertension in patients with diabetes is particularly harmful, since it accelerates the development of cardiovascular disease (CVD) and is estimated to be responsible for up to 75% of diabetic cardiovascular (CV) complications (2), including stroke, coronary artery disease, and peripheral arterial disease.

DIABETIC PATIENTS WITH HYPERTENSION HAVE A SIGNIFICANTLY HIGHER RISK FOR CVD THAN NONDIABETIC PATIENTS

Hypertension increases CV risk in type 2 diabetes mellitus (T2DM) enormously, as clearly demonstrated in the Multiple Risk Factors Intervention Trial, in which 350,000 men between 35 and 57 years of age were followed up for twelve years (3). The absolute risk of CV death was three-fold higher in those who were diabetic, even after adjusting for other common risk factors such as age, race, income, serum cholesterol and smoking. Importantly, the risk at any given level of systolic blood pressure (SBP) was 2.5–3 times higher in those with T2DM than in the non-diabetic patients at every level of SBP assessed (3). Hypertension is also thought to play a major etiologic role in the development of diabetic nephropathy (DN) and diabetic retinopathy (4,5). As a result, many experts and authors have argued that blood-pressure (BP) management is the most critical aspect of the care of patients with T2DM.

Recently, findings from the Strong Heart Study (6) demonstrated that the high risk for CVD associated with BP levels in diabetic patients starts already in the phase of pre-hypertension (Pre-HT) [SBP: 120–139 mm Hg and/or diastolic blood pressure (DBP) of 80–89 mm Hg]. Pre-HT was more prevalent in the diabetic versus nondiabetic patients (59.4% vs. 48.2%; $p = 0.001$). After a follow-up period of twelve years the hazard ratios (HR) of CVD were 3.70 for those with both Pre-HT and diabetes, 2.90 for those with diabetes alone and only 1.80 for nondiabetic patients with Pre-HT. Based on these findings more aggressive interventions (drug treatment for BP control) for prehypertensive individuals with diabetes seem to be warranted.

ABNORMAL DIURNAL VARIATION OF BLOOD PRESSSURE (NONDIPPING)

The mechanism that underpins the increased sensitivity of diabetic subjects to hypertension is not known, but may involve impaired autoregulation or attenuated nocturnal decrease of BP. There is a growing evidence that a decreased nocturnal fall in BP ($< 10\%$ of the daytime level) is associated with a worse prognosis, irrespective of whether nighttime dipping is studied as a continuous or a class variable. Various studies (7–9) indicate that in diabetic patients, measurement of ambulatory 24 h BP is a much better predictor of microvascular and macrovascular complications than conventional BP measurement. An abnormal circadian variation of BP ("nondipping") can be demonstrated in a considerable number of diabetic patients and was found to be related to microalbuminuria and DN (7–9). Nondipping was also found to be associated with glucose intolerance, insulin resistance and enhanced nocturnal sympathetic activity even in nondiabetic patients (10). A disturbed diurnal variation of blood pressure is a predicting marker for progression of both diabetic retinopathy and DN in type 1 diabetes mellitus (T1DM) patients (7–9). A 20-fold risk of dying within the next 5 years was found in those T2DM patients, who had a "reversed" circadian BP profile compared with patients who had a normal decrease in BP during nighttime (11). Interestingly, most sudden deaths or strokes in that study occurred during nighttime or early morning (11). More research is needed to clarify whether the increased risk for end-organ damage can be lowered in diabetic patients with abnormal circadian variation of BP by specific intervention strategies (12).

PATHOPHYSIOLOGY OF HYPERTENSION IS DIFFERENT
IN TYPE 1 AND TYPE 2 DIABETES

There are substantial differences in the causes of hypertension in T1DM and T2DM. In patients with T1DM diabetic nephropathy appears to be the most common cause of hypertension (13). A strong family history of essential hypertension and diabetes mellitus appears to identify those people with T1DM who are most likely to develop renal disease and hypertension (14). Probably an equal number of people with T2DM develop renal disease (15) but hypertension often occurs with normal renal function associated with obesity or older age. Various hypotheses have been suggested to account for the increased prevalence of hypertension particularly in T2DM patients (16). Hypertension may be related, in part to central obesity and increased sympathetic nervous system stimulation and catecholamine production observed in diabetics (16). It is now generally believed that essential hypertension is a part of the insulin resistance syndrome (17), and that hypertension precedes the development of T2DM in a considerable number of patients (18).

NONPHARMACOLOGICAL TREATMENT OF HYPERTENSION IN DIABETIC PATIENTS

The goal of treating hypertension in patients with diabetes mellitus is to prevent associated morbidity and mortality. Lifestyle modification, including weight management, diet, salt reduction, moderation of alcohol intake, increased physical activity and smoking cessation are the cornerstones of therapy. Weight loss in overweight individuals can improve control of both hypertension and diabetes mellitus. Many studies have shown that even modest reduction of body weight can improve BP and glycemic control. Reduction in weight may be associated with BP reductions because of reduction of insulin levels, sympathetic nervous system activity, and vascular resistance.

IMPRESSIVE REDUCTION OF RISK FOR CVD IN DIABETIC PATIENTS
BY ANTIHYPERTENSIVE TREATMENT

There is strong evidence for a beneficial effect of BP reduction on CVD risk in T2DM, and these benefits have been demonstrated with all classes of antihypertensive drugs. In recent years many antihypertensive intervention studies (19–34), which have included a representative number of diabetic patients, have been published. All these intervention studies illustrate that BP lowering is very important for improving the poor prognosis of diabetic patients. Disagreements in the outcome of different clinical trials can easily be explained by heterogeneity of these studies. The included patients showed a wide variation concerning initial BP values and lowering of BP values. Most of the patients had long-standing diabetic disease, however the exact duration of diabetes and/or hypertension was not reported in most of the studies. The follow-up of the hypertensive patients ranged from 2 to 8 years and only newly diagnosed patients were only enrolled in the United Kingdom Prospective Diabetes Study (UKPDS).

In the Systolic Hypertension in Elderly Program (SHEP) the effect of low-dose diuretic-based antihypertensive treatment (19) on major CVD event rates was evaluated in older non-insulin-treated diabetic patients ($n = 583$) with isolated systolic hypertension (ISH) in comparison with nondiabetic patients. There were 4736 patients with ISH (SBP ≥ 160 mm Hg; DBP ≤ 90 mm Hg at baseline) who received either a low dose of chlorthalidone

(2.5–25.0 mm/day) with a step-up to atenolol, a beta-blocker (BB) at 25.0–50.0 mg/day or reserpine (0.05–0.10 mg/day) if needed. The major CVD rate was 34% lower for active treatment compared with placebo, both for diabetic patients and nondiabetic patients. Remarkably, the absolute risk reduction with active treatment compared with placebo was twice as great for diabetic versus nondiabetic patients (101/1000 vs. 51/1000) at the five year follow-up, reflecting the higher risk of diabetic patients. The authors concluded that a low-dose diuretic based treatment is effective in preventing major CVD events—cerebral and cardiac—in both non-insulin treated diabetic and nondiabetic patients with ISH.

In a substudy (20) of the UKPDS 1148 newly detected T2DM patients with a mean BP of 160/94 mm Hg were randomized to either "tight BP control" ($n = 758$) or "usual care" in the BP control ($n = 390$). The mean difference in the achieved BP level of 10/5 mm Hg between the two groups (144/82 vs.154/87 mm Hg) resulted in a significant reduction in diabetes-related endpoints (-24%), diabetes-related death (-32%), stroke (-44%) and microvascular endpoints (-37%). Myocardial infarction or all-cause mortality, however, was not significantly reduced by BP lowering in the UKPDS. The beneficial effects of tight BP control were shown irrespective of whether captopril, an angiotensin-converting-enzyme inhibitor, (ACEi) or atenolol (a BB) was the basis of antihypertensive treatment (21). More patients needed additional antidiabetic drug treatment in the atenolol group compared with the captopril group, which may be explained by the more pronounced weight gain over 9 years in the atenolol group compared with the captopril group (3.4 vs. 1.6 kg).

The Hypertension Optimal Treatment (HOT) Study (22) included 1501 diabetic patients (total number: 18,790 patients) with hypertension who were randomly allocated to three different diastolic BP targets (<90, <85 and <80 mm Hg). As basic treatment the calcium channel blocker (CCB) felodipine was used. The group of diabetic patients ($n = 1501$) with hypertension achieving a mean systolic BP of 139.7 mm Hg and a mean diastolic BP of 81.1 mm Hg had a 51% reduction in major CV events and 67% reduction in CV mortality (Fig. 1) compared with the group with less tight control (143.7 mm Hg, 85.2 mm Hg), although the absolute difference in the diastolic BP was only 4 mm Hg. Remarkably, the enormous risk reduction was seen only in the diabetic patients.

The Systolic Hypertension in Europe (Syst-Eur) trial was initiated to study the effect of the CCB dihydropyridine nitrendipine on the outcome of CV mortality and morbidity in 4695 patients with systolic BP of 160 to 219 mm Hg and diastolic BP below 95 mm Hg. Very positive results were reported for the subgroup of older T2DM patients ($n = 492$) with systolic

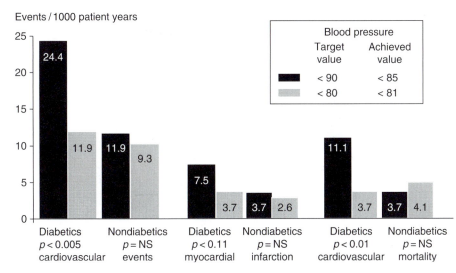

FIGURE 1 Significant relative risk reduction in diabetic patients ($n = 1501$) with target value for diastolic blood pressure ≤80 mm Hg *Abbreviations*: NS, not significant. *Source*: From Ref. 22.

hypertension, randomized to treatment with either the CCB nitrendipine or placebo (23). In the diabetic patients, active treatment reduced overall mortality by 55%, CV events by 76% and strokes by 73%, compared with placebo, although the median follow-up was only two years (Fig. 2). Active treatment with nitrendipine reduced the rate of all CV events by 69% in the diabetic patients but only by 26% in the patients without diabetes.

In the HOPE Study (Heart Outcomes Prevention Evaluation), which lasted 4.5 years, the role of the ACEi ramipril (10 mg per day) versus placebo was assessed in 9297 patients at high risk of CV events (25). In the Micro-HOPE study 3577 diabetic patients (mean age: 65 years; mean duration of diabetes: 11.6 years) were included, who had at least one other CVD risk factor or a history of a previous CV event. Ramipril treatment was associated with a risk reduction of myocardial infarction (22%), stroke (33%), CVD death (37%) and total mortality (24%) compared with placebo (25). Combined microvascular endpoints (overt nephropathy, dialysis or laser therapy for retinopathy) were also significantly reduced (16%). For the interpretation of the Micro-HOPE study, it is important to emphasize that 44% of the included diabetic patients did not have hypertension and that the initial mean BP values of 141.9 mm Hg systolic and 79.6 mm Hg diastolic were only reduced by 2.4 respectively 1.0 mm Hg in the ramipril group. Thus, the benefit could only partly be attributed to the modest mean reduction of blood pressure. In a small subgroup of patients with peripheral arterial disease ($n = 38$), 24-hour ambulatory blood pressure (ABP) measurements were performed before randomization and after one year (26). Although ramipril did not significantly reduce day ABP (6/2 mm Hg), it significantly reduced 24-hour ABP (10/4 mm Hg, $p = 0.03$), mainly because of a more pronounced blood pressure lowering effect during night-time (17/8 mm Hg, $p < 0.001$). Thus, the effects on CV morbidity and mortality seen with ramipril in the HOPE study may, to a larger extent than previously ascribed, relate to effects on blood pressure during nighttime (26).

In the Losartan Intervention For End Point Reduction in Hypertension Study (LIFE) 9153 patients with essential hypertension and left ventricular hypertrophy (LVH) were randomly assigned to either once daily losartan-based or atenolol-based antihypertensive treatment for 4 years (29). As a part of the LIFE study, 1195 patients with diabetes, hypertension and LVH with a mean age of 67 years and a mean blood pressure of 177/96 mm Hg were also included (30). Mean blood pressure fell to 146/79 mm Hg (17/11) in losartan patients and 148/69 mm Hg (19/11) in atenolol patients. Diabetic patients treated with losartan showed a significant reduction of CVD mortality (RR: 36.5%; $p = 0.028$) as well as total mortality (RR: 38.7%; $p = 0.002$) in comparison with patients under atenolol. In addition, myocardial infarction (RR: 17.1%) and stroke (RR: 21.2%) occurred less often in the losartan treated patients, however the difference to atenolol treatment did not reach levels of

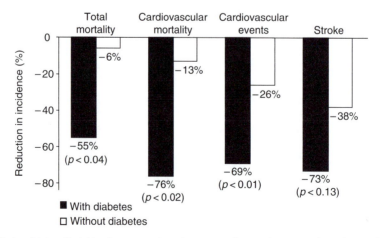

FIGURE 2 Effects of intensified blood pressure lowering on cardiovascular events in patients with and without diabetes. *Source*: From Ref. 23.

significance. Interestingly, losartan was significantly more effective than atenolol in reversing LVH ($p < 0.0001$).

The Antihypertensive and Lipid-Lowering treatment to prevent Heart Attack Trial (ALLHAT) is the largest comparative CV outcomes trial, which compared chlorthalidone, amlodipine and lisinopril in 33,357 patients, including 12,063 T2DM patients, over a 4–8-year follow-up period (33). In the diabetic subgroup, no significant differences were found between the treatment arms in the incidences of the primary outcome (non-fatal myocardial infarction plus coronary heart disease), all-cause mortality, stroke, coronary heart disease or overall CVD. There was a significant benefit in favor of chlorthalidone in the incidence of heart failure, but this result is controversial, as the diagnosis of heart failure was largely based on signs and symptoms and not extensively confirmed by external, independent validation. In addition, compared to the other drugs, diuretics might have had a masking effect on the major clinical signs of heart failure.

In the ASCOT (Anglo-Scandinavian Cardiac Outcomes Trial) blood pressure lowering arm (34) the effect of two different antihypertensive combination therapies (atenolol plus thiazide versus amlodipine plus perindopril) on non-fatal myocardial infarction and fatal coronary heart disease was analyzed in 19,257 hypertensive patients (age range: 40–79 years) who had at least three other CV risk factors. After a follow-up period of 5.5 years, fewer patients treated with the newer drug combination (Fig. 3) reached a primary endpoint (429 vs 474; HR: 0.90; $p = 0.1052$), fatal and non-fatal stroke (327 vs 422; HR: 0.77; $p = 0.0003$), total CVD events and procedures (1362 vs 1602; HR: 0.84; $p < 0.0001$), and all-cause mortality (738 vs 820; HR: 0.89; $p = 0.0247$). In the ASCOT 5345 patients had diabetes, however, risk reduction was not different in diabetic and nondiabetic patients. The incidence of developing diabetes in the nondiabetic patients at baseline was significantly less in the amlodipine-perindopril group compared to the atenolol-thiazide group (567 vs 799; HR: 0.70; $p < 0.0001$).

Table 1 summarizes data for primary outcome of CVD and all-cause mortality in several large placebo-controlled trials, in which representative numbers of diabetic and nondiabetic patients were included. A consistent finding is the marked reduction of the risk for subsequent CV events among diabetic patients on active treatment compared with those on placebo. This finding is consistent for all types of BP-lowering drugs that have been studied. In some studies (SHEP, Syst-Eur and HOT) the risk reduction was much more expressed in the diabetic cohort versus nondiabetic patients. Chosen as the initial drug, the beneficial effect of diuretics, beta-blockers, CCB, and ACEi are well documented. More recently, different antihypertensive drugs have been compared with each other (Table 2). It appears that blockade of the renin-angiotensin-system (RAS) seems to be of particular value, especially when treating hypertension in patients with diabetes at particularly high CV risk.

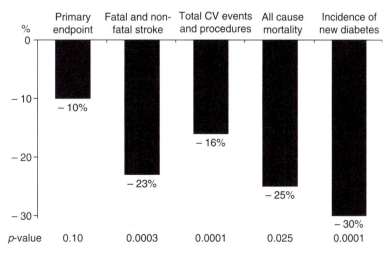

FIGURE 3 Relative risk reduction with the combination of amlodipine and perindopril versus atenolol plus bendroflumethazide (ASCOT). *Source*: From Ref. 34.

TABLE 1 Treatment Effects of Antihypertensive Drugs versus Placebo or Less Intensive Treatment as Reported in Randomized Clinical Trials

| Trial | Treatment comparison | Primary outcome | Risk reduction (%) | | | |
| | | | Relative diabetes | | Absolute diabetes | |
			Yes	No	Yes	No
HDFP (35)	Diuretic vs. standard therapy	All-cause mortality	27	21	4.2	3.0
SHEP (19)	Diuretic vs. placebo	Stroke	54	23	8.8	3.1
Syst-EUR (23)	CCB vs. placebo	Stroke	69	36	18.3	4.5
HOT (22)	<80 vs.<90 mmHg DBP	MI/stroke/CV mortality	51	11	12.5	1.0
HOPE (25, 36)	ACE-I vs. placebo	MI/stroke/CV mortality	25	21	4.5	2.2

Abbreviations: ACE-I, angiotensin-converting-enzyme inhibitor; CCB, calcium channel blocker; CV, cardiovascular; DBP, diastolic blood pressure; MI, myocardial infarction.

PROTECTION OF DIABETIC NEPHROPATHY BY BLOCKADE OF RAS

In most Western countries, diabetic nephropathy (DN) is now the single most common condition (25–45 %) found in patients (15) with end-stage renal disease (ESRD). This is to some extent due to better survival of diabetic patients with renal failure, but mostly due to the dramatic global diabetes epidemic. Alarming data were recently reported also from Asia indicating a dramatic increase in the prevalence of T2DM in this region (41) and that most patients in this region who have ESRD have T2DM (42). About 70 percent of T2DM patients with renal failure suffer from nodular glomerulosclerosis (Kimmelstiel-Wilson). Classical DN evolves in a sequence of stages: after a period of glomerular hyperfiltration, increased urinary albumin excretion (AER; microalbuminuria i.e. 30–300 mg/day) indicates the onset of overt DN. Poor glycemic control and elevated SBP (>135 mm Hg) interact in enhancing the risk of DN; proteinuria and smoking are major promoters of progression. The risk of onset of microalbuminuria can be reduced by lowering of BP and specifically by blockade of the RAS. In patients with established DN, the target SBP should be <130 mm Hg and RAS blockade is obligatory. It was generally believed that chronic kidney disease (CKD) among adults with T2DM follows the same clinical course as in T1DM and that increased AER is the earliest clinical evidence of kidney disease in this population. However, increasing epidemiological evidence suggests that population patterns of chronic kidney disease (CKD) among adults

TABLE 2 Treatment Effects Expressed in Hazard Ratios (95% CI) in Randomized Clinical Trials Comparing Different Antihypertensive Treatments in Hypertensive Patients with T2DM

Trial	Treatment Comparison	No. of patients	Coronary artery disease	Stroke	All-cause mortality	Cardiovascular mortality
UKPDS (21)	ACEi vs BB	1148	ns	ns	ns	ns
FACET (37)	ACEi vs CCB	380	ns	ns	ns	ns
ABCD (38)	ACEi vs CCB	470	0.18 (0.07,0.48)	ns	ns	ns
CAPPP (39)	ACEi vs BB/TZ	572	0.34 (0.17,0.67)	ns	0.54 (0.31,0.96)	0.48 (0.21,1.10)
STOP-2 (31)	ACEi vs BB/TZ	488	0.51 (0.28,0.92)	ns	ns	ns
STOP-2 (31)	CCB vs BB/TZ	484	ns	ns	ns	ns
NORDIL (28)	ACEi vs BB/TZ	727	ns	ns	ns	ns
INSIGHT (40)	CCB vs BB/TZ	1302	ns	ns	ns	ns
ALLHAT (33)	ACEi vs TZ	6929	ns	ns	ns	ns
ALLHAT (33)	CCB vs TZ	7162	ns	ns	ns	ns
LIFE (30)	ARB/TZ vs BB/TZ	1195	ns	0.79 (0.55,1.14)	0.61 (0.45,0.84)	0.63 (0.42,0.95)
ASCOT (34)	CCB/ACEi vs BB/TZ	5145	nr	Combined major CV events	0.86 (0.76,0.98)	

Abbreviations: ACE-i, angiotensin-converting-enzyme inhibitor; ARB, angiotensin II receptor blocker; BB, beta-blocker; CAD, coronary artery disease (mainly myocardial infarction); CCB, calcium channel blocker; CV, cardiovascular; nr, not reported; ns, not significant; TZ, thiazide (or thiazide-like) diuretic.

with T2DM are not as uniform as those noted among adults with T1DM (43). In a recent cross-sectional survey (44), using data from the Third National Health and Nutrition Examination Survey (NHANES III), 33% of diabetic adults with a glomerular filtration rate (GFR) <60 ml/min per $1.73\,m^2$ showed no evidence of microalbuminuria, microalbuminuria, or retinopathy. Findings obtained from T2DM patients with non-albuminuric renal insufficiency (45) suggest that patients with T2DM can commonly progress to a significant degree of renal impairment while remaining normo-albuminuric.

The two main treatment strategies for primary prevention of diabetic nephropathy are improved glycemic control and BP lowering, particularly using drugs such as ACEi. Megatrials and meta-analyses have clearly demonstrated the beneficial effect of both treatment modalities. Antihypertensive treatment of patients with overt diabetic nephropathy induces a reduction in albuminuria, a reduction in the rate of glomerular filtration rate, delays development of ESRD and improves survival of the patients. These benefits have been demonstrated with a variety of BP lowering agents, including BB, CCB, diuretics and ACEi.

Lewis and co-workers (46) compared captopril with placebo over 3 years in 409 T1DM patients with mild renal insufficiency due to DN (proteinuria >500 mg/24h, serum creatinine level <2.5 mg/dl). Captopril treatment nearly halved the rate of increased serum creatinine levels, requirement of dialysis or transplantation or death. The difference in the median DBP during the study was less than 4 mm Hg. Unfortunately, no long-term study has been published concerning the effects of ACEi on the progression of DN in T2DM patients.

RENAL PROTECTION BY ANGIOTENSIN II RECEPTOR BLOCKERS

In recent years several large long-term intervention studies (47–54) in T2DM patients with early or advanced DN have been performed with different angiotensin II receptor blocker agents (ARB; irbesartan, losartan, telmisartan). In recent years, 2 large clinical trials (47,48) have been performed with the intent of determining whether angiotensin-receptor blockade is associated with retardation of the progression of renal disease in type 2 diabetic nephropathy by a mechanism independent of blood pressure control.

In the IDNT (Irbesartan Diabetic Nephropathy Trial) 1715 patients with hypertension and T2DM nephropathy were randomized to daily treatment with 300 mg irbesartan, 10 mg amlodipine, or placebo in a prospective double masked trial (47). BP control was to the same target $<135/85$ mm Hg in all groups. Primary endpoint was a composite of time of doubling of entry serum creatinine, development of ESRD or all-cause mortality. Treatment with irbesartan was associated with a 20% risk reduction of the primary composite endpoint events when compared to placebo ($p = 0.024$) and a 23% risk reduction versus amlodipine ($p = 0.006$). There was a 33% risk reduction with respect to doubling of serum creatinine favoring irbesartan when compared to placebo ($p = 0.003$), and a 37% reduction versus amlodipine ($p = 0.001$). A 23% risk reduction of ESRD for irbesartan relative to both placebo ($p = 0.074$) and to amlodipine ($p = 0.074$) was observed (Table 3). Proteinuria was significantly reduced in the irbesartan group throughout the study, but not in the amlodipine or placebo groups. However, there were no significant differences in the risk of all cause mortality or in the CV composite endpoint. From these data it can be concluded that irbesartan is an effective protective agent against the progression of type 2 DN and that this renoprotection is independent of BP reduction. The post-hoc analysis of the IDNT (50,51) clearly indicated that optimal lowering of systolic BP is very critical for these patients. An SBP >149 mmHg was associated with a 2.2-fold increase in the risk for doubling serum creatinine or ESRD compared with SBP <134 mm Hg (50). Progressive lowering of SBP to 120 mm Hg was associated with improved renal and patient survival, an effect independent of baseline renal function. An additional renoprotective effect of irbesartan (Fig. 4), independent of achieved SBP, was observed down to 120 mm Hg (51). Remarkably, SBP lower than 120 mm Hg was associated with increased all-cause mortality (Fig. 5). Based on these findings a SBP target between 120 and 130 mmHg was recommended for optimal renoprotection, in conjunction with blockade of the RAS in patients withT2DM nephropathy (51). There was no correlation between DBP and renal outcomes. Achieved DBP <85 mmHg was associated with a trend to increase in all-cause mortality, significant increase in myocardial infarction, but

TABLE 3   Comparison of Major Endpoints in the IDNT & RENAAL

| | Relative risk reduction (%) | | | |
| | RENAAL | IDNT | | |
	Losartan vs control	Irbesartan vs control	Irbesartan vs amplodipine	Amlodipine vs control
Doubling of creatinine, ESRD, or death	16 ($p=0.02$)	20 ($p=0.02$)	23 ($p=0.006$)	−4 ($p=0.69$)
Doubling of creatinine	25 ($p=0.006$)	33 ($p=0.003$)	37 ($p<0.001$)	−6 ($p=0.60$)
ESRD	28 ($p=0.002$)	23 ($p=0.07$)	23 ($p=0.07$)	0 ($p=0.99$)
Death	−2 ($p=0.88$)	8 ($p=0.57$)	−4 ($p=0.8$)	12 ($p=0.4$)
CV morbidity & mortality	10 ($p=0.26$)	9 ($p=0.4$)	−3 ($p=0.79$)	12 ($p=0.29$)

Abbreviations: ESRD, end-stage-renal-disease, CV, cardiovascular; IDNT, irbesartan diabetic nephropathy trial; RENAAL, reduction of endpoints in non-insulin dependent diabetes mellitus with the angiotensin II antagonist losartan; vs, versus.
Source: From Refs. 47 and 48.

decreased risk for stroke. Increased pulse pressure predicted increased all-cause mortality, CV mortality, myocardial infarction, and chronic heart failure (50). The IDNT investigators concluded that achieved SBP approaching 120 mmHg and DBP of 85 mmHg are associated with the best protection against CV events in these patients, whereas BP <or = 120/85 may be associated with an increase in CV events.

    In the RENAAL (Reduction of Endpoints in Non-Insulin Dependent Diabetes mellitus with the Angiotensin II Antagonist Losartan) Study (48) the renal protective effect of Losartan (50 to 100 mg/day) was studied in comparison with placebo in 1513 hypertensive T2DM patients with proteinuria. In both treatment groups conventional antihypertensive drugs like CCB, diuretics, BB and α_1 specific blockers were used. In comparison with the control group treatment with losartan (48) reduced the risk (Table 3) for progression to ESRD by 28% ($p=0.002$) and the risk for doubling of serum creatinine by 25% ($p=0.006$). By contrast, the death risk did not significantly differ between the two groups (21.0 vs. 20.3%). A recently published post-hoc analysis of the RENAAL study (52) showed that treatment-induced changes in SBP and albuminuria do not run parallel in a substantial proportion of patients. Among patients with a reduced SBP during treatment, a lack of albuminuria reduction was observed in 37%, 26%, and 51% (total, losartan, and placebo, respectively) at 6 months. SBP or albuminuria reduction was associated with a lower risk for ESRD, whereas combined SBP and albuminuria reduction was associated with the lowest risk for events. Antihypertensive treatment that is aimed at improving renal outcomes in patients with DN may therefore require a dual strategy, targeting both SBP and albuminuria reduction.

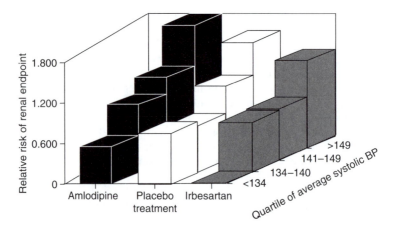

FIGURE 4   Simultaneous impact of quartile of achieved systolic BP and treatment modality on the relative risk for reaching a renal endpoint. *Source*: From Ref. 51.

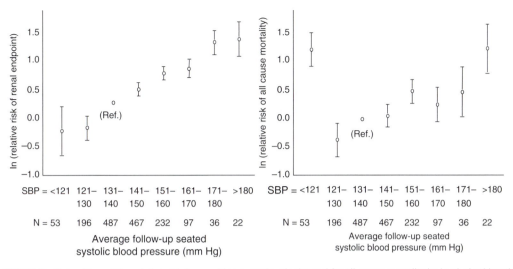

FIGURE 5 Natural log of the relative risk for reaching a renal endpoint and for all-cause mortality by level of achieved follow-up SBP. *Abbreviations*: n, number; Ref, reference; SBP, systolic blood pressure. *Source*: From Ref. 51.

The IRMA-2 (Irbesartan Microalbuminuria Type-2) was a 2-year multicenter, randomized, double-blind trial (49) in 590 T2DM patients with hypertension and microalbuminuria comparing irbesartan (150 or 300 mg once daily) versus placebo. The primary endpoint was onset of overt nephropathy. Treatment with irbesartan resulted in a 70% relative risk reduction ($p = 0.0004$) for the progression from early to a late and more serious stage of kidney disease compared with patients who did not receive the ARB (49). Interestingly, irbesartan treatment yielded significant changes (53) in high sensitive C-reactive protein with a 5.4% decrease per year versus a 10% increase per year in the placebo group ($p < 0.001$). Fibrinogen decreased 0.059 g/l per year from baseline versus placebo's 0.059 g/l increase per year ($p = 0.027$). Interleukin-6 showed a 1.8% increase per year compared with placebo's 6.5% increase per year ($p = 0.005$) and changes in interleukin-6 were associated with changes in albumin excretion ($p = 0.04$). Irbesartan (300 mg once daily) reduced low-grade inflammation in this high-risk population, and this could be relevant for reducing the risk of micro-and macrovascular disease.

In the DETAIL (Diabetics Exposed to Telmisartan and Enalapril) study the renoprotective effects of an ARB (telmisartan 80 mg/day) or an ACEi (enalapril 20 mg/day) were studied in 250 patients with T2DM (54). After five years, the change in glomerular filtration rate (primary end point) was very similar in both groups, -17.5 ml/min in the telmisartan-treated compared with -15.0 ml/min in the enalapril-treated patients. Thus, the DETAIL study showed equivalence of ARB and ACEi in the long-term renoprotection over 5 years, since the effects of the two agents on the primary and secondary end points were not significantly different. Unfortunately, a similar direct comparison of drugs of the two different classes in patients with more advanced nephropathy is not available.

In the (Bergamo Nephrologic Diabetes Complications Trial) BENEDICT study the preventive effect of either ACEi (trandolapril 2mg/day) or non-dihydro-pyridine CCB (verapamil 240 mg/day), alone or in combination on microalbuminuria was studied in 1204 T2DM patients with hypertension and normal urinary albumin excretion (55). The target BP was 120/80 mm Hg. Significantly fewer patients reached the primary end of persistent microalbuminuria when trandolapril was used: 5.7% of patients on both trandolapril plus verapamil and 6.0% in those on trandolapril alone, but 11.9% of patients on verapamil, and 10.0% of those on placebo. In T2DM patients with hypertension but with normoalbuminuria, the use of trandolapril alone or in combination with verapamil decreased the incidence of microalbuminuria to a similar extent, whereas the effect of verapamil alone was not better than that of placebo.

BLOCKADE OF RAS BY HIGH DOSE OF ARB OR DOUBLE BLOCKADE BY ARB AND ACEI

High doses of ARB that are in excess of the usual range have been used to decrease proteinuria to levels that are less than those achieved at approved doses and also concomitantly decrease systemic blood pressure (56). Ultrahigh dosing of irbesartan (900 mg once daily) was generally safe and offered additional renoprotection independent of changes in SBP and GFR in comparison to the currently recommended dose of 300 mg. However, it is difficult to discern whether these results can be attributed to specific proteinuria decreasing effects, more effective antihypertensive effects, or other mechanisms promoting renoprotection (57). The combination of ACEi and ARB together in their usual therapeutic doses also have led to reports of decreasing of proteinuria levels beyond that shown by either of these agents alone in some but not all studies (58–65). Unfortunately, conclusions often are confounded by the inability to equalize blood pressure control in the randomized groups (57).

META-ANALYSES COMPARING THE EFFECTS OF ACEI OR ARB FOR PREVENTING THE DEVELOPMENT AND PROGRESSION OF DIABETIC KIDNEY DISEASE

Recently, several meta-analyses (66–69) comparing the effects of ACEi and ARB for preventing the development and progression of DN were published. Surprisingly, these reports reached totally different conclusions indicating the well known discrepancies between meta-analyses and subsequent large randomized, controlled trials (70). In 2004, Strippoli GF, et al. (66) analyzed 43 trials with a total of 7545 patients; 36 of 43 identified trials compared ACEi with placebo (4008 patients), 4 compared ARB with placebo (3331 patients), and 3 compared ACEi with ARB (206 patients). Both agents had similar effects on renal outcomes. ACEi significantly reduced all-cause mortality [risk reduction (RR) 0.79] compared with placebo but ARB did not (RR 0.99). In 2006 the Australian group reported two further detailed analyses (67,68). Based on one of these (67) they concluded that ACEi are the only agents with proven renal benefit in patients who have diabetes with no nephropathy and the only agents with proven survival benefit in patients who have diabetes with nephropathy. This statement was criticized (57) since they failed to take into account the possibility that their results could be explained by the fact that the majority of trials using ACEi were performed in relatively young patients (mean age 35 years) with type 1 diabetic nephropathy, whereas the treatment trials using ARB were performed mainly in patients with type 2 diabetic nephropathy (mean age 60 years). Thus, it could well be that the difference in CV events and mortality was driven by the population studied and not the therapeutic agent used (57). In their last Cochrane analysis (68, see Table 4) fifty studies (13,215 patients) were identified; 38 compared ACEi with placebo, 5 compared ARB with placebo and 7 compared ACEi and ARB directly. The effects of ACEi and ARB on renal outcomes (ESRD, doubling of creatinine, prevention of progression of micro- to macroalbuminuria, remission of micro- to normoalbuminuria) were similarly beneficial (Table 4). There was no significant difference in the risk of all-cause mortality for ACEi versus placebo (RR 0.91) and ARB versus placebo (RR 0.99). A subgroup analysis of studies using full-dose ACEi versus studies using half or less than half the maximum tolerable dose of ACEi showed a significant reduction in the risk of all-cause mortality with the use of full-dose ACEi (RR 0.78).

Another misleading meta-analysis was reported by Casas, et al. (69), which concluded that ACEi and ARB were no more effective than other antihypertensive drugs with respect to renoprotection. Serious questions have been raised regarding the validity (70,71) of the Casas report, which was primarily an analysis of the ALLHAT patient population (85% of all patients) rather than a meta-analysis. The ALLHAT study excluded patients with severe renal disease and neglected to measure proteinuria. In fact, there was no similarity between the patient populations in the ALLHAT trial when compared with the existing valid DN trials in the literature. The ALLHAT trial itself has been the subject of considerable controversy from many points of view. A secondary analysis by Rahman M, et al. (72) concluded that hypertensive patients with a reduced GFR who were entered into the ALLHAT trial were not protected from the development of ESRD by the use of lisinopril

TABLE 4 The Effects of ACEi and ARB on Renal Outcomes and All-Cause Mortality in Diabetic Patients

Outcome title	ACEi vs. placebo			ARB vs. ACEi			ARB vs. placebo		
	No. of studies	No. of patients	Effect size	No. of studies	No. of patients	Effect size	No. of studies	No. of patients	Effect size
All-cause mortality	21	7295	0.91 [0.71,1.17]	3	307	0.92 [0.31,2.78]	5	3409	0.99 [0.85,1.17]
Cardiovascular mortality			STO	3	307	0.62 [0.10,3.62]			TNS
Doubling of serum creatinine	9	6780	0.68 [0.47,1.00]	0	0	NE	3	3251	0.79 [0.67,0.93]
End-stage kidney disease	10	6819	0.60 [0.39,0.93]	0	0	NE	3	3251	0.78 [0.67,0.91]
Micro- to macroalbuminuria	17	2036	0.45 [0.29,0.69]	3	307	TNS	3	761	0.49 [0.32,0.75]
Micro-to normoalbuminuria	16	1910	3.06 [1.76,5.35]	2	65	1.22 [0.76,1.94]	2	670	1.42 [1.05,1.93]

Abbreviations: ACEi, angiotensin-converting-enzyme inhibitor; ARB, angiotensin II-receptor-blocker; CD, cochrane database; NE, not estimateable; STO, subtotals only; TNS, totals not selected.
Source: From Ref. 68.

when compared with patients receiving amlodipine or chlorthalidone. A serious weakness of ALLHAT is the fact that 50% of the patients in the ACEi group were either not receiving the medication or were receiving a dose so low (only 10 mg lisinopril) that renoprotection might not be expected in the study (73,74).

LONG-TERM RISK OF ESRD IN DIABETIC PATIENTS TREATED WITH DIFFERENT ANTIHYPERTENSIVE DRUGS

The incidence of ESRD in diabetic patients has continued to increase despite the extensive use of ACEi to prevent DN. Recently, Suissa, et al. (75) have assessed the long-term effect of ACEi on the risk of ESRD in a population-based cohort of all diabetic patients treated with antihypertensive drugs between 1982 and 1986. The cohort of 6102 patients, in which 102 cases developed ESRD until 1997, were matched to 4129 controls. Relative to thiazide diuretic use, the adjusted rate ratio of ESRD associated with the use of ACEi was 2.5, whereas it was 0.8 for BB and 0.7 for CCB. The rate ratio of ESRD with the use of ACEi was 0.8 during the first 3 years of follow-up, but increased to 4.2 after 3 years. The authors concluded that ACEi use does not appear to decrease the long-term risk of ERSD in diabetes. The finding of an elevated risk may have at least two possible explanations. First, it could be that ACEi prolong life, thus increasing the opportunity for ESRD incidence. Alternatively, ACEi, while apparently providing an early benefit to the kidney, could damage the kidney in the longer term by mechanisms still unknown. In proteinuric rats (76) and in experimental renal transplantation (77), ACEi regimens induced renal fibrosis in spite of a reduction in proteinuria and blood pressure, that is, an improvement of the established clinical criteria for a good response to therapy.

NEW AMERICAN AND EUROPEAN JOINT GUIDELINES FOR STRICT BLOOD PRESSURE CONTROL: ESC-EASD AND ADA-AHA

Although a number of monotherapies and multidrug therapies are available for the treatment of hypertension, current guidelines provide evidence-based recommendations for the use of specific antihypertensive agents in patients with diabetes. The guidelines from the seventh report of the Joint National Committee on Prevention, Detection, Evaluation, and Treatment of High Blood Pressure (JNC-7) recommend the use of either ACEi or ARB as initial therapy to achieve the BP target in patients with T2DM (78). If one class is not tolerated, the other should be substituted if it is not contraindicated. According to the JNC-7, starting therapy with 2 drugs, separately or as fixed dose combinations, may be considered when SBP is >20 mm Hg or diastolic BP is >10 mm Hg above the desired goal for the individual patient (78). Neither ACEi nor ARB appear to produce any clinically significant changes in metabolic measurements, such as blood glucose and the lipid profile, which is an important consideration in the presence of diabetes. Based on the studies discussed above, ACEi or ARB are specified as the preferred first-line agents for the treatment of patients with hypertension, T2DM, and microalbuminuria as both drug classes delay progression to macroalbuminuria. A recent study (79) provides strong clinical evidence implying that a reduction of microalbuminuria in type 2 diabetic patients is an integrated indicator for renal and CV risk reduction.

Very recently, new joint guidelines (80,81) were published from both the American Heart Association (AHA) and the American Diabetes Association (ADA) as well as from the European Society of Cardiology (ESC) and the European Association for Study of Diabetes (EASD) for reducing the high vascular risk of diabetic patients. Strict blood pressure control and antihypertensive combination therapy is in the center of both recommendations. The joint ESC-EASD guidelines (80) recommend for patients with diabetes and hypertension a target BP level of 130/80 mm Hg. In addition, combination of several anti-hypertensive drugs is recommended for satisfactory BP control and a RAS-inhibitor should be part of the BP-lowering treatment. The joint AHA-ADA guidelines (81) recommend that all patients with diabetes and hypertension should be treated with a regimen that includes either an ACEi or an ARB. If one class is not tolerated, the other should be substituted. Other drug classes demonstrated to reduce CV events in patients with diabetes (BB, thiazide diuretics, and CCB) should be added as needed to achieve BP targets. Multiple-drug therapy generally is required to achieve blood pressure targets.

COMBINATION THERAPY IS MANDATORY FOR MOST PATIENTS TO REACH TARGET VALUES

As clearly stated by recent guidelines (80,81) most patients with diabetes will require two or more antihypertensive therapies from different classes with complementary mechanisms of action to control their blood pressure. Thiazide diuretics, BB, or CCB can be added to ACEi or ARB treatment to achieve target BP, either as an individual drug component or as part of a fixed-dose combination product. Combining an ACEi or an ARB with a thiazide diuretic may be particularly effective, as such combinations provide additive reductions in blood pressure compared with individual monotherapies, and counteract many of the adverse events that may be associated with the use of high doses of thiazide diuretics (82,83), and abolish any interracial differences in the response to ACEi or ARB monotherapy (84,85). For example, coadministration of irbesartan and hydrochlorothiazide, either as individual components or in a fixed dose combination, leads to additive reductions in blood pressure in a diverse patient population compared with individual monotherapies, and the drug treatment is well tolerated (86). Certain BB may be preferred as add-on antihypertensive medications for patients with diabetes because of their glycemic and metabolic effects. Carvedilol, a nonselective BB, has more favourable effects on HbA1c levels, insulin sensitivity, total cholesterol levels, and triglyceride levels than metoprolol in patients with T2DM and hypertension already receiving an ACEi or ARB despite similar effects on BP (87). Moreover, studies with carvedilol demonstrate attenuated increases in albuminuria compared with metoprolol as well as reduction in CV events in chronic kidney disease patients with hypertension (88).

BLOOD PRESSURE TARGET VALUES ARE NOT REACHED IN MOST OF THE INTERVENTION STUDIES

Although in most of the antihypertensive intervention studies two, three or even more drugs of antihypertensive classes were used, the necessary target values were not reached in the majority of studies. In the INSIGHT study (40,90) patients with diabetes were the most resistant to treatment, requiring second and third drugs 40% and 100% more frequently than patients without diabetes and achieving marginally the highest final BP, for any risk group, of $141+/-13/82+/-8$ mm Hg. Figure 6 shows the effects of antihypertensive drug treatment on SBP and DBP in diabetic hypertensive patients of 10 different trials. Values at trial entry and during treatment are shown for each trial. Dashed horizontal lines refer to goal BP values indicated by international guidelines to be achieved during treatment. Unfortunately, an SBP of 130 mm Hg was not reached in any of the 10 intervention studies. Likewise studies in diabetic patients with a specific focus on diabetic nephropathy also failed to reach the SBP target values (Fig. 7) despite the fact that for these patients even lower BP values were recommended by some groups.

RISK FOR DEVELOPMENT OF NEW DIABETES IN RELATION TO ANTIHYPERTENSIVE DRUG THERAPY

Because hypertension is often associated in large populations with impaired glucose tolerance, insulin resistance, and obesity, many patients with hypertension develop diabetes even when treated with placebo. Since in most diabetic patients combination therapy with two, or even three antihypertensive agents is likely to be required, the choice of which antihypertensive class should be given seems to be less problematic. When it comes to nondiabetic hypertensive patients, it seems to be more crucial. A meta-analysis of hypertension trials (91) involving about 116,000 patients, two-thirds of whom did not have diabetes at baseline, found an overall 25% reduction by RAS inhibition (27% for ACEi and 23% for ARB) in new-onset diabetes compared with other antihypertensive classes or placebo (91). Table 5 shows the

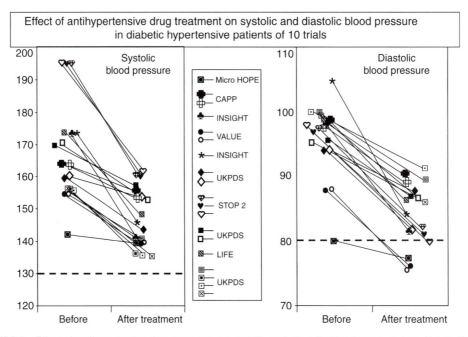

FIGURE 6   Effect of antihypertensive drug treatment on systolic and diastolic blood pressure (mm Hg) in diabetic hypertensive patients in 10 different trials. *Source*: Modified from Ref. 89.

impressive consistency of findings into the direction of reducing the risk for the development of T2DM in almost all studies (24,25,29,33,34,92–100). The clinical relevance of increased incidence of T2DM associated with the use of diuretics or BB is widely unknown. One longitudinal cohort study from Italy (101) showed a significant increase of CVD in people who

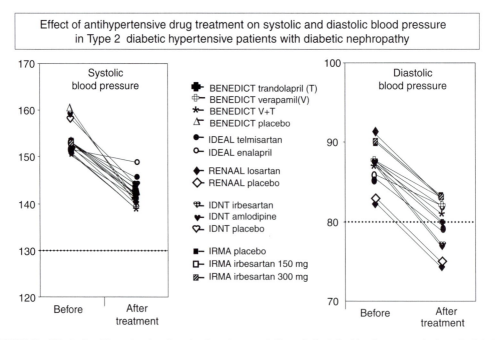

FIGURE 7   Effect of antihypertensive drug treatment on systolic and diastolic blood pressure in type 2 diabetic patients in studies with focus on diabetic nephropathy. *Source*: Modified from Ref. 89.

developed diabetes after randomization to antihypertensive drug therapy, whereas other studies (ALLHAT, SHEP, VALUE) showed no increase (33,100,102). Studies with longer follow-up might help define the time taken for incident diabetes to be associated with increased CV risk.

In the DREAM study (95) among patients with impaired fasting glucose or impaired glucose tolerance, the use of ramipril for three years did not significantly reduce the incidence of diabetes but did significantly increase regression to normoglycemia. In the DREAM study mean BP at baseline was relatively low (136/83 mm Hg) and subjects with CVD and heart failure were excluded in contrast to previous studies. Moreover, subjects were about ten years younger than in previous studies, 55 versus about 65 years. It is possible that the degree of activation of the RAS is higher in people who are older or have known CVD or hypertension and that ACE inhibition may thus have a greater effect in these people than in others.

Very recently, a network meta-analysis (103), which accounts for both direct and indirect comparisons to assess the effects of antihypertensive agents on incident T2DM, was published. In this systematic review, 48 randomized groups of 22 clinical trials with 143,153 participants who did not have T2DM at randomization were included into the analysis. The main outcome was the proportion of patients who developed T2DM. With an initial diuretic as the standard of comparison (8 groups), the following odds ratios were found: ARB (5 groups) 0.57 ($p < 0.0001$); ACEi (8 groups) 0.67 ($p < 0.0001$), CCB (9 groups) 0.75 ($p = 0.002$), placebo (9 groups) 0.77 ($p = 0.009$) and BB (9 groups) 0.90 ($p = 0.30$). Thus, the association of antihypertensive drugs with incident diabetes was lowest for ARB and ACEi followed by CCB and placebo, BB and diuretics in rank order (Fig. 8). Individual pair-wise comparisons between diuretic vs BB ($p = 0.30$), placebo vs CCB (0.72), ACE inhibitor vs ARB (0.16) did not achieve significance ($p < 0.05$).

SUMMARY

Hypertension and diabetes are common, additive risk factors for CV risk. Early, aggressive reduction of blood pressure in diabetics is of fundamental importance, and is possibly the most important aspect of treatment in these patients. Increasing evidence suggests that the choice of antihypertensive is important, with RAS blockade appearing to offer superior renal protection for a given level of blood pressure reduction. However, given the difficulty of reducing blood pressure to goal levels in diabetics, combination therapy with two, or even three antihypertensive agents is likely to be required in most diabetic patients. RAS blockade prevents not only CVD and renal events in diabetic patients, but, also delays or avoids the onset of T2DM in hypertensive patients, who are often obese and insulin-resistant and have therefore a high risk for the later development of type 2 diabetes. Due to the global epidemic of

TABLE 5 Prevention of New-Onset Type 2 Diabetes Mellitus

Trial (Ref.)	No. of patients	Drugs	Statistical method	Effect Size
ALPINE (92)	392	ARB ± CCB vs BB ± diuretic	Risk ratio (95% CI)	0.13 [0.03,0.99]
ALLHAT (33)	33,357	ACE vs diuretic	Risk ratio (95% CI)	0.70 [0.56,0.86]
ANBP2 (93)	6083	ACE vs diuretic	Risk ratio (95% CI)	0.66 [0.54,0.85]
ASCOT-BLPA (34)	19,257	CCB ± ACE vs BB ± diuretic	Odds ratio (95% CI)	0.68 [0.61,0.76]
CAPPP (24)	10,985	ACE vs diuretic/BB	Risk ratio (95% CI)	0.79 [0.67,0.94]
CHARM (94)	7599	ARB vs placebo	Risk ratio (95% CI)	0.78 [0.64,0.96]
DREAM (95)	5269	ACE vs placebo	Hazard ratio (95% CI)	0.91 [0.80–1.03]
HOPE (25)	9297	ACE vs placebo	Risk ratio (95% CI)	0.66 [0.51,0.85]
LIFE (29)	9193	ARB vs BB	Risk ratio (95% CI)	0.75 [0.63,0.88]
PEACE (96)	8290	ACE vs placebo	Risk ratio (95% CI)	0.83 [0.72,0.96]
SCOPE (97)	4937	ARB vs placebo	Risk ratio (95% CI)	0.81 [0.61,1.02]
SOLVD (98)	4228	ACE vs placebo	Risk ratio (95% CI)	0.26 [0.13,0.53]
STOP-2 (99)	6614	ACE vs diuretic/BB	Risk ratio (95% CI)	0.96 [0.72,1.27]
VALUE (100)	15,245	ARB vs CCB	Risk ratio (95% CI)	0.77 [0.69,0.86]

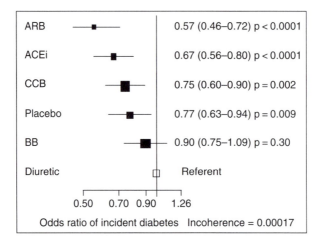

FIGURE 8   Results of network meta-analysis of 22 clinical trials *Abbreviations*: ACEi, angiotensin-converting-enzyme-inhibitor; ARB, angiotension II-receptorablocker; BB, beta-blocker; CCB, calcium channel blocker. *Source*: From Ref. 103.

T2DM, decreasing the risk of diabetes represents a crucial treatment advantage beyond BP reduction, as new-onset diabetes increases vascular risk comparably to pre-existing diabetes and is associated with considerable morbidity and costs.

ADDENDUM AFTER PRESS

After preparation of this review the important findings of the ADVANCE study were published (104). In this randomized controlled trial the routine administration of an ACE inhibitor-diuretic combination on serious vascular events in patients with diabetes, was evaluated in 11,140 patients with type 2 diabetes irrespective of initial blood pressure levels or the use of other blood pressure lowering drugs. Compared with patients assigned placebo, those assigned active therapy had a mean reduction in systolic blood pressure of 5.6 mm Hg and diastolic blood pressure of 2.2 mm Hg. After a mean follow-up period of 4.3 years the relative risk of a major macrovascular or microvascular event was reduced by 9% (861 [15.5%] active versus 938 [16.8%] placebo; hazard ratio 0.91, 95% CI 0.83–1.00, $p = 0.04$). The relative risk of death from cardiovascular disease was reduced by 18% (211 [3.8%] active versus 257 [4.6%] placebo; 0.82, 0.68–0.98, $p = 0.03$) and death from any cause was reduced by 14% (408 [7.3%] active versus 471 [8.5%] placebo; 0.86, 0.75–0.98, $p = 0.03$). The important results of ADVANCE indicate that the routine administration of a fixed combination of perindopril and indapamide to a broad range of patients with diabetes reduces the risks of death and major macrovascular or microvascular complications, irrespective of initial blood pressure level or ancillary treatment with the many other preventive treatments typically provided to diabetic patients today.

REFERENCES

1. Bild D, Teutsch SM. The control of hypertension in persons with diabetes: a public health approach. Public Health Rep. 1987; 102:522–9.
2. Sowers JR. Treatment of hypertension in patients with diabetes. Arch Intern Med. 2004; 164: 1850–1857.
3. Stamler J, Vaccaro O, Neaton JD, et al. Diabetes, other risk factors, and 12-yr cardiovascular mortality for men screened in the Multiple Risk Factor Intervention Trial. Diabetes Care 1993; 16: 434–444.
4. Clermont A, Bursell SE, Feener EP. Role of the angiotensin II type 1 receptor in the pathogenesis of diabetic retinopathy: effects of blood pressure control and beyond. J Hypertens Suppl. 2006; 24: S73–80.
5. Giunti S, Barit D, Cooper ME. Mechanisms of diabetic nephropathy: role of hypertension. Hypertension 2006; 48:519–526.
6. Zhang Y, Lee ET, Devereux RB, et al. Prehypertension, diabetes, and cardiovascular disease risk in a population-based sample: the Strong Heart Study Hypertension 2006; 47:410–4.

7. Equiluz-Bruck S, Schnack C, Kopp HP, et al. Nondipping of nocturnal blood pressure is related to urinary albumin excretion rate in patients with type-2 diabetes mellitus. Am J Hypertension 1996; 9:1139–43.
8. Poulsen PL, Beck T, Ebbehoi E, et al. 24h ambulatory blood pressure and retinopathy in normoalbuminuric IDDM patients. Diabetologia 1998; 41:105–10.
9. Farmer CK, Goldsmith DJ, Quin JD, et al. Progression of diabetic nephropathy–is diurnal blood pressure rhythm as important as absolute blood pressure level? Nephrol Dial Transplant. 1998; 13: 635–9.
10. Chen JW, Jen SL, Lee WL, et al. Differential glucose tolerance in dipper and nondipper essential hypertension. Diabetes Care 1998; 21:1743–1748.
11. Nakano S, Fukuda M, Hotta F, et al: Reversed circadian blood pressure rhythm is associated with occurences of both fatal and nonfatal vascular events in NIDDM subjects. Diabetes 1998; 47:1501–6.
12. Schernthaner G, Ritz E, Philipp T, et al. Night time blood pressure in diabetic patients - the submerged portion of the iceberg? Nephrol.Dial Transplant 1999; 14:1061–1064.
13. Andersen AR, Christiansen JS, Andersen JK, et al. Diabetic nephropathy in type 1 (insulin-dependent) diabetes: an epidemiological study. Diabetologia 1983; 25:496–501.
14. Viberti GC, Keen H, Wiseman MJ. Raised arterial pressure in parents of proteinuric insulin-dependent diabetics. Br Med J. 1987; 295:575–577.
15. Ritz E, Orth SR. Nephropathy in patients with type 2 diabetes mellitus. N Engl J Med 1999; 341: 1127–33.
16. Reaven GM, Lithell H, Landsberg L. Hypertension and associated metabolic abnormalities. The role of insulin resistance and the sympathoadrenal system. N Engl J Med 1996; 334:374–81.
17. DeFronzo RA, Ferrannini E: Insulin resistance - a multifaceted syndrome responsible for NIDDM, obesity, hypertension, dyslipidemia and atheroslerotic disease. Diabetes Care 1991; 14:173–94.
18. Gress TW, Nieto FJ, Shahar E, et al. Hypertension and antihypertensive therapy as risk factors for type 2 diabetes mellitus: N Engl J Med 2000; 342:905–12.
19. Curb JD, Pressel SL, Cutler JA, et al. Effect of diuretic-based Antihypertensive treatment on cardiovascular disease risk in older diabetic patients with isolated systolic hypertension. Systolic Hypertension in the Elderly Program Cooperative Research Group. JAMA 1996; 276:1886–92.
20. UK Prospective Diabetes Study (UKPDS) Group. Tight blood pressure control and risk of macrovascular and microvascular complication in type-2 diabetes: UKPDS 38. BMJ 1998; 317:703–13.
21. UK Prospective Diabetes Study (UKPDS) Group. Efficacy of atenolol and captopril in reducing risk of macrovascular and microvascular complications in type-2 diabetes: UKPDS 39. BMJ 1998; 317:713–20.
22. Hansson L, Zanchetti A, Carruthers SG, et al. Effects of intensive blood-pressure lowering and low-dose aspirin in patients with hypertension: Principal results of the hypertension optimal treatment (HOT) randomised trial. Lancet 1998; 351:1755–62.
23. Tuomilehto J, Rastenyte D, Birkenhager WH, et al. Effects of calcium-channel blockade in older patients with diabetes and systolic hypertension. Systolic Hypertension in Europe Trial Investigators. N Engl J Med 1999; 340:677–84.
24. Hansson L, Lindholm LH, Niskanen L, et al. Effect of angiotensin-converting-enzyme inhibition compared with conventional therapy on cardiovascular morbidity and mortality in hypertension: the Captopril Prevention Project (CAPPP) randomised trial. Lancet 1999; 353:611–16.
25. Heart Outcomes Prevention Evaluation (HOPE) Study Investigators. Effects of ramipril on cardiovascular and microvascular outcomes in people with diabetes mellitus: results of the HOPE study and MICRO-HOPE substudy. Lancet 2000; 355:253–9.
26. Svensson P, de Faire U, Sleight Pz, et al. Comparative effects of ramipril on ambulatory and office blood pressures: a HOPE Substudy. Hypertension 2001; 38:E28–32.
27. Brown MJ, Palmer CR, Castaigne A et al. Morbidity and mortality in patients randomised to double-blind treatment with a long-acting calcium-channel blocker or diuretic in the International Nifedipine GITS study: Intervention as a goal in hypertension treatment (INSIGHT). Lancet 2000; 356:366–72.
28. Hansson L, Hedner T, Lund-Johanson P, et al. Randomized trial of effects of calcium-antagonists compared with diuretics and beta-blockers on cardiovascular morbidity and mortality in hypertension: The Nordic Diltiazem (NORDIL) Study. Lancet 2000; 356:359–65.
29. Dahlof B, Devereux RB, Kjeldsen SE, et al. Cardiovascular morbidity and mortality in the Losartan Intervention for endpoint reduction in hypertension study (LIFE): a randomised trial against atenolol. Lancet 2002; 359:995–1003.
30. Lindholm LH, Ibsen H, Dahlöf B, et al. Cardiovascular morbidity and mortality in patients with diabetes in the Losartan Intervention for endpoint reduction in hypertension study (LIFE): a randomised trial against atenolol. Lancet 2002; 359:1004–10.
31. Lindholm LH, Hansson L, Ekbom T, et al. Comparison of antihypertensive treatments in preventing cardiovascular events in elderly diabetic patients: results from the Swedish Trial in Old Patients with Hypertension-2. STOP Hypertension-2 Study Group. J Hypertens 2000; 18:1671–75.
32. Adler AI, Stratton M, Neil HAW, et al. Association of systolic blood pressure with macrovascular complications of type-2 diabetes (UKPDS 36): prospective observational study. BMJ 2000; 321:412–9.

33. The ALLHAT Officers and Coordinators for the ALLHAT Collaborative Research Group. Major outcomes in high-risk hypertensive patients randomized to angiotensin-converting enzyme inhibitor or calcium channel blocker vs diuretic: The Antihypertensive and Lipid-Lowering Treatment to Prevent Heart Attack Trial (ALLHAT). JAMA 2002; 288:2981–97.

34. Dahlof B, Sever PS, Poulter NR, et al. Prevention of cardiovascular events with an antihyper-tensive regimen of amlodipine adding perindopril as required versus atenolol adding bendroflumethiazide as required, in the Anglo-Scandinavian Cardiac Outcomes Trial-Blood Pressure Lowering Arm (ASCOT-BPLA): a multicentre randomised controlled trial. Lancet 2002; 366:895–906.

35. The Hypertension Detection and Follow-up Programme Cooperative Research Group. Mortality findings for stepped-care and referred-care participants in the hypertension detection and follow-up programme, stratified by other risk factors. Prev Med 1985; 14:312–35.

36. Yusuf S, Sleight P, Pogue J, et al. Heart Outcomes Prevention Evaluation Study Investigators. Effects of an angiotensin-converting-enzyme inhibitor, ramipril, on cardiovascular events in high-risk patients. N Engl J Med 2000; 342:145–53.

37. Tatti P, Pahor M, Byington RP, et al. Outcome results of the Fosinopril versus Amlodipine Cardiovascular Events Randomized Trial (FACET) in patients with hypertension and NIDDM. Diabetes Care 1998; 21:597–603.

38. Estacio RO, Jeffers BW, Hiatt WR, et al. The effect of nisoldipine as compared with enalapril on cardiovascular outcomes in patients with non-insulin-dependent diabetes and hypertension. N Engl J Med 1998; 338:645–52.

39. Niskanen L, Hedner T, Hansson L, et al. Reduced cardiovascular morbidity and mortality in hypertensive diabetic patients on first-line therapy with an ACE inhibitor compared with a diuretic/ beta-blocker-based treatment regimen: a subanalysis of the Captopril Prevention Project. Diabetes Care 2001; 24:2091–6.

40. Mancia G, Brown M, Castaigne A, et al. Outcomes with nifedipine GITS or Co-Amizolide in hypertensive diabetics and nondiabetics in intervention as a goal in hypertension (INSIGHT). Hypertension 2003; 41:431–6.

41. Yoon KH, Lee JH, Kim JW et al. Epidemic obesity and type 2 diabetes in Asia. Lancet 2006; 368: 1681–8.

42. United State Renal Data System. 2005 Annual data report; atlas of end-stage renal disease in the United States. Bethesda, MD, USA: National Institutes of Health, National Institute of Diabetes and Digestive and Kidney Diseases, 2006.

43. Schernthaner G. Kidney disease in Diabetology. Nephrol Dial Transplant. 2007; 22:703–7.

44. Kramer HJ, Nguyen QD, Curhan G, et al. Renal insufficiency in the absence of albuminuria and retinopathy among adults with type 2 diabetes mellitus. JAMA 2003; 289:3273–7.

45. MacIsaac RJ, Tsalamandris C, Panagiotopoulos S, et al. Nonalbuminuric renal insufficiency in type 2 diabetes. Diabetes Care 2004; 27:195–200.

46. Lewis EJ, Hunsicker LG, Bain RP, et al. The effect of angiotensin-converting-enzyme inhibition on diabetic nephropathy. N Engl J Med 1993; 329:1456–62.

47. Lewis EJ, Hunsicker LG, Clarke WR, et al. Renoprotective effect of the angiotensin-receptor antagonist Irbesartan in patients with nephropathy due to type 2 diabetes. N Engl J Med 2001; 345: 851–60.

48. Brenner BM, Cooper ME, De Zeeuw D, et al. Effects of losartan on renal and cardiovascular outcomes in patients with type 2 diabetes and nephropathy. N Engl J Med 2001; 345:861–9.

49. Parving H-H, Lehnert H, Bröchner-Mortensen J, et al. The effect of Irbesartan on the development of diabetic nephropathy in patients with type 2 diabetes N Engl J Med 2001; 345:870–8.

50. Berl T, Hunsicker LG, Lewis JB, et al. Impact of achieved blood pressure on cardiovascular outcomes in the Irbesartan Diabetic Nephropathy Trial. J Am Soc Nephrol. 2005; 16:2170–9.

51. Pohl MA, Blumenthal S, Cordonnier DJ, et al. Independent and additive impact of blood pressure control and angiotensin II receptor blockade on renal outcomes in the irbesartan diabetic nephropathy trial: clinical implications and limitations. J Am Soc Nephrol. 2005; 16:3027–37.

52. Eijkelkamp WB, Zhang Z, Remuzzi G, et al. Albuminuria Is a Target for Renoprotective Therapy Independent from Blood Pressure in Patients with Type 2 Diabetic Nephropathy: Post Hoc Analysis from the Reduction of Endpoints in NIDDM with the Angiotensin II Antagonist Losartan (RENAAL) Trial. J Am Soc Nephrol. 2007; 18:1540–6.

53. Persson F, Rossing P, Hovind P, et al. Irbesartan treatment reduces biomarkers of inflammatory activity in patients with type 2 diabetes and microalbuminuria: an IRMA 2 substudy. Diabetes 2006; 55:3550–5.

54. Barnett AH, Bain SC, Bouter P, et al. Angiotensin-receptor blockade versus converting-enzyme inhibition in type 2 diabetes and nephropathy. N Engl J Med. 2004; 351:1952–61.

55. Ruggenenti P, Fassi A, Ilieva AP, et al. Preventing microalbuminuria in type 2 diabetes. Bergamo Nephrologic Diabetes Complications Trial (BENEDICT) Investigators. N Engl J Med. 2004; 351: 1941–51.

56. Rossing K, Schjoedt KJ, Jensen BR, et al. Enhanced renoprotective effects of ultrahigh doses of irbesartan in patients with type 2 diabetes and microalbuminuria. Kidney Int. 2005; 68:1190–1198.
57. Lewis EJ. Treating hypertension in the patient with overt diabetic nephropathy. Semin. Nephrol. 2007; 27:182–94.
58. Azizi M, Menard J. Combined blockade of the rennin angiotensin system with angiotensin-converting enzyme inhibitors and angiotensin II type I receptor antagonists. Circulation 2004; 109: 2492–9.
59. Mogensen CE, Neldam S, Tikkanen I, et al. Randomized controlled trial of dual blockade of renin-angiotensin system in patients with hypertension, microalbuminuria, and non-insulin dependent diabetes: the candesartan and lisinopril microalbuminuria (CALM) study. BMJ 2003; 321:1440–4.
60. Rossing K, Christensen PK, Jensen BR, et al. Dual blockade of the renin-angiotensin system in diabetic nephropathy: a randomized double-blind crossover study. Diabetes Care 2002; 25:95–100.
61. Jacobsen P, Andersen S, Rossing K, et al. Dual blockade of the renin-angiotensin system in type 1 patients with diabetic nephropathy. Nephrol Dial Transplant. 2002; 17:1019–24.
62. Jacobsen P, Andersen S, Jensen BR, et al. Addictive effect of ACE inhibition and angiotensin II receptor blockade in type 1 diabetic patients with diabetic nephropathy. J Am Soc Nephrol. 2003; 14:992–999.
63. Jacobsen P, Andersen S, Rossing K, et al. Dual blockade of the renin-angiotensin system versus maximal recommended dose of ACE inhibition in diabetic nephropathy. Kidney Int. 2003; 874–880.
64. Rossing K, Jacobsen P, Pietraszek L, et al. Renoprotective effects of adding angiotensin II receptor blocker to maximal recommended doses of ACE inhibitor in diabetic nephropathy: a randomized double-blind crossover trial. Diabetes Care 2003; 26:2268–74.
65. Andersen NH, Poulsen PL, Knudsen ST, et al. Longterm dual blockade with candesartan and lisinopril in hypertensive patients with diabetes: the CALM II study. Diabetes Care 2005; 28: 273–277.
66. Strippoli GF, Craig M, Deeks JJ, et al. Effects of angiotensin converting enzyme inhibitors and angiotensin II receptor antagonists on mortality and renal outcomes in diabetic nephropathy: systemic review. BMJ 2004; 329:828–32.
67. Strippoli GF, Craig MC, Schena FP, et al. Role of blood pressure targets and specific antihypertensive agents used to prevent diabetic nephropathy and delay its progression. J Am Soc Nephrol. 2006; 17:S153-S155.
68. Strippoli GFM, Bonifati C, Craig M, et al. Angiotensin converting enzyme inhibitors and angiotensin II receptor antagonists for preventing the progression of diabetic kidney disease. Cochrane Database of Systematic Reviews 2006, Issue 4. Art. No.: CD006257. DOI: 10.1002/14651858.
69. Casas JP, Chua W, Loukogeorgakis S. Effect of inhibitors of the renin-angiotensin system and other antihypertensive drugs on renal outcomes: systemic review and meta-analysis. Lancet 2005; 366: 2026–2033.
70. LeLorier J, Gregoire G, Benhaddad A et al. Discrepancies between meta-analyses and subsequent large randomized, controlled trials. N Engl J Med 1997; 337:536–542.
71. Levey AS, Uhlig K. Which antihypertensive agents in chronic kidney disease? Ann Intern Med. 2006; 144:213–215.
72. Rahman M, Pressel S, Davis BR, et al. Renal outcomes in high-risk hypertensive patients treated with an angiotensin-converting enzyme inhibitor or a calcium channel blocker vs a diuretic: a report from the Antihypertensive and Lipid-Lowering Treatment to Prevent Heart Attack Trial (ALLHAT). Arch Intern Med. 2005; 165:936–946.
73. Hollenberg NK. Omission of drug dose information. Arch Intern Med. 2006; 166:368.
74. Rahman M, Pressel SL, Davis BR. Omission of drug information. Arch Intern Med. 2006; 166: 368–369.
75. Suissa S, Hutchinson T, Brophy JM, Kezouh A. ACE-inhibitor use and the long-term risk of renal failure in diabetes. Kidney Int. 2006; 69:913–919.
76. Hamming I, Navis G, Kocks M, et al. ACE inhibition has adverse renal effects during dietary sodium restriction in proteinuric and healthy rats. J Pathol 2006; 209:129–139.
77. Smit-van Oosten A, Navis G, Stegeman CA, et al. Chronic blockade of angiotensin II action prevents glomerulosclerosis, but induces graft vasculopathy in experimental kidney transplantation. J Pathol 2001; 194:122–129.
78. Chobanian AV, Bakris GL, Black HR, et al. The seventh report of the Joint National Committee on Prevention, Detection, Evaluation, and Treatment of High Blood Pressure: the JNC-7 report. JAMA 2003; 289:2560–2572.
79. Araki S, Haneda M, Koya D, et al. Reduction in microalbuminuria as an integrated indicator for renal and cardiovascular risk reduction in patients with type 2 diabetes. Diabetes 2007; 56: 1727–1730.
80. Ryden L, Standl E, Bartnik M, et al. Task Force on Diabetes and Cardiovascular Diseases of the European Society of Cardiology (ESC); European Association for the Study of Diabetes (EASD).

Guidelines on diabetes, pre-diabetes, and cardiovascular diseases: executive summary. Eur Heart J. 2007; 28:88–136.

81. Buse JB, Ginsberg HN, Bakris GL, et al. American Heart Association; American Diabetes Association. Primary prevention of cardiovascular diseases in people with diabetes mellitus: a scientific statement from the American Heart Association and the American Diabetes Association. Circulation 2007; 115:114–126.

82. Klauser R, Prager R, Gaube S, et al. Metabolic effects of isradipine versus hydrochlorothiazide in diabetes mellitus. Hypertension 1991; 17:15–21.

83. Kjeldsen SE, Os I, Hoieggen A, et al. Fixed-dose combinations in the management of hypertension: defining the place of angiotensin receptor antagonists and hydrochlorothiazide. Am J Cardiovasc Drugs 2005; 5:17–22.

84. Douglas JG, Bakris GL, Epstein M, et al. Management of high blood pressure in African Americans: consensus statement of the Hypertension in African Americans Working Group of the International Society on Hypertension in Blacks. Arch Intern Med. 2003, 163:525–41.

85. Cushman WC, Reda DJ, Perry HM, et al. Regional and racial differences in response to antihypertensive medication use in a randomized controlled trial of men with hypertension in the United States. Arch Intern Med. 2000; 160:825–31.

86. Raskin P, Guthrie R, Flack J, et al. The long-term antihypertensive activity and tolerability of irbesartan with hydrochlorothiazide. J Hum Hypertens. 1999; 13:683–7.

87. Bakris GL, Fonseca V, Katholi RE, et al. Metabolic effects of carvedilol vs metoprolol in patients with type 2 diabetes mellitus and hypertension: a randomized controlled trial. JAMA 2004; 292: 2227–36.

88. Bakris GL, Hart P, Ritz E. Beta blockers in the management of chronic kidney disease. Kidney Int. 2006; 70:1905–13.

89. Mancia G, Grassi G. Systolic and diastolic blood pressure control in antihypertensive drug trials. J Hypertens 2002; 20:1461–4.

90. Brown MJ, Castaigne A, De Leeuw PW, et al. Influence of diabetes and type of hypertension on the response to antihypertensive treatment. Hypertension 2000; 35:1038–42.

91. Abuissa H, Jones PG, Marso SP, et al. Angiotensin-converting enzyme inhibitors or angiotensin receptor blockers for prevention of type 2 diabetes:a meta-analysis of randomized clinical trials. J Am Coll Cardiol 2005; 46:821–6.

92. Lindholm LH, Persson M, Alaupovic P, et al. Metabolic outcome during 1 year in newly detected hypertensives: results of the Antihypertensive Treatment and Lipid Profile in a North of Sweden Efficacy Evaluation (ALPINE study). J Hypertens 2003; 21:1563–74.

93. Reid CM, Johnston CI, Ryan P, et al. Diabetes and cardiovascular outcomes in elderly subjects treated with ACE-inhibitors or diuretics: findings from the 2nd Australian National Blood Pressure Study (abtrs). Am J Hypertens 2003; 16:11A.

94. Pfeffer MA, Swedberg K, Granger CB, et al. Effects of candesartan on mortality and morbidity in patients with chronic heart failure: the CHARM-Overall programme. Lancet 2003; 362:759–766.

95. DREAM Trial Investigators. Bosch J, Yusuf S, Gerstein HC, et al. Effect of ramipril on the incidence of diabetes. N Engl J Med. 2006; 355:1551–62.

96. Braunwald E, Domanski MJ, Fowler SE, et al. Angiotensin-converting-enzyme inhibition in stable coronary artery disease. N Engl J Med 2004; 351:2058–68.

97. Lithell H, Hansson L, Skoog I, et al. The Study on Cognition and Prognosis in the Elderly (SCOPE): principal results of a randomized double-blind intervention trial. J Hypertens 2003; 21:875–86.

98. Vermes E, Ducharme A, Bourassa MG, et al. Enalapril reduces the incidence of diabetes in patients with chronic heart failure: insight from the Studies Of Left Ventricular Dysfunction (SOLVD). Circulation 2003; 107:1291–6.

99. Hansson L. Results of the STOP-Hypertension-2 trial. Blood Press Suppl. 2000; 2:17–20.

100. Julius S, Kjeldsen S E, Weber M, et al, for the VALUE trial group. Outcomes in hypertensive patients at high cardiovascular risk treated with regimens based on valsartan or amlodipine: the VALUE randomised trial. Lancet 2004; 363:2022–31.

101. Verdecchia P, Reboldi G, Angeli F, et al. Adverse prognostic significance of new diabetes in treated hypertensive subjects. Hypertension 2004; 43:963–9.

102. Kostis JB, Wilson AC, Freudenberger RS, et al. Long-term effect of diuretic-based therapy on fatal outcomes in subjects with isolated systolic hypertension with and without diabetes. Am J Cardiol 2005; 95:29–35.

103. Elliott WJ, Meyer PM. Incident diabetes in clinical trials of antihypertensive drugs: a network meta-analysis. Lancet 2007; 369:201–07.

104. ADVANCE Collaborative Group. Effects of a fixed combination of perindopril and indapamide on macrovascular and microvascular outcomes in patients with type 2 diabetes mellitus (the ADVANCE trial): a randomised controlled trial. Lancet 2007; 370:829–40.

29 | The Evaluation of Cardiac and Peripheral Arterial Disease in Patients with Diabetes Mellitus

Rhuna Shen, Susan E. Wiegers, and Ruchira Glaser
Department of Medicine, Cardiovascular Medicine Division, Hospital of the University of Pennsylvania, Philadelphia, Pennsylvania, U.S.A

Cardiovascular disease is a leading cause of death in the diabetic population, accounting for close to 80% of the mortality in diabetic patients in North America (1,2). Patients with diabetes mellitus have both a significantly higher risk for, and a higher mortality from, coronary artery disease (CAD). The diabetic patient has a two-to four-fold increase in the risk for development of coronary artery disease (2–6). Furthermore, diabetes accounts for 10% of the population attributable risk of first myocardial infarction (MI) (7).

Diabetic patients are not only over-represented among those patients with myocardial infarction, but also have a worse prognosis than non-diabetic patients with myocardial infarction (8–10). Several large studies, including the thrombolysis and angioplasty in myocardial infarction (TAMI) trial, have shown that even in the thrombolytic era, in-hospital mortality rates in diabetic patients remain 1.5 to 2 times higher than in non-diabetic patients (2,11–16). In the Finnish monitoring international cardiovascular disease (FINMONICA) trial, the one-year case fatality rate for a first myocardial infarction, including pre-hospital mortality, was 45% in diabetic men and 39% in diabetic women. These case fatality rates were significantly higher than those of non-diabetic subjects (38% and 25% for men and women, respectively) (9). In addition, many studies have demonstrated that, among survivors of myocardial infarction, diabetic patients have higher late mortality rates than do non-diabetic patients (8,10,17–22).

In addition to a higher prevalence of and mortality from symptomatic cardiovascular disease, diabetic patients also have a higher rate of asymptomatic coronary disease and coronary calcification (23,24). Diabetic patients without a history of myocardial infarction have as high a risk of myocardial infarction as do non-diabetic patients with previous myocardial infarction. In a Finnish population cohort study, the seven-year incidence of both fatal and nonfatal myocardial infarction, among over one thousand non-diabetic patients without prior history of myocardial infarction was 3.5%. In those non-diabetic patients with a prior history of myocardial infarction, the incidence was 18.8%. This incidence was comparable to that of diabetic patients without any prior history of myocardial infarction (20%) (25). These data underscore the need for screening asymptomatic diabetic patients in a manner similar to that of non-diabetic patients with previous infarction.

UNIQUE CHARACTERISTICS OF CORONARY ARTERY DISEASE IN THE DIABETIC POPULATION

Several features distinguish coronary artery disease in the diabetic population from the non-diabetic population. Factors such as premature presentation, greater extent of disease, coagulation abnormalities, and autonomic dysfunction may contribute to the higher morbidity and mortality of coronary heart disease in the diabetic patients (Table 1).

Premature Presentation

Diabetic patients often present with premature coronary artery disease. In type 1 diabetic patients, the duration of diabetes is the most important predictor of premature coronary artery disease, and coronary artery disease may present as early as the third or fourth decade of life.

TABLE 1 Unique Characteristics of Cardiovascular
Disease in the Diabetic Patient

Premature presentation
Extensive disease upon initial presentation
Multiple coronary arteries diseased
Distal coronary artery disease
Small vessel disease
Impaired autoregulation in vessels
Increased risk of developing heart failure
Acceleration of coronary thrombosis
Endothelial dysfunction
Platelet dysfunction
Coagulation abnormalities
Plaque composition
Autonomic dysfunction
Impaired vagal activity and increased sympathetic tone
Increased risk for ischemic events
Increased risk for sudden cardiac death
Impaired pain response to ischemia
Atypical symptoms of ischemia
Absence of symptoms of ischemia

These patients often lack other traditional coronary artery disease risk factors such as hypercholesterolemia, hypertension, tobacco use, and family history of premature coronary artery disease. In contrast, type 2 diabetes patients typically have several cardiovascular risk factors and present in the fifth or sixth decade of life, or later (26).

Extent of Disease

Diabetic patients often have more extensive coronary artery disease at the time of diagnosis. Multi-vessel coronary artery disease is common. The thrombolysis and angioplasty in TAMI trial included 148 diabetic and 923 non-diabetic patients, in whom cardiac catheterizations were performed at 90 min and in seven to ten days after thrombolytic therapy. Diabetic patients had a significantly higher incidence of multi-vessel disease (66% vs. 46%) and a greater number of diseased vessels as compared to non-diabetic patients (12). Pathological and angiographic evidence indicate that the coronary arteries are more diffusely and distally diseased in diabetic patients (2,26–30). Recognition of the propensity for severe coronary artery disease in patients presenting with myocardial infarction is especially important because the presence of multi-vessel coronary disease predicts short-term mortality in patients with acute myocardial infarction (31,32). Multi-vessel disease also contributes significantly to the increased rates of recurrent ischemic episodes and infarction in diabetic patients. This is true for severe (<70% obstruction) and less severe lesions. Plaque disruption leading to infarction most often occurs in vessels with mild to moderate stenoses (33,34). Thus, recurrent ischemic events in diabetics are results of not only the more extensive disease, but also the increased number of vessels with mild to moderate disease (Fig. 1).

In addition to a greater extent of epicardial coronary artery disease, there may be generalized endothelial dysfunction and abnormalities of small vessels in the diabetic patient. Dilatation of the coronary arteries in response to hypoxia is mainly dependent upon endothelium relaxing factor (2,35). Impaired endothelium-dependent relaxation is present in the vascular beds of diabetic patients, including coronary arteries (36–38). The auto-regulatory responses in the microcirculation also appear to be impaired (2).

Increased Risk for the Development of Congestive Heart Failure

The Framingham Study established a strong association between diabetes and heart failure (39). Such association has been confirmed in subsequent studies (40–53). Diabetes alone predicted heart failure independent of coexisting hypertension or coronary artery disease, the relative risk was 3.8 in diabetic men and 5.5 in diabetic women. The frequency of

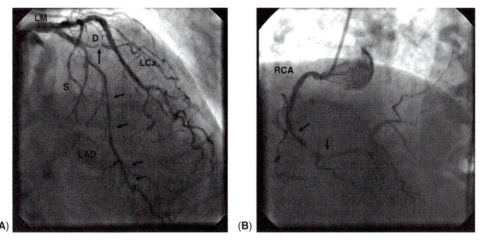

FIGURE 1   Coronary angiogram of a patient with type 2 diabetes mellitus and angina. (**A**) Left coronary angiogram with left anterior oblique and cranial angulation showed a mildly diseased left main (LM) artery that bifurcates to the diffusely diseased left anterior descending artery (LAD) and the left circumflex artery (LCx). The LAD tapers to a smaller vessel after the first major septal perforator (S). There are several moderate stenoses in the mid- to distal LAD (*arrow*). There is a high-grade stenosis at the proximal portion of a diagonal branch (D). The LCx is diffusely diseased, particularly in the more distal segment. (**B**) Right coronary angiogram with left anterior oblique angulation showed a moderate-sized right coronary artery (RCA) with a moderate stenosis in the mid- to distal portion, and a high-grade stenosis (*arrow*).

heart failure in elderly diabetics was even higher. The prevalence of heart failure among Medicare beneficiaries with diabetes was 22.3% in 1994, with a subsequent incidence of newly diagnosed heart failure of 12.6% per year until 1999 (40). The incidence of heart failure after revascularization with angioplasty or bypass surgery is also greater in diabetics (54). This increase in heart failure causes much of the excess in in-hospital mortality of diabetic patients with acute myocardial infarction (2,12,21,45–53). The higher incidence of heart failure after myocardial infarction in the diabetic patient is related to a higher degree of diffuse atherosclerotic disease. Inadequate tissue perfusion to the non-infarcted myocardium leads to not only greater underlying global systolic dysfunction, but also the inability of the non-infarcted myocardium to adequately compensate for the dysfunction of the acutely infarcted region (2,26). In the TAMI trials, ventricular function assessed in the catheterization laboratory by left ventriculography was worse in non-infarcted areas in diabetic patients, as compared with non-diabetic patients (12). Factors associated with heart failure in diabetics include: age, duration of diabetes, insulin use, ischemic heart disease, peripheral arterial disease, elevated serum creatinine, poor glycemic control and microalbuminemia (40,42,44,55,56).

Diastolic dysfunction in diabetic patients can also occur in the absence of significant coronary artery disease, and it is likely an important contributor to worse patient outcomes (21,26,57,58). In fact, on initial presentation with congestive failure symptoms, diabetic patients more often have diminished left ventricular compliance and normal systolic function when compared with non-diabetic patients (2,59–65). The higher incidence of coexistent hypertension in diabetic patients may account for a large part of the diastolic dysfunction observed, although patients without hypertension have manifested diastolic impairment (2). Left ventricular hypertrophy is present in 28% of non-hypertensive type 2 diabetic patients, as compared with >10% of matched patients without diabetes (66).

Mechanisms of Increased Atherosclerosis in Diabetes

A number of mechanisms may contribute to the increased atherosclerosis in diabetics in addition to conventional risk factors such as hypertension and hypercholesterolemia. These mechanisms include endothelial dysfunction, increased platelet activation and aggregation, coagulation abnormalities and abnormal plaque composition.

Endothelial Dysfunction

Hyperglycemia can induce endothelial damage by a variety of molecular mechanisms, (67,68) thereby decrease the bioavalability of nitric oxide and prostacyclin, increase the synthesis of vasoconstrictor prostanoids and endothelin and promote atherosclerotic plaque formation (69). Insulin resistance alone may be associated with coronary endothelial dysfunction (70,71). Although endothelial function can be improved by thiazolidinedion (71) metformin (72) and atorvastatin treatment, (73) whether these improvements result in better outcome remains unknown.

Platelet Dysfunction

Diabetics have altered platelet function, including increased platelet aggregation and activation, (74–77) and enhanced binding of fibrinogen to the glycoprotein IIb/IIIa complex. The platelet abnormalities may be in part mediated by elevated blood glucose, but not plasma insulin level (78). In recent trials of acute coronary syndrome and percutaneous coronary interventions, diabetic patients have benefited from aggressive platelet inhibition from platelet glycoprotein IIb/IIIa antagonists (79,80).

Coagulation Abnormalities

Coagulation abnormalities associated with diabetes include an increase in plasma fibrinogen, (81–83) a reduction in fibrinolytic activity,(84,85) elevations in plasminogen activator inhibitor (PAI-1), (86) and increase in tissue factors and blood thrombogenicity (87). These coagulation disturbances may also decrease the efficacy of thrombolytic therapy in the treatment of ST segment elevation myocardial infarction. The TAMI trials failed to show a difference in angiographic patency rates in diabetic as compared with non-diabetic patients (12). However, non-invasive measures of reperfusion have suggested that reperfusion is achieved less frequently in diabetic patients.

Plaque Composition

Plaque composition may be different in diabetics. Both macrophage infiltration and lipid-rich atheroma are greatly increased in coronary plaques in atherectomy specimens from diabetic patients (88). Both features are associated with a greater risk for plaque rupture and a higher incidence of thrombosis (88). This observation was confirmed by a recent autopsy study (89). Aggressive lipid lowering can reduce cardiovascular events by 22% independent of baseline lipid levels, therefore, it has become a cornerstone of diabetic treatment (90).

Autonomic Dysfunction

The autonomic innervations of the heart may be affected in diabetic patients. Diminished heart rate variability and elevated resting heart rate are often present in early autonomic neuropathy in diabetic patients (2,66). Increased sympathetic activity or decreased vagal activity may contribute to sudden cardiac death. In addition, increased sympathetic activity may facilitate ischemic events.

Autonomic neuropathy may also impair the pain response to ischemia in diabetic patients. This can complicate the detection of coronary artery disease, since the diabetic patient may be asymptomatic or manifest atypical symptoms, such as dyspnea, increased fatigue, or indigestion (26). Langer et al., observed that the uptake of metaiodobensyl- guanidine (MIBG), a norepinephrine analog, is reduced in diabetic patients with silent ischemia (91). This finding supports the notion that silent ischemia in diabetics may be caused by autonomic denervation of the heart. Similar findings have been demonstrated with positron emission tomography (92,93).

INCIDENCE OF ASYMPTOMATIC CORONARY ARTERY DISEASE IN THE DIABETIC PATIENT

It is not surprising that the incidence of asymptomatic coronary disease in the diabetic population is significant. Diabetic patients have more silent ST depression and more perfusion abnormalities during exercise stress testing and thallium scintigraphy (24,94–96). The Milan study on atherosclerosis and diabetes (MiSAD) group found that 12% of the 925 asymptomatic patients with type 2 diabetes had ST depression consistent with ischemia during treadmill stress testing. Approximately half of these patients had nuclear scans consistent with coronary artery disease (94,97). Additional smaller studies have reported asymptomatic coronary artery disease by coronary angiography in approximately 8 to 12% of diabetic patients. In addition to silent ischemia, diabetic patients also have a higher incidence of silent MI (98–100). The utility of non-invasive screening was examined in a study of 1900 asymptomatic diabetic patients, in which stress testing with dipyridamole myocardial contrast echocardiography followed by coronary angiography in those with perfusion defects, was performed. The positive predictive value of stress testing was best in those patients with two or more risk factors (as compared to patients with one or less risk factor), with significantly higher rates of three-vessel disease (33% vs. 8%), diffuse disease (55% vs. 18%), and vessel occlusion (31% vs. 4%) in those with additional risk factors (24). However, overall, studies have demonstrated a fairly low positive predictive value of noninvasive stress testing in the general diabetic population, raising concern about the utility of noninvasive screening of the asymptomatic diabetic population (24,97,101,102).

BENEFITS OF EARLY DETECTION OF CORONARY ARTERY DISEASE

The benefits of early detection of coronary artery disease in the diabetic population include implementation of medical therapy targeted at prevention of further morbidity and mortality from coronary artery disease, identification of patients who would gain survival benefits from revascularization, and modification of lifestyle and other factors which may impact on disease progression.

Implementation of Medical Therapy

Modification of Other Cardiovascular Risk Factors
Modification of cardiovascular risk factors beside diabetes may reduce morbidity and mortality from future events. Perhaps the most striking example is the recent demonstration of mortality reduction in lipid lowering trials. In the Scandinavian Simvastatin Survival Study, 2200 patients with coronary artery disease receiving simvastatin were compared to patients receiving placebo. Lowering cholesterol was associated with a 42% reduction in cardiovascular mortality and a 30% reduction in overall mortality. In the 5% of patients in the trial with diabetes, simvastatin treatment was associated with a 55% reduction in major coronary events (26,103). In the cholesterol and recurrent events (CARE) trial, in which diabetic patients comprised approximately 14% of the study population, there was a 25% reduction in coronary heart disease events (104). Based on secondary prevention trials such as these, the present National Cholesterol Education Program guidelines distinguish lipid-lowering therapy goals based upon the presence of coronary disease in the general population (105). Prospective studies of lipid lowering specifically in the diabetic population, including primary prevention trials, are presently underway (106).

In addition, angiotensin converting enzyme (ACE) inhibitor therapy is indicated in diabetic patients with hypertension with proteinuria, coronary artery disease and left ventricular dysfunction (26). Thus, the demonstration of coronary artery disease or left ventricular systolic dysfunction may impact upon the ideal antihypertensive regimen in diabetic patients.

Implementation of Anti-Ischemic Therapy
The presence of asymptomatic coronary disease should prompt more aggressive anti-ischemic therapy. Agents such as ACE inhibitors, beta-blockers and aspirin may reduce adverse cardiovascular outcomes in patients with coronary artery disease and diabetes.

Recent evidence suggests further benefit to ACE inhibitor therapy in diabetic patients. The heart outcomes prevention evaluation (HOPE) study examined over 9000 patients over the age of 55 who had evidence of vascular disease or diabetes plus one other cardiovascular risk factor. Approximately 38% of the study population had diabetes. Treatment with the ACE inhibitor ramipril reduced the composite endpoint of myocardial infarction, stroke or death from cardiovascular causes at mean follow-up of 5 years by 22%

as compared with placebo. In addition, the rates of cardiovascular death and myocardial infarction were reduced by 26% and 20%, respectively. In a subgroup analysis, the incidence of other complications related to diabetes was also significantly decreased in those receiving ramipril (107). There was less need for dialysis for nephropathy and laser therapy for retinopathy in this patient population.

Beta-blocker therapy effectively reduces re-infarction and sudden death in diabetic patients post myocardial infarction (2,108–111), In the Bezafibrate Infarction Prevention Study, type 2 diabetes patients treated with beta-blocker therapy had close to a 50% reduction in mortality as compared with those patients not treated with beta-blocker therapy (26,112). Thus, knowledge of prior silent myocardial infarction may impact upon the decision to use beta-blocker therapy in the asymptomatic diabetic patient.

Aspirin therapy for secondary prevention of coronary artery disease in diabetics and non-diabetics is also beneficial. In a meta-analysis of 145 prospective studies of the use of aspirin compared with placebo, diabetics and non-diabetics had similar reductions in myocardial infarction, stroke, transient ischemic attacks, or signs of coronary artery disease (113). In addition to secondary prevention for large vessel disease, the American diabetes association (ADA) has recommended consideration of aspirin therapy for primary prevention in high-risk men and women (26,114).

Thus, the early detection of coronary disease in diabetic patients may significantly influence medication use targeted at both modification of cardiovascular risk factors and prevention of further ischemic events.

Referral for Revascularization

The bypass angioplasty revascularization investigation (BARI) trial showed improved 5 year survival in symptomatic diabetic patients with multi-vessel coronary artery disease who underwent coronary artery bypass grafting (CABG) compared with medical management. (115). Furthermore, the outcomes in patients who underwent surgical revascularization were superior to that of diabetic patients who had multi-vessel percutaneous transluminal coronary angioplasty (115,116)]. The 8 year follow-up analysis of the Emory Angioplasty versus Surgery Trial had similar findings (117). In addition, a recent subgroup analysis of the diabetic population in the Arterial Revascularization Therapy Study confirmed that those patients who received multi-vessel coronary stenting had lower event free survival rates at 1 year when compared with those patients receiving CABG (118). Thus, identification of severe multi-vessel coronary disease is paramount because surgical revascularization may significantly lower mortality and event-free survival.

The Asymptomatic Cardiac Ischemia Pilot study addressed broader indications for revascularization in asymptomatic coronary artery disease. 13 to 19% of patients in each treatment strategy had diabetes. Five hundred and fifty eight patients with ischemia during stress testing and ambulatory ECG monitoring who had coronary anatomy suitable for revascularization were randomized to angina guided drug therapy, angina plus ischemia guided drug therapy, or revascularization by angioplasty or bypass surgery. Two years after randomization, the total mortality was 6.6% in the angina-guided group, compared with 4.4% in the ischemia-guided group, and 1.1% in the revascularization group (119). Although further data are needed to confirm whether more liberal indications for revascularization are warranted, these pilot data support a role for revascularization of asymptomatic patients. In this regard, the NIH-sponsored bypass angioplasty revascularization investigation in type 2 diabetes (BARI 2D) trial, aims to determine the optimal five-year treatment for patients with type II diabetes mellitus and documented stable coronary artery disease in the setting of uniform glycemic control and intensive management of other risk factors. With respect to coronary revascularization, it hypothesizes that a strategy of initial elective revascularization (surgical or catheter-based), combined with aggressive medical therapy, will result in lower long-term mortality compared with a strategy of aggressive medical therapy alone. Type 2 diabetic patients with single vessel or more, stable CAD, either symptomatic or asymptomatic with ischemia will be studied for five years, with follow-up anticipated to be completed by 2009 (120).

Lifestyle and Other Risk Modification

Finally, there may be some benefit in more aggressive nutrition control and exercise in diabetic patients with cardiovascular disease. Although they may already be counseled on proper nutrition and exercise, the added concern about known coronary heart disease may motivate these patients further.

In type I diabetes, intensive glucose control has been demonstrated to have cardiovascular benefit with a reduction in the risk of any cardiovascular event by 42%, and the risk of nonfatal myocardial infarction, stroke or death from cardiovascular disease by 57% during follow-up, when compared with conventional treatment in the diabetes control and complication trial (DCCT) and the Observational Epidemiology of Diabetes Interventions and Complications Study (121,122). While microvascular complications are reduced with strict glycemic control in type I diabetic patients, the high dose exogenous insulin and insulin resistance syndromes characteristic of type 2 diabetes may have differential effects on the macrovasculature. Currently, it remains unclear whether control of glycemia alone is sufficient to reduce morbidity and mortality and whether insulin infusion plays a role. The diabetes mellitus insulin-glucose infusion acute myocardial infarction (DIGAMI) study found that hospital use of insulin glucose infusion, followed by 3 months of intensive insulin therapy in patients with acute myocardial infarction, reduced cardiovascular mortality by 29% at one year in type 2 diabetic patients (123). In the CREATE-ECLA trial, glucose-insulin-potassium (GIK) infusion in diabetic patients with acute ST elevation myocardial infarction had no effect on mortality at thirty days, suggesting that insulin administration alone was of no benefit in acute myocardial infarction (124,125). In DIGAMI-2 trial, the role of intensive insulin therapy was further addressed. Type 2 diabetic patients with acute myocardial infarction were randomly assigned to one of three glucose management strategies: group1, inpatient insulin infusion/outpatient intensive subcutaneous insulin treatment; group 2, inpatient insulin infusion/outpatient standard treatment; group 3, inpatient/outpatient glucose management according to local practice. Glycemic control and mortality rates were similar in all three groups. The study, unfortunately did not recruit adequate patient numbers, and therefore had reduced statistical power to detect difference among the three groups (126). The 2004 ACC/AHA guidelines gave a Class I recommendation to the use of an insulin infusion to normalize blood glucose in all patients with an acute myocardial infarction and a complicated course (127).

TARGET SUBGROUPS FOR SCREENING

One of the challenges facing the clinician caring for the diabetic patient is the determination of when testing for coronary artery disease is warranted (Table 2). Given the high incidence and impact of cardiovascular disease in diabetic patients, it is clear that patients with symptoms, either typical or atypical, should undergo a noninvasive evaluation. Patients presenting with symptoms consistent with unstable angina should be referred urgently to cardiology care for a potential invasive evaluation. In addition, previously sedentary diabetic patients who are initiating an exercise program should undergo a noninvasive evaluation, in order to identify those patients at high risk of an acute ischemic event while beginning the new exercise regimen.

Diabetic patients undergoing procedures with high cardiovascular risk benefit from preoperative evaluation for ischemia (Table 3). Further, patients with reduced functional capacity undergoing intermediate risk procedures should undergo preoperative stress testing (128). Patients undergoing renal transplantation especially benefit from peri-operative stress testing because of the high likelihood of concomitant coronary atherosclerosis. In fact, the ADA recommends that all diabetic patients over the age of 35, with either persistent microalbuminuria or overt nephropathy, should undergo cardiac testing (26). However, the indications for testing are less clear in patients who do not complain of symptoms, and are not about to undergo surgery or have changes in exertion.

In their guidelines regarding exercise testing, the American College of Cardiology (ACC) has stated that, in asymptomatic patient without known coronary artery disease, there is no

TABLE 2 Indications for Noninvasive Screening for Coronary Artery Disease
in the Diabetic Patient

Symptomatic
Presence of typical or atypical symptoms of stable angina
Asymptomatic
Age >35 years and initiation of a new exercise program in a previously sedentary lifestyle
Preoperative evaluation prior to high or intermediate risk surgery in a patient with
decreased functional capacity
Evidence of myocardial infarction or ischemia on baseline electrocardiogram
Presence of 2 or more of the following concomitant risk factors:[a]
Total cholesterol >240 mg/dL, LDL cholesterol >160 mg/dL, or HDL cholesterol <35 mg/dl
Blood pressure >140/90 mm Hg
Smoking
Family history of premature coronary artery disease
Positive micro/macroabluminuria test

[a] According to American Diabetes Association guidelines.
Source: From Ref. 26.

class I indication for routine stress testing. However, the ACC notes that, given data from trials such as the ACIP study and the Coronary Artery Surgery Study, a subgroup of asymptomatic patients with multiple risk factors may benefit from stress testing (129). The ADA recommended testing asymptomatic diabetics with an abnormal resting ECG or with evidence of peripheral or carotid artery occlusive disease (26). The rate of high-risk SPECT sans in a study from Mayo Clinic was 43% among diabetic patients with Q waves on ECG, 26% among patients with an abnormal resting ECG, and 28% among those with peripheral arterial disease (130). The ADA also recommended testing in patients with atypical symptoms suspicious of coronary artery disease (e.g. atypical chest pain, dyspnea or fatigue). In patients with no symptoms or evidence of cardiac or peripheral vascular disease, the ADA recommended testing those diabetic patients with two or more of the following risk factors listed in Table 2.

However, the evidence for this indication is less compelling. In the detection of ischemia in asymptomatic diabetics (DIAD) study, 22% of diabetic patients with two or more risk factors had evidence of ischemia on SPECT scans, a rate identical to that among those with fewer than two risk factors (96).

Thus, although there is sufficient evidence supporting noninvasive testing of diabetics with an abnormal ECG or with evidence of vascular disease in the peripheral and carotid arteries, achieving adequate yield of abnormal SPECT in asymptomatic diabetics without overt symptoms is a greater challenge. It has been suggested that by utilizing certain approaches, both the clinical and cost effectiveness of the screening tests can be potentially enhanced. These approaches include the use of an aggregate score incorporating and weighing multiple risk factors rather than counting the number of risk factors present (131,132); the use of valsalva heart ratio as a marker of autonomic function, which was the strongest prediction of an abnormal scan in the DIAD study; (96) incorporating a clinical score into a testing strategy; (133–135) and the use of a calcium score threshold (e.g. >400) (136,137). Further investigation of such strategies is needed in order to identify efficient means for screening this patient population.

METHODS OF DETECTION OF CORONARY ARTERY DISEASE

Several modalities may be used for detection of coronary artery disease once the decision to screen a patient has been made. Stress testing, either exercise or pharmacologic, and either with or without perfusion imaging techniques, ambulatory electrocardiography, and electron beam computed tomography (EBCT) may be used.

Stress Testing

The choice of initial stress test modality should be based on several factors, including the resting electrocardiogram, ability of the patient to exercise, and local expertise and availability. In general, patients should exercise when able. Knowledge of the patient's exercise capacity

TABLE 3 Cardiac Risk[a] Stratification for Noncardiac Surgical Procedures

High
  (Reported cardiac risk often >5%)
  Emergent major operations, particularly in the elderly
  Aortic and other major vascular
  Peripheral vascular
  Anticipated prolonged surgical procedures associated with large fluid
    shifts and/or blood loss

Intermediate
  (Reported cardiac risk generally <5%)
  Carotid endarterectomy
  Head and neck
  Intraperitoneal and intrathoracic
  Orthopedic
  Prostate

Low[b]
  (Reported cardiac risk generally <1%)
  Endoscopic procedures
  Superficial procedure
  Cataract
  Breast

[a] Combined incidence of cardiac death and nonfatal myocardial infarction.
[b] Do not generally require further preoperative cardiac testing.
Source: From Ref. 208.

provides an independent assessment of prognosis. The results of a patient's stress test should be interpreted in light of the exercise capacity. Measures of exercise capacity include maximal exercise duration, maximal metabolic equivalent (MET) level achieved, maximum workload achieved, and maximum heart rate and heart rate-blood pressure product (129).

Exercise electrocardiography, the least expensive noninvasive test for myocardial ischemia is two times less expensive than stress echocardiography and five times less expensive than stress single-photon-emission computed tomography (SPECT). Drugs such as digoxin may cause false positive results in the exercise electrocardiogram (138). Data pooled from 132 studies show that the sensitivity and specificity of routine exercise electrocardiography are 68% and 77%, respectively (139,140). However, there is wide variability in the studies, depending upon the diagnostic criteria used, and the patient population. For example, women have increased false positive rates on routine treadmill testing as compared with men. Inability to achieve 85% of maximum predicted heart rate may influence the results of the test. Negative inotropic medications such as beta blockers and calcium channel blockers may decrease the sensitivity of the test, resulting in false negative tests.

When patients have pre-excitation (Wolff-Parkinson-White), ventricularly paced rhythm, significant ST segment depressions, and left bundle branch block on the baseline electrocardiogram, they require additional nuclear imaging or echocardiography to detect ischemia. The American Diabetes Association recommends that those diabetic patients with typical anginal symptoms or resting Q waves on electrocardiogram undergo a stress perfusion study. In either case, the exercise portion of the test remains a valuable component.

If patients are unable to exercise because of other limitations such as arthritis, amputations, other orthopedic problems, symptomatic peripheral vascular disease, or severe pulmonary disease, they should undergo pharmacologic testing with nuclear imaging or echocardiography. Dobutamine is a positive ionotropic agent that provokes ischemia by increasing myocardial work and thus oxygen demand. Adenosine and dipyridamole are vasodilators that cause relative increases in flow in non-diseased coronary arteries compared to arteries with significant stenoses.

SPECT has a higher sensitivity for the detection of coronary artery disease than does exercise electrocardiography alone (138). However, estimates of the perfusion imaging performance, in terms of sensitivity and specificity, are highly variable. The sensitivity of stress echocardiography is likely in the same range or slightly lower than that of radionuclide perfusion imaging (138). This technique's success is also highly dependent upon the experience of the operator and center. Special technique considerations may be needed in women, obese patients, or patients with emphysema; they may require attenuation correction during SPECT to accommodate artifactual defects from diaphragmatic or breast and tissue attenuation. Similarly, the potentially limited echocardiographic image quality in obese patients or patients with severe pulmonary disease may preclude the use of stress echocardiography in certain patients.

As previously discussed, some small studies suggest decreased positive predictive value of the routine exercise test, as well as nuclear imaging testing, in the diabetic population. (97,101,102) However, a number of recent studies have confirmed that stress SPECT achieves adequate risk stratification in diabetic population (141–144). These reports and others have also consistently shown that normal and abnormal SPECT in diabetics have different prognostic values as compared to non-diabetics. Diabetic patients with a normal stress SPECT are at significantly greater risk than non-diabetics patients with a normal SPECT (130,141,142,144,145). Similarly, the risk conferred by any given extent and severity of an abnormal SPECT scan, is far greater in diabetic patients than non-diabetic patients. Furthermore, the risk is greater for insulin-dependent versus non-insulin-dependent diabetics. The American College of Cardiology presently recommends that, if feasible, in most cases the initial screening of the asymptomatic patient be done with routine exercise electrocardiograph (129). The American Diabetes Association does make the distinction that in certain high risk diabetic patients, as already outlined, perfusion imaging or stress echocardiography is warranted as the initial screening test (26).

Ambulatory Electrocardiogram

At this time, the data on the ambulatory electrocardiogram are insufficient to justify the routine use of this modality to detect coronary artery disease in the asymptomatic diabetic patient (26). Furthermore, in the ACIP trial, those patients with diabetes had less demonstrable ischemia on ambulatory electrocardiography than non-diabetic patients. This was despite more extensive coronary artery disease in that population (146). However, asymptomatic patients with abnormal resting ECG should be referred for further testing.

Electron Beam Computed Tomography

Coronary artery calcification has been correlated with coronary artery atherosclerosis, but also increases with age. Proponents have advocated this method to detect "sub clinical" disease in asymptomatic patients. Current data are insufficient to justify the use of EBCT alone as a general screening modality. Nevertheless, EBCT may be a useful adjunct to stress SPECT in screening certain subset of diabetic patients as discussed above. In a recent series comparing the outcome of asymptomatic diabetic and non-diabetic patients who were referred for EBCT, the average coronary calcium score, as well as the overall death rate was significantly higher for diabetic patients when compared to non-diabetic patients. In a risk-factor-adjusted model, for every increase in coronary calcium score there was a greater increase in mortality for diabetics than for non-diabetics (147). In addition, diabetics without coronary calcium have a survival similar to non-diabetics patients. Therefore, although coronary artery calcium screening is not recommended for risk prediction in asymptomatic patients, among patients who have already undergone testing, an Agaston score <400 to 1000, or a score above the seventy-fifth percentile for age and sex, may warrant further risk stratification testing.

MANAGEMENT OF A POSITIVE SCREENING TEST

The outcome of an indeterminate, sub maximal stress test in the diabetic patient should prompt repetition of the test with pharmacologic stress and perfusion imaging. Many diabetic patients may not experience typical chest pain during exercise, for the reasons previously discussed. Autonomic dysfunction may affect their ability to achieve an adequate heart rate as well (Fig. 2).

Pre-test risk	ETT results			
	Normal	Mildly positive	Moderately positive	Markedly positive
High 4–5 risk factors**	√√	√√√	√√√√	√√√√
Moderate 2–3 risk factors	√	√√√	√√√	√√√√
Low 0–1 risk factors	√	√√√	√√√	√√√√

√ Routine follow-up
√√ Close follow-up
√√√ Imaging
√√√√ Cardiology referral/possible catheterization

FIGURE 2 Appropriate follow-up after screening exercise treadmill test (ETT). When initial exercise stress testing is done in asymptomatic diabetic patients, the type of follow-up depends on the pretest risk and the degree of abnormality on the stress test. Normal follow-up indicates annual reevaluation of symptoms and signs of CHD and ECG. A repeat ETT should be considered in 3–5 years if clinical status is unchanged. Close follow-up means shorter intervals between evaluation and follow-up ETT, i.e., 1–2 years. Pretest risk is assigned based on the presence of other vascular disease and risk factors. *Source*: Reprinted from Ref. 209.

On the other hand, a negative exercise electrocardiographic test at a high workload provides reassurance that the likelihood of advanced coronary artery disease is extremely low. It is important to interpret the findings of stress testing in light of the clinical pre-test probability of disease, as well as the extent of disease found on testing. The maximal value of stress testing is seen in those patients with an intermediate pre-test suspicion for disease.

A positive exercise electrocardiographic test should prompt either repetition with perfusion imaging or direct cardiac catheterization if the patient has high-risk clinical features, such as hypotension, bradycardia, ventricular dysrhythmmias or pulmonary edema, on the initial test. Patients should also be referred directly for cardiac catheterization if ischemia is induced by low-level exercise (<4 METs or heart rate <100 BPM or <70% age predicted) and manifested by one or more of the following:

1. Horizontal or downsloping ST depression >0.1 mV.
2. ST-segment elevation >0.1 mV in a noninfarct lead.
3. Five or more abnormal leads.
4. Persistent ischemic response >3 min after exertion, and
5. Typical angina (128)

Patients with moderate or large perfusion defects on imaging, or defects representative of multiple vascular territories, should be referral for cardiac catheterization in almost all circumstances. The identification of left main coronary disease, proximal left anterior descending artery disease, and multi-vessel disease is especially important, given the proven benefits of revascularization in diabetic patients with severe anatomy (27,115).

Conversely, in a patient with low suspicion for disease and relatively small, distal perfusion defects suggestive of distal coronary artery disease, it is often reasonable to manage the patient medically and follow-up closely.

PERIPHERAL ARTERIAL DISEASE IN THE DIABETIC POPULATION

Peripheral arterial disease (PAD) is a common clinical feature that impacts significantly on the prognosis and health care costs in the diabetic population. Diabetic patients comprise a significant proportion of those patients hospitalized with PAD. In the United Kingdom, of all admissions for PAD during a four-year period from 1991 to 1995, 15.4% of patients were diabetic. This represents an age standardized relative risk of admission of 7.6 and 6.9 for diabetic men and women, respectively, when compared with non-diabetic patients. Furthermore, the relative risk of hospital mortality was 2.8, and the relative risk of surgery was 31.1 when compared with non-diabetics. Eighty Seven percent of the cost of hospitalization was attributable to the diabetic state (148). Further, among diabetic patients, PAD is common, with reported prevalence rate as high as 22% (149). In addition, the risk of developing lower extremity PAD is proportional to the severity and duration of diabetes (150,151).

FEATURES OF PAD IN DIABETIC PATIENTS

Diabetic patients with PAD have several distinct features when compared with non-diabetic patients with PAD. A greater proportion of diabetic patients with PAD have concomitant hypertension (152). In addition, diabetic patients have more distal disease, (152,153) more progressive and severe disease, and they are more likely to undergo surgery and amputation for critical limb ischemia (148,152,153). The rates of gangrene or amputation of lower limbs are as much as 10 to 20 times more frequent in diabetic than in control subjects (154,155). The risk of amputation also increases with age. The annual amputation rates were 14 per 10,000 in patients less than forty-five years of age, 45 per 10,000 in diabetics between age forty-five and sixty-four, and 101 per 10,000 in those over sixty-five. Not surprisingly, duration of diabetes has been found to be a strong risk factor for amputation (155). Interestingly, the type of vessels affected may vary compared with non-diabetic patients with PAD; recent evidence suggests that diabetes was the only significant risk factor for small vessel PAD progression, whereas smoking, dyslipidemia and elevated CRP level, were risk factors for large vessel PAD progression (156).

The risks of fatal and non-fatal MI and stroke are also increased in both diabetic and non-diabetic PAD subjects (148,152,155,157) Cirqui et al., found vascular mortality was five times higher in patients with claudication over a period of ten years, while another group reported an annual rate of fatal and non-fatal cardiovascular events ranging from 3.5 to 8% per year (158,159). One study found that 67% of diabetic patients dying from cardiovascular causes within the five-year observation had PAD at baseline, compared with 15% in those who survived (160). Therefore, diabetic patients with claudication are at high risk of future stroke, MI and premature death.

Evaluation in the Primary Care Setting

All diabetic patients should be screened for peripheral vascular disease including components targeted toward detection of signs and symptoms in the routine history and physical exam. In a workshop examining PAD in diabetes, the American Diabetes Association and American Heart Association made the following joint recommendations for annual screening (161). The history should include questions about the presence and degree of claudication or ischemic rest pain. The physical exam should include inspection of the legs and feet for ulcers and skin changes. The tibialis posterior and the dorsalis pedis pulses should be examined and the femoral pulse auscultated for bruits.

Claudication

Diabetic patients should be asked annually about the presence of exercise-induced calf leg pain. Although the most common site for exercise-induced pain is the calf, it can also develop in the thigh, hip, or buttock when the disease is localized above the inguinal ligament. Often the pain will start in the calf and then progress to the thigh and/or buttock if exercise is continued despite the onset of pain. The Rose intermittent claudication questionnaire, allowed for standardization of many of these features of claudication (162). A typical history of claudication has low sensitivity, but a high specificity for PAD (163,164). A large scale PAD screening study has demonstrated that only one-third of patients with documented PAD had classic claudication symptoms. The remainder patients had either atypical symptoms or no symptom (163,164). Therefore, a thorough physical examination should include blood pressure measurement, palpation of peripheral pulses, and auscultation of pulses and bruits. Severe claudication most often results from multilevel arterial disease, which can be evaluated in the noninvasive laboratory. Patients with lifestyle limiting exercise-induced calf pain should be referred for specialist vascular assessment. Measurement of an Ankle brachial index (ABI) or referral for specialist vascular assessment should also be considered for patients with any leg pain not clearly ascribed to a nonvascular cause.

Signs of Critical Ischemia

Critical ischemia is defined as clinical presentation that is likely to result in an amputation if not reversed. Ischemic rest pain occurs in the toes and forefoot will be relieved by dependency during its early phases. If it does not improve with development of collateral circulation, amputation will be necessary unless some form of intervention, either surgical or endovascular, is performed. When a break in the skin occurs at any location of the foot or lower leg, healing of the ulceration may not occur unless some form of intervention is carried out. When tissue death involves one or more toes or the forefoot, the extent of the amputation may be limited to the involved areas if direct intervention can bring more blood to the ischemic area. Although not as definitive as ischemic rest pain, ulceration and gangrene, skin atrophy, nail changes, and dependent rubor in some patients may require further evaluation. This is particularly true if the ABI is found to be abnormal.

Palpation of Peripheral Pulses

Palpation of leg pulses should be performed on an annual basis for all adult patients with diabetes. Palpation of peripheral pulses should include an assessment of femoral, popliteal and pedal vessels. Pulse should be graded as absent, diminished or normal. Dorsalis pedis pulse abnormalities are less sensitive for PAD, since up to 30% of these abnormalities may be due to a congenital absence of the dorsalis pedis artery (165). An absent or decreased tibialis posterior pulse is an indication for performing an ABI. Since the sensitivity and positive predictive value are moderate for detection, a significant number of cases will be identified by detection of a reduction or absence of these pulses. The presence of these pulses in low-risk diabetic subjects helps to confirm the absence of significant disease.

Femoral Bruits

The detection of femoral bruits is an indication for performing an ABI. Although auscultation for femoral bruits has similar difficulties to those described for pulse palpation, it nonetheless has sufficient sensitivity to merit annual performance.

SCREENING METHODS

The clinical exam and Rose questionnaire are useful though unfortunately fairly insensitive tools for the diagnosis of lower extremity vascular disease (163). Ancillary modalities include the ABI, toe systolic blood pressure, ultrasound duplex scanning, tissue PO_2 measurement, and arteriography.

Ankle Brachial Index (ABI)

The ABI is a ratio of Doppler recorded systolic arterial blood pressures in the lower and upper extremities, (166) and is normally between 1.00 and 1.40 (167). PAD is defined as an ABI less than 0.9. Lower ABI values indicate more severe PAD.

The ADA consensus statement on PAD recommends that a screening ABI be performed in the following situations:

- Individuals 49 and younger with type 1 diabetes mellitus and one other risk factor;
- All diabetic individuals >50 years of age;
- Any patients with symptoms of PAD.

The results of ankle brachial index measurements help to guide further management. An ABI less than 0.50 in any vessel should prompt expeditious referral for specialist vascular assessment, since these patients almost certainly have severe peripheral vascular disease. An ABI between 0.50 and 0.90 warrants a follow-up evaluation within 3 months, because these patients are likely to have mild to moderate peripheral vascular disease. If the subsequent ABI is less than 0.90, intensive risk factor modification and annual ABI follow-up is recommended. If the repeat ABI is greater than 0.90, further follow-up ABI may be performed every 2 or 3 years. Similarly if an initial ABI is greater than 0.90, repeat testing need only be done every 2 to 3 years since these patients are unlikely to have peripheral arterial disease.

ABI may have limited use in certain diabetic patients, such as those in whom the medial wall calcification may render the arteries non-compressible, resulting in unusually high ABI values (>1.40), even in the presence of occlusive disease (167). Under these conditions, the ABI is unreliable (165,168). However, an elevated ABI is still predictive of an increased risk of cardiovascular events, and other non-invasive tests should be considered to diagnose PAD (169).

Noninvasive Imaging Techniques

In patients with a confirmed diagnosis of PAD, further investigation of segmental pressures to localize the diseased vessel, and morphological features of the diseased area, usually in the context of a planned revascularization procedure is needed. This can be achieved by several non-invasive imaging modalities, such as ultrasound duplex scanning, pulse volume recording, MRA or CTA. Ultrasound duplex scanning can directly visualize vessels, providing information on arterial wall thickness, degree of flow turbulence and flow velocity (170). Contrast enhanced MRA produces images that are compatible with conventional angiography (171). Recent development in CTA has also dramatically improved image quantity, replacing conventional angiography in many centers (172,173).

Arteriography

Invasive arteriography has been the definitive procedure for diagnosing PAD. (Fig. 3) However, it is being replaced by noninvasive imaging methods in many centers as discussed before. Arteriography remains an important modality, particularly in the context of endovascular revascularization.

Management of PAD

Intensive Risk Factor Modification

The major cause of PAD is atherosclerosis. Atherosclerotic risk factors for PAD include cigarette smoking, diabetes, dyslipidemia and hypertension. Intensive risk factor modification is an essential component of PAD management.

Smoking Cessation

Cigarette smoking is the most important risk factor for the development of PAD. The amount and duration of tobacco use correlate directly with the development and progression of PAD (174). The effect of smoke cessation on the long-term survival should not be underestimated. In one study, the ten-year survival in former smokers was 82% as compared to 46% in active smokers (175). In a more recent study, the long-term mortality was improved by utilizing the following smoke cessation methods: physician advice, nicotine replacement therapy and counseling (176).

Diabetes

In the UKPDA study, each 1% reduction in the mean glycosalated hemoglobin (HbA_{1C}) was associated with 21% reduction in risk for any endpoint related to diabetes, and 21% reduction in death related to diabetes, 14% reduction in MI and 37% reduction in microvascular complications (177). There is also strong evidence of an association between the duration of diabetes and the risk of PAD in men (178). However, direct evidence supporting aggressive glycemic control to reduce the risk associated with PAD is lacking. Current ADA guidelines recommended a target glycosylated hemoglobin level of <7.0% in diabetic individual (179).

Dyslipidemia

It has been well established that lipid lowering therapy decrease cardiovascular events in diabetic patients (103,104,180,181). However, there is a lack of direct evidence on treating dyslipidemia in patients with both diabetes and PAD. The Heart Protection Study randomized over 20,000 UK adults with occlusive arterial disease including coronary, cerebral and peripheral arterial disease and/or diabetes mellitus and a total cholesterol level greater than 135 mg/dL to simvastatin or placebo (182). Among the 6748 patients with PAD, a 25% risk reduction over five years of follow-up was observed in the simvastatin group. In the classification system of the National Cholesterol Education Program/Adult Treatment Panel

III (NCEP/ATP III), individuals with lower extremity PAD are classified as either "high risk" or "very high risk" depending on associated risk factors. Based on these findings, the ACC/ AHA recommends that treatment with a hydroxymethyl glutaryl (HMG) coenzyme-A reductase inhibitor (statin) medication is indicated for all patients with PAD to achieve a target LDL cholesterol level of less than 100 mg/dL. When the risk is very high, such as for patients with PAD and diabetes, an LDL goal of less than 70 mg/dL is a therapeutic option.

Hypertension
Although the role of intensive blood pressure control in patients with diabetes and PAD has not been well studied, sufficient evidence supports the benefit of a lower target blood pressure. The UKPDA study showed that although diabetes end points were significantly reduced by strict blood pressure control, there was no effect on the risk of amputation due to PAD (183). Nevertheless, a significant reduction in vascular events in diabetic patients treated with aggressive hypertension management has been demonstrated in the hypertension optimal treatment (HOT) trial (184) and the appropriate blood pressure control in diabetes (ABCD) trial (185). In a more recent study, lowering blood pressure in normotensive diabetic patients with PAD was effective in preventing cardiovascular events (186).

Antiplatelet Therapy

Aspirin
Data from secondary prevention trials in non-diabetic subjects indicate that aspirin has a protective effect on subsequent cardiovascular mortality and morbidity (187). However, the only prospective study evaluating the efficacy of five-year aspirin treatment in diabetic patients with PAD is the Veterans Administration Cooperative Study. This study assessed the efficacy of aspirin (650 mg/day) and dipyridamole in preventing the progression of cardiovascular and PAD in 231 diabetic men with limb gangrene or recent amputation for

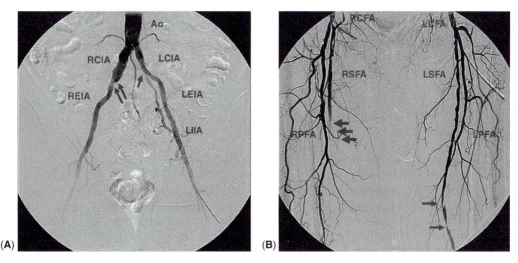

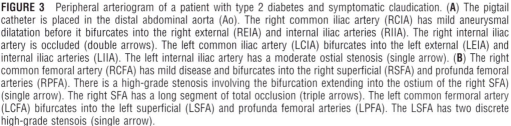

FIGURE 3 Peripheral arteriogram of a patient with type 2 diabetes and symptomatic claudication. (**A**) The pigtail catheter is placed in the distal abdominal aorta (Ao). The right common iliac artery (RCIA) has mild aneurysmal dilatation before it bifurcates into the right external (REIA) and internal iliac arteries (RIIA). The right internal iliac artery is occluded (double arrows). The left common iliac artery (LCIA) bifurcates into the left external (LEIA) and internal iliac arteries (LIIA). The left internal iliac artery has a moderate ostial stenosis (single arrow). (**B**) The right common femoral artery (RCFA) has mild disease and bifurcates into the right superficial (RSFA) and profunda femoral arteries (RPFA). There is a high-grade stenosis involving the bifurcation extending into the ostium of the right SFA (single arrow). The right SFA has a long segment of total occlusion (triple arrows). The left common fermoral artery (LCFA) bifurcates into the left superficial (LSFA) and profunda femoral arteries (LPFA). The LSFA has two discrete high-grade stensois (single arrow).

ischemia. There were no differences in major endpoints such as atherosclerotic vascular death (22% vs. 19%, respectively), in treated and control subjects, or amputation of the opposite extremity (20% vs. 24% in treatment and control subjects) (188). Aspirin has been shown to significantly improve vascular graft patency by the Antiplatelet Trialsts' Collaboration (113). Aspirin is recommended for all diabetic individuals older than 21 years of age (189). However, its role in patients with either diabetes or PAD, but without clinical evidence of CAD or stroke, has not been established. A large secondary prevention trial of aspirin and/or other antiplatelet drugs in diabetic subjects with PAD is therefore needed (190).

Clopidogrel
Based on the results from the Clopidogrel versus aspirin in patients at risk for ischemic events (CAPRIE) study, the ADA consensus recommends that patients with diabetes should be treated with an antiplatelet agent, and those with PAD may benefit more by taking clopidogrel than Aspirin (191). The CAPRIE study evaluated aspirin 325 mg daily versus clopidogrel 75 mg daily in 19,000 patients with recent stroke, recent MI or established PAD (approximately 20% were diabetics). There was a significant 8.7% relative risk reduction in the annual risk of stroke, MI and vascular death in the clopidogrel arm as compared to the aspirin arm (192). In a subset analysis of 6452 patients with PAD, clopidogrel recipients had an annual event rate of 4.86% compared with 7.71% in aspirin recipients, representing a 23.8% relative risk reduction. Furthermore, in the PAD subgroup, clopidogrel was superior to aspirin in diabetic patients (193).

Pentoxifylline and Cilostazol
Pentoxifylline and cilostazol are the two medications currently approved in the U.S. for symptomatic treatment of intermittent claudication. Pentoxifylline is a hemorrheologic agent that decreases blood viscosity and improves erythrocytes flexibility (194). Evidence demonstrating the efficacy of pentoxifylline in improving treadmill walking distance has been equivocal, and therefore its general use in PAD cannot be justified (195). On the other hand, cilostazol, a phosphodiesterase inhibitor, has been shown to improve maximal walking distance by 40% to 50% when compared with placebo (196). In a study directly comparing pentoxifylline and cilostazol for treating claudication, patients treated with cilostazol for 24 weeks had significantly greater walking distance as compared to patients treated with pentoxifylline or placebo (197). Cilostazol is contraindicated in systolic or diastolic heart failure because of concerns about the potential risk of mortality (191).

Various trials have studied prostacyclin or prostacyclin analogues (iloprost and beraprost), and intravenous infusion of prostaglandin E1 for the treatment of claudication. However the results have been inconsistent, and therefore prostaglandin cannot be recommended for the treatment of PAD (198–200).

Endovascular and Surgical Revascularization Therapy
In patients with advance PAD resulting in critical limb ischemia, revascularization is the preferred treatment. Two methods of revascularization techniques include endovascular interventions and open surgical bypasses. In recent years, endovascular revascularization has increased more than five-fold from 1980 to 2000 (201). An endovascular procedure may be more appropriate in patients with relatively focal disease in the arteries above the knee; the best results have been achieved in the aorto-iliac vessels, where one-year patency rate has been reported to be 80 to 90% (202,203). Endovascular procedures carry generally low risk for complications and provide an excellent alternative to surgery in selected patients, particularly those deemed to be poor surgical candidate (204). However, because of its greater durability, surgical therapy remains the definitive therapeutic option in many diabetic patients (205). In addition, diabetes does not adversely affect the surgical treatment of aortoiliac disease (206).

Although most ischemic limbs can be revascularized, some cannot. Amputation is indicated when there is overwhelming infection or significant tissue loss. Despite increased rates of surgical and endovascular revascularization procedures, in the 1990s, there was no decrease in the rates of major amputation in the general population (207).

FUTURE GOALS

Given the unique characteristics and tremendous impact of cardiovascular and peripheral vascular disease in the diabetic population, large prospective studies specifically examining pathophysiology, screening, and efficacy of therapy in this population are warranted. The BARI 2D trial will likely answer whether medical therapy alone, percutaneous coronary intervention, or coronary artery bypass grafting in the setting of strict blood glucose control is the optimal treatment for individuals with type 2 diabetes mellitus with stable CAD. In addition, trials examining the role of HMG–CoA reductase inhibitors, as well as gemfibrozil and other fibrate drugs, specifically in the diabetic population have been proposed or are ongoing. Studies such as these should provide further insight to guide prevention strategies in this high-risk population.

In the meantime, it is important to recognize both the considerable potential for, and serious adverse effects of cardiovascular and peripheral vascular disease in the diabetic population. There is justification to have a lower threshold to screen for cardiovascular disease and to aggressively modify other cardiovascular risk factors, when faced with the challenges of managing the diabetic patient.

REFERENCES

1. Role of cardiovascular risk factors in prevention and treatment of macrovascular disease in diabetes. American Diabetes Association. Diabetes Care 1989; 12:573–9.
2. Aronson D, Rayfield EJ, Chesebro JH. Mechanisms determining course and outcome of diabetic patients who have had acute myocardial infarction. Ann Intern Med 1997; 126:296–306.
3. Kannel WB, McGee DL. Diabetes and glucose tolerance as risk factors for cardiovascular disease: the Framingham study. Diabetes Care 1979; 2:120–6.
4. Pyorala K, Laakso M, Uusitupa M: Diabetes and atherosclerosis: an epidemiologic view. Diabetes Metab Rev 1987; 3:463–524.
5. Stamler J, Vaccaro O, Neaton JD, Wentworth D. Diabetes, other risk factors, and 12-year cardiovascular mortality for men screened in the multiple risk factor intervention trial. Diabetes Care 1993; 16:434–4.
6. B-CE Winngard DL. Heart disease and diabetes. In: Diabetes in America Edited by G NDD, 2nd ed. Washington, DC: Government Printing Office, 1995:429-48.
7. Yusuf S, Hawken S, Ounpuu S, et al. Effect of potentially modifiable risk factors associated with myocardial infarction in 52 countries (the INTERHEART study): case-control study. Lancet 2004; 364:937–52.
8. Abbott RD, Donahue RP, Kannel WB, Wilson PW. The impact of diabetes on survival following myocardial infarction in men vs women. The Framingham Study. J Am Med Assoc 1988; 260: 3456–60.
9. Miettinen H, Lehto S, Salomaa V, et al. Impact of diabetes on mortality after the first myocardial infarction. The FINMONICA Myocardial Infarction Register Study Group. Diabetes Care 1998; 21: 69–75.
10. Herlitz J, Karlson BW, Edvardsson N, Emanuelsson H, Hjalmarson A. Prognosis in diabetics with chest pain or other symptoms suggestive of acute myocardial infarction. Cardiology 1992; 80: 237–45.
11. Barbash GI, White HD, Modan M, Van de Werf F. Significance of diabetes mellitus in patients with acute myocardial infarction receiving thrombolytic therapy. Investigators of the International Tissue Plasminogen Activator/Streptokinase Mortality Trial. J Am Coll Cardiol 1993; 22:707–13.
12. Granger CB, Califf RM, Young S, et al. Outcome of patients with diabetes mellitus and acute myocardial infarction treated with thrombolytic agents. The Thrombolysis and Angioplasty in Myocardial Infarction (TAMI) Study Group. J Am Coll Cardiol 1993; 21:920–5.
13. Hillis LD, Forman S, Braunwald E. Risk stratification before thrombolytic therapy in patients with acute myocardial infarction. The Thrombolysis in Myocardial Infarction (TIMI) Phase II Co-Investigators. J Am Coll Cardiol 1990; 16:313–5.
14. Klein HH, Hengstenberg C, Peuckert M, Jurgensen R. Comparison of death rates from acute myocardial infarction in a single hospital in two different periods (1977 1978 versus 1988 1989). Am J Cardiol 1993; 71:518–23.
15. Mueller HS, Cohen LS, Braunwald E, et al. Predictors of early morbidity and mortality after thrombolytic therapy of acute myocardial infarction. Analyses of patient subgroups in the Thrombolysis in Myocardial Infarction (TIMI) trial, phase II. Circulation 1992; 85:1254–64.
16. Murphy JF, Kahn MG, Krone RJ. Prethrombolytic versus thrombolytic era risk stratification of patients with acute myocardial infarction. Am J Cardiol 1995; 76:827–9.

17. Herlitz J, Malmberg K, Karlson BW, Ryden L, Hjalmarson A. Mortality and morbidity during a five-year follow-up of diabetics with myocardial infarction. Acta Med Scand 1988; 224:31–8.
18. Jacoby RM, Nesto RW. Acute myocardial infarction in the diabetic patient: pathophysiology, clinical course and prognosis. J Am Coll Cardiol 1992; 20:736–44.
19. Karlson BW, Herlitz J, Hjalmarson A. Prognosis of acute myocardial infarction in diabetic and non-diabetic patients. Diabet Med 1993; 10:449–54.
20. Smith JW, Marcus FI, Serokman R. Prognosis of patients with diabetes mellitus after acute myocardial infarction. Am J Cardiol 1984; 54:718–21.
21. Stone PH, Muller JE, Hartwell T, et al. The effect of diabetes mellitus on prognosis and serial left ventricular function after acute myocardial infarction: contribution of both coronary disease and diastolic left ventricular dysfunction to the adverse prognosis. The MILIS Study Group. J Am Coll Cardiol 1989; 14:49–57.
22. Ulvenstam G, Aberg A, Bergstrand R, et al. Long-term prognosis after myocardial infarction in men with diabetes. Diabetes 1985; 34:787–92.
23. Hoff JA, Quinn L, Sevrukov A, et al. The prevalence of coronary artery calcium among diabetic individuals without known coronary artery disease. J Am Coll Cardiol 2003; 41:1008–12.
24. Scognamiglio R, Negut C, Ramondo A, Tiengo A, Avogaro A. Detection of coronary artery disease in asymptomatic patients with type 2 diabetes mellitus. J Am Coll Cardiol 2006; 47:65–71.
25. Haffner SM, Lehto S, Ronnemaa T, Pyorala K, Laakso M. Mortality from coronary heart disease in subjects with type 2 diabetes and in nondiabetic subjects with and without prior myocardial infarction. N Engl J Med 1998; 339:229–34.
26. Consensus development conference on the diagnosis of coronary heart disease in people with diabetes: 10–11 February 1998, Miami, Florida. Am Diabetes Assoc. Diabetes Care 1998; 21:1551–9.
27. Barzilay JI, Kronmal RA, Bittner V, Eaker E, Evans C, Foster ED. Coronary artery disease and coronary artery bypass grafting in diabetic patients aged > or = 65 years (report from the Coronary Artery Surgery Study (CASS] Registry). Am J Cardiol 1994; 74:334–9.
28. Stein B, Weintraub WS, Gebhart SP, et al. Influence of diabetes mellitus on early and late outcome after percutaneous transluminal coronary angioplasty. Circulation 1995; 91:979–89.
29. Vigorito C, Betocchi S, Bonzani G, et al. Severity of coronary artery disease in patients with diabetes mellitus. Angiographic study of 34 diabetic and 120 nondiabetic patients. Am Heart J 1980; 100: 782–7.
30. Waller BF, Palumbo PJ, Lie JT, Roberts WC. Status of the coronary arteries at necropsy in diabetes mellitus with onset after age 30 years. Analysis of 229 diabetic patients with and without clinical evidence of coronary heart disease and comparison to 183 control subjects. Am J Med 1980; 69: 498–506.
31. The effects of tissue plasminogen activator, streptokinase, or both on coronary-artery patency, ventricular function, and survival after acute myocardial infarction. The GUSTO Angiographic Investigators. N Engl J Med 1993; 329:1615–22.
32. Muller DW, Topol EJ, Ellis SG, Sigmon KN, Lee K, Califf RM. Multi-vessel coronary artery disease: a key predictor of short-term prognosis after reperfusion therapy for acute myocardial infarction. Thrombolysis and Angioplasty in Myocardial Infarction (TAMI) Study Group. Am Heart J 1991; 121:1042–9.
33. Fuster V, Badimon L, Badimon JJ, Chesebro JH. The pathogenesis of coronary artery disease and the acute coronary syndromes (2). N Engl J Med 1992; 326:310–8.
34. Libby P. Molecular bases of the acute coronary syndromes. Circulation 1995; 91:2844–50.
35. Umans JG, Levi R. Nitric oxide in the regulation of blood flow and arterial pressure. Annu Rev Physiol 1995; 57:771–90.
36. Cohen RA, Vanhoutte PM. Endothelium-dependent hyperpolarization. Beyond nitric oxide and cyclic GMP. Circulation 1995; 92:3337–49.
37. Johnstone MT, Creager SJ, Scales KM, Cusco JA, Lee BK, Creager MA. Impaired endothelium-dependent vasodilation in patients with insulin-dependent diabetes mellitus. Circulation 1993; 88: 2510–6.
38. Tesfamariam B. Free radicals in diabetic endothelial cell dysfunction. Free Radic Biol Med 1994; 16: 383–91.
39. Kannel WB, Hjortland M, Castelli WP. Role of diabetes in congestive heart failure: the Framingham study. Am J Cardiol 1974; 34:29–34.
40. Bertoni AG, Hundley WG, Massing MW, Bonds DE, Burke GL, Goff DC Jr. Heart failure prevalence, incidence, and mortality in the elderly with diabetes. Diabetes Care 2004; 27:699–703.
41. Bertoni AG, Tsai A, Kasper EK, Brancati FL. Diabetes and idiopathic cardiomyopathy: a nationwide case-control study. Diabetes Care 2003; 26:2791–5.
42. Iribarren C, Karter AJ, Go AS, et al. Glycemic control and heart failure among adult patients with diabetes. Circulation 2001; 103:2668–73.
43. Nichols GA, Gullion CM, Koro CE, Ephross SA, Brown JB. The incidence of congestive heart failure in type 2 diabetes: an update. Diabetes Care 2004; 27:1879–84.

44. Nichols GA, Hillier TA, Erbey JR, Brown JB. Congestive heart failure in type 2 diabetes: prevalence, incidence, and risk factors. Diabetes Care 2001; 24:1614–9.
45. Czyzk A, Krolewski AS, Szablowska S, Alot A, Kopczynski J. Clinical course of myocardial infarction among diabetic patients. Diabetes Care 1980; 3:526–9.
46. Jaffe AS, Spadaro JJ, Schechtman K, Roberts R, Geltman EM, Sobel BE. Increased congestive heart failure after myocardial infarction of modest extent in patients with diabetes mellitus. Am Heart J 1984; 108:31–7.
47. Kouvaras G, Cokkinos D, Spyropoulou M. Increased mortality of diabetics after acute myocardial infarction attributed to diffusely impaired left ventricular performance as assessed by echocardiography. Jpn Heart J 1988; 29:1–9.
48. Lomuscio A, Castagnone M, Vergani D, et al. Clinical correlation between diabetic and non diabetic patients with myocardial infarction. Acta Cardiol 1991; 46:543–54.
49. Malmberg K, Ryden L. Myocardial infarction in patients with diabetes mellitus. Eur Heart J 1988; 9: 259–64.
50. Rytter L, Troelsen S, Beck-Nielsen H. Prevalence and mortality of acute myocardial infarction in patients with diabetes. Diabetes Care 1985; 8:230–4.
51. Savage MP, Krolewski AS, Kenien GG, Lebeis MP, Christlieb AR, Lewis SM. Acute myocardial infarction in diabetes mellitus and significance of congestive heart failure as a prognostic factor. Am J Cardiol 1988; 62:665–9.
52. Tansey MJ, Opie LH, Kennelly BM. High mortality in obese women diabetics with acute myocardial infarction. Br Med J 1977; 1:1624–6.
53. Yudkin JS, Oswald GA. Determinants of hospital admission and case fatality in diabetic patients with myocardial infarction. Diabetes Care 1988; 11:351–8.
54. Halon DA, Merdler A, Flugelman MY, et al. Late-onset heart failure as a mechanism for adverse long-term outcome in diabetic patients undergoing revascularization (a 13-year report from the Lady Davis Carmel Medical Center registry). Am J Cardiol 2000; 85:1420–6.
55. Barzilay JI, Kronmal RA, Gottdiener JS, et al. The association of fasting glucose levels with congestive heart failure in diabetic adults > or =65 years: the Cardiovascular Health Study. J Am Coll Cardiol 2004; 43:2236–41.
56. Carr AA, Kowey PR, Devereux RB, et al. Hospitalizations for new heart failure among subjects with diabetes mellitus in the RENAAL and LIFE studies. Am J Cardiol 2005; 96:1530–6.
57. Arvan S, Singal K, Knapp R, Vagnucci A. Subclinical left ventricular abnormalities in young diabetics. Chest 1988; 93:1031–4.
58. Vered A, Battler A, Segal P, et al. Exercise-induced left ventricular dysfunction in young men with asymptomatic diabetes mellitus (diabetic cardiomyopathy). Am J Cardiol 1984; 54:633–7.
59. Raev DC. Which left ventricular function is impaired earlier in the evolution of diabetic cardiomyopathy? An echocardiographic study of young type I diabetic patients. Diabetes Care 1994; 17:633–9.
60. Riggs TW, Transue D. Doppler echocardiographic evaluation of left ventricular diastolic function in adolescents with diabetes mellitus. Am J Cardiol 1990; 65:899–902.
61. Paillole C, Dahan M, Paycha F, Solal AC, Passa P, Gourgon R. Prevalence and significance of left ventricular filling abnormalities determined by Doppler echocardiography in young type I (insulin-dependent) diabetic patients. Am J Cardiol 1989; 64:1010–6.
62. Uusitupa M, Mustonen J, Laakso M, et al. Impairment of diastolic function in middle-aged type 1 (insulin-dependent) and type 2 (non-insulin-dependent) diabetic patients free of cardiovascular disease. Diabetologia 1988; 31:783–91.
63. Zarich SW, Arbuckle BE, Cohen LR, Roberts M, Nesto RW. Diastolic abnormalities in young asymptomatic diabetic patients assessed by pulsed Doppler echocardiography. J Am Coll Cardiol 1988; 12:114–20.
64. Mildenberger RR, Bar-Shlomo B, Druck MN, et al. Clinically unrecognized ventricular dysfunction in young diabetic patients. J Am Coll Cardiol 1984; 4:234–8.
65. Shapiro LM, Leatherdale BA, Mackinnon J, Fletcher RF. Left ventricular function in diabetes mellitus. II: relation between clinical features and left ventricular function. Br Heart J 1981; 45: 129–32.
66. Bloomgarden ZT. The European Association for the Study of Diabetes Annual Meeting, 1998: complications of diabetes. Diabetes Care 1999; 22:1364–70.
67. Creager MA, Luscher TF, Cosentino F, Beckman JA. Diabetes and vascular disease: pathophysiology, clinical consequences, and medical therapy: Part I. Circulation 2003; 108:1527–32.
68. Du X, Matsumura T, Edelstein D, et al. Inhibition of GAPDH activity by poly(ADP-ribose) polymerase activates three major pathways of hyperglycemic damage in endothelial cells. J Clin Invest 2003; 112:1049–57.
69. Ceriello A, Motz E. Is oxidative stress the pathogenic mechanism underlying insulin resistance, diabetes, and cardiovascular disease? The common soil hypothesis revisited. Arterioscler Thromb Vasc Biol 2004; 24:816–23.

70. Hsueh WA, Lyon CJ, Quinones MJ. Insulin resistance and the endothelium. Am J Med 2004; 117: 109–17.

71. Quinones MJ, Hernandez-Pampaloni M, Schelbert H, et al. Coronary vasomotor abnormalities in insulin-resistant individuals. Ann Intern Med 2004; 140:700–8.

72. Mather KJ, Verma S, Anderson TJ. Improved endothelial function with metformin in type 2 diabetes mellitus. J Am Coll Cardiol 2001; 37:1344–50.

73. Mullen MJ, Wright D, Donald AE, Thorne S, Thomson H, Deanfield JE. Atorvastatin but not L-arginine improves endothelial function in type I diabetes mellitus: a double-blind study. J Am Coll Cardiol 2000; 36:410–6.

74. Calverley DC, Hacker MR, Loda KA, et al. Increased platelet Fc receptor expression as a potential contributing cause of platelet hypersensitivity to collagen in diabetes mellitus. Br J Haematol 2003; 121:139–42.

75. Davi G, Catalano I, Averna M, et al. Thromboxane biosynthesis and platelet function in type II diabetes mellitus. N Engl J Med 1990; 322:1769–74.

76. Davi G, Ciabattoni G, Consoli A, et al. In vivo formation of 8-iso-prostaglandin f2alpha and platelet activation in diabetes mellitus: effects of improved metabolic control and vitamin E supplementation. Circulation 1999; 99:224–9.

77. Winocour PD. Platelet abnormalities in diabetes mellitus. Diabetes 1992; 41 Suppl 2:26-31.

78. Shechter M, Merz CN, Paul-Labrador MJ, Kaul S. Blood glucose and platelet-dependent thrombosis in patients with coronary artery disease. J Am Coll Cardiol 2000; 35:300–7.

79. Bhatt DL, Marso SP, Lincoff AM, Wolski KE, Ellis SG, Topol EJ. Abciximab reduces mortality in diabetics following percutaneous coronary intervention. J Am Coll Cardiol 2000; 35:922–8.

80. Theroux P, Alexander J Jr, Pharand C, et al. Glycoprotein IIb/IIIa receptor blockade improves outcomes in diabetic patients presenting with unstable angina/non-ST-elevation myocardial infarction: results from the Platelet Receptor Inhibition in Ischemic Syndrome Management in Patients Limited by Unstable Signs and Symptoms (PRISM-PLUS) study. Circulation 2000; 102: 2466–72.

81. Ostermann H, van de Loo J. Factors of the hemostatic system in diabetic patients. A survey of controlled studies. Haemostasis 1986; 16:386–416.

82. Saito I, Folsom AR, Brancati FL, Duncan BB, Chambless LE, McGovern PG. Nontraditional risk factors for coronary heart disease incidence among persons with diabetes: the Atherosclerosis Risk in Communities (ARIC) Study. Ann Intern Med 2000; 133:81–91.

83. Stec JJ, Silbershatz H, Tofler GH, et al. Association of fibrinogen with cardiovascular risk factors and cardiovascular disease in the Framingham Offspring Population. Circulation 2000; 102:1634–8.

84. Badawi H, el-Sawy M, Mikhail M, Nomeir AM, Tewfik S. Platelets, coagulation and fibrinolysis in diabetic and non-diabetic patients with quiescent coronary heart disease. Angiology 1970; 21:511–9.

85. Small M, Lowe GD, MacCuish AC, Forbes CD. Thrombin and plasmin activity in diabetes mellitus and their association with glycaemic control. Q J Med 1987; 65:1025–31.

86. Sobel BE, Woodcock-Mitchell J, Schneider DJ, Holt RE, Marutsuka K, Gold H. Increased plasminogen activator inhibitor type 1 in coronary artery atherectomy specimens from type 2 diabetic compared with nondiabetic patients: a potential factor predisposing to thrombosis and its persistence. Circulation 1998; 97:2213–21.

87. Sambola A, Osende J, Hathcock J, et al. Role of risk factors in the modulation of tissue factor activity and blood thrombogenicity. Circulation 2003; 107:973–7.

88. Moreno PR, Murcia AM, Palacios IF, et al. Coronary composition and macrophage infiltration in atherectomy specimens from patients with diabetes mellitus. Circulation 2000; 102:2180–4.

89. Burke AP, Kolodgie FD, Zieske A, et al. Morphologic findings of coronary atherosclerotic plaques in diabetics: a postmortem study. Arterioscler Thromb Vasc Biol 2004; 24:1266–71.

90. Collins R, Armitage J, Parish S, Sleigh P, Peto R. MRC/BHF Heart Protection Study of cholesterol-lowering with simvastatin in 5963 people with diabetes: a randomised placebo-controlled trial. Lancet 2003; 361:2005–16.

91. Langer A, Freeman MR, Josse RG, Armstrong PW. Metaiodobenzylguanidine imaging in diabetes mellitus: assessment of cardiac sympathetic denervation and its relation to autonomic dysfunction and silent myocardial ischemia. J Am Coll Cardiol 1995; 25:610–8.

92. Di Carli MF, Bianco-Batlles D, Landa ME, et al. Effects of autonomic neuropathy on coronary blood flow in patients with diabetes mellitus. Circulation 1999; 100:813–9.

93. Stevens MJ, Raffel DM, Allman KC, et al. Cardiac sympathetic dysinnervation in diabetes: implications for enhanced cardiovascular risk. Circulation 1998; 98:961–8.

94. Prevalence of unrecognized silent myocardial ischemia and its association with atherosclerotic risk factors in noninsulin-dependent diabetes mellitus. Milan Study on Atherosclerosis and Diabetes (MiSAD) Group. Am J Cardiol 1997; 79:134–9.

95. Nesto RW, Watson FS, Kowalchuk GJ, et al. Silent myocardial ischemia and infarction in diabetics with peripheral vascular disease: assessment by dipyridamole thallium-201 scintigraphy. Am Heart J 1990; 120:1073–7.

96. Wackers FJ, Young LH, Inzucchi SE, et al. Detection of silent myocardial ischemia in asymptomatic diabetic subjects: the DIAD study. Diabetes Care 2004; 27:1954–61.

97. Nesto RW. Screening for asymptomatic coronary artery disease in diabetes. Diabetes Care 1999; 22: 1393–5.

98. Kannel WB. Lipids, diabetes, and coronary heart disease: insights from the Framingham Study. Am Heart J 1985; 110:1100–7.

99. Margolis JR, Kannel WS, Feinleib M, Dawber TR, McNamara PM. Clinical features of unrecognized myocardial infarction–silent and symptomatic. Eighteen year follow-up: the Framingham study. Am J Cardiol 1973; 32:1–7.

100. Niakan E, Harati Y, Rolak LA, Comstock JP, Rokey R. Silent myocardial infarction and diabetic cardiovascular autonomic neuropathy. Arch Intern Med 1986; 146:2229–30.

101. Naka M, Hiramatsu K, Aizawa T, et al. Silent myocardial ischemia in patients with non-insulin-dependent diabetes mellitus as judged by treadmill exercise testing and coronary angiography. Am Heart J 1992; 123:46–53.

102. Koistinen MJ. Prevalence of asymptomatic myocardial ischaemia in diabetic subjects. Bmj 1990; 301: 92–5.

103. Pyorala K, Pedersen TR, Kjekshus J, Faergeman O, Olsson AG, Thorgeirsson G. Cholesterol lowering with simvastatin improves prognosis of diabetic patients with coronary heart disease. A subgroup analysis of the Scandinavian Simvastatin Survival Study (4S). Diabetes Care 1997; 20:614–20.

104. Sacks FM, Pfeffer MA, Moye LA, et al. The effect of pravastatin on coronary events after myocardial infarction in patients with average cholesterol levels. Cholesterol and Recurrent Events Trial investigators. N Engl J Med 1996; 335:1001–9.

105. Executive summary of the third report of The National Cholesterol Education Program (NCEP) expert panel on detection, evaluation, and treatment of high blood cholesterol in adults (Adult Treatment Panel III). J Am Med Assoc 2001; 285:2486–97.

106. Steiner G. Lipid intervention trials in diabetes. Diabetes Care 2000; 23 Suppl 2:B49-53.

107. Yusuf S, Sleight P, Pogue J, Bosch J, Davies R, Dagenais G. Effects of an angiotensin-converting-enzyme inhibitor, ramipril, on cardiovascular events in high-risk patients. The heart outcomes prevention evaluation study investigators. N Engl J Med 2000; 342:145–53.

108. Kjekshus J, Gilpin E, Cali G, Blackey AR, Henning H, Ross J Jr. Diabetic patients and beta-blockers after acute myocardial infarction. Eur Heart J 1990; 11:43–50.

109. Kendall MJ, Lynch KP, Hjalmarson A, Kjekshus J. Beta-blockers and sudden cardiac death. Ann Intern Med 1995; 123:358–67.

110. Malmberg K, Herlitz J, Hjalmarson A, Ryden L. Effects of metoprolol on mortality and late infarction in diabetics with suspected acute myocardial infarction. Retrospective data from two large studies. Eur Heart J 1989; 10:423–8.

111. Gundersen T, Kjekshus J. Timolol treatment after myocardial infarction in diabetic patients. Diabetes Care 1983; 6:285–90.

112. Jonas M, Reicher-Reiss H, Boyko V, et al. Usefulness of beta-blocker therapy in patients with non-insulin-dependent diabetes mellitus and coronary artery disease. Bezafibrate Infarction Prevention (BIP) Study Group. Am J Cardiol 1996; 77:1273–7.

113. Collaborative overview of randomised trials of antiplatelet therapy–II: Maintenance of vascular graft or arterial patency by antiplatelet therapy. Antiplatelet Trialists' Collaboration. Br Med J 1994; 308:159–68.

114. Aspirin therapy in diabetes. American Diabetes Association. Diabetes Care 1997; 20:1772–3.

115. Influence of diabetes on 5-year mortality and morbidity in a randomized trial comparing CABG and PTCA in patients with multivessel disease: the Bypass Angioplasty Revascularization Investigation (BARI). Circulation 1997; 96:1761–9.

116. Chaitman. BR, Rosen AD, Williams DO, et al. Myocardial infarction and cardiac mortality in the Bypass angioplasty revascularization investigation (BARI) randomized trial. Circulation 1997; 96: 2162–70.

117. King SB 3rd, Kosinski AS, Guyton RA, Lembo NJ, Weintraub WS. Eight-year mortality in the Emory Angioplasty versus Surgery Trial (EAST). J Am Coll Cardiol 2000; 35:1116–21.

118. Abizaid A, Costa MA, Centemero M, et al. Clinical and economic impact of diabetes mellitus on percutaneous and surgical treatment of multivessel coronary disease patients: insights from the Arterial revascularization therapy study (ARTS) trial. Circulation 2001; 104:533–8.

119. Davies RF, Goldberg AD, Forman S, et al. Asymptomatic Cardiac Ischemia Pilot (ACIP) study two-year follow-up: outcomes of patients randomized to initial strategies of medical therapy versus revascularization. Circulation 1997; 95:2037–43.

120. Sobel BE, Frye R, Detre KM. Burgeoning dilemmas in the management of diabetes and cardiovascular disease: rationale for the Bypass Angioplasty Revascularization Investigation 2 Diabetes (BARI 2D) Trial. Circulation 2003; 107:636–42.

121. Effect of intensive diabetes management on macrovascular events and risk factors in the Diabetes Control and Complications Trial. Am J Cardiol 1995; 75:894–903.

122. Nathan DM, Cleary PA, Backlund JY, et al. Intensive diabetes treatment and cardiovascular disease in patients with type 1 diabetes. N Engl J Med 2005; 353:2643–53.
123. Malmberg K, Ryden L, Efendic S, et al. Randomized trial of insulin-glucose infusion followed by subcutaneous insulin treatment in diabetic patients with acute myocardial infarction (DIGAMI study): effects on mortality at 1 year. J Am Coll Cardiol 1995; 26:57–65.
124. Califf RM. Simple principles of clinical trials remain powerful. J Am Med Assoc 2005; 293:489–91.
125. Mehta SR, Yusuf S, Diaz R, et al. Effect of glucose-insulin-potassium infusion on mortality in patients with acute ST-segment elevation myocardial infarction: the CREATE-ECLA randomized controlled trial. J Am Med Assoc 2005; 293:437–46.
126. Malmberg K. Prospective randomized study of intensive insulin treatment on long term survival after acute myocardial infarction in patients with diabetes mellitus. DIGAMI (Diabetes Mellitus, Insulin Glucose Infusion in Acute Myocardial Infarction) Study Group. Br Med J 1997; 314:1512–5.
127. Antman EM, Anbe DT, Armstrong PW, et al. ACC/AHA guidelines for the management of patients with ST-elevation myocardial infarction executive summary: a report of the American College of Cardiology/American Heart Association Task Force on Practice Guidelines (Writing Committee to Revise the 1999 Guidelines for the Management of Patients With Acute Myocardial Infarction). Circulation 2004; 110:588–636.
128. Eagle KA, Brundage BH, Chaitman BR, et al. Guidelines for perioperative cardiovascular evaluation for noncardiac surgery. Report of the American College of Cardiology/American Heart Association Task Force on Practice Guidelines. Committee on Perioperative Cardiovascular Evaluation for Noncardiac Surgery. Circulation 1996; 93:1278–317.
129. Gibbons RJ, Balady GJ, Beasley JW, et al. ACC/AHA guidelines for exercise testing: executive summary. A report of the American College of Cardiology/American Heart Association Task Force on Practice Guidelines (Committee on Exercise Testing). Circulation 1997; 96:345–54.
130. Rajagopalan N, Miller TD, Hodge DO, Frye RL, Gibbons. RJ. Identifying high-risk asymptomatic diabetic patients who are candidates for screening stress single-photon emission computed tomography imaging. J Am Coll Cardiol 2005; 45:43–9.
131. Diamond GA, Staniloff HM, Forrester JS, Pollock BH, Swan HJ. Computer-assisted diagnosis in the noninvasive evaluation of patients with suspected coronary artery disease. J Am Coll Cardiol 1983; 1:444–55.
132. Pryor DB, Harrell FE Jr, Lee KL, Califf RM, Rosati RA. Estimating the likelihood of significant coronary artery disease. Am J Med 1983; 75:771–80.
133. Berman DS, Hachamovitch R, Kiat H, et al. Incremental value of prognostic testing in patients with known or suspected ischemic heart disease: a basis for optimal utilization of exercise technetium-99m sestamibi myocardial perfusion single-photon emission computed tomography. J Am Coll Cardiol 1995; 26:639–47.
134. Hachamovitch R, Berman DS, Kiat H, Cohen I, Friedman JD, Shaw LJ. Value of stress myocardial perfusion single photon emission computed tomography in patients with normal resting electrocardiograms: an evaluation of incremental prognostic value and cost-effectiveness. Circulation 2002; 105:823–9.
135. Poornima IG, Miller TD, Christian TF, Hodge DO, Bailey KR, Gibbons RJ. Utility of myocardial perfusion imaging in patients with low-risk treadmill scores. J Am Coll Cardiol 2004; 43:194–9.
136. Berman DS, Wong ND, Gransar H, et al. Relationship between stress-induced myocardial ischemia and atherosclerosis measured by coronary calcium tomography. J Am Coll Cardiol 2004; 44:923–30.
137. He ZX, Hedrick TD, Pratt CM, et al. Severity of coronary artery calcification by electron beam computed tomography predicts silent myocardial ischemia. Circulation 2000; 101:244–51.
138. Lee TH, Boucher CA. Clinical practice. Noninvasive tests in patients with stable coronary artery disease. N Engl J Med 2001; 344:1840–5.
139. Garber AM, Solomon NA. Cost-effectiveness of alternative test strategies for the diagnosis of coronary artery disease. Ann Intern Med 1999; 130:719–28.
140. Gianrossi R, Detrano R, Mulvihill D, et al. Exercise-induced ST depression in the diagnosis of coronary artery disease. A meta-analysis. Circulation 1989; 80:87–98.
141. Berman DS, Kang X, Hayes SW, et al. Adenosine myocardial perfusion single-photon emission computed tomography in women compared with men. Impact of diabetes mellitus on incremental prognostic value and effect on patient management. J Am Coll Cardiol 2003; 41:1125–33.
142. Giri S, Shaw LJ, Murthy DR, et al. Impact of diabetes on the risk stratification using stress single-photon emission computed tomography myocardial perfusion imaging in patients with symptoms suggestive of coronary artery disease. Circulation 2002; 105:32–40.
143. Kang X, Berman DS, Lewin HC, et al. Incremental prognostic value of myocardial perfusion single photon emission computed tomography in patients with diabetes mellitus. Am Heart J 1999; 138:1025–32.
144. Zellweger MJ, Hachamovitch R, Kang X, et al. Prognostic relevance of symptoms versus objective evidence of coronary artery disease in diabetic patients. Eur Heart J 2004; 25:543–50.

145. Hachamovitch R, Hayes S, Friedman JD, et al. Determinants of risk and its temporal variation in patients with normal stress myocardial perfusion scans: what is the warranty period of a normal scan? J Am Coll Cardiol 2003; 41:1329–40.
146. Caracciolo EA, Chaitman BR, Forman SA, et al. Diabetics with coronary disease have a prevalence of asymptomatic ischemia during exercise treadmill testing and ambulatory ischemia monitoring similar to that of non-diabetic patients. An ACIP database study. ACIP investigators. Asymptomatic cardiac ischemia pilot investigators. Circulation 1996; 93:2097–105.
147. Raggi P, Shaw LJ, Berman DS, Callister TQ. Prognostic value of coronary artery calcium screening in subjects with and without diabetes. J Am Coll Cardiol 2004; 43:1663–9.
148. Currie CJ, Morgan CL, Peters JR. The epidemiology and cost of inpatient care for peripheral vascular disease, infection, neuropathy, and ulceration in diabetes. Diabetes Care 1998; 21:42–8.
149. Vigilance JE, Reid HL, Richards-George P. Peripheral occlusive arterial disease in diabetic clinic attendees. West Indian Med J 1999; 48:143–6.
150. Katsilambros NL, Tsapogas PC, Arvanitis MP, et al. Risk factors for lower extremity arterial disease in non-insulin-dependent diabetic persons. Diabet Med 1996; 13:243–6.
151. Beks PJ, Mackaay AJ, de Neeling JN, de Vries H, Bouter LM, Heine RJ. Peripheral arterial disease in relation to glycaemic level in an elderly Caucasian population: the Hoorn study. Diabetologia 1995; 38:86–96.
152. Jude EB, Oyibo SO, Chalmers N, Boulton AJ. Peripheral arterial disease in diabetic and nondiabetic patients: a comparison of severity and outcome. Diabetes Care 2001; 24:1433–7.
153. Calle-Pascual AL, Duran A, Diaz A, et al. Comparison of peripheral arterial reconstruction in diabetic and non-diabetic patients: a prospective clinic-based study. Diabetes Res Clin Pract 2001; 53:129–36.
154. Hughson WG, Mann JI, Tibbs DJ, Woods HF, Walton I. Intermittent claudication: factors determining outcome. Br Med J 1978; 1:1377–9.
155. Bild DE, Selby JV, Sinnock P, Browner WS, Braveman P, Showstack JA. Lower-extremity amputation in people with diabetes. Epidemiology and prevention. Diabetes Care 1989; 12:24–31.
156. Aboyans V, Criqui MH, Denenberg JO, Knoke JD, Ridker PM, Fronek A. Risk factors for progression of peripheral arterial disease in large and small vessels. Circulation 2006; 113:2623–9.
157. Coffman JD. Intermittent claudication and rest pain: physiologic concepts and therapeutic approaches. Prog Cardiovasc Dis 1979; 22:53–72.
158. Prevention of atherosclerotic complications: controlled trial of ketanserin. Prevention of atherosclerotic complications with ketanserin trial group. Br Med J 1989; 298:424–30.
159. Criqui MH, Langer RD, Fronek A, et al. Mortality over a period of 10 years in patients with peripheral arterial disease. N Engl J Med 1992; 326:381–6.
160. Janka HU, Standl E, Mehnert H. Peripheral vascular disease in diabetes mellitus and its relation to cardiovascular risk factors: screening with the doppler ultrasonic technique. Diabetes Care 1980; 3: 207–13.
161. Orchard TJ, Strandness DE Jr. Assessment of peripheral vascular disease in diabetes. Report and recommendations of an international workshop sponsored by the American Diabetes Association and the American Heart Association September 18 20, 1992 New Orleans, Louisiana. Circulation 1993; 88:819–28.
162. Murabito JM, D'Agostino. RB, Silbershatz H, Wilson WF. Intermittent claudication. A risk profile from The Framingham Heart Study. Circulation 1997; 96:44–9.
163. Criqui MH, Fronek A, Klauber MR, Barrett-Connor E, Gabriel S. The sensitivity, specificity, and predictive value of traditional clinical evaluation of peripheral arterial disease: results from noninvasive testing in a defined population. Circulation 1985; 71:516–22.
164. Wang JC, Criqui MH, Denenberg JO, McDermott MM, Golomb BA, Fronek A. Exertional leg pain in patients with and without peripheral arterial disease. Circulation 2005; 112:3501–8.
165. Mohler ER 3rd. Peripheral arterial disease: identification and implications. Arch Intern Med 2003; 163:2306–14.
166. McDermott MM. Ankle brachial index as a predictor of outcomes in peripheral arterial disease. J Lab Clin Med 1999; 133:33–40.
167. Hiatt WR, Hoag S, Hamman RF. Effect of diagnostic criteria on the prevalence of peripheral arterial disease. The San Luis Valley Diabetes Study. Circulation 1995; 91:1472–9.
168. Weitz JI, Byrne J, Clagett GP, et al. Diagnosis and treatment of chronic arterial insufficiency of the lower extremities: a critical review. Circulation 1996; 94:3026–49.
169. Resnick HE, Lindsay RS, McDermott MM, et al. Relationship of high and low ankle brachial index to all-cause and cardiovascular disease mortality: the Strong Heart Study. Circulation 2004; 109: 733–9.
170. Hiatt WR, Jones DN. The role of hemodynamics and duplex ultrasound in the diagnosis of peripheral arterial disease. Curr Opin Cardiol 1992; 7:805–10.
171. Ouriel K. Peripheral arterial disease. Lancet 2001; 358:1257–64.

172. Fishman E. CT Angiography: the State of the Art in 2004. In: Book CT ed. Angiography: the State of the Art in 2004. Vol. 2004. City; 2004.

173. Hoffmann U, Ferencik M, Cury RC, Pena AJ. Coronary CT angiography. J Nucl Med 2006; 47: 797–806.

174. Freund KM, Belanger AJ, D'Agostino RB, Kannel WB. The health risks of smoking. The Framingham Study: 34 years of follow-up. Ann Epidemiol 1993; 3:417–24.

175. Jonason T, Bergstrom R. Cessation of smoking in patients with intermittent claudication. Effects on the risk of peripheral vascular complications, myocardial infarction and mortality. Acta Med Scand 1987; 221:253–60.

176. Anthonisen NR, Skeans MA, Wise RA, Manfreda J, Kanner RE, Connett JE. The effects of a smoking cessation intervention on 14.5-year mortality: a randomized clinical trial. Ann Intern Med 2005; 142: 233–9.

177. Stratton IM, Adler AI, Neil HA, et al. Association of glycaemia with macrovascular and microvascular complications of type 2 diabetes (UKPDS 35): prospective observational study. Br Med J 2000; 321:405–12.

178. Al-Delaimy WK, Merchant AT, Rimm EB, Willett WC, Stampfer MJ, Hu FB. Effect of type 2 diabetes and its duration on the risk of peripheral arterial disease among men. Am J Med 2004; 116:236–40.

179. Standards of medical care in diabetes 2006. Diabetes Care 2006; 29 Suppl 1:MS4-42.

180. Cannon CP, Braunwald E, McCabe CH, et al. Intensive versus moderate lipid lowering with statins after acute coronary syndromes. N Engl J Med 2004; 350:1495–504.

181. Pedersen TR, Kjekshus J, Pyorala K, et al. Effect of simvastatin on ischemic signs and symptoms in the Scandinavian simvastatin survival study (4S). Am J Cardiol 1998; 81:333-5.

182. MRC/BHF Heart Protection Study of cholesterol lowering with simvastatin in 20,536 high-risk individuals: a randomised placebo-controlled trial. Lancet 2002; 360:7–22.

183. Tight blood pressure control and risk of macrovascular and microvascular complications in type 2 diabetes: UKPDS 38. UK Prospective Diabetes Study Group. Br Med J 1998; 317:703–13.

184. Hansson L, Zanchetti A, Carruthers SG, et al. Effects of intensive blood-pressure lowering and low-dose aspirin in patients with hypertension: principal results of the Hypertension Optimal Treatment (HOT) randomized trial. HOT Study Group. Lancet 1998; 351:1755–62.

185. Estacio RO, Jeffers BW, Hiatt WR, Biggerstaff SL, Gifford N, Schrier RW. The effect of nisoldipine as compared with enalapril on cardiovascular outcomes in patients with non-insulin-dependent diabetes and hypertension. N Engl J Med 1998; 338:645–52.

186. Mehler PS, Coll JR, Estacio R, Esler A, Schrier RW, Hiatt WR. Intensive blood pressure control reduces the risk of cardiovascular events in patients with peripheral arterial disease and type 2 diabetes. Circulation 2003; 107:753–6.

187. Collaborative overview of randomised trials of antiplatelet therapy–I: Prevention of death, myocardial infarction, and stroke by prolonged antiplatelet therapy in various categories of patients. Antiplatelet Trialists' Collaboration. Br Med J 1994; 308:81–106.

188. Colwell JA, Bingham SF, Abraira C, et al. Veterans Administration Cooperative Study on antiplatelet agents in diabetic patients after amputation for gangrene: II. Effects of aspirin and dipyridamole on atherosclerotic vascular disease rates. Diabetes Care 1986; 9:140–8.

189. Colwell JA. Aspirin therapy in diabetes. Diabetes Care 2003; 26 Suppl 1:S87–8.

190. Cimminiello C, Milani M. Diabetes mellitus and peripheral vascular disease: is aspirin effective in preventing vascular events? Diabetologia 1996; 39:1402–4.

191. Peripheral arterial disease in people with diabetes. Diabetes Care 2003; 26:3333–41.

192. A randomized, blinded, trial of clopidogrel versus aspirin in patients at risk of ischaemic events (CAPRIE). CAPRIE Steering Committee. Lancet 1996; 348:1329–39.

193. Bhatt DL, Marso SP, Hirsch AT, Ringleb PA, Hacke W, Topol EJ. Amplified benefit of clopidogrel versus aspirin in patients with diabetes mellitus. Am J Cardiol 2002; 90:625–8.

194. Angelkort B, Spurk P, Habbaba A, Mahder M. Blood flow properties and walking performance in chronic arterial occlusive disease. Angiology 1985; 36:285–92.

195. Jackson MR, Clagett GP. Antithrombotic therapy in peripheral arterial occlusive disease. Chest 2001; 119:283S–299S.

196. Money SR, Herd JA, Isaacsohn JL, et al. Effect of cilostazol on walking distances in patients with intermittent claudication caused by peripheral vascular disease. J Vasc Surg 1998; 27:267–74. discussion 274–5.

197. Dawson DL, Cutler BS, Hiatt WR, et al. A comparison of cilostazol and pentoxifylline for treating intermittent claudication. Am J Med 2000; 109:523–30.

198. Loosemore TM, Chalmers TC, Dormandy JA. A meta-analysis of randomized placebo control trials in Fontaine stages III and IV peripheral occlusive arterial disease. Int Angiol 1994; 13:133–42.

199. Mohler ER 3rd, Hiatt WR, Olin JW, Wade M, Jeffs R, Hirsch AT. Treatment of intermittent claudication with beraprost sodium, an orally active prostaglandin I2 analogue: a double-blinded, randomized, controlled trial. J Am Coll Cardiol 2003; 41:1679–86.

200. Reiter M, Bucek RA, Stumpflen A, Minar E. Prostanoids for intermittent claudication. Cochrane Database Syst Rev 2004:CD000986.
201. Anderson PL, Gelijns A, Moskowitz A, et al. Understanding trends in inpatient surgical volume: vascular interventions, 1980-2000. J Vasc Surg 2004; 39:1200–8.
202. Dormandy JA, Rutherford RB. Management of peripheral arterial disease (PAD). TASC Working Group. TransAtlantic Inter-Society Concensus (TASC). J Vasc Surg 2000; 31:S1-S296.
203. Sullivan TM, Childs MB, Bacharach JM, Gray BH, Piedmonte MR. Percutaneous transluminal angioplasty and primary stenting of the iliac arteries in 288 patients. J Vasc Surg 1997; 25:829–38. discussion 838–9.
204. Isner JM, Rosenfield K. Redefining the treatment of peripheral artery disease. Role of percutaneous revascularization. Circulation 1993; 88:1534–57.
205. Beckman JA, Creager MA, Libby P. Diabetes and atherosclerosis: epidemiology, pathophysiology, and management. J Am Med Assoc 2002; 287:2570–81.
206. Faries P, LoGerfo F, Hook S. The Impact of diabetes on arterial reconstructions for multilevel arterial occlusive disease. Surg Gynecol Obstet 2001; 181:251.
207. Feinglass J, Brown JL, LoSasso A, et al. Rates of lower-extremity amputation and arterial reconstruction in the United States, 1979 to 1996. Am J Public Health 1999; 89:1222–7.
208. Eagle KA, et al. Guidelines for perioperative cardiovascular evaluation for non-cardiac surgery. Report of the American College of Cardiology/American Heart Association Task Force on Practice Guidelines. Committee on Perioperative Cardiovascular Evaluation for Noncardiac Surgery. Circulation, 1996. 93(6): p. 1278–317.
209. Consensus Development Conference. Diabetes Care, Volume 21(9). September 1998.1551–1559.

30 Acute Coronary Syndrome, Myocardial Infarction, Heart Failure, and Stable Coronary Artery Disease—Specific Considerations in Diabetes

Christian A. Schneider and Erland Erdmann
Clinic III of Internal Medicine, University of Cologne, Cologne, Germany

Coronary artery disease (CAD) and heart failure (HF) are the leading causes of morbidity and mortality among patients with diabetes mellitus. Patients with diabetes are more likely to have more severe CAD (including three vessel diseases), they are more likely to experience episodes of silent ischemia, the outcome of which is worse than that of non-diabetic patients with coronary artery disease. This chapter focuses on therapeutic options for stable coronary artery disease, acute coronary syndromes, and heart failure.

Revascularization of Coronary Artery Disease in Patients with Diabetes Mellitus and Stable Coronary Artery Disease

The indications for revascularization in diabetic patients with stable angina are generally similar to those in patients without diabetes. These indications include angina not responding to medical treatment (beta-blocker, nitrates), extensive myocardial ischemia, or multivessel coronary artery disease with depressed left ventricular function. A post-hoc analysis from the MASS II trial of patients with stable angina randomly assigned to medical therapy, CABG, or percutaneous coronary intervention (PCI), (1) has shown the outcome of diabetic and non-diabetic patients. While no difference in mortality among the treatment strategies in diabetic and non-diabetic patients was found at one year, the mortality thereafter was significantly lower with either revascularization strategy, compared to medical treatment in diabetic patients (8 and 11 vs. 23 %). The procedural success rate is similar in patients with and without diabetes. This is illustrated by a large series of 10,433 patients undergoing elective PCI without stenting (1133 had diabetes) (2). Although the diabetic patients had worse clinical characteristics, there were no differences in initial angiographic success or complication rates between diabetic and non-diabetic patients. However, patients with diabetes have lower rates of event-free survival and freedom from restenosis than non-diabetic patients after PCI. Despite the comparable procedural success of PCI in diabetes, the event-free survival is poorer (3). This was illustrated in an analysis of 1005 diabetic and 3457 non-diabetic patients who underwent PCI with stenting (4,5). The patients with diabetes had significant reductions in event-free survival (72 vs. 79%) and overall mortality (8.3 vs. 3.8%) compared to non diabetics (4). Several diabetes-related factors seem to play a role in the adverse outcome of patients after PCI. These include nephropathy (6,7), the use of sulfonylureas (8), prior less strict glycemic control (9), and the higher incidence of restenosis (10). To reduce the incidence of restenosis, drug-eluting stents are now preferred to bare-metal stents because they are associated with a marked reduction in the incidence of restenosis. In the SIRIUS trial that compared sirolimus-eluting stents to bare-metal stents (11), sirolimus-eluting stents significantly reduced the rate of target lesion revascularization (7 vs. 22 %). Similarly, the paclitaxel-eluting stents in the TAXUS IV trial (12) reduced the rates of binary angiographic restenosis at nine months (6.4 vs. 34.5%). A direct comparison of sirolimus and bare-metal stenting was performed in the DIABETES trial in 160 patients with diabetes (13). Again, the in-segment late lumen loss and the binary restenosis were significantly reduced at nine month follow-up by the drug-eluting stent (Fig. 1).

There are no proven oral drugs to reduce the restenosis rate in patients with diabetes. Recent data were published showing that thiazolidinediones inhibit vascular smooth muscle

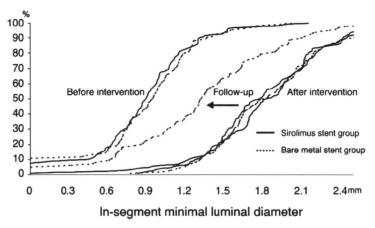

FIGURE 1   Cumulative frequency distribution curves for minimal luminal diameter in the group that received sirolimus-eluting stent and in the group that received standard stent before and immediately after the intervention and at 270 days. Bare-metal stents had higher restenosis rate (arrow).

cell proliferation and migration and reduce intimal proliferation after vascular injury. The potential efficacy of thiazolidinediones to reduce restenosis was evaluated in a randomized trial of 54 patients with type 2 diabetes who underwent PCI with bare-metal stents (14). Pioglitazone (30 mg once daily) reduced compared to controls the late lumen loss (0.30 vs. 1.43 mm) and the binary angiographic restenosis (8 vs. 57%) at six months significantly. Similar results have been shown with rosiglitazone (15). *Glycoprotein (GP) IIb/IIIa inhibitors* reduce the risk of ischemic complications in most patients undergoing coronary artery stenting, including those with an acute coronary syndrome and higher risk patients with stable angina. ISAR-SWEET randomly assigned 701 diabetic patients (16) who were undergoing elective PCI to abciximab plus heparin or placebo plus heparin with additional clopidogrel treatment. The primary endpoint of death or myocardial infarction (MI) at one year was similar in both groups (8.3 vs. 8.6% with placebo); there was also no difference in mortality at one year (4.8 vs. 5.1%). However, follow-up angiography found a moderately reduced rate of angiographic restenosis with abciximab (29 vs. 38 % with placebo).

CABG

Short- and long-term survival after CABG is significantly reduced in diabetic patients (17,18). In several large observational studies, diabetic patients had higher mortality rates at 30 days (5 vs. 2.5 %) (17), at five years (22 vs. 12%), and at 10 years (and 50 vs. 29 %) (18). Reasons for this observation include differences in the comorbidities of diabetic and non-diabetic patients undergoing CABG. For example, diabetic patients are generally older, have more severe three vessel disease, lower ejection fraction, and more often proteinuria, which are all independent risk factors for cardiovascular complications and death (19).

PTCA versus CABG

Most randomized trials comparing PTCA with CABG have reported similar overall outcomes for these two revascularization methods. However, subgroup analysis of randomized trials and prospective nonrandomized studies suggest that diabetes may be an exception, as the outcome is better after CABG, particularly in patients with three vessel disease (20–22). This was demonstrated by the BARI trial (21,23). Among diabetic patients CABG was associated with a significantly higher survival rate compared to PTCA at 5.4 years (81 vs. 66 %) (21) and at seven years (76 vs. 56 %) (24). The difference was entirely due to a lower cardiac mortality in the CABG group (5.8 vs. 20.6% for PTCA at 5.4 years) (23). The cardiac mortality was 2.9% when at least one internal mammary graft was used. Diabetic patients who have undergone CABG may have a better outcome after a subsequent MI than those who have undergone PTCA or were treated medically (25,26). This was suggested in a report from the BARI trial, which evaluated patients with and without diabetes who had undergone revascularization with CABG or PTCA within three months after study entry (25). Among the patients with diabetes, CABG significantly reduced the mortality after a subsequent MI (relative risk 0.09 compared to angioplasty). BARI trial data and results from three other trials that reported results for patients with diabetes (EAST, CABRI, and RITA) were analyzed in a meta-analysis (27). All-cause mortality was significantly lower with CABG than PTCA at four years (absolute risk difference 8.6%) but not longer at six years.

Stenting versus CABG in Multivessel Disease

Diabetics with multivessel disease undergoing coronary stenting may have a worse outcome compared to those undergoing CABG. This was illustrated in the ARTS I trial in which 1205 patients with stable or unstable angina and multivessel disease were randomly assigned to PCI with a bare-metal stent or CABG (28). The 208 patients with diabetes had a lower event-free survival with stenting than with CABG at one year (63 vs. 84% for CABG) and at three years (53 vs. 81%), primarily because of a higher incidence of repeat revascularization (29). In contrast to these findings, the AWESOME trial in patients at high risk for CABG was not able to detect a difference between PCI and CABG in diabetic patients (30). A total of 454 patients with medically refractory angina, who had one or more risk factors for an adverse outcome, were evaluated by an interventional cardiologist and a cardiac surgeon after coronary angiography and found to be acceptable candidates for either CABG or PCI. Of this group, 144 had diabetes: 79 were randomly assigned to CABG and 65 to PCI. Survival at 30 days, six months and 36 months was not significantly different with CABG or PCI. In this trial, 54% of patients received stents and 11% glycoprotein inhibitors. The use of drug-eluting stents may further improve this situation, as it is suggested by data of the ARTS II registry showing a reduced risk of revascularisation with drug-eluting stents (29,31).

Given the current use of stents, particularly drug-eluting stents, and GP IIb/IIIa inhibitors, PCI seems a reasonable first choice in patients with appropriate anatomy who do not have heart failure. In the light of the recently observed higher number of late thrombosis of drug-eluting stents, particularly if clopidogrel is not taken anymore, long-term results are needed in this respect (32).

THERAPY OF ACUTE CORONARY SYNDROMES

Antiplatelet Drugs

All patients with an acute MI are given aspirin indefinitely and clopidogrel for at least nine months. Intravenous glycoprotein (GP) IIb/IIIa inhibitors are used in both ST elevation and non-ST elevation acute coronary syndromes. In a meta-analysis of six randomized trials that enrolled 6458 diabetic patients, therapy with the GP IIb/IIIa inhibitors was associated with a significant reduction in the 30-day mortality (6.2 vs. 4.6% for placebo, odds ratio 0.74) (33). A significant reduction in 30-day mortality was also seen in those undergoing a percutaneous coronary intervention (4.0 vs. 1.2%, odds ratio 0.3).

Beta Blockers

Beta blocker therapy after MI reduces the infarct size, the incidence of reinfarction, and cardiac mortality. This benefit was clearly shown in a report from the National Cooperative Cardiovascular Project, which reviewed the records of 45,308 patients 65 years of age or older, 26% of whom had diabetes (34). The multivariate analysis showed that the use of beta blockers was associated with lower one-year mortality (relative risk reduction between 13 and 27%).

ACE Inhibitors

After acute myocardial infarction, ACE inhibitors reduce infarct size, limit ventricular remodelling, and reduce mortality. ACE inhibitors may be of particular benefit in diabetic patients, as illustrated by data from the GISSI-3 trial. The GISSI-3 trial of patients with acute MI included 2790 diabetic patients, showed that six weeks of treatment with lisinopril reduced the six-month mortality among diabetics (12.9 vs. 16.1% for no lisinopril) (Fig. 2) (35).

Glycemic Control

Suboptimal glycemic control in diabetics and stress hyperglycemia in non diabetics are associated with worse in-hospital outcomes after acute MI. Intense glycemic control may be beneficial (show Fig. 3). Hence, the 2004 ACC/AHA guidelines on STEMI, which should also be applicable to non–ST elevation MI (NSTEMI), gave a Class I recommendation to the use of an insulin infusion to normalize blood glucose in patients with a complicated course (36). A Class IIa recommendation was given to the use of an insulin infusion in all MI patients with hyperglycemia.

Interventional Therapy

Immediate coronary reperfusion is recommended in all patients with an acute ST elevation MI, which is usually achieved by primary PCI. Whenever possible PCI should be attempted, as it has a lower incidence of side effects and complications compared to thrombolytic therapy. In patients with NSTEMI, coronary angiography should be performed within 48 hours as long-term outcome improves with early coronary angiography. Limited data are consistent with diabetics having a better outcome with primary PCI (37,38). This was shown in the GUSTO-IIb angioplasty substudy in which patients with an acute STEMI were randomly assigned to primary PCI or accelerated alteplase; the study included 1138 patients including 177 diabetic patients (37). Diabetics undergoing PCI, compared to those receiving thrombolysis, had the same relative reduction in the 30-day incidence of cardiovascular endpoints as the non diabetics (0.70 vs. 0.62). The value of primary PCI with stenting compared to PTCA alone was analyzed in the CADILLAC trial in which 2082 patients with acute STEMI (almost 17% diabetic) were randomly assigned to PCI alone, PCI and abciximab, stenting alone, or stenting and abciximab (39). The outcomes were significantly better with stenting and the relative benefit was similar in diabetics and non diabetics (odds ratio 0.56 and 0.52, respectively). However, at six months, the rate of the primary combined cardiovascular end-point was higher in diabetic patients (e.g., 14.1 vs. 9.7% with stenting).

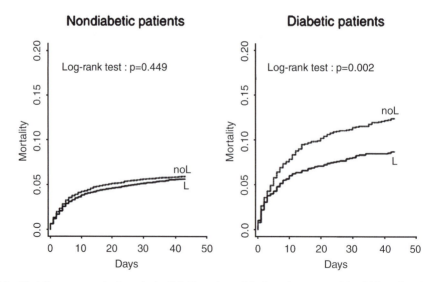

FIGURE 2   Mortality curves up to 6 weeks in diabetic and nondiabetic patients treated (*solid line; L*) and not treated (*dotted line; No L*) with lisinopril.

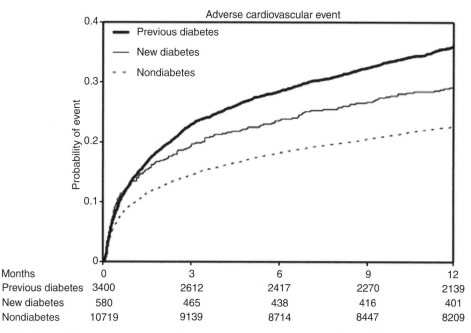

FIGURE 3 Kaplan-Meier curves for composite outcome of cardiovascular mortality/morbidity at 1 year by diabetic status. $p=0.005$ for previous versus new diabetes diagnosis; $p<0.001$ for previous versus no diabetes diagnosis; $p<0.001$ for new versus no diabetes diagnosis.

PROGNOSIS

ST Elevation MI

Significant increases in post-MI mortality have been described in diabetic patients treated with thrombolysis compared to those without diabetes (40). This increase in mortality is largely the result of reinfarction and heart failure (40–42). In GUSTO-I, the 30-day mortality was 6.2% in nondiabetics compared to 9.7 and 12.5% in non–insulin-treated and insulin-treated diabetics (40). Diabetes remained an independent predictor of mortality at one year (14.5 vs. 8.9% in non diabetics). The incidence of nonfatal cardiac events is also increased in patients with diabetes after an MI (43,44). This was recently shown in an analysis from the VALIANT trial of 14,703 patients with an acute MI complicated by left ventricular dysfunction (43). At one year, the rate of composite cardiovascular endpoints was higher for those with previously known or newly diagnosed diabetes than for those without (36 and 29 vs. 23%) (Fig. 3).

NSTEMI/Unstable Angina

The long-term outcome in diabetics who present with a NSTEMI or unstable angina is worse than for non diabetics (42,45,46). This was evaluated in the OASIS registry of 8013 patients, 21% of whom had diabetes (46). After a two year follow-up, diabetes was an independent predictor of mortality (18 vs. 10% for non diabetics, relative risk 1.57, 95% CI 1.38 1.81).

HEART FAILURE

Epidemiology

The Framingham study established the epidemiologic link between diabetes and HF (47) showing that the relative risk of HF remained elevated at 3.8-fold in diabetic men and 5.5-fold in diabetic women even after exclusion of patients with coronary artery disease. Current studies show similar data. In a report of 9591 subjects with type 2 diabetes and matched controls, HF was more frequent at baseline in diabetics (11.8 vs. 4.5%) (48). Among those free of HF at baseline, HF developed more often in diabetics during a 30-month follow-up (7.7 vs. 3.4%). In elderly diabetic patients the incidence is even higher as shown in a national sample of Medicare claims from 1994 to 1999; this population included over 150,000 registered Medicare patients with diabetes who were $\geq$ 65 years of age (49). The prevalence of HF was 22.3% in 1994, with a subsequent incidence of newly diagnosed HF of 12.6% per year. Factors associated with HF in adult diabetic patients are age, duration of diabetes, insulin use, peripheral arterial disease, ischemic heart disease, and poor glycemic control. The importance of glycemic control was shown in an analysis from Kaiser Permanente health maintenance organization. They evaluated almost 50,000 adult patients with type 2 diabetes and no HF at the beginning who were followed for a mean of 2.2 years (50). Each 1% increase in hemoglobin (Hb) A1c was associated with an 8% increased risk of heart failure.

Etiology

The etiology of heart failure in patients with diabetes is diverse and involves systolic heart failure due to coronary artery disease, diastolic heart failure due to hypertension, and left ventricular hypertrophy and the diabetic cardiomyopathy, which may contribute to other etiologies. The ventricular dysfunction due to diabetic cardiomyopathy is manifested by systolic and/or diastolic dysfunction. Several pathologic changes have been described in the myocardium in diabetics including fibrosis, infiltration of the interstitium with periodic acid–Schiff-positive material, and alterations in the myocardial capillary basement membrane. Several clinical features were found in diabetic patients who may be interpreted as early signs of developing heart failure: Diabetic patients had higher left ventricular mass, wall thickness, and arterial stiffness and reduced systolic function compared to normals in the Strong Heart study. Abnormal diastolic function has been noted in 27 to 70% of asymptomatic diabetic patients, which may be due in part to increased left ventricular mass. Diastolic dysfunction is more abnormal in those with worse glycemic control and in those who are also hypertensive. Autonomic neuropathy may play a role in the development of left ventricular dysfunction. Microcirculatory dysfunction in diabetics may be due to downregulation of the expression of vascular endothelial growth factor (VEGF). Local replenishment of VEGF via DNA gene therapy was associated with increased capillary density and a significant improvement in cardiac function in an animal model (51).

Prognosis

Among patients with HF, those with diabetes have higher mortality rates (Fig. 4). This relationship was demonstrated in a report from studies of left ventricular dysfunction (SOLVD) which enrolled 6791 patients, including 1310 with diabetes (52). Compared to nondiabetics, diabetic patients were significantly more likely to be admitted for heart failure (risk ratio 1.6) and had higher rates at one year of all-cause mortality (32 vs. 22%). The increase in all-cause mortality associated with diabetes in SOLVD was limited to patients with an ischemic cardiomyopathy (adjusted relative risk 1.37 compared to 0.98 in patients with non-ischemic cardiomyopathy) (53). In the presence of coronary disease, diabetes was independent of other risk factors for predicting worsening of heart failure. Among patients with diabetes, those who develop HF have poorer prognosis than those who do not develop heart failure. In an analysis of Medicare patients, the mortality rates were 32.7 and 3.7% per year, respectively (hazard ratio [HR] 10.6) (49). The five-year survival rate for diabetics with HF was 12.5%.

Therapy

Diabetic patients with systolic heart failure are treated in the same way as nondiabetics, with ACE inhibitors and beta-blockers. A meta-analysis of beta blocker trials in HF (including 1883 diabetics) showed a relative risk reduction in mortality of 23% with beta-blocker treatment (54). Both the SOLVD and SAVE trials also showed that diabetics benefit from angiotensin-converting enzyme (ACE) inhibitors (52,55). In a meta-analysis of ACE inhibitor trials in HF that included 2398 diabetics, the survival benefit with ACE inhibitor therapy was the same for those with diabetes as for those without (relative risk 0.84) (54). The optimal therapy for diabetic patients with diastolic heart failure is not known, as no prospective randomized

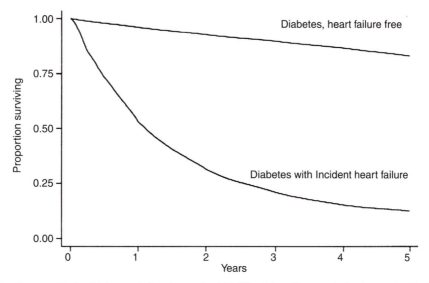

FIGURE 4   Five-year Kaplan–Meier survival estimates for 115,803 adults ≥ 65 years in fee-for-service Medicare with diabetes by incident heart failure status.

studies exist. Considering hypertension and diabetic cardiomyopathy as the principal cause for diastolic heart failure in diabetics, an optimized treatment for these risk factors seems to be a reasonable recommendation.

Glucose-Lowering Agents

The optimum choice of glucose lowering drugs in diabetic patients with symptomatic heart failure is not known, as no prospective randomized studies exist that have included exclusively this important patient population. Neither insulin nor sulfonyureas have been shown to be safe in diabetic patients with heart failure. There are mixed data for thiazolidinediones and metformin.

Thiazolidinediones

Thiazolidinediones (TZDs) increase insulin sensitivity. In both randomized and observational studies, TZD use has been associated with worsening HF and pulmonary edema (56,57). Weight gain and fluid retention are more common with concomitant insulin therapy. The PROactive trial randomly assigned 5238 patients with type 2 diabetes and either coronary artery disease, stroke, or peripheral arterial disease to pioglitazone or placebo (58). The primary endpoint was a composite of all-cause mortality, nonfatal MI (including silent myocardial infarction), stroke, acute coronary syndrome, endovascular or surgical intervention in the coronary or leg arteries, and amputation above the ankle. At a mean follow-up of almost three years, there was a 10% non-significant difference between the two groups in this endpoint (hazard ratio [HR] 0.90, 95% CI 0.80–1.02). There was a significant improvement with pioglitazone in a principal secondary endpoint of all-cause mortality, nonfatal MI, and stroke that were components of the primary endpoint (HR 0.84, 95% CI 0.72–0.98). Pioglitazone use was also associated with improved glycemic control and a significant increase in hospital admissions for HF (6 vs. 4%) but no increase in mortality due to HF. Despite these concerns, TZDs are being used with increasing frequency in diabetic patients with HF and may be associated with improved outcomes (46,47). This was documented in a retrospective study of 16,417 Medicare members with diabetes who were discharged from the hospital with a primary discharge diagnosis of HF; 2226 patients (13.6%) were treated with a TZD (59). At one year, the crude one-year mortality rate was significantly lower in these patients than in the 12,069 treated with neither a TZD nor metformin (30.1 vs. 36.0%, multivariable adjusted hazard ratio 0.87, 95% CI 0.80–0.94) (Fig. 5). Based upon all of these findings, TZDs should be

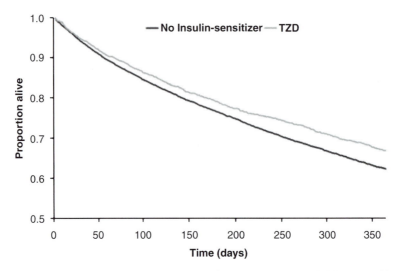

FIGURE 5 Adjusted mortality curves for patients hospitalized with heart failure and diabetes receiving prescription for thiazolidinedione (TZD) at hospital discharge and patients not treated with insulin-sensitizing drug.

avoided in patients with symptomatic congestive HF unless prospective studies will have shown treatment benefits. Possibly the often occurring sodium and water retention increases preload and aggravates underlying left ventricular dysfunction.

Metformin

According to the U.S. Food and Drug Administration, metformin is contraindicated in patients with HF treated with drugs (60). However, as metformin is an effective and useful agent in the management of diabetes mellitus it is prescribed in many patients with heart failure. The safety of metformin and its possible prognostic benefit was shown in the Medicare study described above; 1861 (11.3%) were treated with metformin (59). At one year, the crude one-year mortality rate was significantly lower in these patients than in the 12,069 treated with neither metformin nor a TZD (24.7 vs. 36.0%, hazard ratio 0.87, 95% CI 0.78–0.97).

In summary, patients with type 2 diabetes and HF have a poor prognosis. Optimal treatment for these patients is not known. Therefore they should be treated as non diabetics with ACE inhibitors, beta blockers, and diuretics. Certainly, tight glucose control does not harm these patients.

REFERENCES

1. Soares PR, Hueb WA, Lemos PA, et al. Coronary revascularization (surgical or percutaneous) decreases mortality after the first year in diabetic subjects but not in nondiabetic subjects with multivessel disease: an analysis from the Medicine, Angioplasty, or Surgery Study (MASS II). Circulation 2006; 114:I420.
2. Stein B, Weintraub W, King, S. Influence of diabetes mellitus on early and late outcome after percutaneous transluminal coronary angioplasty. Circulation 1995; 91:979.
3. Mehran R, Dangas GD, Kobayashi Y, et al. Short- and long-term results after multivessel stenting in diabetic patients. J Am Coll Cardiol 2004; 43:1348.
4. Elezi S, Kastrati A, Pache J, et al. Diabetes mellitus and the clinical and angiographic outcome after coronary stent placement. J Am Coll Cardiol 1998; 32:1866
5. Ahmed JM, Hong MK, Mehran R, et al. Influence of diabetes mellitus on early and late clinical outcomes in saphenous vein graft stenting. J Am Coll Cardiol 2000; 36:1186.
6. Marso SP, Ellis SG, Tuzcu EM, et al. The importance of proteinuria as a determinant of mortality following percutaneous coronary revascularization in diabetics. J Am Coll Cardiol 1999; 33:1269.
7. Reeder GS, Holmes DR, Lennon RJ, et al. Proteinuria, serum creatinine, and outcome of percutaneous coronary intervention in patients with diabetes mellitus. Am J Cardiol 2002; 89:760.

8. Garratt KN, Brady PA, Hassinger NL, et al. Sulfonylurea drugs increase early mortality in patients with diabetes mellitus after direct angioplasty for acute myocardial infarction. J Am Coll Cardiol 1999; 33:119.

9. Corpus RA, George PB, House JA, et al. Optimal glycemic control is associated with a lower rate of target vessel revascularization in treated type II diabetic patients undergoing elective percutaneous coronary intervention. J Am Coll Cardiol 2004; 43:8.

10. West NE, Ruygrok PN, Disco CM, et al. Clinical and angiographic predictors of restenosis after stent deployment in diabetic patients. Circulation 2004; 109:867.

11. Moussa I, Leon MB, Baim DS, et al. Impact of sirolimus-eluting stents on outcome in diabetic patients: a SIRIUS (SIRolImUS-coated Bx Velocity balloon-expandable stent in the treatment of patients with de novo coronary artery lesions) substudy. Circulation 2004; 109:2273.

12. Hermiller JB, Raizner A, Cannon L, et al. Outcomes with the polymer-based paclitaxel-luting TAXUS stent in patients with diabetes mellitus: the TAXUS-IV trial. J Am Coll Cardiol 2005; 45: 1172.

13. Sabate M, Jimenez-Quevedo P, Angiolillo DJ, et al. Randomized comparison of sirolimus-eluting stent versus standard stent for percutaneous coronary revascularization in diabetic patients: the diabetes and sirolimus-eluting stent (DIABETES) trial. Circulation 2005; 112:2175.

14. Nishio K, Sakurai M, Kusuyama T, et al. A randomized comparison of pioglitazone to inhibit restenosis after coronary stenting in patients with type 2 diabetes. Diabetes Care 2006; 29:101.

15. Choi D, Kim SK, Choi SH, et al. Preventative effects of rosiglitazone on restenosis after coronary stent implantation in patients with type 2 diabetes. Diabetes Care 2004; 27:2654.

16. Mehilli J, Kastrati A, Schuhlen H, et al. Randomized clinical trial of abciximab in diabetic patients undergoing elective percutaneous coronary interventions after treatment with a high loading dose of clopidogrel. Circulation 2004; 110:3627.

17. Cohen Y, Raz I, Merin G, Mozes B. Comparison of factors associated with 30-day mortality after coronary artery bypass grafting in patients with versus without diabetes mellitus. Israeli Coronary Bypass (ISCAB) Study Consortium. Am J Cardiol 1998; 81:7.

18. Thourani VH, Weintraub WS, Stein, B, et al. Influence of diabetes mellitus on early and late outcome after coronary artery bypass grafting. Ann Thorac Surg 1999; 67:1045.

19. Marso SP, Ellis SG, et al. Proteinuria is a key determinant of death in patients with diabetes after isolated coronary artery bypass graft surgery. Am Heart J 2000; 139:939.

20. Weintraub WS, Stein B, Kosinski A, et al. Outcome of coronary bypass surgery versus coronary angioplasty in diabetic patients with multivessel coronary artery disease. J Am Coll Cardiol 1998; 31: 10.

21. BARI 1996 Comparison of coronary bypass surgery with angioplasty in patients with multivessel disease. The bypass angioplasty revascularization investigation (BARI) investigators. N Engl J Med 1996; 335:217.

22. Niles NW, McGrath PD, Malenka D, et al. Survival of patients with diabetes and multivessel coronary artery disease after surgical or percutaneous coronary revascularization: results of a large regional prospective study. Northern New England Cardiovascular Disease Study Group. J Am Coll Cardiol 2001; 37:1008.

23. BARI 1997. Influence of diabetes on 5-year mortality and morbidity in a randomized trial comparing CABG and PTCA in patients with multivessel disease: the Bypass Angioplasty Revascularization Investigation (BARI). Circulation 1997; 96:1761.

24. BARI 2000. Seven-year outcome in the Bypass Angioplasty Revascularization Investigation (BARI) by treatment and diabetic status. J Am Coll Cardiol 2000; 35:1122.

25. Detre KM, Lombardero MS, Brooks MM, et al. The effect of previous coronary-artery bypass surgery on the prognosis of patients with diabetes who have acute myocardial infarction. Bypass angioplasty revascularization investigation investigators. N Engl J Med 2000; 342:989.

26. Peduzzi P, Detre K, Murphy ML, et al. Ten-year incidence of myocardial infarction and prognosis after infarction. Department of Veterans Affairs Cooperative Study of Coronary Artery Bypass Surgery. Circulation 1991; 83:747.

27. Hoffman SN, TenBrook JA, Wolf MP. A meta-analysis of randomized controlled trials comparing coronary artery bypass graft with percutaneous transluminal coronary angioplasty: one- to eight-year outcomes. J Am Coll Cardiol 2003; 41:1293.

28. Serruys PW, Unger F, Sousa JE, et al. Comparison of coronary-artery bypass surgery and stenting for the treatment of multivessel disease. N Engl J Med 2001; 344:1117.

29. Abizaid A, Costa MA, Centemero M, et al. Clinical and economic impact of diabetes mellitus on percutaneous and surgical treatment of multivessel coronary disease patients: insights from the Arterial Revascularization Therapy Study (ARTS) trial. Circulation 2001; 104:533.

30. Sedlis, SP, Morrison, DA, Lorin, JD, et al. Percutaneous coronary intervention versus coronary bypass graft surgery for diabetic patients with unstable angina and risk factors for adverse outcomes with bypass. outcome of diabetic patients in the AWESOME randomized trial and registry. J Am Coll Cardiol 2002; 40:1555.

31. Macaya C, Garcia H, Serruys P, et al. Sirolimus-eluting stents versus surgery and bare metal stenting in the treatment of diabetic patients with multivessel disease—a comparison between ARTS I and ARTS II (abstract). Circulation 2005; 112:II-655.

32. Smith SC Jr, Feldman TE, Hirshfeld, JW Jr, et al. ACC/AHA/SCAI 2005 guideline update for percutaneous coronary intervention a report of the American College of Cardiology/American Heart Association Task Force on Practice Guidelines (ACC/AHA/SCAI Writing Committee to Update the 2001 Guidelines for Percutaneous Coronary Intervention). J Am Coll Cardiol 2006; 47:e1.

33. Roffi M, Chew DP, Mukherjee D, et al. Platelet glycoprotein IIb/IIIa inhibitors reduce mortality in diabetic patients with non-ST-segment-elevation acute coronary syndromes. Circulation 2001; 104: 2767.

34. Chen J, Marciniak TA, Radford MJ, et al. Beta-blocker therapy for secondary prevention of myocardial infarction in elderly diabetic patients. Results from the National Cooperative Cardiovascular Project. J Am Coll Cardiol 1999; 34:1388.

35. Zuanetti G, Latini R, Maggioni AP, et al. Effect of the ACE inhibitor lisinopril on mortaltiy in diabetic patients with acute myocardial infarction: data from the GISSI-3 study. Circulation 1997; 96:4239.

36. Antman EM, Anbe T, Armstrong PW, et al. ACC/AHA guidelines for the management of patients with ST-Elevation myocardial infarction. J Am Coll Cardiol 2004; 44:671–719.

37. Hasdai D, Granger CB, Srivatsa SS, et al. Diabetes mellitus and outcome after primary coronary angioplasty for acute myocardial infarction: lessons from the GUSTO-IIb Angioplasty Substudy. Global Use of Strategies to Open Occluded Arteries in Acute Coronary Syndromes. J Am Coll Cardiol 2000; 35:1502.

38. Hsu LF, Mak, KH, Lau, KW, et al. Clinical outcomes of patients with diabetes mellitus and acute myocardial infarction treated with primary angioplasty or fibrinolysis. Heart 2002; 88:260.

39. Stone GW, Grines CL, Cox DA, et al. Comparison of angioplasty with stenting, with or without abciximab, in acute myocardial infarction. NEJM 2002; 346(13):957–66.

40. Mak KH, Moliterno DJ, Granger CB, et al. Influence of diabetes mellitus on clinical outcome in the thrombolytic era of acute myocardial infarction. GUSTO-I Investigators. Global Utilization of Streptokinase and Tissue Plasminogen Activator for Occluded Coronary Arteries. J Am Coll Cardiol 1997 (1):171–9.

41. Berger AK, Breall JA, Gersh BJ, et al. Effect of diabetes mellitus and insulin use on survival after acute myocardial infarction in the elderly (the Cooperative Cardiovascular Project). Am J Cardiol 2001; 87:272.

42. Murcia AM, Hennekens CH, Lamas GA, et al. Impact of diabetes on mortality in patients with myocardial infarction and left ventricular dysfunction. Arch Intern Med 2004; 164:2273.

43. Aguilar D, Solomon SD, Kober L, Rouleau JL, Skali H; McMurray JJ; Francis GS; Henis M; O'Connor CM; Diaz R; Belenkov YN; Varshavsky S; Leimberger JD; Velazquez EJ; Califf RM; Pfeffer MA Newly diagnosed and previously known diabetes mellitus and 1-year outcomes of acute myocardial infarction: the VALsartan In Acute myocardial iNfarcTion (VALIANT) trial. Circulation 2004 Sep 21; 110(12):1572–8. Epub 2004 Sep 13.

44. Gilpin E, Ricon F, Dittrich H, et al. Factors associated with recurrent myocardial infarction within one year after acute myocardial infarction. Am Heart J 1991; 121:457.

45. Franklin K, Goldberg RJ, Spencer F, Klein W, et al. Implications of diabetes in patients with acute coronary syndromes. The Global Registry of Acute Coronary Events. Arch Intern Med 2004 Jul 12;164(13):1457–63.

46. Malmberg K, Yusuf S, Gerstein HC, et al. Impact of diabetes on long-term prognosis in patients with unstable angina and non-Q-wave myocardial infarction. Results of the OASIS (Organization to Assess Strategies for Ischemic Syndromes) Registry. Circulation 2000; 102:1014.

47. Kannel W, Hjortland M, Castelli W. Role of diabetes in congestive heart failure. The Framingham Study. Am J Cardiol 1974; 34:29.

48. Nichols GA, Hillier TA, Erbey JR, Brown JB. Congestive heart failure in type 2 diabetes: prevalence, incidence, and risk factors. Diabetes Care 2001; 24:1614.

49. Bertoni AG, Hundley WG, Massing MW, et al. Heart failure prevalence, incidence, and mortality in the elderly with diabetes. Diabetes Care 2004; 27:699.

50. Iribarren C, Karter AJ, Go AS, et al. Glycemic control and heart failure among adult patients with diabetes. Circulation 2001; 103:2668.

51. Yoon YS, Uchida S, Masuo O, et al. Progressive attenuation of myocardial vascular endothelial growth factor expression is a seminal event in diabetic cardiomyopathy: restoration of microvascular homeostasis and recovery of cardiac function in diabetic cardiomyopathy after replenishment of local vascular endothelial growth factor. Circulation 2005; 111:2073.

52. Shindler DM, Kostis JB, Yusuf S, et al. for the SOLVD Investigators. Diabetes mellitus, a predictor of morbidity and mortality in the studies of left ventricular dysfunction (SOLVD) Trials and Registry. Am J Cardiol 1996; 77:1017.

53. Dries DL, Sweitzer NK, Drazner MH, et al. Prognostic impact of diabetes mellitus in patients with heart failure according to the etiology of left ventricular systolic dysfunction. J Am Coll Cardiol 2001; 38:421.

54. Shekelle PG, Rich MW, Morton SC, et al. Efficacy of angiotensin-converting enzyme inhibitors and beta-blockers in the management of left ventricular systolic dysfunction according to race, gender, and diabetic status: a meta-analysis of major clinical trials. J Am Coll Cardiol 2003; 41:1529.

55. Moye LA, Pfeffer MA, Wun CC, et al. Uniformity of captopril benefit in the SAVE Study: subgroup analysis. Survival and Ventricular Enlargement Study. Eur Heart J 1994; 15Suppl B:2.

56. Hirsch IB, Kelly J, Cooper S. Pulmonary edema associated with troglitazone therapy. Arch Intern Med 1999; 159:1811.

57. Thomas ML Lloyd, SJ. Pulmonary edema associated with rosiglitazone and troglitazone. Ann Pharmacother 2001; 35:123.

58. Dormandy JA, Charbonnel B, Eckland DJ, et al. Secondary prevention of macrovascular events in patients with type 2 diabetes in the PROactive Study (PROspective pioglitAzone Clinical Trial In macroVascular Events): a randomised controlled trial. Lancet 2005; 366:1279.

59. Masoudi FA, Inzucchi SE, Wang Y, et al. Thiazolidinediones, metformin, and outcomes in older patients with diabetes and heart failure: an observational study. Circulation 2005; 111:583.

60. FDA. Available from the US Food and Drug Administration website at www.fda.gov/medwatch/safety/1997/nov97.htm#glucop (Accessed 3/7/05).

31 | Anesthesia and Surgery in the Diabetic Patient

Jeffrey I. Joseph
Department of Anesthesiology, The Artificial Pancreas Center, Jefferson Medical College, Thomas Jefferson University, Philadelphia, Pennsylvania, U.S.A.

APPROACH TO THE SURGICAL PATIENT WITH HYPERGLYCEMIA

Diabetic and non-diabetic patients develop hyperglycemia during surgery and medical illness due to enhanced hepatic gluconeogenesis, relative insulin deficiency, and decreased sensitivity of the liver, skeletal muscle, and adipose tissue to the actions of insulin (1–3). While clinical evidence suggests a direct association between hyperglycemia and adverse outcome in patients undergoing vascular and cardiac surgery, there is little prospective data available to indicate that glucose control improves outcome in the average hyperglycemic patient undergoing other types of surgical procedures (4–13). The adverse effects of hyperglycemia are mediated in large part by enhanced oxidative stress, which is not counter-balanced by endogenous antioxidants.

The optimal range of blood glucose (BG) control in a specific patient population remains controversial. The fear of hypoglycemia (change in mental status, seizure, coma, myocardial ischemia, arrhythmia, and death) dictates the psychology of diabetes management in the hospital setting. Nurses and physicians err on the side of hyperglycemia to avoid the consequences of low BG levels (14–17). Current therapeutic methods that attempt to maintain tight control (80–110 mg/dL) are associated with fluctuation in BG levels beyond the desired range and a high incidence of hypoglycemia (4,5,18). The incidence and severity of hypoglycemia are significantly increased when attempting to achieve tight BG control using intensive insulin therapy (5,19).

The BG range 100 to 180 mg/dL has traditionally been recommended to minimize the risk for hypoglycemia and the sequellae of hyperglycemia. Levels above 180 mg/exceed the renal threshold for glucose and increase the risk for dehydration and electrolyte imbalance (14–17). Levels above 200 mg/dL increase the risk of infection and worst clinical outcome following cerebral and myocardial ischemia. Even brief periods of hyperglycemia have been shown to adversely effect cellular and humoral immunity (7–8). Acute hyperglycemia delays gastric emptying and may increase the risk for aspiration pneumonia (21). Recent evidence suggests that high glycemic variability may be associated with increased morbidity and mortality (18).

The results of a landmark study performed by Van den Berghe et al. highlighted the importance of glucose control in an ICU population of medical and postoperative cardiac surgical patients. The prospective randomized trial was designed to determine a difference in clinical outcome resulting from an intravenous infusion of insulin titrated to achieve normal BG control (<110 mg/dL) versus insulin titrated to achieve moderate hyperglycemia (180–200 mg/dL). End-organ complications were decreased and long-term survival increased when BG levels were maintained <110 mg/dL. Mortality in the group of patients who required ICU care for more than five days decreased from 20.2% in the conventional-treatment group to 10.6% in the intensive-treatment group at 12 months post discharge. Death in the intensive care unit decreased from 8.0% to 4.6% (43% relative reduction). Intensive insulin therapy and tight glucose control provided the greatest protection from death by decreasing the incidence and severity of systemic infection (multiple-organ failure with a proven septic focus). The intensive-treatment group had an overall 34% reduction in hospital mortality, 46% reduction in bloodstream infections, 41% reduction in renal failure requiring dialysis, 50% reduction in the median number of red blood cell transfusions, and a reduction in the need for prolonged mechanical ventilation. Hypoglycemia, defined as a BG level less than 40 mg/dL, occurred in 39 patients in the intensive-treatment group ($N=765$) and six patients in the conventional-treatment group ($N=783$) (4).

Van den Berghe performed an identical prospective study in a cohort of medical patients requiring long-term intensive care. Similar to the original study, major adverse events were significantly reduced in patients treated aggressively with insulin. Mortality was significantly reduced in those hyperglycemic patients treated intensively with insulin (BG < 110 mg/dL) for three of more days. Although hypoglycemia (BG < 40 mg/dL) occurred in 22% of the patients treated with intensive insulin therapy, serious adverse events related to hypoglycemia were not reported (5).

A retrospective review of medical and surgical inpatients by Umpierrez et al. found a 38% prevalence of hyperglycemia. Patients that developed hyperglycemia had an 18-fold increase in (in-hospital) mortality, increased rate of infection, length of stay, and overall cost (22). A retrospective study of medical and surgical ICU patients by Krinsley et al. showed a close association between hyperglycemia and mortality. A follow-up prospective study by the same investigators documented a marked decrease in mortality, organ dysfunction, length of stay, and cost in ICU patients treated with intensive insulin therapy and tight BG control (10,11).

Furnary et al. studied the effects of intensive insulin therapy and tight BG control over 15 years in more than 3500 cardiac surgery patients. Subcutaneous tissue insulin injections were replaced by intravenous infusions of insulin, resulting in a decrease in the average BG from > 180 mg/dL to < 120 mg/dL. Risk-adjusted mortality was decreased significantly when the three-day average BG level was maintained < 150 mg/dL. The incidence of atrial fibrillation, deep sternal wound infection, length of stay, and overall cost were significantly reduced when glucose levels were aggressively controlled with intravenous insulin in the SCCU and surgical floor (6,7).

Two retrospective studies of patients undergoing cardiac surgery using an IV insulin infusion protocol revealed a close association with hyperglycemia and increased morbidity/mortality (8,9). Kalin et al studied CABG patients treated with an intravenous infusion of insulin. In-hospital mortality in the intensively managed group was similar to the mortality rate in a matched group of 876 patients without diabetes (1.75% vs. 1.71%) (23).

A position statement released by the American College of Clinical Endocrinologists in 2005 endorsed the prevention of hyperglycemia in all hospitalized patients, regardless of prior diabetic status. The multidisciplinary team of physicians recommended that insulin be aggressively titrated to keep BG levels < 110 mg/dL in medical ICU patients and cardiac surgery patients. Non-ICU patients should be maintained < 110 mg/dL pre-prandial and < 180 mg/dL post-prandial. The team also recommended that BG levels be maintained < 100 mg/dL during labor and delivery of term pregnancies (24). The risk/benefit ratio of tight BG control should be determined on an individual patient basis.

Tight glucose control has been achieved with a variety of regimens. A variable-rate intravenous infusion of regular insulin has been shown to be the most effective method of providing tight BG control in surgical patients with diabetes and stress induced hyperglycemia (4–11). Insulin dose algorithms are based upon physiological principles and the pharmacokinetic/dynamic profiles of intravenous insulin. An accurate bedside glucose meter, properly trained nurses, and frequent glucose monitoring are mandatory for the safe and effective application of intensive-insulin therapy. Higher glycemic goals are required in patients that experience hypoglycemia unawareness and when nursing issues prevent an adequate frequency of BG monitoring and bedside vigilance (14–17).

THE DIABETIC SURGICAL POPULATION

Approximately 4.0 million individuals with diabetes are admitted to U.S. hospitals each year. The majority of hospitalizations are related to the micro and macrovascular complications of diabetes, rather than the acute control of blood glucose. Diabetics require surgical procedures on the eye (laser retina), heart (coronary artery bypass surgery, PTCA), and major blood vessels (carotid endarterectomy, peripheral artery bypass surgery, AAA repair) more frequently than the non-diabetic population. Procedures related to the management of chronic renal failure (kidney transplantation, hemodialysis/peritoneal dialysis access formation) and other microvascular complications (limb amputation, I&D infection, penile prosthesis) are also required more frequently as a consequence of long-term hyperglycemia (25,26).

It is estimated that 6.0 million patients develop significant hyperglycemia each year while in the hospital. Many of these patients will have a prior diagnosis of type 1, type 2, gestational, or secondary diabetes. Approximately half of the hyperglycemic patients will have previously undiagnosed diabetes and will require insulin or oral hypoglycemic therapy following discharge from the hospital (27–29). A significant number of non-diabetic patients will develop hyperglycemia due to the metabolic effects of anesthesia, tissue trauma, pain, systemic illness, and infection (1–3). Although insulin is often required during the stressful event, medication is often not required following hospital discharge. The number of surgical patients with diabetes and impaired glucose tolerance (IGT) is expected to increase over the next 15 years, due to the aging baby-boom population, the sedentary lifestyle of the US population, and the increasing incidence of obesity (26,29).

It is important to identify patients that do not produce endogenous insulin (type 1 diabetes, ketosis prone) and those with limited endogenous insulin production (type 2 diabetes with severely impaired beta-cell function). This group of patients has the potential to develop clinically significant ketosis, acidosis, and unstable glucose metabolism. Type 2 diabetics previously treated by diet, exercise, and oral hypoglycemic agents should not develop ketosis, because sufficient endogenous insulin is produced to inhibit lipolysis and partial oxidation of free fatty acids (15–17).

THE METABOLIC STRESS RESPONSE

The clinical course of the surgical patient can be characterized by predictable physiological changes (hormonal, metabolic, and hemodynamic) that occur along a continuum (Table 1). Perioperative complications can be avoided with timely recognition of an inadequate compensatory response (deviations from the expected pattern) followed by appropriate supportive care.

Cellular metabolism, core temperature, and peripheral blood flow decrease during anesthesia, and remain low in the immediate postoperative period. Physiological processes not essential to the survival of the patient decrease to basal levels. Blood flow is preferentially diverted to the vital organs and wound. The disruption of capillaries and tissue edema within the surgical wound requires increased blood flow for the delivery of essential cellular

TABLE 1   The Metabolic Stress Response to Anesthesia and Major Surgery in Patients with Type 2 Diabetes

	Preop. Fasting	Anesthesia	Evening surgery	Postoperative day 1	Postoperative day 3
Insulin secretion	−	−	±	±	±
Insulin sensitivity	−	−	−	−	−
Glucagon	+	−	−	±	±
Epinephrine	+	++	+++	++	+
Norepinephrine	+	++	+++	+++	++
Cortisol	+	++	+++	++	++
Growth hormone	−	+	+	+	+
Glycogenolysis	+++	++	++	+	+
Gluconeogenesis	−	++	+++	+++	++
Proteolysis	+	+	++	++	+
Lipolysis	+	±	±	±	±
Ketogenesis	++	+	±	±	±
Heart rate	±	±	+++	++	++
Respiratory rate	±	−	++	++	++
Cardiac contractility	±	−	++	++	++

Abbreviations: + increased effect, − decreased effect, +/− variable effect. Effects may be attenuated by anesthetic/analgesic techniques and cardiovascular medications.

nutrients. The wound requires elevated levels of oxygen, glucose, free fatty acids, amino acids, lactic acid, and ketone bodies to satisfy the nutritional needs of neutrophils, macrophages, and fibroblasts. Blood levels of catecholamines (epinephrine, norepinephrine), catabolic hormones (glucagon, cortisol, growth hormone), and cytokines (interleukin-1, tumor necrosis factor) increase in proportion to the degree of tissue injury and the number of white blood cells invading the surgical wound (1–3). Insulin resistance and enhanced hepatic/renal gluconeogenesis are most pronounced immediately after surgery and decrease over several days. The hyperdynamic and catabolic response (proteolysis, lipolysis, and gluconeogenesis) slowly resolve once new capillaries form within the healing wound. A prolonged stress response suggests inadequate nutrient delivery to the wound or infection (3,12,13). Still unanswered is whether hyperglycemia is a mechanism to optimize wound homeostasis or an unwanted side effect of the stress response?

PREOPERATIVE EVALUATION OF THE DIABETIC PATIENT

A surgical procedure cannot be considered successful unless the patient recovers with an equal or improved quality of life and long-term survival. Patients with long standing diabetes are at increased risk for developing complications. The goal of preoperative assessment is to identify patient risk factors and quantify risk, in order to decide the appropriateness of the planned surgical procedure and the timing of surgery. History, physical, and selective tests are used to identify the presence and severity of co-existing disease. The patient's condition can then be optimized prior to anesthesia and surgery. Procedures of short duration with minimal tissue trauma, blood loss, and fluid shifts are usually well tolerated (even by the high-risk patient). Elderly patients requiring emergency surgery (especially on the heart and great vessels) experience the highest risk. Successful outcomes require surgical skill and close communication between the physicians, nurses, and patient. A well-developed and implemented treatment plan remains the key to avoiding complications that may lead to decreased quality of life and premature death.

Patients with diabetes are at increased risk for developing chronic renal failure. Diabetic nephropathy progresses to renal insufficiency/failure in 35% of type 1 and 10% of type 2 diabetics. The duration of diabetes, degree of glycemic control, and level of proteinuria are useful to estimate the severity of preexisting nephropathy. The highest incidence of perioperative renal failure has been documented in older diabetics following cardiac and vascular surgery. Renal parenchyma may be injured by decreased renal blood flow (low cardiac output, prolonged hypotension, or surgical clamp), atherosclerotic emboli, free hemoglobin, nephrotoxic antibiotics, radiographic contrast agents, and sepsis. Chronic use of ACE inhibitors has been associated with an increased risk of perioperative renal insufficiency. Modern anesthetic agents rarely cause direct renal tissue damage. Adequate hydration (optimal renal blood flow) is mandatory to decrease the risk for acute renal failure (30).

Patients with diabetic neuropathy may be at increased risk for developing a peripheral nerve injury during surgery. Diabetic nerves may be more susceptible to ischemia from stretch and compression, leading to permanent disability. The brachial plexus, ulnar nerve, and sciatic nerve are most commonly affected (31). Whether transient hyperglycemia increases the incidence of perioperative nerve injury is unknown.

Although uncommon, aspiration pneumonia may lead to prolonged mechanical ventilation and death. The risk for aspiration may be increased in the diabetic patient due to gastroparesis (solid food remains in stomach >12 h) and increased difficulty placing an endotracheal tube (obesity and stiff cervical spine). Transient hyperglycemia is known to reduce gastric motility and delay gastric emptying. Pro-motility agents and proton pump inhibitors may be indicated in select diabetics (31,32). Patients should be weaned as quickly as possible from mechanical ventilation to minimize the risk of nosocomial pneumonia.

The risk of infection is increased in diabetic surgical patients. Proven methods to decrease the risk of infection include maintaining normal body temperature, normal nutritional status, and near-normal blood glucose control. Intravenous and urinary catheters should be inserted using strict aseptic technique and removed as quickly as possible (12,13,30).

Diabetes and impaired glucose tolerance are major risk factors for the development of atherosclerotic vascular disease (33–36). Diabetics have a nearly six-fold greater risk for developing a first-time myocardial infarction (20.2% vs. 3.5%) and a higher rate of re-infarction (45% vs. 18.8 %) when compared to non-diabetics (37). Associated risk factors (hypertension, dyslipidemia, family history, central obesity, and smoking) greatly increase the risk of a diabetic dying from cardiovascular disease (34,35). Myocardial infarction (MI) continues to be the leading cause of mortality in hospitalized patients with diabetes. The incidence of perioperative MI (<7 days after non-cardiac surgery) in patients without a history of previous MI, has been reported in the range of 0.13% to 0.66%. A higher incidence has been confirmed in patients with diabetes. Patients that have experienced a previous MI have an increased risk of acute MI in the perioperative period (4.3–15.9%). The incidence of myocardial ischemia and MI peaks during the 24 to 72 h after surgery. The risk of perioperative MI increases significantly for 3 to 6 months following an acute MI (range 6–54% risk). After 6 months, the risk for perioperative MI decreases to approximately 4% to 6%. Elective surgery should be delayed 6 months following an acute MI, especially if non-invasive studies reveal significant myocardium at risk (33–41).

Perioperative MI is associated with a high mortality (27–69%) compared to acute MI not associated with surgery (15–20%), with the greatest mortality occurring in diabetic patients that develop congestive heart failure (38). Diabetic hearts have decreased coronary flow reserve, decreased contractile reserve, and decreased compensatory response of the non-infarcted myocardial segments (40). The pathophysiology of perioperative MI is the same as acute MI in the non-surgical setting (41). In addition, surgery and diabetes produce a hyperdynamic and mildly prothrombotic state, making the diabetic coronary artery more prone to fissure and thrombosis. Myocardial ischemia and infarction are almost always silent in the perioperative period, and may not be associated with Q-waves or ST-segment elevation (31,32).

A number of clinical scoring systems have been developed to more accurately define cardiovascular risk in the perioperative setting (33,39). Recent scoring systems place more emphasis on active co-existing conditions and the location/complexity of the proposed surgical procedure (36). The American Heart Association's Task Force on Practice Guidelines has defined perioperative risk based upon end-organ pathology and whether the disease process is stable or unstable. Long-standing diabetes was judged an intermediate predictor of cardiovascular risk. Coronary angiography may be useful to define therapy in high-risk patients, or intermediate-risk patients about to undergo a high-risk surgical procedure (42). The benefit of pre-operative angioplasty with stent placement has not been evaluated in a controlled trial. Successful CABG surgery has been shown to decrease the risk of MI following subsequent non-cardiac surgery (32). Emergent CABG surgery prior to urgent non-cardiac surgery cannot be recommended due to excessive risk.

Intra- and postoperative beta-blockade has been shown to protect the myocardium from ischemia/infarction and improve long-term outcome. Beta-blockade has been used in many surgical patients with diabetes and heart failure without adverse effect (31,37,39).

Diabetic patients with a prior stroke are at increased risk for stroke in the perioperative period. The highest incidence of cerebral ischemia and stroke follows cardiac and vascular surgery. Focal ischemia occurs when atherosclerotic emboli travel from the thoracic and cerebral arteries to the brain (43). The area of cerebral ischemia at risk of infarction may increase due to enhanced coagulation and decreased fibrinolysis. Hemodynamic instability due to anesthetics, dehydration, autonomic neuropathy, cardiopulmonary bypass, and heart failure may increase the risk for global cerebral ischemia (31,32,40).

RATIONALE FOR CONTROL OF BLOOD GLUCOSE

Normal metabolism should be mimicked as closely as possible. Therapeutic goals include the avoidance of hypoglycemia, hyperglycemia, lipolysis, ketogenesis, proteolysis, dehydration, and electrolyte imbalance. Type 1 diabetic patients should receive a continuous supply of insulin to avoid ketosis. Sufficient insulin should be supplied to counterbalance the hyperglycemic effects epinephrine, norepinephrine, cortisol, glucagon, and growth hormone

(1,4,7). High rates of glucose infusion often exceed the body's ability to utilize glucose and cause hyperglycemia in both diabetic and non-diabetic surgical patients.

HYPOGLYCEMIA

Factors that predispose the surgical patient to hypoglycemia include prolonged fasting, inadequate/delayed food intake, changing insulin sensitivity, variability in subcutaneous insulin absorption, and changing renal function (5,19,44,45). The danger of hypoglycemia may be increased because the signs and symptoms of neuroglycopenia are masked by sedatives, anesthetics, and cardiovascular medications (16). Signs of hypoglycemia (diaphoresis, tachycardia, arrhythmia, and hypertension) may be mistaken for inadequate levels of analgesia or anesthesia (31). Changes in mental status, including focal neurological symptoms, may persist for hours to days following even a single episode of severe neuroglycopenia.

Frequent blood glucose monitoring is the key to avoiding hypoglycemia. Although the optimal frequency of monitoring has not been determined, many experts recommend hourly blood glucose measurements during and immediately following major surgery (5,7,14,16). Less frequent monitoring (every 2–6 h) has been recommended following the return of metabolic stability (5,7). Diabetics with high insulin sensitivity and hypoglycemia unaware-ness should be monitored more closely. Unfortunately, many clinicians do not monitor glucose levels with the recommended frequency. Golden et al. studied 411 adult diabetics undergoing CABG surgery. Only six capillary blood glucose measurements were taken during the 36-h period following surgery. The mean blood glucose level exceeded 200 mg/dL in more than 75% of the patients and one patient experienced severe hypoglycemia (12). Other reports document a low frequency of blood glucose monitoring in the perioperative period (16,17,46).

Many experts recommend an infusion of glucose to minimize the risk of hypoglycemia (8,14,15,16). Approximately 100 to 125 g of exogenous glucose per day are required to meet the basal caloric needs of the surgical patient, prevent ketosis, and prevent excessive protein breakdown. The additional calories required in the post-operative period can be provided with an infusion of glucose averaging 1.2 to 2.4 mg/kg/min (515 g/h for an adult) (17,27,47)]. Higher rates of glucose infusion often exceed the body's ability to utilize glucose and cause hyperglycemia.

Anesthesiologists commonly infuse non-glucose containing fluids during surgery to avoid hyperglycemia. Withholding glucose has been justified by the high incidence of hyperglycemia and low incidence of hypoglycemia during surgery (31). Controlled studies are needed to more clearly define the clinical importance of exogenous glucose (and other nutrients) during and after major surgery. Intravenous glucose should be used in the post-operative period rather than glucagon to treat hypoglycemia due to depleted hepatic glycogen stores.

DIABETIC KETOACIDOSIS

Increased catecholamine and catabolic hormone levels combine with an absolute or relative insulin deficiency to cause lipolysis and ketoacidosis (DKA). Clinically significant ketosis and acidosis can occur even when blood glucose levels are only modestly elevated. Many cases of DKA have occurred in patients with plasma glucose concentrations < 300 mg/dL. Euglycemic DKA (100 mg/dL glucose range) has been reported in surgical patients (2). Patients with DKA caused by a medical etiology often present with symptoms resembling an acute surgical abdomen. Surgery should be delayed until the underlying cause is identified, because abdominal symptoms often resolve following hydration and improved metabolic control (31). Although much more common in patients with type 1 diabetes, DKA can occur in type 2 diabetics with insulin resistance and limited endogenous insulin production (14,15,16,17).

HYPEROSMOLAR NONKETOTIC SYNDROME

Surgical patients with diabetes and impaired glucose tolerance are susceptible to volume depletion and electrolyte imbalance leading to the hyperosmolar nonketotic syndrome. Intravenous fluids are required to replace the pre-existing volume deficient, hemorrhage, third-space losses, GI losses, and the ongoing osmotic diuresis. Appropriate attention to intravascular volume will facilitate hepatic/renal blood flow and correction of the hyperosmolar condition. Placement of a pulmonary artery catheter and/or transesophageal endoscope (TEE) may provide useful data to guide fluid management, especially in the diabetic with renal insufficiency or decreased cardiac reserve (31).

NOSOCOMIAL INFECTION

Hyperglycemia has been firmly established as an independent risk factor for the development of infection. In animal and human studies, even brief periods of hyperglycemia interfere with leukocyte chemotaxis, opsinization, and phagocytosis (20). Furnary et al. demonstrated in a prospective, controlled study of coronary artery bypass patients, that tight glucose control can decrease the incidence of deep sternal wound infection (2.0–0.8%) (6). Other perioperative studies have demonstrated an association between tight blood glucose control and decreased risk for bacteremia, pneumonia, sepsis, cystitis, and wound infection (12,13,20).

WOUND STRENGTH

Hyperglycemia may affect fibroblast function during the period of granulation tissue formation and maturation. Decreased levels and cross-linking of collagen may impair wound healing and wound strength. Animal and human studies have demonstrated impaired wound healing/strength when blood glucose levels exceed 200 mg/dL in the days following surgery.

PERIOPERATIVE MI, CHF, STROKE

Controlled studies have tried to define whether tight glucose control using intensive insulin therapy can improve long-term outcome following acute MI. The diabetes insulin glucose in acute myocardial infarction (DIGAMI) study randomized acute MI patients to receive either conventional diabetes care or tight glucose control using an intravenous infusion of glucose-insulin-potassium (GIK) followed by multiple daily subcutaneous insulin injections. In-hospital mortality decreased 58%, one-year mortality decreased 52%, and three-year mortality decreased 25% in diabetics managed with intensive therapy (48). Glucose-insulin-potassium infusions have been recommended to promote myocardial utilization of glucose for energy production (12,35). Fatty acids are preferentially utilized by the myocardium when insulin levels are deficient, leading to enhanced oxygen consumption, and an increased incidence of myocardial ischemia, arrhythmias, and contractile dysfunction (1,2,3).

Capes et al. performed a retrospective meta-analysis of 15 clinical studies of acute MI patients. Non-diabetics with stress hyperglycemia following an acute MI (above 109–124 mg/dL) had a four-fold increased rate of in-hospital mortality. Diabetic patients with hyperglycemia (above 124–180 mg/dL range) had a two-fold increased rate of in-hospital mortality. Hyperglycemia was also associated with an increased incidence of post MI congestive heart failure and cardiogenic shock (49).

Independent of previous cardiac disease, diabetes, or other co morbidities, McGirt et al. determined that hyperglycemia at the time of carotid endarterectomy (CEA) was associated with an increased risk of perioperative stroke or transient ischemic attack, myocardial infarction, and death. The authors suggested that strict glucose control be attempted before surgery to minimize the risk of morbidity and mortality after CEA (50). Hyperglycemia is associated with increased infarct size and worsened long-term outcome following cerebral ischemia (51). Elevated HbA_{1c} and blood glucose levels at the time of hospital admission have been shown to correlate with cerebral infarct size and long-term prognosis (43). Controlled trials are underway to determine whether tight glucose control can improve outcome following cerebral ischemia, stroke, or spinal cord injury.

GLYCEMIC GOALS

Although AACE guidelines recommend that glucose levels be controlled in all hyperglycemic inpatients, regardless of previous diabetes status, glycemic goals in the perioperative period remain controversial (5,7,9,11,18,19,24). Previous reviews recommend target glucose levels in the 100 to 180 mg/dL range. This level of glycemia was selected to prevent dehydration (osmotic diuresis) and infection and to minimize the risk of hypoglycemia (14–17). Recent outcome studies have advocated tighter glucose control. The prospective, controlled studies by Van Den Berge et al. in medical and surgical ICU patients demonstrate that intravenous insulin therapy aggressively titrated to achieve BG control < 110 mg/dL, significantly reduced morbidity and mortality. Unfortunately, intensive insulin therapy has been associated with a high incidence of hypoglycemia (4,5).

METHODS TO ACHIEVE NEAR-NORMAL GLUCOSE CONTROL

Treatment regimens should focus on safety and simplicity to minimize the risk for errors that may cause hypoglycemia. A program established by the United States Pharmacopoeia to track hospital drug errors reported that errors involving insulin delivery ranked second in number, and ranked first as the leading cause of patient morbidity (52). Simplicity is also required because overworked nurses and junior physicians often undertake bedside management. A variety of insulin delivery algorithms are currently used to manage blood glucose levels in the perioperative setting.

Variable-Rate Intravenous Insulin Infusion Regimen

A variable-rate intravenous infusion of regular insulin is the safest and most versatile way to manage blood glucose levels during and after major surgery (Table 2). The safety of an intravenous infusion regimen has been demonstrated in the operating room, intensive care unit, and general surgical floor (2,9,11,42). The usual starting dose for a variable-rate insulin infusion is 1.0 U/h, with smaller starting doses recommended in patients with high insulin sensitivity (athletes and thin women). Higher starting doses of insulin (2.0–4.0 U/h) are recommended in patients with insulin resistance and to increase the time to metabolic decompensation should there be an interruption of insulin delivery (53). The majority of

TABLE 2   Variable-Rate, Intravenous Infusion of Regular Insulin

Replace Chlorpropamide 5 days before surgery with short-acting sulphonylurea. Discontinue Metformin 48 h before procedures associated with renal dysfunction (risk for lactic acidosis).
Withhold oral hypoglycemic agent(s) the morning of surgery.
If non-emergent surgery, control BG prior to procedure (90 to 180 mg/dL).
Hold solid food for > 8 h (longer with history gastroparesis). Clear liquids permitted until 2 h before surgery.
Antihypertensive and antianginal medication taken with water.
Measure fasting BG level with calibrated bedside glucose monitor.
Provide usual dose of intermediate-acting insulin at bedtime, the evening before surgery.
Insist upon early admission to hospital. Start intravenous infusion of 10% glucose in water or 0.45 N saline (510 g/h) around 7:00 AM. Infuse isotonic saline solution if dehydrated due to bowel prep, prolonged fast, or osmotic diuresis.
Prepare an insulin solution that contains 250 Units short-acting (regular) insulin in 250 ml 0.9% saline (1 U/ml). Flush tubing with 50 ml insulin solution to minimize the effects of surface binding on insulin delivery.
Start intravenous infusion of insulin around 7:00 AM using a separate calibrated pump. Choose an initial insulin infusion rate, typically 1.0 U/h. Insulin and glucose infusions may be piggy-backed into the same intravenous catheter.
Measure BG at least once every hour during and following major surgery.
Titrate variable-rate insulin infusion to hourly BG measurements, intravenous glucose infusion rate, and anticipated level of metabolic stress (Table 3).
Determine optimal glycemic range for individual patient. Maintain blood glucose levels in 90 to 180 mg/dL range for average control, and 90 to 110 mg/dL for tight control. Frequent BG monitoring and aggressive insulin titrations are required to avoid hypoglycemia.
Inject 15 to 25 ml 50% glucose solution for symptomatic hypoglycemia.
Measure electrolytes daily. Hyponatremia and hypokalemia are common in the postoperative period.
Measure urine for glucose and ketones when BG > 200 mg/dL.
Convert variable-rate intravenous insulin regimen to a subcutaneous insulin regimen once the patient is tolerating solid food. Discontinue insulin infusion 30 to 60 min after injecting subcutaneous insulin (Table 6).
Adjust subcutaneous insulin-dosage schedule and reinstitute oral hypoglycemic agent(s) doses prior to hospital discharge.

clinicians use a variable-rate insulin infusion and a fixed-rate glucose infusion. The rate of insulin delivery is typically adjusted once per hour (0.5–4.0 U/h increase or decrease) based upon frequent blood glucose measurements and an algorithm (Table 3). Recent protocols base each adjustment in the rate of insulin delivery upon the absolute BG value, the direction of BG change, and the amount of change from the previous BG measurement (5,7,11,54,55). An algorithm using a variable-rate glucose infusion has also been described (Table 4).

Watts et al. were able to achieve tight glucose control (mean glucose 136 ± 15 mg/dL) with a low incidence of hypoglycemia using separate infusions of insulin and glucose. In contrast, patients managed with conventional therapy (subcutaneous sliding-scale insulin or fixed-rate insulin infusion) were not able to achieve near-normal BG control (mean glucose 208 ± 20 mg/dL, 30–306 mg/dL range) (47).

In general, diabetic surgical patients require 0.3 to 0.4 Units of insulin per gram of infused glucose per hour (0.3–0.4 U g^{1}/h^{1}) (14,15,16,17). Higher doses of insulin are required for patients with pre-existing or acquired insulin resistance due to obesity, systemic infection, hypothermic cardiopulmonary bypass, certain anesthetics, elevated catecholamine levels, and steroid therapy. Patients with renal, hepatic, and heart failure may require decreased insulin doses (44,56).

Glucose-Insulin-Potassium Intravenous Infusion Regimen

An alternative intravenous insulin regimen contains a fixed concentration of glucose, potassium, and regular insulin in one solution bag. The "GIK regimen" gained widespread clinical acceptance in the 1970s because of its simplicity and safety. Insulin and glucose are delivered in balanced proportions at a constant rate (100 ml/h) without the need for an electronic pump. Unfortunately, this method lacks flexibility and often fails to achieve desired glucose control, compared to the variable-rate method. Any significant change in the requirement for insulin, glucose, or potassium would necessitate a change from the original mixture to a new solution bag with the appropriate proportions (Table 5) (27,56).

Intermittent Intravenous Insulin Bolus Injection Regimen

The bolus intravenous injection of regular insulin is the most common method used by anesthesiologists to control blood glucose levels (44,46,47). This method is without physiological basis and cannot be recommended. The short pharmacokinetic (4–7 min) and

TABLE 3 Variable-Rate Insulin Infusion Regimen for Tight Blood Glucose Control (Fixed-Rate Glucose Infusion)

Blood glucose measurement (mg/dL)	Intravenous insulin dose
< 80	Discontinue infusion for 30 min; administer 20 to 30 ml 50% dextrose;
	Re-measure BG in 30 min
	Restart insulin infusion at 0.5 U/h after blood glucose > 100 mg/dL
81–120	Decrease rate by 0.3 U/h
121–180	No change in insulin infusion rate
181–240	Increase by 0.3 U/h
241–300	Increase by 0.6 U/h
> 300 mg/dL	Increase by 1 U/h

Note: Typical initial infusion rate 0.02 U kg^{-1} h^{-1} (~1.0–1.5 U^{-1}h^{-1}) may be adjusted higher for patients with insulin resistance, and lower for insulin-sensitive patients. Surgical patients generally require 0.3 to 0.4 U of insulin per gram of glucose infused per hour. Higher infusion rates are required in some patients with liver disease (0.5–0.6 U g^{-1} h^{-1}), sepsis (0.6–0.8 U g^{-1} h^{-1}), obesity (0.4–0.6 U g^{-1} h^{-1}), and those receiving catecholamine or glucocorticoid therapy (0.5–0.8 U g^{-1} h^{-1}). Lower infusion rates may be required with hepatic, renal, or congestive heart failure. Large doses of insulin are often required during anesthesia and surgery (especially hypothermic cardiopulmonary bypass) to counter the effects of insulin resistance. Frequent BG monitoring is required in the immediate postoperative period to avoid hypoglycemia following the resolution of insulin resistance.
Source: From Refs. 14, 15, 16, 17, 48, 54, 55, 56.

TABLE 4   Variable-Rate Insulin/Variable-Rate Glucose Infusion Regimen for Tight Blood Glucose Control

Blood glucose (mg/dL)	Intravenous insulin dose (U/h)	10% Glucose infusion rate (ml/h)
< 70	discontinue infusion[a]	75 ml/h
71–100	1.0 U/h	65 ml/h
101–150	1.5 U/h	50 ml/h
151–200	2.0 U/h	50 ml/h
201–250	3.0 U/h	50 ml/h
251–300	4.0 U/h	40 ml/h
> 300	12.0 U/h	25 ml/h

[a] Discontinue insulin infusion for 30 min; administer 10 to 20 ml 50% dextrose; re-measure blood glucose in 30 min, and restart insulin infusion after blood glucose > 100 mg/dL. Although this regimen is more difficult to implement in the clinical setting (two variables changed simultaneously), it has the potential to provide superior glycemic control with less risk for hypoglycemia.
Source: From Ref. 63.

biological half-life (< 60 min) of an IV insulin bolus produces extremely high (but short-lived) plasma and tissue insulin levels (15,45). Large bolus doses of insulin may saturate all of the insulin receptors, leading to a prolonged hypoglycemic effect (57,58).

Subcutaneous Injections of Insulin Regimen

Subcutaneous tissue injection continues to be the most common route for insulin delivery in the pre and post-operative period. Absorption of regular insulin from the subcutaneous tissue is often slow and variable. The coefficient of variation between patients has been shown to exceed 50% and intra-individual coefficient of variation exceeds 25% (45). Greater variability of absorption should be expected in the hospitalized patient.

Sliding-scale insulin regimens based upon retrospective hyperglycemia often fail to achieve the desired degree of glycemic control (12,16,27,44). This technique does not consider

TABLE 5   Fixed-Rate Glucose-Insulin-Potassium (GIK) Infusion Regimen

Replace Chlorpropamide 5 days before surgery with short-acting sulphonylurea. Discontinue Metformin 48 h before procedures associated with renal dysfunction (risk for lactic acidosis).
Withhold oral hypoglycemic agent(s) the morning of surgery.
If non-emergent surgery, control BG prior to procedure (90–180 mg/dL).
Hold solid food for > 8 h (longer with history gastroparesis). Clear liquids permitted until 2 h before surgery.
Antihypertensive and antianginal medication taken with water.
Measure fasting BG level with calibrated bedside glucose monitor.
Inject one-half usual morning dose of intermediate-acting insulin upon awakening. Inject one-half of usual morning dose of short-acting insulin if fasting BG level exceeds 200 mg/dL. Hold insulin for fasting BG levels < 100 mg/dL.
Insist upon early admission to hospital. Start intravenous infusion of 10% glucose in water or 0.45% saline (5 to 10 g/h) around 7:00 AM. Infuse isotonic saline solution if dehydrated due to bowel prep, prolonged fast, or osmotic diuresis.
Monitor BG hourly until the induction of anesthesia and surgery.
Replace glucose infusion with "GIK" solution, two hours prior to surgery. Mix glucose (5000 mg), regular insulin (15 Units), and potassium (10 mmol KCl) in 500 ml water to form a 10% dextrose "GIK" solution. Infuse at 100 ml/h through a peripheral vein.
Measure BG once-hourly during and immediately following major surgery. Frequency of BG monitoring may be decreased to every 2 to 4 h in fasting patients with residual endogenous insulin production, average insulin sensitivity, and no history of hypoglycemia unawareness.
Determine optimal glycemic range for individual patient. Maintain BG levels within 100 to 200 mg/dL range. Tight BG control (90 to 110 mg/dL) may be difficult to achieve with this regimen.
If BG > 200 mg/dL, change "GIK" solution to 20 Units insulin per 500 ml.
If BG < 90 mg/dL, change "GIK" solution to 5 Units insulin per 500 ml.
Inject 25 to 50 ml 50% glucose solution for symptomatic hypoglycemia.
Measure electrolytes daily and change "GIK" solution as necessary. Hyponatremia and hypokalemia are common in the postoperative period.
Measure urine for glucose and ketones when BG > 200 mg/dL.
Convert "GIK" to a subcutaneous insulin regimen once the patient is able to tolerate solid food. Discontinue "GIK" infusion 30 to 60 min after injecting subcutaneous insulin (Table 6).
Adjust subcutaneous insulin-dosage schedule and reinstitute oral hypoglycemic agent(s) prior to hospital discharge.

events that produce an increase in metabolic stress, the timing of meals, and the differences in insulin requirements at different times of the day (12). Despite its lack of recommendation in the recent medical literature, the sliding-scale method remains the most common technique for managing blood glucose levels in the perioperative period (44,59).

In contrast, insulin algorithms take into account patient and surgery specific information. The total amount of daily insulin is based upon the previous 24-h insulin requirement, carbohydrate load, degree of stress, level of patient activity, and presence of gluconeogenic medications (14–17,44). An intermediate-acting or long-acting insulin formulation (NPH or Glargine) is typically injected once to twice per day to supply approximately 50% of the patient's daily needs. Short-acting (Regular) or rapid-acting (Lispro) insulin is typically injected into the subcutaneous tissue prior to each meal or snack. The algorithm recommends small correction doses of short-acting insulin to fine-tune BG control. Regular insulin should be used with caution (or avoided) at bedtime to decrease the risk for early morning hypoglycemia (Table 6) (44,51,53).

Conversion of Intravenous Insulin Infusion to Subcutaneous Injections

Surgical patients are typically converted from an intravenous infusion of insulin to intermediate injections of insulin once tolerating a liquid diet. The morning dose of basal insulin (NPH or Glargine) and prandial insulin (Regular or Lispro) are injected prior to breakfast, according to the amount of insulin delivered over the prior 24-h, the anticipated carbohydrate composition of the meal, and the fasting BG measurement. The IV infusion of regular insulin is typically discontinued 60 min after injection of the sc insulin (16,17,44).

IN-HOSPITAL ARTIFICIAL ENDOCRINE PANCREAS

An artificial endocrine pancreas (AP) was commercialized in the 1970s (Biostator, Miles Laboratory) to automate the process of blood glucose monitoring and insulin delivery. The device contained a flow-through glucose sensor connected to an intravenous catheter. Glucose was measured every few minutes with accuracy similar to a laboratory glucometer. Insulin and glucose were infused according to a preprogrammed computer algorithm. The subsequent dose of insulin (or glucose) was based upon the absolute glucose concentration and the rate of change of blood glucose over time. Tight glucose control could be achieved without hypoglycemia in the majority of clinical situations. Unfortunately, the device was too large and complex for routine clinical application. The sensor required frequent manual re-calibration and greater than 200 ml blood loss per day (60). Researchers are attempting to develop more accurate glucose monitoring systems and a modern version of the AP that is safe and easy to use in the clinical setting.

TABLE 6 Postoperative Blood Glucose Management when Patient Tolerates Solid Food (Algorithm for Variable Subcutaneous Insulin Injections)

Blood Glucose (mg/dL)	Breakfast	Lunch	Dinner	2200
<70 mg/dL	3 U	2 U	2 U	0
71–100 mg/dL	4 U	3 U	3 U	0
101–150 mg/dL	6 U	4 U	4 U	0
151–200 mg/dL	8 U	6 U	6 U	0
201–250 mg/dL	10 U	8 U	8 U	1 U
251–300 mg/dL	12 U	10 U	10 U	2 U
>300 mg/dL	14 U	12 U	12 U	3 U

Note: Administer 10 to 15 U intermediate-acting or long-acting insulin upon awakening and/or bedtime.
Reduce NPH dose if hypoglycemia present at 0330.
Administer oral glucose or 20 to 40 ml 50% glucose solution (IV) for hypoglycemia. Continue glucose/insulin infusions until the patient is metabolically stable and tolerating solid food. Discontinue insulin/glucose infusions 30 to 60 min after the administration of subcutaneous insulin. Measure BG level before each meal, at 2200, and at 0300. Provide 3 meals and 3 small snacks per day (20 to 30 kcal/kg/day). Administer short-acting insulin 30 min before each meal. Make sure meals provided at appropriate time interval. Rapid-acting insulin may be given immediately prior to the meal. Dose insulin according to the above schedule.
Abbreviation: U, subcutaneous close of short-acting insulin.
Source: From Refs. 63,64.

PERIOPERATIVE MANAGEMENT OF THE TYPE 2 DIABETIC: MAJOR SURGERY

Type 2 diabetics unable to increase endogenous insulin secretion may behave metabolically in the perioperative period similar to the classic patient with type 1 diabetes (1,14,44). Insulin therapy and frequent blood glucose monitoring are required to minimize the risk for ketoacidosis and hypoglycemia (16,17). A variable-rate insulin infusion/fixed-rate glucose infusion method provides the greatest flexibility, safety, and degree of glycemic control.

Surgery should be scheduled as early in the morning as possible. A solution of glucose should be started around 7:00 AM and infused at a rate of 5 to 10 g/h. Patients that normally take NPH and regular insulin before breakfast may take one-half to two-thirds of their usual dose (of each type of insulin) on the morning of surgery. Regular insulin should be withheld if the fasting glucose measurement detects hypoglycemia. The dose should be increased if fasting glucose exceeds 200 mg/dL. Alternatively, patients may be given NPH or Glargine insulin at bedtime the night before surgery. Upon awakening, the patient can receive one-half to two-thirds of their usual morning dose of NPH insulin (with little or no regular insulin) or their full dose of Glargine. The NPH insulin dose from the evening before will peak around 6:00 to 9:00 AM and the morning dose will attenuate post-operative hyperglycemia (16,17,44). When early morning surgery is not feasible, the morning dose of subcutaneous insulin should be withheld and intravenous infusions of insulin and glucose started around 7:00 am and titrated to hourly glucose measurements. The infusions can be discontinued once the patient is able to tolerate food, or restarted if the patient experiences prolonged nausea and emesis (15). Following satisfactory return of GI function, subcutaneous regular insulin can be carefully titrated according to meals and the clinical situation (44).

Patients with type 2 diabetes previously managed by diet, exercise, and oral hypoglycemic agents should have sufficient endogenous insulin production to avoid ketosis and excessive hyperglycemia. Subcutaneous insulin regimens may be considered when the clinician anticipates a brief period of fasting in a patient with well-controlled BG levels. Short-acting sulfonylurea agents are typically held the day of surgery while the longer-acting agent Chlorpropamide is held for 2 to 3 days prior to surgery. The biguanide Metformin is typically held prior to surgery in patients at risk for renal or hepatic dysfunction due to the uncommon occurrence of lactic acidosis. Glucose levels must be monitored frequently if oral hypoglycemia agents are continued up until the day of surgery (14,44,61,62). Post-operative type 2 diabetic patients that require <24 units of insulin per day can be converted to oral agents once tolerating food. A significant number of diabetic patients previously on oral agents will require insulin following discharge from the hospital.

Patients using an external insulin pump with rapid-acting insulin (CSII) should continue basal rate therapy until the time of surgery. The pump should be removed prior to surgery, followed immediately by an intravenous infusion of regular insulin. Insulin should never be withheld in patients with suspected type 1 diabetes because ketoacidosis can develop while the patient is waiting for surgery.

PERIOPERATIVE MANAGEMENT OF THE TYPE 2 DIABETIC: OUTPATIENT SURGERY

Post operative glucose levels are often increased above 250 mg/dL when insulin or oral agents are withheld in type 2 diabetics undergoing outpatient surgery. This data has led to the recommendation that insulin therapy be considered for all type 2 diabetics managed with an oral hypoglycemic agent. Alternatively, type 2 diabetics well controlled by diet and exercise can be managed without insulin in the ambulatory surgical setting (61,62). Patients previously treated with insulin should receive subcutaneous insulin or an intravenous infusion of insulin. Oral hypoglycemic agents that are withheld prior to the surgical procedure should be given with the first post-operative meal. Patients that take an oral hypoglycemic agent while fasting should be started on an intravenous infusion of glucose (5–10 g/h) that can be titrated to hourly BG measurements. Patients that experience post-operative nausea and emesis are at increased risk for hypoglycemia and metabolic decompensation. Admission to the hospital may be required (16,17,44).

REFERENCES

1. McCowen KC, Malhotra A, Bistian BR. Endocrine and metabolic dysfunction syndromes in the critically ill: Stress-induced hyperglycemia. Critical Care Clinics 2001; 17:1:793–894.
2. Foster K, Alberti K, Binder C, et al. Lipid metabolism and nitrogen balance after abdominal surgery in man. Br J Surg 1979; 66:242–5.
3. Werb MR, Zinman B, Teasdale SJ, Goldman BS, Skully HE, Marliss EB. Hormone and metabolic responses during coronary artery bypass surgery: Role of infused glucose. J Clin Endocrinol Metab 1989; 69:1010–8.
4. Van den Berghe G, Wouters P, Weekers F, et al. Intensive insulin therapy in critical ill patients. N Engl J Med 2001; 345(19):1359–67.
5. Van den Berghe G, Wilmer A, Hermans G, Intensive insulin therapy in the medical ICU. N Engl J Med 2006; 354:449–61.
6. Furnary AP, Zerr KJ, Grunkemeier GL, Starr A. Continuous intravenous insulin infusion reduces the incidence of deep sternal wound infection in diabetic patients after cardiac surgical procedures. Ann Thoracic Surgery 1999; 67(2):352–60.
7. Furnary AP. Continuous insulin infusion reduces mortality in patients with diabetes undergoing coronary artery bypass grafting. J Thor Cardiovasc Surg 2003; 125(5):1007–21.
8. Outtara A. Poor intraoperative blood glucose control is associated with a worst hospital outcome after cardiac surgery in diabetic patients. Anesthesiology 2005; 103:687–94.
9. Gandi GJ. Intraoperative hyperglycemia and perioperative outcomes in cardiac surgery patients. Mayo Clin Proc 2005; 80:862–6.
10. Krinsley JS. Association of hyperglycemia and increased hospital mortality in a heterogeneous population of critically ill patients. Mayo Clin Proc 2003; 78:1471–9.
11. Krinsley JS. Effect of intensive glucose management protocol on the mortality of critically ill adult patients. Mayo Clin Proc 2004; 79(8):992–1000.
12. Golden SH, Peart-Vigilance C, Kao WH, Brancati FL. Perioperative glycemiac control and the risk of infectious complications in a cohort of adults with diabetes. Diabetes Care 1999; 22(9):1408–14.
13. Pomposelli JJ, Baxter JK 3rd, Babineau TJ, et al. Early postoperative glucose control predicts nosocomial infection rate in diabetic patients. J Parenteral & Enteral Nutrition 1998; 22(2):77–81.
14. Jacober SJ, Sowers JR. An update on perioperative management of diabetes. Arch of Intern Med 1999; 159:2405–11.
15. Hirsch IB, McGill JB. Role of insulin in management of surgical patients with diabetes mellitus. Diabetes Care 1990; 13:980–91.
16. Hirsch IB, McGill JB, Cryer PE, White PF. Perioperative management of Surgical Patients with Diabetes Mellitus. Anesthesiology 1991; 74:346–59.
17. Levetan CS, Magee MF. Hospital management of diabetes. Endocrinology clinics of North America 2000; 29(4):745–70.
18. Egi M, Bellomo R, Stachowski E, French C, Hart G. Variability of blood glucose concentrations and short-term mortality in critically ill patients. Anesthesiology 2006; 105(2):381–93.
19. Cryer P, Hypoglycemia is the limiting factor in the management of diabetes. Diabetes Met Res Rev. 1999; 15:42–6.
20. Rassias AJ, Marrin CA, Arruda J, Whalen PK, Beach M, Yeager MP. Insulin infusion improves neutrophil function in diabetic cardiac surgery patients. Anesth Anal 1999; 88(5):1011–6.
21. Hjortrup A, Sorensen C, Dyremose E, Hjortso N, Kehlet H. Influence of diabetes on operative risk. Br J Surg 1985; 72:785–7.
22. Umpierrez GE, Isaacs SD, Bazargan N. Hyperglycemia: an independent marker of in-hospital mortality in patients with undiagnosed diabetes. J Clin Endocrinol Metab 2002; 87:978–82.
23. Kalin MF, Tranbaugh RF, Salas J. Intensive intervention by a diabetes team diminishes excess hospital mortality in patients with diabetes who undergo coronary artery bypass graft. Diabetes 1998; 47:A87.
24. American College of Endocrinology Position Statement on Inpatient Diabetes and Metabolic Control. Endocrine Practice 2004; 10(1):77–82. (www.aace.org)
25. American Diabetes Association: Direct and indirect costs of diabetes in the United States. American Diabetes Association web site. Accessed November 2006. (www.diabetes.org/main).
26. National Center for Health Statistics web site. Center for Disease Control, U.S. Department of Health and Human Services. Accessed November 2006. (www.cdc.gov).
27. Pezzarossa A, Taddei F, Cimicchi MG, et al. Perioperative management of diabetic subjects: Subcutaneous versus intravenous insulin administration during glucose-potassium infusion. Diabetes Care 1988; 11:52–58.
28. Levetan CS, Passaro M, Jablonski K, Ratnere R. Unrecognized diabetes among hospitalized patients. Diabetes Care 1998; 21:246–9.
29. Diagnosis and classification of diabetes mellitus. Diabetes Care 2005; 28(supp 1):S37–42.

30. Mangano CM, Diamondstone LS, Ramsay JG, Aggarwal A, Herskowitz A, Mangano DT. Renal dysfunction after myocardial revascularization: risk factors, adverse outcomes, and hospital resource utilization. The Multicenter Study of Perioperative Ischemia Research Group. Ann Int Med 1998; 128(3):194–203.

31. Barash PG, Cullen BF, Stoelting RK. Clin Anesth. 3rd edn. Lippincott-Raven, 1997.

32. Mangano DT, Perioperative cardiac morbidity. Anesthesiology 1990; 72:153–84.

33. Cooperman M, Pflug B, Martin EW Jr, Evans WE. Cardiovascular risk factors in patients with peripheral vascular disease. Surgery 1978; 84(4):505–9.

34. Daviglus ML, Stamler J. Major risk factors and coronary heart disease: Much has been achieved but crucial challenges remain. J Am Coll Cardiol 2001 Oct; 38(4):1012–7.

35. Harris MI. Health care and health status and outcomes for patients with type 2 diabetes. Diabetes Care 2000; 23(6):754–8.

36. Ashton CM, Wray NP. Preoperative assessment of patients with coronary disease. New England J Med 1996; 334(16):1064–5.

37. Haffner SM, Lehto S, Ronnemaa T, Pyorala K, Laakso M. Mortality from coronary heart disease in subjects with type 2 diabetes and in nondiabetic subjects with and without prior myocardial infarction. N Engl J Med. 1998 Dec 3; 339(23):1714–5.

38. Steen PA, Tinker JH, Tarhan S. Myocardial reinfarction after anesthesia and surgery. J Am Med Assoc 1978: 239:256.

39. Goldman L. Assessing and reducing cardiac risks of non-cardiac surgery. Am J Med. 2001 Mar; 110 (4):260–6.

40. Roghi A, Palmieri B, Crivellaro W, Faletra F, Puttini M. Relationship of unrecognized myocardial infarction, diabetes mellitus and type of surgery to postoperative cardiac outcomes in vascular surgery. Eur Vascular Endovasc Surg 2001; 21(1):9–16.

41. Dawood MM, Gutpa DK, Southern J, Walia A, Atkinson JB, Eagle KA. Pathology of fatal perioperative myocardial infarction: implications regarding pathophysiology and prevention. Interna J Cardiol 1996; 57(1):37–44.

42. Scanlon PJ, Faxon DP, Audet AM, et al. ACC/AHA guidelines for coronary angiography. A report of the American College of Cardiology/American Heart Association Task Force on practice guidelines (Committee on Coronary Angiography). J Amer College of Cardiol 1999; 33(6):1756–824.

43. Kiers L, Davis S, Larkins R. Stroke topography and outcome in relation to hyperglycemia and diabetes. J Neurol Neurosurg Psychiatry 1992; 55:263–70.

44. Clement S, Braithwaite S, Magee M, et al. : Management of diabetes and hyperglycemia in hospitals. Diabetes Care 2004; 27:253–591.

45. Galloway JA, Spradlin CT, Howey DC, Dupre J. Intrasubject differences in pharmacokinetics and pharmacodynamic responses: the immutable problem of present-day treatment? Diabetes. Excerpta Medica 1986; 877–86.

46. Farkas-Hirsch R, Boyle PJ, Hirsch IB. Glycemic control of the surgical patient with IDDM. Diabetes 1989; (Suppl 2):39A.

47. Watts NB, Gebhart SP, Clark RV, Phillips RS. Perioperative management of diabetes mellitus: steady-state glucose control with bedside algorithm for insulin adjustment. Diabetes Care 1987; 10:722–8.

48. Malmberg K, Ryden L, Efendic S. Randomized trial of insulin-glucose infusion followed by subcutaneous insulin treatment in diabetic patients with acute myocardial infarction (DIGAMI study): effects on mortality at 1 year. J Am Coll Cardiol 1995; 26:57–65.

49. Capes SE, Hunt D, Malmberg K, Gerstein HC. Stress hyperglycemia and increased risk of death after myocardial infarction in patients with and without diabetes: a systematic overview. Lancet 2000; 355 (9206):773–8.

50. McGirt M, Woodworth Brooke G, Coon B, et al. Hyperglycemia independently increases the risk of perioperative stroke, myocardial infarction, and death after carotid endarterectomy. Neurosurgery 2006; 58(6):1066–73.

51. Golden S, Hill-Briggs F, Williams K, Stolka K, Mayer S. Management of diabetes during acute stroke and inpatient stroke rehabilitation. Arch Phys Med Rehab 2005; 86(12):2377–84.

52. US Pharmacopoeia report: Summary of 1999 information submitted to MedMARx. A national database for hospital medication error reporting (www.USPharmacopoeia.gov).

53. Gill GV. Surgery in patients with diabetes mellitus. Textbook of Diabetes. Blackwell Science 1997; Chapter 71:71.1–7.

54. Goldberg P, Siegal M, Sherwin R. Implementation of a safe and effective insulin infusion protocol in a medical intensive care unit. Diabetes Care 2004; 27(2):461–7.

55. Vora A, Improved perioperative glycemic control by continuous insulin infusion under supervision of an endocrinologist does not increase costs in patients with diabetes. Endocrine Practice 2004; 10 (2):112–8.

56. Alberti KG, Gill GV, Elliott MJ. Insulin delivery during surgery in the diabetic patient. Diabetes Care 1982; 5(Suppl 5):65–77.

57. King GL, Johnson SM. Receptor-mediated transport of insulin across endothelial cells. Science 1985; 277:1583–6.
58. Steil GM, Ader M, Moore DM, Rebrin K, Bergman RN. Transendothelial insulin transport is not saturable in vivo. J Clin Invest 1996; 97:1497–503.
59. Genuth SM. The automatic (regular insulin) sliding scale or 2, 4, 6, 8- call HO. Clin Diabetes 1994; 12: 40–2.
60. Albisser AM, Leibel BS, Ewart TG, Davidovac Z, Botz CK, Zingg W. An artificial endocrine pancreas. Diabetes 1974; 23(5):389–96.
61. Husband DJ, Tahi AC, Alberti KG. Management of diabetes during surgery with glucose-insulin-potassium infusion. Diabetic Med 1986; 3:69–74.
62. Malling B, Knudsen L, Christiansen BA, Schurizek BA, Hermansen K. Insulin treatment in non-insulin-dependent diabetic patients undergoing minor surgery. Diabetes Nutr Metab 1989; 2:125–31.
63. Rosenstock J, Raskin P. Surgery: practical guidelines for diabetes management. Clin Diabetes 1987; 5: 49–61; Gill GV. Surgery in patients with diabetes mellitus. In: Pickup J, Williams eds. Textbook of Diabetes. Oxford: Blackwell Science, 1997:71.1–7.

32 | Type 2 Diabetes: Geriatric Considerations

Jill P. Crandall
Diabetes Research and Training Center, Institute for Aging Research,
Albert Einstein College of Medicine, Bronx, New York, U.S.A.

INTRODUCTION

The dramatic increase in the incidence and prevalence of type 2 diabetes affects all age groups and has led to a notable increase in type 2 diabetes in children and young adults. Nonetheless, diabetes remains very much a disease of the elderly. The prevalence of known cases of diabetes increases from 6% for persons aged 45 to 64 years, to 15% for those aged 65 and older, with an additional 7% to 12% having undiagnosed diabetes (Fig. 1) (1,2). In addition, up to 30% of people over age 65 have impaired glucose regulation (IGR) [impaired glucose tolerance (IGT) or impaired fasting glucose (IFG)], a condition that increases the risk of diabetes as well as cardiovascular disease (3). In total, abnormal glucose regulation affects almost half of older adults and has substantial impact on public health and clinical care. Medical care for patients with diabetes is costly; approximately two-thirds of all medical costs related to diabetes are attributable to the elderly (4). As the U.S. population ages, the burden of diabetes care will undoubtedly increase and it is essential that healthcare providers be prepared to address the specific needs of elderly patients with diabetes.

Diabetes is not only more common among the elderly, but also has distinct and characteristic clinical presentations. Older adults with long-duration diabetes ("survivors of middle-aged diabetes") frequently have a high burden of microvascular complications, multiple co-morbidities such as hypertension and coronary heart disease, and often require insulin treatment to achieve adequate glucose control (5). On the other hand, new-onset diabetes in the elderly may be relatively mild and is often undetected unless vascular complications or acute metabolic decompensation occur. Recognition of this heterogeneity of diabetes in the elderly is a key factor in the planning and implementation of appropriate treatment.

AGE-RELATED CHANGES IN GLUCOSE METABOLISM

There is substantial evidence that age-related impairment in both insulin action and beta cell function are key factors in the high incidence of diabetes in the elderly (6,7). Typical changes in body composition, including an increase in overall adiposity, but especially visceral adipose tissue appear to be the major factors responsible for the resistance to insulin action (8). This effect is, at least in part, mediated by alterations in fat-derived peptides (adiponectin, TNF-alpha, leptin) and increased circulating free fatty acid levels (9). Reduction in skeletal muscle mass (sarcopenia) and infiltration of muscle tissue by fat may also contribute to impaired insulin-mediated glucose disposal (10). Defective inhibition of hepatic glucose production by insulin is an additional contributor to glucose intolerance with aging (11).

Insulin secretion in response to an oral glucose challenge, including reduction in both first and second phase insulin secretion (12,13), is characteristically impaired, even in normal aging. Similar alterations in insulin secretion following a mixed meal have also been reported (6) and suggest there is an intrinsic alteration in beta cell function. Beta cell mass may decline with age, but functional defects in insulin processing and exocytosis likely make a greater contribution to the age-related secretory defect. Hepatic insulin extraction is greater in the elderly and whole-body insulin clearance is lower, factors that reflect the complexity of changes in insulin and glucose metabolism with aging (6).

Additional factors contribute to the high rate of diabetes in the elderly, including medication use (glucocorticoids, thiazide diuretics, atypical anti-psychotics, etc.), sedentary lifestyle and dietary habits.

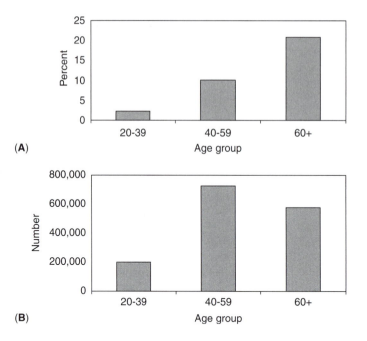

FIGURE 1 (**A**) Estimated total prevalence of diabetes in people aged 20 years or older by age group in the United States, 2005. (**B**) Estimated number of new cases of diagnosed diabetes in people aged 20 years or older by age group in the United States, 2005. *Source*: From Ref. 1.

CLINICAL PRESENTATION OF TYPE 2 DIABETES IN THE ELDERLY

Diagnosis

Criteria for the diagnosis of diabetes by American Diabetes Association (ADA) or World Health Organization (WHO) criteria do not differ by age (14,15). However, there are important differences in the characteristic glucose profile of older adults. Fasting glucose levels increase modestly with age, but a more dramatic increase in post-challenge (or postprandial) glucose levels has been reported in most studies (Fig. 2) (16,17). In fact, the increased prevalence of undiagnosed diabetes and IGR in the elderly population is primarily a consequence of the substantial increase in post-challenge, rather than fasting, hyperglycemia. New cases of diabetes (which account for approximately half of diabetes cases in people ≥65 years) may be missed if fasting glucose levels alone are used for diagnosis (18). Screening for diabetes using an oral glucose tolerance test (OGTT) has the added advantage of detecting the presence of IGT, thus allowing for appropriate interventions aimed at reducing diabetes and cerebrovascular disease (CVD) risk. Universal screening with OGTT has not been recommended, but should be considered in selected patients.

Spectrum of Clinical Presentation

Type 2 diabetes is a heterogeneous disorder and is especially apparent among the elderly. Many survivors of middle-age onset diabetes have established micro and macrovascular complications and other co-morbidities. As is usual with a long duration of disease, these patients often require insulin treatment and may display labile glucose levels more typical of insulin-deficient or type 1 diabetes. Other patients with many years of diabetes have more stable glycemia, possibly because of preserved endogenous insulin production, and may be well controlled on simple oral therapy regimens. Need for anti-diabetic treatment may actually decline in some older patients because of weight loss, anorexia and declining renal function.

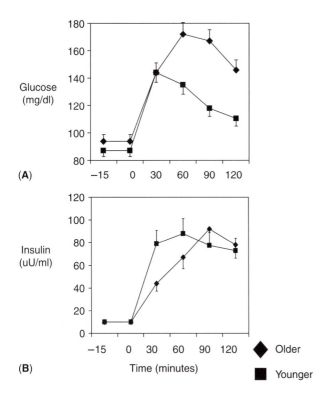

(A)

(B)

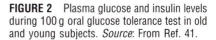

Older

Younger

FIGURE 2 Plasma glucose and insulin levels during 100 g oral glucose tolerance test in old and young subjects. *Source*: From Ref. 41.

Incident diabetes in the elderly also may present in a variety of ways, from mild asymptomatic hyperglycemia detected on a random glucose measurement to profound hyperglycemia with dehydration and coma. The elderly appear to be at greatest risk of hyperglycemic hyperosmolar state (HHS) for a variety of reasons, including altered thirst, inability to obtain adequate hydration due to dementia or immobility, concomitant use of diuretics and impaired renal concentrating ability. This serious disorder constitutes a true medical emergency requiring intensive care and has a high mortality rate.

Incident diabetes in the elderly may also present as mild, typically postprandial (or post-challenge) hyperglycemia that is generally asymptomatic, unrecognized and untreated. Although the degree of hyperglycemia may be modest, there is substantial evidence that CVD risk is increased (19,20) and appears to be equivalent to those with middle-age onset diabetes (5). Modification of CVD risk factors (lipids, hypertension, smoking) is indicated, but the role of anti-hyperglycemic therapy in reducing CVD risk in these patients remains uncertain.

DIABETES AND NEUROPSYCHIATRIC DISORDERS

There is an emerging body of evidence that diabetes may accelerate age-related cognitive decline and leads to an almost twofold increase in the risk of both vascular and Alzheimer's dementia (21,22). An association with cognitive impairment has also been observed in "pre-diabetic" states of IFG (23), the metabolic syndrome (24) and insulin resistance (25). Diabetes may accelerate global cognitive decline, but psychomotor slowing has been reported as a characteristic finding in patients with diabetes (26). Although the increased prevalence of CVD may be a contributing factor, diabetes-associated dementia may occur independently of clinically significant micro or macrovascular disease (22,27). Proposed biological mechanisms for diabetes-associated central nervous system dysfunction include free radical-mediated oxidative stress, formation of advanced glycation end-products and alterations in neuronal insulin signaling pathways. In addition, a direct relationship between insulin metabolism (via insulin degrading enzyme) and formation of beta amyloid (pathogenic for Alzheimer's dementia) has been proposed (27,28).

Regardless of its pathogenesis, the presence of cognitive impairment has substantial implications for diabetes management in affected patients. Even mild, unrecognized cognitive impairment has been associated with poor diabetes control in older adults (29). Complex tasks related to diabetes self-management, including attention to medication schedules, blood glucose monitoring and nutritional factors, become more difficult as cognition (especially memory and executive function) declines. Thus, treatment goals (i.e., less stringent glucose control in order to avoid hypoglycemia) and patient education efforts (medication reminders, pill boxes, etc.) should be modified as cognitive status declines. Ultimately, responsibility for care may need to be shifted to others.

Unrecognized depression is common among elderly diabetic patients (30) and may co-exist with (or masquerade as) dementia. The presence of depression can have significant impact on diabetes control through changes in appetite, lack of attention to treatment regimen and use of psychoactive substances such as sedatives or ethanol.

VASCULAR COMPLICATIONS

Elderly patients with diabetes are at risk for both typical microvascular complications (retinopathy, nephropathy, neuropathy) and cardiovascular disease.

Microvascular

Data from cross-sectional studies indicate that older diabetic patients (middle-age onset) have greater rates of retinopathy and neuropathy than younger diabetics (5), which is likely due to longer duration of disease and greater glycemic exposure. Screening and treatment of these conditions are similar in older and younger patients, but with special considerations such as the potential for adverse effects of drug therapy [e.g., angiotensin converting enzyme-inhibitors (ACE-I)] and drug–drug interactions. Elderly patients with compromised renal function should be evaluated for other renal abnormalities, including genitourinary tract obstructions and infections, which may be common in this population. Older patients with diabetes are also at increased risk of vision loss as a result of glaucoma, cataracts and macular degeneration, so regular examination by an ophthalmologist is essential. Routine podiatric care is also important, since impaired vision and mobility and concomitant peripheral vascular disease may combine to increase risk of ulceration and eventual amputation in older patients with neuropathy.

Macrovascular

An increased risk of CVD represents the most common and serious consequence of diabetes in the elderly. CVD risk is increased similarly in both "middle-age onset" and "elderly onset" diabetes (5), and is almost twofold higher when compared with age-mates without diabetes. Similar increased CVD risk has also been reported with isolated post-challenge hyperglycemia (IPH), compared with controls having normal glucose tolerance (18,19) and risk is also elevated in older adults with IGT (31). Hyperglycemia in the elderly often co-exists with other metabolic defects that promote vascular disease risk, leading to metabolic syndrome (MS) prevalence as high as 45% in adults age 60 and older (32). Among older adults without known CVD, the presence of the MS remains a significant predictor of CVD events (hazard rate of approximately 2.0), even after adjusting for conventional CVD risk factors (33).

Although reports of CVD treatment and prevention in elderly diabetic patients are limited, many statin trials have included sizable numbers of elderly subjects, and subgroup analyses suggest that older patients do benefit from lipid-lowering therapy (34,35). However, no primary or secondary CVD prevention studies have been reported specifically in elderly diabetic patients. Recent evidence-based guidelines (36) have recommended a standard approach to lipid-lowering therapy in elderly diabetics, with consideration of overall health status and life expectancy. Likewise, hypertension should be actively treated to a minimum target of <140/80, but blood pressure should be lowered gradually to enhance tolerance and avoid complications.

HYPOGLYCEMIA RISK

Elderly diabetic patients treated with glucose-lowering drugs are at particular risk for iatrogenic hypoglycemia. Multiple factors contribute to this risk, including declining renal function, polypharmacy and frailty-associated anorexia (37,38). In addition, cognitive impairment may alter the behavioral response to hypoglycemia and predispose to errors in medication use. It is unclear if hypoglycemia counter-regulation is impaired as a function of aging, but type 2 patients with long-standing insulin-deficient diabetes appear to be at particular risk. Hypoglycemic symptoms may be attenuated by use of adrenergic-blocking drugs and the presence of multiple co-morbidities may lead to uncertainty over the cause of symptoms such as dizziness, fatigue or confusion. Prevention of hypoglycemia may require modification of glycemic goals, regular home glucose monitoring and cautious use of drugs, particularly long-acting sulfonylureas (SU), ACE-I and ethanol, which are commonly associated with hypoglycemia.

TREATMENT

The population of older adults with diabetes is heterogeneous and treatment goals must be individualized and periodically re-evaluated (36). Age alone should not lead to a reduction in treatment intensity, since many older patients have substantial life expectancy and are at risk for diabetic microvascular complications, which are preventable with careful control of glycemia. Factors such as concomitant illnesses, functional status, remaining life expectancy, finances and patient preference all need to be considered when planning treatment. Minimal treatment goals ("basic care") should include prevention of acute metabolic decompensation (i.e., maintenance of mean plasma glucose <200 mg/dL and avoidance of hypoglycemia) and treatment of cardiovascular risk factors, such as hypertension, dyslipidemia and smoking. Optimal treatment goals are consistent with guidelines for younger patients (i.e., $HbA_{1c} < 7\%$, preprandial glucose 80 to 120 mg and postprandial glucose <160 mg/dL), but generally require active patient participation in all aspects of diabetes care. Diabetes self-management training may be especially useful for older patients and many such services are reimbursable under Medicare (39).

Nutrition Therapy

Many, if not most, older diabetics are overweight or obese and nutrition therapy remains a key component of diabetes management in the elderly. Weight loss can be remarkably effective in improving insulin sensitivity (40) in older adults and may also lead to improved beta cell function (41). Moderation of carbohydrate intake alone, without reducing calories, may have substantial benefit in reducing postprandial hyperglycemia (42).

Weight loss that occurs in old age has been associated with increased mortality and this had led some to advise against weight reduction diets in the elderly. However, unintentional weight loss frequently occurs in the context of a serious disease (i.e., cancer, congestive heart failure) and could confound the interpretation of weight loss effects on mortality. In fact, data suggest that intentional weight loss reduces mortality in older patients with diabetes (43,44) and that obesity itself is a cause of frailty and functional decline (45). Nonetheless, nutritional deficiencies are common in the elderly, despite obesity (46,47), because altered taste perception and poor dentition may lead to inadequate intake of micronutrients, fiber and protein. Weight loss diets can exacerbate the age-related decline in fat-free body mass (sarcopenia), but this effect can be attenuated by inclusion of a program of regular exercise (48). The presence of multiple co-morbidities (hypertension, congestive heart failure, diverticulosis, anticoagulant therapy, etc.) may also impose additional dietary restrictions on older patients. Individualization of dietary goals and meal planning by a qualified dietician is beneficial in many cases.

Exercise

Reduced muscle mass and deconditioning are common among older patients, but there is substantial evidence that exercise can be beneficial in enhancing insulin sensitivity and improving glycemic control (49). Resistance training may be more effective in this regard than aerobic exercise (50,51) and may also be easier to implement for patients with orthopedic limitations, such as arthritis. Because of the high frequency of CVD in elderly patients with diabetes, cardiac evaluation should be considered before institution of any vigorous exercise program.

Lifestyle Modification and Diabetes Prevention

Lifestyle modification programs, with the combined goal of modest weight reduction and increased physical activity, have been shown to reduce the development of type 2 diabetes by 55% to 58% in high-risk populations with impaired glucose tolerance (52,53). In the U.S. Diabetes Prevention Program (DPP), lifestyle modification was effective in all age groups, but had the greatest impact among older participants, ages 60 to 85 at baseline (54). This robust effect was largely attributable to the greater weight loss and activity levels achieved by the older group. An additional benefit of the DPP lifestyle intervention was a reduction of the occurrence of urinary incontinence among women (55), a problem that has been linked to obesity and is a frequent complaint of the elderly. The DPP cohort was highly selected, generally healthy and motivated, so some caution is necessary when applying these results to frail or disabled older adults. Nonetheless, the DPP lifestyle intervention was both feasible and well-tolerated by older participants and can be recommended for older individuals at risk for type 2 diabetes.

Medications

For patients who do not meet glycemic goals with dietary modification and exercise, the choice of medication is in large part determined by side effect profile and cost (56,57). Despite the large number of elderly patients with diabetes, relatively few pharmaceutical trials have been conducted in older adults. Elderly patients with diabetes may be at increased risk of drug-related adverse effects because of altered renal or hepatic drug metabolism or the existence of concomitant medical conditions, such as congestive heart failure. All classes of oral and parenteral drugs may be used in older diabetics—what follows are special considerations when these drugs are used in the elderly.

Metformin

The biguanide metformin works primarily by suppression of hepatic glucose production and it indirectly improves insulin action. Although gastrointestinal side effects (dyspepsia, diarrhea) are common, hypoglycemia rarely occurs. However, metformin should be used with caution in elderly patients because of the risk of lactic acidosis. Metformin is contraindicated with even mild renal insufficiency (serum creatinine $\geq 1.5\,mg/dL$ in men, $\geq 1.4\,mg/dL$ in women) and in patients age 80 and above unless normal creatinine clearance is demonstrated on a 24-h urine collection. Metformin also should not be used in patients with clinically significant (pharmacologically treated) congestive heart failure. Metformin is most effective at lowering fasting glucose levels, but may contribute less to reducing postprandial hyperglycemia. Metformin was not effective in preventing diabetes among the older participants of the DPP (54).

Thiazolidendiones (Glitazones)

Thiazolidenediones (TZD), including pioglitazone and rosiglitazone, work by enhancing insulin-mediated glucose uptake; however, their effects are pleiotropic and their mechanisms of action are incompletely understood. Weight gain (5 to 10 kg) is common with TZD therapy. Fluid retention and edema formation can occur and TZD may precipitate clinical deterioration in patients with congestive heart failure. This adverse effect appears to occur more frequently when TZD are used in combination with insulin. Since hypoglycemia does not occur with monotherapy, TZD therapy may be particularly useful for patients who are at high risk for hypoglycemia.

Sulfonylureas

The SU insulin secretagogues have a long history of use, with predictable action and side effect profile. The major adverse effect of SUs is hypoglycemia and elderly patients are at increased risk because age-related decline in renal function impairs drug metabolism and clearance. All members of this drug class can cause hypoglycemia, but glyburide appears to be associated with the greatest risk (58). When SU therapy is initiated in recent onset diabetes, low doses should be used (1.25 mg glyburide, 2.5 mg glipizide or 1 mg glimepiride), with cautious dose titration. In contrast, patients with long standing type 2 diabetes may no longer respond to SU treatment, despite maximal doses.

Meglitinides

The meglitinides, repaglinide and nateglinide, are short-acting insulin secretagogues that bind to an identical beta cell receptor as do SU. However, onset and duration of action are much shorter and consequently, hypoglycemia risk is reduced (59). Meglitinides are dosed preprandially (tid), which may affect adherence for some patients and the cost is substantially greater than SU. Although direct comparison studies are limited, it appears that repaglinide is equipotent to SU, with nateglinide being somewhat less effective. Meglitinides may be particularly useful in elderly patients with predominantly postprandial hyperglycemia or those who have experienced excessive hypoglycemia with the use of SU.

Incretin-Based Therapies

Recently, a new class of pharmacologic agents that augment or mimic the effects of endogenous insulin secretagogues (incretins) were introduced. These include the parenteral drug exenatide, a glucagon-like peptide-1 (GLP-1) receptor agonist and oral drugs that inhibit the enzyme that degrades GLP-1, called DPP-IV inhibitors. Because these drugs enhance glucose-mediated insulin secretion, the risk of hypoglycemia appears to be small. The anorectic effect of exenatide, desirable for younger obese patients, has led to some concern about its use in the frail or malnourished elderly. The DPP-IV inhibitors (sitagliptin, vildagliptin) are weight neutral, with less pronounced effect on appetite and might be preferable for those patients.

Alpha-Glucosidase Inhibitors

Alpha-glucosidase inhibitors (AGI), including miglitol and acarbose, work by inhibiting enzymatic degradation of complex carbohydrates, thus slowing their intestinal absorption. The effect of AGI is essentially limited to reduction of postprandial hyperglycemia, but this may be sufficient for some older patients with mild diabetes. However, many older patients are intolerant to the gastrointestinal side effects (bloating, flatulence), which may limit the drug's usefulness. AGIs have also been reported to reduce the development of diabetes in a middle-aged high-risk population with IGT (60), but effectiveness among older patients has not been reported.

Insulin

Although in many cases, use of insulin to control hyperglycemia is considered a "last resort", there are advantages to earlier initiation of insulin therapy in the elderly. Insulin's action is generally predictable, side effects well understood and drug interactions few. For some patients, a simple basal insulin regimen may be just as effective, and substantially cheaper, than combination oral therapy. Nonetheless, practical barriers (i.e., need for injection) and misconceptions about insulin use (i.e., acceleration of vascular complications) lead many patients and practitioners to avoid this therapy.

The general principle for insulin therapy in the elderly is to use the simplest regimen that achieves glycemic goals. For some patients, basal insulin alone—such as neutral protamine hagedorn (NPH), glargine or detemir may be adequate. Others, especially those with long duration of diabetes, may require the addition of rapid-acting insulin at mealtimes. Fixed insulin combinations (i.e., 70/30, 50/50, etc.) can be considered for patients unable to manage more complex regimens, but may be associated with greater hypoglycemia risk. Insulin pen devices may be especially useful for patients with limited vision or problems with manual dexterity and may be more readily accepted by patients than the conventional vial and syringe method.

Insulin is also indicated for patients with acute metabolic decompensation, including hyperosmolar hyperglycemic coma, and during time of unusual stress, such as hospitalization, surgery and infection. Many elderly patients who require insulin therapy during an episode of glycemic decompensation are ultimately able to control glucose with oral medications or lifestyle measures alone.

Combination Therapy

Experience, such as in the UKPDS (61), has shown that over time, most patients require treatment with more than a single diabetes medication in order to maintain adequate glycemic control. This is especially true of the elderly with long-duration diabetes, who may require multiple oral medications and insulin. The combination of drugs that enhance insulin action (TZD, metformin) with drugs that promote insulin secretion (SU-, megltinides-, incretin-based treatment) is a popular and effective approach.

SUMMARY

Type 2 diabetes and IGR are extremely common among older adults and result in significant acute and chronic morbidity. Recognition of the heterogeneous nature of diabetes in the elderly will allow individualization of treatment goals and therapies. Older adults with long-standing diabetes often have a substantial burden of vascular complications and require treatment with combination oral medications and/or insulin, whereas incident diabetes in the elderly is often mild and unrecognized. Periodic reassessment of metabolic and cognitive status is essential as aging progresses.

REFERENCES

1. http://diabetes.niddk.nih.gov/dm/pubs/statistics/index.htm, accessed 9 February 2007.
2. Cowie CC, Rust KF, Byrd-Holt D, et al. Prevalence of diabetes and impaired fasting glucose in adults–United States, 1999–2000. MMWR 2003; 52:833–37.
3. Harris M, Flegal K, Cowie C, et al. Prevalence of diabetes, impaired fasting glucose and impaired glucose tolerance in US adults. Diabetes Care 1998; 21:518–24.
4. Roman SH, Harris MI. Management of diabetes mellitus from a public health perspective. Endocrinol Clin N Am 1997; 26:443–74.
5. Selvin E, Coresh J, Brancati F. The burden and treatment of diabetes in elderly individuals in the US. Diabetes Care 2006; 29:2415–19.
6. Basu R, Breda E, Oberg A. Mechanisms of the age-associated deterioration in glucose tolerance: contribution of alterations in insulin secretion, action and clearance. Diabetes 2003; 52:1738–48.
7. Chen M, Bergman R, Pacini G, et al. Pathogenesis of age-related glucose intolerance in man: insulin resistance and decreased β-cell function. J Clin Endocrinol Metab 1985; 60:13–20.
8. Utzschneider K, Carr D, Hull K, et al. Impact of intra-abdominal fat and age on insulin sensitivity and beta cell function. Diabetes 2004; 53:2867–72.
9. Bevilaqua S, Bonaddona R, Buzzigoli G, et al. Acute elevation of FFA levels leads to hepatic insulin resistance in obese subjects. Metabolism 1987; 36:502–6.
10. Cree MG, Newcomer BR, Katsanos CS, et al. Intramuscular and liver triglycerides are increased in the elderly. J Clin Endocrinol Metab 2004; 89:3864–71.
11. Meneilly G, Elliott T. Metabolic alterations in middle-aged and elderly obese patients with type 2 diabetes. Diabetes Care 1999; 22:112–8.
12. Bourey RE, Kohrt MW, Kirwan JP, et al. Relationship between glucose tolerance and glucose-stimulated insulin response in 65-year-olds. J Gerontol 1993; 48:M122–7.
13. Gumbinar B, Polonsky KS, Beltz WF, et al. Effects of aging on insulin secretion. Diabetes 1989; 38: 1549–56.
14. American Diabetes Association. Diagnosis and classification of diabetes mellitus. Diabetes Care 2006; 29:S43–8.
15. World Health Organization. Diabetes mellitus: Report of a WHO study group. Geneva, World Health Organization, 1985 (Tech. Rep. Ser. No. 727).

16. Resnick H, Harris M, Brock D, et al. American Diabetes Association diabetes diagnostic criteria, advancing age and cardiovascular disease risk profile. Diabetes Care 2000; 23:176–80.
17. The DECODE Study Group. Age and sex-specific prevalence of diabetes and impaired glucose regulation in 13 European cohorts. Diabetes Care 2003; 26:61–9.
18. Wahl P, Savage P, Psaty B, et al. Diabetes in older adults: comparison of 1997 American Diabetes Association classification of diabetes mellitus with 1985 WHO classification. Lancet 1998; 352: 1012–1015.
19. The DECODE Study Group. Glucose tolerance and cardiovascular mortality. Comparison of fasting and 2-hour diagnostic criteria. Arch Intern Med 2001; 161:397-404.
20. Barrett-Connor E, Ferrara A. Isolated post-challenge hyperglycemia and the risk of fatal cardiovascular disease in older women and men. Diabetes Care 2000; 23:176–80.
21. Yaffe K, Blackwell T, Kanaya AM, et al. Diabetes, impaired fasting glucose and development of cognitive impairment in older women. Neurology 2004; 63:658–63.
22. Arvanitakis Z, Wilson R, Bienas J, et al. Diabetes Mellitus and risk of Alzheimer disease and decline of cognitive function. Arch Neurol 2004; 61:661–6.
23. Yaffe K, Kanaya A, Lindquist K, et al. The metabolic syndrome, inflammation and risk of cognitive decline. JAMA 2004; 292:2237–42.
24. Vanhanen M, Koivisto K, Moilanen L, et al. Association of metabolic syndrome with Alzheimer disease: a population-based study. Neurology 2006; 67:843–7.
25. Kalmijin S, Feskens EJ, Launer LJ, et al. Glucose intolerance, hyperinsulinemia and cognitive function in a general population of elderly men. Diabetologia 1995; 38:1096–102.
26. Ryan C. Diabetes, aging and cognitive decline. Neurobiol Aging 2005; 26S:S21–25.
27. Farris W, Mansourian S, Chang Y, et al. Insulin degrading enzyme regulates the levels of insulin, amyloid β-protein and the β-amyloid precursor protein intracellular domain in vivo. Proc Natl Acad Sci USA 2003; 100:4162–7.
28. Boyt AA, Taddei TK, Hallmayer J, et al. The effect of insulin and glucose on the plasma concentration of Alzheimer's amyloid precursor protein. Neuroscience 2000; 95:727–34.
29. Munshi M, Grande K, Hayes M, et al. Cognitive dysfunction is associated with poor diabetes control in older adults. Diabetes Care 2006; 29:1794–9.
30. Finkelstein EA, Bray JW, Chen H, et al. Prevalence and costs of major depression among elderly claimants with diabetes. Diabetes Care 2003; 26:415–20.
31. Hanefeld M, Koehler C, Schaper F, et al. Postprandial plasma glucose is an independent risk factor for increased carotid intima-media thickness in non-diabetic individuals. Atherosclerosis 1999; 144: 229–35.
32. Ford ES, Giles WH, Dietz WH. Prevalence of the metabolic syndrome among US adults: findings from the third National Health and Nutrition Examination Survey. JAMA 2002; 287:356–9.
33. Scuteri A, Najjar S, Morrell C, Lakatta E. The metabolic syndrome in older individuals: prevalence and prediction of cardiovascular events. Diabetes Care 2005; 28:882–7.
34. Neil HA, DeMicco D, Luo D, et al. Analysis of efficacy and safety in patients aged 65–75 years at randomization: Collaborative Atorvastatin Diabetes Study (CARDS). Diabetes Care 2006; 29: 2378–84.
35. Miettinen TA, Pyorala K, Olsson AG, et al. Cholesterol lowering therapy in women and elderly patients with myocardial infarction or angina pectoris: findings from the Scandinavian Simvastatin Survivial Study (4S). Circulation 1997; 96:4211–18.
36. Brown AF, Mangione CM, Saliba D, Sarkisian CA, the California Healthcare Foundation/American Geriatrics Society. Guidelines for improving the care of the older person with diabetes mellitus. J Am Geriatr Soc 2003; 51:S265–80.
37. Chelliah A, Burge MR. Hypoglycemia in elderly patients with diabetes mellitus: causes and strategies for prevention. Drugs Aging 2004; 21:511–30.
38. Greco D, Angileri G. Drug-induced severe hypoglycemia in type 2 diabetic patients aged 80 years or older. Diab Nutr Metab 2004; 17:23–6.
39. http://www.medicare.gov.health/diabetes.as.p.
40. Colman E, Katzel LI, Rogus E, et al. Weight loss reduces abdominal fat and improves insulin action in middle-aged and older men with impaired glucose tolerance. Metabolism 1995; 44:1502–8.
41. Utzschneider K, Carr D, Barsness S, et al. Diet-induced weight loss is associated with an improvement in beta cell function in older men. J Clin Endocrinol Metab 2004; 89:2704–10.
42. Chen M, Halter J, Porte D. The role of dietary carbohydrate in the decreased glucose tolerance of the elderly. J Am Geriatr Soc 1987; 35:417–24.
43. Villareal D, Apovian C, Kushner R, Klein S. Obesity in older adults: Technical review and position statement of the American Society for Nutrition and NAASO, The Obesity Society. Obes Res 2005; 13:1849–63.
44. Newman A, Yanez D, Harris T, et al. Weight change in old age and its association with mortality. J Am Geriatr Soc 2001; 49:1309–18.

45. Blaum CS, Xue QL, Micheline E, et al. The association between obesity and the frailty syndrome in older women: The Women's Health JAGS 2005; 53:927–34.
46. Ledikwe JH, Smiciklas-Wright H, Mitchell DC, et al. Nutritional risk assessment and obesity in rural older adults: a sex difference. Am J Clin Nutr 2003; 77:551–8.
47. Millen BE, Silliman RA, Cantey-Kiser J, et al. Nutritional risk in an urban homebound older population. The nutrition and healthy aging project. J Nutr Health Aging 2001; 5:269–77.
48. Dziura J, Mendes deLeon C, Kasl S, et al. Can physical activity attenuate aging-related weight loss in older people? The Yale Health and Aging Study, 1982–1994. Am Epidemiol 2004; 159:759–67.
49. Miller J, Pratley R, Goldberg A, et al. Strength training increases insulin action in healthy 50–65 year old men. J Appl Physiol 1994; 77:1122–7.
50. Dunstan D, Daly R, Owen N, et al. High intensity resistance training improves glycemic control in older patients with type 2 diabetes. Diabetes Care 2002; 25:1729–36.
51. Holten M, Zacho M, Gaster M, et al. Strength training increases insulin-mediated glucose uptake, GLUT4 content and insulin signaling in skeletal muscle in patients with type 2 diabetes. Diabetes 2004; 53:294–305.
52. The DPP Research Group. Reduction in the incidence of type 2 diabetes with lifestyle intervention or metformin. N Engl J Med 2002; 346:393–403.
53. Tuomilehto J, Lindstrom J, Eriksson JG, et al. Prevention of type 2 diabetes mellitus by changes in lifestyle among subjects with impaired glucose tolerance. N Engl J Med 2001; 344:1343–50.
54. The DPP Research Group. The influence of age on the effects of lifestyle modification and metformin in prevention of diabetes. J Gerontol/Med Sci 2006; 61:1075–81.
55. Brown JS, Wing R, Barrett-Connor E, et al. for the Diabetes Prevention Program Research Group. Lifestyle intervention is associated with lower prevalence of urinary incontinence: The Diabetes Prevention Program. Diabetes Care 2006; 29(2):385–90.
56. Inzucchi S. Oral antihyperglycemic therapy for type 2 diabetes. JAMA 2002; 287:360–72.
57. Crandall J, Barzilai N. Treatment of diabetes mellitus in older people: oral therapy options. J Am Geriatr Soc 2003; 51:272–4.
58. Szoke E, Gosmanov NR, Sinklin JC, et al. Effects of glimepiride and glyburide on glucose counter regulation and recovery from hypoglycemia. Metabolism 2006; 55:78–83.
59. Papa G, Fedele V, Rizzo M, et al. Safety of Type 2 diabetes treatment with repaglinide compared with glibenclamide in elderly people. Diabetes Care 2006; 29:1918–19.
60. Chaisson J, Josse R, Gomis R, et al. for the STOP-NIDDM Trial Research Group. Acarbose for prevention of type 2 diabetes mellitus: the STOP-NIDDM randomized trial. Lancet 2002; 359: 2072–77.
61. Turner RC, Cull CA, Frighi V, Holman R. Glycemic control with diet, sulfonylurea, metformin or insulin in patients with type 2 diabetes mellitus: progressive requirement for multiple therapies (UKPDS 49). JAMA 1999; 281:2005–12.

33 | Diabetes in High-Risk Ethnic Populations

Ebenezer A. Nyenwe and Samuel Dagogo-Jack
Division of Endocrinology, Diabetes, and Metabolism, University of Tennessee Health Science Center, Memphis, Tennessee, U.S.A.

Diabetes mellitus is a chronic debilitating disease currently estimated to affect 7% (over 20 million) of the total population of the United States (1). Type 2 diabetes accounts for 90% to 95% of all cases of diabetes. Studies show that the prevalence of diabetes is disproportionately higher among ethnic minority groups, including African Americans, Asian Americans, Pacific Islanders, Hispanic Americans, and Native Americans compared with Caucasians (1). Compared with white Americans, the relative increase in the prevalence of diabetes is 2.2-fold in American Indians and Alaskan indigenous peoples, twofold in Asian Americans and Pacific Islanders, 1.8-fold in African Americans and 1.7-fold in Hispanic/Latino Americans (1). Whereas the prevalence rate of diabetes is 8.7% in non-Hispanic white adults, it rises to 13.3% in African Americans and 27.6% in American Indians in Arizona (Fig. 1a). Furthermore, the incidence of new cases of diabetes in ethnic minority groups continues to increase. Whereas age-adjusted incidence of diabetes in subjects aged 18 to 79 years in the United States in 2004 was six per 1000 among whites, it was approximately 10 per 1000 in African American and Hispanic subjects (Fig. 1b) (1). A similar trend in the prevalence of diabetes has been demonstrated in the United Kingdom (UK). The prevalence of diabetes among Europeans in north-west London is 4%, compared to 30% in South Asian populations living in the same location, and 14% to 29% in people of African descent living in different locations in the United Kingdom (2).

Ethnic disparity in prevalence is accompanied by higher risk for diabetic complications, hospitalization rates and disability in minority groups (1,3). Again, in comparison with Caucasians, diabetes-related mortality rate is also higher in African Americans and other ethnic minority groups (Fig. 2) (3,4). Despite these disparities in prevalence and complications of diabetes, the efficacy of interventions for the prevention and control of diabetes remains the same in all ethnic groups. The ethnic differences in morbidity and mortality disappear when Caucasians and the minority populations are maintained at comparable glycemic levels (3,5). It becomes imperative therefore, that barriers to optimum care in high-risk populations be identified and corrected, in order to achieve better disease control, and to ameliorate physical and economic burden of diabetes. This chapter discusses the etiology of ethnic disparity in the prevalence and complications of type 2 diabetes and also identifies practical ways of achieving better disease control in high-risk ethnic populations.

COMPLICATIONS OF DIABETES IN HIGH-RISK POPULATIONS

Acute Metabolic Complications

The age-adjusted hospital admission rate for diabetic ketoacidosis (DKA) has remained high in African Americans since 1980 (1,6). In 2003, the age-adjusted DKA rate was 28.6 per 1000 blacks with diabetes compared to 21.4 per 1000 whites with diabetes (1). DKA appears to be a more aggressive disease in black males when compared with the whites. Mortality from DKA is about threefold higher in black males compared with whites. Cessation of insulin therapy is the major precipitating cause for DKA in African-American and Hispanic patients (7,8). In many cases, omission of insulin therapy was due to lack of resources in the economically disadvantaged patient (7).

Over the years, increasing number of patients from ethnic minority populations with type 2 diabetes, particularly African Americans and Hispanics have been noted to present with DKA (9–11). About 50% of such patients present with DKA as initial manifestation of

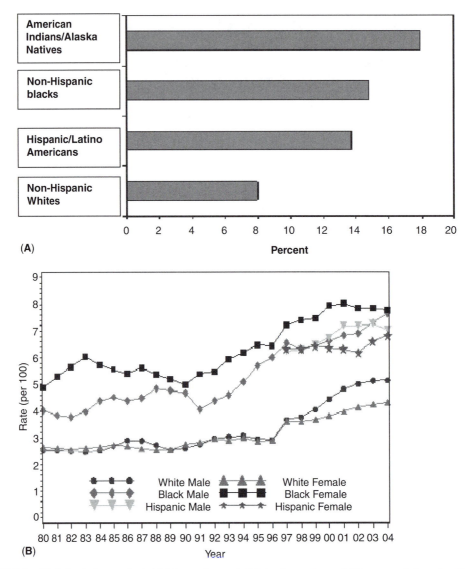

FIGURE 1 (**A**) Estimated age-adjusted total prevalence of diabetes in people aged 20 years and above by ethnicity/race, U.S. 2005. (**B**) Trend in the prevalence of diabetes by race/ethnicity and sex, 1980–2004. *Source*: From Ref. 1.

type 2 diabetes (9,10). Patients with this entity known as ketosis-prone type 2 diabetes, exhibit initial profound impairment in insulin secretion and action, which resolves with correction of DKA and hyperglycemia using insulin therapy. After a 10-year follow-up period, 40% of patients with ketosis-prone diabetes have remained well controlled without insulin (10). This finding is of significant therapeutic implication in ethnic minority patients with type 2 diabetes. The precise etiology of acute severe but transient β-cell failure is uncertain. Postulated mechanisms include glucotoxicity, lipotoxicity and genetic predisposition. A genetic association between glucose-6-phosphate dehydrogenase deficiency and ketosis-prone type 2 diabetes has been reported (11).

Chronic Complications

Diabetes is a leading cause of cardiovascular disease, stroke, blindness, end-stage renal disease (ESRD) and non-traumatic amputation across populations. Current estimates show that it

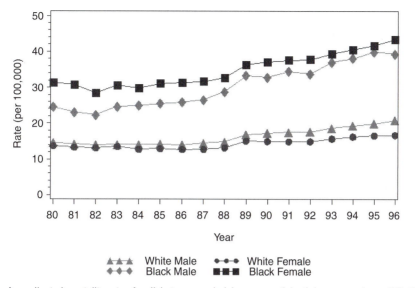

FIGURE 2   Age-adjusted mortality rates for diabetes as underlying cause of death by race and sex, U.S. 1980–1996. *Source*: From Ref. 1.

accounts for 44% of all new cases of ESRD, 60% to 70% of cases of neuropathy and more than 60% of non-traumatic lower limb amputations in the United States (1,12). Ethnic disparity in the prevalence of type 2 diabetes translates to increased burden of diabetic complications in minority populations. Long-term complications of diabetes can be classified into micro-vascular and macrovascular complications. Diabetes-specific microvascular complications, which include, retinopathy, nephropathy and neuropathy require chronic hyperglycemia to occur. About 25% of patients with type 2 diabetes already have evidence of microvascular complications at the time of diagnosis (3). Data from the third National Health and Nutrition Examination Survey (NHANES III) showed that prevalence of diabetic retinopathy was 46% higher in African Americans and 84% higher in Mexican Americans, compared with non-Hispanic whites. Ethnic minority populations also had more advanced retinopathy and higher levels of putative risk factors compared with Caucasians (7). However, the age-adjusted prevalence of visual impairment is 19.5% for whites, 16.7% for Hispanics and 19.1% for African Americans (1).

The rates of ESRD are approximately threefold higher in African Americans, Latinos and Native Americans compared with Caucasians (13). Between 1984 and 2002, the incidence of treatment for ESRD attributable to diabetes was highest among African-American males (1). Diabetic nephropathy is heralded by microalbuminuria, which can be reversed by tight glycemic control and blood pressure control using angiotensin-converting enzyme-inhibitors or angiotensin-receptor blockers. Moreover, microalbuminuria may precede ESRD by nearly two decades, thus affording a window of opportunity for the prevention of ESRD in diabetic patients (3).

Diabetic neuropathy occurs in nearly 30% of patients with diabetes aged 40 years or more (1). It results in impaired sensation, which manifests as numbness, parasthesia and pain in the feet and hands. Diabetic autonomic neuropathy leads to delayed digestion of food due to gastroparesis. Neuropathy, sometimes acting in concert with peripheral vascular disease is a major contributor to diabetes-related non-traumatic lower extremity amputation. Loss of protective pain sensation predisposes to injury, polymicrobial infection and gangrene, which may require amputation to preserve life. Although the rates of hospitalization for lower extremity ulcers are similar in all ethnic groups, amputation rates are two to three times higher in African Americans and Hispanic patients compared with American whites (14). In 2002, the age-adjusted lower extremity amputation rate per 1000 persons with diabetes was 5.3 in

African-Americans and 4.1 in Caucasians (1). Gangrene and amputation in patients with established diabetic neuropathy can be prevented by screening using 5.07 monofilament, to identify patients at high-risk, who would benefit from diligent foot care (15).

Macrovascular Complications

The macrovascular complications of diabetes include coronary artery disease (CAD), stroke and peripheral vascular disease. About 65% of deaths in diabetic patients are attributable to heart disease and stroke. Mortality from cardiac disease in diabetic patients is two to fourfold higher than that in non-diabetic individuals (1). Furthermore, diabetic patients have a two to four times higher risk for developing a stroke compared with their non-diabetic counterparts. The risk of macrovascular complications has not been shown to be higher in ethnic minority populations (16,17); despite a higher prevalence of diabetes and hypertension, especially in African Americans. A similar observation has been made in Africans in developing countries (18) and the UK (3), where the incidence of CAD is low in diabetic patients. Although cerebrovascular disease is a common cause of death in African diabetic patients, especially those with concomitant hypertension, CAD is uncommon (18). For instance, in Nigeria where the prevalence of diabetes may be more than 7% in some urban centers (19), the prevalence of CAD (by autopsy) in patients who died suddenly from cardiac causes is only 4% (20). There may be a mitigating factor protecting the minority patient from excess CAD burden as may be predicted from the disparate prevalence of diabetes and hypertension. The etiology of this discordance is not known with certainty, although it is thought to be due to less atherogenic lipid profile in African Americans. Understanding the nature of this factor may hold a promise for reducing the incidence of CAD. Even though the prevalence rates of macrovascular complications are similar among the ethnic groups, mortality from CAD is higher in the high-risk ethnic populations, particularly African-American women (21). The reason for this disparity, which merits further study, remains unclear.

ETIOLOGY OF DISPARITY IN THE PREVALENCE OF DIABETES

In 1893, William Osler described diabetes with the following words "hereditary influences play an important role. It is a disease of adult life, a majority of cases occur from the third to the sixth decade … in a considerable proportion of these cases of diabetes the subjects have been excessively fat at the beginning of, or prior to the onset of the disease … The combination of over-indulgence in food and drink, with sedentary life, seem particularly prone to induce the disease". This description summarizes the basic elements of type 2 diabetes (22). The precise reasons for racial disparities in the prevalence of diabetes are not entirely clear, but the balance of available evidence indicates that the higher propensity for developing diabetes in ethnic minority populations is driven by an interaction between a heritable genetic predisposition and environmental precipitants. Some postulated explanations for this disparity would be examined below.

GENETIC FACTORS

The clustering of type 2 diabetes in families, and certain ethnic populations implies that there is a strong genetic influence on the disease. To explain this genetic influence Neel proposed the "thrifty genotype" hypothesis. He postulated that the genotype which is now diabetogenic conferred some survival advantage in the primeval times. People with such genotype were metabolically more efficient at storing energy as fat during times of abundance. Such stores were vital for survival in times of famine, war or other disasters, which were frequent in the past. As a result of plentiful food supply and sedentary lifestyle, the thrifty genotype, which was protective has become detrimental by contributing to a diabetic genotype (23). The thrifty genotype hypothesis is accepted as a plausible explanation for obesity, since it served the purpose of preserving life, but its extension to explain the epidemic of type 2 diabetes has been challenged (24). Considering that diabetes reduces the average life span of an individual by a decade, the teleological reason for conservation and propagation of the thrifty genotype is very unclear. Secondly, the development of diabetes in migrant populations such as the Japanese (25) or the Ethiopian Jews (26) occurs almost immediately, and does not wait for many generations. Thirdly, the thrifty gene hypothesis does not explain the lower prevalence of type 2 diabetes in persons of European ancestry as compared to the ethnic minority groups. Obesity is prevalent in the European populations, which also were not exempted from scarcity of food in the past.

Owing to these shortcomings of the thrifty gene hypothesis, alternative theories have been postulated. These include the "antagonistic pleiotropy" (27) and the "genetic trash can" hypotheses (28). The Former posits that thriftiness at a younger age ensured survival and reproductive viability of the individual, but after middle age, the thrifty genes become a predisposing factor for diabetes. This theory is weakened by the lack of empirical examples in nature. The "genetic trash can" hypothesis holds that the preservation, propagation and concentration of multiple individually neutral gene mutations, which confer aggregate risks for type 2 diabetes is the origin of excess prevalence in some ethnic groups (28,29). In support of this is the fact that aboriginal societies with higher prevalence rates have experienced fewer admixtures or exogamy compared with European populations.

Another postulation, "the thrifty phenotype" hypothesis is based on the observation that people with low birth weight have a higher likelihood for developing diabetes in adult life, possibly because they would have developed with fewer pancreatic β-cells (30). It proposes that inadequate nutrition in utero programs the fetus to develop insulin resistance in adult life. It is also possible that a genetically determined defect in insulin action may also manifest as low birth weight and as insulin resistance later on in life, especially in those who become obese.

Despite the flaws in these hypotheses, some concrete evidence incriminating certain genetic constitution in the etiology of type 2 diabetes is beginning to emerge. Recent studies have shown an association between common polymorphisms of the transcription factor 7-like 2 gene (TCF7L2) and type 2 diabetes (31). Genetic analysis of the subjects in the Diabetes Prevention Study (DPP) revealed that subjects who were homozygous for the risk-conferring gene were about one-and-half times more likely to progress from impaired glucose tolerance (IGT) to type 2 diabetes, they also demonstrated impaired β-cell function (decreased insulin secretion) but not insulin resistance (31). The DPP study did not show any ethnic differences in the rate of conversion from IGT to diabetes.

ENVIRONMENTAL FACTORS

The role of the environment in unmasking latent genetic predisposition, thus leading to diabetes has been well known (32). Studies of Japanese immigrants to the US showed a threefold increase in the prevalence rate of diabetes compared with native Japanese (25), due to change of diet and lifestyle. The environmental triggers associated with increased prevalence of type 2 diabetes are called risk factors. These include obesity, physical inactivity, history of gestational diabetes or big babies and others shown in Table 1. Although the distribution of these risk factors differs among ethnic groups, the aggregate risk factor burden in the various populations must overlap considerably. Therefore, the marked disparity in diabetes prevalence cannot be explained by ethnic differences in the risk factors alone (29). Obesity is the strongest modifiable risk factor for type 2 diabetes, however; only a susceptible minority of people with obesity develop diabetes. Nevertheless, obesity has been found to be a strong risk factor among African Americans (33), and Hispanics (34) compared with Caucasians. National surveys have shown low levels of physical activity across all populations in the US, especially young African-American women (29); this no doubt would contribute to high prevalence of type 2 diabetes.

Cultural factors are of importance in the etiology of ethnic disparity in type 2 diabetes. Attitudes and belief about physical activity, ideal body size and diet will impact on the prevalence of diabetes. Cultural practices that encourage large physique will inadvertently make for increased diabetes prevalence (29). Neuropsychiatric factors including stress and atypical anti-psychotic agents may alter glucoregulation, thus predisposing to diabetes. It is possible that differential susceptibility to environmental stress may play a role in the disparate prevalence of diabetes (29).

TABLE 1   Risk Factors for Type 2 Diabetes

Age 45 years
Overweight (BMI > 25 kg/m^2)^a
Family history of diabetes (i.e., parents or siblings with diabetes)

Habitual physical inactivity

Race/ethnicity (e.g., African Americans, Hispanic Americans, Native Americans, Asian
   Americans, and Pacific Islanders)
Previously identified IFG or IGT

Hypertension (<140/90 mmHg in adults)

HDL cholesterol 35 mg/dL (0.90 mmol/L) and/or a triglyceride level 250 mg/dL (2.82 mmol/L)

Polycystic ovary syndrome

History of vascular disease

^{a}May not be correct for all ethnic groups. The WHO recommends a cut-off BMI of 22 kg/m^2 for Asians.
Source: From Diabetes Care 2004; 27:S11–4.

PATHOPHYSIOLOGY OF TYPE 2 DIABETES IN HIGH-RISK POPULATIONS

The fundamental defects in type 2 diabetes include insulin resistance and impaired pancreatic
β-cell function. Insulin resistance is said to occur when there is reduced sensitivity of the
tissues (liver, muscle and fat) to the metabolic actions of insulin, thus the pancreas secretes an
increasing amount of insulin to meet the demands of the body (hyperinsulinemia). Overtime
pancreatic β-cell failure ensues and diabetes manifests. This pathogenetic mechanism has been
confirmed in a longitudinal study in Pima Indians (35). Studies have demonstrated higher
degrees of insulin resistance in people of African descent (36) and Hispanics (37), compared
with whites, independent of age, gender, obesity and physical activity score. Decreased insulin
clearance, which contributes to hyperinsulinemia (36), and low-insulin secretory responses in
offsprings of diabetic subjects (38) have been reported in subjects of West African ancestry.
These studies support a role for genetically propagated insulin resistance and pancreatic β-cell
functional abnormality as underlying defects producing ethnic disparities in type 2 diabetes.

ETIOLOGY OF DISPARITY IN THE COMPLICATIONS OF DIABETES

The reasons for high prevalence of diabetic complications in the high-risk ethnic populations
may be attributable to genetic and acquired factors. The observation of familial clustering of
diabetic microvascular complications, particularly nephropathy, has raised the possibility of a
heritable genetic predisposition in the minority patients as the underlying cause of disparity in
diabetic complications. However, the Diabetes Control and Complications Trial showed
conclusively that proper glycemic control (hemoglobin A1c <7%) resulted in 50% to 70%
reduction in the risk of microvascular complications (39). Similarly, the United Kingdom
Prospective Diabetes Study (UKDPS) demonstrated that good glycemic control diminished the
risk of doubling of serum creatinine by 74% (40). These findings were further substantiated in
Japan by the Kumamoto study (41). The robust effect of glycemic control on the incidence of
target organ damage in diabetes clearly indicates that genetic predisposition may be
permissive, but not an obligate determinant of the risk for developing microvascular
complications. In the NHANES III retinopathy data (7), the disparity in the prevalence of
retinopathy became insignificant after adjusting for risk factors for retinopathy such as
chronicity of diabetes, hemoglobin A1c level and blood pressure.

   Acquired factors that may contribute to the excess burden of diabetic complications in
minority populations include non-adherence to therapeutic recommendations, low socioeconomic status and suboptimal quality of care. It may appear plausible that poor compliance
with therapeutic recommendations would account for the excess burden of diabetic
complications in high-risk groups, but studies have not shown any evidence of racial
differences in adherence to medications and lifestyle modification (42), or compliance with

TABLE 2   Diabetes Management: Patient Compliance and Practices by Ethnicity[a]

	Hispanic (%)	African American (%)	Caucasian (%)
Missed clinic	1.4	1.9	1.5
Non-compliance	34	27	26
Alcoholism	3.4	2.2	2.5
Missed foot clinic	0	2.7	5.6
Missed weight visit	17	15	9
Missed eye clinic	0	2	7

[a] There were no significant radical/ethnic differences in compliance behavior.
Source: From Ref. 51.

other diabetes-related tasks (43) (Table 2). Although another study (6), found a lower rate of self-monitoring of blood glucose (SMBG) in African Americans compared with whites and Hispanics, it is worthy of mention that the frequency of monitoring was suboptimal in all three ethnic groups. It may be attractive to label a patient as non-compliant in an attempt to explain poor treatment outcome. However, it should be emphasized that a positive interaction between patients and physicians is an indispensable element in the successful management of chronic disorders like diabetes. Therefore, before a conclusion of poor compliance or adherence is drawn every effort should be made to ascertain that this is truly so, as this "diagnosis" could create prejudice in other health-care providers and undermine dedicated therapeutic action. This obviously portends tragedy for diabetes management. Health-care providers should identify and make diligent efforts to correct barriers to delivery of optimal care.

Low socioeconomic status, limitations in access to health care, lack of health insurance or underinsurance, and other socioeconomic barriers contribute significantly to the increased burden of diabetic complications in ethnic minority groups (44). Cessation of insulin therapy is a major precipitating cause of DKA in African Americans, occurring in nearly 70% of the cases (7). Omission of insulin was either due to lack of means to replenish stock in 43% of patients or poor understanding of sick day management in another 25%. The importance of socio-economic factors in the genesis of disparity in diabetes complications is demonstrated very succinctly by a study which showed that the marked disparity in lower extremity amputation rates observed in the general population was not evident in an ethnically diverse population with uniform health care coverage. Even the frequency of SMBG among African Americans was not different from that of Whites and Hispanics (17).

Delivery of suboptimal care has been explored to explain the excess morbidity from diabetes in high-risk populations. It is noteworthy that the general level of diabetes control in the US is currently below expected goals. Saadine et al. (45) documented the quality of diabetes care in the US between 1988 and 1995 and found deficiency between recommended care and actual care received. It was further observed that after controlling for age, sex, ethnicity, level of education, insulin use and duration of diabetes, African Americans were more likely to have poorly controlled blood glucose and blood pressure. National surveys have not demonstrated any disparity in care between ethnic minority populations and the Caucasians (Table 3). It may be that the excess morbidity from diabetes in the minority groups is due to interaction between low general level of care and other factors such as low socioeconomic status, rather than a systematic under-treatment of minority patients.

STRATEGIES FOR MANAGEMENT AND PREVENTION OF DIABETES IN HIGH-RISK ETHNIC POPULATIONS

The ethnic disparity observed in the rates of diabetic nephropathy, neuropathy and retinopathy disappears when the ethnic groups are maintained at a comparable level of glycemic control. Response to lifestyle or pharmacological intervention was also similar among the ethnic groups in the DPP study (46). These findings raise hope and confidence that the high morbidity of diabetes in the ethnic minority groups can be ameliorated provided the barriers to the delivery of optimal care are identified and dealt with effectively.

TABLE 3 Medical Care for Black Adults and White adults with
Type 2 Diabetes[a]

	Black (%)	White (%)
≥4 physician visits/yr	62.4	58.9
Insulin	51.9	35.9
Oral agents	50.1	39.9
Following diet	88.9	88.2
SMBG	18	35
Visit dietician	28	19
Diabetes education	43	32
Eye examination	64	60
Visit podiatrist	19	16

[a]National Diabetes Data Group. Analysis based on 1989 clinical data.
Abbreviation: SMBG, self-monitoring of blood glucose.
Source: From Ref. 51.

Non-Pharmacologic Measures

The mnemonic **MEDEM** (**m**onitoring, **e**ducation, **d**iet, **e**xercise, **m**edications) can be used to represent the major elements of diabetes management (29). SMBG is a very useful tool in the management of diabetes, the performance of which is associated with better glycemic control (12). Patients should be encouraged to monitor their blood glucose levels regularly, and also to maintain a logbook, which is reviewed by the physician, with feedback given to the patient. Diabetes education, dietary counseling and exercise are effective in ethnic minority groups and should be promoted vigorously as indispensable adjuncts to pharmacological agents. Using this approach, Ziemer et al. (47) obtained hemoglobin A1c reduction of 2% in 6 to 12 months. Referral to certified diabetes educators and dieticians is worthwhile in achieving this goal. Exercise programs, which should be tailored to individual patient's physical condition improves insulin sensitivity and lipid profile and also reduces obesity and blood pressure, caloric restriction and weight loss also contribute to reducing insulin resistance. Aerobic exercise such as walking, cycling and swimming at approximately 60% of maximum oxygen utilization for 30 min, three or more times a week have been found to be effective (29). Cardiac evaluation with stress electrocardiogram (ECG) is recommended for patients 35 years or older, especially if they have other risk factors for CAD.

Pharmacologic Measures

The ideal therapy for type 2 diabetes should correct insulin resistance, normalize hepatic glucose production, improve pancreatic β-cell function, normalize blood glucose level and prevent the development of acute and chronic complications of diabetes (3,29,48). Since the major underlying pathophysiologic mechanism for type 2 diabetes is insulin resistance and abnormal β-cell function, drugs that correct these abnormalities should be effective in controlling type 2 diabetes.

Thiazolidindiones

Thiozolidindiones (TZDs–Rosiglitazone and Piogitazone) induce peripheral tissue sensitization to insulin by binding to nuclear peroxisome proliferators-activated receptor-γ or PPAR-γ, thus stimulating the transcription of genes that regulate carbohydrate and lipid metabolism. Studies have shown reduction of insulin resistance by up to 33% (49) with the use of TZDs. Furthermore, recent data suggest that TZDs improve β-cell function by as much as 65% (48). Remarkable response to the metabolic effects of rosiglitazone has been noted in ethnic minority groups including African Americans, Hispanics and Chinese patients (12,29,48). TZDs may cause fluid retention, heart failure, and weight gain, which may make them less attractive for obese patients, however the metabolic gains of these agents outweigh these side effects in most patients.

Metformin

Metformin, a biguanide with insulin sensitizing effects in the liver (but rather inconsistent peripheral effects), acting by unclear mechanism results in the reduction of hepatic glucose production by suppressing gluconeogenesis. Metformin also results in weight loss. Thus, metformin should be a reasonable choice in ethnic minority patients with type 2 diabetes if there is no contraindication to its use, particularly if they are obese. It can be combined with TZDs for better metabolic control while at the same time mitigating against weight gain induced by TZDs.

Incretin Mimetics and Agonists

Incretins are local gut hormones released in response to food ingestion which modulate glucose homeostasis. Glucagon-like peptide-1 (GLP-1) and glucose-dependent insulinotropic polypeptide (GIP) are the two major incretins. Exanetide is a synthetic analogue of GLP-1 that is resistant to degradation by dipeptidyl peptidase-4 (DPP-4) enzyme. Exanetide is approved for subcutaneous injection. Orally active incretin agents are designed to inhibit DPP-4, thereby boosting postprandial levels of endogenous GLP-1 and GIP. These oral agents include Sitagliptin (recently approved) and Vidagliptin, which is awaiting FDA approval. The incretin agents improve glycemic control, augment insulin secretion, suppress glucagon secretion and are often associated with no weight gain or even weight loss (exanitide).

Other anti-diabetic agents also have their place in the treatment of ethnic minority patients with type 2 diabetes. They include insulin secretagogue (sulfonylureas, repaglinide and metiglinide), α-glucosidase inhibitors (acarbose and miglitol). The initial agent for treatment of type 2 diabetes is largely dependent on clinical judgment. The insulin secretagogues, metformin and TZDs are equipotent in their glucose-lowering effects. Additional considerations in choosing oral agents are their cost, tolerability and effects on non-glycemic metabolic profile, especially on cardiovascular risk factors (12). Most patients with type 2 diabetes ultimately require combination therapy as was shown by the UKPDS study, where only 50% of the patients could maintain hemoglobin A1c of 7% or lower after 3 years (49). Owing to the high rate of complications, early use of combination therapy should be considered in ethnic minority groups to achieve strict glycemic control. Considering the underlying pathophysiologic defect in type 2 diabetes, especially in high-risk ethnic populations, it would be prudent to include at least one insulin sensitizing agent in every combination regimen. Fixed-dose combination agents may encourage compliance and should be used in patients that would benefit from them.

With continued deterioration of β-cell function, some patients with type 2 diabetes would require insulin therapy to achieve good glycemic control. Again, because of high rate of complications in ethnic minority patients, exogenous insulin should be used without hesitation when indicated. This is usually not well received by patients initially, but education of the patient, and hope for improvement in general well being as well as the incentive of reduced complications, all help to overcome this resistance. Adequate control of blood pressure and dyslipidemia are very important components of diabetes management as well.

PRIMARY PREVENTION OF DIABETES

Early detection by screening remains the solution to the high rate of undiagnosed diabetes in ethnic minority populations. For the general US population, screening is recommended for all persons at age 45 years or older; normal tests should be repeated every 3 years. Screening should be done at an earlier age and more frequently in high-risk populations. (Table 1). Fasting blood glucose or oral glucose tolerance test could be used for screening. Individuals with IGT or prediabetes progress to type 2 diabetes over several years and have cardiovascular risk profile between that of patients with type 2 diabetes and normoglycemia. Aggressive lifestyle modification should be pursued in patients with IGT. Obesity should be treated by caloric restriction and exercise, which are effective in reducing the risk for progression from IGT to type 2 diabetes (46). A weight reduction of 5% to 7% could reduce the risk of diabetes by more than 50%. The anti-diabetic agents metformin and acarbose have also been shown to reduce the risk of progression from IGT to diabetes. A recent study demonstrated that resiglitazone reduced the risk of type 2 diabetes by 60% and induced reversion from prediabetes to normal glucose tolerance (50).

In the DPP study (46), the rate of progression from IGT to diabetes (approximately 11%) was similar in all the ethnic groups. The ethnic disparity in type 2 diabetes was not evident among over 3000 DPP cohort from diverse ethnic background who were followed for over 2 years. This finding indicates that progression from IGT to diabetes is independent of ethnic or racial influences. The genetic predisposition in ethnic minority populations would have exerted its full influence before the transition from euglycemia to IGT. Studies are currently underway to determine the nature of these early influences.

BARRIERS TO OPTIMAL DIABETES CARE

Although many effective treatment modalities are available for the control of diabetes, glycemic control is still below national guidelines. Suboptimal treatment of diabetes in ethnic groups may be due to barriers that hinder effective treatment. The barriers at the level of the patient include poor diabetes-specific knowledge, lack of self-management skills and non-adherence to lifestyle modification such as diet and exercise. Others include, negative belief and attitudes about diabetes, low literacy rates, language barriers as well as poor patient–physician communication, which may derive from differential socioeconomic levels. These obstacles need to be addressed in order to achieve good diabetes control especially in ethnic minority patients (20). Overcoming these obstacles can be quite challenging but not insurmountable. Diabetes education on the part of the patient as well as understanding and patience on the part of the physician are necessary ingredients for achieving this goal.

There are also barriers at the level of the providers, such as perceived complexity and difficulty of treating diabetes, lack of adequate time and resources for diabetes treatment. The barriers at the level of the health system include health insurance coverage, reimbursement levels and formulary restrictions, accessibility, availability and convenience of appointments. Identification and correction of these factors would improve diabetes care not only in ethnic minority groups, but also in all and sundry.

CONCLUSION

Ethnic minority groups (African Americans, Asian Americans and Pacific Islanders, Hispanic Americans, and Native Americans) are disproportionately affected by higher prevalence, complication and mortality from type 2 diabetes compared with Caucasians. Insulin resistance and β-cell failure play important roles in the evolution of type 2 diabetes in ethnic minority patients. Anti-diabetic agents, particularly those that correct insulin resistance are effective in patients from ethnic minority populations. Adequate glycemic control is the key to preventing complications of diabetes. Barriers to effective diabetes care should be identified and corrected in patients who are not optimally controlled. Primary prevention of type 2 diabetes is achievable and should be pursued vigorously in ethnic minority populations.

REFERENCES

1. Centers for Disease Control and Prevention. National Diabetes Surveillance System. Atlanta, GA: US Department of Health and Human Services. 2005; available at www.cdc.gov/diabetes/statistics/index.htm, accessed 5 July 2006.
2. Cappuccino FP. Ethnicity and cardiovascular risk: variations in people of African and South Asian origin. J Human Hypertens 1999; 11:571–6.
3. Dagogo-Jack S, Gavin JR. Diabetes. In: Multicultural Medicine and Health Disparities. McGraw-Hill Medical Publishing, 2005; 181–96.
4. Centers for Disease Control, Division of Diabetes Translation. Diabetes Surveillance, 1980–1987. Policy Program Research Annual Report DHHS9-12, 1990.
5. Harris MI, Klein R, Cowie CC, et al. Is the risk of diabetic retinopathy greater in non-Hispanic blacks and Mexican Americans than in non-Hispanic whites with type 2 diabetes? A U.S. population study. Diabetes Care 1998; 21(8):1230–5.

6. Tull E, Roseman J. Diabetes in African Americans. In: Diabetes in America, 2nd ed. Bethesda: National Institute of Health, 1995; 613–29. Available at http//diabetes.niddk.nih.gov/dm/pubs/America/pdf/chapter31.pdf.

7. Musey VC, Lee JK, Crawford R, et al. Diabetes in urban African Americans. Cessation of insulin therapy is the major precipitating cause of diabetes ketoacidosis. Diabetes Care 1995; 18(4): 483–9.

8. Nyenwe EA, Loganathan RS, Blum S, et al. Active use of cocaine: an independent risk factor for recurrent diabetic ketoacidosis in a city hospital. Endocr Pract 2007; 13(13):22–9.

9. Umpierrez GE, Smiley D, Kitabchi AE. Ketosis-prone type 2 diabetes mellitus. Ann Int Med 2006; 144(5):350–7.

10. Mauvais-Jarvis F, Sobngwi E, Porcher R, et al. Ketosis-prone type 2 diabetes in patients of sub-Saharan African origin: clinical pathophysiology and natural history of beta-cell dysfunction and insulin resistance. Diabetes 2004; 53:645–53.

11. Sobngwi E, Gautier JF, Kevorkian JP, et al. High prevalence of glucose 6-phosphate dehydrogenase deficiency without gene mutation suggests a novel genetic mechanism predisposed to ketosis-prone diabetes. J Clin Endocr Metab 2005; 90:4446–51.

12. Egede LE, Dagogo-Jack S. Epidemiology of type 2 diabetes: focus on ethnic minorities. Med Clin N Am 2005; 89:949–75.

13. Rostand SG, Kirk KA, Rutky EA, et al. Racial differences in the incidence of treatment for end stage renal disease. N Engl J Med 1982; 306(21):1276–9.

14. Lavery LA, Ashry HR, van Houtum W, et al. Variation in the incidence and proportion of diabetes-related amputations in minorities. Diabetes Care. 1996; 19(1):48–52.

15. Dagogo-Jack S. Preventing diabetes-related morbidity and mortality in the primary care setting. J Natl Med Assoc 2002; 94(7):549–60.

16. Lowe LP, Liu K, Greenland P, et al. Diabetes, asymptomatic hyperglycemia, and 22-year mortality in Black and White men. The Chicago Heart Association Detection Project in industry study. Diabetes Care 1997; 20(2):163–9.

17. Karter AJ, Ferrara A, Liu JY, et al. Ethnic disparities in diabetic complications in an insured population. JAMA 2002; 287(19):2519–27.

18. Mclarty DC, Pollitt C, Swai ABM. Diabetes in Africa. Part.2. Pract Diabetes Digest 1992; 3(2):35–40.

19. Nyenwe EA, Odia OJ, Ihekwaba AE, Ojule A, Babatunde S. Type 2 diabetes in adult Nigerians: a study of its prevalence and risk factors in Port Harcourt, Nigeria. Diab Res Clin Pract. 2003; 62: 177–85.

20. Rotimi O, Ajayi AA, Odesanmi WO. Sudden unexpected death from cardiac causes in Nigerians: a review of 50 autopsied cases. Int J Cardiol 1998; 63(2):111–5.

21. Tofler GH, Stone PH, Muller JE, et al. Effects of gender and race on prognosis after myocardial infarction: adverse prognosis for women, particularly black women. Am J Coll Cardiol 1987; 9(3): 473–82.

22. Weir GC, Leahy JL. Pathogenesis of non-insulin dependent diabetes mellitus. In: Kahn RC, Weir GC (eds), Joslin's Diabetes Mellitus, 13th ed. Philadelphia: Lea and Febiger, 1994; 240–64.

23. Neel JV, Weder AB, Julius S. Type 2 diabetes, essential hypertension and obesity as "syndromes of impaired genetic homeostasis: The thrifty genotype" hypothesis enters the 21st century. Perspect Biol Med 1998; 42(1):44–74.

24. Lev-Ran A. Thrifty genotype: how applicable is it to obesity and type 2 diabetes? Diabetes Rev 1999; 7:1–22.

25. Fujimoto W, Diabetes in Asian and Pacific Islander Americans. In: Harris MI, Cowie CC, Stern MP, et al. (eds), Diabetes in America, 2nd ed. Bethesda: National Diabetes Data Group, National Institute of Health, 1995; 661–81.

26. Cohen MP, Stern E, Rusecki Y, Zeidlre A. High prevalence of diabetes in young adult Ethiopian immigrants to Israel. Diabetes 1988; 37(6):824–8.

27. Curtsinger JW, Service PM, Prout T. Antagonistic pleiotropy, reversal of dominance, and genetic polymorphism. Am Nat 1994; 144:210–28.

28. Turnner RC, Levy JC, Clark A. Complex genetic of type 2 diabetes: thrifty genes and previously neural polymorphisms. Q J Med 1993; 86:413–7.

29. Dagogo-Jack S. Ethnic disparities in type 2 diabetes: pathophysiology and implications for prevention and management. J Natl Med Assoc 2003; 95(9):774,779–89.

30. Hales CN, Barker DJ. Type 2 (non-insulin-dependent) diabetes mellitus: the thrifty phenotype hypothesis. Diabetologia 1992; 35(7):595–601.

31. Florez JC, Jablonski KA, Bailey N, et al. TCF7L2 polymorphisms and progression to diabetes in the Diabetes Prevention Program. N Engl J Med 2006; 355:241–50.

32. Groop LC, Yuomi T. Non-insulin-dependent diabetes mellitus: a collision between thrifty genes and affluent society. Ann Med 1997; 29:37–53.

33. Harris MI. Non-insulin-dependent diabetes mellitus in black and white Americans. Diabetes Metab Rev 1990; 6:71–90.

34. Stern MP, Gaskill SP, Hazuda HP, Gardner LI, Haffner SM. Does obesity explain excess prevalence of diabetes among Mexican Americans? Result of the San Antonio Heart Study. Diabetologia 1983; 24: 272–7.

35. Weyer C, Tatarani PA, Borgadus C, et al. Insulin resistance and insulin secretory dysfunction are independent predictors of worsening of glucose tolerance during each stage of type 2 diabetes development. Diabetes Care 2000; 24:89–94.

36. Osei K, Schuster DP, Owusu SK, et al. Race ethnicity determine serum insulin and C-peptide concentrations and hepatic insulin extraction and insulin clearance: comparative studies of three populations of West African ancestry and white Americans. Metabolism 1997; 46:53–8.

37. Haffner SM, D'Agostino R, Saad MF, et al. Increased insulin resistance and insulin secretion in nondiabetic African Americans and Hispanics compared with non-Hispanic whites. Diabetes 1996; 45:742–8.

38. Mbanya JC, Pani LN, Mbanya DN, et al. Reduced insulin secretion in offspring of African type 2 diabetic parents. Diabetes Care 2003; 23(12):1761–5.

39. Cowie CC, Harris MI. Physical and metabolic characteristics of persons with diabetes. In: Harris MI, Cowie CC, Stern MP, et al. (eds), Diabetes in America, 2nd ed. Bethesda: National Diabetes Data Group, National Institute of Health, 1995; 117–64.

40. The Diabetes and Complications trial Research Group. The effect of intensive treatment of diabetes on the development and progression of long-term complications in insulin-dependent diabetes mellitus. N Engl J Med 1993; 329:978–86.

41. Shichiri M, Kishikawa H, Okhubo Y, Wake N. Long-term results of the Kumamoto study on optimal diabetes control in type 2 diabetic patients. Diabetes Care 2000; 23(Suppl. 2):B21–9.

42. Egede LE. Lifestyle modification to improve blood pressure control in individuals with diabetes: is physician advice effective? Diabetes Care 2003; 26:602–7.

43. Martin TI, Selby JV, Zhang D. physician and patient preventive practices in NIDDM in a large urban managed-care organization. Diabetes Care 1995; 18:1124–32.

44. Harris MI. Racial and ethic differences in health care access and health outcomes for adults with type 2 diabetes. Diabetes Care 2001; 24:454–949.

45. Saadine JB, Engelgau MM, Beckles GL, et al. A diabetes report card for the United States: quality of care in the 1990s. Ann Intern Med 2002; 136:565–74.

46. The Diabetes Control and Complications Trial Research Group. The effect of intensive treatment of diabetes on the development and progression of long-term complications in insulin-dependent diabetes mellitus. N Engl J Med 1993; 329:977–86.

47. Ziemer DC, Goldschmid MG, Musey VC, et al. Diabetes in urban African Americans, III: management of type II diabetes in a municipal hospital setting. Am J Med 1996; 101:25–33.

48. Umpierrez GU, Dagogo-Jack S. Role of thiazolidindiones in the management of type 2 diabetes: a focus on ethnic minority populations. Ethnicity Dis 2006; 16:51–7.

49. Turner RC, Cull CA, Frighi V, et al. Glycemic control with diet, sulfonylurea, metformin or insulin in patients with type 2 diabetes mellitus: progressive requirement for multiple therapies (UKPDS 49). JAMA 1999; 281:2005–12.

50. DREAM trial investigators. Effect of rosiglitazone on the frequency of diabetes in patients with impaired glucose tolerance and impaired fasting glucose: a randomized controlled trial. Lancet. 2006; 6736(06):69420–8; Published online September 15, doi:10.1016/S0140.

51. Tull ES, Roseman JM. Diabetes in African Americans. In: Diabetes In America. 2nd ed. Bethesda, MD: National Diabetes Data Group, NIH; 1995:613–29.

34 | Drug-Induced Hyperglycemia and Diabetes Mellitus

Mary Kate McCullen and Intekhab Ahmed
Division of Endocrinology, Diabetes and Metabolic Diseases, Department of Medicine, Thomas Jefferson University, Philadelphia, Pennsylvania, U.S.A.

INTRODUCTION

Diabetes mellitus (DM) has emerged as one of the most common diseases of this century. Its incidence is on the rise and the numbers are projected to reach a dreaded level by the year 2030 (1). In the United States alone, 4000 cases of diabetes are diagnosed every day (2). Most of them are type 2 diabetes mellitus (T2DM), and overall 8% of the population carries this diagnosis (3). Hyperglycemia is the sine qua non for diabetes. It results from the disturbance of normal glucose homeostasis. Under normal physiological conditions, plasma glucose concentrations are maintained within a narrow range, despite wide fluctuations in supply and demand, through a tightly regulated and dynamic interaction between tissue sensitivity to insulin and insulin secretion (4). Several pathologic processes can result in the disturbance of this balance. These range from autoimmune destruction of the β-cells of the pancreas with consequent insulin deficiency in T1DM to abnormalities that result in insulin resistance in the majority of T2DM. Impairment of insulin secretion and defects in insulin action frequently coexist in the same patient with T2DM. It is often difficult to decipher which abnormality, if either alone, is the primary cause of hyperglycemia (5).

A wide variety of frequently prescribed medications are known to cause glucose intolerance and can precipitate overt diabetes in non-diabetic individuals or worsen glycemic control in subjects with established diabetes.

This diabetogenic effect may occur even in people with normal metabolism as an undesired side effect with a great number of drugs, during an illness, or secondary to another disease process. Particularly with already existing glucose tolerance disturbances, or hereditary disposition, a further deterioration can lead to DM that may not always disappear after discontinued use of the drug or resolution of illness. Diabetes that develops in association with illness, drugs or other endocrinological disturbances is classified as secondary diabetes. Despite the rather large number of drugs known to worsen glucose tolerance, in relation to the total number of diabetics, drug-induced diabetes can be considered a rare cause of diabetes.

MECHANISMS OF DRUG-INDUCED DIABETES

Multiple mechanisms have been postulated to explain drug-induced diabetes (6). Some of these mechanisms have been confirmed while others are conflicting. It is important to remember that a drug can act through more than one mechanism. In general, these mechanisms can be classified into four categories: effects on insulin release, effects on insulin sensitivity, effects on liver, and effects on peripheral blood flow (Figure 1).

i.   Inhibition of insulin release will result in hyperglycemia, and medications that result in destruction of beta cells like pentamidine (7) or beta-blockers (8) which have long been considered to inhibit insulin release through pancreatic beta-cell blockade. Diuretics have also been associated with impaired insulin release through depletion of serum potassium (9).

ii. Insulin sensitivity can be altered through effects on insulin receptors or post-receptor disturbance of signaling. Hypokalemia has been linked to reduced insulin-receptor sensitivity. Various medications are involved in the alteration of glucose transport proteins (GLUT-1 and GLUT-4), tyrosine kinase activity or insulin receptor-binding affinity (10).

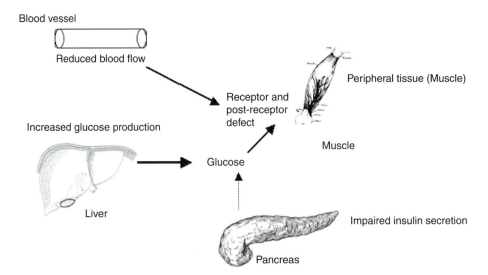

FIGURE 1   Possible mechanism of drug-induced diabetes.

iii.   Drugs like steroids (11) are associated with hepatic insulin resistance in addition to increasing glucagons release that further causes hyperglycemia by increasing glycogenolysis.

iv.   Finally, medications that reduce peripheral blood flow could direct blood flow away from the sites of glucose uptake, reducing glucose disposal (12). Non-selective beta-blockers are known to act via this mechanism as well (8). This mechanism is documented by reduced capillary density in skeletal muscles and increased risk of beta-blocker-induced hyperglycemia.

This chapter reviews commonly used prescribing agents that are associated with hyperglycemia (Table 1).

Anti-Hypertensive Medications

Thiazides

Thiazides have been associated with glycemic disturbance for many decades. In 1981, a randomized, controlled trial from the Medical Research Council suggested that patients receiving bendrofluazide developed more impaired glucose tolerance (IGT) than those receiving propranolol (15.4 vs. 4.8 cases patient–years, respectively) (13). This study was criticized for using extremely high dose of bendrofluazide. There are, however, many prospective clinical trials that have demonstrated definite adverse effects of thiazide diuretics on glucose homeostasis (14). In a post hoc analysis of the Systolic Hypertension in the Elderly Program (SHEP) trial, 3 years of low-dose chlorthalidone was associated with a significant elevation in fasting glucose compared to placebo (0.51 mmol/L vs. 0.31 mmol/L, respectively; $P<0.01$) (15). This trail also demonstrated a clinically significant increase in the incidence of diabetes (13% vs. 8.7%, respectively; $P<0.001$). In anti-hypertensive and lipid-lowering treatment to prevent Heart Attack Trial (ALLHAT), over 42,000 hypertensive patients received chlorthalidone, amlodipine, lisinopril or doxazosin as treatment for control of blood pressure. After 4 years, the incidence of diabetes was significantly higher in the chlorthalidone group (11.6%) than other treatment groups; amlodipine (9.8%) and lisinopril (8.1%) (16).

It is logical to conclude that diuretics appear to have a dose-dependent unfavorable effect on glycemic control, which may not be apparent, in short term. There are multiple mechanisms through which thiazide diuretics may worsen glycemic control. The hypokalemic effect of diuretics may blunt the release of insulin from the pancreas (17), elevations in fatty

TABLE 1 Drugs With Potential Adverse Effects on Glucose Homeostasis

Anti-hypertensive drugs
Thiazide diuretics
Beta-blockers
Calcium-channel blockers
Minoxidil
Diazoxide
Alpha-agonist
Lipid-lowering agents
Niacin
Beta adrenoreceptor agonists
Corticosteroids
Immunosupressive and immune modulating drugs
Tacrolimus
Cyclosporine
Interleukins
Thyroid hormones
Growth hormone
Oral contraceptives
Drugs for HIV treatment
Psychiatric agents
Miscellaneous
Glucosamine sulphate
Interferon
Phenytoin
Lithium

acids and lipids as a result of their use can cause hyperglycemia (18). Other mechanisms that may result in hyperglycemia include decreased insulin sensitivity (19), increased hepatic glucose production (20), a direct inhibitory effect on insulin secretion (21) and enhanced catecholamine secretion and action (22).

Beta-Blockers

Beta-blockers are known to impair glucose tolerance or even precipitate overt diabetes in non-diabetic individuals. These deleterious effects are more pronounced with nonspecific beta agonists like propranolol or beta-1 selective like metoprolol (23) compared to beta-blockers with alpha-blocking activity like carvedilol (24). In Atherosclerosis Risk In Communities (ARIC) study, a prospective study of 12,550 adults by Gress et al. (25), beta-blockers increased the risk for subsequent diabetes by 28% among hypertensive patients compared with hypertensive patients not receiving any therapy. Moreover, in the recent trials, the incidence of diabetes was highest with the use of beta-blockers, Atenolol vs. Losartan in LIFE (The Losartan Intervention (26) For End point Reduction trial, Verapamil vs. conventional therapy i.e., beta-blockers in COVINCE (Controlled Onset Verapamil Investigation of Cardiovascular End Points) (27) and INVEST (International Verapamil SR-Trandopril Study) (28). Table 2 provides a summary of 11 randomized clinical outcome trials where development of new-onset diabetes was evaluated as a secondary endpoint.

The mechanisms by which beta-blockers impair glucose tolerance are not completely understood. The degree of lipophilicity seems to be an important determinant factor (29). Other contributing factors may include weight gain (30), alterations in insulin clearance (31), reduced first-phase insulin secretion (32) and reduced peripheral blood flow due to increased peripheral vascular resistance (33).

Calcium-Channel Blockers (CCBs)

Insulin release from pancreas depends on an increase in cytosolic calcium in vitro (34) and CCBs have been used in the treatment of insulinoma (35). It appears that induction of glucose intolerance by CCBs is dose-dependent and clinically used dosages do not pose any major threat, though few reports implicate therapeutic use of verapamil with marked hyperglycemia (36).

TABLE 2   Randomized Trials that Examined Incidence of New-Onset Diabetes

Trial	Primary treatment	Increase in new-onset diabetes by primary treatment	Comparator
SHEP	Placebo	↓5%	Thiazide diuretic ± BB
STOP-2	BB/thiazide diuretic	No difference from comparator	ACE-I/CCB
CAPPP	Thiazide diuretic/BB	↑13%	ACE-I
HOPE	Placebo ± BB/thiazide diuretic	↑52%	ACE-I
INSIGHT	Thiazide diuretic/BB	↑43%	DHP-CCB
LIFE	BB/thiazide diuretic	↑32%	ARB ± thiazide diuretic
ALLHAT	Thiazide diuretic	↑16%/30%	DHP-CCB/ACE-I
INVEST	BB ± thiazide diuretic	↑17%	Non-DHP-CCB based
CHARM	Placebo ± BB/thiazide diuretic	↑17%	ARB ± BB/thiazide diuretic
VALUE	DHP-CCB	↑25%	ARB based
ASCOT	BB ± thiazide diuretic	↑32%	DHP-CCB based

Abbreviations: ACE-I, ACE-inhibitor; ARB, angiotensin II receptor blocker; ASCOT, Anglo-Scandinavian Cardiac Outcomes Trial; BB, beta-blocker; CAPP, Captopril Prevention Project; CHARM, Candesartan Cilexetil (Candesartan)in Heart Failure: Assessment of Reduction in Mortality and Morbidity; DHP, dihydropyridine; HOPE, Heart Outcomes Prevention Evaluation; INSIGHT, Intervention as a Goal in Hypertension Treatment; INVEST, International Verapamil-Trandolapril Study; LIFE, Losartan Intervention For Endpoint reduction in hypertension; VALUE, Valsartan Antihypertensive Long-Term Use Evaluation.

Minoxidil

Minoxidil can lead to rise in plasma glucose especially in diabetic individuals and patients with glucose intolerance (37). No plausible mechanism has been identified for this glucose rise.

Diazoxide

It is considered an orphan drug and is available in liquid form for the treatment of insulinoma. Short-term use of this agent for the treatment of hypertension has been associated with hyperglycemia and hyperosmolar non-ketotic coma (38). Direct inhibition of insulin secretion may be the primary mechanism responsible for the hyperglycemia (39) Other possible mechanisms may include direct stimulation of hepatic glucose production, increased epinephrine secretion, decreased insulin sensitivity and increased insulin clearance (40).

Nicotinic Acid and Niacin

Traditionally, diabetes has been regarded as a relative contraindication to the use of niacin secondary to its worsening effect on glucose homeostasis. There are case reports of severe hyperglycemia resulting from use of niacin (41). Most recent studies have shown that hyperglycemic effect of niacin is dose-dependent (42). Severe hyperglycemia with niacin use is seen mostly in patients with established glucose intolerance or with a diagnosis of diabetes (43). The higher use of niacin in non-insulin-dependent diabetic patients has resulted in 16% increase in plasma glucose levels and a 21% increase in glycosylated hemoglobin levels (44).

Mechanism of niacin-induced hyperglycemia appears to be an increased hepatic glucose output due to enhanced gluconeogensis, secondary to rebound increase in the flow of free fatty acids (FFA) to the liver (45).

Beta-Agonists

Interestingly, both beta-agonists and antagonists are implicated in causing diabetes through different mechanisms. Increased beta-receptor stimulation has been shown to increase plasma glucose via increase in glycogenolysis and lipolysis, despite increased insulin secretion (46). Beta-agonist's diabetogenic potential is dose-dependent and more pronounced with intravenous and oral route than subcutaneous route (47). There are case reports of diabetic ketoacidosis after the infusion of beta-2 agonists (48). Multiple mechanisms have been proposed for this diabetogenic potential of beta-agonists: increase in hepatic glucose production, increase in peripheral insulin resistance and increase in plasma glucagons following beta-2 agonists and increase in lipolysis (45).

Steroids

Glucocorticoids are the most common cause of drug-induced DM (49). Factors predisposing to diabetes with the use of steroids include type of steroid, age, weight, family history of diabetes or a personal history of gestational diabetes (11). Patients with decreased insulin secretory reserve are more prone to develop diabetes (50). Not everyone on steroids develop diabetes Abnormal glucose tolerance occurs in up to 90% of patients with Cushing's syndrome, but only 10% to 29% of these patients develop frank DM suggesting that the dose of glucocorticoids may be another factor in the development of diabetes (51). Steroid-induced diabetes is uncommon with topical and nasal use of steroids but high-dose steroids are associated with significant hyperglycemia, including development of hyperglycemic hyperosmolar syndrome (52,53) and even diabetic ketoacidosis in patients with type 1 diabetes mellitus (T1DM) (54).

Several mechanisms contribute to the development of hyperglycemia and steroid-induced diabetes, including decreased peripheral insulin sensitivity, increased hepatic glucose production and inhibition of pancreatic insulin production and secretion (55–57). Although all glucocorticoids can induce glucose intolerance, the glucocorticoids that are oxygenated in the 11- and 17-positions, such as hydrocortisone and the presence of 1,2 double bond in the A ring (prednisone and prednisolone), have the most diabetogenic effects. Glucocorticoids can also induce hyperglycemia through stimulation of alpha cells, leading to hyperglucogonomia and increased glycogenolysis (58). Mineralocorticoids do not directly influence carbohydrate metabolism, although hypokalemia associated with their use may reduce insulin secretion (59). With discontinuation of steroids, these effects resolve in majority of individuals.

Immunosuppressive and Immune-Modulating Drugs

New-Onset Diabetes After Transplant (NODAT)

With advancement in the field of organ transplantation, NODAT has also increased significantly and adversely affects patient survival, graft survival and quality of life. Multiple factors play an important role in the development of post-transplant diabetes including obesity, age, race, ethnicity, family history, history of hepatitis-C infection, donor source (cadaver vs. living), acute rejection, corticosteroid dose and type of immunosuppressive drugs used (Table 3) (60–62).

Calcineurin inhibitors—tacrolimus and cyclosporine are most commonly used immunosuppressive drugs used in post-transplant population and are associated with an increased incidence of diabetes in transplant individuals though comparative incidence of new-onset diabetes after transplantation induced by tacrolimus vs. cyclosporine remain controversial. In a recent meta-analysis of 16 randomized trials, the incidence of NODAT in all solid organ recipients treated with calcineurin inhibitor-containing regimen was 13.4% with higher incidence in patients receiving tacrolimus than cyclosporine (16.6% vs. 9.8%) (61).

Both tacrolimus and cycosporine reduce insulin release from the beta cells by inhibiting insulin gene transcription (63). Multiple studies have confirmed this mechanism without any change in insulin resistance (64,65).

TABLE 3 Pre-transplant Risk Factors for NODAT

Pre-transplant IGT or IFG
Increasing age (>45 years of age)
Increased body mass index (>25 kg/m^2)
Family history of diabetes
Ethnic background (non-Caucasian > Caucasian)
Smoking
Hypertension
Hyperlipidemia
Hepatitis-C infection
Deceased donor

Thyroid Hormones

Thyroid hormones have variable effects on glucose homeostasis. In hyperthyroid patients, a correlation between plasma levels of triiodothyronine and glycosylated hemoglobin has been found (66). Hyperthyroidism of any etiology in acute phase is associated with glucose intolerance (67,68). The exact mechanisms by which thyroid hormones induce glucose intolerance are controversial. Possible mechanisms include increase in hepatic glucose production (69) and depletion of insulin secretory capacity of beta cells (70,71).

Growth Hormone

Growth hormone (GH) has been used for more than 40 years. GH improves height velocity in many conditions associated with impaired growth and corrects metabolic deficits attributable to GH deficiency (GHD). The approved indications for growth hormone have expanded substantially in the last several years. Now, it is also approved for the treatment of cachexia associated with acquired immunodeficiency syndrome (AIDS) (72). It is also approved as replacement therapy in the elderly with GHD. For all these purposes, the dosages are in excess of those previously recommended. These pharmacological uses have resulted in an increased incidence of glucose intolerance and DM especially among the elderly population as they are likely to be overweight, resulting in increased insulin resistance. An increased incidence of hyperglycemia has also emerged among children receiving GH in the setting of small for gestational age, Prader-Willi syndrome and Turner Syndrome (73). In addition, "off-label" uses of GH is on the rise mainly for cosmetic reasons among elderly, for the treatment of lipodystrophy in AIDS, and for muscle building among athletes.

The effects of GH on carbohydrates are dependent on dosage and the duration of administration. In the short term, GH causes glucose oxidation to decline as a result of an increase in lipid oxidation, while muscular glucose uptake is suppressed (74). GH not only decreases the release of insulin from the beta-cells (75,76), but also induces insulin resistance at a post-receptor level in cells (77). There is no correlation between GH-induced diabetes and levels of adiponectin, leptin or resistin (78). In patients with acromegaly, a natural example of GH excess, incidence of diabetes is 20% to 30% (79).

Oral Contraceptives

Alterations in carbohydrate metabolism have been reported with long-term use of oral contraceptives and are known to be secondary to progesten component of the oral contraceptive (80–82). The exact etiology of glucose intolerance is not clear as literature is filled with conflicting data (83). Contraceptives with high doses of progestogen are more likely to cause glucose intolerance (84), though several studies have shown counterintuitive results regarding low-dose vs. high-dose use of oral contraceptives. In a study comparing low-dose vs. high-dose oral contraceptives containing norgestrel, the subjects on low-dose exhibited more glucose disturbance and beta cell dysfunction compared to subjects on high-dose and controls (85). Another possible mechanism of increased insulin resistance in oral contraceptive users may be the weight gain that is associated with their long-term use (86).

It is important to emphasize that low-dose oral contraceptives, and especially triphasic pill have minimal effect on carbohydrate metabolism (87). Although monitoring of plasma glucose levels may be prudent, diabetes has not been shown to be an important impediment to hormone-based contraception (83).

HIV Drugs

Disorders of glucose metabolism have been reported in patients infected with HIV (88,89). Cross-sectional studies estimate prevalence of diabetes to be 2% to 7% in HIV individuals receiving protease inhibitors (PIs) (90–92), and an additional 16% having IGT (91).

Protease Inhibitors (PI)

The introduction of highly active antiretroviral therapy (HAART) has significantly improved the survival and quality of life of HIV-infected individuals. However, HARRT-regimen, especially those including PIs have also resulted in increased incidence of metabolic syndrome and diabetes. Eleven PIs are now available in US and at least eight of them are clearly associated with disturbance in glucose homeostasis. It is estimated that up to 40% of patients receiving PI-based regimen show glucose intolerance and 6% to 7% develop new-onset diabetes (92). One of the early reports of PI-induced diabetes was in 1997 by Visnigarwala et al. (93) when addition of nelfinavir to the patient's regimen resulted in overt diabetes in less than 2 weeks. The duration of PI therapy preceding the onset of hyperglycemia or overt diabetes is still debatable, timing of onset has been seen as early as 2 weeks (94) to as late as up to 24 months (95). Some investigators have shown the biochemical abnormalities with even a single dose of indinavir (96).

Currently, mechanisms responsible for hyperglycemia and onset of overt diabetes with use of PI include onset of insulin resistance (97), presence of beta cell dysfunction (98) and effect of dyslipidemia on both peripheral resistance and beta-cells (99).

Several studies have shown that use of PI results in decreased activity of GLUT4, a major transporter for glucose uptake by the peripheral tissues, especially in skeletal muscle resulting in insulin resistance (100).

Literature is also rife with data showing direct effect of PIs on beta cells resulting in decreased release of insulin in the setting of insulin resistance (101). In addition, recent literature also proposes the role of lipotoxicity in the insulin resistance. A study by Yarasheski et al. (102) presented data from a cross-sectional study of 22 non-obese, HIV-infected individuals in whom insulin sensitivity was assessed with hyperinsulinemic euglycemic clamp. Author found an inverse correlation between insulin sensitivity and hepatic and soleus muscle lipid content.

The newer PIs—atazanavir, tipranavir, mozenavir and amprenavir—do not seem to have any hyperglycemic effects.

Didanosine

A commonly used antiretroviral agent is also known to cause hyperglycemia and diabetes (103). Incidence of didanosine-induced pancreatitis is much higher in elder patients than young (10% vs. 5%) (104). Some reports indicate reversible hyperglycemia and diabetes without any evidence of pancreatitis (105). Albrecht et al. (106) prospectively followed 12 patients who at the beginning of didanosine treatment had normal glucose tolerance; six developed IGT, which reverted to normal glucose tolerance on discontinuation of didanosine.

Pentamidine

An anti-parasitic agent used to treat infections with *Pnemocystis carinii* (107). It is well known for causing hypoglycemia, IGT and overt DM (108). Diabetes has been observed in more than 100 patients, sometimes with ketoacidosis or lactic acidosis (109–114). Hypoglycemia and diabetes have also been reported after pentamidine isethionate (115) and pentamidine aerosol therapies (116,117). Inappropriate plasma insulin levels were sometimes determined: they were excessive in the presence of hypoglycemia, and lower than normal in the diabetic patients treated with pentamidine (110). It has been suggested that a dose-dependent toxicity of pentamidine to the islets of Langerhans can account for these opposite adverse metabolic effects: an early excessive insulin leakage from lesioned B-cells as a cause of hypoglycemia, and then B-cell death and insulinopenia causing diabetes.

Megestrol Acetate (Megace)

An oral progestational agent frequently used in the treatment of AIDS-related cachexia (118). Cases of reversible hyperglycemia and diabetes have been reported with its use (119). Most of these cases are dose-dependent. The drug appears to have glucocorticoids like activity, which may lead to peripheral insulin resistance and increased caloric intake (120). There are cases of Cushingoid state associated with its use as well (121).

Antipsychotic Agents/Psychiatric Drugs

Patients with psychiatric illness are known to suffer from diabetes more often than the general population (122). A recent Italian study (123) found an overall incidence of diabetes in 95 schizophrenic patients to be 15.8% compared to 3% prevalence in the general Italian population. This increased incidence in diabetes was independent of antipsychotic drug administration (124,125). Apart from genetic predisposition, environmental influences also play a significant role in increased incidence of diabetes as most of the patients with psychiatric illness generally lack insight and do not recognize or complain of the physical symptoms of diabetes. These observations have further increased the concern about the occurrence of diabetes associated with the use of atypical antipsychotic (AAP) drugs. Such a concern is justifiable as diabetes carries a considerable risk of morbidity and mortality.

The first account of disturbance of glucose metabolism in schizophrenic patients dates from 1879 (126) and has been confirmed by many authors (127–129) in the first half of the 20th century. The introduction of neuroleptics also brought a rapid increase in the incidence of type 2 diabetes in these patients. The atypical or second generation antipsychotic drugs, introduced in 1990s, showed less extrapyramidal side effects but seemed to have a stronger diabetogenic effect than classical anti-psychotics (130).

Patients on olanzapine and clozapine carry the highest risk of developing hyperglycemia, ketoacidosis and new-onset diabetes than other second-generation antipsychotic agents (131). The risk of developing diabetes with antipsychotic agents is around 4.7%. The risk is lowest with risperidone (132), whereas quetiapine, olanzapine and clozapine are not different in their risk from first-generation antipsychotics.

The mechanisms responsible for the increased diabetes risk with antipsychotic agents are hard to decipher for a number of reasons: (1) most of the patients receive multiple medications simultaneously that makes it difficult to identify a particular drug as a causative agent, and (2) untreated schizophrenic patients have a higher rate of diabetes than general population. However, a number of mechanisms have been postulated to explain this association:

a. Receptor action: It is possible that AAP drugs induce diabetes by blocking dopamine D2 receptors in certain areas of the brain and secondarily increasing neurotensin. Neurotensin causes both antipsychotic as well as diabetogenic actions (133,134).
b. Chemical structure: The fact that all four thieno-benzodiazepine drugs-clozapine, olanzapine, loxitane and amoxapine induce diabetes implies that the three-ring chemical structure may be responsible for it (135).
c. Leptin: The hormone leptin synthesized by adipocytes plays a key role in the regulation of appetite, food intake and body weight by acting in the hypothalamus at leptin receptors. In olanzapine-and clozapine-treated patients, serum leptin levels increase more rapidly than with other AAP drugs. This rapid increase in leptin levels may be a potential mechanism of causing insulin resistance (136–139).
d. Low insulin-like growth factor-I: The insulin-like growth factor-I (IGF-I) and insulin-like growth factor binding protein-I (IGFBP-I) are important for glucose homeostasis. Circulating IGF-I is dependent on growth hormone, insulin levels and nutrition. The median level of IGF-I was significantly lower in patients treated with clozapine compared with the patients on neuroleptics. Therefore, decreased IGF-I may be responsible for diabetes in patients treated with AAP drugs (140).
e. Hyperlipidemia: AAP drugs cause hyperlipidemia of variable degrees. Clozapine causes hypertriglyceridemia as much as 37% from the baseline. It is possible that hypertriglyceridemia contributes to insulin resistance with these agents (141,142).
f. Genetic predisposition: Since only a small fraction of patients treated with AAP drugs develop diabetes and, in addition, African-American patients treated with AAP agents develop diabetes more often than similarly treated Caucasian patients. This indicates the possible role of genetic predisposition to the adverse effects of these agents (143,144).

Miscellaneous

Glucosamine Sulphate

The use of glucosamine sulphate is on the rise in industrialized nations secondary to increased incidence of obesity and resulting in osteoarthritis (145). Multiple studies have observed a dose-dependent hyperglycemia with the use of glucosamine sulphate (146).

Glucosamine induces insulin resistance by increasing glucose flux through hexosamine biosynthetic pathway (147). Furthermore, it also inhibits glucose-induced release of insulin from beta cells (148).

Interferons

Interferons (IFNs) comprise a group of related proteins whose effects include antiviral activity, growth regulatory properties, inhibition of angiogenesis, regulation of cell differentiation, enhancement of major histocompatibility complex antigen expression and a wide variety of immunomodulatory activities. They were originally classified according to their source and have subsequently been renamed: Alpha-IFN (formerly known as leukocyte IFN), beta-IFN (formerly known as fibroblast IFN) and gamma-IFN (formerly known as immune IFN). Use of IFN therapy especially IFN-alpha in the treatment of hepatitis-C is common. They are commonly used in the management of hepatitis-C. There have been some reports of it causing IGT or DM. In some cases the presence of immunological data suggests DM1 (149–152) while in others the need for insulin is only temporary (153). This diabetogenic effect is perhaps unsurprising since: (i) IFN is a cytokine involved in the immunopathology that leads to β-cell destruction (154–156), and (ii) its administration is related to other autoimmune processes, including thyroiditis. The impact of IFN on glucose metabolism has been studied with contradictory results (157–160). Epidemiological studies have related hepatitis C virus (HCV) infection to DM, implicating a different pathophysiological effect (161). Thus the link between IFN-α treatment and the development of DM in chronic hepatitis C is unclear.

Lithium

The effects of lithium on carbohydrate metabolism are complex, and improvement and worsening of glucose tolerance have both been observed in patients receiving lithium (162–164). Studies in rats show that lithium exerts anti-diabetic effects by increasing glycogenesis, either through an insulin-sensitizing action or through direct activation of enzymes involved in hepatic glycogenesis (165). Clinically, therapeutic use of lithium does not pose any significant threat in patients.

Diphenylhydantoin (Phenytoin)

It is a commonly used anti-convulsant and also used frequently for diabetic neuropathy. Phenytoin is known to cause hyperglycemia (166) and pancreatitis (167). It inhibits both first and second phases of insulin release (168). In a study of patients with previous myocardial infarction, a tendency of diphenylhydantoin to impair the insulin response to glucose was confirmed (169). Diabetes usually resolves with discontinuation of phenytoin.

CONCLUSION

Drug-induced hyperglycemia occurs due to the use of a wide variety of drugs and mechanisms. Despite the ever-increasing number of diabetics and use of multiple medications, especially in the elderly to manage their health, the entity of drug-induced diabetes does not appear to be very common. However, since strict goals of hyperglycemic control have a proven beneficial effect on the well-being of patients, we should be very vigilant in our choice of medicines. An understanding of the drug and its possible mechanisms in causing hyperglycemia is a helpful tool in selecting the right approach to drug-induced diabetes. Drug-induced diabetes secondary to insulin secretory defect can be managed by sulfonylurea or insulin. The thiazolidinedeione drugs can be very promising in cases where insulin resistance by a drug has resulted in diabetes.

REFERENCES

1. CDC Diabetes Program. Available at http://www.cdc.gov/diabetes/pubs/estimates.htm.
2. Cowie C, Rust F Keith, Eberhardt M, Flegal K, Engelgau M, Geiss L, Gregg WE. Prevalence of Diabetes and Imapired Fasting Glucose in adults in the U.S. Population: National Health and Nutrition Examination Survey. 1999–2002 Diabetes Care 2006; 29:1263–1268.

3. Nathan DM. Initial management of glycemia in type-2 diabetes mellitus. N Engl J Med 2002; 347: 1342–9. Rickheim P, et al. Type 2 Diabetes BASICS Curriculum Guide, 2nd ed. 2004.

4. Stumvoll M, Goldstein BJ Van Haeften TW, Pollare T, Lithell H, Selinus I, Berne C. Type 2 diabetes: principles of pathogenesis and therapy. Lancet 2005; 365(9467):1333–46.

5. Blackburn DF, Wilson TW. Antihypertensive medications and blood sugar: theories and implications. Can J Cardiol 2006; 22(3):229–33.

6. Coyle P, Carr AD, Depczynski BB, Chisholm DJ. Diabetes mellitus associated with pentamidine use in HIV-infected patients. Med J Aust 1996; 165(10):587–8.

7. Pollare T, Litbell H, Selirius I. Sensitivity to insulin during treatment with atenolol and metroprolol: a randomized, double blind study of effects on carbohydrate and lipoprotein metabolism in hypertensive patients. BMJ 1989; 298:1152–7.

8. Hunrer SJ, Harper R, et al. Effects of combination therapy with an angiotensin converting enzyme inhibitor and thiazide diuretic on insulin action in essential hypertension. J Hypertens 1998; 16: 103–9.

9. Dominguez LJ, Barbbagallo M, Jacober SJ, Sowers JR. Bisoprolol and captopril effects on insulin receptor tyrosine kinase activity in essential hypertension. Am J Hypertens 1997; 309:226–30.

10. Trence DL. Management of patients on chronic glucocorticoids therapy: an endocrine perspective. Prim Care Clin Office Pract 2003; 30:593–605.

11. Reaven GM, Lithell H, Landsberg L. Hypertension and associated metabolic abnormalities—the role of insulin resistance and the sympathoadrenal system. N Engl J Med 1996; 334:374–81.

12. Medical Research Council. Adverse reactions to bendrofluazide and propranolol for the treatment of mild hypertension. Report of the Medical Research Council Working party on Mild to Moderate Hypertension. Lancet 1981; 2:254–549.

13. Zanchetti A, Ruilope LM. Antihypertensive treatment in patients with type-2 diabetes mellitus: what guidance from recent controlled randomized trials? J Hypertens 2002; 20:2099–110.

14. Sowers JR. Hypertension in type 2 diabetes: update on therapy. J Clin Hypertens 1994; 1:41–7.

15. Sierra C, Ruilope LM. New-onset diabetes and antihypertensive therapy: comments on ALLHAT trial. J Renin-Angiotensin-Aldosterone Syst 2003; 4(3):169–70.

16. Zillich AJ, Garg J, Basu S, Bakris GL, Carter BL. Thiazide diuretics, potassium, and the development of diabetes: a quantitative review. Hypertension 2006; 48(2):219–24.

17. Gulliford MC, Charlton J, Latinovic R. Trends in antihypertensive and lipid lowering therapy in subjects with type II diabetes: clinical effectiveness or clinical discretion? J Human Hypertens 2005; 19(2):111–7.

18. Weir MR, Moser M. Diuretics and beta-blockers: is there a risk for dyslipidemia? Am Heart J 2000; 139(1 Pt 1):174–83.

19. Bell DS. Insulin resistance: an often unrecognized problem accompanying chronic medical disorders. Postgrad Med 1993; 93(7):99–103, 106–7.

20. Davies DM, Textbook of Adverse Reactions. New York: Oxford University Press, 1985; 352–69.

21. Flamenbaum W. Metabolic consequences of antihypertensive therapy. Ann Intern Med 1983; 98: 875–80.

22. Micossi P, Pollavini G, Raggi U, et al. Effects of metoprolol and propranolol on glucose tolerance and insulin secretion in diabetes mellitus. Horm Metab Res 1984; 16:59–63.

23. Bakris GL, Fonseca V, Katholi RE, McGill JB, Messerli FH, Phillips RA, Raskin P, Wright JT Jr, Oakes R, Lukas MA, Bell DS: Metabolic effects of carvedilol vs. metoprolol in patients with type 2 diabetes mellitus and hypertension: a randomized controlled trial. JAMA 2004; 292:2227–36.

24. Gress TW, Nieto FJ, Shahar E, Wofford MR, Brancati FL. Hypertension and antihypertensive therapy as risk factors for type 2 diabetes mellitus. N Engl J Med 2000; 342:905–12.

25. Dahlof B, Devereux RB, Kjeldsen SE, et al. Cardiovascular morbidity and mortality in the Losartan Intervention For Endpoint reduction in hypertension study (LIFE): a randomized trial against atenolol. Lancet 2002; 359(9311):995–1003.

26. Black HR, Elliott WJ, Grandtts G, et al. Principal results of the controlled Onset Verapamil Investigation of Cardiovascular End Points (CONVINCE) trial. JAMA 2003; 289:2073–82.

27. Pepine CJ, Handeberg EM, Cooper-Dehoff RM, et al. AAA calcium antagonist versus a non-calcium antagonist hypertension treatment strategy for patients with coronary artery disease. The International Verapamil-Trandolapril Study (INVEST): a randomized controlled trial. JAMA 2003; 290:2805–16.

28. Whitcroft I, Wilkinson N, Rawthorne A, Thomas J, Davies JB. Beta-adrenoceptor antagonist impair long-term glucose control in hypertensive diabetics: role of beta-adrenoceptor selectivity and lipid solubility. Br J Clin Pharm 1986; 22:236P–7P.

29. Pischon T, Sharma AM. Use of beta-blockers in obesity, hypertension: potential role of weight gain. Obes Rev 2001; 2(4):275–80.

30. Jacob S, Rett K, Henriksen EJ. Antihypertensive therapy and insulin sensitivity: do we have to redefine the role of beta-blocking agents? Am J Hypertens 1998; 11(10):1258–65.

31. Chan JC, Cockram CS, Critchley JA. Drug-induced disorders of glucose metabolism: mechanisms and management. Drug Safety 1996; 15(2):135–57.
32. Van Bortel LM, Ament AJ. Selective versus nonselective beta adrenoceptor antagonists in hypertension. 1995; 8(6):513–23.
33. Wollheim CB, Kikuchi M, Renold AE, Sharp CW. The roles of intracellular and extracellular Ca++ in glucose-stimulated biphasic insulin release by rat islets. J Clin Invest 1978; 62(2):451–8.
34. Owecki M, Sowinski J. Successful pharmacological treatment of hyperinsulinemic hypoglycemia with verapamil and amlodipine—case report. Polski Merkuriusz Lekarski 2005; 19(110):196–8.
35. Roth AM, Belhassen B, Laniado S. Slow-release verapamil and hyperglycemic metabolic acidosis. Ann Intern Med 1989; 110(2):171–2.
36. Lederballe Pedersen O. Long-term experience with minoxidil in combination treatment of severe arterial hypertension. Acta Cardiol 1977; 32:283–93.
37. Levine SN, Sanson TH. Treatment of hyperglycemic hyperosmolar non-ketotic syndrome. Drugs 1989; 38(3):462–72.
38. Hansen JB, Arkhammar PO, Bodvarsdottir TB, Wahl P. Inhibition of insulin secretion as a new drug target in the treatment of metabolic disorders. Curr Med Chem 2004; 11(12):1595–615.
39. Knapp MS, Cove-Smith R, Hall G, McIllmurray M. Dangers of diazoxide. BMJ 1972; 4(5834):229–30.
40. Schwartz ML. Severe reversible hyperglycemia as a consequence of niacin therapy. Arch Int Med 1993; 153(17):2050–2.
41. Tornvall P, Walldius D. A comparison between nicotinic acid and acipimox in hypertryglyceridemia—effects on serum lipids, lipoproteins, glucose tolerance and tolerability. J Intern Med 1991; 230:415–21.
42. Henkin Y, Oberman A, Hurst DC, Segrest JP. Niacin revisited: clinical observation on an important but underutilized drug. Am J Med 1991; 91:239–46.
43. Garg A, Grundy SM. Nicotinic acid as therapy for dyslipidemia in non-insulin dependent diabetes mellitus. JAMA 1990; 264:723–6.
44. Mohan RJ, Mohan R. Drug induced diabetes mellitus. JAPI 1997; 45(11):876–8.
45. O'Byrne S, Feely J. Effects of drugs on glucose tolerance in non-insulin dependent diabetics (Part II). Drugs 1990; 40:6–18.
46. Leslie D, Coats PM. Salbutamol-induced diabetic ketoacidosis (letter). BMJ 1977; 2:768.
47. Barnewolt BA, Walter FG, Bey TA. Metabolic effects of metaproterenol overdose: hypokalemia, hyperglycemia, and hyperlactatemia. Vet Human Toxicol 2001; 43(3):158–60.
48. Bressler P, De Fronzo RA. Drugs and diabetes. Diabetes Rev 1994; 2:25–84.
49. Mokshagundam SP, Peiris AN. Drug induced disorders of glucose metabolism. In: Leahy JL, Clark NG, Cefalu WT (eds), Medical Management of Diabetes Mellitus. New York: Marcel Decker; 2000, 201–15.
50. Welbourn RB, Montgomery DA, Kennedy TL. The natural history of treated Cushing's syndrome. Br J Surg 1971; 58:1–16.
51. Terence DL, Hirsch IB. Hyperglycemic crises in diabetes mellitus type 2. Endocrinol Metab Clin North Am 2001; 30:817–31.
52. Heazell AE, Shina A, Bhatti NR. A case of gestational diabetes arising following treatment with glucocorticoids for pemphigoid gestations. J Maternal-Fetal Neonatal Med 2005; 18(5):353–5.
53. Bedalov A, Balasurbramanyam A. Glucocorticoid-induced ketoacidosis in gestational diabetes: sequelae of the acute treatment of preterm labor. Diabetes Care 1997; 20:922–4.
54. Pagano G, Cavallo-Perin, Cassader M, et al. An in vivo and in vitro study of the mechanism of prednisone induced insulin resistance in healthy subjects. J Clin Invest 1983; 72:1814–20.
55. Shamoon H, Soman V, Sherwin R. The influence of acute physiological increments of cortisol on fuel metabolism and insulin binding to monocytes in normal humans. J Clin Endorinol Metab 1980; 50:495–501.
56. Andrews RC, Herlihy O, Livingstone DE, Andrew R, Walker BR. Abnormal cortisol metabolism and tissue sensitivity to cortisol in patients with glucose intolerance. J Clin Endocriol Metab 2002; 87(12):5587–93.
57. Chan JC, Cockram CS. Drug-induced disturbances of carbohydrate metabolism. Adverse Drug React Toxicol Rev 1991; 10:1–29.
58. Fallo F, Veglio F, Bertello C, et al. Prevalence and characteristics of the metabolic syndrome in primary aldosteronism. J Clin Endocrinol Metab 2006; 91(2):454–9.
59. Ojo AO, Hansen JA, Wolfe Ra, et al. Long-term survival in renal transplant recipients with graft function. Kidney Int 2000; 57:307–13.
60. Heisel O, Heisel R, Keown P. New onset diabetes mellitus in patients receiving calcineurin inhibitors. Am J Transplant 2004; 4:583–95.
61. Vesco L, Busson M, Bedrossian J, et al. Diabetes mellitus after renal transplantation: characteristics, outcomes, and risk factors. Transplantation 1996; 61:1475–8.

62. Nam JH, Mun JI, Kim SI, et al. Beta-cell dysfunction rather than insulin resistance is the main contributing factor for the development of post-renal transplantation diabetes mellitus. Transplantation 2001; 71:1417–23.

63. Oetjen E, Baun D, Beimesche S, et al. Inhibition of human insulin gene transcription by the immunosuppressive drugs cyclosporine and tacrolimus in primary, mature islets of transgenic mice. Mol Pharmacol 2003; 63:1289–95.

64. Redmon JB, Olson LK, Armstrong MB, et al. Effects of tacrolimus on human insulin gene expression, insulin mRNA levels, and insulin secretion in HIT-T15 cells. J Clin Invest 1996; 98: 2786–93.

65. Saito T, Sato T, Yamamoto M, et al. Hemoglobin A1c levels in hyperthyroidism. Endocrinol Jpn 1982; 29:137–40.

66. Paul DT, Mollah FH, Alam MK, Fariduddin M, Azad K, Arsalan MI. Glycemic status in hyperthyroid subjects. Mymensingh Med J 2004; 13(1):71–5.

67. Moon SW, Hahm JR, Lee GW, et al. A case of hyperosmolar state associated with Graves' hyperthyroidism. J Korean Med Sci 2006; 21(4):765–7.

68. Pandolfi C, Pellegrini L, Dede A. Blood glucose and insulin responses to oral glucose in hyperthyroidism. Minerva Endocrinol 1996; 21(2):63–5.

69. Muller MJ, Von Schutz B, Huhnt HJ, et al. Glucoregulatory function of thyroid hormones: interaction with insulin depends on the prevailing glucose concentration. J Clin Endocrinol Metab 1986; 63(1):62–71.

70. Karlander SG, Khan A, Wajngot A, Torring O, Vranic M, Efendic S. Glucose turnover in hyperthyroid patients with normal glucose tolerance. J Clin Endocrinol Metab 1989; 68:780–6.

71. Medical Economics Co., Physician's Desk reference. Montvale, NJ: Medical Economics Co., 2001.

72. Statement from the Growth Hormone Research Society. Critical evaluation of the safety of recombinant human growth hormone administration. J Clin Endocrinol Metab 2001; 86: 1868–70.

73. Czernichow P. Growth hormone administration and carbohydrate metabolism. Horm Res 1993; 39: 102–3.

74. Wiesli P, Schaffler E, Seifert B, Schmid C, Donath MY. Islets secretory capacity determines glucose homoeostasis in the face of insulin resistance. Swiss Med Weekly 2004; 134(37–38):559–64.

75. Steffin B, Gutt B, Bidlingmaier M, Schophol J, et al. Effects of the long-acting Somatostatin analogue Lanreotide Autogel on glucose tolerance and insulin resistance in acromegaly. Eur J Endocrinol 2006; 155(1):73–8.

76. Watanabe A, Komine F, Nirei K, et al. A case of secondary diabetes mellitus with acromegaly improved by pioglitazone. Diabetes Med 2004; 12(9):1049–50.

77. Silha JV, Krsek M, Hana V, Marek J, Jezkova J, Murphy LJ. Perturbations in adiponectin, leptin, and resistin levels in acromegaly: lack of correlation with insulin resistance. Clin Endocrinol 2003; 58(6): 736–42.

78. Krisht AF, Tindall GT. Pituitary Disorders: Comprehensive Management. Lippincott Williams & Wilkins; 1999. New Zealand: Drugs & Aging; 2000, 17(6):453–61.

79. Fineberg, SE. Glycemic control and hormone replacement therapy: implications of the postmenopausal Estrogen/Progestogen Intervention (PEPI) Study. Drugs Aging 2000; 17(6): 453–61.

80. Xiang AH, Kawakubo M, Kjos SL, Buchanan TA. Long acting injectable progestin contraception and risk of type 2 diabetes in Latino women with prior gestational diabetes. Diabetes Care 2006; 29 (3):613–7.

81. Shawe J, Lawrenson R. Hormonal contraception in women with diabetes mellitus: special consideration. 2003; 2(5):321–30.

82. Van Bortel LM, Ament AJ. Selective versus nonselective beta adrenoceptor antagonists in hypertension. Pharmacoeconomics 1995; 8(6):513–23.

83. Rosenthal AD, Shu Xo, Jin F, Yang G, Elasy TA, Li Q, Xu HX, Gao YT, Zheng W. Oral contraceptive use and risk of diabetes among Chinese women. Contraception 2004; 69(3):251–7.

84. Gallo MF, Lopez Lm, Grimes DA, Schulz KF, Helmerhorst FM. Combination contraceptives: effects on weight. Cochrane Database Syst Rev 2003; 3(2):CD003987.

85. Spellacy WN, Tsibris JC, Ellindson AB. Carbohydrate metabolic studies in women using a levonorgestrel/ethinyl estradiol containing triphasic oral contraceptive for eighteen months. Int J Gynaecol Obstet 1991; 35:69–71.

86. Spellacy WN. Carbohydrate metabolism during treatment with estrogen, progestrogen and low-dose oral contraceptives. Am J Obstet Gynecol 1982; 142:732–4.

87. Dube MP, Johnson DL, Currier JS, et al. Protease inhibitor associated hyperglycemia. Lancet 1997; 350:713–4.

88. Dever LL, Oruwari PA, Figueora W, et al. Hyperglycemia associated with protease inhibitors in an urban HIV-infected minority patient population. Ann Pharmacother 2000; 34:580–4.

89. Karr A, Samaras K, Thorisdottir A, et al. Diagnosis, prediction, and natural course of HIV-I protease inhibitor-associated lipodystrophy, hyperlipidemia, and diabetes mellitus: a cohort study. Lancet 1999; 353:2093–9.

90. Currier J, Boyd F, Kawabata H, et al. Diabetes mellitus in HIV infected individuals (Abstract 677-T). Presented at the 9th Conference on Retrovirus and Opportunistic Infections, Seattle, 2002.

91. Hammer SM, Squires KE, Hughes MD, et al. A trial of two nucleosides analogues plus indinavir in persons with human immunodeficiency virus infections and CD cell count of 200 per cubic millimeter or less. N Engl J Med 1997; 337:725–33.

92. Visnegarwala F, Krause KL, Musher DM, et al. Severe diabetes associated with protease inhibitor therapy. Ann Intern Med 1997; 127(10):947.

93. Hughes C, Taylor G. Metformin in an HIV infected patient with protease inhibitor-induced diabetic ketoacidosis. Ann Pharmacother 2001; 35:877–80.

94. Saves M, Raffi S, Capeau J, et al. Factors related with lipodystrophy and metabolic alterations in patients with human immunodeficiency virus infection receiving highly active antiviral therapy. Clin Infect Dis 2002; 34:1396–1405.

95. Noor AM, Seneviratne T, Aweeka FT, et al. Indinavir acutely inhibits insulin-stimulated glucose disposal in humans: a randomized placebo controlled study. AIDS 2002; 16:F1–8.

96. Yarasheski K, Tebas P, Sigmund C, et al. Insulin resistance in HIV-protease inhibitor-associated diabetes. J Acquire Immune Def Syndr 1999; 21:209–16.

97. Woerle H, Mariuz P, Meyer C, et al. Mechanism for deterioration in glucose tolerance associated with HIV protease inhibitor regimens. Diabetes 2003; 52:918–25.

98. Gan SK, Samaras K, Thompson C, et al. Altered myocellular and abdominal fat partitioning predicts disturbance in insulin action in HIV protease inhibitor-associated lipodystrophy. Diabetes 2002; 51:3163–9.

99. Murata H, Hruz PW, Mueckler M. The mechanism of insulin resistance caused by HIV protease inhibitors. J Biol Chem 2000; 275:20251–4.

100. Saint-Marc T, Touraine JL. Effects of metformin on insulin resistance and central adiposity in patients receiving effective protease inhibitor therapy. AIDS 1999; 13:1000–02.

101. Yarasheski K, Reeds D, Schulte J, et al. Impaired insulin sensitivity in HIV infected patients is associated with higher hepatic lipid content and visceral adiposity. (Abstract 757). Tenth Conference on Retroviruses and Opportunistic Infections, 2003.

102. Garcia-Benayas T, Rendon AL, Rodriguez-Novoa S, Barrios A, Maida I, Blanco F, Barreiro P, Rivas P, Soriano V. Higher risk of hyperglycemia in HIV-infected patients treated with didanosine plus tenofovir. AIDS Res Human Retroviruses 2006; 22(4):333–7.

103. Kakuda TN. Pharmacology of the nucleoside and nucleotide reverse transcriptase inhibitor-induced mitochondrial toxicity. Clin Therapeut 2000; 22(6):685–708.

104. Vittecoq D, Zucman D, Auperin I, Passeron J. Transient insulin dependent diabetes mellitus in an HIV-infected patient receiving didanosine. AIDS 1994; 8(9):1351.

105. Albrecht H, Stellbrink HJ, Araseth K. Didanosine induced disorders of glucose tolerance. Ann Intern Med 1993; 119:1050.

106. Izzedine H, Launay-Vacher V, Deybach C, Bourry E, Barrou B, Deray G. Drug-induced diabetes mellitus. Expert Opin Drug Saf 2005; 4(6):1097–109.

107. Bressler P, De Fronzo RA. Drugs and diabetes. Diabetes Rev 1994; 2:53–84.

108. Naafs B. Pentamidine-induced diabetes mellitus. Trans R Soc Trop Med Hyg 1985; 79:141.

109. Lambertus MW, Murthy AR, Nagami P, Bidwell P, Goetz M. Diabetic ketoacidosis after pentamidine therapy in a patient with the acquired immunodeficiency syndrome. West J Med 1988; 149:602–4.

110. Collins RJ, Pien FD, Houk JH. Insulin-dependent diabetes mellitus associated with pentamidine. Am J Med Sci 1989; 297:174–5.

111. Perronne C, Bricaire F, Leport C, Assan D, Vilde JL, Assan R. Hypoglycemia and diabetes mellitus after parenteral pentamidine mesylate treatment in AIDS patients. Diabetic Med 1990; 7:585–9.

112. Herchline TE, Plouffe JR, Para MF. Diabetes mellitus presenting with ketoacidosis, after pentamidine therapy in patients with acquired immunodeficiency syndrome. J Infect Dis 1991; 22:41–4.

113. Morin D, Dumas ML, Valette H, Dumas R. Transitory acute kidney insufficiency and insulin-dependent diabetes after treatment of kala-azar with pentamidine and N-methylglucamine antimony. Arch Fr Pediatr 1991; 48:349–51.

114. Anderson R, Boedicker M. Adverse reactions associated with pentamidine isethionate in AIDS patients: recommendations for monitoring therapy. Drug Intell Clin Pharm 1986; 20:862–8.

115. Hart CC. Aerosolized pentamidine and pancreatitis (Letter). Ann Intern Med 1989; 111:691.

116. Chen JP, Braham RL, Squires KE. Diabetes after aerosolized pentamidine. Ann Intern Med 1991; 114:913–4.

117. Kilby JM, Taberaux PB. Severe hyperglycemia in an HIV clinic: preexisting versus drug-associated diabetes mellitus. J Acquire Immune Def Syndr Human Retrovirology 1998; 17(1):46–50.

118. Salinas I, Lucas A, Clotet B. Secondary diabetes induced by megestrol therapy in a patient with AIDS-associated cachexia. AIDS 1993; 7(6):894.
119. Mann M, Koller E, Murgo A, Malozowski S, Bacsanyi J, Leinung M. Glucocorticoid-like activity of megestrol: a summary of Food and Drug administration experience and review of the literature. Arch Intern Med 1997; 157(15);1651–6.
120. Steer KA, Kurtz AB, Honour JW. Megestrol-induced Cushing's syndrome. Clin Endocrinol 1995; 42 (1):91–3.
121. Newcomer JW. Medical risk in patients with bipolar disorder and schizophrenia. J Clin Psych 2006; 9(Suppl. 67):25–30.
122. Mukerjee S, Decina P, Bocola V, et al. Diabetes mellitus in schizophrenic patients. Compr Psychiatry 1996; 37:68–73.
123. Keskiner A, El-Toumi A, Bousquet T. Psychotropic drugs, diabetes, and chronic mental patient. Psychosomatics 1973; 14:176–81.
124. Schwarz L, Munoz R. Blood sugar levels in patients treated with chloropromazine. Am J Psychiatry 1968; 125:2523–525.
125. Maudsley H. The Pathology of Mind, 3rd ed. London: Macmillan and Co; 1879, 113–18.
126. Singer HD, Clark SN. Psychoses associated with diabetes mellitus J Nerv Mental Dis 1917; 46:421–8.
127. Appel KE, Farr CB. The blood sugar reaction to insulin in psychoses. Arch Neurol Psychiatry 1929; 21:145–8.
128. Freeman H. Resistance to insulin in mentally disturbed soldiers. Arch Neurol Psychiatry 1946; 56: 74–8.
129. Gianfrancesco F, White R, Wang RN, Nasrallah HA. Antipsychotic-induced type 2 diabetes: evidence from a large health plan database. J Clin Psychopharmacol 2003; 23:328–35.
130. Sumiyoshi T, Roy A, Anil AE, Jayathilake K, Ertugrul A, Meltzer HY. A comparison of incidence of diabetes mellitus between atypical antipsychotic drugs. J Clin Psychopharm 2004; 24:345–8.
131. Smith RC, Lindenmayer JP, Bark N, Warner-Cohen J, Vaidhyanathaswamy S, Khandat A. Clozapine, risperidone, olanzapine, and conventional antipsychotic drug effects on glucose, lipids, and leptin in schizophrenic patients. Int J Neuropsychopharmcol 2005; 8:183–94.
132. Stone JM, Pilowsky LS. Antipsychotic drug action: targets for drug discovery with neurochemical imaging. Expert Rev Neuorotherapeut 2006; 6(1):57–64.
133. Merchant KM, Dorsa DM. Differential induction of neurotensin and c-fos gene expression by typical versus atypical antipsychotics. Proc Natl Acad Sci USA 1993; 90(8):3447–51.
134. Tollefson G, Lesar T. Nonketotic hyperglycemia associated with loxapine and amoxapine: case report. J Clin Psychiatry 1983; 44:347–8.
135. Woods SC, Kaiyala K, Porte D, Schwartz MW. Food intake and energy balance. In: Porte D, Sherwin R (eds), Diabetes Mellitus, 5th ed. Stanford: Appleton and Lange, 1997; 175–92.
136. Aiston S, Agius L. Leptin enhances glycogen storage in hepatocytes by inhibition of the phosphorylase and exerts an additive effect with insulin. Diabetes 1999; 49:15–20.
137. Seufert J, Kieffer TJ, Leech CA, Holz GG, Mortiz W, Ricordi C Habner JF. Leptin suppression of insulin secretion and gene expression in human pancreatic islets: implications of the development of adipogenic diabetes mellitus. J Clin Endocrinol Metab 1999; 84:670–6.
138. Bromel T, Blum WF, Zeigler A, et al. Serum leptin levels increase rapidly after initiation of clozapine therapy. Mol Psychiatry 1998; 3:76–80.
139. Melkersson KI, Hulting A-L, Brismar KE. Different influences of classical antipsychotic and clozapine on glucose-insulin homeostasis in patients with schizophrenia or related psychoses. J Clin Psychiatry 1999; 60:783–91.
140. Osser DN, Najarian DM, Dufresne RL. Olanzapine increases weight and serum triglyceride levels. J Clin Psychiatry 1999; 60:767–70.
141. Ghaeli P, Dufresne RL. Elevated serum triglycerides on clonazapine resolve with resperidone. Pharmacotherapy 1995; 15:382.
142. Vaxillaire M, Phillippi A, Frougel P, et al. A gene for maturity onset diabetes of the young (MODY) maps to chromosome 12q. Nat Genet 1995; 9:418–23.
143. Yamagata K, Oda N, Kaisaki PJ, et al. Mutation in hepatocyte nuclear factor-1 alpha gene in maturity onset diabetes of the young (MODY 3). Nature 1996; 384:455–8.
144. Reginester JY, Deroisy R, Rovati LC, et al. Long-term effects of glucosamine sulphate on osteoarthritis progression: a randomized, placebo-controlled trial. Lancet 2001; 357:251–6.
145. Monauni T, Zenti MG, Cretti A, et al. Effects of glucosamine infusion on insulin secretion and insulin action in humans. Diabetes 2000; 49:926–35.
146. Giaccari A, Morviducci L, Zoretta D, et al. In vivo effects of glucosamine on insulin secretion and insulin sensitivity in rat: possible relevance to the maladaptive responses to chronic hyperglycemia. Diabetalogia 1995; 38:518–24.
147. Anello M, Spampinato D, Piro S, Purrello F, Rabuazzo AM. Glucosamine-induced alterations of mitochondria function in pancreatic beta-cells: possible role of protein glycosylation. Am J Physiol-Endocrinol Metab 2004; 287(4):E602–8.

148. Fabris O, De Floreani A, Lazzari F, Betterle C, Naccarato R, Chiaramonte M. Development of type 1 diabetes mellitus during IFN alpha therapy for chronic HCV hepatitis. Lancet 1992; 340;548.

149. Imagawa A, Itoh N, Hanafusa M, Kuwajima M, Matsuzawa Y. Antibodies to glutamic acid decarboxylase induced by interferon alpha therapy for chronic viral hepatitis. Diabetologia 1996; 39:126.

150. Fabris P, Betterle C, Greggio NA, et al. Insulin-dependent diabetes mellitus during alpha interferon therapy for chronic viral hepatitis. J Hepatol 1998; 28:514–7.

151. Tohda G, Oida K, Higashi S, Miyamori I. Interferon alpha and development of type 1 diabetes mellitus. Diabetes Care 1998; 21:1774.

152. Chedin P, Cahen-Varsaux J, Boyer N. Non-insulin dependent diabetes mellitus development during interferon alpha therapy for chronic viral hepatitis. Ann Intern Med 1996; 125:521.

153. Foulis AK, Farquharson MA, Meager A. Immunoreactive alpha-interferon in insulin secreting beta-cells in type 1 diabetes mellitus. Lancet 1987; 2:1423–7.

154. Stewart TA, Hultgren B, Huang X, Pitts-Meek S, Hully J, MacLanchlan NJ. Induction of type 1 diabetes mellitus by interferon α in transgenic mice. Science 1993; 260:1942–6.

155. Pankewycz OG, Guan J-X, Benedict JF. Cytokines as mediators of autoimmune diabetes and diabetic complications. Endocrine Rev 1995; 16:164–71.

156. Kolacinsky JW, Taskinen M-R, Hilden H, Kiviluoto T, Cantell K, Koivisto VA. Effects of interferon alpha on insulin binding and glucose transport in human adipocytes. Eur J Clin Invest 1992; 22:292–9.

157. Konrad T, Zeuzem S, Vicini P, et al. Evaluation of factors controlling glucose tolerance in patients with HCV infection before and after 4 months therapy with interferon-alpha. Eur J Clin Invest 2000; 30:111–21.

158. Pusztay M, Nemesanszky E. Effect of interferon therapy on carbohydrate metabolism in chronic hepatitis C patients. Orv Hetil 1999; 140:1579–81.

159. Ozylikau E, Arslan M. Increased prevalence of diabetes mellitus in patients with chronic hepatitis C virus infection. Am J Gastroenterol 1997; 91:1480–1.

160. Sobngwi E, Mauvais-Jarvis F, Vexiau P, Mbanya JC, Gautier JF. Diabetes in Africans. Part 2: ketosis-prone atypical diabetes mellitus. Diabetes Metab 2002; 28:5–12.

161. Okosieme OE, Campbell A, Patton K, Evans ML. Transient diabetes associated with withdrawal of lithium therapy. Diabetes Care 2006; 29(5):1181. Waziri R. Nelson J. Lithium in diabetes mellitus: a paradoxical response. J Clin Psychiatry 1978; 39(7):623–5. Rodriguez-Gil JE, Fernandez-Novell JM, Barbera A, Guinovart JJ. Lithium's effects on rat liver glucose metabolism in vitro. Arch Biochem Biophys 2000; 375:377–84. Carter BL, Small RE, Mandel MD, Stakman MT. Phenytoin-induced hyperglycemia. Am J Hosp Pharm 1981; 38(10):1508–12. Pezzilli R, Billi P, Fontana G. Anticonvulsant-induced chronic pancreatitis: a case report. Ital J Gastroenterol 1992; 24(5):245–6. Nabe K, Fujimoto S, Shimodahira M, et al. Diphenlhydantoin suppresses glucose induced insulin release by decreasing cytoplasmic H+ concentration in pancreatic islets. Endocrinology 2006; 147 (6):2717–27.

162. Perry-Keene DA, Larkins RG, Heyma P, Peter CT, Ross D, Sloman JG. The effect of long-term diphenylhydantoin therapy on glucose tolerance and insulin secretion: a controlled trial. Clin Endocrinol 1980; 12:575–80.

35 | MODY: Lessons from Monogenetic Diabetes Forms

Birgit Knebel
Institute of Clinical Biochemistry and Pathobiochemistry, German Diabetes Center, Heinrich-Heine-University Düsseldorf and Leibniz-Center for Diabetes-Research, Düsseldorf, Germany

Dirk Müller-Wieland
Division of General Internal Medicine, Department of Endocrinology, Diabetes and Metabolism, Asklepios Clinic St. Georg and Teaching Hospital of the University of Hamburg, Hamburg, Germany

DIABETES MELLITUS TYPE-2 IS A MULTIFACTORIAL DISEASE WITH STRONG GENETIC SUSCEPTIBILITY

Diabetes mellitus type 2 is the most common endocrine-metabolic disorder and affects at least 5% of Western society. According to the persisting trends for increasing obesity, the amount of newly diagnosed patients will increase dramatically over the next decades. Unfortunately, lifestyle in combination with affluent alimentation does not spare the young, and increasing obesity in this group is already observed. Usually diabetes mellitus occurs at ages over 40 but we now observe a shift in the age of onset towards younger patients. In Germany diabetes mellitus type 2 is the major cause for blindness, kidney failure and amputation of lower extremities. Patients with diabetes not only develop microangiographical vascular complications but also have a three to five times increased risk for cardiovascular complications. According to the expected long period of the disease duration especially within young patients, the diabetic complications must be treated with great efforts, and a fast diagnosis of the underlying diabetes sub-classification is necessary for best treatment.

The key to developing diabetes is the genetic predisposition. The concordance rate of monozygotic twins is over 75% for developing diabetes type 2 even when they grow up in different environmental and social backgrounds (1). Certain populations like the Pima Indians have a higher risk of developing diabetes (2). This indicates that in contrast to the general public opinion, diabetes is a complex genetic disorder with strong genetic predisposition. So in diabetes, like in every other complex multifactorial disease, e.g. cancer, the personal genetic predisposition determines whether a person would develop the syndrome or not. The individual life style determines the age and the severity of diabetes onset.

GENETIC BASIS OF DIABETES

The genetic basis of the common late-onset diabetes mellitus type 2 is rather polygenic than monogenic. Clinically overt diabetes is characterized by two pathophysiological phenomenon, i.e., reduced insulin sensitivity or insulin resistance and a β-cell dysfunction with diminished insulin secretion. Even if impaired insulin sensitivity is the earliest detectable parameter, diabetes generally manifests when insulin secretion is decreased (2–4). On the survey for genetic factors responsible for an impaired insulin secretion no specific gene or mutation has been identified for late-onset diabetes mellitus type 2 up to now. Nevertheless, during the past decades a great effort has been made to identify monogenic sub-classifications of diabetes as the cause for β-cell dysfunction. The identification of these monogenetic forms of diabetes lead to a paradigm change influencing especially the pediatric physicians to determine the genetic cause of early-onset diabetes and distinguish between type I diabetes and the early-onset monogenetic diabetes forms.

MATURITY-ONSET DIABETES OF THE YOUNG

Maturity-Onset Diabetes of the Young (MODY) is the classical example of monogenic disease with autosomal dominant inheritance. MODY represents a group of clinically and genetically heterogeneous familial disorders with clinical appearance similar to non-insulin-dependent type 2 (5,6). MODY is characterized by autosomal dominant inheritance and early-onset of diabetes, typically but not exclusively before the age of 25 (7). There are at least six different forms of MODY, each resulting from heterozygous mutations in six different genes encoding the key regulator of the glycolytic pathway the glucokinase gene (GCK/MODY2) (8) and transcription factors genes hepatic nuclear factor (HNF)-4α (MODY1) (9), HNF-1α (MODY3) (10), HNF-1β (MODY5) (11), insulin promoter factor (IPF)-1 (MODY4) (12) and NEURO D1/β2 (MODY6) (13). MODY2 and MODY3 have the highest prevalence in most populations (Table 1).

MUTATIONS IN THE GLUCOKINASE GENE (MODY2)

MODY2 presents with mild, dietary manageable hyperglycemia and in the case of a positive family anamnesis, this MODY form is especially seen in children with the highest prevalence. Usually affected subjects are free of symptoms at diagnosis and are identified in routine health examinations (Table 2). Approximately half of the female mutation carriers present for the first time with gestation diabetes. The molecular causes of MODY2 are mutations in the glucokinase (GCK) gene and more than 200 mutations have been identified up to now (14). While heterozygous mutations of GCK are associated with MODY2, homozygous mutations of the enzyme that lead to a complete loss of function are one cause of permanent neonatal diabetes but also of neonatal lethality (15). Heterozygous mutations result in a mild form of non-progressive hyperglycemia. GCK catalyses the first and rate-limiting step of the glycolytic pathway, the phosphate transfer from ATP to glucose to generate glucose-6-phosphate. Glucose-6-phospate enters the Krebs' cycle to cause the degeneration of glucose and energy production within the cell. It has been shown that pancreatic β-cell and liver have the highest expression levels of GCK. GCK expressed in liver is mainly involved in converting glucose to glycogen for storage in the postprandial state. In the β-cell, GCK is the rate-limiting enzyme for glucose catabolism and as a consequence couples glucose to insulin secretion. Therefore, GCK expressed in β-cells has the function of a glucose sensor for insulin secretion. This represents the link that mutations in GCK lead to a diminished insulin secretion by mainly affecting the glucose-induced feedback loop of the β-cell.

Accepting in advance the function of GCK as key regulator in glucose sensitivity and the insulin secretion of the β-cell, the mild and non-progressive outcome of MODY2 is somehow surprising. Probably, a physiological adaptation of the β-cell to the mild but relatively stable and unaltered hyperglycemia by increasing insulin secretion occurs, limiting the existing hyperglycemia. So the β-cell can compensate by slightly increasing insulin secretion. In MODY2, diabetic complications can be expected to only a minor degree, but cannot be completely excluded. Patients should be monitored routinely at least twice a year for stable blood glucose levels or further markers like HbA$_{1c}$-levels. In a family suspected of MODY2, a genetic investigation should be considered to exclude other MODY subtypes and to sensitize the patient for the positive family history, thus taking more care in identifying affected family members at an early age. One further major aspect should not be neglected. Female MODY2 patients are at risk to develop gestation diabetes and therefore are at risk for having offspring with reduced birth weight (16). Reduced birth weight of the newborn will increase its risk to develop type 2 diabetes during its lifetime even without the inheritance of the GCK mutation (17). Next to this, hyperglycemia of the newborn might be misdiagnosed as type 1 diabetes.

MUTATIONS IN HNF (MODY1, MODY3 AND MODY5)

Besides MODY2 other forms of MODY are caused by mutations in transcription factors of the HNF family that regulate gene expression of genes involved in the development and the maintenance of the pancreatic β-cell, i.e., (HNF)-1α (MODY3), HNF-1β (MODY5) and HNF-4α (MODY1).

Investigations of tissue-specific gene regulation in the liver resulted in the identification of the transcription factors HNF-1α and HNF-1β members of the basic-helix-loop-helix leucine

TABLE 1 Molecular Genetics and Clinical Phenotypes in MODY

MODY	Gene	Clinical phenotype at heterozygous state	Treatment	Prevalence (% of MODY-families)	Age of onset
MODY1	HNF-4α	Diabetes, microvascular complications (often); reduced serum concentrations of triglycerides, Apolipoprotein AII ans CIII, and Lp(a) lipoprotein	Oral hypoglycemic agent, insulin	Rare	Postpubertal
MODY2	Glucokinase	Impaired fasting glucose tolerance, diabetes, normal proinsulin-insulin ratio in serum	Diet and exercise	8–63	Childhood
MODY3	HNF-1α	Diabetes, microvascular complications (often); renal glucosuria, increased sensitivity to sulfonylurea drugs increased proinsulin-insulin ratio in serum	Oral hypoglycemic agent, insulin	21–64	Postpubertal
MODY4	IPF-1/PDX-1	Diabetes	Oral hypoglycemic agent	Rare	Early adulthood
MODY5	HNF-1β	Diabetes, renal cysts and other abnormalities of renal development; progressive non-diabetic renal dysfunction, leading to chronic renal insufficiency and failure; internal genital abnormalities (females)	Insulin	Unknown	Postpubertal
MODY6	NeuroD1 bzw. Neuroβ 2	Diabetes	Insulin	Rare	Early adulthood
MODY-X	Unknown	Unknown/heterogeneous?	–	10–20% in Europe	Heterogenous

zipper superfamily and HNF-4α, a nuclear orphane receptor (18). These transcription factors are expressed in the liver, pancreatic β-cells, kidney and reproductive organs and are central factors in the transcriptional network of these cells (Fig. 1). There is an integrative regulation of these factors in embryogenesis and also in adult tissues. Next to the insulin gene expression itself these transcription factors regulate genes that have key functions in glucose transport or metabolism in pancreatic β-cells (19,20).

The direct association of the genetic mutations and the MODY phenotype have been examined and proven in certain transgenic mouse models. For example mice with a

TABLE 2 Criteria for MODY Diagnosis

Strict criteria	Considerations
Mild, non-ketotic diabetes	Patient might not present with symptoms
No auto-antibodies	In rare cases low levels of antibodies can be detected
Lean BMI< 25	Ethical consideration; increased BMI possible
Non-insulin dependent diabetes within 5 years after diagnosis; significant circulating C-peptide	Parameters show-up in combination or only one parameter
Early-onset usually <25 years	Onset can occur 10–60 years (30); >35 years should be accepted (mild symptoms)
Heredity over three generations	Undiagnosed family members, due to mild diabetes; patients' family history unknown/unclear; rare spontaneous mutations, therefore no family history

Source: From Ref. 7.

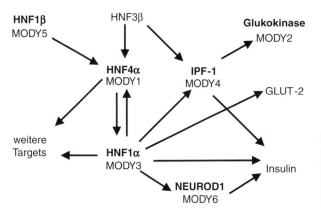

FIGURE 1 Scheme of the hierarchical transcription factor network of the pancreatic β-cell. The diagram shows the regulation of gene expression. The arrows indicate the interaction. Genes responsible for MODY are indicated. *Source*: From Ref. 15.

heterozygous deficiency of HNF-1α show impaired insulin secretion and develop diabetes. HNF-4α models show impaired hepatic differentiation and reduced HNF-1α expression.

In most ethnic groups only MODY3 is next to MODY2 with the highest prevalence, whereas all other forms are rare. Up to now more than 150 HNF-1α mutations are known (21). Like patients with MODY2, patients with MODY3 first develop a mild form of diabetes mellitus type 2. It has been shown that despite a slight elevation of fasting blood glucose levels comparable with the one of MODY2 patients, in MODY3 patients the postprandial glucose levels are markedly increased 2 h after glucose load. Hyperglycemia is very progressive in MODY3 patients, and treatment with anti-diabetic agents or insulin is necessary. Patients with MODY3 show a reduced glucose re-absorption in combination with diminished nephritic barrier for glucose. Because the clinical outcome is much more aggressive, tight medical control is necessary. It has been shown that there is a direct correlation between the manifestation of diabetic complications and the appropriate treatment of the patients. MODY3 patients can develop all possible diabetes complications and the patients directly benefit from being treated as soon as possible with adequate medication to prevent or delay complications (22,23).

Mutations in HNF-4α resembling MODY1 might affect the regulation of the insulin gene by HNF-4α via HNF-1α, so that the pathogenetic mechanisms for MODY1 and MODY3 are quite similar. Moreover, HNF-4α also regulates metabolic key enzymes like the glucose transporter GLUT2, glyceroaldehyd-3-phosphate dehydrogenase or pyruvate kinase. So in families with MODY1 a progressive loss of insulin secretion can be observed (24–26), whereas a compensation of the altered physiological situation does not seem to occur in MODY1 patients (27,28). Next to a defect in insulin secretion, a reduced β-cell function exists in MODY1 patients (24–26). There is also evidence for further pancreatic deficiencies in MODY1 patients as arginine-induced glucagon secretion and the pancreatic polypeptide response to hyperglycemia are deficient.

Mutations in HNF-1β are responsible for the very rare MODY5. HNF-1β can form heterodimers with HNF-1α and directly regulates HNF-4α. Heterozygote HNF-1β mutation can be associated with a broad clinical spectrum, but MODY5 has similar features to MODY1 and is characterized by diabetes mellitus, renal cysts, proteinuria, and renal failure. As a consequence of renal cysts, hypoplastic glomerulocystic kidney disease can develop in the affected patients. Female patients can exhibit malformation of the inner genitals (29–32).

RARE FORMS OF MODY (MODY4 AND MODY6)

Transcription factors specifically regulate the temporal and spatial expression of their defined target genes and are thereof responsible for specificity and maintenance of tissue diversity. Models with depletion of transcription factor, insulin promoter factor (IPF)-1 (also called PDX-1) (MODY4) are characterized by reduced insulin gene expression and impaired pancreatic development and remodeling during neogenesis. The transcription factor IPF-1/PDX-1 was the first transcription factor identified that directly regulates the expression of the insulin gene and the somatostatin gene in the pancreatic β-cell. Further examinations indicate its pivotal role in the development, general gene expression and maintenance of the β-cell. Examples of IPF-1/PDX-1 regulated genes are glucokinase or GLUT2 and the glucose-regulated expression of the insulin gene is regulated by IPF-1/PDX-1 (33,34). Mutations in IPF-1/PDX-1 are the molecular cause of MODY4 but the prevalence of MODY4 is still low (35,36).

Mouse models deficient in the transcription factor NeuroD1/Beta2 (MODY6) show reduced β-cell number, altered β-cell morphology and develop neonatal diabetes as well as die within the first week after delivery (35,37–43). Like IPF-1/PDX-1 NeuroD1/Beta2 is a direct regulator of the insulin gene (41) and furthermore involved in pancreatic development. Mutations in NeuroD1/Beta2 have been identified in one Icelandic and one European family fulfilling the diagnostics criteria for MODY (13,36). Recently, in certain populations HNF-4α or NeuroD1/Beta2 mutations have been suspected to be also involved in late-onset type 2 diabetes (13,30).

Although a clear association of a mutation in one of the MODY genes with the respective clinical phenotype has been identified, it still remains unclear how these misfunctions of genes involved can result in a disturbed insulin secretion. Interestingly, approximately 20% of patients with clinical features of MODY do not carry a mutation in one of the known MODY genes indicating further subtypes of MODY X with different genetic mutations in genes unidentified up to know.

GENETIC TESTING FOR MODY?

The genetic characterization of the diverse MODY forms is necessary to decide the patient's therapy and helps to predict the pathogenesis of the syndrome. Therefore, testing can be very beneficial, e.g., if the patient can switch to tablets instead of injections. The predominant question in genetic testing is whether a mutation identified has a functional relevance and therefore a meaning for the clinical phenotype. In most cases an analysis of family members is essential and should be ideally performed for several generations. A clinically relevant mutation must be carried by all affected family members, whereas healthy family members must not be carriers. The interpretation might bare inconsistencies because type 2 diabetes can develop for multiple reasons. If no association can be detected it is reasonable that the questioned mutation is functionally apparent and does not alternate gene expression or functionality. It is tremendously important to have sequence information of the ethnic group of the patient investigated. These data are provided in public databases and can be used in any case where no relative is available or willing to be examined. Nevertheless, it is important to have data available from a healthy control population that should be chosen according to ethnic group and genetic admixture. Allelic heterogeneity (several mutations identical phenotype) or phenotypical heterogeneity (one variation several phenotypes) mainly depending on further genetic background effects should be considered. Non-allelic heterogeneity depicts a situation where a phenotype is the result of several different sequence variations. Gene ontology data might be helpful, too. An amino acid conserved during evolution from yeast to humans is more likely to be of functional relevance than the one that differs even in comparison with, for example, a chimp. This question should be considered in cooperation with physicians and genetics resembling the idea of bench to bedside for optimal patient care.

REFERENCES

1. Medici F, Hawa M, Inari A, Leslie RDG. Concordance rate for type II diabetes mellitus in monozygotic twins: actual analysis. Diabetologia 1999; 42:146–50.
2. Bennett PH, WC Knowler, DJ Pettitt, MJ Carraher, Vasquez B. Longitudinal studies in the development of diabetes in Pima Indians. In: Eschwege E, (ed.), Advances in Diabetes Epidemiology. Amsterdam, Netherlands: Elsevier, 1982; 65–74.
3. Martin BC, Warram JHT, Krolewski AS, Bergmann RN, Soeldner JS, Kahn CR. Role of glucose and insulin resistance in development of type 2 diabetes mellitus: results of a 25-year follow-up study. Lancet 1992; 340:925–9.

4. Ferrannini E, Nannipieri M, Williams K, Gonzales C, Haffner SM, Stern MP. Mode of onset of type 2 diabetes from normal or impaired glucose tolerance. Diabetes 2004; 53:160–5.
5. Fajans SS, Bell GI, Polonsky KS. Molecular mechanisms and clinical pathophysiology of maturity-onset diabetes of the young. N Engl J Med 2001; 345:971–80.
6. Velho G, Robert JJ. Maturity-onset diabetes of the young (MODY): genetic and clinical characteristics. Horm Res 2002; 57:29–33.
7. Hattersley AT, Tattersall RB. Maturity onset diabetes of the young. In: Pickup J, William G (eds), Textbook of Diabetes (2nd ed.). Oxford: Blackwell, 1997; 22.1–10.
8. Froguel P, Zouali H, Vionnet N, et al. Familial hyperglycemia due to mutations in glucokinase. Definition of a subtype of diabetes mellitus. N Engl J Med 1993; 328(10):697–702.
9. Yamagata K, Furuta H, Oda N, Kaisaki PJ, Menzel S, Cox NJ, Fajans SS, Signorini S, Stoffel M, Bell GI. Mutations in the hepatocyte nuclear factor-4alpha gene in maturity-onset diabetes of the young (MODY1). Nature 1996; 5; 384(6608):458–60.
10. Yamagata K, Oda N, Kaisaki PJ, et al. Mutations in the hepatocyte nuclear factor-1alpha gene in maturity-onset diabetes of the young (MODY3). Nature 1996; 5; 384(6608):455–8.
11. Horikawa Y, Iwasaki N, Hara M, Furuta H, Hinokio Y, Cockburn BN, Lindner T, Yamagata K, Ogata M, Tomonaga O, Kuroki H, Kasahara T, Iwamoto Y, Bell GI. Mutation in hepatocyte nuclear factor beta gene (TCF2) associated with MODY. Nat Genet 1997; 17:384–5.
12. Stoffers DA, Ferrer J, Clarke WL, Habener JF. Early-onset type-II diabetes mellitus (MODY4) linked to IPF1. Nat Genet 1997; 17(2):138–9.
13. Maleki MT, Jhala US, Antonellis A Fields L, Doria A, Orban T, Saad M, Warram JH, Montminy M, Krolewski AS. Mutations in NeuroD1 are associated with the development of type 2 diabetes mellitus. Nat Genet 1999; 23:323–8.
14. Gloyn AL. Glucokinase (GCK) mutations in hyper- and hypoglycemia: maturity-onset diabetes of the young, permanent neonatal diabetes, and hyperinsulinemia of infancy. Hum Mutat 2003; 22: 353–62.
15. Niølstad PR, Søvik O, Cuesta-Munoz A. Neonatal diabetes mellitus due to complete glucokinase deficiency. N Engl J Med 2001; 344:1588–92.
16. Hattersley AT, Beards F, Ballantyne E, Appleton M, Harvey R, Ellard S. Mutations in the glucokinase gene of the fetus result in reduced birth weight. Nat Genet 1998; 19:268–70.
17. Newsome CA, Shiell AW, Fall CHD, Phillips DI, Shier R, Law CN. Is birth weight related to later glucose and insulin metabolism?-a systematic review. Diab Med 2003; 20:339–48.
18. Cereghini S, Liver enriched transcription factors and hepatocyte differentiation. FASEB J 1996; 10: 267–82.
19. Shih DQ, Stoffel M. Dissecting the transcriptional network of pancreatic islets due development and differentiation. Proc Natl Acad Sci USA 2001; 98:14481–6.
20. Kulkarni RN, Kahn CR. HNFs: linking the liver and pancreatic islets in diabetes. Science 2004; 303: 1311–2.
21. Ellard S. Hepatocyte nuclear factor alpha (HNF-1α) mutations in maturity-onset diabetes of the young. Hum Mutat 2000; 16:377–85.
22. Isomaa B, Henricsson M, Letho M, Forsblom C, Karanko S, Sarelin L, Haggblom M, Groop L. Chronic diabetic complications in patients with MODY3 diabetes. Diabetologia 1998; 41:467–573.
23. Frayling TM, Bulamn MP, Ellard S, Appleton M, Dronsfield MJ, Mackie AD, Baird JD, Kaisaki PJ, Yamagata K, Bell GI, Bain SC, Hattersley AT. Mutations in hepatocyte nuclear factor 1α gene are a common cause of maturity onset diabetes of the young in the UK. Diabetes 1997; 46:720–5.
24. Odom DT, Zizlsperger N, Gordon DB, Bell GW, Rinaldi NJ, Murray HL, Volkert TL, Schreiber J, Rolfe PA, Gifford DK, Fraenkel E, Bell GI, Young RA. Control of pancreas and liver gene expression by HNF transcription factors. Science 2004; 303:1378–81.
25. Herman WH, Fajans SS, Ortiz FJ, Smith MJ, Sturis J, Bell GI, Polonsky KS, Halter JB. Abnormal insulin secretion not insulin resistance, is the genetic or primary defect of MODY in the RW pedigree. Diabetes 1994; 43:40–6.
26. Byrne MM, Sturis J, Fajans SS, Ortiz FJ, Stoltz A, Stoffel M, Smith MJ, Bell GI, Halter JB, Polonsky KS. Altered insulin secretory responses to glucose in subjects with a mutation in the MODY1 gene on chromosome 20. Diabetes 1995; 44:699–704.
27. Byrne MM, Sturis J, Menzel S, Yamagata K, Fajans SS, Dronsfield MJ, Bain SC, Hattersley AT, Velho G, Froguel P, Bell GI, Polonsky KS. Altered insulin secretory responses to glucose in diabetic and nondiabetic subjects with a mutation in the diabetes susceptibility gene MODY3 on chromosome 12. Diabetes 1996; 45:1503–10.
28. Letho M, Tuomi T, Mahtanti MM, Widen E, Forsblom C, Sarelin L, Gullstrom M, et al. Characterization of the MODY3 phenotype: early-onset diabetes caused by an insulin secretion defect. J Clin Invest 1997; 99:582–91.
29. Nishigori H, Yamada S, Kohama T, Tomura H, Sho K, Horikawa Y, Bell GI, Takeuchi T, Takeda J. Frameshift mutation, A263fsinsGG, in hepatocyte nuclear factor 1β gene associated with diabetes and renal dysfunction. Diabetes 1998; 47:1354–5.

30. Lindner TH, Njolstad PR, Horikawa Y, Bostad L, Bell GI, Sovik O. A novel syndrome of diabetes mellitus, renal dysfunction and genital malformation associated with a partial deletion of the pseudo POU domain of the hepatocyte nuclear factor 1β. Hum Mol Genet 1999; 8:2001–8.

31. Iwasaki N, Okabe I, Momoi MY, Ohashi H, Ogata M, Iwamoto Y. Splice site mutation in the hepatocyte nuclear factor 1β gene, IVS2nt+1G>A, associated with maturity onset diabetes of the young, renal dysplasia and bicornuate uterus. Diabetologia 2001; 44:387–8.

32. Bingham C, Bulman MP, Ellard S, Allen LI, Lipkin GW, Hoff WG, Woolf AS, Rizzoni G, Novelli G, Nicholls AJ, Hattersley AT. Mutations in the hepatocyte nuclear factor 1β gene are associated with familial hypoplastic glomerulocystic kidney disease. Am J Hum Genet 2001; 68:219–24.

33. St-Onge L, Wehr R, Gruss P. Pancreatic development and diabetes. Curr Opin Genet Dev 1999; 9: 295–300.

34. Marshak S, Totary H, Cerasi E, Melloul D. Purification of the beta cell glucose sensitive factor that transactivates the insulin gene differentially in normal and transformed island cells. Proc Natl Acad Sci USA 1996; 93:15057–62.

35. Clocquet AR, Eagan JM, Stoffers DA, Muller DC, Wideman L, Chin GA, Clarke WL, Hanks JB, Habener JF, Elahi D. Impaired insulin secretion and increased insulin sensitivity in familial maturity-onset diabetes of the young 4 (insulin promoter factor 1 gene). Diabetes 2000; 49:1856–64.

36. Kristinsson SY, Thorolfsdottir ET, Talseth B, Steingrimsson E, Thorsson AV, Helgason T, Hreidarsson AB, Arngrimsson R. MODY in Iceland is associated with mutations in HNF-1alpha and a novel mutation in NeuroD1. Diabetologia 2001; 44(11):2098–2103.

37. Pontoglio M, Sreenan S, Roe M, Pugh W, Ostrega D, Doyen A, Pick AJ, Baldwin A, Velho G, Froguel P, Levisetti M, Bonner-Weir S, Bell 0GI, Yaniv M, Polonsky KS. Defective insulin secretion in hepatocyte nuclear factor 1alpha-deficient mice. J Clin Invest 1998; 101:2215–22.

38. Shih DQ, Screenan S, Munoz KN, Philipson L, Pontoglio M, Yaniv M, Polonsky KS, Stoffel M. Loss of HNF-1α function in mice leads to abnormal expression of genes involved in pancreatic islet development and metabolism. Diabetes 2001; 50:2472–80.

39. Duncan SA, Navas MA, Dufort D, Rossant J, Stoffel M. Regulation of a transcription factor network required for differentiation and metabolism. Science 1998; 281(5377):692–5.

40. Li J, Ning G, Duncan SA. Mammalian hepatocyte differentiation requires the transcription factor HNF-4alpha. Genes Dev 2000; Feb 15; 14(4):464–74.

41. Ahlgren U, Jonsson J, Edlund H. The morphogenesis of the pancreatic mesenchyme is uncoupled from that of the pancreatic epithelium in IPF1/PDX1-deficient mice. Development 1996; 122(5): 1409–16.

42. Offield MF, Jetton TL, Labosky PA, Ray M, Stein RW, Magnuson MA, Hogan BL, Wright CV. PDX-1 is required for pancreatic outgrowth and differentiation of the rostral duodenum. Development 1996; 122(3):983–95.

43. Naya FJ, Huang HP, Qui Y, Mutoh H, DeMayo FJ, Leiter AB, Tsai MJ. Diabetes, defective pancreatic morphogenesis, and abnormal enteroendocrine differentiation in BEAT2/NeuroD1 deficient mice. Genes Dev 1997; 11:2323–34.

36 | Polycystic Ovary Syndrome and the Metabolic Syndrome

Onno E. Janssen, Susanne Tan, and Tiina Dietz
Department of Medicine, Division of Endocrinology, University Hospital of Essen Medical School, University of Duisburg-Essen, Essen, Germany

Susanne Hahn
Endokrinologikum Ruhr, Center for Metabolic and Endocrine Diseases, Bochum-Wattenscheid, Germany

INTRODUCTION

Polycystic ovary syndrome (PCOS) is a common endocrine disorder characterized by hyperandrogenism and chronic anovulation that affects at least 6% of women at reproductive age (1). PCOS patients suffer from infertility, hirsutism, acne, seborrhoea, alopecia, and obesity (2,3). A significant proportion of PCOS patients has been found to have defective insulin secretion and insulin resistance (4). Accordingly, PCOS patients may be expected to have a higher morbidity and mortality from the sequelae of the metabolic syndrome (MBS) (5,6).

Historical Perspective

With their eponymous paper of 1935, describing seven patients with polycystic ovaries (PCO), amenorrhea, hirsutism, and obesity, Stein and Leventhal are credited for defining the syndrome later to be known as PCOS (7), although others had reported case reports with similar ovarian pathology as early as 1721 (8–10). With a paper published in 1921, Achard and Thiers are considered to be the first to report on the association of hyperandrogenism and diabetes mellitus in a 71-year-old bearded obese woman (11). However, this disorder, which they called "diabète des femmes à barbe", was likely to be caused by adrenocortical pathology, rather than representative of PCOS. In 1980, with the development of standardized methods to measure insulin, Burghen et al. (12) demonstrated a correlation of hyperandrogenism with hyperinsulinemia in PCOS. With the first report on the amelioration of PCOS symptoms with the insulin sensitizer metformin by Velazquez et al. (13) in 1994, insulin resistance and its metabolic consequences have been established as an integral part of the syndrome (14).

Definition and Epidemiology

PCOS is a diagnosis of exclusion, requiring the elimination of other causes of androgen excess or related disorders (15). To facilitate better comparability of clinical studies, a 1990 NIH conference defined PCOS as the presence of both (1) hyperandrogenism and/or hyperandrogenemia and (2) oligo- or anovulation (16). As this definition did not include ovarian morphology, a 2003 conference in Rotterdam (re-)introduced PCO as a third criterion and defined PCOS as the presence of at least two of the three above features (17). These two definitions, usually referred to as the 1990 NIH and the 2003 Rotterdam criteria, have recently been challenged by a task force report from the Androgen Excess Society, requiring the presence of hyperandrogenism and/or hyperandrogenemia as a condition sine qua non, and either oligo-/anovulation or PCO or both, in addition to the exclusion of other disorders (18).

In spite of the multitude of definitions and the resulting difficulty in ascertaining the prevalence of PCOS, recent data suggest that it affects between 6% and 8% of women worldwide, using the 1990 NIH criteria (1,19–22).

Etiology and Clinical Presentation

The etiology of PCOS, most likely a combination of genetic disposition and environmental factors, is not completely understood (23,24). While familial clustering of PCOS has been well documented, even including a male factor with higher androgen levels in first degree relatives of affected patients (25,26), the search for candidate genes has not come up with obvious culprits (27,28).

While not its cause, insulin resistance plays a pathogenic role in the development of PCOS. Hyperinsulinemia increases ovarian and adrenal steroid hormone production, alters luteinizing hormone (LH) and follicle-stimulating hormone (FSH) release, and decreases hepatic sex hormone-binding globulin (SHBG) production, thus increasing free androgen and estrogen levels (Fig. 1) (29). The unopposed estrogens stimulate the proliferation of adipose tissue, which is a source of aromatase and thus vice versa converts androgens into estrogens, further increasing their serum levels and leading to inappropriate gonadotropin secretion (30). Treatment to improve insulin sensitivity should thus be useful in PCOS patients, and, indeed, diet/lifestyle modifications, metformin, glitazone and D-chiro-inositol treatment are effective approaches (2).

The clinical appearances (hirsutism, acne, alopecia, obesity) and biochemical features of PCOS are highly variable in affected women. A case–control cross-sectional study of South Asian and Caucasian PCOS women (31) revealed ethnic differences, presenting more severe clinical manifestations (hirsutism, acne) and a higher insulin resistance in young Asian women, supporting the hypothesis, of ethnic variations in clinical and biochemical features of PCOS. A population of Indian women with PCOS also showed a higher insulin response to a glucose load than age-matched Caucasian PCOS patients (32). Significant differences related to ethnicity were also found in Caribbean–Hispanic and non-Hispanic white PCOS women (33). Hispanic women had an increased insulin resistance and a reduced metabolic clearance rate of insulin compared with non-Hispanics in euglycemic clamp tests. Mexican American women were also shown to be more insulin resistant than white women (34). Another study comparing Maori, Pacific Island and Europeans, found European PCOS women less obese, less insulin-resistant and less prone to present with lipid abnormalities than the two other ethnic groups (35). In addition, Pacific Island women only had little or no acne. A German PCOS cohort was comparable to other Caucasian populations (3).

Diagnosing a woman as having PCOS implies an increased risk for several severe health problems, including endometrial carcinoma, T2DM, dyslipidemia, hypertension and possibly cardiovascular disease (CVD). Furthermore, it has important familial implications for her mother (36) and sisters (37). The diagnosis of PCOS should thus not be assigned lightly, as it

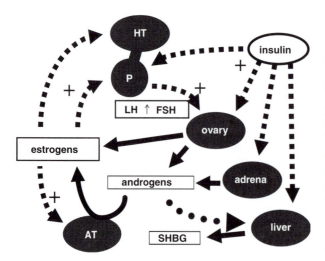

FIGURE 1 Pathopysiology of PCOS. Hyperinsulinemia augments elevated luteinizing hormone (LH) secretion by the pituitary (P), ovarian and adrenal steroid hormone production, and the androgen-induced decrease in hepatic sex hormone binding-globulin (SHBG) synthesis, thus increasing the free fraction of estrogens and androgens. The elevated estrogens increase the proliferation of adipose tissue (AT), which converts androgens to estrogens with its aromatase activity. The unopposed estrogens further disturb gonadotropin regulation of the hypothalamus (HT) and the pituitary, thus creating a vicious cycle of hormonal dysregulation.

could imply life-long treatment and may negatively affect her ability to access healthcare coverage.

PCOS AND THE METABOLIC SYNDROME

Insulin resistance and hyperinsulinemia have been extensively studied in PCOS. While obese patients have a more pronounced phenotype, even lean PCOS patients have a reduced insulin-mediated glucose disposal and elevated basal hepatic glucose production (38). The hyperinsulinemia first described by Burghen et al. (12) was subsequently confirmed, including studies showing higher fasting insulin levels resulting from a higher basal insulin secretion rate (39), higher insulin responses during an oral glucose tolerance test (OGTT) independently of body weight (40), defects in insulin secretion (41) and combined beta-cell dysfunction (42). In about half of the affected patients, insulin resistance can be correlated with an augmented serine rather than tyrosine phosphorylation of insulin receptor-substrate 1 (IRS-1), causing impaired insulin signaling (43). The resulting hyperinsulinemia in turn induces more serine phosphorylation, propagating a vicious circle that continues until hyperinsulinemia fails to compensate for insulin resistance (44). This, and possibly other similar mechanisms may be the reason for the high conversion rate of insulin resistance to impaired glucose tolerance (IGT) and overt T2DM in PCOS patients (45).

Obesity

The increase in body weight is the main reason for the increase in the prevalence of both the MBS and T2DM in men (46) and women (47). Apart from a genetic predisposition, the main culprit of this development is the modern, sedentary lifestyle with too little physical activity and constant availability of high energy food.

Worldwide, PCOS patients have higher body weight, body mass index (BMI), waist and/or hip circumference and an elevated intra-abdominal fat mass than age-matched controls (48). The prevalence of affected PCOS patients correlates with the degree of obesity in the general population of their country of residence and thus likely reflects life style factors such as high calorie diet, composition of diet and lack of exercise, as well as ethnic components (2,49). In the U.S. 42% to 50% of PCOS patients are obese, with an average BMI around 35–38 kg/m^2 (1,50,51). However, in other countries, women with PCOS tend to be leaner, with mean BMIs of 25 kg/m^2 in England (52), 28 kg/m^2 in Finland (53), 29 kg/m^2 in Italy (54) and 31 kg/m^2 in Germany (3). In a study of blood donors in Spain, 30% of the women were overweight, but only 10% were obese (22). In any case, weight gain after adolescence and abdominal obesity are associated with an increased prevalence of PCOS (55).

The importance of obesity in PCOS is also supported by the finding that obesity can profoundly affect quality-of-life (QoL) independent of the presence of other clinical symptoms in otherwise healthy subjects (56). Interestingly, obesity is linked strongly to the physical dimension of QoL, rather than with psychosocial status (57) and social adjustment (58). A variety of studies demonstrated that BMI and hirsutism are the primary mediators in the relationship between PCOS and the reductions in QoL (59–62). In addition, in obese patients the impact of weight reduction on QoL has been well established (58). On the basis of the data documenting the psychological and emotional consequences of changes in outer appearance, clinical interventions in PCOS women that influence obesity, hirsutism, acne, menstrual disturbances or infertility would be expected to improve overall QoL (63).

Insulin Resistance

It is a common assumption that all women with PCOS are insulin resistant, although this can be demonstrated only in about 70% of them with available tests (64–66), the main reason being that no generally accepted method for the quantification of insulin resistance exists (67,68). Clinically, in PCOS as well as other patients suspected of suffering from insulin resistance, the standard 2-h OGTT measuring both insulin and glucose yields the highest amount of information for a reasonable cost and risk, providing an assessment of both the degrees of hyperinsulinemia and glucose tolerance (69). In addition to obesity and family history of diabetes, ethnicity adversely affects the prevalence of insulin resistance, and generally minority populations with PCOS tend to be more insulin-resistant than Caucasians (33).

Impaired Glucose Tolerance and Diabetes Mellitus

IGT and overt T2DM occur when the pancreatic β-cell is unable to compensate insulin resistance with hyperinsulinemia. In the U.S., PCOS is associated with a prevalence of IGT in excess of 30% and of T2DM in excess of 8%, while 27% of female T2DM patients have PCOS (Fig. 2) (69–71). In Italy and Germany, IGT is found in <15% and T2DM in <4% of PCOS patients, most likely due to the lower mean BMI of European women (3,54,72,73).

The Nurses' Health Study showed an increased risk of T2DMin women with oligomenorrhea, of whom about 80% were likely to have had PCOS (74). In a British study, 82% of T2DM women had PCO on ultrasound (75). A Swedish study found a high prevalence of PCO in women with previous gestational diabetes (76). A Spanish study reported a high prevalence of ovarian hyperandrogenism and PCOS among women with Type 1 DM (77), and suggested that it is not insulin resistance that is primarily responsible for the ovarian hyperandrogenism, but rather hyperinsulinemia (78).

While obesity contributes to insulin resistance and thus plays a determining role in the development of diabetes, almost all lean and most obese insulin-resistant PCOS women still have normal glucose tolerance. On the other hand, PCOS women with IGT or T2DM are significantly more insulin-resistant and hyperinsulinemic than those with normal glucose tolerance, regardless of the presence of obesity (72). Risk factors for glucose intolerance in women with PCOS include a family history of diabetes, low birth weight, early menarche, age, obesity and especially a centripetal fat distribution (69,71,79,80). Several prospective studies from Australia, Italy and the U.S. with up to 10 years of follow-up have found that insulin resistance tends to worsen over time, with the development of both IGT and T2DM in a significant portion of PCOS patients (45,81,82).

Metabolic Syndrome

The metabolic syndrome [MBS, aka syndrome X or insulin resistance syndrome, recently referred to as syndrome XX for PCOS patients (83)] describes a cluster of specific cardiovascular risk (CVR) factors whose underlying pathophysiology is thought to be related to insulin resistance (84). Since the introduction of the concept of insulin resistance as a predictor of CVD by Reaven in his famous 1988 Banting lecture (85), the definition of MBS underwent significant changes (86,87). The commonly used 2001 ATP III criteria of the National Cholesterol Education Program were developed to predict coronary heart disease (CHD) and to identify patients who would benefit from a lipid-lowering therapy (88).

While it is generally accepted that the individual risk factors including central obesity, hypertriglyceridemia, low HDL cholesterol levels, hypertension and elevated fasting plasma glucose predict morbidity and mortality from CVD (88,89), the usefulness of the term MBS has recently been challenged (90) to be imprecisely defined, with arbitrary thresholds and a CVD risk no greater than the sum of its parts. Also, at present, treatment of the syndrome is identical to treatment of its components.

Several recent studies have found a much higher prevalence of the MBS in PCOS patients than in the general population (3,91–95), even after controlling for the increased

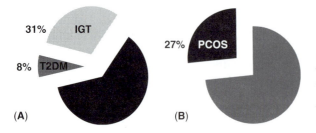

FIGURE 2 Association of PCOS and T2DM. In two studies from the United States, **(A)** Legro et al. found that out of 254 PCOS patients 31% had IGT and 8% T2DM, while **(B)** Peppard et al. found that 27% of their T2DM patients had PCOS. *Source*: From Refs. 69,70.

prevalence of obesity among affected women (37). A higher prevalence of MBS has also been found in PCOS-affected adolescents in comparison to age and BMI-matched control groups (96,97). There is intriguing evidence that this increased risk may be conferred not only by insulin resistance but also by hyperandrogenemia (93,98), in agreement with the higher bioavailable testosterone levels of postmenopausal women with rather than without MBS (99). The components of the MBS, namely obesity, dyslipidemia, insulin resistance and less commonly, hypertension, may be important determinants of overall, long-term health in PCOS patients (48,100).

Dyslipidemia is a primary target for therapeutic intervention in patients with MBS and CVD (101). A multitude of studies have shown elevated levels of total, LDL and VLDL cholesterol and triglycerides, as well as low HDL cholesterol in PCOS patients in excess of values expected from their obesity (102–108). Furthermore, total and LDL cholesterol were increased in hyperandrogenemic and PCOS-affected sisters and mothers of PCOS patients, consistent with a heritable trait (36,37).

Results concerning hypertension and PCOS are conflicting. While several studies have reported a higher prevalence of hypertension in PCOS patients (109–111), others have not (3). In 24-h ambulatory Holter-monitoring, women with PCOS had higher systolic blood pressure in comparison with BMI-, body fat-, and insulin sensitivity-matched controls in a study from Sweden (112), but not in a study from Canada (113).

Low-grade chronic inflammation is involved in the pathogenesis of the MBS and atherosclerosis (114). Hyperinsulinemia is associated with low-grade inflammation, which can be demonstrated by the elevation of C-reactive protein (CRP). CRP is an independent predictor for the development of T2DM (115) and a prognostic factor for cardiovascular events (116). Studies from Israel (117) and Turkey (118) found higher CRP levels in PCOS patients compared to controls, while a German study found a correlation of CRP levels with BMI unrelated to the presence of PCOS (119). Cytokines, which stimulate hepatic CRP production via induction of tumor necrosis factor-α (TNF-α), have also been correlated with MBS and CVD (114). In PCOS patients, Escobar-Moreale et al. found elevated interleukin-18 levels, which correlated with total testosterone and several indexes of global and visceral adiposity and with insulin resistance (120), while interleukin-6 was correlated with obesity rather than PCOS (119,121). An elevated white blood cell count has been proposed as a marker of subclinical inflammation and predictor of future cardiovascular events (114). This putative marker of CVR has recently been shown to correlate with other risk factors in PCOS patients (122). While elevated homocysteine levels appear to be correlated to CVD, therapeutic intervention with folate and B-vitamin substitution did not reduce morbidity or mortality in the HOPE-2 trial (123). Several studies have reported elevated homocysteine levels in PCOS, with a positive correlation with the degree of insulin resistance (124–126). Endothelin-1, a marker of vascular dysfunction, was found to be elevated in PCOS patients and could be reduced by metformin treatment both in lean (127) and obese patients (128).

Two studies have linked insulin resistance to endothelial dysfunction in PCOS patients by showing diminished vasodilatation to methacholine infusion (129) or reduced pulse wave velocity (130). However, a study using ultrasound to examine brachial arterial diameters as marker for vasodilatation found no difference between women with and without PCOS (131). In PCOS women older than 45 years, increased carotid intima media thickness (132,133) and coronary calcification on electron beam computed tomography (6) as surrogate markers of CVD have been reported. Recently, increased intima media thickness has also been reported for younger PCOS patients and was found to correlate with age, BMI, insulin resistance, dyslipidemia and family history of CVD and T2DM (134).

Concurrent with the increased prevalence of PCOS with obesity, the prevalence of the MBS is substantially higher in women with PCOS, ranging in the U.S. from 33% to more than 50% (93). However, in some other countries, the prevalence of the MBS in patients with PCOS is lower than that observed in the U.S. (3,54), most likely due to differences in body weight, environmental factors and food composition (Fig. 3). In contrast to the 1990 NIH criteria, which predict a higher prevalence of the MBS in PCOS patients, the use of PCO as a screening parameter does not identify PCOS patients at increased risk for the MBS (Fig. 4) (95).

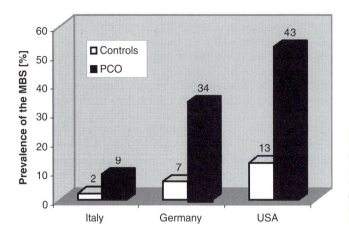

FIGURE 3 The prevalence of MBS is higher in PCOS and depends on BMI. Compared to age-matched controls, PCOS patients have a higher prevalence of the MBS, which also depends on the average BMI—Italy 29 kg/m²; Germany 31 kg/m²; USA 35–38 kg/m². *Source*: From Refs. 3,54,94.

Available data reporting higher cardiovascular morbidity and mortality are limited to studies which interpolate the diagnosis of PCOS from the presence of one symptom, either PCO or menstrual disorders. A four- to sevenfold increase in myocardial infarction has been found among women who had ovarian wedge resection for PCO (109). A history of irregular menses was found to be associated with increased risks of CHD and fatal myocardial infarction (135). In a study by Birdsall et al., 42% of 143 patients 60 years and older who underwent cardiac catheterization had PCO, the presence of which was correlated with a higher rate of hemodynamic relevant stenosis (136). On the other hand, a retrospective study with morbidity data of 319 PCOS patients identified by discharge records, diagnostic indexes, histopathological records and operating theatre records of wedge resection or ovarian biopsy, and compared to 1060 controls, found an increase of non-fatal CVD, T2DM and hypertension, but no increase in PCOS-associated CVD morbidity or mortality (111).

TREATMENT

As long-term prospective studies on the intervention of MBS in PCOS are not available, no clear therapeutic recommendations can be made. In analogy to the prevention and treatment of T2DM, lifestyle modifications aimed to reduce weight, optimize diet and encourage exercise are the primary goals to beware affected women from possible adverse metabolic consequences of PCOS. Diabetes Prevention Program targets for weight loss (≥7% of body

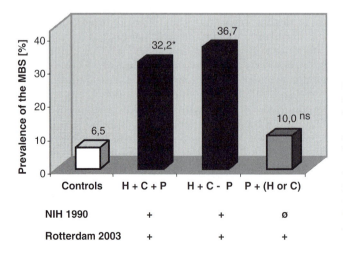

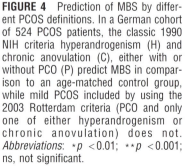

FIGURE 4 Prediction of MBS by different PCOS definitions. In a German cohort of 524 PCOS patients, the classic 1990 NIH criteria hyperandrogenism (H) and chronic anovulation (C), either with or without PCO (P) predict MBS in comparison to an age-matched control group, while mild PCOS included by using the 2003 Rotterdam criteria (PCO and only one of either hyperandrogenism or chronic anovulation) does not. *Abbreviations*: *p < 0.01; **p < 0.001; ns, not significant.

weight), and fitness (>150 min of physical activity per week) are probably appropriate but difficult to reach (137). Early identification of IGT and T2DM is important, and screening has indeed been recommended by the American Association of Clinical Endocrinologists for all PCOS patients 30 years or older (84). As there is no specific treatment of the MBS, its components should be treated individually according to the current guidelines for dyslipidemia, hypertension and diabetes. Insulin sensitizers, especially metformin, are promising, but their usefulness in the prevention of T2DM and CVD has not yet been shown in long-term studies.

Lifestyle Changes

For obese PCOS patients, there is a world-wide agreement that dietary-induced weight loss should always represent the first line therapeutic advice (138,139). Hypocaloric diet has been shown to improve the endocrine profile, facilitate weight loss, normalize menstrual cycles and increase the likelihood of ovulation and a healthy pregnancy (139–143).

Studies by Clark et al. (144,145), demonstrated that weight loss achieved by an exercise schedule, combined with a hypocaloric diet over a 6-month period, improved insulin sensitivity, endocrine parameters, menstrual regularity, the frequency of spontaneous ovulation and the chance of pregnancy. Even a modest weight loss of 2% to 5% of total body weight restored ovulation in overweight women with PCOS and achieved a reduction of central fat and an improvement in insulin sensitivity (143). The study by Crosignani et al. also found that women with anovulatory PCOS who lost weight experienced an improvement in ovarian function, ovulation and anthropometric indices (146). However, Kiddy et al. (141) found that insulin sensitivity and androgen concentrations were unlikely to improve in patients who lost <5% of their initial weight.

Pasquali et al. (147) studied two groups of 20 obese women either with or without PCOS who were given a low-calorie diet (1200–1400 kcal/day) for 1 month, after which they were randomized to receive metformin 850 mg twice daily or placebo for 6 months. Metformin treatment reduced body weight and BMI significantly more than placebo in both PCOS and control women. Fasting insulin decreased significantly in both PCOS women and controls and testosterone concentrations decreased only in PCOS women treated with metformin.

A study by Hoeger et al. (148) randomizing 38 women with a mean BMI of >39 kg/m^2 to receive either advice on lifestyle modification aiming for 500–1000 calorie deficit per day combined with exercise or no advice with either metformin (850 mg twice daily) or placebo found the greatest effect on weight and hyperandrogenism in the combination group, yet irrespective of treatment the greatest improvement in ovulation rate was achieved by those who lost weight.

Lifestyle modification is thus a key component for the improvement of reproductive function for overweight, anovulatory women with PCOS (138,149–151). Weight loss should be encouraged prior to ovulation induction treatments, since these are less effective when BMI is >28–30 kg/m^2 (152). Monitoring treatment is also harder in the obese as visualization of the ovaries is more difficult which raises the risk of multiple ovulations and pregnancies. Furthermore, pregnancy carries greater risks in the obese, such as miscarriage, gestational diabetes and hypertension (153–156). The main component of diet should be calorie restriction (157,158), with an additional effect from diet composition (49).

Insulin Sensitizers

Treatment options with insulin sensitizers (51,159–161) and anti-androgens (162–164) or their combination (147,165) have shown to be effective in the treatment of all aspects of PCOS. However, in dieting obese PCOS women, improvement of insulin sensitivity and hyperinsulinemia were mostly dependent on hypocaloric diet, rather than on pharmacological treatment (139,147,165).

In women with PCOS, metformin administered at doses of up to 2550 mg/day decreases insulin, testosterone, LH levels, triglyceride and HDL-cholesterol concentrations, favors weight loss and improves QoL (166,167). Some studies showed an improvement of pro-inflammatory markers, such as PAI-1, endothelin and CRP (166).

Moreover, metformin significantly improves menstrual cycles, ovulation and pregnancy rates (166,168,169). Metformin also appears to be more effective than laparoscopic ovarian diathermy in overall reproductive outcomes in overweight infertile clomiphene-resistant women with PCOS (170). Two studies have shown that metformin may reduce the rate of first trimester spontaneous abortions (171,172), which is threefold higher in PCOS women than in the general population. Another study has indicated that metformin may also be effective in controlling glucose metabolism and preventing gestational diabetes (173). To further decrease androgen levels, metformin may be used in combination with oral contraceptives (174,175) or with anti-androgens (164,176–178). However, the effect of metformin in women with PCOS requires an adequate, weight-adapted dose (139,179–183) and a sufficient duration of treatment (184).

Most clinical studies evaluating the effect of glitazones on PCOS have been performed with troglitazone, subsequently withdrawn because of its hepatotoxicity. Troglitazone has been shown to improve insulin resistance, glucose tolerance, hyperandrogenemia (free testosterone, androstenedione, DHEA-S) and ovulation rates (51,185). Moreover, the use of troglitazone in clomiphene-resistant patients resulted in ovulation and pregnancy rates of 83% and 39%, respectively (186).

Similar data regarding improvement in insulin resistance and hyperinsulinemia, hyperandrogenism and ovulation rates were subsequently reported in smaller studies in which obese PCOS women underwent treatment with rosiglitazone or pioglitazone (161). Rosiglitazone was found to increase ovulatory frequency and improve hyperandrogenemia even in non-obese women with PCOS with normal insulin sensitivity, but metformin treatment was even better (187). In another study, pioglitazone and metformin decreased insulin resistance and hyperandrogenemia in a group of obese women with PCOS to the same extent (188). A sequential treatment with pioglitazone for 10 months in 13 dieting obese women not responsive to a 12-month treatment with metformin reduced insulin, insulin resistance, glucose and DHEA-S, increased HDL cholesterol and SHBG, and improved menstrual regularity with respect to the previous metformin administration (189). However, a 6-month combination of rosiglitazone and metformin was not more potent than the monotherapies in improving ovulation and hyperandrogenemia in another study of normal weight non-insulin-resistant PCOS women (187), suggesting that glitazones might be useful only in a subset of PCOS patients not responsive to metformin.

REFERENCES

1. Azziz R, Woods KS, Reyna R, Key TJ, Knochenhauer ES, Yildiz BO. The prevalence and features of the polycystic ovary syndrome in an unselected population. J Clin Endocrinol Metab 2004; 89(6): 2745–9.
2. Ehrmann DA. Polycystic ovary syndrome. N Engl J Med 2005; 352(12):1223–36.
3. Hahn S, Tan S, Elsenbruch S, et al. Clinical and biochemical characterization of women with polycystic ovary syndrome in North Rhine-Westphalia. Horm Metab Res 2005; 37(7):438–44.
4. Venkatesan AM, Dunaif A, Corbould A. Insulin resistance in polycystic ovary syndrome: progress and paradoxes. Recent Prog Horm Res 2001; 56:295–308.
5. Talbott EO, Zborowski JV, Sutton-Tyrrell K, McHugh-Pemu KP, Guzick DS. Cardiovascular risk in women with polycystic ovary syndrome. Obstet Gynecol Clin North Am 2001; 28(1):111–133, vii.
6. Christian RC, Dumesic DA, Behrenbeck T, Oberg AL, Sheedy PFn, Fitzpatrick LA. Prevalence and predictors of coronary artery calcification in women with polycystic ovary syndrome. J Clin Endocrinol Metab 2003; 88(6):2562–8.
7. Stein I, Leventhal M. Amenorrhoea associated with bilateral polycystic ovaries. Am J Obstet Gynecol 1935; 29:181–5.
8. Vallisneri A. Istoria della Generazione dell'Uomo, e degli Animali, se sia da' vermicelli spermatici, o dalle uova. Venezia: Appreso Gio Gabbriel Hertz; 1721.
9. Chereau A. Mémoires pour servir à l'étude des maladies des ovaries. Paris: Fortin, Masson & Cie; 1844.
10. Rokitanski C. A Manual of Pathological Anatomy. Philadelphia: Blanchard & Lea; 1855.
11. Achard C, Thiers J. Le virilisme pilaire et son association a l'insuffisance glycolytique (diabete des femmes a barbe). Bull Acad Natl Med 1921; 86:51–64.
12. Burghen GA, Givens JR, Kitabchi AE. Correlation of hyperandrogenism with hyperinsulinism in polycystic ovarian disease. J Clin Endocrinol Metab 1980; 50(1):113–6.

13. Velazquez EM, Mendoza S, Hamer T, Sosa F, Glueck CJ. Metformin therapy in polycystic ovary syndrome reduces hyperinsulinemia, insulin resistance, hyperandrogenemia, and systolic blood pressure, while facilitating normal menses and pregnancy. Metabolism 1994; 43(5):647–54.

14. Baillargeon JP, Nestler JE. Commentary: polycystic ovary syndrome: a syndrome of ovarian hypersensitivity to insulin? J Clin Endocrinol Metab 2006; 91(7):22–4.

15. Hahn S, Bering van Halteren W, Kimmig R, Mann K, Gärtner R, Janssen OE. Diagnostic procedures in polycystic ovary syndrome. J Lab Med 2003; 27(1/2):53–9.

16. Zawadski JK, Dunaif A. Diagnostic criteria for polycystic ovary syndrome: towards a rational approach. In: Dunaif A, Givens JR, Haseltine FP, Merriam GR (eds), Polycystic Ovary Syndrome. Boston: Blackwell Scientific Publications; 1992, 377–84.

17. ESHRE/ASRM. Revised 2003 consensus on diagnostic criteria and long-term health risks related to polycystic ovary syndrome. Fertil Steril 2004; 81(7):19–25.

18. Azziz R, Carmina E, Dewailly D, et al. Criteria for defining polycystic ovary syndrome as a predominantly hyperandrogenic syndrome: an androgen excess society guideline. J Clin Endocrinol Metab 2006; 91(11):4237–45.

19. Knochenhauer ES, Key TJ, Kahsar-Miller M, Waggoner W, Boots LR, Azziz R. Prevalence of the polycystic ovary syndrome in unselected black and white women of the southeastern United States: a prospective study. J Clin Endocrinol Metab 1998; 83(9):3078–82.

20. Diamanti-Kandarakis E, Kouli CR, Bergiele AT, et al. A survey of the polycystic ovary syndrome in the Greek island of Lesbos: hormonal and metabolic profile. J Clin Endocrinol Metab 1999; 84(11): 4006–11.

21. Michelmore KF, Balen AH, Dunger DB, Vessey MP. Polycystic ovaries and associated clinical and biochemical features in young women. Clin Endocrinol (Oxf) 1999; 51(6):779–86.

22. Asuncion M, Calvo RM, San Millan JL, Sancho J, Avila S, Escobar-Morreale HF. A prospective study of the prevalence of the polycystic ovary syndrome in unselected Caucasian women from Spain. J Clin Endocrinol Metab 2000; 85(7):2434–8.

23. Dunaif A, Thomas A. Current concepts in the polycystic ovary syndrome. Annu Rev Med 2001; 52: 401–19.

24. Escobar-Morreale HF, Luque-Ramirez M, San Millan JL. The molecular-genetic basis of functional hyperandrogenism and the polycystic ovary syndrome. Endocr Rev 2005; 26(2):251–82.

25. Legro RS, Kunselman AR, Demers L, Wang SC, Bentley-Lewis R, Dunaif A. Elevated dehydroepiandrosterone sulfate levels as the reproductive phenotype in the brothers of women with polycystic ovary syndrome. J Clin Endocrinol Metab 2002; 87(5):2134–8.

26. Yildiz BO, Yarali H, Oguz H, Bayraktar M. Glucose intolerance, insulin resistance, and hyperandrogenemia in first degree relatives of women with polycystic ovary syndrome. J Clin Endocrinol Metab 2003; 88(5):2031–6.

27. Urbanek M, Spielman RS. Genetic analysis of candidate genes for the polycystic ovary syndrome. Curr Opin Endocrinol Diab 2002; 9:492–501.

28. Diamanti-Kandarakis E, Piperi C. Genetics of polycystic ovary syndrome: searching for the way out of the labyrinth. Hum Reprod Update 2005; 11(6):631-43.

29. Nestler JE, Powers LP, Matt DW, et al. A direct effect of hyperinsulinemia on serum sex hormone-binding globulin levels in obese women with the polycystic ovary syndrome. J Clin Endocrinol Metab 1991; 72(1):83–9.

30. Bulun SE, Noble LS, Takayama K, et al. Endocrine disorders associated with inappropriately high aromatase expression. J Steroid Biochem Mol Biol 1997; 61(3–6):133–9.

31. Wijeyaratne CN, Balen AH, Barth JH, Belchetz PE. Clinical manifestations and insulin resistance (IR) in polycystic ovary syndrome (PCOS) among South Asians and Caucasians: is there a difference? Clin Endocrinol (Oxf) 2002; 57(3):343–50.

32. Norman RJ, Mahabeer S, Masters S. Ethnic differences in insulin and glucose response to glucose between white and Indian women with polycystic ovary syndrome. Fertil Steril 1995; 63 (1):58–62.

33. Dunaif A, Sorbara L, Delson R, Green G. Ethnicity and polycystic ovary syndrome are associated with independent and additive decreases in insulin action in Caribbean-Hispanic women. Diabetes 1993; 42(10):1462–8.

34. Kauffman RP, Baker VM, Dimarino P, Gimpel T, Castracane VD. Polycystic ovarian syndrome and insulin resistance in white and Mexican American women: a comparison of two distinct populations. Am J Obstet Gynecol 2002; 187(5):1362–9.

35. Williamson K, Gunn AJ, Johnson N, Milsom SR. The impact of ethnicity on the presentation of polycystic ovarian syndrome. Aust N Z J Obstet Gynaecol 2001; 41(2):202–6.

36. Sam S, Legro RS, Essah PA, Apridonidze T, Dunaif A. Evidence for metabolic and reproductive phenotypes in mothers of women with polycystic ovary syndrome. Proc Natl Acad Sci USA 2006; 103(18):7030–5.

37. Sam S, Legro RS, Bentley-Lewis R, Dunaif A. Dyslipidemia and metabolic syndrome in the sisters of women with polycystic ovary syndrome. J Clin Endocrinol Metab 2005; 90(8):4797–4802.

38. Dunaif A, Segal KR, Futterweit W, Dobrjansky A. Profound peripheral insulin resistance, independent of obesity, in polycystic ovary syndrome. Diabetes 1989; 38(9):1165–74.
39. O'Meara NM, Blackman JD, Ehrmann DA, et al. Defects in beta-cell function in functional ovarian hyperandrogenism. J Clin Endocrinol Metab 1993; 76(5):1241–7.
40. Dunaif A. Insulin resistance and the polycystic ovary syndrome: mechanism and implications for pathogenesis. Endocr Rev 1997; 18(6):774–800.
41. Ehrmann DA, Sturis J, Byrne MM, Karrison T, Rosenfield RL, Polonsky KS. Insulin secretory defects in polycystic ovary syndrome. Relationship to insulin sensitivity and family history of non-insulin-dependent diabetes mellitus. J Clin Invest 1995; 96(1):520–7.
42. Dunaif A, Finegood DT. Beta-cell dysfunction independent of obesity and glucose intolerance in the polycystic ovary syndrome. J Clin Endocrinol Metab 1996; 81(3):942–7.
43. Dunaif A, Xia J, Book CB, Schenker E, Tang Z. Excessive insulin receptor serine phosphorylation in cultured fibroblasts and in skeletal muscle. A potential mechanism for insulin resistance in the polycystic ovary syndrome. J Clin Invest 1995; 96(2):801–10.
44. Rui L, Aguirre V, Kim JK, et al. Insulin/IGF-1 and TNF-alpha stimulate phosphorylation of IRS-1 at inhibitory Ser307 via distinct pathways. J Clin Invest 2001; 107(2):181–9.
45. Norman RJ, Masters L, Milner CR, Wang JX, Davies MJ. Relative risk of conversion from normoglycaemia to impaired glucose tolerance or non-insulin dependent diabetes mellitus in polycystic ovarian syndrome. Hum Reprod 2001; 16(9):1995–8.
46. Chan JM, Rimm EB, Colditz GA, Stampfer MJ, Willett WC. Obesity, fat distribution, and weight gain as risk factors for clinical diabetes in men. Diabetes Care 1994; 17(9):961–9.
47. Colditz GA, Willett WC, Rotnitzky A, Manson JE. Weight gain as a risk factor for clinical diabetes mellitus in women. Ann Intern Med 1995; 122(7):481–6.
48. Faloia E, Canibus P, Gatti C, et al. Body composition, fat distribution and metabolic characteristics in lean and obese women with polycystic ovary syndrome. J Endocrinol Invest 2004; 27(5):424–9.
49. Carmina E, Legro RS, Stamets K, Lowell J, Lobo RA. Difference in body weight between American and Italian women with polycystic ovary syndrome: influence of the diet. Hum Reprod 2003; 18 (11):2289–93.
50. Yen SS. The polycystic ovary syndrome. Clin Endocrinol (Oxf) 1980; 12(7):177–207.
51. Azziz R, Ehrmann D, Legro RS, et al. Troglitazone improves ovulation and hirsutism in the polycystic ovary syndrome: a multicenter, double blind, placebo-controlled trial. J Clin Endocrinol Metab 2001; 86(4):1626–32.
52. Balen AH, Conway GS, Kaltsas G, et al. Polycystic ovary syndrome: the spectrum of the disorder in 1741 patients. Hum Reprod 1995; 10(8):2107–11.
53. Taponen S, Martikainen H, Jarvelin MR, et al. Metabolic cardiovascular disease risk factors in women with self-reported symptoms of oligomenorrhea and/or hirsutism: Northern Finland Birth Cohort 1966 Study. J Clin Endocrinol Metab 2004; 89(5):2114–8.
54. Carmina E, Chu MC, Longo RA, Rini GB, Lobo RA. Phenotypic variation in hyperandrogenic women influences the findings of abnormal metabolic and cardiovascular risk parameters. J Clin Endocrinol Metab 2005; 90(5):2545–9.
55. Laitinen J, Taponen S, Martikainen H, et al. Body size from birth to adulthood as a predictor of self-reported polycystic ovary syndrome symptoms. Int J Obes Relat Metab Disord 2003; 27(6):710–5.
56. Stunkard AJ, Faith MS, Allison KC. Depression and obesity. Biol Psychiatry 2003; 54(3):330–7.
57. Mannucci E, Ricca V, Barciulli E, et al. Quality of life and overweight: the obesity related well-being (Orwell 97) questionnaire. Addict Behav 1999; 24(3):345–57.
58. Swallen KC, Reither EN, Haas SA, Meier AM. Overweight, obesity, and health-related quality of life among adolescents: the National Longitudinal Study of Adolescent Health. Pediatrics 2005; 115 (2):340–7.
59. Hashimoto DM, Schmid J, Martins FM, et al. The impact of the weight status on subjective symptomatology of the polycystic ovary syndrome: a cross-cultural comparison between Brazilian and Austrian women. Anthropol Anz 2003; 61(3):297–310.
60. McCook JG, Reame NE, Thatcher SS. Health-related quality of life issues in women with polycystic ovary syndrome. J Obstet Gynecol Neonatal Nurs 2005; 34(1):12–20.
61. Trent M, Austin SB, Rich M, Gordon CM. Overweight status of adolescent girls with polycystic ovary syndrome: body mass index as mediator of quality of life. Ambul Pediatr 2005; 5(2): 107–11.
62. Hahn S, Janssen OE, Tan S, et al. Clinical and psychological correlates of quality-of-life in polycystic ovary syndrome. Eur J Endocrinol 2005; 153(6):853–60.
63. Elsenbruch S, Hahn S, Kowalsky D, et al. Quality of life, psychosocial well-being, and sexual satisfaction in women with polycystic ovary syndrome. J Clin Endocrinol Metab 2003; 88(12): 5801–7.
64. Carmina E, Koyama T, Chang L, Stanczyk FZ, Lobo RA. Does ethnicity influence the prevalence of adrenal hyperandrogenism and insulin resistance in polycystic ovary syndrome? Am J Obstet Gynecol 1992; 167(6):1807–12.

65. Legro RS, Finegood D, Dunaif A. A fasting glucose to insulin ratio is a useful measure of insulin sensitivity in women with polycystic ovary syndrome. J Clin Endocrinol Metab 1998; 83(8):2694–8.

66. DeUgarte CM, Bartolucci AA, Azziz R. Prevalence of insulin resistance in the polycystic ovary syndrome using the homeostasis model assessment. Fertil Steril 2005; 83(5):1454–60.

67. Gennarelli G, Holte J, Berglund L, Berne C, Massobrio M, Lithell H. Prediction models for insulin resistance in the polycystic ovary syndrome. Hum Reprod 2000; 15(10):2098–102.

68. Legro RS, Castracane VD, Kauffman RP. Detecting insulin resistance in polycystic ovary syndrome: purposes and pitfalls. Obstet Gynecol Surv 2004; 59(2):141–54.

69. Legro RS, Kunselman AR, Dodson WC, Dunaif A. Prevalence and predictors of risk for type 2 diabetes mellitus and impaired glucose tolerance in polycystic ovary syndrome: a prospective, controlled study in 254 affected women. J Clin Endocrinol Metab 1999; 84(1):165–9.

70. Peppard HR, Marfori J, Iuorno MJ, Nestler JE. Prevalence of polycystic ovary syndrome among premenopausal women with type 2 diabetes. Diabetes Care 2001; 24(6):1050–2.

71. Ehrmann DA, Kasza K, Azziz R, Legro RS, Ghazzi MN. Effects of race and family history of type 2 diabetes on metabolic status of women with polycystic ovary syndrome. J Clin Endocrinol Metab 2005; 90(1):66–71.

72. Gambineri A, Pelusi C, Manicardi E, et al. Glucose intolerance in a large cohort of mediterranean women with polycystic ovary syndrome: phenotype and associated factors. Diabetes 2004; 53(9): 2353–8.

73. Pasquali R, Patton L, Pagotto U, Gambineri A. Metabolic alterations and cardiovascular risk factors in the polycystic ovary syndrome. Minerva Ginecol 2005; 57(1):79–85.

74. Solomon CG, Hu FB, Dunaif A, et al. Long or highly irregular menstrual cycles as a marker for risk of type 2 diabetes mellitus. JAMA 2001; 286(19):2421–6.

75. Conn JJ, Jacobs HS, Conway GS. The prevalence of polycystic ovaries in women with type 2 diabetes mellitus. Clin Endocrinol (Oxf) 2000; 52(1):81–6.

76. Holte J, Gennarelli G, Wide L, Lithell H, Berne C. High prevalence of polycystic ovaries and associated clinical, endocrine, and metabolic features in women with previous gestational diabetes mellitus. J Clin Endocrinol Metab 1998; 83(4):1143–50.

77. Escobar-Morreale HF, Roldan B, Barrio R, et al. High prevalence of the polycystic ovary syndrome and hirsutism in women with type 1 diabetes mellitus. J Clin Endocrinol Metab 2000; 85(11):4182–7.

78. Roldan B, Escobar-Morreale HF, Barrio R, et al. Identification of the source of androgen excess in hyperandrogenic type 1 diabetic patients. Diabetes Care 2001; 24(7):1297–9.

79. Ehrmann DA, Barnes RB, Rosenfield RL, Cavaghan MK, Imperial J. Prevalence of impaired glucose tolerance and diabetes in women with polycystic ovary syndrome. Diabetes Care 1999; 22(1):141–6.

80. Ibanez L, Jaramillo A, Enriquez G, et al. Polycystic ovaries after precocious pubarche: relation to prenatal growth. Hum Reprod 2006.

81. Pasquali R, Gambineri A, Anconetani B, et al. The natural history of the metabolic syndrome in young women with the polycystic ovary syndrome and the effect of long-term oestrogen—progestrogen treatment. Clin Endocrinol (Oxf) 1999; 50(4):517–27.

82. Legro RS, Gnatuk CL, Kunselman AR, Dunaif A. Changes in glucose tolerance over time in women with polycystic ovary syndrome: a controlled study. J Clin Endocrinol Metab 2005; 90(6):3236–42.

83. Sam S, Dunaif A. Polycystic ovary syndrome: syndrome XX? Trends Endocrinol Metab 2003; 14(8): 365–70.

84. ACE. ACE position statement on the insulin resistance syndrome. Endocr Pract 2003; 9(3):240–52.

85. Reaven GM. Banting lecture 1988. Role of insulin resistance in human disease. Diabetes 1988; 37 (12):1595–607.

86. Alberti KG, Zimmet P, Shaw J. Metabolic syndrome: a new world-wide definition. A Consensus Statement from the International Diabetes Federation. Diabetes Med 2006; 23(5):469–80.

87. Eckel RH, Grundy SM, Zimmet PZ. The metabolic syndrome. Lancet 2005; 365(9468):1415–28.

88. NCEP. Third Report of the National Cholesterol Education Program (NCEP) Expert Panel on Detection, Evaluation, and Treatment of High Blood Cholesterol in Adults (Adult Treatment Panel III) final report. Circulation 2002; 106(25):3143–421.

89. Girman CJ, Dekker JM, Rhodes T, et al. An exploratory analysis of criteria for the metabolic syndrome and its prediction of long-term cardiovascular outcomes: the Hoorn study. Am J Epidemiol 2005; 162(5):438–47.

90. Kahn R, Buse J, Ferrannini E, Stern M. The metabolic syndrome: time for a critical appraisal: joint statement from the American Diabetes Association and the European Association for the Study of Diabetes. Diabetes Care 2005; 28(9):2289–304.

91. Bloomgarden ZT. American Association of Clinical Endocrinologists (AACE) Consensus Conference on the Insulin Resistance Syndrome, 25–26 August 2002, Washington, DC. Diabetes Care 2003; 26(4):1297–303.

92. Glueck CJ, Papanna R, Wang P, Goldenberg N, Sieve-Smith L. Incidence and treatment of metabolic syndrome in newly referred women with confirmed polycystic ovarian syndrome. Metabolism 2003; 52(7):908–15.

93. Apridonidze T, Essah PA, Iuorno MJ, Nestler JE. Prevalence and characteristics of the metabolic syndrome in women with polycystic ovary syndrome. J Clin Endocrinol Metab 2005; 90(4): 1929–35.

94. Ehrmann DA, Liljenquist DR, Kasza K, Azziz R, Legro RS, Ghazzi MN. Prevalence and predictors of the metabolic syndrome in women with polycystic ovary syndrome (PCOS). J Clin Endocrinol Metab 2005.

95. Carmina E, Napoli N, Longo RA, Rini GB, Lobo RA. Metabolic syndrome in polycystic ovary syndrome (PCOS): lower prevalence in southern Italy than in the USA and the influence of criteria for the diagnosis of PCOS. Eur J Endocrinol 2006; 154(1):141–5.

96. Cook S, Weitzman M, Auinger P, Nguyen M, Dietz WH. Prevalence of a metabolic syndrome phenotype in adolescents: findings from the third National Health and Nutrition Examination Survey, 1988–1994. Arch Pediatr Adolesc Med 2003; 157(8):821–7.

97. de Ferranti SD, Gauvreau K, Ludwig DS, Neufeld EJ, Newburger JW, Rifai N. Prevalence of the metabolic syndrome in American adolescents: findings from the Third National Health and Nutrition Examination Survey. Circulation 2004; 110(16):2494–7.

98. Coviello AD, Legro RS, Dunaif A. Adolescent girls with polycystic ovary syndrome have an increased risk of the metabolic syndrome associated with increasing androgen levels independent of obesity and insulin resistance. J Clin Endocrinol Metab 2005.

99. Golden SH, Ding J, Szklo M, Schmidt MI, Duncan BB, Dobs A. Glucose and insulin components of the metabolic syndrome are associated with hyperandrogenism in postmenopausal women: the atherosclerosis risk in communities study. Am J Epidemiol 2004; 160(6):540–8.

100. Legro RS. Polycystic ovary syndrome and cardiovascular disease: a premature association? Endocr Rev 2003; 24(3):302–12.

101. Baigent C, Keech A, Kearney PM, et al. Efficacy and safety of cholesterol-lowering treatment: prospective meta-analysis of data from 90,056 participants in 14 randomised trials of statins. Lancet 2005; 366(9493):1267–78.

102. Mattsson LA, Cullberg G, Hamberger L, Samsioe G, Silfverstolpe G. Lipid metabolism in women with polycystic ovary syndrome: possible implications for an increased risk of coronary heart disease. Fertil Steril 1984; 42(4):579–84.

103. Wild RA, Painter PC, Coulson PB, Carruth KB, Ranney GB. Lipoprotein lipid concentrations and cardiovascular risk in women with polycystic ovary syndrome. J Clin Endocrinol Metab 1985; 61(7): 946–51.

104. Talbott E, Guzick D, Clerici A, et al. Coronary heart disease risk factors in women with polycystic ovary syndrome. Arterioscler Thromb Vasc Biol 1995; 15(1):821–6.

105. Talbott E, Clerici A, Berga SL, et al. Adverse lipid and coronary heart disease risk profiles in young women with polycystic ovary syndrome: results of a case–control study. J Clin Epidemiol 1998; 51 (4):415–22.

106. Mather KJ, Kwan F, Corenblum B. Hyperinsulinemia in polycystic ovary syndrome correlates with increased cardiovascular risk independent of obesity. Fertil Steril 2000; 73(1):150–6.

107. Dejager S, Pichard C, Giral P, et al. Smaller LDL particle size in women with polycystic ovary syndrome compared to controls. Clin Endocrinol (Oxf) 2001; 54(4):455–62.

108. Legro RS. Diabetes prevalence and risk factors in polycystic ovary syndrome. Obstet Gynecol Clin North Am 2001; 28(1):99–109.

109. Dahlgren E, Johansson S, Lindstedt G, et al. Women with polycystic ovary syndrome wedge resected in 1956 to 1965: a long-term follow-up focusing on natural history and circulating hormones. Fertil Steril 1992; 57(3):505–13.

110. Conway GS, Agrawal R, Betteridge DJ, Jacobs HS. Risk factors for coronary artery disease in lean and obese women with the polycystic ovary syndrome. Clin Endocrinol (Oxf) 1992; 37(2):119–25.

111. Wild S, Pierpoint T, McKeigue P, Jacobs H. Cardiovascular disease in women with polycystic ovary syndrome at long-term follow-up: a retrospective cohort study. Clin Endocrinol (Oxf) 2000; 52(5): 595–600.

112. Holte J, Gennarelli G, Berne C, Bergh T, Lithell H. Elevated ambulatory day-time blood pressure in women with polycystic ovary syndrome: a sign of a pre-hypertensive state? Hum Reprod 1996; 11 (1):23–8.

113. Zimmermann S, Phillips RA, Dunaif A, et al. Polycystic ovary syndrome: lack of hypertension despite profound insulin resistance. J Clin Endocrinol Metab 1992; 75(2):508–13.

114. Hansson GK. Inflammation, atherosclerosis, and coronary artery disease. N Engl J Med 2005; 352 (16):1685–95.

115. Spranger J, Kroke A, Mohlig M, et al. Inflammatory cytokines and the risk to develop type 2 diabetes: results of the prospective population-based European Prospective Investigation into Cancer and Nutrition (EPIC)-Potsdam Study. Diabetes 2003; 52(3):812–7.

116. Ridker PM, Buring JE, Cook NR, Rifai N. C-reactive protein, the metabolic syndrome, and risk of incident cardiovascular events: an 8-year follow-up of 14-719 initially healthy American women. Circulation 2003; 107(3):391–7.

117. Boulman N, Levy Y, Leiba R, et al. Increased C-reactive protein levels in the polycystic ovary syndrome: a marker of cardiovascular disease. J Clin Endocrinol Metab 2004; 89(5):2160–5.
118. Tarkun I, Arslan BC, Canturk Z, Turemen E, Sahin T, Duman C. Endothelial dysfunction in young women with polycystic ovary syndrome: relationship with insulin resistance and low-grade chronic inflammation. J Clin Endocrinol Metab 2004; 89(11):5592–6.
119. Mohlig M, Spranger J, Osterhoff M, et al. The polycystic ovary syndrome per se is not associated with increased chronic inflammation. Eur J Endocrinol 2004; 150(4):525–32.
120. Escobar-Morreale HF, Botella-Carretero JI, Villuendas G, Sancho J, San Millan JL. Serum interleukin-18 concentrations are increased in the polycystic ovary syndrome: relationship to insulin resistance and to obesity. J Clin Endocrinol Metab 2004; 89(2):806–11.
121. Escobar-Morreale HF, Villuendas G, Botella-Carretero JI, Sancho J, San Millan JL. Obesity, and not insulin resistance, is the major determinant of serum inflammatory cardiovascular risk markers in pre-menopausal women. Diabetologia 2003; 46(5):625–33.
122. Orio F, Jr., Palomba S, Cascella T, et al. The increase of leukocytes as a new putative marker of low-grade chronic inflammation and early cardiovascular risk in polycystic ovary syndrome. J Clin Endocrinol Metab 2005; 90(1):2–5.
123. Lonn E, Yusuf S, Arnold MJ, et al. Homocysteine lowering with folic acid and B vitamins in vascular disease. N Engl J Med 2006; 354(15):1567–77.
124. Loverro G, Lorusso F, Mei L, Depalo R, Cormio G, Selvaggi L. The plasma homocysteine levels are increased in polycystic ovary syndrome. Gynecol Obstet Invest 2002; 53(3):157–62.
125. Schachter M, Raziel A, Friedler S, Strassburger D, Bern O, Ron-El R. Insulin resistance in patients with polycystic ovary syndrome is associated with elevated plasma homocysteine. Hum Reprod 2003; 18(4):721–7.
126. Kilic-Okman T, Guldiken S, Kucuk M. Relationship between homocysteine and insulin resistance in women with polycystic ovary syndrome. Endocr J 2004; 51(5):505–8.
127. Orio F Jr, Palomba S, Cascella T, et al. Improvement in endothelial structure and function after metformin treatment in young normal-weight women with polycystic ovary syndrome: results of a 6-month study. J Clin Endocrinol Metab 2005; 90(11):6072–6.
128. Diamanti-Kandarakis E, Alexandraki K, Protogerou A, et al. Metformin administration improves endothelial function in women with polycystic ovary syndrome. Eur J Endocrinol 2005; 152(5): 749–56.
129. Paradisi G, Steinberg HO, Hempfling A, et al. Polycystic ovary syndrome is associated with endothelial dysfunction. Circulation 2001; 103(10):1410–5.
130. Kelly CJ, Speirs A, Gould GW, Petrie JR, Lyall H, Connell JM. Altered vascular function in young women with polycystic ovary syndrome. J Clin Endocrinol Metab 2002; 87(2):742–6.
131. Mather KJ, Verma S, Corenblum B, Anderson TJ. Normal endothelial function despite insulin resistance in healthy women with the polycystic ovary syndrome. J Clin Endocrinol Metab 2000; 85 (5):1851–6.
132. Orio F, Jr., Palomba S, Cascella T, et al. Early impairment of endothelial structure and function in young normal-weight women with polycystic ovary syndrome. J Clin Endocrinol Metab 2004; 89 (9):4588–93.
133. Talbott EO, Zborowski JV, Boudreaux MY, McHugh-Pemu KP, Sutton-Tyrrell K, Guzick DS. The relationship between C-reactive protein and carotid intima-media wall thickness in middle-aged women with polycystic ovary syndrome. J Clin Endocrinol Metab 2004; 89(12):6061–7.
134. Vryonidou A, Papatheodorou A, Tavridou A, et al. Association of hyperandrogenemic and metabolic phenotype with carotid intima-media thickness in young women with polycystic ovary syndrome. J Clin Endocrinol Metab 2005; 90(5):2740–6.
135. Solomon CG, Hu FB, Dunaif A, et al. Menstrual cycle irregularity and risk for future cardiovascular disease. J Clin Endocrinol Metab 2002; 87(5):2013–7.
136. Birdsall MA, Farquhar CM, White HD. Association between polycystic ovaries and extent of coronary artery disease in women having cardiac catheterization. Ann Intern Med 1997; 126(1):32–5.
137. Knowler WC, Barrett-Connor E, Fowler SE, et al. Reduction in the incidence of type 2 diabetes with lifestyle intervention or metformin. N Engl J Med 2002; 346(6):393–403.
138. Pasquali R, Gambineri A. Treatment of the polycystic ovary syndrome with lifestyle intervention. Curr Opin Endocrinol Diab 2002; 9:459–68.
139. Tang T, Glanville J, Hayden CJ, White D, Barth JH, Balen AH. Combined lifestyle modification and metformin in obese patients with polycystic ovary syndrome. A randomized, placebo-controlled, double-blind multicentre study. Hum Reprod 2006; 21(1):80–9.
140. Pasquali R, Antenucci D, Casimirri F, et al. Clinical and hormonal characteristics of obese amenorrheic hyperandrogenic women before and after weight loss. J Clin Endocrinol Metab 1989; 68(1):173–9.
141. Kiddy DS, Hamilton-Fairley D, Bush A, et al. Improvement in endocrine and ovarian function during dietary treatment of obese women with polycystic ovary syndrome. Clin Endocrinol (Oxf) 1992; 36(1):105–11.

142. Jakubowicz DJ, Nestler JE. 17 alpha-Hydroxyprogesterone responses to leuprolide and serum androgens in obese women with and without polycystic ovary syndrome offer dietary weight loss. J Clin Endocrinol Metab 1997; 82(2):556–60.

143. Huber-Buchholz MM, Carey DG, Norman RJ. Restoration of reproductive potential by lifestyle modification in obese polycystic ovary syndrome: role of insulin sensitivity and luteinizing hormone. J Clin Endocrinol Metab 1999; 84(4):1470–4.

144. Clark AM, Ledger W, Galletly C, et al. Weight loss results in significant improvement in pregnancy and ovulation rates in anovulatory obese women. Hum Reprod 1995; 10(10):2705–12.

145. Clark AM, Thornley B, Tomlinson L, Galletley C, Norman RJ. Weight loss in obese infertile women results in improvement in reproductive outcome for all forms of fertility treatment. Hum Reprod 1998; 13(6):1502–5.

146. Crosignani PG, Colombo M, Vegetti W, Somigliana E, Gessati A, Ragni G. Overweight and obese anovulatory patients with polycystic ovaries: parallel improvements in anthropometric indices, ovarian physiology and fertility rate induced by diet. Hum Reprod 2003; 18(9):1928–32.

147. Pasquali R, Gambineri A, Biscotti D, et al. Effect of long-term treatment with metformin added to hypocaloric diet on body composition, fat distribution, and androgen and insulin levels in abdominally obese women with and without the polycystic ovary syndrome. J Clin Endocrinol Metab 2000; 85(8):2767–74.

148. Hoeger KM, Kochman L, Wixom N, Craig K, Miller RK, Guzick DS. A randomized, 48-week, placebo-controlled trial of intensive lifestyle modification and/or metformin therapy in overweight women with polycystic ovary syndrome: a pilot study. Fertil Steril 2004; 82(2):421–9.

149. Norman RJ, Davies MJ, Lord J, Moran LJ. The role of lifestyle modification in polycystic ovary syndrome. Trends Endocrinol Metab 2002; 13(6):251–7.

150. Norman RJ, Noakes M, Wu R, Davies MJ, Moran L, Wang JX. Improving reproductive performance in overweight/obese women with effective weight management. Hum Reprod Update 2004; 10(3): 267–80.

151. Pasquali R, Gambineri A. Role of changes in dietary habits in polycystic ovary syndrome. Reprod Biomed Online 2004; 8(4):431–9.

152. Hamilton-Fairley D, Kiddy D, Watson H, Paterson C, Franks S. Association of moderate obesity with a poor pregnancy outcome in women with polycystic ovary syndrome treated with low dose gonadotrophin. 0Br J Obstet Gynaecol 1992; 99(2):128–31.

153. Gjonnaess H. The course and outcome of pregnancy after ovarian electrocautery in women with polycystic ovarian syndrome: the influence of body-weight. Br J Obstet Gynaecol 1989; 96(6): 714–9.

154. Sebire NJ, Jolly M, Harris JP, et al. Maternal obesity and pregnancy outcome: a study of 287,213 pregnancies in London. Int J Obes Relat Metab Disord 2001; 25(8):1175–82.

155. Cedergren MI. Maternal morbid obesity and the risk of adverse pregnancy outcome. Obstet Gynecol 2004; 103(2):219–24.

156. Linne Y. Effects of obesity on women's reproduction and complications during pregnancy. Obes Rev 2004; 5(3):137–43.

157. Moran LJ, Noakes M, Clifton PM, Tomlinson L, Norman RJ. Dietary composition in restoring reproductive and metabolic physiology in overweight women with polycystic ovary syndrome. J Clin Endocrinol Metab 2003; 88(2):812–9.

158. Stamets K, Taylor DS, Kunselman A, Demers LM, Pelkman CL, Legro RS. A randomized trial of the effects of two types of short-term hypocaloric diets on weight loss in women with polycystic ovary syndrome. Fertil Steril 2004; 81(3):630–7.

159. Nestler JE, Jakubowicz DJ, Evans WS, Pasquali R. Effects of metformin on spontaneous and clomiphene-induced ovulation in the polycystic ovary syndrome. N Engl J Med 1998; 338(26): 1876–80.

160. Moghetti P, Castello R, Negri C, et al. Metformin effects on clinical features, endocrine and metabolic profiles, and insulin sensitivity in polycystic ovary syndrome: a randomized, double-blind, placebo-controlled 6-month trial, followed by open, long-term clinical evaluation. J Clin Endocrinol Metab 2000; 85(1):139–46.

161. Pasquali R, Gambineri A. Insulin-sensitizing agents in women with polycystic ovary syndrome. Fertil Steril 2006; 86(Suppl. 1):S28–9.

162. De Leo V, Lanzetta D, D'Antona D, la Marca A, Morgante G. Hormonal effects of flutamide in young women with polycystic ovary syndrome. J Clin Endocrinol Metab 1998; 83(1):99–102.

163. Eagleson CA, Gingrich MB, Pastor CL, et al. Polycystic ovarian syndrome: evidence that flutamide restores sensitivity of the gonadotropin-releasing hormone pulse generator to inhibition by estradiol and progesterone. J Clin Endocrinol Metab 2000; 85(11):4047–52.

164. Ibanez L, Potau N, Marcos MV, de Zegher F. Treatment of hirsutism, hyperandrogenism, oligomenorrhea, dyslipidemia, and hyperinsulinism in nonobese, adolescent girls: effect of flutamide. J Clin Endocrinol Metab 2000; 85(9):3251–5.

165. Gambineri A, Pelusi C, Genghini S, et al. Effect of flutamide and metformin administered alone or in combination in dieting obese women with polycystic ovary syndrome. Clin Endocrinol (Oxf) 2004; 60(2):241–9.
166. De Leo V, la Marca A, Petraglia F. Insulin-lowering agents in the management of polycystic ovary syndrome. Endocr Rev 2003; 24(5):633–67.
167. Hahn S, Benson S, Elsenbruch S, et al. Metformin treatment of polycystic ovary syndrome improves health-related quality-of-life, emotional distress and sexuality. Hum Reprod 2006; 21(7):1925–34.
168. Lord JM, Flight IH, Norman RJ. Metformin in polycystic ovary syndrome: systematic review and meta-analysis. BMJ 2003; 327(7421):951–3.
169. Kashyap S, Wells GA, Rosenwaks Z. Insulin-sensitizing agents as primary therapy for patients with polycystic ovarian syndrome. Hum Reprod 2004; 19(11):2474–83.
170. Palomba S, Orio F Jr, Nardo LG, et al. Metformin administration versus laparoscopic ovarian diathermy in clomiphene citrate-resistant women with polycystic ovary syndrome: a prospective parallel randomized double-blind placebo-controlled trial. J Clin Endocrinol Metab 2004; 89(10): 4801–9.
171. Glueck CJ, Phillips H, Cameron D, Sieve-Smith L, Wang P. Continuing metformin throughout pregnancy in women with polycystic ovary syndrome appears to safely reduce first-trimester spontaneous abortion: a pilot study. Fertil Steril 2001; 75(1):46–52.
172. Jakubowicz DJ, Iuorno MJ, Jakubowicz S, Roberts KA, Nestler JE. Effects of metformin on early pregnancy loss in the polycystic ovary syndrome. J Clin Endocrinol Metab 2002; 87(2):524–9.
173. Glueck CJ, Wang P, Goldenberg N, Sieve-Smith L. Pregnancy outcomes among women with polycystic ovary syndrome treated with metformin. Hum Reprod 2002; 17(11):2858–64.
174. Elter K, Imir G, Durmusoglu F. Clinical, endocrine and metabolic effects of metformin added to ethinyl estradiol-cyproterone acetate in non-obese women with polycystic ovarian syndrome: a randomized controlled study. Hum Reprod 2002; 17(7):1729–37.
175. Morin-Papunen L, Vauhkonen I, Koivunen R, Ruokonen A, Martikainen H, Tapanainen JS. Metform in versus ethinyl estradiol-cyproterone acetate in the treatment of nonobese women with polycystic ovary syndrome: a randomized study. J Clin Endocrinol Metab 2003; 88(1):148–56.
176. Diamanti-Kandarakis E, Mitrakou A, Hennes MM, et al. Insulin sensitivity and antiandrogenic therapy in women with polycystic ovary syndrome. Metabolism 1995; 44(4):525–31.
177. Diamanti-Kandarakis E, Mitrakou A, Raptis S, Tolis G, Duleba AJ. The effect of a pure antiandrogen receptor blocker, flutamide, on the lipid profile in the polycystic ovary syndrome. J Clin Endocrinol Metab 1998; 83(8):2699–705.
178. Gambineri A, Patton L, Vaccina A, et al. Treatment with flutamide, metformin, and their combination added to a hypocaloric diet in overweight-obese women with polycystic ovary syndrome: a randomized, 12-month, placebo-controlled study. J Clin Endocrinol Metab 2006; 91 (10):3970–80.
179. Crave JC, Fimbel S, Lejeune H, Cugnardey N, Dechaud H, Pugeat M. Effects of diet and metformin administration on sex hormone-binding globulin, androgens, and insulin in hirsute and obese women. J Clin Endocrinol Metab 1995; 80(7):2057–62.
180. Fleming R, Hopkinson ZE, Wallace AM, Greer IA, Sattar N. Ovarian function and metabolic factors in women with oligomenorrhea treated with metformin in a randomized double blind placebo-controlled trial. J Clin Endocrinol Metab 2002; 87(2):569–74.
181. Maciel GA, Soares Junior JM, Alves da Motta EL, Abi Haidar M, de Lima GR, Baracat EC. Nonobese women with polycystic ovary syndrome respond better than obese women to treatment with metformin. Fertil Steril 2004; 81(2):355–60.
182. Kumari AS, Haq A, Jayasundaram R, Abdel-Wareth LO, Al Haija SA, Alvares M. Metformin monotherapy in lean women with polycystic ovary syndrome. Reprod Biomed Online 2005; 10(1): 100–4.
183. Goldenberg N, Glueck CJ, Loftspring M, Sherman A, Wang P. Metformin-diet benefits in women with polycystic ovary syndrome in the bottom and top quintiles for insulin resistance. Metabolism 2005; 54(1):113–21.
184. Eisenhardt S, Schwarzmann N, Henschel V, et al. Early effects of metformin in women with polycystic ovary syndrome: a prospective randomized, double-blind, placebo-controlled trial. J Clin Endocrinol Metab 2006; 91(3):946–52.
185. Dunaif A, Scott D, Finegood D, Quintana B, Whitcomb R. The insulin-sensitizing agent troglitazone improves metabolic and reproductive abnormalities in the polycystic ovary syndrome. J Clin Endocrinol Metab 1996; 81(9):3299–306.
186. Mitwally MF, Kuscu NK, Yalcinkaya TM. High ovulatory rates with use of troglitazone in clomiphene-resistant women with polycystic ovary syndrome. Hum Reprod 1999; 14(11):2700–3.
187. Baillargeon JP, Jakubowicz DJ, Iuorno MJ, Jakubowicz S, Nestler JE. Effects of metformin and rosiglitazone, alone and in combination, in nonobese women with polycystic ovary syndrome and normal indices of insulin sensitivity. Fertil Steril 2004; 82(4):893–902.

188. Ortega-Gonzalez C, Luna S, Hernandez L, et al. Responses of serum androgen and insulin resistance to metformin and pioglitazone in obese, insulin-resistant women with polycystic ovary syndrome. J Clin Endocrinol Metab 2005; 90(3):1360–5.
189. Glueck CJ, Moreira A, Goldenberg N, Sieve L, Wang P. Pioglitazone and metformin in obese women with polycystic ovary syndrome not optimally responsive to metformin. Hum Reprod 2003; 18(8):1618–25.

37 | Nonalcoholic Fatty Liver Disease and Diabetes Mellitus

Leon A. Adams
School of Medicine, The University of Western Australia, Sir Charles Gairdner Hospital, Perth, Australia

INTRODUCTION

The risk of death from liver disease is 2.5-fold higher among patients with type 2 diabetes mellitus compared to the general population (1). The most common liver disease among diabetics is non-alcoholic liver disease (NAFLD), which refers to the presence of hepatic steatosis not associated with excessive ethanol consumption. NAFLD occurs as a histological and clinical spectrum of disease; "simple steatosis" has a relatively benign course that rarely leads to advanced liver disease, whereas steatosis plus inflammation and/or fibrosis (non-alcoholic steatohepatitis or NASH) has the potential to lead to cirrhosis.

NAFLD may be categorized as primary or secondary depending on the underlying pathogenic factors (Table 1). Primary NAFLD is the most common form and is associated with insulin-resistant states such as diabetes mellitus and obesity, and thus is a common condition presenting to diabetologists and endocrinologists. Multiple mechanisms are implicated in secondary forms of NAFLD, including disturbances of hepatic lipid transport as in Wolman's disease; defective mitochondrial oxidation as seen in mushroom toxin exposure and acute fatty liver of pregnancy; or induction of metabolic risk factors as observed with corticosteroid administration. Distinction from secondary types is important, as these have differing treatment and prognoses (2).

EPIDEMIOLOGY

NAFLD is highly prevalent across a range of ethnicities and age groups. A large population-based study of 2287 subjects from the United States using the highly sensitive technique of magnetic resonance spectroscopy found the prevalence of NAFLD to be 32% (3). Using the less-sensitive diagnostic tool of ultrasound, population studies from Japan, China, and Italy have found a prevalence between 13% and 25% (4–7). NAFLD occurs in 2.6% of children and becomes more prevalent with increasing age, with a peak prevalence as determined by ultrasound of 25.6% among subjects older than 40 years (6,8).

Insulin resistance is present in 66% to 83% of subjects with NAFLD and is a strong risk factor for NAFLD among normoglycemic non-obese individuals (9). Concordantly, metabolic risk factors are present in the majority (85%) of subjects with NAFLD, with 56% to 79% being overweight [body mass index $(BMI > 25 \, kg/m^2)$] and one-third of individuals having the complete metabolic syndrome (3,10,11). The prevalence of diabetes or impaired fasting glycemia (>110)mg/dL) among the subjects with NAFLD ranges between 18% and 33% (3,4). Conversely, NAFLD is common among patients with type 2 diabetes with the prevalence ranging between 49% and 62% (5,12). The degree of glucose intolerance increases the risk of NAFLD, with NAFLD affecting 43% of those with impaired fasting glycemia and up to 62% with type 2 diabetes mellitus (5). In contrast, patients with type 1 diabetes mellitus having low insulin levels and without significant insulin resistance infrequently develop NAFLD (13).

Patients with type 2 diabetes mellitus are more likely to have the histologically more aggressive form of NASH, with a prevalence of 12.2% among those with diabetes compared to 4.7% among non-diabetics (14). The presence of obesity compounds the effects of diabetes, with NAFLD almost universally present and NASH occurring in 21% to 50% (2,14).

TABLE 1 Primary and Secondary Types of NAFLD

Primary NAFLD	
Metabolic features	Obesity, glucose intolerance, hypertension, hypertriglyceridemia, low HDL cholesterol
Secondary NAFLD	
Drugs	Corticosteroids, tamoxifen, tormifene, synthetic oestrogens, diltiazem, nifedipine, verapamil, methyldopa, choloroquine, zidovudine, tetracycline, didanosine, stavudine, aspirin, valproate, cocaine, amiodarone, perhexilene, methotrexate, irinotecan, oxaliplatin
Infections	Hepatitis C, human immunodeficiency virus, small bowel diverticulosis with bacterial overgrowth, gram-negative sepsis
Metabolic conditions	Hypobetalipoproteinemia, lipodystrophy, Weber-Christian syndrome, acute fatty liver of pregnancy, Reyes syndrome, cholesterol ester storage disease, Wolman's disease, Wilson's disease, Dorfman Chanarin syndrome, adult onset type 2 citrullinemia
Toxins	Organic solvents, mushroom toxins (*Aminanta phalloides, Lepiota*), phosphorus poisoning, petrochemical exposure, *Bacillus cereus* toxin
Nutritional	Rapid weight loss, intestinal bypass surgery, starvation, protein calorie malnutrition, coeliac disease, inflammatory bowel disease, total parenteral nutrition, choline deficiency

PATHOGENESIS AND PATHOPHYSIOLOGY

The pathogenic mechanisms that lead to NAFLD are complex and not completely understood. Insulin resistance and accompanying metabolic abnormalities appear pivotal in the development of hepatic steatosis as well as contributing to hepatic inflammation and fibrosis.

Accumulation of hepatic triglyceride occurs when lipid influx and de novo synthesis in the liver exceeds lipid export and oxidation. Insulin resistance promotes lipolysis of peripheral adipose tissue, which increases free-fatty acid (FFA) influx into the liver, subsequently driving hepatic triglyceride production (15). In addition, hyperinsulinemia and hyperglycemia promote de novo hepatic lipogenesis by up-regulating lipogenic transcription factors such as sterol regulatory element binding protein-1c (SREBP-1c) and carbohydrate response element binding protein (16). FFA oxidation is inhibited by increased levels of malonyl-CoA, which also occurs as a result of insulin-mediated activation of SREBP-1c, thereby favoring hepatic triglyceride accumulation (16). Furthermore, lipid export from the liver in the form of very low-density lipoproteins may be impaired because of defective incorporation of triglyceride into apolipoprotein B or reduced apolipoprotein B synthesis or excretion (17).

Hepatic triglyceride accumulation subsequently leads to hepatic insulin resistance by interfering with tyrosine phosphorylation of insulin receptor substrates 1 and 2 (18). This may potentially exacerbate systemic insulin resistance creating an escalating cycle of insulin resistance leading to NAFLD, which worsens insulin resistance providing further stimulus for hepatic fat accumulation.

Hepatic lipid accumulation does not universally result in hepatocellular injury, indicating that additional secondary insults are important (19). Insulin resistance and associated metabolic disturbances in adipose-derived factors including FFA, tumor necrosis factor-α (TNF-α), leptin and adiponectin have been implicated in contributing to liver damage in NAFLD. Hyperinsulinemia and hyperglycemia may directly stimulate fibrosis by up-regulation of fibrogenic growth factor produced by hepatic stellate cells (20,21). Increased hepatic FFA oxidation can generate oxygen radicals with subsequent lipid peroxidation, cytokine induction and mitochondrial dysfunction (22). FFA may also lead to hepatocyte apoptosis, which is a prominent mechanism of cellular injury among NAFLD patients (23). Genetic polymorphisms of inflammatory and fibrogenic cytokines such as TNF-α, tumor growth factor-β, angiotensinogen have been implicated to influence progression to NASH, as has polymorphisms of manganese superoxide dismutase, which is protective against reactive oxygen species (15). Pro-inflammatory TNF-α levels may also be increased secondary to gut-derived bacterial lipopolysaccharide and increased fat mass (23–25). Increased hepatic necroinflammation and cytokine levels may stimulate a family of proteins named "suppressors of cytokine signaling," which exacerbate insulin resistance and up-regulate SREBP-1c potentially leading to a vicious cycle of cytokine induction, suppression, insulin resistance and hepatic steatosis (26).

Adipocytokine metabolism may be altered in patients with NAFLD. Insulin sensitizing and potentially hepatoprotective cytokines such as adiponectin are inappropriately low among NASH patients, potentially predisposing to the development of NAFLD and the progression to NASH (27). Leptin is required for hepatic fibrogenesis in animal models (28) and leptin-deficient *ob/ob* mice develop a phenotype of obesity, insulin resistance and fatty liver (29). However, the pathogenic association in humans between leptin and NAFLD remains to be fully elucidated.

Finally, with progressive lipid accumulation, hepatocytes become swollen and distorted, which in conjunction with sinusoidal fibrosis may lead to microvascular insufficiency. Subsequent impairment of hepatocyte oxygen and nutrient exchange may lead to an inflammatory response that has been hypothesized to lead to further venous obstruction and eventual development and progression of fibrosis (30).

HISTOLOGY

The histological changes of NAFLD are similar to that produced by alcohol (31). Thus the diagnosis of NAFLD cannot be made by histological means alone and requires the clinical exclusion of excessive alcohol intake. The histological hallmark of NAFLD is hepatocellular triglyceride accumulation, which is predominantly macrovescicular, although may be mixed with microvescicular fat, which implies defective mitochondrial FFA oxidation. Steatohepatitis requires the presence of lobular inflammation, which is usually a mixed mononuclear/ neutrophilic infiltrate and is frequently associated with hepatocyte ballooning and less commonly Mallory's hyaline (32). Hepatocellular ballooning, disarray and fibrosis are typically predominant in zone three of the hepatic lobule. Fibrosis is typically pericellular and perisinusoidal giving a "chickenwire" appearance. Eventually, fibrotic septae form between the hepatic vein and portal tract and nodules may form heralding the onset of cirrhosis. Interestingly, as fibrosis progresses, steatosis may diminish and become absent in the setting of cirrhosis (33). Thus, the diagnosis of NAFLD may be difficult in the setting of cirrhosis and thus may be the underlying cause of a substantial proportion of subjects previously diagnosed as having 'cryptogenic' cirrhosis.

Less common histological findings among patients with diabetes mellitus include diabetic hepatosclerosis and glycogenic hepatopathy (34,35). These conditions appear to occur more frequently in patients with type 1 diabetes mellitus. Diabetic hepatosclerosis refers to sinusoidal basement membrane thickening and fibrosis in the absence of NAFLD and often occurs concomitantly with evidence of other microvascular disease (35). Abundant cytoplasmic glycogen in the setting of poorly controlled type 1 diabetes is termed glycogenic hepatopathy. Although rarely causing fibrosis, it may present with hepatomegaly, elevated transaminases, growth retardation and delayed puberty (Mauriac syndrome) (34).

CLINICAL FEATURES

Patients with NAFLD are generally asymptomatic although may have abdominal discomfort and hepatomegaly. Clinical examination may reveal signs of portal hypertension such as splenomegaly or ascites if cirrhosis is present. Children may have acanthosis nigricans reflecting underlying insulin resistance.

Liver enzymes may be normal in up to 78% of patients including those with cirrhosis, and thus are insensitive for both the detection of NAFLD and the exclusion of advanced liver disease (3). When present, liver enzyme elevations are generally modest and restricted to alanine aminotransaminase (ALT) and aspartate aminotransaminase (AST). Elevations of ALT and AST greater than five times the upper limit of normal are uncommon and should prompt investigation for an alternative cause. A ratio of AST/ALT > 1 may signify advanced fibrosis (36). Iron studies are also frequently elevated with elevated ferritin observed in 20% to 50% of patients and raised transferrin saturation in 5% to 10% of cases (2). This is presumably secondary to hepatic inflammation or low-grade systemic inflammation that may accompany the metabolic syndrome.

Imaging studies such as ultrasound, computed tomography and magnetic resonance imaging can be used to confirm the diagnosis of NAFLD and are accurate for detecting moderate to severe hepatic steatosis. The sensitivity and specificity of ultrasound for detecting >33% steatosis is between 60% to 94% and 88% to 95% respectively, although falls with increasing BMI to 49% and 75%, respectively, among morbidly obese individuals (37). Thus mild steatosis is difficult to exclude by ultrasound, particularly in the setting of obesity.

Localized proton magnetic resonance spectroscopy is able to accurately quantify hepatic triglyceride content in the liver whereas ultrasound, computed tomography and magnetic resonance are semi-quantitative at best (38). However, no imaging modality is able to differentiate between the histological subtypes of relatively benign non-alcoholic hepatic steatosis or more aggressive NASH. Nor is imaging able to stage the degree of liver fibrosis (39).

Liver biopsy is able to stage the disease and thus is valuable for prognostic reasons. In addition, histological evaluation can be useful to exclude other liver disease, particularly in the setting of potential concomitant drug hepatotoxicity, elevated iron studies or positive auto-antibodies (2,40). Importantly, monitoring disease progression or response to therapy requires a liver biopsy as aminotransaminase levels improve over time regardless of whether hepatic fibrosis progresses or improves (33). The potential benefits of liver biopsy must be weighed against the small risk of complications including pain, bleeding and rarely death. The decision to pursue biopsy needs to be discussed and individualized with each patient.

NATURAL HISTORY

Overall, patients with diabetes mellitus compared to the general population, have a greater relative risk of death from cirrhosis (2.5-fold) than cardiovascular disease (1.3-fold) (1). Death from chronic liver disease or hepatoma is the fourth most common cause of death among diabetics, accounting for approximately 1 in 20 deaths (1). The relative risk of death from cirrhosis increases as the severity of diabetes increases with those requiring oral hypoglycemic medications having a 4.9-fold increased risk and those on insulin having a 6.8-fold increased risk compared to those treated with diet alone (1).

The prognosis of patients with diabetes mellitus and concomitant NAFLD is not well defined. No population-based studies exist, however one study from a tertiary referral centre found cirrhosis developed in 25% of diabetics with NAFLD and liver related death occurred in 18% (41). Although there was no control group, it would be reasonable to predict that the incidence of cirrhosis and liver-related death among patients with diabetes but not NAFLD would be substantially lower.

The natural history of patients diagnosed with NAFLD (with and without diabetes mellitus) is better characterized with these patients having an increased (1.3-fold) mortality rate compared to the general population (42), most likely due to complications of insulin resistance such as vascular disease and NAFLD cirrhosis (43). Liver disease among patients with NAFLD is characteristically slowly progressive with a 3.1% incidence of cirrhosis over 7.6 years (43). Over decades, this may be complicated by hepatocellular carcinoma in a small number (0.5% to 2%) (43,44) and lead to death from liver disease in up to 13% of those with NAFLD.

The prognosis of patients with NAFLD can be stratified according to their histology; those with bland steatosis without evidence of steatohepatitis, have a relatively benign liver-related prognosis with 1.5% developing cirrhosis and 1% dying from liver-related causes over one to two decades (45,46). In contrast, the liver-related death rate among patients from tertiary care centers with biopsy proven NASH is up to 11% (46).

Metabolic disease and in particular diabetes mellitus, is an adverse prognostic factor among patients with NAFLD. The risk of advanced fibrosis increases in the presence of diabetes mellitus as well as with obesity and age (36,41,47). Furthermore, diabetes mellitus is associated with an increased rate of hepatic fibrosis progression (33). Consequently, diabetes is a risk factor for liver-related death (up to 22-fold) as well as overall death (2.6- to 3.3-fold) in patients with NAFLD (41).

NAFLD AS A RISK FACTOR FOR DIABETES

The liver plays a key role in glucose homeostasis in the body and thus may contribute to the development of diabetes mellitus. Accumulation of hepatic steatosis impairs insulin signaling resulting in hepatic insulin resistance (18). Consequently, patients with NAFLD are more insulin-resistant than age-, gender- and BMI-matched controls (48). Raised aminotransaminases (a marker of NAFLD) are well-established to increase the risk of developing diabetes three to sixfold (49). Similarly, patients who gain weight tend to develop abnormal liver tests before glucose intolerance is detected (50). Thus, accumulation of visceral and hepatic fat may be important and sequential steps in the development of type 2 diabetes.

NAFLD AS A CARDIOVASCULAR RISK FACTOR

Data is emerging that NAFLD is an independent risk factor for vascular disease, which is the most common cause of death among patients with diabetes (1). Patients with NAFLD have a greater carotid intima-media thickness as well as a higher prevalence of carotid atheromatous plaques (51). The presence of NAFLD among patients with type 2 diabetes is associated with an increased risk of developing vascular disease, which is only partly associated with the presence of the metabolic syndrome (52,53). Similarly, ALT is independently predictive of the development of coronary heart disease (54). The mechanisms through which NAFLD may result in increased vascular disease are unclear and it is difficult to distinguish whether this is an association with the abnormal metabolic milieu that occurs in association with NAFLD or whether it is related to the increased lipid oxidation, inflammation and abnormal hepatic lipid metabolism that occurs with NAFLD. Certainly, lipid profiles among diabetics with NAFLD are more atherogenic with lower HDL-cholesterol levels and higher levels of small LDL cholesterol (55). In addition, hepatic steatosis in diabetics is associated with myocardial insulin resistance and lower coronary flow reserve, which increases susceptibility to myocardial injury (56).

TREATMENT

Treatment strategies for NAFLD aim to improve insulin sensitivity and modify underlying metabolic risk factors, or protect the liver from oxidative stress and further insults (Table 2). Liver transplantation may be required for patients with decompensated cirrhosis or liver cancer. Pharmacotherapy should probably be reserved for those patients with risk factors for developing complications, i.e. those with NASH, diabetes and obesity. The lack of adequately powered randomized controlled trials of sufficient duration and with histological endpoints make definitive recommendations difficult at this time.

Diet and exercise improve liver biochemistry and hepatic steatosis (57). It is unknown whether the low (5% to 10%) carbohydrate (Atkins diet) versus standard (40% to 60%) carbohydrate diet is more beneficial, with benefits reported from both (57,58). Uncontrolled

TABLE 2 Potential Treatments for NAFLD

Treatment	Mechanism of action	Trial type	Liver enzymes	Liver histology
Weight loss	Improve insulin sensitivity	Pilot	Improve	Improve
Metformin	Improve insulin sensitivity	Pilot, RCT	Improve	Improve[a]
Thioglitazones	Improve insulin sensitivity	Pilot	Improve	Improve
Vitamin E	Antioxidant	Pilot, RCT	No change	Improve[a]
Ursodeoxycholic acid	Hepatoprotective	RCT	No change	No change
Pentoxifylline	Hepatoprotective	Pilot	Improve	NA
Betaine	Hepatoprotective	Pilot	Improve	Improve
Losartan	Hepatoprotective	Pilot	Improve	No change
Statins	Lipid metabolism	Pilot	Improve	No change
Clofibrate	Lipid metabolism	Pilot	No change	No change

[a] Improvement in histology compared to baseline but not compared to control group.
Abbreviation: RCT, randomized controlled trial.

series have demonstrated improvement in liver histology with bariatric surgery (59), although very rapid weight loss associated with very low calorie diets (<500 kcal/day) can worsen hepatic inflammation and fibrosis (2).

Of the insulin-sensitizing agents, metformin significantly improves aminotransaminases and reduces the prevalence of the metabolic syndrome, compared to either diet therapy or vitamin E (60). Several uncontrolled pilot trials have shown that the thiazolidinediones rosiglitazone and pioglitazone are associated with an improvement of histological features (61). However, concern exists regarding hepatotoxicity as 2% to 5% of patients were withdrawn because of rising aminotransaminases.

Vitamin E has not been shown to convincingly improve liver biochemistry or histology. Other hepatoprotective and anti-fibrotic agents such as betaine, pentoxifylline and losartan have shown promise in small pilot trials (62). Statins appear to be safe among patients with NAFLD and may have some benefit in lowering liver enzyme levels (63).

CONCLUSIONS

NAFLD is pathogenically associated with insulin resistance and thus affects a significant proportion of individuals with type 2 diabetes mellitus. These patients are at increased risk of progressing to cirrhosis and its complications, with obesity and insulin requirements increasing the risk of developing advanced liver disease. In addition, NAFLD exacerbates hepatic insulin resistance and may predispose to the development of diabetes and cardio-vascular disease. NAFLD is generally asymptomatic and often associated with normal liver enzymes and thus may be under-recognized. Diagnosis requires confirmation by hepatic steatosis, which can generally be done by imaging studies. Staging of NAFLD requires a liver biopsy. A diagnosis of NAFLD should prompt attention to management of metabolic risk factors. Further studies are required to identify pharmacotherapeutic agents that alter the natural history of the disease as well as to identify patients who will benefit most from treatment.

REFERENCES

1. De Marco R, Locatelli F, Zoppini G, et al. Cause-specific mortality in type 2 diabetes. The Verona Diabetes Study. Diabetes Care 1999; 22:756–61.
2. Angulo P. Nonalcoholic fatty liver disease. N Engl J Med 2002; 346(16):1221–31.
3. Browning JD, Szczepaniak LS, Dobbins R, et al. Prevalence of hepatic steatosis in an urban population in the United States: impact of ethnicity. Hepatology 2004; 40(6):1387–95.
4. Fan JG, Zhu G, Li XJ, et al. Prevalence of and risk factors for fatty liver in a general population of Shanghai China. J Hepatol 2005; 43:508–13.
5. Jimba S, Nakagami T, Takahashi M, et al. Prevalence of non-alcoholic fatty liver disease and its association with impaired glucose metabolism in Japanese adults. Diabetic Med. 2005; 22(9):1141–5.
6. Nomura H, Kashiwagi S, Hayashi J, et al. Prevalence of fatty liver in a general population of Okinawa, Japan. Jpn J Med 1988; 27(2):142–9.
7. Bedogni G, Miglioli L, Masutti F, et al. Prevalence of and risk factors for nonalcoholic fatty liver disease: the Dionysos nutrition and liver study. Hepatology 2005; 42(1):44–52.
8. Tominaga K, Kurata JH, Chen YK, et al. Prevalence of fatty liver in Japanese children and relationship to obesity. An epidemiological ultrasonographic survey. Dig Dis Sci 1995; 40(9):2002–9.
9. Marchesini G, Brizi M, Morselli-Labate AM, et al. Association of nonalcoholic fatty liver disease with insulin resistance. Am J Med 1999; 107(5):450–5.
10. Marchesini G, Bugianesi E, Forlani G, et al. Nonalcoholic fatty liver, steatohepatitis, and the metabolic syndrome. Hepatology 2003; 37(4):917–23.
11. Bugianesi E, Manzini P, D'Antico S, et al. Relative contribution of iron burden, HFE mutations, and insulin resistance to fibrosis in nonalcoholic fatty liver. Hepatology 2004; 39(1):179–87.
12. Gupte P, Amarapurkar D, Agal S, et al. Non-alcoholic steatohepatitis in type 2 diabetes mellitus. J Gastroenterol Hepatol 2004; 19(8):854–8.
13. Perseghin G, Lattuada G, De Cobelli F, et al. Reduced intrahepatic fat content is associated with increased whole-body lipid oxidation in patients with type 1 diabetes. Diabetologia 2005; 48(12): 2615–21.
14. Wanless IR, Lentz JS. Fatty liver hepatitis (steatohepatitis) and obesity: an autopsy study with analysis of risk factors. Hepatology 1990; 12(5):1106–10.

15. Adams LA, Angulo P, Lindor KD. Nonalcoholic fatty liver disease. CMAJ 2005; 172(7):899–905.
16. Browning JD, Horton JD. Molecular mediators of hepatic steatosis and liver injury. J Clin Invest 2004; 114(2):147–52.
17. Charlton M, Sreekumar R, Rasmussen D, et al. Apolipoprotein synthesis in nonalcoholic steatohepatitis. Hepatology 2002; 35(4):898–904.
18. Schattenberg JM, Wang Y, Singh R, et al. Hepatocyte CYP2E1 overexpression and steatohepatitis lead to impaired hepatic insulin signaling. J Biol Chem. 2005; 280(11):9887–94.
19. Day CP, James OF. Steatohepatitis: a tale of two "hits"? Gastroenterology 1998; 114(4):842–5.
20. Paradis V, Perlemuter G, Bonvoust F, et al. High glucose and hyperinsulinemia stimulate connective tissue growth factor expression: a potential mechanism involved in progression to fibrosis in nonalcoholic steatohepatitis. Hepatology 2001; 34(4 Pt 1):738–44.
21. Sugimoto R, Enjoji M, Kohjima M, et al. High glucose stimulates hepatic stellate cells to proliferate and to produce collagen through free radical production and activation of mitogen-activated protein kinase. Liver Int 2005; 25(5):1018–26.
22. Haque M, Sanyal AJ. The metabolic abnormalities associated with non-alcoholic fatty liver disease. Best Pract Res Clin Gastroenterol 2002; 6(5):709–31.
23. Feldstein AE, Werneburg NW, Canbay A, et al. Free fatty acids promote hepatic lipotoxicity by stimulating TNF-alpha expression via a lysosomal pathway. Hepatology 2004; 40(1):185–94.
24. Valenti L, Fracanzani AL, Dongiovanni P, et al. Tumor necrosis factor alpha promoter polymorphisms and insulin resistance in nonalcoholic fatty liver disease. Gastroenterology 2002; 122(2):274–80.
25. Wigg AJ, Roberts-Thomson IC, Dymock RB, et al. The role of small intestinal bacterial overgrowth, intestinal permeability, endotoxaemia, and tumour necrosis factor alpha in the pathogenesis of non-alcoholic steatohepatitis. Gut 2001; 48(2):206–11.
26. Ueki K, Kondo T, Tseng YH, et al. Central role of suppressors of cytokine signaling proteins in hepatic steatosis, insulin resistance, and the metabolic syndrome in the mouse. Proc Natl Acad Sci USA 2004; 101(28):10422–7.
27. Hui JM, Hodge A, Farrell GC, et al. Beyond insulin resistance in NASH: TNF-alpha or adiponectin? Hepatology 2004; 40(1):46–54.
28. Leclercq IA, Farrell GC, Schriemer R, et al. Leptin is essential for the hepatic fibrogenic response to chronic liver injury. J Hepatol 2002; 37(2):206–13.
29. Anania FA. Leptin, liver, and obese mice: fibrosis in the fat lane. Hepatology 2002; 36(1):246–8.
30. Wanless IR, Shiota K. The pathogenesis of nonalcoholic steatohepatitis and other fatty liver diseases: a four-step model including the role of lipid release and hepatic venular obstruction in the progression to cirrhosis. Semin Liver Dis 2004; 24(1):99–106.
31. Diehl AM, Goodman Z, Ishak KG. Alcohol-like liver disease in nonalcoholics. A clinical and histologic comparison with alcohol-induced liver injury. Gastroenterology 1988; 95(4):1056–62.
32. Brunt EM, Janney CG, Di Bisceglie AM, et al. Nonalcoholic steatohepatitis: a proposal for grading and staging the histological lesions. Am J Gastroenterol 1999; 94(9):2467–74.
33. Adams LA, Sanderson S, Lindor KD, et al. The histological course of nonalcoholic fatty liver disease: a longitudinal study of 103 patients with sequential liver biopsies. J Hepatol 2005; 42(1):132–8.
34. Torbenson M, Chen YY, Brunt E, et al. Glycogenic hepatopathy: an underrecognized hepatic complication of diabetes mellitus. Am J Surg Pathol 2006; 30(4):508–13.
35. Harrison SA, Brunt EM, Goodman ZD, et al. Diabetic hepatosclerosis: diabetic microangiopathy of the liver. Arch Pathol Lab Med 2006; 130(1):27–32.
36. Angulo P, Keach JC, Batts KP, et al. Independent predictors of liver fibrosis in patients with nonalcoholic steatohepatitis. Hepatology 1999; 30(6):1356–62.
37. Joy D, Thava VR, Scott BB. Diagnosis of fatty liver disease: is biopsy necessary? Eur J Gastroenterol Hepatol 2003; 15(5):539–43.
38. Szczepaniak LS, Nurenberg P, Leonard D, et al. Magnetic resonance spectroscopy to measure hepatic triglyceride content: prevalence of hepatic steatosis in the general population. Am J Physiol Endocrinol Metab 2005; 288(2):E462–8.
39. Saadeh S, Younossi ZM, Remer EM, et al. The utility of radiological imaging in nonalcoholic fatty liver disease. Gastroenterology 2002; 123(3):745–50.
40. Van Ness MM, Diehl AM. Is liver biopsy useful in the evaluation of patients with chronically elevated liver enzymes? Ann Intern Med 1989; 111(6):473–8.
41. Younossi ZM, Gramlich T, Matteoni CA, et al. Nonalcoholic fatty liver disease in patients with type 2 diabetes. Clin Gastroenterol Hepatol 2004; 2(3):262–5.
42. Jepsen P, Vilstrup H, Mellemkjaer L, et al. Prognosis of patients with a diagnosis of fatty liver: a registry-based cohort study. Hepatogastroenterology 2003; 50(54):2101–4.
43. Adams LA, Lymp JF, St Sauver J, et al. The natural history of nonalcoholic fatty liver disease: a population-based cohort study. Gastroenterology 2005; 129(1):113–21.
44. Powell EE, Cooksley WG, Hanson R, et al. The natural history of nonalcoholic steatohepatitis: a follow-up study of forty-two patients for up to 21 years. Hepatology 1990; 11(1):74–80.

45. Dam-Larsen S, Franzmann M, Andersen IB, et al. Long term prognosis of fatty liver: risk of chronic liver disease and death. Gut 2004; 53(5):750–5.
46. Matteoni CA, Younossi ZM, Gramlich T, et al. Nonalcoholic fatty liver disease: a spectrum of clinical and pathological severity. Gastroenterology 1999; 116(6):1413–9.
47. Ratziu V, Giral P, Charlotte F, et al. Liver fibrosis in overweight patients. Gastroenterology 2000; 118 (6):1117–23.
48. Pagano G, Pacini G, Musso G, et al. Nonalcoholic steatohepatitis, insulin resistance, and metabolic syndrome: further evidence for an etiologic association. Hepatology 2002; 35(2):367–72.
49. Wannamethee SG, Shaper AG, Lennon L, et al. Hepatic enzymes, the metabolic syndrome, and the risk of type 2 diabetes in older men. Diabetes Care 2005; 28(12):2913–8.
50. Suzuki A, Angulo P, Lymp J, et al. Chronological development of elevated aminotransferases in a nonalcoholic population. Hepatology 2005; 41(1):64–71.
51. Targher G, Bertolini L, Padovani R, et al. Relations between carotid artery wall thickness and liver histology in subjects with nonalcoholic fatty liver disease. Diabetes Care 2006; 29(6):1325–30.
52. Targher G, Bertolini L, Padovani R, et al. Increased prevalence of cardiovascular disease in Type 2 diabetic patients with non-alcoholic fatty liver disease. Diabetes Med 2006; 23(4):403–9.
53. Targher G, Bertolini L, Poli F, et al. Nonalcoholic fatty liver disease and risk of future cardiovascular events among type 2 diabetic patients. Diabetes 2005; 54(12):3541–6.
54. Schindhelm RK, Dekker JM, Nijpels G, et al. Alanine aminotransferase predicts coronary heart disease events: a 10-year follow-up of the Hoorn Study. Atherosclerosis 2007;191(2):391–6.
55. Toledo FG, Sniderman AD, Kelley DE. Influence of hepatic steatosis (fatty liver) on severity and composition of dyslipidemia in type 2 diabetes. Diabetes Care 2006; 29(8):1845–50.
56. Lautamaki R, Borra R, Iozzo P, et al. Liver steatosis coexists with myocardial insulin resistance and coronary dysfunction in patients with type 2 diabetes. Am J Physiol Endocrinol Metab 2006; 291(2): E282–90.
57. Huang MA, Greenson JK, Chao C, et al. One-year intense nutritional counseling results in histological improvement in patients with non-alcoholic steatohepatitis: a pilot study. Am J Gastroenterol 2005; 100(5):1072–81.
58. Browning JD, Davis J, Saboorian MH, et al. A low-carbohydrate diet rapidly and dramatically reduces intrahepatic triglyceride content. Hepatology 2006; 44(2):487–8.
59. Dixon JB, Bhathal PS, Hughes NR, et al. Nonalcoholic fatty liver disease: Improvement in liver histological analysis with weight loss. Hepatology 2004; 39(6):1647–54.
60. Bugianesi E, Gentilcore E, Manini R, et al. A randomized controlled trial of metformin versus vitamin E or prescriptive diet in nonalcoholic fatty liver disease. Am J Gastroenterol 2005; 100(5): 1082–90.
61. Caldwell SH, Argo CK, Al-Osaimi AM. Therapy of NAFLD: insulin sensitizing agents. J Clin Gastroenterol 2006; 40(3 Suppl. 1):S61–6.
62. Chang CY, Argo CK, Al-Osaimi AM, et al. Therapy of NAFLD: antioxidants and cytoprotective agents. J Clin Gastroenterol 2006; 40(3 Suppl. 1):S51–60.
63. Chalasani N. Statins and hepatotoxicity: focus on patients with fatty liver. Hepatology 2005; 41(4): 690–5.

38 | Future Management Approaches: New Devices on the Horizon for Glucose Monitoring and Medication Delivery

Jeffrey I. Joseph
Department of Anesthesiology, The Artificial Pancreas Center, Jefferson Medical College, Thomas Jefferson University, Philadelphia, Pennsylvania, U.S.A.

INTRODUCTION

Current methods of blood glucose (BG) control are labor-intensive, expensive and prone to human error (1,2). The clinical success of self-monitoring of blood glucose levels (SMBG) and self-titration of anti-diabetes medication has shifted the responsibility of BG control to the patient and family caregivers (3). Hypoglycemia continues to be the factor that limits tight BG control in all diabetic patients, whether they use insulin or oral medications (4). The risk of hypoglycemia can be reduced or eliminated by the appropriate application of BG monitoring techniques (5).

The complications of diabetes (myocardial infarction, stroke, blindness, kidney failure, limb amputation, congestive heart failure and death) can be prevented or delayed by controlling fasting BG, postprandial BG and average BG in the normal range (70 to 80 mg/dL, <140 mg/dL, $HbA_{1c} < 6.5\%$) or near-normal range (70 to 126 mg/dL, <140 to 180 mg/dL, $HbA_{1c} < 7.5\%$) (6–8). Unfortunately, the incidence of moderate to severe hypoglycemia is markedly increased in patients who are intensively managed with insulin and/or multiple oral hypoglycemia drug regimens (4,6).

It is difficult for the average person with diabetes to consistently maintain the high degree of motivation and vigilance required to achieve near-normal BG control. Primary-care physicians and general internists often lack the time, resources, funding and expertise in their offices to provide the education and close medical supervision required for intensive glucose control. Medical devices have great potential to help the diabetic patient tighten their BG control and decrease the risk for hypoglycemia, while improving the everyday burden of diabetes management.

The following is a brief review of the evolving field of medical device innovation related to the management of diabetes. Current methods of diabetes management require active participation by the patient. For example, patients self-administer insulin and oral medication based upon their estimate of meal size, meal composition, effect of prior drug delivery, and finger-stick BG measurements (SMBG) (9). Computer algorithms are being developed that assist the patient make decisions that are safe and appropriate for the clinical situation. Insulin pumps now have smart algorithms that recommend an optimal basal/bolus dose of insulin, based upon meal size, meal composition, an estimate of insulin sensitivity and the pharmacokinetics and dynamics of rapid-acting insulin delivered into the subcutaneous tissue. Pumps and glucose meters wirelessly communicate vital information to each other, to a family member or to a diabetes educator via the internet. Totally automated systems are being developed that safely and effectively deliver insulin during meals, exercise, sleep and illness. These so-called artificial pancreas systems integrate a continuous glucose monitoring system (CGM), an insulin delivery system (pump) and a computer algorithm that controls the level of BG with minimal patient supervision or intervention. The reader is referred to the web journal Diabetes Science and Therapeutics (http://www.journalofdst.org), the journal Diabetes Technology and Therapeutics (http://www.liebertpub.com/publications) and the website Diabetes Mall (http://www.mendosa.com/mall.html) for updated information.

SELF-MONITORING OF BLOOD GLUCOSE LEVELS

Frequent SMBG monitoring has been shown to correlate closely with improved long-term BG control and decreased risk for hypoglycemia in patients with type 1 diabetes (8). The clinical benefit of frequent SMBG in patients with type 2 diabetes managed with diet and oral agents remain controversial (7,10). HbA$_{1c}$ levels decline when type 2 diabetics monitor their blood-glucose levels more than once per day and aggressively self-regulate their doses of insulin (11).

Current recommendations of the American Diabetes Association (ADA) call for individuals with type 1 diabetes to SMBG four or more times per day (before each meal and 10 pm) and at least one SMBG per day (before breakfast) in persons with type 2 diabetes treated with insulin or oral agents (1,3). In actual clinical practice, as many as 56% of type 2 diabetics never practice SMBG. About 8% to 9% practice SMBG only once per week, 15% to 22% practice SMBG one to six times per week and 11% to 17% practice SMBG more than once per day (9). Reasons for infrequent self-monitoring include finger stick pain, inconvenience, cost and lack of knowledge about the importance of SMBG for tight glucose control.

Older BG meters did not consistently achieve either the ADA or the Food and Drug Administration goals for BG meter accuracy (± 15 mg/dL below 90 mg/dL and $\pm 20\%$ above 90 mg/dL) (1,12). Modern meters provide a more accurate SMBG measurement using a smaller sample volume (0.3–5 µL), more consistent sample delivery to the site of assay, membrane technology that minimizes the effects of interfering substances and more rapid measurement time.

Recent meters allow testing from an alternate site, such as the forearm or palm, for the purpose of decreasing pain. Controversy continues regarding a circulatory time delay and bias when SMBG forearm/palm measurements are compared with the fingertip. Human trials, however, have shown a small difference that is not considered to be clinically significant (13).

Glucose level, time of day and meal data can be downloaded to a PC computer and displayed for the patient and clinician to perform trend analysis. Strowig et al. (14) demonstrated that HbA1C could be lowered 0.5% by merely providing the diabetic patient with accurate SMBG trend data from a meter memory. It is important to confirm that the meter has been programmed with the correct time to optimize trend analysis. Several devices have simplified the process of SMBG by integrating the test strip and lancet into a single, miniature hand-held device (http://abbottdiabetescare.com, http://www.bayerdiabetes.com, http://www.rochediagnostics.com.au/accu-chek, http://www.lifescan.com).

NON-INVASIVE SMBG TECHNOLOGY

It is thought that by eliminating the discomfort of finger-stick sampling, patients would SMBG more frequently. To be clinically useful, non-invasive glucose monitoring systems would have to be small, light weight, portable, safe and accurate. A variety of optical methods have been devised to measure glucose in blood, interstitial fluid (ISF) and eye fluid (15,16). The prototype devices require sophisticated optics and electronics for stability and high signal-to-noise. Unfortunately, there continues to be great variability in the optical signal when attempting to couple the light source and detector to the sample tissue. Complex signal processing and analytical techniques are required to extract the glucose information from the optical spectra. Recent technologies that are promising involve shinning a near-infrared light through the tongue (transmission spectroscopy) (15) and measuring the change in light polarization across the anterior chamber of the eye (optical rotation) (16).

CONTINUOUS GLUCOSE MONITORING (CGM) SYSTEMS: REAL-TIME GLUCOSE SENSORS

It is not possible to perform SMBG frequently enough to accurately identify all major BG excursions. Real-time glucose sensors, also called CGM systems, measure the concentration of glucose in blood and/or interstitial tissue fluid every 1–5 min. Currently available sensors are inserted into the subcutaneous tissue and measure glucose in the tissue fluid for 3 to 7 days. The implanted sensor must be calibrated to a finger-stick SMBG, and recalibrated two or more times per day, to make sure the sensor output signal accurately reflect the BG concentration.

The BG trend data provides a real-time appreciation of the glucose direction of change (increasing or decreasing); and the glucose rate of change (±0.5, ±1.0, ±1.5, ±2.0, ±2.5, ±3.0 mg/dL/min) (Fig. 1). CGM systems display two up-arrows or an arrow that moves from 3 o'clock to 12 o'clock to denote a rapidly rising glucose level. Two down-arrows or an arrow that moves from 3 o'clock to 6 o'clock denotes a rapidly falling glucose level. The displayed trend data can be used by the patient, physician and diabetes educator to enhance BG control through a better understanding of the relationship between meals, exercise and sleep with the amount/timing of insulin and oral hypoglycemic drug therapy (Fig. 2A– 2C) (17–23).

CGM TREND DATA USED TO MINIMIZE POSTPRANDIAL HYPERGLYCEMIA AND AVOID HYPOGLYCEMIA

Patients use the real-time glucose trend data displayed on the hand-held CGM monitor to make more appropriate clinical decisions regarding BG control (20,22,23). The Food and Drug Administration (FDA), however, does not currently allow the patient with diabetes to initiate a change in medical therapy (insulin or oral hypoglycemia medication) based solely upon CGM glucose sensor data. Diabetic patient are therefore required to adjust drug therapy according to traditional SMBG measurements. This limitation was imposed by the FDA to prevent the unsafe administration of insulin, due to the potential for inaccurate CGM sensor data (www.fda.gov).

However, patients given real-time access to CGM glucose sensor information have quickly learned to utilize the trend data to minimize postprandial hyperglycemia and avoid hypoglycemia. Most patients have not required extensive education to utilize the real-time BG data safely and effectively (22–24). In a randomized, prospective clinical trial using the

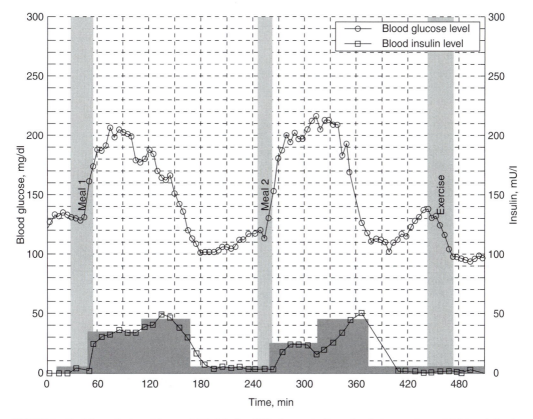

FIGURE 1   Real-time display of frequent BG data (mg/dL), demonstrating rate of glucose rise and fall in relation to meals and exercise, measured using the Metracor VIA-GLU enzyme-based electrochemical sensor.

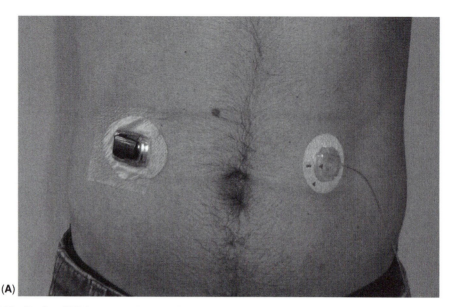

(A)

FIGURE 2A DexCom STS Continuous Glucose Monitor attached to the skin of abdomen (*left*) with sensor tip inserted into the subcutaneous tissue. Insulin pump catheter attached to the skin of abdomen (*right*) with tip inserted into the subcutaneous tissue.

Medtronic Guardian RT System, patients with type 1 diabetes were able to significantly decrease their HbA_{1c} levels by changing their medications and meals according to real-time glucose trend information. Fifty percent of the patients who used the CGM data continuously for 3 months achieved a significant reduction of HbA_{1c} level ≥1%, and 26% achieved reductions ≥2% (significantly lower % HbA_{1c} than control group patients, and patients who utilized CGM intermittently) (24). FDA approval should be granted shortly, for patients to utilize real-time CGM glucose sensor information to titrate medical therapy.

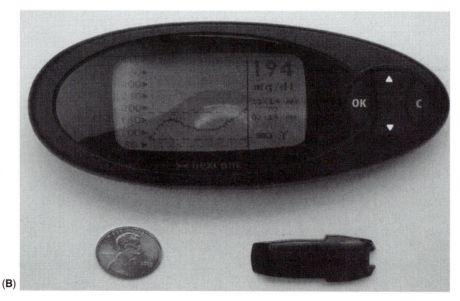

(B)

FIGURE 2B DexCom STS Continuous Glucose Monitor displaying glucose measurement (194 mg/dL) on *y*-axis and time (min) on *x*-axis. Data from patient-worn sensor/transceiver (*lower right*) is transmitted wirelessly to hand-held monitor with flat-panel display. Monitor is able to display 1, 3, and 9-hour trend data.

Glucose Trend

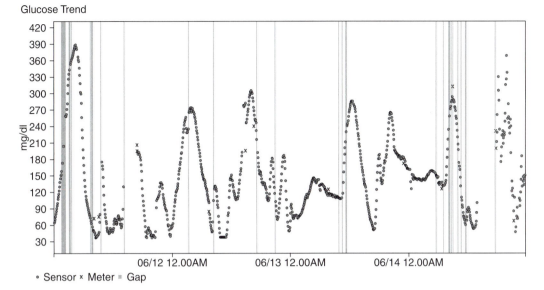

• Sensor × Meter ▒ Gap

FIGURE 2C Seventy-two hour glucose profile using the DexCom STS CGM. Note the dynamic nature of glucose fluctuations and relationship between continuous sensor measurements and intermittent SMBG measurements.

Computer algorithms are being developed that analyze glucose sensor data in real-time to diagnose hypoglycemia. The CGM algorithm alerts the patient when the concentration of glucose falls below a programmable threshold (<90, <80, <70 and <60 mg/dL) or when the BG levels is predicted to decrease into the hypoglycemia range within the subsequent 20 to 30 min time period (25–27).

Future medical devices may automatically deliver glucagon, glucose or epinephrine to prevent or treat impending or established hypoglycemia. This type of system would be most beneficial to patients who have recurrent hypoglycemia or hypoglycemia unawareness (reduced glucagon and/or epinephrine response to low BG levels). Most clinicians would advocate intensive drug therapy and tight BG control if a CGM system was able to automatically detect and prevent hypoglycemia, prior to the onset of CNS or cardiovascular symptoms (1–8,27).

Algorithms currently being tested in the research setting, utilize glucose trend data and insulin delivery data to minimize hyperglycemia following consumption of a meal. The CGM system algorithms often consider: time since last meal, onset time of current meal, meal size, meal composition, estimated time of gastric emptying/intestinal absorption, time/dose of previously delivered insulin, time/intensity of previous exercise and an estimate of insulin sensitivity (19,20,28–30).

Postprandial hyperglycemia can be minimized by injecting rapid-acting insulin into the subcutaneous (sc) tissue 0 to 20 min before a meal. Moderate hyperglycemia will occur when the insulin bolus is delayed until after the onset of the meal, because of the slow and variable absorption of "rapid" acting insulin from the sc tissue into the circulation (31,32–35). Optimal BG control may be achieved by delivering 60% to 70% of the total meal insulin dose prior to the meal, and 30% to 40% of the total meal insulin dose over the subsequent 2–4 h. CGM algorithms will utilize CGM glucose trend data and an estimate of rapid-acting insulin's pharmacodynamic glucose-lowering effect, to determine the optimal duration of the extended square wave bolus. A meal bolus that is prematurely stopped may lead to postprandial hyperglycemia, while an excessively long meal bolus can lead to hypoglycemia (4,5,20,23,24,28,29,36,37).

MINIMALLY INVASIVE CGM: NEEDLE-TYPE TISSUE FLUID GLUCOSE SENSOR

Miniature needle-type glucose sensors continuously measure the concentration of glucose in the ISF of sc tissue. Thin, flexible sensing electrodes are inserted through the skin into the sc adipose tissue by the patient (Fig. 2A). This classic electrochemical sensor uses a small amount of glucose oxidase enzyme to covert ISF glucose to hydrogen peroxide. Electrons generated by the chemical reaction are measured as an electric current. The sensor's electrodes are connected to a battery and transmitter that relays the averaged output signal to a patient-worn display every 1–5 min (Figs. 2B and 2C). The sensor output signal (milliamp current) is correlated to the BG concentration using two or more finger-stick SMBG and a calibrated glucose meter.

The electrodes and glucose oxidase enzyme are protected beneath a biocompatible porous membrane (Fig. 3) that is permeable only to small molecules such as oxygen and glucose. Following insertion, the pores of the membrane become fouled with plasma proteins and white blood cells, causing a dynamic change in sensitivity (decreased sensor output in response to a change in glucose concentration). Initial calibration is typically performed after a run-in period of 2–10 h following sc tissue insertion.

A second calibration is typically performed 2–6 h later, and then once every 6–12 h, in an attempt to compensate for sensor instability and drift. Recalibration should be performed when the ISF glucose concentration and BG concentration are changing slowly. A close

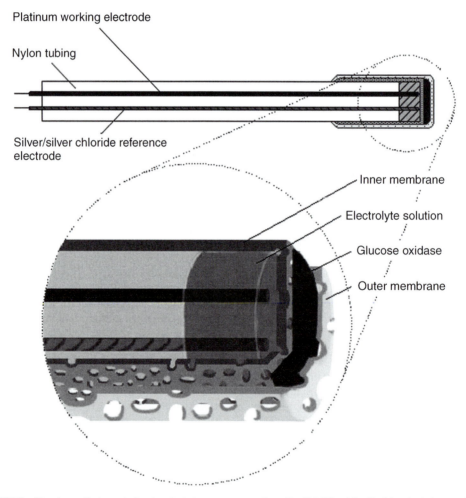

FIGURE 3 Classic needle-type electrochemical glucose sensor where the distal tip of the flexible wire is inserted for 3 to 7 days within the loose connective tissue under the skin. Glucose and oxygen molecules within the ISF diffuse through the outer membrane to interact with the enzyme glucose oxidase. The hydrogen peroxide that is produced travels through the inner membrane and electrolyte solution to interact with the working electrode. An increase or decrease in the number of glucose molecules reaching the enzyme correlates directly with an increase or decrease in the electric current output signal of the glucose sensor. *Source*: Courtesy of Brian Hipszer.

correlation between blood and ISF glucose typically occurs before meals and several hours after an insulin bolus. When properly inserted and calibrated, the needle-type CGM sensors exhibit satisfactory sensitivity, specificity, accuracy and precision over the physiological range (40–400 mg/dL). Long-term sensor function is limited owing to foiling of the enzyme and electrodes (38,39). The risk of infection necessitates the placement of a new sensor at an alternate location every three to seven days (http://www.fda.gov; 17–19,21,22,24,26).

The needle-type CGM systems developed by Medtronic Diabetes, DexCom Corporation and Abbott Diabetes have received FDA approval for glucose monitoring by adult ambulatory patient with type 1 and type 2 diabetes (http://www.medtronicdiabetes.com, http://www.dexcom.com, http://www.abbottdiabetescare.com). CGM monitors display the current ISF glucose level, the direction of glucose change (stable, rising or falling) and the rate of glucose change over time.

MINIMALLY INVASIVE CGM: DIALYSIS CATHETER-TYPE ISF GLUCOSE SENSOR

Dialysis catheter-type glucose sensors consist of a flexible catheter that the patient inserts through the skin into the sc tissue. The small pore dialysis catheter is connected to a fluidics system that transports a salt solution (dialysate) into and out of the body. Glucose-free dialysate is infused into the dialysis catheter previously inserted into the sc tissue, and allowed to equilibrate with ISF glucose. Glucose containing dialysate is pumped out of the body to an external electrochemical glucose sensor at a slow rate (5–10 μL/min) to optimize equilibration and recovery of glucose from tissue fluids. The glucose sensor is automatically calibrated and recalibrated using liquid glucose standards obtained from the manufacturer. Sensor drift is less of a problem because the enzyme and electrodes are not in direct contact with the body tissues. Limitations include large size, long sample acquisition time (10–15 min), inaccuracy due to incomplete glucose equilibration, infection and cost (Fig. 4)(39).

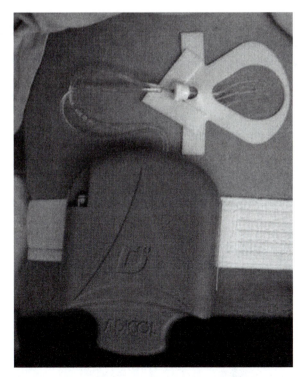

FIGURE 4 Dialysis catheter-type CGM system. Flexible small-pore catheter is connected to an external flow through electrochemical glucose sensor, following insertion into the subcutaneous loose connective tissue (www.ADICOL.com).

NONINVASIVE CGM: USES REVERSE IONOPHORESIS TO SAMPLE TISSUE FLUID

A noninvasive CGM system called the Glucowatch Biographer utilizes an electric current (reverse ionophoresis) to extract glucose-containing ISF from the skin (Animas Corporation, West Chester, PA, USA, http://www.animas.com). Tissue fluid collected within a gel pad under the Glucowatch is analyzed for glucose using an enzyme-based, electrochemical technique. The system displays the absolute glucose concentration and the rate/direction of change, every 10–15 minutes for patient interpretation. Programmable alarms are designed to warn the patient of impending hypo and hyperglycemia. The technology is limited by inadequate accuracy, long extraction time, long warm-up period (2 h), short gel pad lifetime (12 h), irritation of the skin and cost (37).

LONG-TERM IMPLANTABLE CGM: ENZYME-BASED TISSUE FLUID GLUCOSE ELECTROCHEMICAL SENSOR

The implantable tissue fluid glucose sensor developed by DexCom Corporation has been tested long-term in ambulatory patients with type 1 diabetes (http://www.DexCom.com). Patients successfully used the real-time glucose sensor data to improve fasting and postprandial glucose control while virtually eliminating hypoglycemia. A surgeon can easily implant the miniature sensor within the sc tissue of the abdomen or chest wall. The sensor contains the enzyme glucose oxidase and electrodes covered by a multi-layered porous membrane, a power source, microprocessor and transceiver. An external electronics module receives and displays the absolute glucose concentration and glucose trend data in real-time (Fig. 5). Key to the clinical success of this long-term implantable sensor is an engineered sensor-tissue interface that remains vascular for the life of the sensor. Unfortunately, there is a decrease in vascularity and increase in fibrous tissue that surrounds the sensor following long-term implantation in diabetic humans. This foreign body response to device implantation produces a barrier to the diffusion of glucose, and premature sensor failure (38,39).

LONG-TERM IMPLANTABLE CGM: ENZYME-BASED BLOOD GLUCOSE ELECTROCHEMICAL SENSOR

Medtronic Diabetes has developed an electrochemical sensor for long-term implantation in the superior vena cava called the Vascular Glucose Monitoring System (http://www.medtronicdiabetes.com). The distal tip of the flexible vascular catheter contains an oxygen

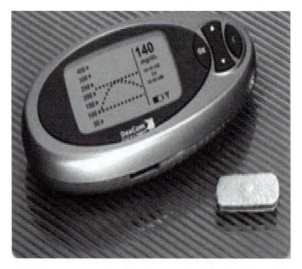

FIGURE 5 Electrochemical ISF glucose sensor designed for long-term implantation within the subcutaneous tissue. ISF glucose data is transmitted wirelessly to the patient-worn display (mg/dL versus time) (www.DexCom.com).

electrode that is covered with the enzyme glucose oxidase. A second oxygen electrode is used to measure the partial pressure of oxygen in central venous blood. The concentration of glucose is calculated by comparing the oxygen concentration adjacent to the enzyme (change in local oxygen concentration due to oxidation of glucose) to the oxygen concentration in blood. Porous membranes protect the enzyme from fouling and ensure an adequate supply of oxygen.

The catheter is attached to an electronics module that is implanted within the subcutaneous tissue below the clavicle, similar to a pacemaker. The implanted module contains the power source, microprocessor and transceiver for receiving calibration data from an external reference glucose meter, and transmitting glucose data to an external display (Fig. 6). Excellent accuracy and sensor stability have been demonstrated in animal and human trials. Unfortunately, the harsh chemical environment of the bloodstream has caused premature sensor failure from membrane fouling and enzyme degradation, limiting long-term clinical application (38,39,40).

LONG-TERM IMPLANTABLE CGM: OPTICAL BLOOD GLUCOSE SENSOR

Animas Corporation is developing a long-term implantable sensor that uses near-infrared spectroscopy to measure the concentration of glucose in blood. The system resembles a pacemaker with an sc electronics/optical module and a miniature sensor head that is surgically implanted around a blood vessel. A universal calibration algorithm has been developed that allows glucose to be accurately predicted from the optical spectra. The system has been designed to overcome the biocompatibility limitations of other electrochemical sensors because near-infrared light can easily pass through any layer of cells and the protein that coat the optical windows following implantation (http://www.animas.com) (41).

DEVICES FOR INSULIN DELIVERY

Inhaled Insulin

Inhaled insulin therapy was recently approval by the FDA for clinical use in patients with type 1 and type 2 diabetes. Dry powder or liquid insulin formulations are aerosolized within an inhaler and delivered into the distal airways for alveolar absorption. Insulin is typically inhaled immediately before a meal because the peak glucose-lowering effect occurs 30–60 min post-inhalation. Studies in type 2 diabetics demonstrate postprandial BG control similar to rapid-acting insulin injected into the sc tissue (42).

Routine use of inhaled insulin appears to be safe and effective when used by patients who do not smoke cigarettes or have chronic obstructive pulmonary disease. The long-term

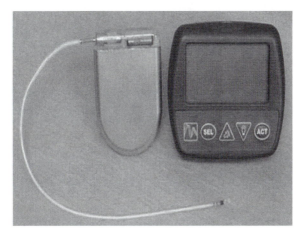

FIGURE 6   Enzyme-based electrochemical/oxygen blood glucose sensor with flexible catheter designed to float freely long-term in the superior vena cava (www.MedtronicDiabetes.com).

health effects of delivering large doses of insulin deep in the lung, however, are unknown. Only 20% to 30% of the inhaled dose is absorbed into the pulmonary bloodstream, whereas 70% to 80% is metabolized within the alveoli and bronchi. Clinical trials have revealed a mild decrease in lung function (forced expiratory volume and lung volume), increase in insulin antibodies and increase in the incidence of pulmonary thromboses (43).

Insulin Pens

Insulin pens provide increased convenience, improve accuracy of dose and overall safety. One-half unit incremental dosing is now possible. The most common therapeutic regimen consists of multiple daily injections of rapid-acting insulin (prior to meals) and intermediate-acting insulin at bedtime. Pens using a mixture of rapid- and intermediate-acting insulin provide convenience and improve BG control when compared with oral hypoglycemic agent therapy (44).

CONTINUOUS SUBCUTANEOUS INSULIN INFUSION (CSII) THERAPY USING AN EXTERNAL INSULIN PUMP

External insulin pumps have gained popularity because of increased flexibility of dosing, improved glycemic control and a lower incidence of hypoglycemia when compared with traditional insulin injection methods (5,6,45–48). However, CSII requires that patients count carbohydrates, SMBG frequently and carefully control caloric intake to avoid hypoglycemia and excessive weight gain. Failure to deliver rapid-acting insulin (due to pump malfunction, catheter occlusion or catheter disconnection) can lead to hyperglycemia and ketoacidosis within several hours, because of the small depot of sc insulin (two to four units) during typical basal CSII therapy (25,33,45).

Although pumps can deliver basal and bolus doses of rapid-acting insulin (insulin Lispro or insulin Aspart in the USA) into the sc tissue with great precision, initial absorption into the circulation can be delayed up to 20 min, with 30% to 50% intra-subject variability (31,32,34,35). Large bolus doses and high basal rates are associated with a four to 10 unit depot of sc insulin. Once delivered into the sc tissue, the depot of rapid-acting insulin may not be completely absorbed into the circulation for 2–4 h. This highlights a major limitation of CSII insulin therapy; plasma insulin levels will continue to rise for several hours even if the patient attempts to decrease the actions of insulin by stopping the delivery of insulin (35,45).

Doyle et al. performed a prospective randomized clinical trial in patients with type 1 diabetes comparing pump therapy with Lispro insulin (CSII) and multiple dose therapy using Lispro and Glargine insulin (MDI). Fifty percent of the patients managed with CSII achieved near-normal BG control (HbA$_{1c}$ < 7%), compared to only 12% of patients managed with MDI (46). In another randomized clinical trial, Rudolph et al. (49) demonstrated a 74% reduction in the incidence of severe hypoglycemia in type 1 diabetic patients managed with CSII compared to MDI.

Modern pumps are small, light weight, water-resistant, reliable and highly programmable. Advanced pumps manufactured by Medtronic Diabetes and Smiths-Medical communicate wirelessly with a patient's SMBG meter, while an Animas Corporation pump has a detailed library of meals and an algorithm that calculates an optimal meal bolus dose of rapid-acting insulin. Improved estimation of meal carbohydrate content leads to decreased postprandial hyperglycemia (36). Several pumps have an "insulin on board" feature that estimates the future glucose-lowering effect of delivered insulin to prevent the patient from injecting additional insulin when a large amount is already present in the subcutaneous depot. The inadvertent stacking of meal or correction boluses of rapid-acting insulin often leads to hypoglycemia (28,33,46,47).

Medtronic Diabetes recently received FDA approval for a device that combines the Guardian RT continuous glucose monitoring system with an insulin pump (Fig. 7). Patients are able to utilize the real-time glucose and insulin trend data to improve BG control with meals, exercise and sleep (19,20,22). This exciting technology is limited because the patient must frequently look at the CGM display, thus clinical decisions about therapy are made intermittently. Future devices may "close the loop" during sleep or continuously throughout the day.

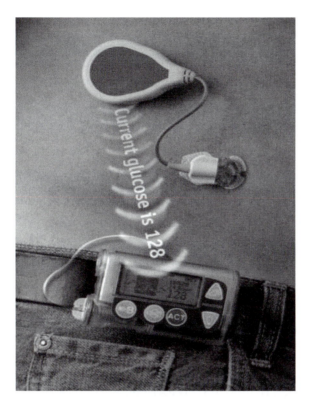

FIGURE 7 Medtronic Diabetes (Guardian REAL-Time) CGM System. Distal tip of needle-type glucose sensor is implanted into the subcutaneous tissue of the abdomen. Glucose data is sent wirelessly from telemetry module to insulin pump. Glucose data displayed on *y*-axis and time of day on *x*-axis. CGMS is open-loop system, requiring patient initiated SMBG for change in insulin dose (www.medtronicdiabetes.com).

Insulet Corporation recently commercialized an insulin pump that separates the insulin delivery system from the programmer and display. The small, lightweight and disposable insulin "pod" attaches to the skin with an adhesive and self-inserts the infusion needle with minimal discomfort. Patient comfort and convenience are improved by eliminating the need for an infusion catheter and tubing (Fig. 8). (www.animas.com, www.medtronicdiabetes.com, www.roche.com, www.smiths-medical.com, www.insulet.com.)

IMPLANTABLE INSULIN PUMPS: CONTINUOUS PERITONEAL INSULIN INFUSION

The safety and efficacy of continuous peritoneal insulin infusion (CPII) therapy using a programmable implantable insulin pump have been demonstrated in patients with type 1 and type 2 diabetes. An external programmer is used to control the basal rate and timing/amount of a regular insulin bolus infused prior to meals. Peritoneal insulin delivery significantly reduces the risk of hypoglycemia, an advantage that may be due to portal delivery of insulin and a more physiological ratio of portal to systemic insulin levels. The sc pump reservoir can be easily refilled (with U-400 insulin) every 2–3 months in the physician's office. Limitations include the need for a surgical procedure for implantation, localized infection, catheter failure due to fibrous tissue obstruction and cost (50).

ARTIFICIAL ENDOCRINE PANCREAS (FOR AMBULATORY PATIENTS)

An artificial endocrine pancreas (AP) consists of a real-time glucose sensor, an insulin infusion pump and a computer control algorithm (controller). The integrated system can automatically determine the appropriate dose and timing of insulin based upon the absolute glucose measurement and recent glucose trends, integrating the rate of increase or decrease, and the recent dose of delivered insulin. Predictive and adaptive control algorithms use a model of patient physiology, insulin pharmacokinetics and insulin dynamics to determine the appropriate dose of insulin for subsequent delivery (51). Closed-loop control algorithms

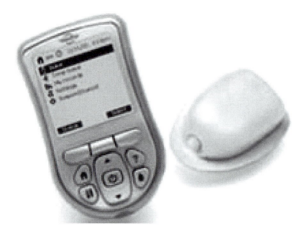

FIGURE 8 Omni-Pod insulin pump manufactured by Insulet Corporation has separate patient-worn insulin delivery system (*right*) connected wirelessly to hand-held glucose meter/controller (*left*). The insulin delivery system is able to deliver a variety of basal and bolus doses of insulin, according to finger-stick SMBG measurements (www.insulet.com).

have been developed that automatically regulate the delivery of insulin without patient intervention. It is difficult for closed-loop systems to achieve normal BG control because of time delays in the CGM recognizing an increase in glucose due to food, and delays in insulin absorption from the sc tissue. Semi-closed-loop algorithms overcome this limitation by utilizing data input from the patient regarding meal timing/composition, and the onset of exercise. Inadequate glucose sensor accuracy and robustness remains the major obstacle to routine application of an AP system in the clinical setting (28–30).

ARTIFICIAL ENDOCRINE PANCREAS (FOR HOSPITALIZED PATIENTS)

In a landmark study, Van den Berghe et al. (52) demonstrated that control of glucose to near normal levels (90 to 110 mg/dL) decreased morbidity and mortality following surgery and major illness in hospitalized patients. Numerous clinical trials have demonstrated the clinical advantage of controlling glucose levels in the near-normal range during major surgery and severe illness (53–55). Current hospital methods require frequent bedside glucose monitoring and careful titration of an intravenous insulin infusion to achieve tight BG control. Despite these precautions, the incidence of wide swings in BG and episodes of hypoglycemia remains high (4,52,54,55).

A closed-loop AP system was developed in the 1970s called the Biostator, to control BG levels in hospitalized patients during surgery and critical illness. Venous blood was acquired from an intravenous catheter, anti-coagulated with heparin and then transported to a flow-through electrochemical sensor that used the enzyme glucose oxidase to measure the concentration of BG. An algorithm used BG trend data to determine the appropriate intravenous infusion dose of insulin or glucose to maintain BG levels in a predetermined range. Although the bedside device successfully automated the process of glucose monitoring and insulin delivery, it did not achieve routine clinical utility because the sensor required frequent recalibration, sample acquisition was unreliable and phlebotomy caused >150 mL blood loss per day. Modern glucose sensors are being developed that sample the blood, measure the glucose level and return the blood to the patient with a small volume of flush solution, as frequently as every few minutes (56). Although this method avoids blood loss, large volumes of flush solution may not be appropriate for hospitalized patients with decreased cardiac reserve.

REFERENCES

1. American Diabetes Association. Standards of medical care for patients with diabetes mellitus (Position Statement) Diabetes Care 1998; 21(Suppl. 1):S23–31.
2. Klein R, Klein BE, Moss SE, Cruikshanks KJ. The medical management of hyperglycemia over a 10-year period in people with diabetes. Diabetes Care 1996; 19:744–50.

3. American Diabetes Association. Self-monitoring of blood glucose (Consensus statement). Diabetes Care 1996; 19(Suppl. 1):562–6.
4. Cryer PE, Fisher JN, Shamoon. Hypoglycemia (technical review) Diabetes Care 1994; 17:734–55.
5. DCCT Research Group. Hypoglycemia in the Diabetes Control and Complications Trial. Diabetes 1997; 46:271–86.
6. The Diabetes Control and Complications Trial Research Group. The effect of intensive treatment of diabetes on the development and progression of long-term complications in insulin-dependent diabetes mellitus. N Engl J Med 1993; 329:977–86.
7. UK Prospective Diabetes Study (UKPDS) Group. Intensive blood-glucose control with sulfonylureas or insulin compared with conventional treatment in patients with type 2 diabetes (UKPDS 33). Lancet 1998; 352:837–53.
8. Edelman SV. Importance of glucose control. Med Clin N Am 1998; 82(4):665–87.
9. Harris MI, Eastman RC, Cowie CC, Flegal KM, Eberhardt MS. Racial and ethnic differences in glycemic control of adults with type 2 diabetes. Diabetes Care 1999; 22:403–13.
10. Faas A, Schellevis FG, van Eijk JT. The efficacy of self-monitoring of blood glucose in NIDDM subjects: a criteria-based literature review, Diabetes Care 1997; 20(9):1482–6.
11. Franciosi M, Pellegrini F, De Berardis G, Belfiglio M, Cavaliere D, Di Nardo B, Greenfield S, Kaplan S, Sacco M, Tognoni G, Valentini M, Nicolucci A. The impact of blood glucose self-monitoring on metabolic control and quality of life in type 2 diabetic patients. Diabetes Care 2001; 24 (11):1870–7.
12. Food and Drug Administration. Review criteria assessment of portable blood glucose monitoring in vitro diagnostic devices using glucose oxidase, dehydrogenase or hexokinase methodology. Draft Guidance Document, 1997 (www.fda.gov).
13. Feldman B, McGarrraugh G, Heller A, Bohannon N, Skler J, DeLeeuw E, Clarke DF. A small-volume electrochemical glucose sensor for home blood glucose testing. Diab Technol Therapeut 2000; 2(2): 221–9.
14. Strowig SM, Raskin P. Improved glycemic control in intensively treated type 1 diabetic patients using blood glucose meters with storage capacity and computer-assisted analyses. Diabetes Care 1998; 21(10):1694–8.
15. Burmeister JJ, Arnold MA, Small GW. Non-invasive blood glucose measurements by near-infrared transmission spectroscopy across human tongues. Diab Technol Therapeut 2000; 2(1):5–16.
16. Cameron B, Gorde H, Satheesan B, Cote G. The use of polarized laser light through the eye for noninvasive glucose monitoring. Diab Technol Therapeut 1999; 1(1):135–43.
17. Mastrototaro JJ. The MiniMed continuous glucose monitoring system. Diab Technol Therapeut 2000; 2(S.1):S-13–8.
18. Gross TM, Ter Veer A. Continuous glucose monitoring in previously unstudied population subgroups. Diab Technol Therapeut 2000; 2(Suppl. 1):27–34.
19. Bode BW, Gross TM, Thornton KR, Mastrototaro JJ. Continuous glucose monitoring used to direct diabetes therapy improves glycosylated hemoglobin; a pilot study. Diabetes Res Clin Pract 1999; 46 (3):183–90.
20. Ludvigsson J, Hanes R. Continuous subcutaneous glucose monitoring improved metabolic control in pediatric patients with type 1 diabetes: a controlled cross over study. Pediatrics 2003; 111(5):933–8.
21. Steil G, Rebrin K, Mastrototaro J, Barnaba B, Saad M. Determination of plasma glucose excursions with subcutaneous glucose sensor. Diabet Technol Therapeut 2003; 5(1):27–31.
22. Garg S, Zisser H, Schwartz S, Bailey T, Kaplan R, Ellis S, Jovanovic L. Improvement in glycemic excursions with a transcutaneous, real-time continuous glucose sensor: a randomized controlled trial. Diabetes Care 2006; 29(1):44–50.
23. Deiss D, Bolinder J, Rivelin JP, Battelino T, Bosi E, Tubiana-Rufi N, Kerr D, Phillip M. Improved glycemic control in patients with type 1 diabetes using real-time continuous glucose monitoring. Diabetes Care 2006; 29(12):2625–31.
24. Bode BW, Gross TM, Thornton KR, et al. Continuous glucose monitoring used to adjust diabetes therapy improves glycosylated hemoglobin: a pilot study. Diab Res Clin Pract 1999; 46:183–90.
25. Bode B, Gross K, Rikalo N, et al. Alarms based on real-time sensor glucose values alert patients to hypo- and hyperglycemia: the guardian continuous glucose monitoring system. Diab Technol Ther 2004; 6(2):105–13.
26. Caplin NJ, O'Leary P, Bulsara M, et al. Subcutaneous glucose sensor values closely parallel blood glucose during insulin-induced hypoglycemia. Diabetes Med 2003; 20:238–41.
27. Klonoff D. Continuous Glucose Monitoring. Diabetes Care 2005; 28:1231–39.
28. Rebrin K, Fischer U, von Woedtke T, Abel P, Brunstein E. Automated feedback control of subcutaneous glucose concentration in diabetic dogs. Diabetologia 1989; 32(8):573–6.
29. Steil G, Panteleon AE, Rebrin K. Closed-loop insulin delivery: the path to physiological glucose control. Adv Drug Deliv Rev 2004; 56(2):125–44.
30. Shichiri M, Sakakida M, Nishida K, Shimoda S. Enhanced, simplified glucose sensors: long-term clinical application of wearable artificial endocrine pancreas. Artif Organs 1998; 22:32–42.

31. Heinemann L. Variability of insulin absorption and insulin action [Review]. Diab Technol Therapeut 2002; 4(5):673–82.

32. Mudaliar SR, Lindberg FA, Joyce M, et al. Insulin aspart (B28 asp-insulin): a fast-acting analog of human insulin: absorption kinetics and action profile compared with regular human insulin in healthy non-diabetic subjects. Diabetes Care 1999; 22(9):1501–6.

33. Farkas-Hirsch R, Hirsch IB. Continuous subcutaneous insulin infusion: A review of the past and its implementation for the future. Diab Spec 1994; 7(2):136–8.

34. Saudek CD. Novel forms of insulin delivery. Current therapies for diabetes. Endocrinol Metab Clin N Am 1997; 26(3):599–610.

35. Heinemann L, Anderson Jr, JH. Measurement of insulin absorption and insulin action [Review]. Diab Technol Therapeut 2004; 6(5):698–718.

36. Gross T, Kayne D, King A, et al. A bolus calculator is an effective means of controlling postprandial glycemia in patients on insulin pump therapy. Diab Technol Ther 2003; 5(3):365–9.

37. Tierney MJ, Tamada JA, Potts RO, Eastman RC, Pitzer K, Ackerman NR, Fermi SJ. The GlucoWatch Biographer: a frequent, automatic, and non-invasive glucose monitor. Ann Med 2000; 32:632–41.

38. Wisniewski N, Moussy F, Reichert WM. Characterization of implantable biosensor membrane biofouling. Fresn J Anal Chem 2000; 366(6–7):611–21.

39. Joseph JI, Torman MC. Implantable glucose sensors. In Encyclopedia of Biomaterials. NY: Dekker 2004.

40. Armour JC, Lucisano JY, McKean BD, Gough DA. Application of chronic intravascular blood glucose sensor in dogs. Diabetes 1990; 39:1519–26.

41. Joseph JI, Torjman MC, Moritz M, Liu JB, Murphy ME, De Stefano M. Long-term vessel patency following perivascular sensor implantation. Biomater Suppl 2000; S-231.

42. Weiss SR, Berger S Cheng S, Kourides IA, Landschulz WH, Gelfand RA: for the Phase II Inhaled Insulin Study Group. Adjunctive therapy with inhaled human insulin in type 2 diabetic patients failing oral agents: a multi-center phase II trial. Diabetes 1999; 48(Suppl. 1):A12.

43. Cefalu W, Skyler J, Kourides I, Landschulz W, Balagtas C, Cheng S, Gelfand, R; for the Inhaled Insulin Study Group. Inhaled human insulin treatment in patients with type 2 diabetes mellitus. Ann Int Med 2001; 134(3):203–7.

44. Wikby A, Stenstrom U, Andersson PO, Hornquist J. Metabolic control, quality of life, and negative life events: a longitudinal study of well-controlled and poorly regulated patients with type 1 diabetes after changeover to insulin pen treatment. Diab Educ 1998; 24(1):61–6.

45. Reichel A, Rietzsch H, Kohler HJ, Pfutzner A, Gudat U, Schulze J. Cessation of insulin infusion at night-time during CSII-therapy: comparison of regular insulin and insulin lispro. Exp Clin Endocrinol Diab 1998; 106(3):168–72.

46. Bode BW, Steed RD, Davidson PC. Reduction in severe hypoglycemia with long-term continuous subcutaneous insulin infusion in type 1 diabetes. Diabetes Care 1996; 19(4):324–7.

47. Doyle (Boland) E. A randomized, prospective trial comparing the efficacy of continuous subcutaneous insulin infusion with multiple daily injections using insulin glargine. Diabetes Care 2004; 27:1554–8.

48. Turner RC, Cull CA, Frighi V, Holman RR; for the U.K. Prospective Diabetes Study Group (UKPDS). Glycemic control with diet, sulfonlyurea, metformin, or insulin in patients with type 2 diabetes mellitus. Progressive requirement for multiple therapies (UKPDS 49). JAMA 1999; 281: 2005–12.

49. Rudolph JW, Hirsch IB. Assessment of therapy with continuous subcutaneous insulin infusion in an Academic Diabetes Clinic. Endocr Pract 2002; 8:401–5.

50. Saudek CD. Novel forms of insulin delivery. Current therapies for diabetes. Endocrinol Metab Clin N Am 1997; 26(3):599–610.

51. Hipszer B, Joseph J, Kam M. Pharmacokinetics of intravenous insulin delivery in humans with type 1 diabetes. Diab Technol Therapeut 2005; 7(1):83–93.

52. van Den Berghe G, Wouters P, Weekers F, Verwaest C, Bruyninckx F, Schetz M, Vlasselaers D, Ferinande P, Lauwers P, Bouillon R. Intensive insulin therapy in critically ill patients. N Engl J Med 2001; 345(19):1359–67.

53. Furnary AP. Continuous insulin infusion reduces mortality in patients with diabetes undergoing coronary artery bypass grafting. J Thorac Cardiovasc Surg 2003; 125(5):1007–21.

54. Krinsley JS. Effect of intensive glucose management protocol on the mortality of critically ill adult patients. Mayo Clin Proc 2004; 79(8):992–1000.

55. Clement S, Braithwaite S, Magee M, Ahmann A, Smith E, Schafer R, Hirsch I, American Diabetes Association Diabetes in Hospitals Writing Committee. Management of diabetes and hyperglycemia in hospitals. Diabetes Care 2004; 27:253–591.

56. Joseph JI, Torjman MC; The Artificial Pancreas Symposium. Glucose monitoring insulin delivery, feedback control. Diab Technol Therapeut 1999; 1(3):323–8.

Index